# Pathology
# of the Female
# Genital Tract

## with contributions by

**Murray R. Abell**
*University of Michigan Medical School*
**Bradley Bigelow**
*New York University Medical Center*
**Ancel Blaustein**
*New York University School of Medicine*
**Rita Blaustein**
*Booth Memorial Medical Center*
**John Bonnar**
*Trinity College Medical School, Rotunda Hospital, Ireland*
**Herbert J. Buchsbaum**
*University of Iowa Medical Center*
**E. Cotchin**
*University of London, England*
**Bernard Czernobilsky**
*Kaplan Hospital, Israel*
*Medical School of the Hebrew University, Israel*
**Charles H. Debrovner**
*New York University School of Medicine*
**Rita Demopoulos**
*New York University School of Medicine*
**Felix de Narvaez**
*New York University*
*Public Health Department, New York*
**Alex Ferenczy**
*Jewish General Hospital, Canada*
**Eduard G. Friedrich, Jr.**
*The Medical College of Wisconsin*
**Arthur L. Herbst**
*University of Chicago*
**Jan Langman**
*University of Virginia*

**June Marchant**
*Queen Elizabeth Medical Centre, England*
**Luigi Mastroianni**
*University of Pennsylvania*
**Lila E. Nachtigall**
*New York University Medical Center*
**Stanley Robboy**
*Massachusetts General Hospital*
**Laszlo Sarkozi**
*The Mount Sinai Hospital*
*Mount Sinai School of Medicine of the City University of New York*
**Robert E. Scully**
*Massachusetts General Hospital*
**Lawrence R. Shapiro**
*Letchworth Village Developmental Center, New York*
*New York Medical College*
*Westchester County Medical Center*
**Lewis Shenker**
*New York University School of Medicine*
**B. L. Sheppard**
*Trinity College Medical School, Rotunda Hospital, Ireland*
**A. Talerman**
*Institute of Radiotherapy, The Netherlands*
**James E. Wheeler**
*Hospital of the University of Pennsylvania*
**A. J. White**
*306 Oak Hills Medical Building, Texas*
**Edward J. Wilkinson**
*The Medical College of Wisconsin*

# Pathology of the Female Genital Tract

Edited by
## Ancel Blaustein

*Clinical Professor of Pathology*
*New York University School of Medicine*
*New York, New York*

**with 1206 illustrations**
**and 39 four-color figures**

## Springer–Verlag
### New York Heidelberg Berlin

**Library of Congress Cataloging in Publication Data**
Main entry under title:

Pathology of the female genital tract.

Includes index.
1. Pathology, Gynecological.    I. Blaustein, Ancel U.
[DNLM:    1. Genitalia, Female—Pathology. WP100 P297]
RG77.P37          618.1'07          76-54630

Printed in the United States of America

© 1977 by Springer–Verlag New York Inc.

ISBN 0-387-90180-9 Springer–Verlag New York
ISBN 3-540-90180-9 Springer–Verlag Berlin Heidelberg

## Dedicated to

*Gynecologists and pathologists, who working together, have contributed to the body of information incorporated in the text.*

*The authors of this book who labored in the presentation of their material.*

*To my wife, Rita Leff Blaustein, M.D., and the families of all the authors, for patience and encouragement.*

# Preface

This text is written for the obstetrician, gynecologist, pathologist, and for residents training in these disciplines. It is a multi-authored book and the editor is aware of the problems this can create, but the expansion of information in the field of gynecologic pathology renders single authorship obsolete.

The format is largely traditional but the contents include topics that have not appeared in past texts. Clear cell adenocarcinoma of the vagina and vaginal and cervical adenoses are discussed in detail in a separate chapter. A chapter on embryology and congenital anomalies is written by an embryologist and the advantage of its inclusion is self evident. Ovarian neoplasms in childhood and adolescence are fortunately rare occurrences, but information concerning them is generally not readily available in existing texts. It is of sufficient importance to deserve a separate chapter. Amniotic fluid analysis for fetal viability is now commonly used and for this reason a detailed discussion of this subject is presented.

A chapter is included on gross description and preparation of gynecologic specimens. It contains the input and review of several directors of gynecologic-pathology laboratories.

The text contains many electron micrographs taken by transmission and scanning electron microscopy. Their inclusion is not an absolute necessity in gynecologic pathology, but is informative because they offer another perspective and are now a commonly used modality for studying tissue. The present day literature is replete with descriptions of specimens by electron microscopy, and it is hoped that the text will enable the readers to familiarize themselves with electron microscopy as used in this specialty.

Experimentation in the field of obstetrics and gynecology has become more sophisticated over the years and for this reason the chapter on animal models of tumors of the ovaries and uterus is included. The contributions that comparative pathology can make to understanding disease mechanisms justify the addition of the chapter on comparative uterine and ovarian tumors in the animal kingdom.

The authors include a mixture of clinicians, pathologists, and basic scientists, and it is hoped that this gives the book the balance between the experience of the clinician and the pathologist.

Ancel Blaustein

# Acknowledgments

The editor wishes to acknowledge the help of Dr. Shirley Driscoll and Dr. William Blanc in providing their indications for examination of the placenta. Dr. Ralph Richart was kind enough to review the chapter on gross description and preparation of surgical specimens as well as the chapter on diseases of the cervix.

Drs. Mastoianni and Wheeler express their gratitude to Drs. H. T. Enterline and R. Bronson for their advice and criticism in preparing the chapter on "Pathology of the Fallopian Tube."

Dr. Czernobilsky is indebted to the excellent assistance in the manuscript preparation of Mrs. Norma Freedman and Miss Danielle Lavergne; the photographic skills of Mr. N. Feiffer and Fabienne Brand; the illustration preparation of Mrs. R. Frischberg and M. Avigdori; and to the secretarial assistance of Mrs. M. Batalion and Mary McFarland-Klein; and expresses his gratitude to Drs. H. T. Enterline and R. Bronson for their advice and criticism.

Mrs. M. Batalion, Mrs. Mollie Grossman, Mrs. Elizabeth Zebelein, Mary McFarland-Klein, Mrs. Norma Freedman and Miss Danielle Lavergne gave of their secretarial and typing talents. Mr. N. Feiffer, Mr. Fabienne Brand, Mrs. R. Frischberg and M. Avigdori were responsible for the preparation of many excellent illustrations. Mrs. Nina Federoff helped the editor to complete and correct reference data. We have been permitted the use of excellent illustrations by numerous individuals, journals and publishers. Each is separately acknowledged.

# Contents

Contents

Contents

Contents

Contents

Contents

## CHAPTER 38
## Animal Models for Tumors of the Ovary and Uterus    797

## CHAPTER 39
## Spontaneous Tumors of the Uterus and Ovaries in Animals    822

Jan Langman, M.D., Ph.D.

# 1

# Embryology and Congenital Malformations of the Female Genital Tract

## Primordial Germ Cells

In mammalian embryos the first indication of sex differentiation appears in the form of the primordial germ cells. Although for a long time considerable controversy has existed on whether these cells arise within the gonad or in an extragonadal site, it is now generally accepted that they originate in the wall of the yolk sac close to the allantois[8,21] (Figure 1.1a). From various experimental and histochemical studies[5,19] it has been concluded that the germ cell line begins with the primordial germ cells and that these cells appear at an early stage of development in the yolk sac entoderm. Subsequently they are incorporated into the wall of the hindgut and finally migrate through the dorsal mesentery to the gonadal ridges. In these ridges they multiply, differentiate, and give rise to the definitive germ cells (Figure 1.1b). Hence, the early primordial germ cells form a continuous cell line from early embryonic development to the definitive germ cells in the adult stages of life.[9]

Although unanimous agreement exists that the primordial germ cells develop in extragonadal sites, it is not certain whether they originate from entodermal or mesodermal cells. Chiquoine[5] and Mintz and Russell,[19] using the alkaline phosphatase technique, concluded that the primordial germ cells originate in the entoderm. Ozdzenski[22] and Spiegelman and Bennett[24] noted that primordial germ cells in the hindgut entoderm resembled

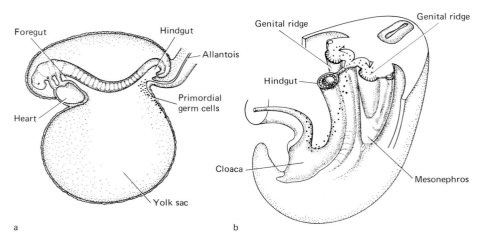

**1.1 a.** Schematic drawing of a 3-week-old embryo showing the primordial germ cells in the wall of the yolk sac, close to the attachment of the allantois. [After E. Witschi, Migration of the germ cells of human embryos from the yolk sac to the primitive gonadal folds, *Contrib. Embryol. Carnegie Inst. 32:67, 1948.*] **b.** Drawing to show the migration path of the primordial germ cells along the wall of the hindgut and the dorsal mesentery into the genital ridge. Note the position of the genital ridge and mesonephros.

splanchnic mesoderm cells and suggested that they might have been migrating in from the mesoderm. This theory has recently won more support from the studies by Clark and Eddy.[6] By examining the primordial germ cells with the electron microscope, they have found evidence that the cells do not originate in the entoderm but probably enter the entoderm shortly after their formation. Although in several points the fine structure of the primordial germ cells differed from the entoderm cells of the yolk sac, they were quite similar to the mesodermal cells adjacent to the yolk sac entoderm. In addition, some primordial germ cells were found between the entoderm and the mesoderm. Whatever their origin may be, the primordial germ cells arise early in development and are found in the posterior wall of the yolk sac very close to the allantois.

A typical characteristic of the primordial germ cells is their migratory ability. According to Witschi[27] the primordial germ cells of human embryos move individually through the tissues into the gonadal ridges. Indeed, when living primordial germ cells were studied, they showed considerable active ameboid movement.[1] Similarly, in fine structural studies the cells were found to have several characteristics of migrating cells.[7,32] In a recent study Clark and Eddy[6] have found that the primordial germ cells in the yolk sac entoderm have the appearance of sedentary cells, and they suggest that they are probably carried into the hindgut by invagination of the surrounding entoderm instead of by independent migration. Once they have arrived in the dorsal mesentery, in contrast, they usually are found to have the morphology of migrating cells. Once in the gonadal ridge, however, the primordial germ cells become round again and have a homogeneous distribution of their organelles.

## Gonadal Primordia

The gonadal primordia appear in the 4-week human embryo as a pair of longitudinal ridges located on each side of the midline between the mesonephros and the dorsal mesentery and closely related to the excretory ductules of the mesonephros (Figure 1.2a,b). When the embryo is about 5 weeks old a number of cellular components can be distinguished in the gonadal ridges. On the surface is found a rather thick, proliferating layer of coelomic epithelium (Figure 1.3). This layer covers the mesenchyme, which extends toward the mesonephros. In the mesenchyme are cellular condensations lying at right angles to the coelomic epithelium and sometimes referred to as primitive sex cords. Finally, a number of primordial germ cells can be distinguished beneath the coelomic epithelium and between the cells of the sex cords. At this

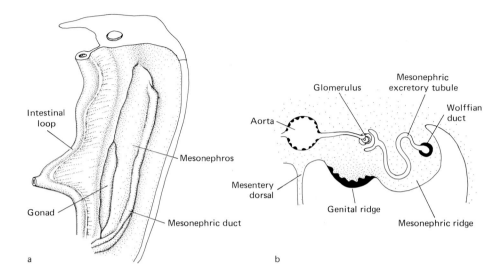

**1.2 a.** Drawing to show the relationship of the genital ridge and the mesonephros. Note the location of the mesonephric or Wolffian duct. **b.** Transverse section through the mesonephros and genital ridge at a level indicated in **a.**

Intestinal loop

Gonad

Mesonephros

Mesonephric duct

a

Glomerulus

Mesonephric excretory tubule

Aorta

Wolffian duct

Mesentery dorsal

Genital ridge

Mesonephric ridge

b

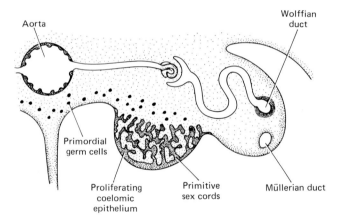

Aorta

Wolffian duct

Primordial germ cells

Proliferating coelomic epithelium

Primitive sex cords

Müllerian duct

**1.3** Schematic transverse section through the lumbar region of a 6-week embryo, showing the indifferent gonad with the primitive sex cords. Some of the primordial germ cells are surrounded by cells of the primitive sex cords.

stage of development the male and female gonad cannot be distinguished from each other and the gonad is therefore referred to as the indifferent gonad. It maintains this stage until the eighth week of development.[10]

According to Witschi,[28,29] the coelomic or germinal epithelium forms the early cortex of the gonad and the cellular condensations and cords seen in the underlying mesenchyme form the medulla. Subsequent condensation of the cells in the medulla brings about connections with the mesonephric tubules, the primordial efferent duc-

tules.[30] Witschi[30] rules out the coelomic epithelium as the source for the medulla and states that the primordial germ cells are first located in or beneath the epithelium and not in the cords. According to more recent theories, the mesenchymal condensations facilitate the ingrowth of the sex cords from the coelomic epithelium. These cords interdigitate with the mesenchymal condensations and it becomes difficult to distinguish the two primordia. The large primordial germ cells are mainly found in the cords close to the coelomic epithelium, whereas the deeper parts of the cords do not contain primordial germ cells. The latter will become the straight tubules and the rete material and the more peripheral parts will form the primary sex cords.

When the embryo is genetically male, the primitive sex cords become well defined and delineated at some distance under the germinative epithelium (Figure 1.4a,b). They consist of germ cells and somatic cells, which ultimately form the Sertoli cells. Toward the hilus of the gland the cords form tiny cell strands that give rise to the tubules of the rete testis. At the beginning of the eighth week they lose contact with the surface epithelium, which then gradually flattens and becomes the superficial layer of the tunica albuginea. The testis differentiates early and when it can be first recognized the gonad in the female is still undifferentiated. At early stages of development, therefore, presumptive ovaries are identified only because they have not differentiated into testes.

The presumptive ovaries maintain their indifferent status until the twelfth week. During this time the primordial germ cells continue multiplying and numerous germ cells are found beneath the coelomic epithelium. The thick

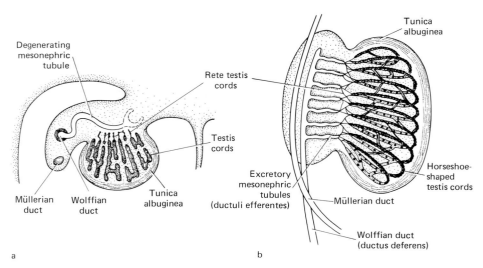

**1.4 a.** Transverse section through the testis in the eighth week of development. Note the tunica albuginea, the testis cords, the rete testis, and the primordial germ cells. The glomerulus and Bowman's capsule of the mesonephric excretory tubule are in regression. **b.** Schematic representation of the testis and the genital ducts in the fourth month of development. The horseshoe-shaped testis cords are continuous with the rete testis cords. Note the ductuli efferentes (excretory mesonephric tubules), which enter the Wolffian duct.

cortical layer remains in continuity with the coelomic epithelium.

With further differentiation of the female gonad the so-called cortical or ovarian cords develop. According to most investigators these new cords develop directly from the coelomic epithelium and penetrate into the underlying mesenchyme (Figure 1.5a,b). Others,[11] however, believe that the cortical cords develop beneath the germinal epithelium and consist of the peripheral parts of the thickened primitive sex cords of the indifferent stage. The deeper parts of the primitive cords (also referred to as the medullary cords) gradually disappear and are replaced by vascular stroma to form the ovarian medulla.

# Factors Influencing Gonad Differentiation

The sex of an embryo is determined at the time of fertilization and depends on whether the spermatocyte carries an X or a Y chromosome. In embryos with an XX sex chromosome configuration, the cords extending into the medulla of the gonad regress and those close to the cortex (cortical cords) come to full development. In embryos with XY chromosomes, the medullary cords develop into testis cords and the secondary cortical cords fail to develop. Because at these early stages of development few, if any, hormones circulate in the embryo, it may be stated that the development of the gonad into testis or ovary is mainly influenced by the sex chromosome complex established at fertilization.

When one of the X chromosomes is lacking, such as in patients with Turner's syndrome (44 + XO), gonad development is abnormal. The primordial germ cells are present and migrate into the undifferentiated gonad as in normal conditions, but few, if any, true follicles develop and during the last half of intrauterine life many of the germ cells degenerate. Six months after birth all germ cells have disappeared and the ovary is hypoplastic.[4,12] Apparently in the absence of the second X or a Y chromosome the undifferentiated gonad begins to develop as an ovary but is unable to fully differentiate or maintain its germ cells.

If the primordial germ cells do not reach the undifferentiated gonad, neither testis nor ovary develops. In these patients with pure gonadal dysgenesis the gonad maintains its early embryonic undifferentiated form and may be found as an undifferentiated streak gonad. Hence, to accomplish full differentiation of the gonad into testis or

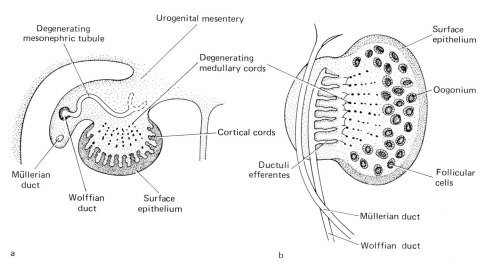

**1.5 a.** Transverse section through the ovary at the seventh week of development, showing the degeneration of the primitive (medullary) sex cords and the formation of the cortical cords. **b.** Schematic drawing of the ovary and genital ducts in the fifth month of development. Note the degeneration of the medullary cords. The excretory mesonephric tubules (ductuli efferentes) do not communicate with the rete. The cortical zone of the ovary contains groups of oogonia surrounded by follicular cells.

ovary, the primordial germ cells must reach the gonads and must have their full chromosomal complement either male or female.

In considering gonadal differentiation the question must be raised whether embryonic "hormones" influence early gonad differentiation. For many years concepts of sex differentiation have been based on the theory of cortico-medullary antagonism.[31] According to this theory, which is based mainly on studies with amphibians, the cortex and the medulla secrete antagonistic inductors. The dominant inductive system (under normal conditions corresponding to the genetic sex of the embryo) determines the sex of the developing gonad. Sex reversal was thought to result from reduced influence of the original dominant system or from an increase in the activity of the opposite (dormant) component. A humoral agent capable of interfering with gonadal development was first found in freemartins.[16,17] (The "freemartin" is the female partner of heterosexual twins in cattle.) Under influence of the male twin the ovaries of the female are inhibited and sterile.[15] The ovarian cortex is suppressed and replaced by a tunica albuginea. Sometimes the medullary part of the ovary contains tubules that resemble seminiferous tubules. Hence, it seems that in cattle the developing testis of the male twin produces a hormone that suppresses cortical

differentiation in the female twin. Similar observations were made in experiments in which rat and rabbit ovaries were grown with fetal testes, as grafts in adult hosts.[14] The only case in which adult sex hormones were capable of influencing gonadal differentiation was in the opossum. When embryos at early stages of development were treated with estradiol dipropionate,[3] the germinal epithelium of the early testis persisted and proliferated (cortical proliferation), but the central medullary part was profoundly inhibited and atrophied. Hence, although in a few experiments and in heterosexual twins in cattle gonadal differentiation is influenced by hormones, at present there is no evidence that in humans hormones play a role in the development of the indifferent gonad into testis or ovary.

## The Duct System

### Indifferent Stage

In the sixth week of development both male and female embryos have two pairs of genital ducts (Figure 1.6a,b). One is the mesonephric duct extending from the meso-nephros to the cloaca and referred to as the Wolffian system; the second duct arises as a longitudinal invagina-

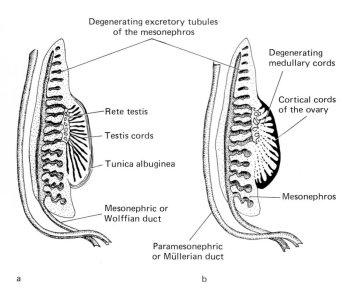

Degenerating excretory tubules
of the mesonephros

Degenerating
medullary cords

Rete testis

Cortical cords
of the ovary

Testis cords

Tunica albuginea

Mesonephros

Mesonephric or
Wolffian duct

Paramesonephric
or Müllerian duct

a

b

**1.6** Diagram of the genital ducts in the sixth week of development in the male **a** and in the female **b.** The Wolffian and Müllerian ducts are present in both the male and female. Note the excretory tubules of the mesonephros and their relationship to the developing gonad.

tion of the coelomic epithelium on the anterolateral surface of the urogenital ridge. This duct runs parallel to the Wolffian duct and is known as the paramesonephric duct or Müllerian duct. It opens into the coelomic cavity with a funnel-like structure. Hence, contrary to the mesonephric duct, which is connected to the mesonephric tissue through the excretory tubules, the Müllerian duct opens widely into the coelomic cavity and does not possess any excretory tubules.

The Müllerian duct first courses laterally to the mesonephric duct but then crosses it ventrally, growing in a caudomedial direction. In the midline the two Müllerian ducts meet. Initially they remain separated by a septum, but in later development they fuse to form a single canal. The caudal tip of the combined ducts grows further caudally until it makes contact with the posterior wall of the urogenital sinus (Figure 1.8a). Where the Müllerian ducts make contact with the sinus, the caudal wall proliferates, forming the Müllerian tubercle. On both sides of the tubercle are the openings of the Wolffian ducts into the urogenital sinus. Hence in early development both sexes possess two Wolffian ducts and two Müllerian ducts.

## Duct Development in the Male

When the embryo is genetically male, the excretory tubules of the mesonephros close to the developing testis lose their glomeruli, become somewhat shortened, and establish contact with the cords of the rete testis, thus forming the ductuli efferentes of the testis (Figure 1.7a,b). The excretory tubules located cranial to the testis disappear almost completely except for vestiges of a few ductuli, known as the paradidymis. The mesonephric duct thus becomes the main duct for the testis and is connected to it through the ductuli efferentes. By the end of the eighth week the paramesonephric or Müllerian duct in the male has degenerated entirely except for a small portion at its cranial end that persists as the appendix testis. According to some authors a small portion of the caudal end of the duct also persists to form the utriculus prostaticus or uterus masculinus, a small diverticulum in the wall of the prostatic urethra. Other authors, however, believe that the caudal parts disappear entirely and that the utriculus prostaticus is formed by an outpocketing of the urogenital sinus.

## Duct Development in the Female

In females the Müllerian duct develops into the main genital duct. Initially, three parts can be recognized. The first part runs vertically and opens into the coelomic cavity; the second portion is horizontal and crosses the Wolffian duct; the third or caudal part fuses with its partner of the opposite side (Figure 1.8a,b). With the descent of the ovary the first two parts obtain a horizontal position and form the oviduct or fallopian tube. The coelomic opening is known as the abdominal ostium. Simultaneously the urogenital ridges change position and gradually occupy a transverse plane. When the two ducts have fused in the midline, a broad transverse fold is established in the pelvis. These peritoneal folds extend from the lateral sides of the fused Müllerian ducts toward the lateral walls of the bony pelvis and are known as the broad ligaments (Figure 1.9). The ovaries are located on the posterior surface of the broad ligaments.

The solid caudal tip of the Müllerian ducts reaches the posterior wall of the urogenital sinus in the ninth week of development (Figure 1.10). Here it meets two solid evaginations from the posterior wall of the urogenital sinus, the sinovaginal bulbs. These bulbs proliferate extensively and form a solid plate, the vaginal plate.[2] This plate enfolds the end of the fused Müllerian ducts and begins to vacuolize at its caudal end in embryos of approximately 11

**1.7 a.** Diagram of the genital ducts in the male in the fourth month of development. The Müllerian duct has degenerated except for the appendix testis and the utriculus prostaticus. **b.** The genital duct after descent of the testis. Note the horseshoe-shaped testis cords, the rete testis, and the ductuli efferentes entering the ductus deferens. The paradidymis is formed by the remnants of the paragenital mesonephric tubules.

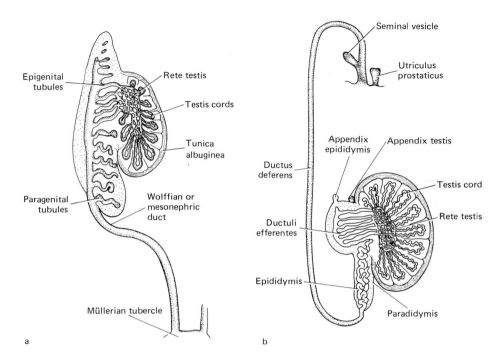

**1.8 a.** Schematic drawing of the genital ducts in the female at the end of the second month of development. Note the Müllerian tubercle and the formation of the uterine canal. **b.** The genital ducts after descent of the ovary. The only parts remaining of the mesonephric system are the epoophoron, the paroophoron, and Gärtner's cyst. Note the suspensory ligament of the ovary, the ligament of the ovary proper, and the round ligament of the uterus.

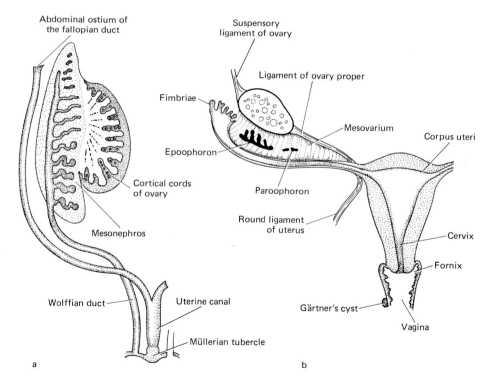

**1.9** Transverse sections through the urogenital ridge at progressively lower levels (**a** through **c**). Note that the Müllerian ducts approach each other in the midline to fuse. As a result of the fusion of the ducts a transverse fold, the broad ligament of the uterus, is formed in the pelvis. The gonads come to lie at the posterior aspect of the transverse fold.

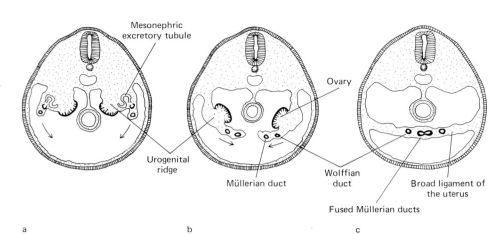

**1.10** Schematic sagittal sections showing the formation of the uterus and vagina at various stages of development (**a** through **c**).

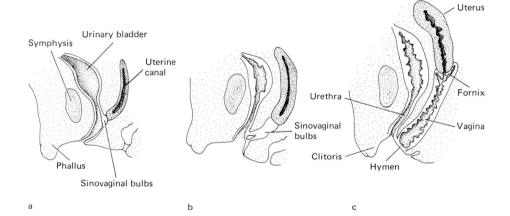

weeks. Proliferation continues at the cranial end of the vaginal plate, and the distance between the caudal tip of the Müllerian ducts (uterus) and the wall of the urogenital sinus increases. By the fifth month the vaginal outgrowth is entirely canalized and forms winglike expansions around the end of the uterus. Hence, according to this theory, the vagina is entirely formed by an outgrowth of the urogenital sinus. Although Müller[20] himself proposed this theory, which was later supported by many investigators, another group favors a dual source in the establishment of the vagina. The upper part of the vagina is thought to be derived from the fused Müllerian ducts, whereas the lower part originates from the sinovaginal bulbs.[18] This theory has the great advantage that it can explain most of the vaginal malformations. Incomplete fusion of the Müllerian ducts results not only in a dual or septate uterus but also in a septum in the upper portion of the vagina. Similarly,

atresia of the lower portion of the vagina and the presence of a small vaginal pouch close to the uterus may be explained by lack of vacuolization in the bulbovaginal portion of the vagina and normal vacuolization in the Müllerian cranial portion of the vagina. The development of a transverse septum can also easily be explained. Unfortunately, it has been difficult to confirm this theory by observations on the development of the vagina in normal fetuses.

As the uterus and vagina are formed, the mesonephric system and the Wolffian ducts disappear except for a few remnants. These are located in the mesovarium and are vestiges of excretory mesonephric tubules and a portion of the Wolffian duct. In the mesosalpinx they form the epoophoron (Figure 1.8b). The more caudally located mesonephric tubules form a remnant known as the paroophoron. On occasion a vestige of the more caudal part of the Wolffian duct may persist in the form of Gärtner's cysts. These cysts are found in the lateral wall of the vagina and sometimes in the wall of the uterus. In summary, in the female embryo the Müllerian system comes to full development, whereas the Wolffian system disappears almost entirely.

# External Genitalia

## Indifferent Stage

Similar to the indifferent stage of the gonads and ducts, the external genitalia are also characterized by an indifferent phase. In the third week of development mesenchyme cells originating in the primitive streak migrate around the cloacal membrane and form a pair of slightly elevated folds, the cloacal folds. Cranial to the membrane the two folds unite and form the genital tubercle (Figure 1.11a,b). When in the sixth week the cloacal membrane is divided into the urogenital and anal membranes, the cloacal folds are likewise subdivided into the urethral folds anteriorly and the anal folds posteriorly. While this occurs, another pair of swellings becomes visible on each side of the urethral folds. These are known as genital swellings and in the female differentiate into the labia majora and in the male into the scrotal swellings. By the end of the sixth week, however, the appearance of the external genitalia is identical in the male and female.

## Further Development of the External Genitalia

The external genitalia of the female change only little from the indifferent stage. The genital tubercle elongates slightly to form the clitoris and the urethral folds develop into the labia minora and the genital swellings in the labia majora. Because in many cases the external genitalia of the female differentiate in a male direction, a brief account of the male development is necessary. It is characterized by the rapid elongation of the genital tubercle, which is now called the phallus. The elongation is such that the urethral folds are pulled forward and temporarily form the lateral walls of a deep urethral or urogenital groove (Figure 1.12a,b). At the end of the third month the two urethral folds close over the groove, thus forming the penis and the penile part of the urethra. The genital swellings, initially located in the inguinal region, move more caudally and closer together. Finally the two fuse in the midline, and each swelling makes up a half of the scrotum. The plane of

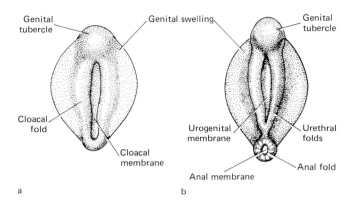

**1.11** The indifferent stage of the external genitalia (**a**) at approximately 4 weeks and (**b**) at approximately 6 weeks.

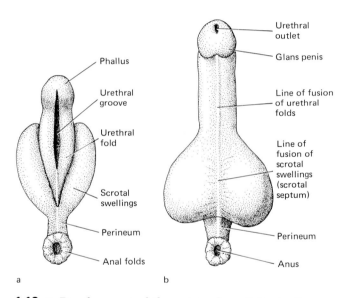

**1.12 a.** Development of the external genitalia in the male at 10 weeks. Note the deep urethral groove flanked by the urethral folds. **b.** In the newborn.

fusion defines the scrotal septum. Hence, in the male the urethral and genital swellings fuse but in the female they remain separated.

## Factors Controlling Development of the Duct System and External Genitalia

It is now generally accepted that the genital ducts and external genitalia develop under the influence of hormones circulating in the fetus during intrauterine life.[15] The fetal testes produce a nonsteroidal substance known as the inducer substance. This substance induces growth and differentiation of the Wolffian duct system but inhibits the development of the Müllerian ducts. For this reason it has also been called the suppressor substance. In addition to the inducer substance, the testes produce androgens that stimulate the development of the external genitalia, such as the growth of the penis, the formation of the penile urethra, the fusion of the scrotal swellings, and the formation of the prostate and seminal vesicles.

In females the Müllerian ducts develop into the oviducts and uterus in response to maternal and placental estrogens circulating in the fetus. Because the male inducer substance is absent, the Wolffian duct system regresses. In the absence of androgens the indifferent external genitalia are stimulated by maternal and placental estrogens and differentiate into labia majora, labia minora, clitoris, and vagina.

## Human Sexual Abnormalities

Considering the above-stated general rules it is evident that in patients with ovarian hypoplasia or dysgenesis the duct system and external genitalia develop in the female direction. No testis is present and hence no inducer substance or androgens are formed. Under the influence of maternal and placental estrogens the Müllerian duct system is stimulated and the external genitalia develop as in the normal female. However, because in these patients the gonads do not produce hormones after birth, further growth of the oviducts, uterus, and vagina, as well as of the external genitalia, ceases and the sex characteristics remain infantile. Hence, in cases in which inducer substance as well as androgens are absent the duct system and external genitalia are of female appearance.

A female appearance, however, does not necessarily indicate a genetic female as is evident from patients with the testicular feminization syndrome. These patients have a $44 + XY$ chromosome complement and a normal female appearance but do have testes. Because in these patients the inducer substance is present, the Müllerian duct system is suppressed and the oviducts and uterus are absent. Frequently the testes are found in the inguinal region, and a ductus deferens (Wolffian duct) is present. No spermatogenesis occurs. The tissues are thought to be unresponsive to androgens and consequently the external genitalia, prostate, and seminal vesicles fail to develop.[25] Instead, the placental and maternal estrogens stimulate the external genitalia to develop in female direction.

A different set of abnormalities is seen in the pseudohermaphrodites. In these patients the genotypic sex is masked by a phenotypic appearance that closely resembles the other sex. When the pseudohermaphrodite has an ovary, the patient is called a female pseudohermaphrodite; when a testis is present, the patient is called a male pseudohermaphrodite. The most common cause of female pseudohermaphroditism is the adrenogenital syndrome. The patient has a $44 + XX$ chromosome complement and has ovaries. The excessive production of androgens by the adrenals, however, causes the external genitalia to develop in a male direction.[23] Frequently the clitoris is considerably hypertrophied and the labia majora are partially fused giving the impression of a scrotum. A small persistent urogenital sinus is usually present. Although this type of pseudohermaphroditism is caused by a recessive gene, progestins administered during pregnancy may cause similar abnormalities as in the adrenogenital syndrome. The great majority of female pseudohermaphrodites fall in the first category.[13,26]

Most of the congenital malformations of the female genital tract can be explained by the action of hormones on the duct system and external genitalia. Another group of abnormalities, however, is caused by faulty morphogenetic processes, similar to those observed in other organs of the embryo. These processes, such as lack of vacuolization of solid outbuddings, absence of cell degeneration in embryonic septa, and lack of fusion of ducts, are seen in many developing organ systems. Some of these faulty morphogenetic processes may result from abnormal hormonal conditions but others are of genetic origin or of unknown etiology.

Under normal conditions the uterus and probably the upper third of the vagina are formed by fusion of the two Müllerian ducts. The ducts not only come together in the midline but, after they have fused, the fused walls disappear as a result of cell degeneration. Hence, two types of abnormalities may be expected. In the first category belongs the uterus bicornis, resulting from a nonfusion of the ducts. In the second category belong those abnormalities which result from the persistence of the fused walls in the form of a septum. In some patients the septum may persist throughout its entire length, resulting in a uterus didelphys with a partially double vagina (Figure 1.13).

Another group of malformations concerns the complete or partial atresia of one or both Müllerian ducts in otherwise normal women. If one side is involved, the only components remaining are the fimbriae and a small muscular mass located at the lateral wall of the pelvis. Sometimes the rudimentary part lies as an appendage to the

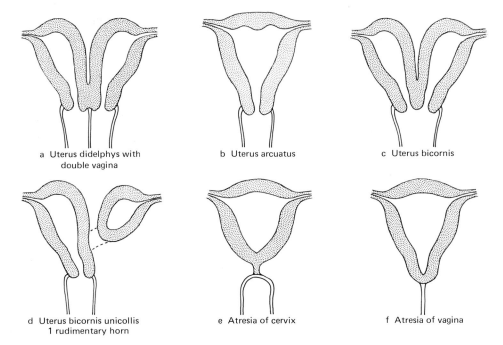

**1.13** Schematic representation of the main abnormalities of the uterus and vagina, caused by persistence of the uterine septum or obliteration of the lumen of the uterine canal.

a Uterus didelphys with double vagina

b Uterus arcuatus

c Uterus bicornis

d Uterus bicornis unicollis 1 rudimentary horn

e Atresia of cervix

f Atresia of vagina

well-developed side (uterus bicornis unicollis with rudimentary horn). In its most severe form the uterus is represented bilaterally by rudimentary, noncanalized, muscular buds located at the lateral pelvic wall. This abnormality is frequently combined with vaginal and upper urinary tract anomalies (Rokitansky–Küster–Houser syndrome), suggesting a severe morphogenetic abnormality of a more general nature and affecting the embryo simultaneously in several organ systems. Hence, although many abnormalities in the female genital system can be explained by abnormal hormonal actions, a large number of anomalies are of totally unknown origin.

# REFERENCES

1. Blandau, R. J., White, B. J., and Rumery, R. E. Observations on the movements of the living primordial germ cells in the mouse. *Fertil. Steril.* 14:482, 1963.

2. Bulmer, D. The development of the human vagina. *J. Anat.* 91:490, 1957.

3. Burns, R. K. Jr. Hormones versus constitutional factors in the growth of embryonic sex primordia in the opossum. *Am. J. Anat.* 98:35, 1956.

4. Carr, D. H., Haggar, R. A., and Hart, A. G. Germ cells in the ovaries of XO female infants. *Am. J. Clin. Pathol.* 49:521, 1968.

5. Chiquoine, A. D. The identification, origin and migration of the primordial germ cells in the mouse embryo. *Anat. Rec.* 118:135, 1954.

6. Clark, J. M., and Eddy, E. M. Fine structural observations on the origin and associations of primordial germ cells of the mouse. *Dev. Biol.* 47:136, 1975.

7. Eddy, E. M., and Clark, J. M. Electron microscopic study of migrating primordial germ cells in the rat, *in* Hess, M., ed.: *Electron Microscopic Concepts of Secretion. The Ultrastructure of Endocrine and Reproductive Organs.* New York, Wiley, 1975, pp. 151–168.

8. Everett, N. B. The present status of the germ cell problem in vertebrates. *Biol. Rev.* 26:45, 1945.

9. Franchi, L. L., Mandl, A. M., and Zuckerman, S. The development of the ovary and the process of oogenesis, *in* Zuckerman, S., Mandl, A. M., and Eckstein, P., eds.: *The Ovary.* London, Academic Press, 1962, Vol. 1, pp. 1–87.

10. Gillman, J. The development of the gonads in man, with a consideration of the role of fetal endocrines and the histogenesis of ovarian tumors. *Contrib. Embryol.* 32:81, 1948.

11. Gropp, A., and Ohno, S. The presence of a common embryonic blastema for ovarian and testicular parenchymal (follicular, interstitial and tubular) cells in cattle, *Bos taurus*. *Z. Zellforsch.* 74:505, 1966.

12. Hamerton, J. L. *Human Cytogenetics. Vol. 1. Clinical Cytogenetics.* New York, Academic Press, 1971.

13. Hayles, A. B., and Nolan, R. B. Masculinization of female fetus, possibly related to administration of progesterone during pregnancy: Report of two cases. *Proc. Staff Meet. Mayo Clin.* 33:200, 1958.

14. Holyoke, E. A., and Beber, B. A. Cultures of gonads of mammalian embryos. *Science* 128:1082, 1958.

15. Jost, A. Embryonic sexual differentiation (morphology,

physiology, abnormalities), *in* Jones, H., Jr., and Scott, W. W., eds.: *Hermaphroditism, Genital Anomalies and Related Endocrine Disorders*, 2nd ed. Baltimore, Williams & Wilkins, 1971, p. 16.

16. Lillie, F. R. The theory of the free-martin. *Science* 43:611, 1916.

17. Lillie, F. R. The etiology of the freemartin. *Vet. Rec.* 2:167, 1922.

18. McKelvey, J. L., and Baxter, J. S. Abnormal development of the vagina and genitourinary tract. *Am. J. Obstet. Gynecol. 29*:267, 1935.

19. Mintz, B., and Russell, E. S. Gene-induced embryological modifications of primordial germ cells in the mouse. *J. Exp. Zool. 134*:207, 1957.

20. Müller, J. *Bildungsgeschichte der Genitalien aus Anatomischen Untersuchungen an Embryonen des Menschen und der Thiere.* Dusseldorf, 1930, Arnz.

21. Nieuwkoop, P. D. The present status of the problem of the "Keimbahn" in the vertebrates. *Experientia 5*:308, 1949.

22. Ozdzenski, W. Observations on the origin of primordial germ cells in the mouse. *Zool. Pol. 17*:367, 1967.

23. Schlegel, R. J., and Gardner, L. I. Ambiguous and abnormal genitalia in infants: Differential diagnosis and clinical management, *in* Gardner, L. I., ed.: *Endocrine and Genetic Diseases of Childhood.* Philadelphia, W. B. Saunders, 1969.

24. Spiegelman, M., and Bennett, D. A light- and electron-microscopic study of primordial germ cells in the early mouse embryo. *J. Embryol. Exp. Morphol., 30*:97, 1973.

25. Wilkins, L. *The Diagnosis and Treatment of Endocrine Disorders in Childhood and Adolescence.* Springfield, Ill., Charles C Thomas, 1950.

26. Wilkins, L. *The Diagnosis and Treatment of Endocrine Disorders in Childhood and Adolescence,* 2nd ed. Springfield, Ill., Charles C Thomas, 1957.

27. Witschi, E. Migration of the germ cells of human embryos from the yolk sac to the primitive gonadal folds. *Contrib. Embryol. Carnegie Inst. 32*:67, 1948.

28. Witschi, E. Embryogenesis of the adrenal and the reproductive glands. *Recent Prog. Horm. Res. 6*:1, 1951.

29. Witschi, E. *Development of Vertebrates.* Philadelphia, W. B. Saunders, 1956.

30. Witschi, E. Embryology of the ovary, *in* Grady, H. G., and Smith, D. E., eds.: *The Ovary.* Baltimore, Williams & Wilkins, 1962, pp. 1–10.

31. Witschi, E. Biochemistry of sex differentiation in vertebrate embryos, *in* Weber, R., ed.: *The Biochemistry of Animal Development.* New York, Academic Press, 1967, Vol. 2, pp. 193–225.

32. Zamboni, L., and Merchant, H. The fine morphology of mouse primordial germ cells in extragonadal locations. *Am. J. Anat. 137*:299, 1973.

Eduard G. Friedrich, Jr.,
    H.A.B., M.D., F.A.C.O.G.,
and Edward J. Wilkinson,
    B.A., M.D., F.A.C.O.G., F.A.S.C.P.

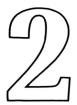

# The Vulva

## Anatomy

### Structure

The external female genitalia include the mons pubis, the labia majora and minora, the clitoris with its prepuce and frenulum, and the vestibule into which open the orifices of Skene's and Bartholin's glands and the urethral meatus (Figure 2.1). All of these structures are easily visualized except for the Bartholin gland orifices, which are normally not seen unless inflamed. With adrenarche, the mons pubis and lateral aspects of the labia majora acquire increased amounts of subcutaneous fat and develop the coarse curly surface hair characteristic of the adult. With maturation of the hair follicle apparatus, there is concomitant maturation and development of the sebaceous and apocrine glands in the hair-bearing regions and also in the labia minora and inner aspect of the prepuce. Other than the areola of the breast, these are the only areas where sebaceous glands routinely develop without concomitant hair formation (Figure 2.2). During adolescence, the labia acquire a characteristic hyperpigmentation and the clitoris undergoes some selective enlargement. The labia majora contain both smooth muscle and fat, whereas the labia minora are devoid of adipose tissue but are rich in elastic fibers and blood vessels. The entire vulva is covered by a keratinized, stratified squamous epithelium. Medially as the vaginal introitus is approached, this epi-

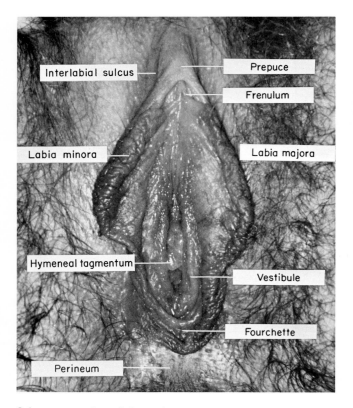

**2.1** Topography of the vulva.

Interlabial sulcus
Prepuce
Frenulum
Labia minora
Labia majora
Hymeneal tagmentum
Vestibule
Fourchette
Perineum

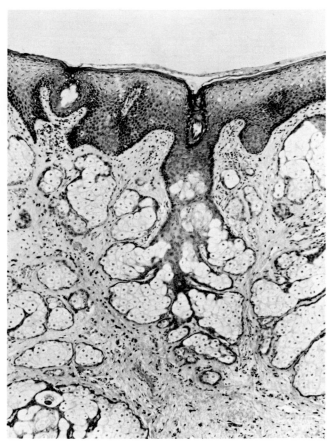

**2.2** Sebaceous glands of the labia minora. Note the absence of hair shafts.

thelium becomes thinner, the rete ridges less prominent, and the keratin layer less pronounced. The hymen is thinly keratinized on its external surface but on the vaginal surface shows a nonkeratinized mucous membrane that is rich in glycogen. The epithelium of the vestibule merges with transitional epithelium at the urethral meatus and the duct openings of the Bartholin glands.

The apocrine glands of the majora, minora, and prepuce (Figure 2.3), like the apocrine glands of the axilla, develop their secretory function at adrenarche, whereas the eccrine sweat glands, primarily involved in heat regulation, function prior to puberty.[70] The apocrine glands are homologous to the scent glands of lower animals and secrete via a process of decapitation.

The paired external openings of the paraurethral glands (Skene's) are found on either side of the urethral meatus but these glandular structures are known to be distributed along the posterior and lateral aspects of the urethra and may indeed have multiple orifices entering into the urethra itself.[69] The ducts are lined with cylindrical epithelium, whereas the glands are composed of pseudostratified columnar epithelium. Involvement of these glands by

inflammation or infection may contribute to the development of suburethral diverticula.

The vulvovaginal glands of Bartholin are racemose, tubular alveolar glands, drained by a duct that measures approximately 2.5 cm in length and is lined with transitional epithelium. The most superficial cells are of the mucous-secreting type.[132] The duct exits at the junction of the hymenal ring and labia minora on the posterolateral aspect of the vaginal orifice. The gland acini are composed of simple columnar mucous-secreting cells (Figure 2.4).

The clitoris is a specialized structure covered with a stratified squamous epithelium that is thinly keratinized. There are no sebaceous, apocrine, or eccrine sweat glands present. Within the stroma of the clitoris are two conjoined corpora cavernosa that branch near the base of the clitoris and lie along the pubic rami as divided crura. They are invested in a loose fibrous tissue sheath with an incomplete center septum. At their insertion, the crura contain

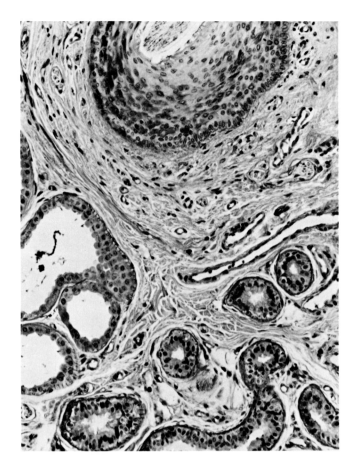

**2.3** Apocrine apparatus. Large gland spaces and narrow ducts coil near a hair shaft.

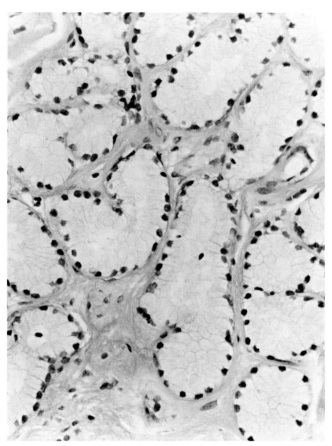

**2.4** Bartholin gland. Mucous-secreting acini in racemose arrangement.

ischiocavernosus muscles. The clitoris is further supported bilaterally and dorsally by suspensory ligaments.

The superficial and deep external pudendal arteries branch from the femoral artery. The internal pudendal arteries branch from the internal iliac arteries. These major branches from the femoral and internal iliac arteries provide the major blood supply to the vulva. The anterior labial branches, from the external pudendal arteries, and the posterior labial branches, from the internal pudendal, supply the labia minora and majora. The clitoris including the crura and corpora cavernosa are supplied by the deep arteries of the clitoris. The anterior vaginal artery supplies blood flow to the vestibule and the Bartholin glands. The venous return parallels the arterial supply.

The femoral and inguinal lymph nodes receive all of the lymphatic drainage from the vulva with the exception of the clitoris. Lymphatic drainage from the glans clitoris can proceed to the upper quadrants of the superficial femoral nodes via the presymphyseal plexus where, within the mons, these channels converge with those from the prepuce and labia.[126,129] The second lymphatic pathway from the glans clitoris proceeds with the lymphatic drainage of the urethra and dorsal vein of the clitoris to course inferior to the symphysis pubis. Traversing the urogenital diaphragm, it merges with the lymphatic plexus on the anterior surface of the bladder. Subsequently, the inferior trunks drain to the interiliac and obturator nodes, whereas the superior trunk terminates in the nodes of the femoral ring or the medial group of the external iliac nodes. The implications of the lymphatic drainage of the vulva, provided the glans clitoris is not involved with malignancy, are that if the superficial lymph nodes are free of tumor, it is highly unlikely that the deep nodes are involved.

The nerve supply to the vulva includes sensory nerves, special receptors, and autonomic nerves to the vessels and various glands. The major nerves of the vulva derive from the anterior (ilioinguinal) and posterior (pudendal) labial nerves. The clitoris is innervated by the dorsal nerve of the clitoris and the cavernous nerves of the clitoris, which also supply the vestibule.[51]

## Developmental Defects

Clitoral enlargement may occur with or without associated hyperplasia of the remaining vulva. Clitoral enlargement in the newborn suggests adrenogenital syndrome, exogenous maternal androgen therapy, or some form of hermaphroditism. Such specimens may come to the attention of the pathologist subsequent to partial removal of the clitoris in an attempt to return the cosmetic appearance of the vulva to normal.

Hypertrophy and asymmetry of the labia minora may occur without demonstrable etiology and may be seen in some cases of multiple sclerosis.

True hypoplasia occurs infrequently and is usually a sign of defective steroidogenesis. Imperforate hymen is remarkably rare, with a reported incidence of 0.014% and is usually discovered sometime after the onset of expected menarche between the ages of 10 and 18.[30]

Labial fusion, like clitoral hypertrophy, may be present with intersex disorders. In these situations, the defect is developmental, but such fusion may also be acquired secondary to inflammation and subsequent adhesion formation.[13]

Duplication of the vulva is extremely rare but has been recorded. Such duplications often involve duplication of the internal Müllerian system and rectum as well[65] (see Figure 2.5, Plate I).

The urethra may open into the vagina instead of into the vestibule; and ectopic urethral orifices are occasionally seen adjacent to the hymen.[24]

Absence of the perineal body is generally secondary to childbirth lacerations. Surgically submitted tissue at the time of plastic repair usually includes portions of the vagina and rectum from the fistulous tract.

In Müllerian agenesis, the hymen and vagina are represented only by a depression in the vestibular area. Congenital absence of the clitoris and mons pubis has also been described.[32,71]

# Infectious Diseases of the Vulva

The infectious lesions of the vulva prevalent in North America include condylomata acuminata, herpes genitalis, syphilis, and molluscum contagiosum. These and other

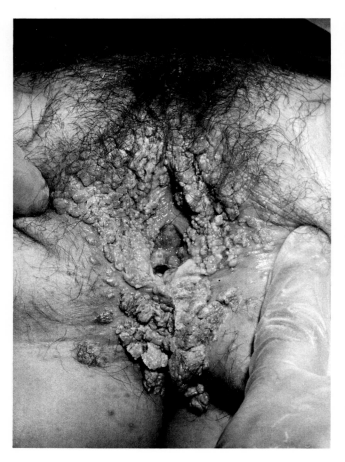

**2.6** Condylomata acuminata. Widespread involvement of the vulva and perianal region.

infectious conditions of the vulva are listed in Table 2.1. It is accepted that the criteria for clinical diagnosis do not necessarily require specific organism characterization in all these conditions.

## Condylomata Acuminata

Condylomata acuminata are benign, contagious, sexually transmitted neoplasms that may involve the vulva, vagina, cervix, and perianal skin and are caused by a virus of the papova group.[123,130] Clinically, condylomata present as papillary or verrucous lesions of the skin and mucous membrane that are nearly always multiple and frequently confluent (Figure 2.6). Except for occasional pruritus, the lesions are asymptomatic unless secondarily infected. The virus causing condyloma acuminatum is believed to be "biotropic," activated in response to a

PLATE I

**2.5** Double vulva.
[Courtesy of Dr. Leonard Wolfe.]

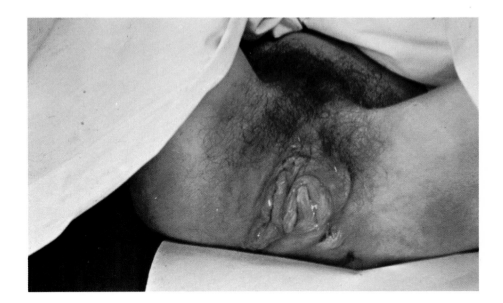

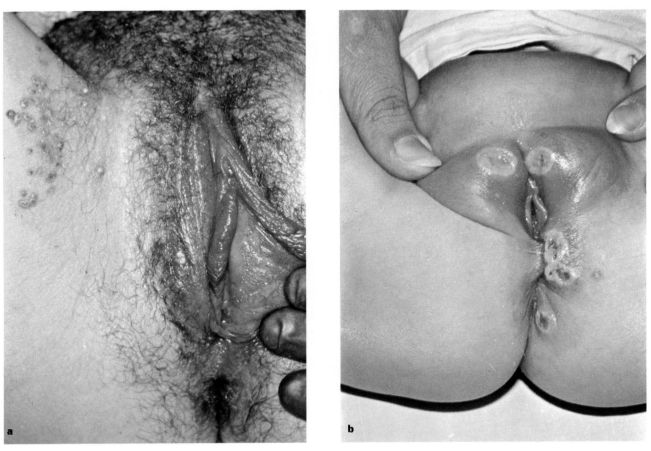

**2.8 a.** Herpes vesicles on labia and thigh. **b.** Herpes ulcers.
[**a** and **b** by courtesy of Dr. Leonard Wolfe.]

PLATE II

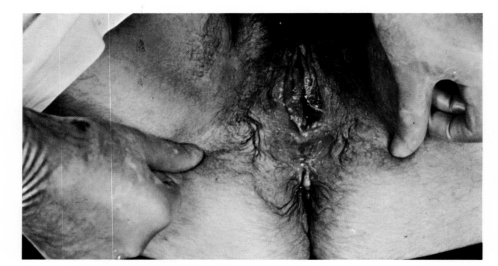

**2.10** Chancre. Painless shallow ulcer.

[Courtesy of Dr. Leonard Wolfe.]

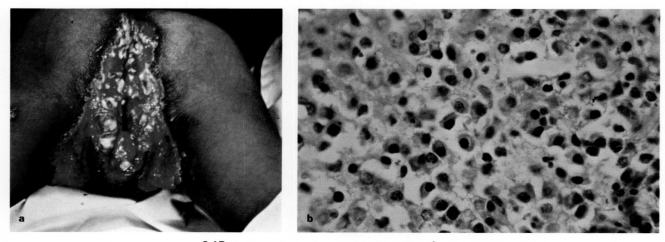

**2.15 a.** Granuloma inguinale ulceration. **b.** Granulation tissue.

**2.19 a.** Behcef's disease, oral lesions. **b.** Behcef's disease, genital ulcers.

[**a** and **b** by courtesy of Dr. Leonard Wolfe.]

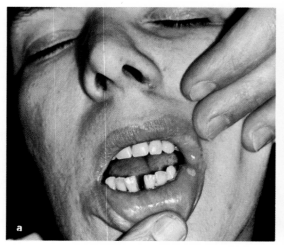
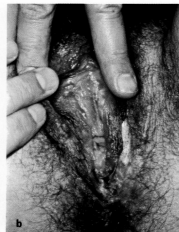

PLATE III

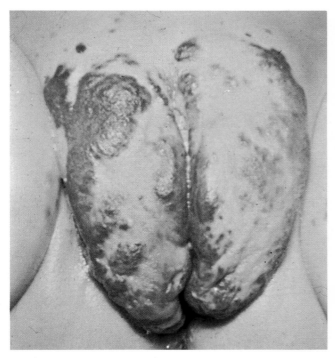

**2.24** Hemangioma of the labia.

[Courtesy of Dr. Leonard Wolfe.]

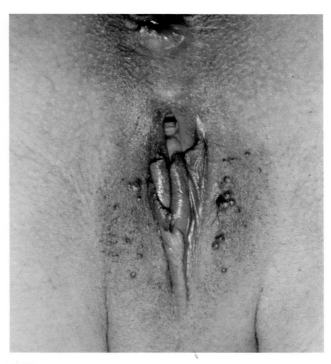

**2.25** Angiokeratoma.

[Courtesy of Dr. Leonard Wolfe.]

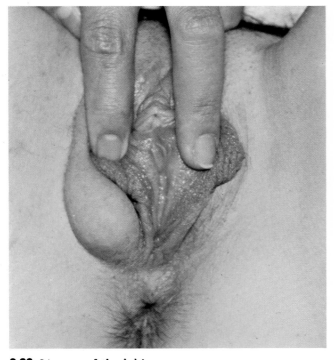

**2.28** Lipoma of the labia.

[Courtesy of Dr. Leonard Wolfe.]

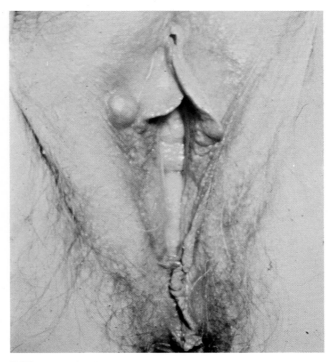

**2.29 a.** Hydradenoma of the vulva.

PLATE IV

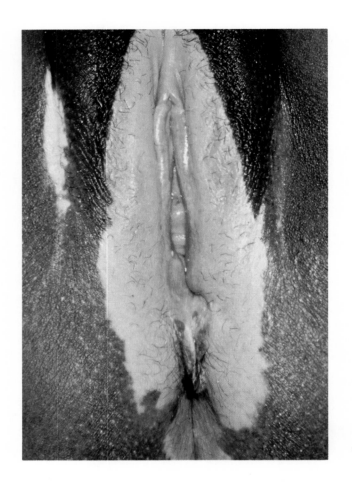

**2.33** Vitiligo.

[Courtesy of Dr. Leonard Wolfe.]

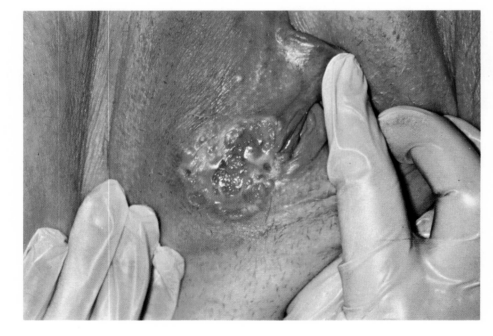

**2.57** Basal cell carcinoma of
the vulva.

[Courtesy of Dr. Leonard Wolfe.]

**Table 2.1**   Infectious diseases of the vulva

| Disease | Cause | Histopathology | Diagnosis |
|---|---|---|---|
| Condyloma acuminatum | DNA papova virus group | Acanthosis, hyperkeratosis, parakeratosis, papillomatosis, perinuclear "halo" | Histopathology |
| Herpes genitalis | Herpes simplex hominis type II | Intranuclear inclusions | Cytopathology, culture, serology |
| Syphilitic chancre | Treponema pallidum | Ulceration, chronic inflammation, vasculitis | Dark field, fluorescence, silver stain, serology |
| Condyloma lata | Treponema pallidum | Like chancre with epithelial hyperplasia | Same as chancre |
| Molluscum contagiosum | DNA pox virus group | Intracytoplasmic inclusions | Cytopathology, histopathology |
| Lymphogranuloma venereum | Chlamydia (TRIC agent) | Granulomatous reaction without caseation | Serology, Frei test |
| Granuloma inguinale | Calymmatobacterium granulomatis | Donovan bodies, granulomatous reaction without caseation, pseudoepitheliomatous hyperplasia | Giemsa stain, silver stain |
| Tuberculosis | Mycobacterium tuberculosis | Acid-fast bacilli, granulomatous reaction with caseation | AFB stain, AFB culture |
| Chancroid | Hemophilus ducrey | Granulomatous reaction without caseation | Culture, gram stain |

stimulus by other organisms. In most cases this stimulus is provided by a concomitant vulvovaginitis, either bacterial or fungal in origin.[45]

On gross inspection, condylomata acuminata are discrete verrucous or papillary growths, which may arise from a central stalk. Alternatively, they may involve a large area in a sessile fashion. Histologically, parakeratosis, acanthosis, and hyperkeratosis are evident. Typical perinuclear cytoplasmic "halos" are commonly seen on the more superficial epithelial cells (Figure 2.7). Within the dermis there is usually a chronic inflammatory infiltrate. No intranuclear or intracytoplasmic inclusions are found. The condition can usually be differentiated histologically from the solitary squamous papilloma or an underlying connective tissue disorder provided a satisfactory biopsy is taken and properly embedded and sectioned. The clinical diagnosis rests on the characteristic histopathology and multiplicity of the lesions. It must be emphasized that the biopsy site should be one which includes the stalk of the condyloma whenever possible to assure that the lesion is examined in its entirety because of potential misinterpretation or confusion with invasive squamous carcinoma or verrucous carcinoma. The marked epithelial atypia second-

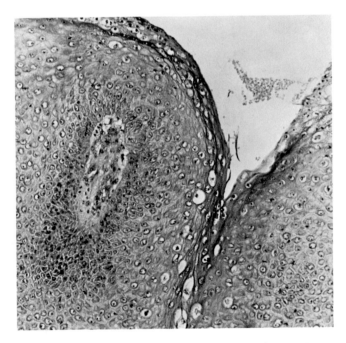

**2.7** Condylomata acuminata. Papillary parakeratotic squamous lesion with typical perinuclear halos.

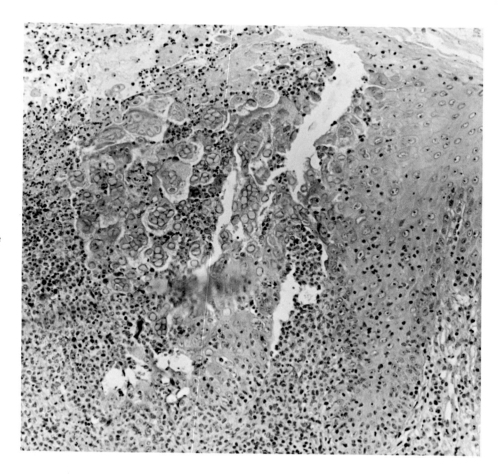

**2.9** *Herpes simplex* ulcer. Crater margin shows multinucleated clusters with distinctive intranuclear homogenization and inclusion bodies.

ary to podophyllin therapy consists of swollen cells, clear cells resembling corps ronds, and numerous mitotic figures. These changes are caused by the colchicine-like effect of the drug and must be differentiated from the features of carcinoma in situ, which they closely resemble.[57,86]

Condylomata acuminata are commonly associated with pregnancy, diabetes mellitus, and poor perineal hygiene. They may, however, occur in any sexually active patient.[122] Such lesions on the vulva at the time of vaginal delivery have been associated with laryngeal papillomas of the newborn. The larynx is presumed to be inoculated and infected with the virus during passage through the birth canal. Once condylomata are established, they follow a protracted course and spontaneous remission is rare, although some lesions regress during the puerperium. Lesions may rarely progress to become giant condylomata of Buschke–Lowenstein.[78,100] Although considered benign, giant condylomata have been associated with vulvar squamous cell carcinoma.[34,140]

## Herpetic Vulvitis

Herpetic vulvitis is an infectious disease characterized by the sequential appearance of vesicles, pustules, and painful shallow ulcers that are often secondarily infected with bacteria. The causative agent is the *Herpes simplex* virus (var. *hominis* type II), although in some instances the type I virus may be involved. The patient often presents with dysuria and vulvar pain, which may be incapacitating. A generalized viremia is frequently present in primary infections resulting in malaise and fever. Vesicles are usually asymptomatic, whereas ulcers are extremely painful and may involve the urethra, bladder, cervix, and vagina as well as the vulva (Figures 2.8a, b, Plate I).[53]

Histopathologic examination of an early intact vesicle demonstrates an extension deep into the epidermis. The characteristic intranuclear inclusions are seen at the periphery of the lesion (Figure 2.9). The histologic transformation of the *Herpes hominis* infected epithelial cell begins with a homogenization of the nuclear chromatin resulting in a "ground-glass" appearance, which then progresses to the more typical eosinophilic intranuclear inclusion body. Subsequently the cells undergo karyorexis and lysis. A biopsy taken in the late ulcerative phase, therefore, may not always show the characteristic intranuclear inclusions.

Viral isolation by culture is necessary in order to distinguish *Herpes* virus type I from type II, although this is relatively unimportant clinically. Isolation of *Herpes simplex* virus, type I or II, can be achieved by the inoculation of tissue culture monolayers, such as WI-38 human embryonic lung fibroblasts. Both types of *Herpes simplex* virus produce characteristic cytopathic changes on this cell line and virus isolation can be achieved within 4 days.[3] Culture swabs, obtained from opened vesicles or clean ulcers, can be transported and stored up to 24 hr in Stuart's transport media, Amies Bacto-transport media, or Eagle's tissue culture media. If a delay over 24 hr is anticipated before inoculation, the inoculated media must be refrigerated. Freezing is unnecessary and may actually decrease the success of isolation. Viral titer substantially decreases if it is not inoculated within 24 hr.[93] Serologic methods are presently the most sensitive and specific for virus typing and include neutralization, complement fixation, passive hemagglutination, counterimmunoelectrophoresis, and immunofluorescence.[3,29,113] Cytologic examination of vesicular aspirate is an effective method of identifying the cytopathologic changes of *Herpes* virus and is almost as sensitive as virus isolation.[112,114] The characteristic cytopathologic changes include multinucleation, giant cell formation, and nuclear "ground-glass" appearance.

## Syphilis

Syphilis is a venereal disease caused by the spirochete *Treponema pallidum.* This organism measures up to 15 $\mu$ in length and 0.20 $\mu$ in thickness. The organism is spiral in shape, with six to 14 coils. Motility, characterized by flexion, rotation about the long axis, and random movement, is noted.

The primary lesion is the chancre, a painless, shallow ucler with raised edges (Figure 2.10, Plate II). The chancre usually presents within 3 weeks after initial contact; however, the range is from 10 to 90 days. If secondarily infected, the chancre may become soft and painful and show an ulcerated surface. Although chancres are generally single, they may be multiple. It must be appreciated that chancres may occur on inconspicuous surfaces, such as the cervix, anal mucosa, or oral pharynx, and in approximately

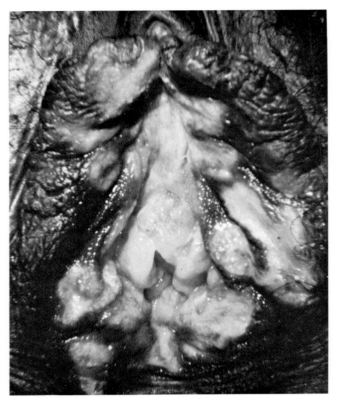

**2.11** Condylomata lata. Broad exudative papules are rich in spirochetes.

50% of females and 30% of males the primary lesion is never seen. Lymphadenopathy presents 3–4 days after the chancre. The nodes are nontender, free, and rubbery.[31]

If it is untreated in the primary phase, the secondary stage of the disease becomes evident within 6 weeks to 6 months. At this point, the patient may present with a skin rash that often involves mucous membranes as well as the palms of the hands and soles of the feet.[157] On occasion, the secondary lesions are papular, especially about the vulva, and present as elevated plaques up to 3 cm in diameter. These are known as condylomata lata (Figure 2.11). Such lesions may also occur on other mucocutaneous borders. The tertiary gumma of syphilis is rarely seen on the vulva.

Chancres are not commonly biopsied on the vulva because the diagnosis can often be made serologically or with the aid of dark field or fluorescent methods. When a biopsy is done, especially if syphilis was not considered in the clinical differential, the diagnosis may be quite difficult from histologic material alone. The histologic picture is

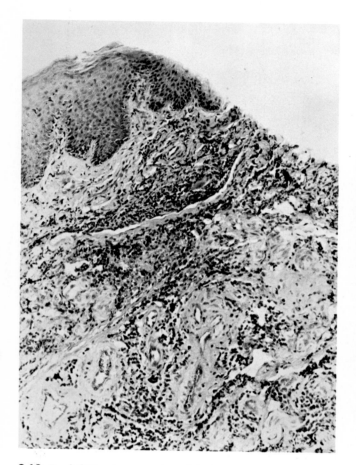

**2.12** Syphilitic chancre. Arteritis is present beneath the chancre margin.

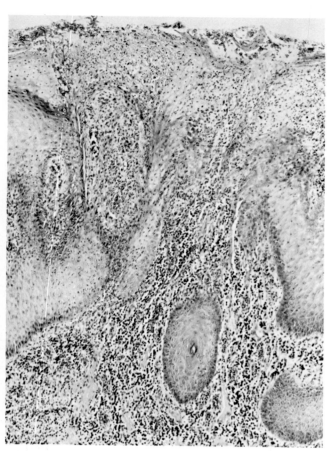

**2.13** Condylomata lata. Epithelial hyperplasia with superficial ulceration and marked inflammatory reaction.

one of ulceration of the epidermis with acute and chronic inflammation within the dermis (Figure 2.12). There is a marked perivascular inflammatory response and large numbers of plasma cells are seen within the tissue. On histologic examination of condylomata lata, marked acanthosis, epithelial hyperplasia, and hyperkeratosis are seen (Figure 2.13). The inflammatory response within the dermis is similar to that in the primary chancre, with a marked chronic inflammatory cell infiltrate containing many plasma cells. The arteritis in both lesions may be sufficiently severe to result in obliteration of the smaller vessels.

The primary chancre, the condyloma latum, and other secondary lesions are rich in spirochetes. When a chancre or secondary lesion of syphilis is suspected therefore, an attempt to identify spirochetes within the lesion should be made. This may be accomplished through either dark field examination of serum expressed from the base of the ulcer or by the fluorescent conjugated antibody technique, which employs a dried smear preparation. These methods are far more sensitive than are silver-stain attempts at identifying spirochetes within paraffin embedded tissue. Because the chancre may present as early as the first week after exposure, it may be present several weeks before the serologic tests become reactive. And yet, over 70% of patients with dark field-positive lesions have a reactive serology at the time of initial diagnosis. The most common serologic testing methods are based on the identification of reagin and these tests become positive approximately 1 month after the disease is contracted. Common reagin testing methods employ microflocculation testing and include the VDRL (venereal disease research laboratory) and RPR (rapid plasma reagin). These two tests have similar specificity and can be quantitated to evaluate the course of the disease and response to therapy. The FTA-ABS (fluorescent *Treponema* antibody, absorbed) is gener-

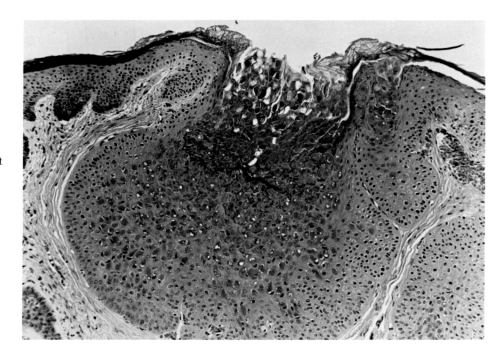

**2.14** Molluscum contagiosum. Cells within the acanthotic nest show increasing density of intracytoplasmic inclusions as the surface umbilication is approached.

ally the next test to be ordered if either of the first two tests are nonreactive or weakly reactive, or if there is a possibility of a false-positive VDRL or RPR. Biologic false positives can occur in lupus erythematosus, virus infection, cirrhosis of the liver, pregnancy, malaria, and other conditions. The FTA-ABS is a more sensitive test early in the disease and can be used to evaluate weak reactions.[121] It is appreciated however that once the FTA-ABS becomes positive, it may remain so for the life of the patient. Therefore, if the FTA-ABS is positive, spinal fluid serologic evaluation become necessary in order to rule out neurosyphilis. A false-positive FTA-ABS is rare and, if detected, requires *T. pallidum* immobilization (TPI) testing and careful followup.[142]

Approximately 30% of patients undergo spontaneous remission of the disease. Those who are not treated or do not achieve spontaneous remission may progress to tertiary syphilis with its well-recognized cardiovascular and central nervous system effects. Untreated syphilis is said to prove fatal in 10% of those so afflicted.

## Molluscum Contagiosum

Molluscum contagiosum is a moderately contagious viral disease which, in adults, is often related to sexual intercourse.[99, 108] The lesions are small, smooth papules (3 to 6 mm in diameter) with a central punctum or umbili-cation. Lesions are generally multiple and separate, although they may be single. Rare plaque formations made up of 50 to 100 individual clustered lesions have also been described. The incubation period varies between 14 and 50 days.

Diagnosis does not usually require biopsy. Cytologic examination of the scrapings of the interior of the molluscum papule are adequate to confirm the diagnosis. When biopsies are submitted, histologic examination demonstrates a marked acanthosis, and the characteristic intracytoplasmic viral inclusions can be seen (Figure 2.14). Young, recently infected cells show an eosinophilic cytoplasmic inclusion. With aging, the inclusion bodies take on a more basophilic appearance, preceding lysis of the cell. The central dimple of the lesion is often seen histologically if care is taken to bisect the lesion at the gross cutting table. Within the dermis there is often a rather marked vascular response with endothelial proliferation and a moderate perivascular inflammation. Electron microscopy has demonstrated that the virus is brick-shaped and contains a DNA core with a two-layered protein coat.[8]

Molluscum contagiosum is usually asymptomatic, yet lesions about the anus frequently become pruritic or secondarily infected. Although most lesions regress spontaneously, untreated lesions may persist for years, during which time they may be spread by close contact.

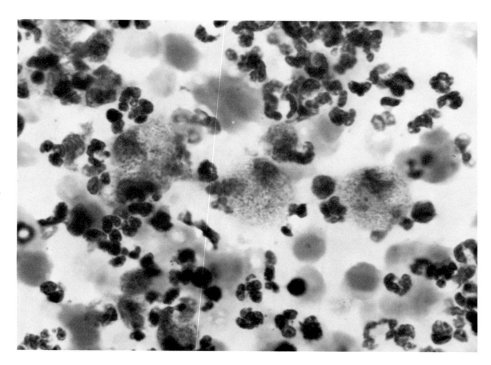

**2.15 c.** Granuloma inguinale. Large histiocytes obtained by smear show numerous intracytoplasmic Donovan bodies.

## Granuloma Inguinale

Granuloma inguinale (GI) is caused by *Calymmatobacterium granulomatis* which is a gram-negative, heavily encapsulated rod considered to be of the bacterial family, Enterobacteriaceae. GI occurs with approximately equal frequency in men and women. Primary lesions may occur on the vulva or cervix and often present as tender or painful papules or ulcers (Figure 2.15a, Plate II).[28] GI extends primarily by local infiltration, although lymphatic permeation may occur with later stages of the disease and chronic lymphatic infiltration and fibrosis frequently results in a massive brawny edema of the external genitalia. There is some controversy as to the true origin of the edema, because dye tests suggest that the lymphatic drainage is intact. With involvement of the cervix, the disease may advance via the cervical lymphatics to involve parametrial tissues.

The clinical diagnosis of GI is dependent on the identification of the Donovan bodies within the tissue. This is best accomplished by preparing smears from the base of a biopsy, taken in an area of primary involvement. Any antibiotic treatment may obscure the diagnosis and additional biopsies at a later date may be necessary to positively confirm the diagnosis. Air-dried smears stained with Giemsa, Wright, or similar stain will demonstrate the

encapsulated rods. These gram-negative bacteria can also be detected on frozen sections by employing methylene blue stain.[54] Histologically, the main portion of the lesion consists of granulation tissue associated with an extensive chronic inflammatory cell infiltrate and endarteritis (Figure 2.15b, Plate II). Within this granulation tissue, large vacuolated histiocytes are found that contain the characteristic Donovan bodies within their cytoplasm (Figure 2.15c). The surface epithelium often demonstrates pseudoepitheliomatous hyperplasia, which may be so exuberant that it mimics squamous carcinoma.

The organism *Calymmatobacterium granulomatis* may be cultured by special techniques and a complement fixation test is available that is believed reliable in titers greater than 1:40.[28]

## Lymphogranuloma Venereum

Lymphogranuloma venereum is caused by a *Chlamydia* organism (TRIC agent) and is approximately three times more frequent in men than in women. This disease is characterized clinically by three phases: the first consists of erosion of the skin, the second is characterized by adenitis, and the third is one of fibrosis and destruction.[28] Lymphogranuloma venereum (LGV) is primarily spread via the lymphatics. The initial ulcers are generally not tender or painful and are often ignored. Adenitis, which may painfully involve the superficial groin nodes (bubos), frequently results in spontaneous rupture through the skin accompanied by exudation of a purulent discharge. The third phase of the disease, the destructive process, often results in stricture and fibrosis of the vagina and rectum.[157] In this phase, chronic lymphatic obstruction is responsible for the characteristic nonpitting edema of the external genitalia.

The histology of LGV is not in itself diagnostic, and to establish a clinical diagnosis it is necessary to have the typical clinical presentation along with positive complement fixation tests. The histology reveals no characteristic viral inclusions or identifiable organisms by the usual modes of investigation. Biopsy is often indicated to rule out carcinoma, and smears of the base of the biopsy should be made to search for the Donovan bodies of granuloma inguinale. Histologically, giant cells may be seen along with lymphocytes and plasma cells. In older lesions there is extensive fibrosis of the dermis, and occasionally the biopsy contains sinus tracts.

## Chancroid

Chancroid is caused by the organism *Hemophilus ducrey,* which is gram-negative and nonmotile and which in culture grows in pairs and chains. Histologic examination of the tissue demonstrates a granulomatous-type reaction with chronic inflammatory cells consisting primarily of lymphocytes and plasma cells. Clinical diagnosis rests on identification of the organism. Gram stains of histologic sections as well as of smears of the tissue may be of value; definitive diagnosis, however, depends on the bacterial isolation of the organism. Primary lesions may be single or multiple and tend to be small, measuring approximately 1–2 mm in diameter. Coalescence of the lesions leads to ulcers approaching 3 cm in diameter.[65] Chancroid is frequently asymptomatic and the incubation period may approach 1 year in length.

## Tuberculosis

Tuberculosis of the vulva is extremely rare. When it occurs it is usually associated with tuberculosis of other genital sites, primarily fallopian tube and endometrium. Autoinoculation by the hematogenous or direct route is therefore the most common method of spread and primary inoculation or sexual transmission of tuberculosis is most uncommon. The usual organism is *Mycobacterium tuberculosis;* however, atypical mycobacteria have also been in-

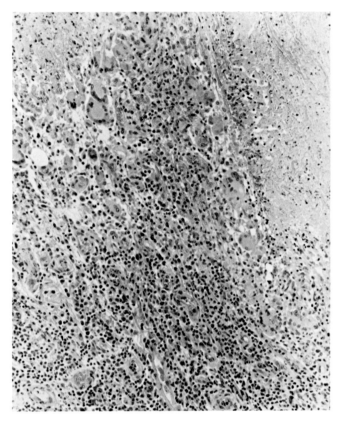

**2.16** Vulvar tuberculosis. Caseating granulomas with Langhan's giant cells.

criminated. The diagnosis can usually be made by biopsy of the involved tissues. Caseating granulomas with Langhans' giant cells are found on histologic section (Figure 2.16). Acid-fast stains may demonstrate the mycobacterium, and culture methods will provide the final identification of the organism.

Giant cells of the foreign body type are frequently encountered in vulvar tissues where a previous biopsy has been performed (Figure 2.17). These giant cells, associated with noncaseating granulomas, often result from embedded suture, which can occasionally be seen in the biopsy area and must be differentiated from the more infrequent tuberculosis.

## Miscellaneous

Chronic inflammatory conditions of the vulvar and perianal skin without concomitant ulceration are often caused by fungal infections. *Candida* and dermatophytes

23

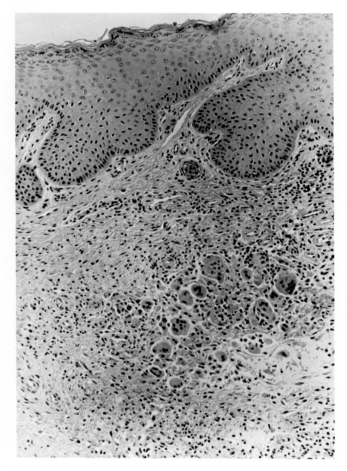

**2.17** Foreign body giant cell reaction. Multinucleated giant cells with diffuse nuclear distribution. Caseation is lacking.

are frequent pathogens. Such conditions rarely require biopsy and accurate diagnosis can generally be accomplished with microscopic examination of KOH smears or the use of cultural identification.

Bacterial infections may produce a picture similar to that seen with fungus infections. Erythrasma is a chronic bacterial infection of the genitocrural area that shows a coral-red fluorescence under Wood's light. The disease is most common in obese diabetics. Scrapings of these lesions, when stained with gram stain, demonstrate the causative gram-positive bacteria (*Corynebacterium minutissimum*) in rods, filaments, and coccoid forms.[135]

Mites are capable of producing local and limited chronic skin infections of the perineal area. Unless specifically considered, they may go unrecognized because they are not demonstrable by the usual skin scraping or culture techniques.[67] Mites, which belong to the order Acari, cause scabies. They differ from lice, which are insects, in that they have a fused head and thorax, are devoid of primary segmentation, and have four pairs of legs. Mites burrow within the epidermis and may induce severe pruritus. The overt skin lesions are papular and, when examined under a magnifying lens, reveal an adjacent burrow. This burrow may be unroofed with a sharp knife blade coated with mineral oil. The scrapings, mixed in the oil, are then mounted on a glass slide.[111] An alternate method of diagnosis, if no papules can be found, is to shake out the patient's clothing into a plastic container to which can be added an alcohol–ether–acetic acid–formalin mixture, which fixes the mites and permits their histologic identification.[67]

Lice are associated with irritation of the skin caused by secondary infection of feeding sites. The pubic louse, *Phthirus pubis,* of the class Insecta, is the usual offender and can be diagnosed by identification of the louse and nits on the hair shaft (Figure 2.18).

*Enterobius vermicularis* (pinworm, seatworm) is a relatively common intestinal parasite. The female worm measures 8 to 13 mm in length and 0.5 mm in diameter. The male is approximately one-fourth as long with the same diameter. Infected children frequently present with complaints of severe vulvovaginal pruritus which may awaken them at night. Other complaints include lower abdominal pains, diarrhea, restlessness, and nocturia. Studies for fungus and bacteria are not diagnostic and examination of the vulvar vestibule and vagina reveal marked inflammation. Occasionally, an adult female helminth is brought to the laboratory after being found on the vestibule or perineal areas. More commonly, the pathologist is presented with a cellulose tape–slide preparation for identification of the typical embryonated eggs of *E. vermicularis.*[45]

## Inflammatory Diseases (Noninfectious)

Behcet's syndrome refers to the triad of oral ulcers, genital ulcers, and various opthalmologic inflammations (Figures 2.19a, b, Plate II).[66] Eye changes may be absent in mild cases. Other findings include acne, cutaneous nodules, thrombophlebitis, encephalopathy, and colitis.[94,107,120] Histologically, necrotizing arteritis is frequently seen and can be considered a cardinal pathologic finding. A chronic inflammatory infiltrate is present about and within the vessel wall with homogenization of the

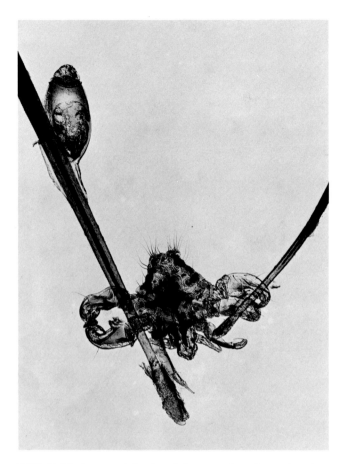

**2.18** Pubic louse with nit. *Phthirus pubis* clings, head down, to a hair shaft with attached egg.

[Courtesy of Mr. Gerald Staut.]

arterial media. There is endothelial cell swelling, which may result in arteriolar occlusion, and venous thrombosis. On the vulva, Behcet's syndrome causes deep ulcerations that may result in fenestration of the labia. We have observed one patient in whom this process has led to gangrene of the labia. These ulcerations are characteristically relapsing and usually associated with simultaneous oral apthosis.

Crohn's disease is a chronic noncaseating granulomatous disease of unknown etiology; it is more common in women. Although it usually involves the distal ileum and colon, it may involve any segment of the gastrointestinal tract from the mouth to the anus. Cutaneous ulcerations are the basis of this disease and generally occur in areas where there is close apposition of skin, such as the vulva and submammary areas.[79] When Crohn's disease involves the vulva, the resulting ulcers are often multiple, deep, and

secondarily infected. Perianal draining sinuses and abscesses may be present and often drain a fluid resembling small bowel content. Histopathology demonstrates noncaseating granulomatous inflammation within the dermis. Studies for acid-fast bacteria and fungi are negative. Marked granulation tissue response is frequently seen about the ulcers. Rarely, however, is there any significant associated lymphadenitis. The differential diagnosis includes vulvar tuberculosis, actinomycosis, lymphogranuloma venereum, granuloma inguinale, and chronic inflammation of the skin appendages, such as hidradenitis suppurativa.

Hidradenitis suppurativa is generally believed to be an apocrine gland disorder.[70] Deep seated, painful, subcutaneous nodules are found in areas with apocrine glands, especially the axilla and vulva. The lesions commonly progress subcutaneously, producing confluent masses that subsequently erode the epidermis and result in draining sinuses and extensive scarring. The condition may coexist with Fox–Fordyce disease. Excision of the involved areas brings the condition to the attention of the pathologist.[21] Histologically hidradenitis suppurativa in its early stages demonstrates a perifolliculitis with an acute and chronic infiltrate within the dermis. In the later stages of the disease, destruction of the epithelial appendages and sinus tract formation results.[94]

Acute single painful ulcers of the medial portion of the labia minora following within 24 hr of coitus have been described.[10] Evaluation of these ulcerations, to date, reveals no causative agent.

Although virtually any dermatologic disease can involve the vulva, Darier's disease, familial benign pemphigus, and psoriasis are discussed because they may be first observed and biopsied by the gynecologist.

Darier's disease (keratosis follicularis) is inherited as an autosomal dominant, although spontaneous cases are recognized. In affected patients, the disease frequently involves the vulva. Patients present anytime after late childhood with crusted, hyperkeratotic papules that often appear darker than the surrounding skin and may be secondarily infected.[94,127,131] Histologically, acantholysis of the suprabasal epithelial cells results in clefts that extend from the basal layer through the granular layer. Acantholytic cells are seen within the clefts. Corps ronds and nuclear grains can be found in the granular layer and individual cell keratinization may be present, reflecting dyskeratosis. Hyperkeratosis, acanthosis, and papillomatosis are seen along with keratotic plugs. Rarely, epithelial cells proliferate into the dermis with resultant basal budding. The inflammatory cell infiltration within the dermis is usually minimal unless the lesions are secondarily infected.[127]

Familial benign pemphigus (Hailey–Hailey disease) is inherited as an autosomal dominant; however, in approximately one-third of patients no family history of the disease exists. Onset of the lesions often occurs during adolescence. Intertriginous areas are usually involved, and several cases confined exclusively to the vulva have been reported.[131] Recurrent clusters of vesicles develop, rupture, and result in crusted and moist papules that later coalesce to form plaques. For diagnostic biopsy, early vesicles should be selected. Histologically, acantholysis occurs with resultant suprabasalar lacunae. Unlike the usual picture of Darier's disease, vesicles and bullae are also found. Acantholytic cells, which maintain their nuclear detail, can be seen within the vesicle and the acantholysis is more marked than in Darier's disease. Basal cells maintain their orientation to the basement membrane. Rarely corps ronds are seen in the granular layer. There is minimal if any dyskeratosis, in contrast to Darier's disease. Strands of epidermal cells may proliferate into the dermis but little dermal inflammatory infiltrate exists unless secondary infection is present.

Darier's disease and familial benign pemphigus must not only be distinguished from one another, they must also be distinguished from pemphigus vulgaris and pemphigus vegitans. These four acantholytic conditions must be considered whenever acantholysis with vesicles is found.[94]

Psoriasis is inherited as a simple autosomal dominant with incomplete penetrance. Psoriasis affects approximately 2% of the population of the United States. On the vulva, the disease involves the lateral aspects of the labia majora and genitocrural areas.[131] The lesions present as silvery topped erythematous papules. When this loose silvery scale is removed, several punctate bleeding points can be seen (Auspitz sign). Coalescence of papules results in plaque formation. The lesions are frequently symmetrical and may persist for years. New psoriatic lesions may develop within 7 to 30 days at sites of trauma (Koebner phenomenon). Histologic findings include hyperkeratosis, parakeratosis, uniform acanthosis (elongation of the rete ridges to an even length), diminution of the granular layer, and collections of polymorphonuclear leukocytes within the epidermis (Munro abscesses). There is increased mitotic activity within the epidermis, reflecting the significantly increased rate of epithelial turnover.[36] The dermal papillae are clubbed and edematous. Prominent vessels are seen within the papillae, and there is a minimal chronic inflammatory cell infiltrate within the dermis.[94]

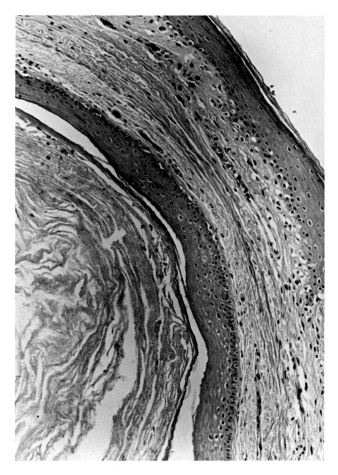

**2.20** Keratinous cyst. Stratified squamous epithelial lining is evident.

# Benign Cystic Tumors

Cystic lesions of the vulva include the Bartholin cyst, keratinous cyst, mucous cyst, mesonephric cyst, cysts of the canal of Nuck, and Fox–Fordyce disease.

## Bartholin Cyst

The Bartholin glands, first described by Bartholin in 1677, are tubular alveolar, paired glands that produce a clear mucoid secretion, which is thought to provide a continuous lubrication for the vestibular surface.[165] These glands do not, as previously thought, contribute significantly to vaginal secretion prior to intercourse.[132,165] Lined by transitional epithelium, the ducts of these glands are prone to obstruction at their vestibular orifice. Such obstruction results in the subsequent accumulation of

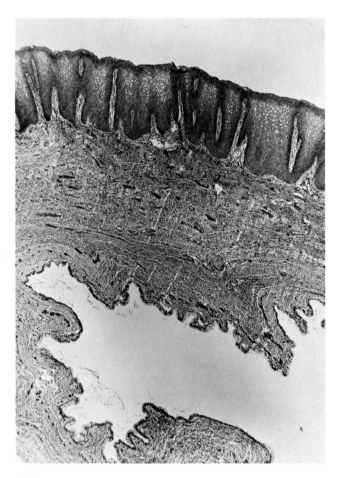

**2.21** Mucous cyst of the vestibule. Irregular folds are frequently noted in the cyst wall.

of the Bartholin duct abscess demonstrates a striking acute inflammatory reaction within the stroma of the duct apparatus. A purulent exudate is present within the lumen of the abscess wall formed by dilatation of the duct.[165] Such abscesses are rarely excised, although portions of abscess wall may be submitted to the laboratory. Occasionally, the infection may subside without abscess formation or become chronic in nature, resulting in chronic Bartholin adenitis. In such cases, Bartholin duct cysts may result from dilatation of the duct secondary to chronic inflammatory obstruction.

## Keratinous Cysts

Although the labia minora and majora are richly endowed with sebaceous glands, the finding of keratinous cysts in this region does not imply that they arise from these glands. Keratinous cysts are frequently seen on the vulva and generally located on the labia majora. They usually contain a white to pale yellow grumous or cheesy material without hair. Giant cells may be seen in the tissue adjacent to the cyst wall. The lining of such cysts is characterized by a relatively flattened stratified squamous epithelium (Figure 2.20). Whether or not these cysts represent primary keratinous cysts, unrelated to sebaceous glands, or are actually occluded sebaceous glands that have undergone squamous metaplasia is debated.[87,118] Such cysts are not considered premalignant, although carcinoma arising in keratinous cysts has been described.[118,152]

## Mucous Cysts (Dysontogenetic Cysts)

Mucous cysts of the vulva are characterized by a lining of tall to cuboidal, mucous-secreting, columnar epithelium, without peripheral muscle fibers or evidence of myoepithelial cells (Figure 2.21). They are usually seen within the vestibule. Histochemical studies demonstrate that the cyst lining stains with both Alcian blue and Mayer's mucicarmine, whereas cysts of mesonephric origin do not exhibit these reactions.[74] Historically, mucous cysts have been related to Müllerian *anlage*. It is now recognized however, that the Müllerian system does not contribute to the formation of the vulvar vestibule where these cysts are usually found. Therefore, they are considered to arise from the urogenital sinus epithelium and represent examples of dysontogenetic formation.[48] The similarity of the mucous lining (Figure 2.22) to the paraurethral and Bartholin gland epithelium, as well as the recognition that the urogenital sinus is the major contributor to the vestibule, strongly recommends this view.

secretion and cystic dilatation of the duct.[165] The content of an uninfected Bartholin cyst is therefore a mucoid, clear, translucent liquid, and cultures of this material fail to grow bacteria. Such cysts generally show minimal, if any, inflammatory response within the stroma of the gland or about the dilated duct. Careful examination of the duct area, if available, may demonstrate variable degrees of synechia formation and duct occlusion. Such cysts may be recurrent and occasionally are associated with primary infection of the Bartholin gland. They may require drainage, but in women over 40 they should be surgically excised. Because of the possibility of concomitant carcinoma of the Bartholin gland, the pathologist must pay special attention to the tissue adjacent to the cystic structure.

Bartholin abscess is an acute process generally associated with a *Neisseria* gonorrheal infection though it may be related to *Staphylococcus* or other organisms. The pathology

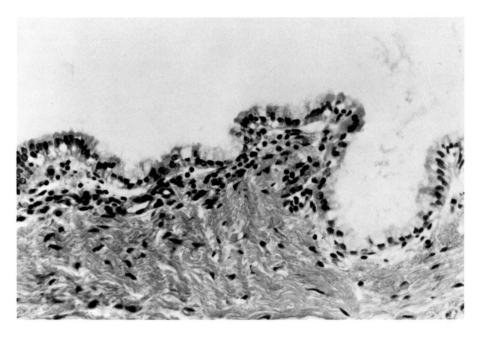

**2.22** Mucous cyst of the vestibule. Simple columnar mucous-secreting cells rest on the basement membrane. Note the absence of an underlying smooth muscle layer.

## Mesonephric Cysts

These cysts, called either Wolffian duct or mesonephric cysts, are generally encountered on the lateral aspects of the vulva and vagina. They are thin-walled and somewhat translucent and contain a clear fluid. On histologic examination the lining epithelium is usually cuboidal, although it may be columnar. Histochemical techniques show smooth muscle in the submucosal areas.[74]

## Cysts of the Canal of Nuck (Peritoneal Lined Cysts)

Such cysts are generally found in the superior aspect of the labia majora or inguinal canal and are believed to arise from inclusions of the peritoneum at the inferior insertion of the round ligament into the labia majora. As such, they are analogous to the hydrocele of the spermatic cord. They may achieve substantial size and must be distinguished from inguinal herniae.

## Fox–Fordyce Disease

Fox–Fordyce disease is a disorder of the apocrine glands. Ninety percent of the cases occur in women. The disease begins at puberty and presents as a pruritic papular eruption usually involving the axillae, vulvar, and perianal regions. The center of the papule often contains a hair follicle and apocrine sweat gland duct, plugged by hyper-

keratosis. There is dilatation of the apocrine gland acini (Figure 2.23). Chronic inflammatory changes in the dermis and epidermal acanthosis and spongiosis are also present. There may be an associated rupture of the interepithelial portion of the duct with subsequent vesicle formation within the epidermis. These vesicles may not be seen unless serial sections are performed.[70] Deposition of mucin may be found in the ducts and glands and may be free in the tissues about the appendages.[109]

# Benign Solid Tumors

Benign solid tumors of the vulva, although rare, comprise a fascinating group. For convenience, the lesions may be divided into those which arise from the vulvar connective tissues and those which are of epithelial origin.

## Connective Tissue Tumors

STRAWBERRY HEMANGIOMA (nevus vasculosis) and cavernous hemangioma rarely appear on the vulva, although their occurrence in young children has been documented (Figure 2.24, Plate III).[82] Far more common are cherry hemangiomata (senile hemangiomata), which are small, red to purple papules with no known clinical significance. Excessive surface trauma may induce bleeding, necessitating excision. Histologically, numerous dilated capillaries are noted in the subepithelial tissue. These vascu-

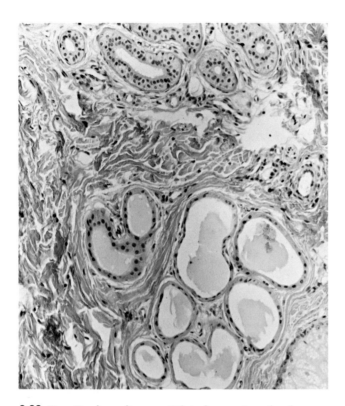

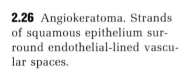

**2.23** Fox–Fordyce disease. Dilated apocrine glands show inspissated section.

lar spaces are lined by a single layer of endothelial cells and are separated by connective tissue that may show collagenization.

ANGIOKERATOMA is a variant of hemangioma and occurs almost exclusively on the scrotum and vulva (Figure 2.25, Plate III). Somewhat larger than cherry angiomata, these lesions are often purple in color and occur primarily in women of childbearing age. Histologically, the dilated endothelial-lined channels are separated by strands and cords of squamous epithelial cells representing downgrowth from the overlying epithelium, which is often hyperkeratotic (Figure 2.26). Varying degrees of acanthosis and papillomatosis are present along with a mild inflammatory reaction in the deep dermis. Again, although the lesions are of no clinical significance, their peculiar appearance often prompts excisional diagnostic biopsy.[7,71]

The PYOGENIC GRANULOMA is a variant of hemangioma that may occur anywhere on the skin. It is analogous to the epulis tumor of pregnancy and most of the pyogenic granulomas that have occurred on the vulva have done so during gestation. Although previously thought to be secondary to a superficial wound infection, this tumor is, in fact, a form of hemangioma characterized by rapid growth. Because the surface is easily traumatized, the lesion is often secondarily infected. Histologically, a thin ulcerated epidermis is noted covering a mass of granulation tissue.

**2.26** Angiokeratoma. Strands of squamous epithelium surround endothelial-lined vascular spaces.

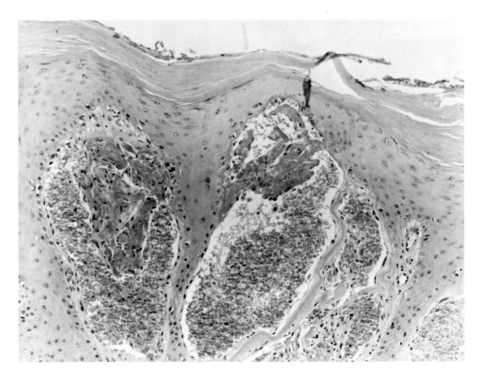

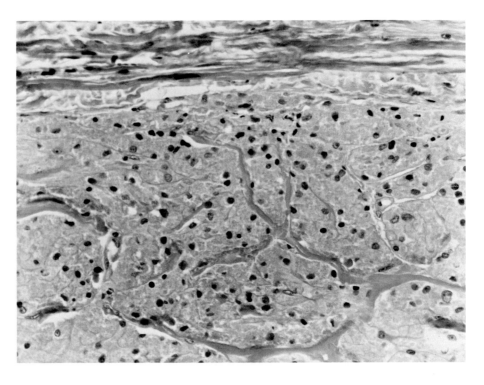

**2.27** Granular cell myoblastoma. Note the nests of polyhedral cells with a grainy cytoplasm separated by collagenous cords.

Capillary proliferation is intense and secondary inflammatory changes are frequently found within the stroma. Around the periphery of the lesion there may be a downward growth of the epidermis, producing a "collarette."

The HEMANGIOPERICYTOMA is an extremely rare tumor, but its occurrence has been reported on the vulva.[103] Histologically, numerous small capillaries are seen to be separated by dense cords of spindle-shaped pericytes. Malignant variants of this tumor do occur and nuclear pleomorphism with numerous mitoses characterize the aggressive lesions. Differentiation from other malignant angiomatous tumors may be facilitated by the use of reticulum stains, which show the pericytes to be external to the reticulum network surrounding the individual blood vessels.[94,118]

Benign LEIOMYOMAS have been reported to arise from the smooth muscle elements surrounding the crura of the clitoris.[145]

The SCHWANNOMA is another rare tumor that is occasionally recognized on the vulva.[19] Such tumors were formerly known as granular cell myoblastomas. Sobel and his colleagues[141] have conclusively shown that the same primitive stem cell is the precursor for both lesions. These tumors are not encapsulated and unless they are treated with wide excision local recurrences are common. The margins of the surgical specimen are, therefore, especially important with this tumor. These tumors may be seen at any age and are generally slow-growing, asymptomatic, small masses arising from the labia majora. Histologically, irregular tracts of large polyhedral cells with indistinct cell borders are noted. The cytoplasm of these cells is packed with numerous eosinophilic granules, and the nuclei are generally small and hyperchromatic (Figure 2.27). In response to this tumor, the overlying squamous epithelium often exhibits the remarkable phenomenon of pseudo-epitheliomatous hyperplasia. Extreme degrees of acanthosis are noted and the nests and cords of hyperplastic squamous cells may mimic the appearance of invasive squamous carcinoma.[82,118]

BENIGN FIBROMAS, caused by the proliferation of mature fibrocytes, may appear as vulvar masses, but these tumors actually arise from the deeper connective tissues surrounding the vaginal introitus or adjacent to the perineal body. Rarely do such tumors undergo malignant degeneration; if left untreated, however, they may grow to excessive size. On cut section, the lesion is firm and smooth with a white or grayish color. Yellow striae and a somewhat softer consistency signify the admixture of a lipomatous element, which is not uncommon. Histologically, parallel bundles of fibrocytes are seen. With large tumors, both hyaline and cystic forms of degeneration have been described.

LIPOMAS (Figure 2.28, Plate III) arising from vulvar

fat pads present as soft, lobulated growths that are generally attached to the labia majora by broad-based pedicles. Histologically, mature fat cells are seen, often interspersed with strands of fibrous connective tissue. When this element is prominent, the tumor should properly be termed a fibrolipoma.[82,96]

HISTIOCYTOMAS appear as firm, brownish nodules that may be clinically confused with large nevi. In the older literature, these tumors were known as dermatofibromas or sclerosing hemangiomas. Histiocytes may act facultatively as fibroblasts and produce an extremely fibrocytic tumor, although most are xanthomatous and exhibit cells with a foamy cytoplasm caused by engulfed lipid or hemosiderin.

NEUROFIBROMATA are usually noted in association with multiple neurofibromatosis and vulvar involvement has been found in 18% of females with von Recklinghausen's disease.[136] Occurrence of neurofibromata is rare prior to puberty, but thereafter they grow rapidly and malignant degeneration may occur. Arising from the nerve sheath, these tumors are made up of whorls and wavy bundles of narrow cells that often exhibit a palisade arrangement of the nuclei. Special nerve stains show long, thin nerve fibers scattered throughout the tumors and occasionally the intervening collagen may undergo a peculiar mucoid degeneration.[94]

The ACROCHORDON, also known as a fibroepithelial polyp or skin tag, is a common tumor with both connective tissue and epithelial elements. These lesions vary in their clinical appearance from small, flesh-colored or hyperpigmented, papillomatous growths resembling condylomata to large, baggy, pedunculated tumors, which are often hypopigmented on their apical surface. Small tumors may be confused with nevi and the larger lesions may present cosmetic problems; generally, however, these tumors are clinically insignificant. On cut section, such tumors are soft and fleshy. Histologically, their epithelial surface varies from a thickened layer with papillomatosis, hyperkeratosis, and acanthosis to an attenuated flattened layer exhibiting multiple primary folds. The connective tissue stalk is composed of loose bundles of collagen with a moderate number of blood vessels.

## Epithelial Tumors

Because the "milk line" extends into the vulva, the occurrence of breast tissue in this location is not strictly ectopic, but accessory. The amount and character of breast tissue reported within the labia majora varies from small, isolated nodules of mammary duct epithelium to large, bilateral structures that have been observed to lactate during the puerperium. Most lesions are clinically amorphous enlargements of the labia, first noted to arise in association with pregnancy. Histologically, accessory breast tissue is identical with that of mammary structures elsewhere, but there is a higher incidence of malignancy developing in accessory sites, and adenocarcinoma of the accessory breast tissue of the vulva[63] has been reported. The complete removal of such areas is therefore advocated. When such tissue is discovered during pregnancy, it is best to delay total excision until after puerperal regression is complete.

PAPILLARY HIDRADENOMA of the vulva has been historically misinterpreted to represent a form of adenocarcinoma. These tumors are small, less than 2 cm in size, and generally arise from the labia majora, interlabial sulci (Figure 2.29a, Plate III), or lateral surface of the labia minora. Extrusion of the pulpy mass of adenomatous tissue through the center of the dome-shaped lesion, or ulceration of the overlying surface, may produce bleeding. As a rule, these tumors are asymptomatic. Papillary hidradenomas have not been described prior to puberty and almost all cases have occurred in Caucasian women. Histologically, under low-power examination, an adenomatous pattern is seen, highly suggestive of adenocarcinoma (Figure 2.29b). Stromal compression often results in the formation of a pseudocapsule, although the adenomatous cells may show infiltration into the surrounding connective tissue. Inflammatory reaction is unusual and not part of the classic picture. The tumor is composed of numerous tubules and acini lined with a single or double layer of cuboidal cells (Figure 2.29c). At times, the cells lining the lumen of the adenomatous structures are large and pale and exhibit the morphologic and staining characteristics of apocrine sweat gland secretory cells (Figure 2.29d). When a double layer of cells is present, the outermost layer is thought to represent the myoepithelial cells, often demonstrable in apocrine gland structures. Woodworth et al.[164] describe a large series of these tumors and point out the similarity of the papillary hidradenoma to the intraductal papilloma of the breast, suggesting that the two tumors may be identical. Most authorities,[68,118] however, feel that the tumor is of sweat gland origin, although the fact that such tumors have not been described in other areas of the body, equally rich in apocrine glands, has never been explained. Clinically, hidradenomas are benign, and their greatest significance lies in the possible pathologic misinterpretation that may occur if only cursory examination is given to the material. Careful high-power microscopy shows a paucity of mitotic figures and only mild degrees of cellular and nuclear pleomorphism.

**2.29 b.** Hidradenoma. Low-power pattern of this adenomatous tumor ulcerating through the skin surface resembles adenocarcinoma.

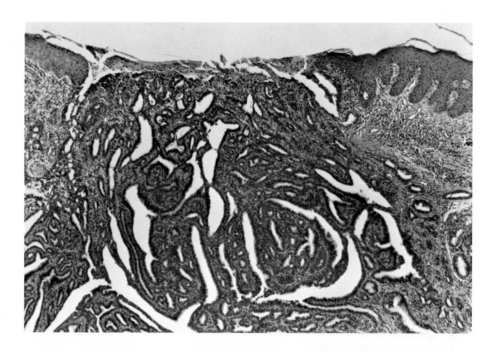

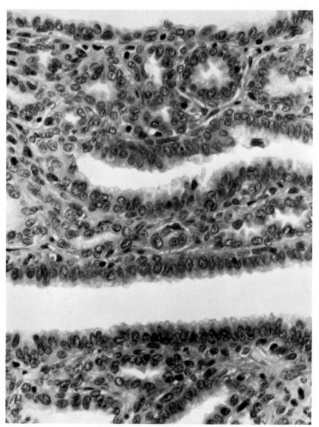

**c.** Hidradenoma. High-power examination shows tubules and acini lined with a single or double layer of cuboidal to columnar cells.

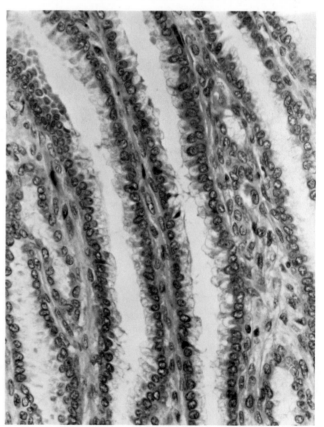

**d.** Hidradenoma. The apocrine-like appearance of many of the cells is striking.

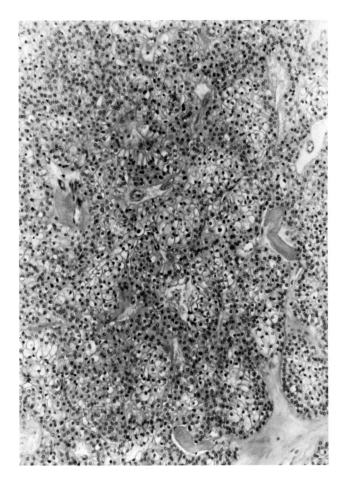

**2.30** Clear cell hidradenoma. The sheets of large clear cells are broken by occasional collagen bands and blood vessels.

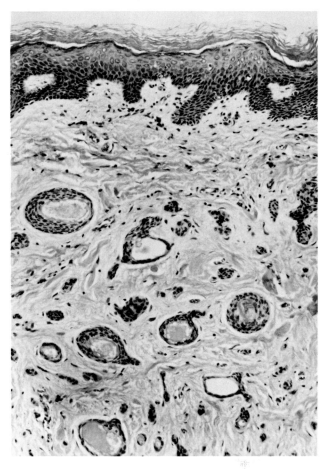

**2.31** Syringoma. The comma pattern of the eccrine structures is easily appreciated.

The CLEAR CELL HIDRADENOMA is not a variant of the papillary hidradenoma but represents a distinctive and unusual tumor of the epidermal adnexa that is most often found on the face, scalp, thoracic wall, and abdomen. Isolated examples of this tumor have occasionally been found on the vulva and we have observed a single case in our own clinic. Kersting[85] is of the opinion that the tumor is derived from the epithelial matrices in eccrine sweat gland primordia and recommends wide local excision. Histologically, the tumor is largely solid and does not resemble the papillary hidradenoma. Lobules or segments of large clear cells are divided by strands of reticular connective tissue. The characteristic cell is large and polygonal and the cytoplasm appears transparent. The relatively small nucleus is round to oval and may exhibit an irregular outline. The chromatin is often clumped and a single nucleolus is often seen. Mitotic figures are unusual (Figure 2.30).

The SYRINGOMA is assumed to be an adenoma of the eccrine ducts. These lesions occur on the vulva as well as the eyelids, cheeks, axillae, and abdomen. Clinically, flesh-colored papules are noted within the deeper skin layers of the labia majora. These are often asymptomatic, although pruritus may be present.[15] Histologically, the tumor lacks a clearly defined border. Within the dermis, numerous small dilated duct spaces are seen. These spaces are usually lined by two rows of epithelial cells, which appear flat secondary to pressure atrophy. The commalike formation of these glandular spaces is characteristic (Figure 2.31). Although an apocrine origin has been suggested, histochemical and electron microscopic studies have established the syringoma as an eccrine derivative. Mixed adnexoid tumors have also been described on the vulva in which a mixture of syringomatous and pilosebaceous elements are noted.[58]

Benign tumors arising directly from the squamous

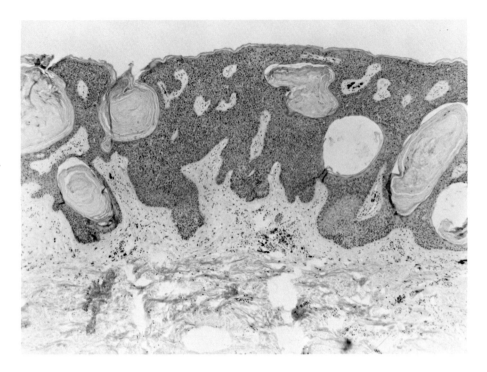

**2.32** Seborrheic keratosis. Keratin cysts and columns of pigmented squamous cells make up this superficial tumor.

epithelium of the vulva include the squamous papilloma, keratoacanthoma, and seborrheic keratosis. SQUAMOUS PAPILLOMAS may be thought of as variants of common skin tags in which the epithelial element predominates. Histologically, papillomatosis, acanthosis, and varying degrees of hyperkeratosis are seen. However, such lesions are usually single and no viral etiology is suspected, although in other respects they may resemble condylomata acuminata.

KERATOACANTHOMAS are rapidly growing, self-limited proliferations of the squamous epithelium in which horny masses of keratin are pushed upward and tongues of squamous epithelium invade the dermis. Lever and Schaumburg–Lever[94] mention that these tumors may occur on any hairy cutaneous site.

SEBORRHEIC KERATOSES are extremely common raised lesions with irregular borders that may occur almost anywhere on the skin. Their color varies from pale brown to brownish black and they appear to be "stuck on" to the skin surface. Although clinically insignificant, their appearance often mimics that of a nevus or melanoma and when present on the vulva, these tumors are often excised for diagnosis. Histologically, hyperkeratosis, acanthosis, and papillomatosis are seen. Often, the entire tumor lies above a straight line that can be drawn from the normal epidermis at one side of the tumor to the normal epidermis at the other side. Both mature squamous cells and basal type cells are noted proliferating in strands and cords that surround numerous horny keratin cysts (Figure 2.32). Varying degrees of hyperpigmentation are present.

VULVAR ENDOMETRIOMAS represent tumors caused by truly ectopic epithelium. Decidua implanted in an episiotomy incision at the time of delivery and menstrual blood implanting in a small area of trauma have both been implicated in the etiology of this unusual condition.[16,33] The clinical appearance is variable, ranging from bluish red cystic masses to amorphous deep-seated nodules that are usually located near the posterior fourchette. Cyclic enlargement and regression are often noted. Histologically, both endometrial glands and stroma are present and a fibrocytic response, with foreign body giant cell reaction, may be noted in cases the onset of which was preceded by recent surgery.

## Pigmentation Disorders

### Hypopigmented Conditions

The vulvar skin is usually more pigmented than is the general body surface. Biopsies of the normal vulva show dendritic melanocytes scattered along the basal layer of the epithelium and squamous keratinocytes containing variable concentrations of melanin granules. Areas of the vulvar

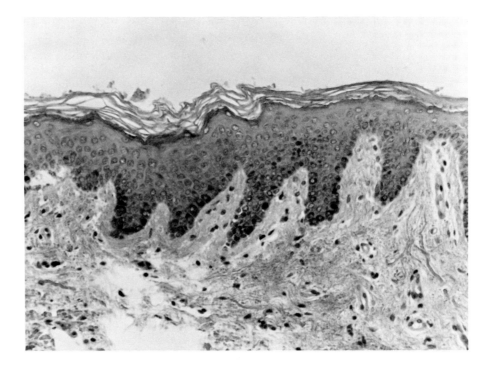

**2.34** Lentigo. There is a heavy concentration of deeply pigmented melanocytes at the tips of the accentuated rete ridges.

skin that appear hypopigmented are therefore clinically remarkable, and biopsies may be submitted from such areas. There are three basic conditions that result in vulvar hypopigmentation: vitiligo, albinism, and postinflammatory depigmentation (leukoderma).

VITILIGO is an inherited disorder in which the melanocytes are lost from areas of skin that previously have been normally pigmented. This condition frequently affects the vulva and biopsies from vitiliginous areas show a remarkable absence of both basilar melanocytes and melanin granules (Figure 2.33, Plate IV).

ALBINISM, also a genetic disorder, is characterized by an inability of the melanocytes to form melanin pigment. Again, there is an absence of melanin granules in the keratinocytes and, in addition, large, pale cells may be present within the basal layer representing the incompetent melanocytes. At times this disorder is confined to small areas of ventral skin in a condition known as piebaldism; however, the histopathology is identical.

Finally, in areas of previous ulcerative inflammation, recently healed skin will temporarily lack a normal population of melanocytes. Such postinflammatory depigmentation, or LEUKODERMA, is common following *Herpes* infections and syphilitic ulcerations. Histologically, the skin appears somewhat thin, metabolically active, and lacking in the usual amount of pigment, although on careful inspection some degree of pigment formation is evident.

## Hyperpigmented Lesions

Freckles (ephelides) do not occur on the vulva, although they are certainly the most common hyperpigmented lesion in other areas of the skin. Freckles represent areas of epidermis in which a normal or decreased melanocytic population is stimulated to an excess of melanin production by actinic radiation. The vulvar skin, however, is rarely exposed to sunlight and as such does not exhibit common freckles. The commonest hyperpigmented lesion occurring on the vulva is that of LENTIGO SIMPLEX, in which isolated areas of epidermis are noted to contain an increased population of functioning melanocytes. Extreme degrees of epidermal pigmentation may be present, with numerous squamous cells exhibiting cytoplasmic melanin granules. There may be mild accentuation of the rete ridges and heavily pigmented melanophages may be present in the upper dermis (Figure 2.34). At times a minimal amount of inflammatory infiltration is noted, but this is by no means constant. Clinically, lentigenes closely resemble junctional nevi and are therefore frequently biopsied. Except for the rare "leopard syndrome," in which thousands of lentigenes are present all over the body, lentigo is essentially devoid of clinical significance.

Juvenile, junctional, compound, and intradermal nevi all occur on the vulva. Rarely are juvenile nevi recognized and biopsied. Therefore, only the latter three types are seen

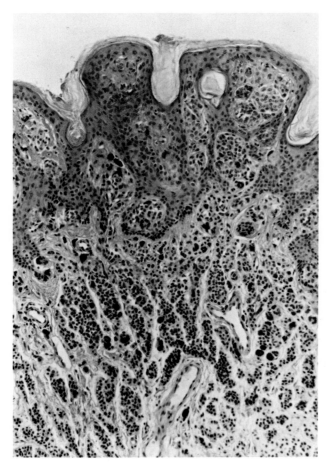

**2.35** Compound nevus. Nests of nevus cells are evident within the epithelium as well as within the dermis.

with any regularity. As described by Pinkus and Merehgan,[127] the typical nevus cell is characterized mainly by its negative attributes. The cells are somewhat larger than melanocytes and have round or ovoid nuclei. Dendrites are not present, nor are intercellular connections visible. The cells may lie singly within the dermis, but more commonly they tend to form nests. Unless they contain melanin, their cytoplasm is clear without granulations or fibrils. In pure junctional nevi, the nevus cells are located within the epidermis and the lower portion of the individual cells or cell nests bulges downward from the tips of the rete ridges. There is no connective tissue noted between the nevus cells and the adjacent squamous keratinocytes. Such lesions are young and somewhat undifferentiated and therefore maintain the possibility of malignant transformation into melanoma. With age, the

**Table 2.2**  Classification of vulvar dystrophies

Hyperplastic
 No atypia
 Atypia (mild, moderate, severe)
Lichen sclerosus
Mixed
 No atypia
 Atypia (mild, moderate, severe)

basement membrane of the epidermis surrounding the nests disappears and reticulum, collagen, and elastic fibers envelop the nests, pushing the epidermis upward. During this process, the lesion is clinically noted to be elevated above the level of the surrounding skin and histologically one notes nevus cells within both the epidermis and the dermis alike. Such lesions are called compound nevi (Figure 2.35). Further differentiation results in complete enclosure of the nevus cells and nests by connective tissue elements such that they lie wholly within the dermis and no activity is seen at the dermoepidermal junction. These, then, are intradermal nevi and are considered to be devoid of premalignant potential.[143,147] Most vulvar nevi are of the compound or intradermal variety.

## Dystrophic Conditions

White lesions of the vulva are not degenerative diseases and the vast majority of them have no premalignant potential. Both the clinician and the pathologist have been confused by such diagnoses as "kraurosis vulvae," "card-like scleroderma," "leukoplakia," "morphea guttata," "atrophic vulvitis," and "white spot disease." Such vague terminology reflects an earlier age of gross morphologic description. A new and more accurate nomenclature has been developed by the International Society for the Study of Vulvar Disease (Table 2.2).[72] This multinational group of pathologists, gynecologists, and dermatologists has recommended that all these lesions be placed under the single heading of dystrophy, and that the older terms be abandoned. The term "dystrophy" was first proposed by Jeffcoate and Woodcock[76] and characterizes those disorders of epithelial growth and nutrition which often present as white lesions of the vulva and result in otherwise unclassified alterations of the epithelial and dermal architecture.

There are two basic varieties of dystrophy: hyperplastic dystrophy and lichen sclerosus. When both coexist on

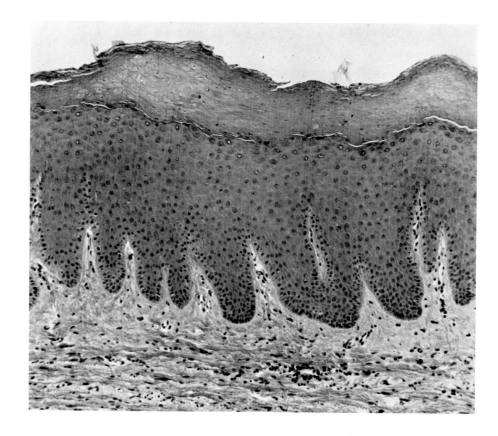

**2.36** Hyperplastic dystrophy, benign. Hyperkeratosis, acanthosis, and mild inflammation characterize this entity.

different areas of the same vulva, a mixed dystrophy is present. Atypical changes are sometimes present in hyperplastic areas. If these are found, they are graded as mild, moderate, or severe. The term "dysplasia" is not used. It is not possible to distinguish the various forms of dystrophy by their gross appearance alone; all may be white, scaly, and fissured. Such changes pose two basic problems for the clinician: "Is this now, or will it become, cancer?" and "What treatment will be effective?" Multiple representative biopsies must be obtained to sample the entire lesion. On the basis of the histologic findings, the pathologist can then provide an accurate response to both clinical questions.

## Hyperplastic Dystrophy

The cardinal feature of hyperplastic dystrophy is elongation, widening, clubbing, or confluency of the rete ridges of the epidermis (acanthosis). Often, hyperkeratosis is present (Figure 2.36). When this thickened layer of keratin is wet, it gives a white appearance to the vulvar tissues. As a rule, a chronic inflammatory infiltrate is noted within the dermis, which is otherwise normal or slightly edematous. At times this infiltrate is predominantly perivascular in location; at other times it is more diffuse. The dermal papillomatosis seen in condylomata acuminata or squamous papilloma is lacking. The individual squamous cells are regular with distinct intercellular bridges. The nuclei are round to oval and contain finely distributed chromatin. Nucleoli may be prominent, and there is progressive maturation of the cells as they approach the superficial layers. Mitotic figures are often quite numerous in the basal layers and, occasionally, inflammatory exocytosis may be seen. The retention of nuclear material in the keratin layer (parakeratosis) is usually associated with loss of the granular zone, whereas in the presence of hyperkeratosis this zone may be accentuated.

Although parakeratosis may be present in otherwise typical areas of hyperplasia (Figure 2.37), its presence should prompt a careful search for signs of cellular atypicality deeper in the epithelium.

Hyperplastic dystrophy may occur at any time but it is most commonly found in women between 30 and 60 years of age. It affects both black and white races equally and accounts for approximately one-half of all vulvar dystrophies.[84] Grossly, the lesions may be white, red, or

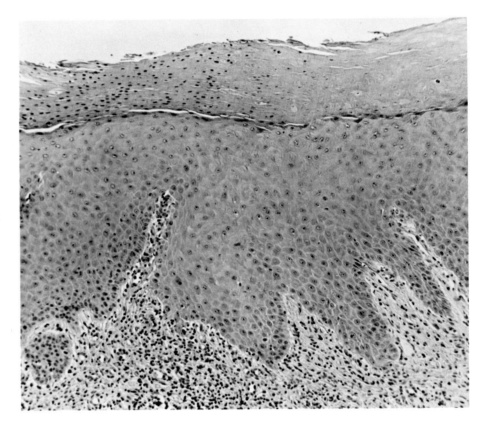

**2.37** Hyperplastic dystrophy, benign. Parakeratosis is present focally.

bright pink. The skin surface may be corrugated and raised or scaly and eczematoid. There is no need to subclassify this disorder on the basis of rete ridge pattern or suspected etiology. "Lichen simplex chronicus," "reactive leuko-keratosis," "neurodermatitis," and so forth all exhibit the same basic histologic features, and all present with indistinguishable clinical findings. The prospective studies by Jeffcoate[75] and Kaufman *et al.*[84] have shown that in the absence of atypia there is no progression of this disorder to carcinoma. It is therefore important for the pathologist to avoid the use of such terms as "leukoplakia" that suggest to the clinician that a premalignant condition exists. Hyperplastic dystrophy is a benign disorder that responds quickly and often dramatically to conservative topical therapy and medical management.[45]

## Lichen Sclerosus

"Lichen sclerosus" is a term that is well entrenched in the literature and that denotes a specific dermatopathologic entity. The principal changes occurring in this form of dystrophy include blunting or loss of the rete ridges and the concomitant development of a homogeneous sub-epithelial layer in the dermis (Figure 2.38). Hyperkeratosis is present in some cases (Figure 2.39). The homogeneous zone has been described as "collagenized" or "edematous" and usually shows a reduction or absence of elastic fibers. Suurmond[146] attributes the blurred outline of the collagen bundles and the decrease of their staining capacities to a swelling and splitting of the bundles into fibers and fibrils, which are subsequently enveloped by the gel-like ground substance. Beneath this layer, a band of chronic inflammatory infiltrate may be noted. The number of cellular layers in the epidermis is decreased and the basal cell layer is often disorganized and hydropic (Figure 2.40). There is both an absence of melanosomes in the keratinocytes and a disappearance of the melanocytes.[101] This lack of pigment contributes to the white clinical appearance. Mitotic figures are rare or absent. In some cases, the mechanical trauma of rubbing and scratching will have produced bullous areas of lymphedema and lacunae filled with erythrocytes (Figure 2.41). Areas of ulceration and acute inflammation may also be seen. All of these features set lichen sclerosus apart from true circumscribed scleroderma, which rarely affects the vulva.[144]

The suffix "et atrophicus" was once applied to this

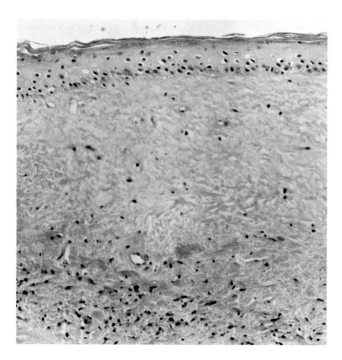

**2.38** Lichen sclerosus. There is thinning of the epithelium with a loss of rete ridges, homogenization of the dermis, and inflammatory infiltrate.

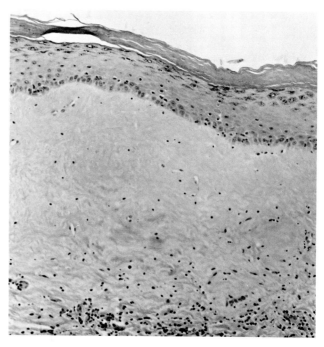

**2.39** Lichen sclerosus. Hyperkeratosis is occasionally present along with the other cardinal findings.

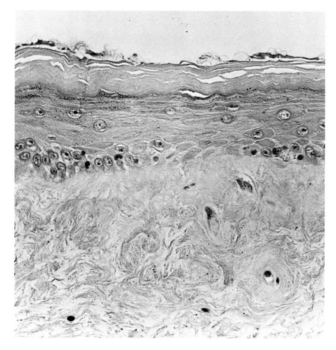

**2.40** Lichen sclerosus. The disorganization and hydropic appearance of the basal layer is evident on high power.

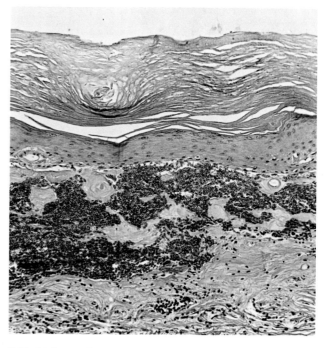

**2.41** Lichen sclerosus. Marked hyperkeratosis with extrasavation of blood in the dermis.

condition but studies of cellular kinetics and metabolism in lichen sclerosus[47,106,159] have demonstrated a remarkable concentration of enzymes and nucleic acids present within the cells of such epithelia. This degree of metabolic activity precludes the epithet "atrophic." Squamous cell atypia is not seen in the areas of pure lichen sclerosus. A careful retrospective analysis of 107 cases from the Armed Forces Institute of Pathology was undertaken by Hart, Norris, and Helwig.[60] Carcinoma developed in only one patient and arose from an isolated area of hyperplasia. They concluded that lichen sclerosus was not a premalignant condition. This fact is borne out by the prospective studies by Oberfield,[119] Jeffcoate and Woodcock,[76] and Kaufman, *et al.*,[84] who also noted the tendency for lichen sclerosus to recur after attempts at surgical excision.

Lichen sclerosus is not confined to aged women; cases are reported occurring in children[17] and patches of this dystrophy can occasionally be found on the vulvas of women during the reproductive years of normal ovarian function. Therefore it is not directly related to estrogen metabolism. Although the vulva is the most frequently affected area, isolated patches of similar skin change are sometimes found on other parts of the body, and males may be affected as well (balanitis xerotica obliterans).

The dystrophy of lichen sclerosus produces gross changes in the vulvar architecture that include flattening and dissolution of the labia minora along with edema and agglutination of the preputial folds. The area appears white because of the diminished superficial vascularity, loss of melanin pigment, and wet keratin covering. The pruritus that accompanies these changes leads to scratching and subsequent irritation and soreness. If sexual intercourse becomes painful and is no longer practiced, a stenosis of the vaginal introitus (kraurosis) can result from lack of regular dilatation. Like hyperplastic dystrophy, lichen sclerosus has been shown to respond to topical medical management, which can arrest and at times reverse the disease process.[45,46]

## Mixed Dystrophy

Both forms of dystrophy may affect different areas of the same vulva at the same time, and multiple biopsies should be taken from various representative sites. If some of these are compatible with hyperplastic dystrophy and others with lichen sclerosus, then a mixed condition exists. Ten to 15% of all dystrophies fall into this category. It is erroneous to surmise that these different but mixed histologic pictures represent different stages of the same disease. Neither is there any evidence for such an interpretation because areas of untreated lichen sclerosus do not become hyperplastic nor vice versa. Instead, the different areas seem to represent clones of cells responding in different ways to the same general but unidentified stimulus. Mixed dystrophy is somewhat more difficult to treat, and foci of atypia are noted in the hyperplastic areas more frequently than in pure hyperplastic dystrophy.

## Atypia

The epidermal keratinocyte usually betrays the presence of an abnormal genome by a disturbance in the maturation process. The cell may retain the juvenile characteristics of mitotic capability, high nuclear/cytoplasmic ratio, and relative cytoplasmic basophilia as it progresses into the upper layers of the epithelium. Alternatively, the cell may show evidence of accelerated maturation with nuclear pyknosis surrounded by a clear perinuclear halo (corps rond formation), keratinization of the individual cell cytoplasm while that cell is still well beneath the granular zone, or the formation of intraepithelial "pearls" within the acanthotic rete ridges. Multinucleation is indicative of the inability of cells to complete their cytoplasmic separation after nuclear reduplication has taken place. Bizarre and giant mitoses attest to a defect occurring early in the mitotic process. Irregular nuclear membranes and coarse clumping of the chromatin are further suggestions of DNA abnormality. Parakeratosis is seen when keratinocytes fail to form granules of prekeratin and retain basophilic nuclear material at the epithelial surface. Any or all of these changes may be seen, and their presence constitutes atypia. When grading the degree of atypia, the quality and quantity of the individual cellular atypicalities are considered along with the relative density of the cell population and overall architecture of the epithelium.

When atypical changes are few in number and confined to the lower third of the epithelium, mild atypia should be reported (Figure 2.42). Moderate atypia is recognized if such changes extend through approximately one-half to two-thirds of the epithelium. Individually keratinized cells and mitoses above the basal layer should be infrequent (Figure 2.43). When cellular atypia involves more than two-thirds of the full thickness of the epithelium (disregarding the keratin layer), then severe atypia should be diagnosed. Juvenile cells of the parabasal type may reach almost to the surface and corps rond formation, individually keratinized cells, and abnormal mitoses are seen with greater frequency (Figure 2.44). Admittedly, the graduations of atypia are somewhat subjective. Mild and moderate atypia may show considerable degrees of overlap, and the borderline between severe atypia and carcinoma in situ is often indistinct.

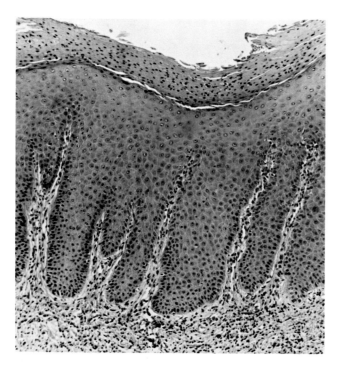

**2.42** Mild atypia. Parakeratosis is present and occasional atypical cells are seen.

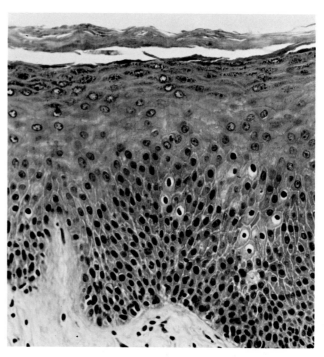

**2.43** Moderate atypia. Basal cell hyperplasia is noted, along with corps ronds formation involving the lower half of the epithelium.

The cause of these atypicalities is essentially unknown. Their natural history and biologic behavior have not been subjected to careful study. Many of these lesions disappear spontaneously, especially if they are noted during pregnancy.[43] Others disappear when the background lesion of hyperplastic dystrophy has been properly treated. Some may progress to carcinoma in situ, but such progression is not inexorable and has not been documented on the vulva as well as it has been on the cervix.[158] The premalignant potential of atypia, then, is an unknown quantity. Published experience suggests that very few such cases (fewer than 10%), actually progress to invasive cancer,[76] and most are adequately managed with conservative therapy. Nonetheless, the only cases of vulvar dystrophy that have eventuated in carcinoma are those in which the initial biopsies have shown atypical changes. Careful, long-term followup and frequent reevaluation is therefore necessary unless complete excision of the lesion is carried out.

# Intraepithelial Neoplasia

Historically, four varieties of intraepithelial neoplasia of the vulvar skin have been recognized.[83] When they occur on the vulva, Bowen's disease, erythroplasia of Queyrat,

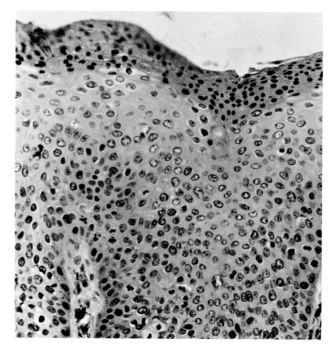

**2.44** Severe atypia. Marked parakeratosis, nuclear pleomorphism, ectopic mitoses, and hyperchromatic nuclei are seen. The upper layers of the epithelium beneath the parakeratosis are normal.

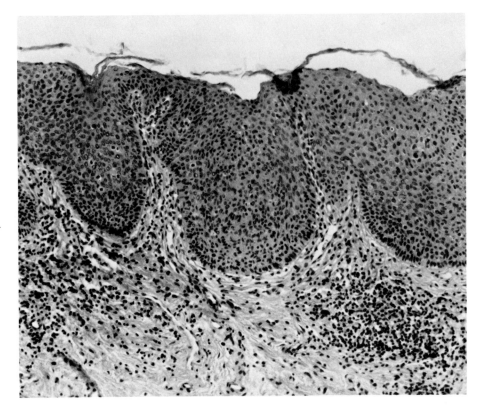

**2.45** Carcinoma in situ. An erythroplastic area with minimal keratin coating and prominent dermal papillae. Full thickness change is evident.

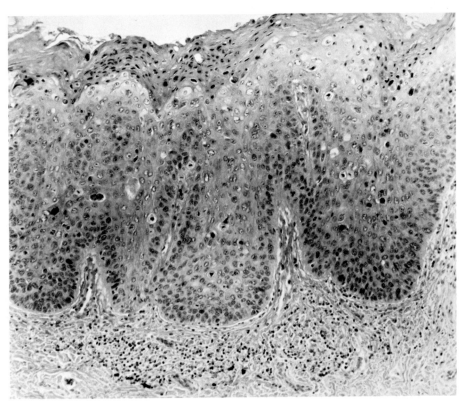

**2.46** Carcinoma in situ. A Bowenoid area with parakeratosis, giant cells, dyskeratotic cells, and multinucleation.

and carcinoma simplex exhibit such marked biologic similarities that the International Society for the Study of Vulvar Disease has recommended that they be grouped under the single heading of "carcinoma in situ."[72] The fourth variety, Paget's disease of the vulva, is a distinct clinicopathologic entity that warrants separate denomination.

## Carcinoma in Situ

Clinically, the lesions of vulvar carcinoma in situ present as papules or macules that may be unifocal or multicentric, coalescent or discrete. Pruritus is present in more than half of the cases. The involved areas of epithelium may appear darkly pigmented, white and lichenified, pink and scaly, or moist and red. The location of the lesion (mucous or cutaneous surface), the quality of local hygiene, and the amount of previous grattage or scratching all affect the surface appearance. A 1% solution of toluidine blue dye may be topically applied to "direct" the clinician's biopsy. If the surface keratin is absent or denuded, or if the lesion is parakeratotic, it retains the blue color after a 1% acetic acid wash.[20]

Histologically, the lesions are characterized by a disorientation of epithelial architecture that extends throughout the full thickness of the epithelium, not including the surface layers above the granular zone (Figure 2.45). Giant cells, multinucleated cells, abnormalities of nuclear/cytoplasmic ratio, dyskeratosis, individual cell keratinization, corps rond formation, abnormal mitoses, mitotic figures above the basal layer, and an increased density of cell population may all be seen in varying degrees (Figure 2.46). The formation of intraepithelial squamous "pearls" in the deep portions of the rete ridges with loss of the normal basal layer is also a sinister pattern and constitutes an unusual form of carcinoma in situ. Both intracellular and extracellular pigment granules may be seen distributed throughout the epidermis. Dermal melanophages are often prominent beneath the basal layer and within the dermal papillae. This is not true pigment incontinence but such lesions often appear hyperpigmented.

Nuclear morphology is abnormal (Figure 2.47). The nuclear borders may be irregular and the chromatin is coarse and often clumped. On an ultrastructural level, this corresponds to an increased number of interchromatinic and perichromatinic granules sometimes clustered in globular structures.[80] The karyotype of these abnormal cells was analyzed in six cases.[81] Twenty-four percent of the cells were peridiploid, whereas 22% were peritriploid and 54% were in the tetraploid range or above. Multiple nuclei

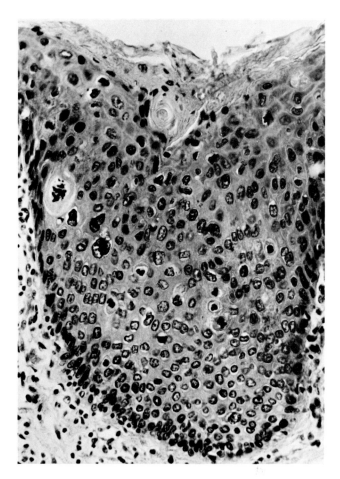

**2.47** Carcinoma in situ. Full thickness change is evident with marked nuclear abnormalities of all types.

are sometimes seen and the overall size of the nucleus is generally increased. Most of the individual cells show little tendency to mature as they approach the surface, but intercellular bridges can usually be recognized. Others begin maturation and degeneration (individual cell keratinization and corps rond formation) while still in the deeper layers of the epithelium. Seiji and Mizuno[138] attribute individual cell keratinization to the presence of aggregated tonofilaments and nuclear substances present in the cytoplasm and suggest that they may be produced in the process of abnormal cell division. At times, these lesions bear a striking resemblance to areas of carcinoma in situ of the cervix, but this is by no means always the case (Figure 2.48).

The edges of the lesion may show benign hyperplastic dystrophy or gradations of atypia. More often, however, the epithelium immediately adjacent to the area of in situ

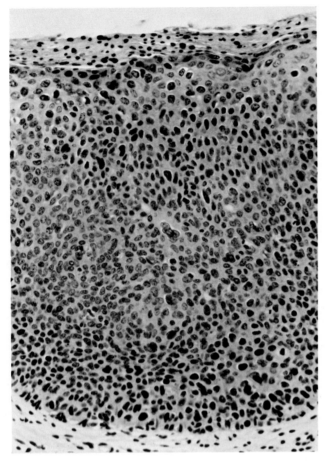

**2.48** Carcinoma in situ. Complete replacement of the epithelium with overlying parakeratosis resembling carcinoma in situ of the cervix. Note the large multinucleated cell in the center.

change appears completely normal and the transition is very abrupt. Although these changes may be recognized and diagnosed with a fair degree of certainty, the pathologist must be aware of the fact that their biologic significance is quite uncertain. That similar changes have been observed adjacent to the frankly invasive squamous cell carcinoma does not prove that the in situ lesion has preceded the invasive disease. Szodoray[148] believes that in the vast majority of cases, cancer appears to develop without the presence of the so-called intraepidermal precarcinomatous lesions. Yet, on the basis of such "guilt by association," many clinicians have been accustomed to perform a total vulvectomy for carcinoma in situ of the vulva. For many cases, this probably represents overtreatment. Woodruff and his colleagues[161] have called attention to the fact that this disease is being found with

increasing frequency. Many patients are quite young, and the median age in our own clinic is only 32. More than half of the cases are unifocal in nature and involve only a small area of the vulva. For such patients, wide local excision has proved to be adequate therapy, and little is gained by the routine excision of an uninvolved clitoris or normal appearing labial tissue.

Two cases of carcinoma in situ of the vulva, occurring in identical twins, were reported to have developed after many years of skin contact with arsenical insecticides.[44] In most patients, however, the etiology is obscure. There is a high incidence of association of carcinoma in situ of the vulva with other genital tract malignancies, especially carcinoma in situ of the cervix.[59,161] Such multicentric foci of carcinoma in situ occur in approximately 10 to 20% of the cases, although they are not necessarily concomitant. In one case of simultaneous occurrence, chromosomal analysis of the cervical and vulvar tumors has shown them to have arisen from completely different cell lines with remarkably dissimilar karyotypes.[160] Although the lesions may arise concomitantly, therefore, they probably represent the response of different sites to a common oncogenic stimulus or else they are both examples of the inability of the immune system to adequately recognize or suppress clones of abnormal cells that have arisen independently of one another, despite their temporal and anatomic proximity. Graham and Helwig[56] noted that 80% of 35 patients with Bowen's disease developed one or more primary internal cancers or primary skin cancers with metastases at an average of 8.5 years after the onset of the in situ lesion. Anderson and his colleagues,[2] however, were unable to corroborate this association in their study of 207 consecutive patients. Nevertheless, the patient with carcinoma in situ of the vulva must be considered at increased risk for the development of other carcinomas elsewhere in the reproductive system. Both cytologic and biopsy material from other sites, especially the cervix and vagina, should be requested and carefully studied in all cases in which carcinoma in situ of the vulva is found.

## Paget's Disease

Paget's disease of the skin is a curious phenomenon generally confined to the integument along the "milk line." It occurs most commonly on the nipple, where its presence signifies an underlying adenocarcinoma of the breast. Genital, perianal, and axillary lesions have also been described, and all these areas are known to be rich in apocrine glands.[4] Early investigators noted underlying apocrine adenocarcinoma of the skin in the vicinity of the

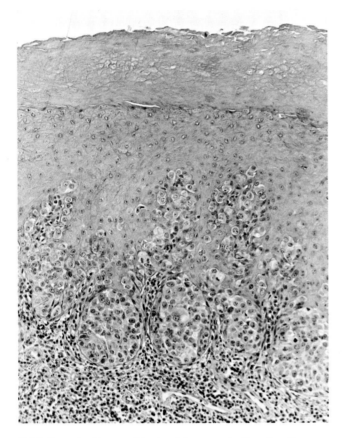

**2.49** Paget's disease. Nests of large pale Paget cells are seen at tips of the rete ridges. Single cells infiltrate upward in the epithelium, which is hyperkeratotic.

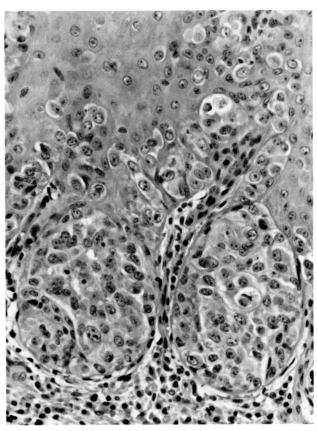

**2.50** Paget's disease. Paget cells are present singly and in nests. Their pale cytoplasm easily differentiates them from surrounding keratinocytes.

superficial Paget's change in many of the extramammary cases. They surmised that the Paget cells in the epidermis had migrated to that site from the underlying carcinoma. Within recent years, a much larger number of cases has been added to the literature and the study of these peculiar cells has been intensified. On the basis of these investigations, it now seems clear that Paget cells arise *de novo* in the epidermis or epidermally derived adnexal structures. When present in extramammary locations, their presence may or may not be associated with a separate and often subjacent, independent carcinoma.

Paget cells often occur in nests surrounded by small hyperchromatic basaloid cells, which are considered to be Paget precursors by some investigators.[62,125] The individual cells within such a nest may surround a central clear area, giving an acinar appearance to the structure. Isolated Paget cells may file upward in the epithelium, where they are surrounded by squamous keratinocytes and are distin-

guished by an absence of intercellular bridges (Figure 2.49). Hair shafts and sweat gland structures, deep in the dermis, may also contain Paget cells. Even in these locations, they must be considered intraepithelial as long as they are bordered by the basement membrane.

The typical Paget cell is large and round or oval in shape. The cytoplasm is pale and occasionally vacuolated. The nuclei are variable in character: Most are vesicular with finely distributed chromatin; others are more hyperchromatic and may be indented. The nucleoli are prominent but not enlarged, and mitotic figures are present only in atypical cases (Figure 2.50). The cytoplasm of Paget cells contains neutral and acid mucopolysaccharides. This accounts for their characteristic staining reactions: PAS positive (diastase resistant), mucicarmine positive, aldehyde–fuchsin positive, and alcian blue positive.[62,149] These reactions distinguish Paget cells from the large pale cells sometimes seen in Bowenoid types of carcinoma in situ or in superficial amelanotic melanomas. The dopa reaction on fresh tissue has been studied and found to be negative in Paget's disease.[163] This indicates an inability of the cell to produce melanin and again distinguishes it from a melanoma cell. Paget cells may contain granules of melanin, demonstrable with Fontana–Masson stain, but these are probably produced by neighboring melanocytes and only secondarily engulfed by the Paget cell. Enzymatic histochemical determinations have shown patterns similar to those present in eccrine sweat gland cells.[6] Extensive work on their ultrastructure has shown some Paget cells to contain the organelles associated with apocrine cells,[116] whereas others resemble eccrine cells[38] and still others resemble squamous keratinocytes.[39] In some instances, more than one type has been identified within the same case. These findings are all consistent with the concept that the Paget cell represents an aberrant differentiation from a multipotent cell derived from the embryonic stratum germinativum of the epidermis. Primitive stem cells that are destined to form basal keratinocytes may differentiate into Paget cells with some of the ultrastructural characteristics of keratinocytes; those stem cells differentiating into apocrine anlage may form Paget cells with apocrine organelles and so forth. Such an interpretation accounts for the observed facts that Paget cells are often first noted just above the basal layer of the epithelium and that they may be located within any of the skin adnexae.

The finding of "Pagetoid" or "Paget-like" cells in foci of metastatic tumors of either squamous or adenomatous origin, then, indicates that the malignant tumor cell is still capable of aberrant differentiation into Paget cells instead of that the Paget cell had become invasive. Whether the Paget cell itself is capable of invasion and metastasis is somewhat controversial. Parmley et al.[125] reported seven examples in which they felt the Paget's disease was "invasive." These cases, however, were associated with invasive tumors that showed foci lacking any differentiation, or, contained areas of other epithelial atypicalities. It is possible that these poorly differentiated carcinomas contained cells capable of Pagetoid differentiation. Other rare instances have been reported in which dermal infiltration of Paget cells has been seen, but this behavior is most unusual.[37] Therefore, although vulvar Paget's disease is properly classified as a form of intraepithelial neoplasia, it is usually a slowly progressive, indolent, localized process.

Of far greater significance is the frequency with which the epidermal changes are associated with separate invasive carcinomas. Approximately one-third of Helwig and Graham's series[62] were found to have an underlying adnexal carcinoma of the skin. Friedrich and his colleagues[49] found that 14% of all reported cases of vulvar Paget's disease were associated with a carcinoma of the breast. Cases with associated adenocarcinoma of the Bartholin gland[151] and squamous cell carcinoma of the vulva[162] have also been reported, and perianal involvement is associated with a high incidence of adenocarcinoma of the rectum.[62] The treatment and prognosis of Paget's disease of the vulva, therefore, depends on the presence or absence of associated invasive carcinoma, and patients may be divided into two groups on this basis.[22,150] Consequently, it is incumbent on the pathologist to make a diligent search through all submitted tissue in order to identify or rule out invasive carcinomas. It is equally incumbent on the surgeon to provide the total vulva, excised to a depth including the subcutaneous fat and fibromuscular tissues, in order that this histologic scrutiny be accomplished. In addition, the clinical workup should provide evidence regarding the status of the breasts and internal organs. If an associated invasive vulvar cancer is present, regional lymphadenectomy is indicated, but the presence of lymph node metastases substantially reduces the prognosis.

Even after wide and total excision, localized recurrences of the Paget's phenomenon are common. The sharply demarcated visible borders of the disease do not correspond to the extent of histologic involvement. At times there may even be deep nests of Paget cells far removed from the visible lesion, lying beneath normal appearing skin.[49] Such occult foci, not recognized or excised at the time of original surgery, probably account for most recurrent episodes. A careful search must therefore be made of all surgical margins; if Paget cells are present, the likelihood of recurrence is great. Even when the margins are free, however, the disease may recur. The ability of the Paget cell to migrate across suture lines within the epithelium may account for these repeated episodes.[1] The recent finding of Paget's disease developing within skin grafted to the vulva and perianal area from the thigh suggests that an unidentified dermal factor may also influence Pagetoid differentiation of the overlying epidermis.[5]

# Malignant Tumors

## Invasive Squamous Cell Carcinoma

The most common malignant tumor afflicting the vulva originates in the squamous epithelium; it accounts for approximately 4% of all female genital malignancy and over 90% of all vulvar malignancies. The incidence of squamous cell carcinoma of the vulva is closely related to age and occurs once in every 75,000 women between the

**Table 2.3** Clinical staging of squamous carcinoma of the vulva (FIGO)

| | |
|---|---|
| Stage I | Tumor confined to the vulva, 2 cm or less in diameter, without suspicious groin nodes |
| Stage II | Tumor confined to the vulva, exceeding 2 cm in diameter, without suspicious groin nodes |
| Stage III | Extension beyond the vulva, without suspicious groin nodes; or lesions of any size with suspicious groin nodes |
| Stage IV | Grossly positive groin nodes, regardless of extent of primary; or evidence of other metastases |

ages of 50 and 60; the incidence rises to 1:25,000 between the ages of 60 and 70, and over the age of 70 years, to 1:22,000. Fewer than 6% of the patients are noted to be premenopausal.[95] Three-dimensional growth is a characteristic clinical hallmark. Approximately one-third are ulcerated endophytic lesions and the remainder are of the exophytic nodular or vegetative type. Pruritus of long duration is generally the first symptom noted, but with ulceration and secondary infection exudation and bleeding may occur. In general, these tumors grow slowly and extend to involve the contiguous skin, urethra, vagina, and rectum. When lymphatic propagation occurs, the inguinal and femoral lymph node groups are the first to be involved: Spread to the pelvic lymph nodes is a late manifestation of the disease.[89,98]

There are no clear-cut precursors to the development of this lesion. Only a small minority show carcinoma in situ at the periphery of the invasive tumor and in most cases, the margins are composed of remarkably normal epithelium. Some investigators have noted a higher incidence of this disease following granulomatous infections of the vulva.[61,91,133] The incidence of diabetes, cardiovascular disease, and previous surgery is consistent with the advanced age of the patients. Many studies have emphasized the frequent occurrence (6 to 15%) of associated neoplasia of the anogenital tract.[12,42,77] The cervix is the most common site of these second primary tumors, a fact that suggests the possibility of a common pathogenetic factor.

Since 1971, a uniform staging system defined by the International Federation of Obstetricians and Gynecologists (FIGO), utilizing the TNM Classification, has been in general use (Table 2.3). Franklin[41] has reviewed the systems used prior to 1971 and has related the current FIGO clinical staging method to a large series. This sys-

tem uses 2-cm diameter as the critical size differentiating stage I from stage II lesions and depends heavily on the clinical assessment of groin node involvement, a practice that has been shown to have an error rate as high as 45 to 50%.[153] Recently, new staging systems have been proposed by Krupp[90] and by Friedrich.[45] Both of these classifications are based on the postoperative histologic assessment of nodal metastases and utilize a 3-cm diameter critical size, which results in a more uniform distribution of cases.

The corrected 5-year survival for all patients treated with radical surgery is approximately 70%. With negative nodes, 90% show no evidence of disease at 5 years; with positive groin nodes this survival drops to below 65%, and for those with positive pelvic nodes the figure is less than 25%.

Histologically, invasive squamous cell carcinomas are usually well-differentiated tumors, but anaplastic varieties are found in 5 to 10% of the cases.[55,153] Most investigators have noted an inverse correlation between the degree of differentiation and the incidence of node involvement.[134] In Way's series,[153] 35% of differentiated tumors had positive nodes, whereas 62% of anaplastic tumors showed these metastases. Although the FIGO staging system makes no allowance for histologic grade, it is clinically useful to differentiate such tumors into those that are well differentiated and those that are anaplastic. Well-differentiated tumors show broad anastomosing masses of atypical squamous cells with prominent intercellular bridges and cytoplasmic inclusions of keratin (Figure 2.51). Whorls and nests of keratin (pearls) are almost constant features of the well-differentiated tumor and nuclear atypicalities and mitotic figures are not outstanding (Figure 2.52). In the poorly differentiated tumors, marked nuclear pleomorphism and low nuclear cytoplasmic ratios are seen, along with minimal keratin formation and numerous mitotic figures (Figure 2.53).

Depth of stromal invasion is of questionable prognostic significance. Wharton et al.[154] reported that of 25 patients with carcinomas of the vulva that had invaded the stroma to a depth of 5 mm or less, none had positive lymph nodes on groin dissection and none developed recurrence or died as a result of their vulvar cancer. Others, however, have documented cases with less than 5 mm of invasion that have resulted in positive lymph node metastases.[25,115] Parker et al.[124] studied 58 patients with 5 mm or less of stromal invasion and noted that 5% (three patients) had pelvic lymph node metastases. In two of these cases, there was recognizable invasion of vascular channels, whereas the third patient's tumor was of an anaplastic variety. They suggested that the degree of tumor anaplasia and vascular channel involvement were more important prognostic parameters than was the simple depth of stromal invasion.

Aberrant hormonal activity has been reported in some gynecologic tumors.[139] The vulva is second only to the ovary in the incidence of hypercalcemia associated with large tumors. Niebyl *et al.*[117] described two cases of well-differentiated squamous carcinoma of the vulva, non-metastatic, without bony involvement, in which toxic levels of hypercalcemia were noted. This hypercalcemia was not responsive to preoperative metabolic therapy; however, once the tumor had been surgically removed, the serum calcium levels returned to normal.

Two other varieties of squamous cell carcinoma of the vulva deserve mention. Lasser[92] described an adenoid squamous type of tumor with rounded spaces or "pseudo-acini" lined by a single layer of squamous cells. Dys-keratotic and acantholytic cells were sometimes present in the central lumen. These changes were focal in most cases, and many histologic investigators have mentioned their occasional presence within otherwise well-differentiated tumors. Although interesting, such foci of adenoid archi-tecture do not appear to be associated with the incidence of node involvement or the clinical course of the tumor.

Verrucous carcinoma is a distinct variant with a unique biologic course.[50] It is a rare and potentially lethal cancer often unrecognized by clinician and pathologist alike. Clinically, these lesions mimic condylomata acuminata, which are unresponsive to the usual methods of therapy,

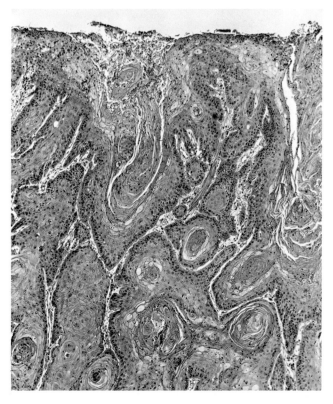

**2.51** Invasive squamous cell carcinoma, well differenti-ated. A typical area of invasive carcinoma showing tongues and islands of mature keratinocytes.

**2.52** Invasive squamous cell carcinoma, well differentiated. Tongues of disorganized squa-mous epithelium are seen and "pearl" formation is evident.

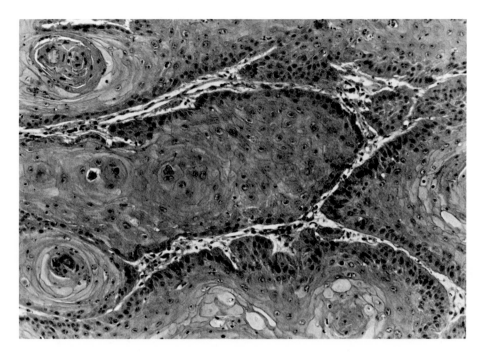

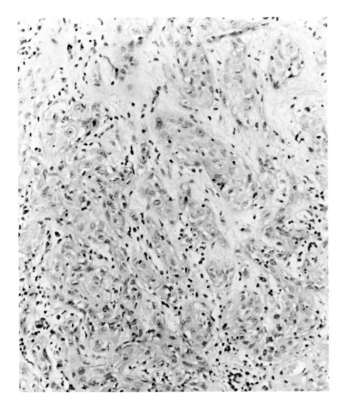

**2.53** Invasive squamous carcinoma, anaplastic. Small nests of invasive cells not clearly squamous in origin show aggressive infiltration.

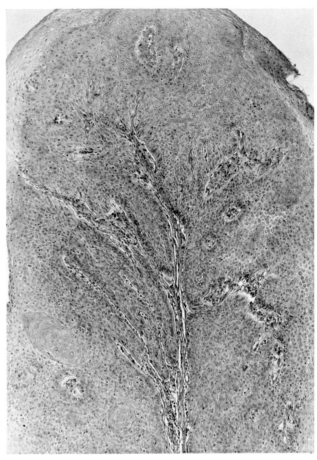

**2.54** Verrucous carcinoma. An overall papillary pattern is evident with parakeratosis resembling condyloma acuminatum. However, islands of abnormal maturation and individually anaplastic cells are present.

and are biopsied only after many attempts at eradication with topical podophyllin, local surgery, or other techniques. With few exceptions,[40] most patients with this disease are postmenopausal. Histologically, these tumors are extremely well differentiated and papillary (Figure 2.54). Intercellular bridges are prominent, mitoses are rare, and the cells have abundant eosinophilic cytoplasm. Invasive infiltration of the underlying tissue is generally accompanied by marked inflammatory response. The tumor invades by local extension and nodal metastases are absent. Ill-advised radiation therapy has often resulted in the development of an aggressive anaplastic tumor, whereas the natural biologic history of the untreated disease is one of local aggression amenable to wide surgical excision.[88,97]

## Melanoma

Melanoma comprises between 2 and 9% of most series of vulvar cancers.[98] The age range of patients with this tumor is wider than that of squamous carcinoma. The mean age at incidence is 54 years, and most cases have occurred during the sixth and seventh decades, but 32% are premenopausal.[18] Although this is a rare tumor, its highly aggressive behavior and low overall survival rate (30%) account for its clinical importance.[73,110,166]

Two major varieties of melanoma occur on the vulva: nodular melanoma, and superficial spreading melanoma. Changes occurring in a preexisting dark lesion of the vulva are rarely noted by the patients, whose presenting complaint is usually that of a "lump" along with bleeding or itching. Attempts at application of the FIGO staging system for squamous cell carcinoma of the vulva to malignant melanoma of the vulva are hampered because of the biologic behavior of the lesion: rapid and aggressive invasion as opposed to slow local enlargement. Mihm *et al.*[104]

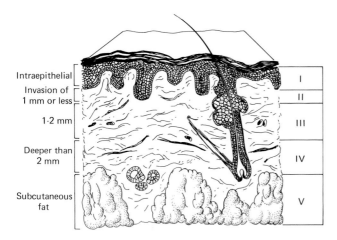

**2.55** Levels of vulvar melanoma invasion. The classical levels translated into measurements by Chung *et al.,* Malignant melanoma of the vulva. *Obstet. Gynecol.* 45:638, 1975.

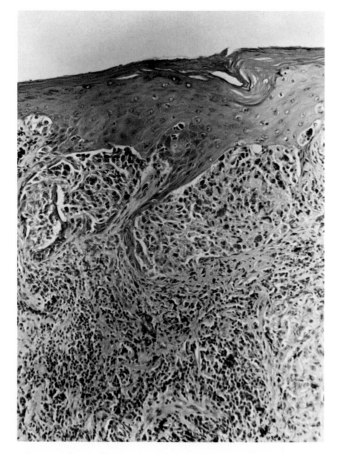

**2.56** Melanoma. Nests of melanoma cells invade the epidermis and diffusely infiltrate the dermal tissue.

have advocated that melanoma be staged according to the level of invasion and five levels are recognized. Chung and his colleagues[18] have applied this system to the vulva (Figure 2.55) and note that patients with level I disease are extremely rare. Of those with level II disease, all survived after adequate surgery. A 40% survival is expected with levels III and IV, whereas only a 20% survival is found after level V has been reached. Patients who die of melanoma generally exhibit widespread metastases, most often to lungs, liver, and brain.

Histologic sections from invasive areas of the superficial spreading variety of melanoma show relatively uniform, large, malignant melanocytes present in the epidermis. The dermis may not be involved. The nuclei are relatively uniform, and there is usually an abundance of "dusty" cytoplasm. In contrast, the nodular melanoma is a tumor in which intraepidermal growth is always associated with dermal invasion. Irregular junctional activity is frequent, and both spindle-shaped and polygonal epithelioid cells are seen (Figure 2.56). The latter, more common cells are large and usually contain a variable concentration of melanin granules. Mitotic figures are almost always present but their absence does not absolutely preclude malignancy. Unlike benign nests of nevus cells, nests of melanoma cells are not surrounded by well-organized bundles of collagen. In addition, an inflammatory reaction of lymphocytes and plasma cells is often seen.[94,127]

## Other Malignancies

Although basal cell carcinomas of the skin are extremely common, they rarely occur on the vulva, a site not often exposed to actinic radiation. Breen *et al.*[11] have shown that when such vulvar tumors arise, they are primarily found in elderly white women whose symptomatology consists of itching or chronic presence of a mass (Figure 2.57, Plate IV). Most lesions are confined to the labia majora and a local recurrence rate of 20% is noted after wide local excision. Yet, the overall prognosis for these tumors is excellent and no patients have been observed to expire from the disease. The histologic pattern resembles that of basal cell carcinomas occurring elsewhere on the skin. Small, elongated cells with deeply basophilic nuclei are present and a large variety of architectural patterns can be recognized, ranging from slight palisading of the basal layer of the epidermis to the formation of large, club-shaped masses of pleomorphic basal cells. The connective tissue response frequently consists of a chronic inflammatory cell infiltrate and occasionally shows a mucoid or myxomatous change. Focal maturation of the malignant basal layer may occur with the formation of mature squamous cells and keratin "pearls." Such keratinization should be regarded as a sign of progressive maturation and not dedifferentiation or anaplasia. Careful histologic study is necessary to distinguish the metatypical basal cell carcinoma or "basosquamous" carcinoma, in which both squamous and basal elements show cytoplasmic and nuclear signs of anaplasia. The clinical significance of such change is unclear.[137] Some investigators, nonetheless, feel that the presence of "basosquamous" change with a mature malignant element should be treated in a manner similar to that of an invasive squamous carcinoma.[9]

Sarcomas of the vulvar connective tissue are unusual tumors. Leiomyosarcoma is the most common type but neurofibrosarcomas, rhabdomyosarcomas, fibrosarcomas, angiosarcomas, and epithelioid sarcomas are among others that have been recorded.[26] Most of these lesions arise from the labia majora, and a wide age range (6 to 64 years) is noted. The clinical course of these lesions is unpredictable and only somewhat dependent on the histologic type of predominant cell. Rhabdomyosarcomas are rapidly growing tumors that metastasize early, whereas leiomyosarcomas are more indolent neoplasms with a tendency to local recurrence after resection. Malignant histiocytes may function facultatively as fibroblasts and result in a desmoplastic growth whose monotonous fibrocytic patterns resemble those of the benign dermatofibrosarcoma protuberans group. However, when such mild appearing tumors are deeply invasive, they may be extremely aggressive and result in early distant metastases.[64] The histogenesis of epithelioid sarcomas is obscure, but they occur in young individuals and are characterized by slow but progressive growth with a marked tendency to recurrence after inadequate excision.[128] Microscopically, they are composed of polygonal cells arranged in sheets and nests. Their abundance of eosinophilic cytoplasm gives some cells an epithelioid appearance. Nuclear pleomorphism and frequent mitotic figures are generally noted.

Adenocarcinoma of the vulva is among the rarest of vulvar malignancies.[98] Many previous reports of this entity have retrospectively been shown to represent benign hidradenomas. Adenocarcinoma of the underlying apocrine glands has been found in approximately 30% of the cases of vulvar Paget's disease, but most adenocarcinomas arise as primary malignant tumors of the Bartholin gland. In the Wharton and Everett series,[155] approximately one-half of Bartholin gland tumors were adenocarcinomas, one-third were of the squamous variety, and the remainder were of indeterminate origin. Bartholin gland malignancies carry a poor prognosis because of the rich lymphatic

supply to the area, the deep and occult site of involvement, and the tendency to dismiss enlargements of the Bartholin area as having a benign cause. The average age of patients with Bartholin gland cancer is 50 years old and 67% of the patients are between the ages of 40 and 69. Accordingly, excision is recommended for all tumors of the Bartholin area in women over the age of 40 in order to obtain histologic documentation of the cause. Dodson et al.[27] noted a racial preponderance among white women and found a previous history of inflammation of the Bartholin gland in only a small minority of cases.

Metastatic and secondary tumors occasionally involve the vulva, and the epidermoid carcinoma of the cervix is the most frequent primary lesion followed by carcinomas of the endometrium, kidney, and urethra.[23] Metastatic adenocarcinomas tend to invade the overlying squamous epithelium, whereas metastases from epidermoid carcinomas often remain within the deeper vulvar tissues. Other primary tumors that have metastasized to the vulva include malignant lesions of the breast, choriocarcinomas, and carcinoma of the lung. In our own clinic, we have observed three cases of vulvar involvement by malignant lymphomas.

# Urethra

No discussion of vulvar pathology is complete without mention of the lesions that afflict the female urethra.

Prolapse of the urethral mucosa may occur at any age but it is most common in children between 8 and 12 years. Redundancy of the mucosa and laxity of the supporting periurethral fascia contribute to the formation of prolapse, which is aggravated by increased abdominal pressure and may be related to relative estrogen lack. Large, red polypoid lesions can protrude between the vulvar folds and mimic the clinical appearance of sarcoma botryoides. Excision is recommended for urethral prolapse. Histologically, the specimen of urethral mucosa may exhibit ulceration and the underlying connective tissue is generally edematous. Vascular engorgement and acute and chronic inflammation is usually present.[14]

The caruncle is by far the most common lesion of the urethra. Marshall and his colleagues[102] found caruncles in 376 of 394 patients with urethral tumors. Caruncles are sessile or polypoid masses that present at the urethral meatus in postmenopausal women. They are often asymptomatic but may cause bleeding or dysuria. Clinical differentiation from urethral carcinoma may be impossible and excision, with hemostatic destruction of the base of the lesion, is the treatment of choice. Histologically the sub-mucosa contains large venous channels, which are often dilated and engorged. A myxomatous or granulomatous pattern is present in the supporting tissue, which is often densely infiltrated with chronic inflammatory cells. At times the appearance is similar to that of a rectal hemorrhoid.

Urethral carcinoma constitutes less than 1% of malignancies affecting the female genitalia.[98] The vast majority of these tumors are squamous in origin and arise from the distal urethra. Urethral bleeding and dysuria are the most frequent presenting complaints. Carcinomas of the urethra that arise distally give rise to symptoms early in their course. Their lymphatic drainage is via the superficial inguinal node groups, and so they are associated with a better prognosis than are carcinomas located more posteriorly, which drain via the deep pelvic lymph node chains.

Suburethral diverticula originate from the upper two-thirds of the posterior urethral wall and may extend cephalad to involve the region beneath the vesicle neck. Although a congenital etiology has been proposed for some cases, most are often thought to begin as an infection in one of the tubular periurethral glands, followed by abscess formation with eventual breakthrough into the urethral lumen. After excision, the surgical specimen consists of fragmented epithelium, either transitional or columnar, with evidence of pressure atrophy and inflammation.[52]

# Processing of Vulvar Specimens in the Surgical Pathology Laboratory

The range of vulvar specimens that are received in the surgical pathology laboratory extends from a skin punch biopsy to a radical vulvectomy specimen with *en bloc* lymph nodes. Regardless of the size of the specimen, the principles of proper labeling, identification, fixation, and sectioning apply. Proper labeling includes the patient's name, hospital number, and date, which should be recorded on the requisition slip along with the surgeon's name and all pertinent clinical data. When multiple biopsies are obtained from a single patient, the site of the biopsy should be noted separately for each specimen and each specimen should be appropriately numbered. The specimen, which is received fresh, should be grossly described and fixed as soon as possible. This assures optimum preservation of histologic characteristics. Unnecessary delay results in autolysis and artifact, which can seriously compromise pathologic interpretation.

## Vulvar Biopsies

Vulvar skin biopsies should be cut at right angles to their epithelial surface in preparing sections. Sections should not be thick and should not exceed 3 mm before they are placed into the cassette for paraffin embedding and subsequent microtome sectioning. A poorly oriented specimen within a paraffin block results in an oblique cut of the epithelium, which can result in erroneous diagnosis. This is especially troublesome when dealing with verrucous lesions or severe epithelial atypias. Simple punch biopsies of the skin generally measure 3 to 5 mm in diameter across their epithelial surface. When placing such specimens into the cassette we have found it best to bisect the specimen, placing the cut surfaces toward the surface that is subsequently to be cut by the microtome sectioning knife. The use of mercurochrome may assist the histotechnologist to orient the specimen within the paraffin. The mercurochrome is painted on the surface that is to be cut by the microtome knife. In this way, the histotechnologist can place the tissue into the paraffin, such that the mercurochrome painted edge is upright. If surgical margins are of concern, India ink can be painted on the surgical margins in question. On histologic sectioning, the ink provides accurate identification of the marginal surface. The surgical pathologist must be able to think in three dimensions. Not only are the width and length important, but the depth of the lesion must also be assessed. Here the use of India ink applied to the deep margin of excision may prove especially useful. This evaluation is extremely important in the complete assessment of malignant lesions.

When malignancy is considered, the entire visible lesion must be submitted for histologic sectioning and the peripheral margins of excision must be adequately evaluated. Prior fixation lessens the distortion made by cutting. It is generally accepted that sections are obtained parallel to the longest axis of the specimen, provided they fit in the cassette, and that these specimens are through and through slices of the excised lesion. The peripheral and deep margins are thus included in the primary sections.

## The Superficial Vulvectomy

In special situations a superficial excision of the vulvar and perianal skin is employed to remove confluent areas of carcinoma in situ of the vulva. Such specimens include the entire labia majora, labia minora, clitoris, perineal body, and perianal tissue without subcutaneous fat (Figure 2.58). The lesions of carcinoma in situ are frequently multi-

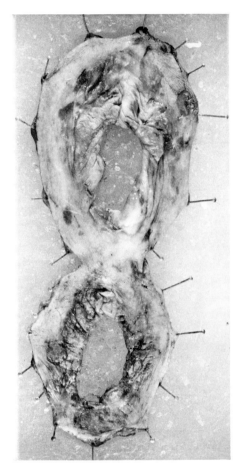

**2.58** Superficial vulvectomy specimen. Circumscribed vulvar and perianal skin pinned out on paraffin.

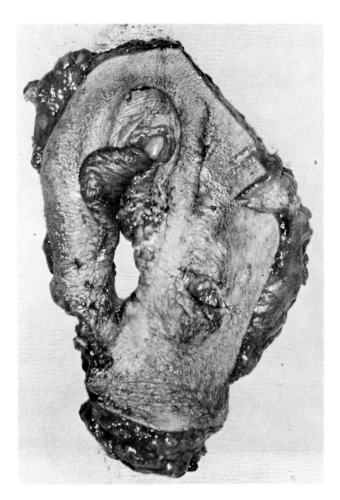

**2.59** Total vulvectomy specimen. Entire vulva includes the deep subcutaneous tissue. Note the extra wide margin around the visible Paget's disease.

centric. Numerous sections must therefore be made through the carcinoma in situ lesions to rule out invasive carcinoma. If foci of invasive cancer are present within the specimen, subsequent radical vulvectomy is required. The surgical margins of such superficial vulvectomy specimens are often quite extensive. Sections parallel to the line of surgical excision evaluate surgical margins more expediently than do multiple radial sections. This not only allows for improved visualization of the surgical margins but also diminishes the number of slides necessary for adequate evaluation.

## Total Vulvectomy

Total vulvectomy is defined as the complete excision of the entire vulva down to the deep fascia (Figure 2.59). Such a specimen includes the subcutaneous fat and is most

often employed in the treatment of Paget's disease. It is necessary to take special care in sectioning the deep tissue because 30% of patients with Paget's disease of the vulva can have underlying sweat gland carcinoma.[62] The total vulvectomy specimen should first be pinned out and fixed. Once it is thoroughly fixed, the specimen is cut through at approximately 0.5-cm parallel intervals to fully assess the underlying dermis. Only with such careful sectioning can underlying sweat gland tumor and occult foci of Paget's involvement be identified.

## The Radical Vulvectomy Specimen

The radical vulvectomy specimen consists of the entire vulva, the inguinal skin and subcutaneous tissue, the femoral and inguinal lymph nodes, and portions of the

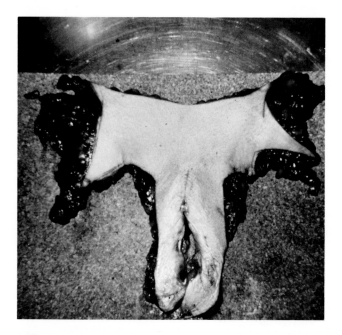

**2.60** Radical vulvectomy specimen. *En bloc* dissection includes bilateral groin node groups with overlying skin.

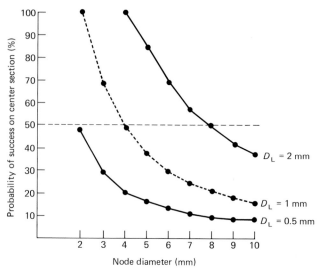

**2.61** Single cut probability. Probability of identifying lesions of varying diameters ($D_L$) in nodes of varying sizes.

[From E. J. Wilkinson and L. Hause, Probability in lymph node sectioning, *Cancer* 33:1269–74, 1974.]

saphenous veins (Figure 2.60). Because of the bulky and fatty nature of the specimen, it is often extremely difficult to palpate or visualize individual lymph nodes. We have found the use of xerography or radiography to be of great assistance in locating the nodes within such specimens[105] (see Chapter 37, Figures 37.12 and 37.13).

The xerography is first performed on receiving the fresh specimen and can be repeated as often as required after dissection until no further nodes are identified. High-contrast x-ray film gives nearly equal results to those of xerography if xerographic equipment is not available. We have observed that if the specimen is immersed in a water bath using a radiolucent container, the marginal contrast edge enhancement effect does not cause confusion while the lymph nodes are being sought. As a rule, the lymph nodes are more radiodense than the surrounding adipose tissue and can generally be seen with ease. The xerographic or radiographic picture is then used as a road map to identify lymph nodes within the specimen and remains as a permanent document of the location of the nodes for future reference. Although the specimen may be fixed in formalin prior to xerographic or radiographic examination, it cannot be fixed in Zenker's solution or any other fixative solution containing heavy metals because these salts produce radiographic density, obscuring the underlying nodes.

After fixation, the node-bearing areas of the specimen should be sliced in parallel 0.5-cm increments. After each slice, the location in relation to the x ray can be evaluated and the entire slice can be palpated for nodes. Simple line drawings of the specimen showing the location of positive lymph nodes and the extent of invasive lesions contribute significantly to the understanding of the distribution of the tumor and its subsequent spread. Careful investigation of such specimens, although tedious, contributes valuable information to the pelvic oncologist who is responsible for planning further care.

The vaginal margins, deep clitoral stumps, and perirectal margins deserve particular consideration, along with the circumferential skin edges of the vulva. Once the lymph nodes are removed from the surgical specimen and properly identified and properly fixed, the method of sectioning of the nodes must assure that metastatic disease to the nodes be identified. To accomplish this a significant surface area of the node must be examined by the pathologist to assure maximal node evaluation. Using lymph node mathematical models it can be shown that the probability of identifying a 1-mm lesion in a 4-mm node on a single center section is only 50% (Figure 2.61).[156] This can be remedied without increase in the number of sections, or casettes, by proper node sectioning. No lymph node slice should exceed 2 mm in thickness, regardless of the node

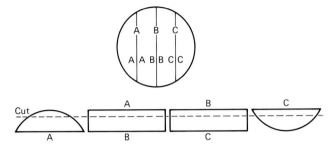

**2.62** Ideal sectioning of lymph node slices. Three cuts provide four tissue segments. There should be arranged such that alternate faces are presented for microtome sectioning. Measurements were made from the granular layer of surface epithelium.

[From E. J. Wilkinson and L. Hause, Probability in lymph node sectioning, *Cancer* 33:1269–74, 1974.]

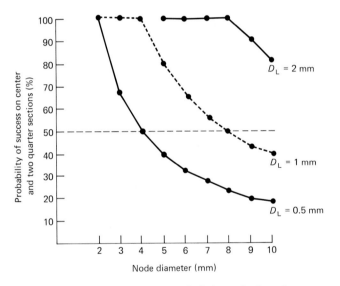

**2.63** Triple cut probability. Probability of identifying lesions of varying diameters ($D_L$) in nodes of varying sizes.

[From E. J. Wilkinson and L. Hause, Probability in lymph node sectioning, *Cancer* 33:1269–74, 1974.]

size. The node slices, to achieve best surface area exposure, should be oriented with alternate cut surfaces up for sectioning (Figure 2.62). In this manner, alternate faces of the lymph node slice are cut by the microtome knife, achieving maximum lymph node exposure. The probability curves for quarter sectioning the node, with proper orientation, demonstrate that the probability of identifying a 1-mm lesion in a 4-mm node with this improved sectioning method approaches 100% (Figure 2.63).

# REFERENCES

1. Adamsons, K., and Reisfield, D. Observations on intradermal migration of Paget cells. *Am. J. Obstet. Gynecol.* 90:1274, 1964.

2. Andersen, S. L., Nielson, A., and Reymann, F. Relationship between Bowen disease and internal malignant tumors. *Arch. Dermatol.* 108:367, 1973.

3. Aurelian, L. The viruses of love and cancer. *Am. J. Med. Technol.* 40:496, 1974.

4. Becker, S. W., Brennan, B., and Weichselbaum, P. K. Genital Paget's disease. *Arch. Dermatol.* 82:857, 1960.

5. Beecham, C. T. Paget's disease of the vulva. *Obstet. Gynecol.* 47(Suppl.):61, 1976.

6. Belcher, R. W. Extramammary Paget's disease. *Arch. Pathol.* 94:59, 1972.

7. Blair, C. Angiokeratoma of the vulva. *Br. J. Dermatol.* 83:409, 1970.

8. Blank, H., Davis, C., and Collins, C. Electron microscopy for the diagnosis of cutaneous viral infections. *Br. J. Dermatol.* 83:69, 1970.

9. Borel, D. M. Cutaneous basosquamous carcinoma. *Arch. Pathol.* 95:293, 1973.

10. Boyce, D. C., and Valpey, J. M. Acute ulcerative vulvitis of obscure etiology. *Obstet. Gynecol.* 38:440, 1971.

11. Breen, J. L., Neubecker, R. D., Greenwald, E., and Gregori, C. A. Basal cell carcinoma of the vulva. *Obstet. Gynecol.* 46:122, 1975.

12. Buchler, D. A. Multiple primaries and gynecologic malignancies. *Am. J. Obstet. Gynecol.* 123:376, 1975.

13. Capraro, V. J. Congenital anomalies. *Clin. Obstet. Gynecol.* 14:988, 1971.

14. Capraro, V. J., Bayonet-Rivera, N. P., and Magoss, I. Vulvar tumor in children due to prolapse of urethral mucosa. *Am. J. Obstet. Gynecol.* 108:572, 1970.

15. Carneiro, S. J. C., Gardner, H. L., and Knox, J. M. Syringoma of the vulva. *Arch. Dermatol.* 103:494, 1971.

16. Catherwood, A. E., and Cohen, E. S. Endometriosis with decidual reaction in episiotomy scar. *Am. J. Obstet. Gynecol.* 62:1364, 1951.

17. Clark, J. A., and Muller, S. A. Lichen sclerosus et atrophicus in children. *Arch. Dermatol.* 95:476, 1967.

18. Chung, A. F., Woodruff, J. M., and Lewis, J. L. Malignant melanoma of the vulva. *Obstet. Gynecol.* 45:638, 1975.

19. Coates, J. B., and Hales, J. S. Granular cell myoblastoma of the vulva. *Obstet. Gynecol.* 41:796, 1973.

20. Collins, C. G., Hansen, L. H., and Theriot, E. A clinical stain for use in selecting biopsy sites in patients with vulvar disease. *Obstet. Gynecol.* 28:158, 1966.

21. Conway, H., Stark, R. B., Climo, S., Weeter, J. C., and Garcia, F. A. The surgical treatment of chronic hidradenitis suppurativa. *Surg. Gynecol. Obstet.* 95:455, 1952.

22. Creasman, W. T., Gallager, H. S., and Rutledge, F. Paget's disease of the vulva. *Gynecol. Oncol.* 3:133, 1975.

23. Dehner, L. P. Metastatic and secondary tumors of the vulva. *Obstet. Gynecol.* 42:47, 1973.

24. Dewhurst, C. J. Congenital malformations of the genital tract in childhood. *J. Obstet. Gynaecol. Br. Commonw.* 75:377, 1968.

25. DiPaola, G. R., Gomez-Rueda, N., and Arrighi, L. Relevance of microinvasion in carcinoma of the vulva. *Obstet. Gynecol.* 45:647, 1975.

26. DiSaia, P. J., Rutledge, F., and Smith, J. P. Sarcoma of the vulva. *Obstet. Gynecol.* 38:180, 1971.

27. Dodson, M. G., O'Leary, J. A., and Averette, H. E. Primary carcinoma of Bartholin's gland. *Obstet. Gynecol.* 35:578, 1970.

28. Douglas, C. P. Lymphogranuloma venereum and granuloma inguinale of the vulva. *J. Obstet. Gynaecol. Br. Commonw.* 69:871, 1962.

29. Dowdle, W. R., Nahmias, A. J., Harwell, R. W., and Pauls, F. P. Association of antigenic type of herpes virus hominis with site of viral recovery. *J. Immunol.* 99:974, 1967.

30. Doyle, J. C. Imperforate hymen. *Calif. West. Med.* 56:242, 1942.

31. Drusin, L. M. The diagnosis and treatment of infectious and latent syphilis. *Med. Clin. N. Am.* 56:1161, 1972.

32. Dunn, J. M. Congenital absence of the external genitalia. *J. Reprod. Med.* 4:66, 1970.

33. Duson, C. K., and Zelenik, J. S. Vulvar endometriosis. *Obstet. Gynecol.* 3:76, 1954.

34. Embrey, M. P. Vulval carcinoma complicating condylomata acuminata. *J. Obstet. Gynaecol. Br. Commonw.* 68:503, 1961.

35. Falk, H. C., and Hyman, A. B. Congenital absence of clitoris. *Obstet. Gynecol.* 38:269, 1971.

36. Farber, E. M., and McClintock, R. P. A current review of psoriasis. *Calif. Med.* 108:440, 1968.

37. Fenn, M. E., Morley, G. W., and Abell, M. R. Paget's disease of vulva. *Obstet. Gynecol.* 38:660, 1971.

38. Ferenczy, A., and Richart, R. M. Ultrastructure of perianal Paget's disease. *Cancer* 29:1141, 1972.

39. Fetherston, W. C., and Friedrich, E. G. The origin and significance of vulvar Paget's disease. *Obstet. Gynecol.* 39:735, 1972.

40. Foye, G., Marsh, M. R., and Minkowitz, S. Verrucous carcinoma of the vulva. *Obstet. Gynecol.* 34:484, 1969.

41. Franklin, E. W. Clinical staging of carcinoma of the vulva. *Obstet. Gynecol.* 40:277, 1972.

42. Franklin, E. W., and Rutledge, F. D. Epidemiology of epidermoid carcinoma of the vulva. *Obstet. Gynecol.* 39:165, 1972.

43. Friedrich, E. G. Reversible vulvar atypia. *Obstet. Gynecol.* 39:173, 1972.

44. Friedrich, E. G. Vulvar carcinoma in situ in identical twins—an occupational hazard. *Obstet. Gynecol.* 39:837, 1972.

45. Friedrich, E. G. *Vulvar Disease.* Philadelphia, W. B. Saunders, 1976.

46. Friedrich, E. G., Lichen Sclerosus. *J. Reprod. Med.* 17:147, 1976.

47. Friedrich, E. G., Julian, C. G., and Woodruff, J. D. Acridine orange fluorescence in vulvar dysplasia. *Am. J. Obstet. Gynecol.* 90:1281, 1964.

48. Friedrich, E. G., and Wilkinson, E. J. Mucous cysts of the vulvar vestibule. *Obstet. Gynecol.* 42:407, 1973.

49. Friedrich, E. G., Wilkinson, E. J., Steingraeber, P. H., and Lewis, D. J. Paget's disease of the vulva and carcinoma of the breast. *Obstet. Gynecol.* 46:130, 1975.

50. Gallousis, S. Verrucous carcinoma. *Obstet. Gynecol.* 40:502, 1972.

51. Gardner, E., Gray, D. J., and O'Rahilly, R. *Anatomy, A Regional Study of Human Structure.* Philadelphia, W. B. Saunders, 1960.

52. Gardner, H. L., and Kaufman, R. H. *Benign Diseases of the Vulva and Vagina.* St. Louis, C. V. Mosby, 1969.

53. Gardner, H. L., and Kaufman, R. H. Viral infections in gynecology and obstetrics. *Clin. Obstet. Gynecol.* 15:856, 1972.

54. Gompel, C., and Silverberg, S. G. *Pathology in Gynecology and Obstetrics.* Philadelphia, J. B. Lippincott, 1969.

55. Gosling, J. R. G. Abell, M. R., Drolette, B. M., and Loughrin, T. D. Infiltrative squamous cell carcinoma of the vulva. *Cancer* 14:330, 1961.

56. Graham, J. H., and Helwig, E. B. Bowen's disease and its relationship to systemic cancer. *Arch. Dermatol.* 80:133, 1959.

57. Gueson, E. T., Liu, C. T., and Emich, J. P. Dysplasia following podophyllin treatment of vulvar condyloma acuminata. *J. Reprod. Med.* 6:159, 1971.

58. Guindi, S. F., Silberberg, B. K., and Evans, T. N. Multifocal mixed adnexoid tumors of the vulva. *Int. J. Gynecol. Obstet.* 12:138, 1974.

59. Hansen, L. H., and Collins, C. G. Multicentric squamous cell carcinomas of the lower female genital tract. *Am. J. Obstet. Gynecol.* 98:982, 1967.

60. Hart, W. R., Norris, H. J., and Helwig, E. B. Relation of lichen sclerosus et atrophicus of the vulva to development of carcinoma. *Obstet. Gynecol.* 45:369, 1975.

61. Hay, D. M., and Cole, F. M. Postgranulomatous epidermoid carcinoma of the vulva. *Am. J. Obstet. Gynecol.* 108:479, 1970.

62. Helwig, E. B., and Graham, J. H. Anogenital (extramammary) Paget's disease. *Cancer* 16:387, 1963.

63. Hendrix, R. C., and Behrman, S. J. Adenocarcinoma arising in a supernumerary mammary gland in the vulva. *Obstet. Gynecol.* 8:238, 1956.

64. Hensley, G. T., and Friedrich, E. G. Malignant fibroxanthoma: a sarcoma of the vulva. *Am. J. Obstet. Gynecol.* 116:289, 1973.

65. Herbut, P. A. *Gynecological and Obstetrical Pathology.* Philadelphia, Lea and Febiger, 1953.

66. Hewitt, A. B. Behcet's disease. *Br. J. Vener. Dis.* 47:52, 1971.

67. Hewitt, M., Barrow, G. I., Miller, D. C., Turk, F., and Turk, S. Mites in the personal environment and their role in skin disorders. *Br. J. Dermatol.* 89:401, 1973.

68. Hobbs, J. E. Sweat gland tumors. *Clin. Obstet. Gynecol.* 8:946, 1965.

69. Huffman, J. W. The detailed anatomy of the paraurethral ducts in the adult human female. *Am. J. Obstet. Gynecol.* 55:86, 1948.

70. Hurley, H. J., and Shelley, W. B. *The Human Aprocine Sweat Gland in Health and Disease.* Springfield, Ill., Charles C Thomas, 1960.

71. Imperial, R., and Helwig, E. B. Angiokeratoma of the vulva. *Obstet. Gynecol.* 29:307, 1967.

72. International Society for the Study of Vulvar Disease. New nomenclature for vulvar disease I. *Obstet. Gynecol.* 47:122, 1976.

73. Janovski, N. A., Marshall, D., and Taki, I. Malignant melanoma of the vulva. *Am. J. Obstet. Gynecol.* 84:523, 1962.

74. Janovski, N. A., and Weir, J. H. Comparative histologic and histochemical studies of mesonephric derivatives and tumors. *Obstet. Gynecol.* 19:57, 1962.

75. Jeffcoate, T. N. A. Chronic Vulval dystrophies. *Am. J. Obstet. Gynecol.* 95:61, 1966.

76. Jeffcoate, T. N. A., and Woodcock, A. S. Premalignant conditions of the vulva, with particular reference to chronic epithelial dystrophies. *Br. Med. J.* 2:127, 1961.

77. Jimerson, G. K., and Merrill, J. A. Multicentric squamous malignancy involving both cervix and vulva. *Cancer 26:*150, 1970.

78. Judge, J. R. Giant condylomata acuminata involving vulva and rectum. *Arch. Pathol. 88:*46, 1969.

79. Kao, M., Paulson, J. D., and Askin, F. B. Crohn's disease of the vulva. *Obstet. Gynecol. 46:*329, 1975.

80. Karasek, J., Smetana, K., Oehlert, W., and Konrad, B. The ultrastructure of Bowen's disease: nuclear and nucleolar lesions. *Cancer Res. 30:*2791, 1970.

81. Katayama, K. P., Woodruff, J. D., Jones, H. W., and Preston, E. Chromosomes of condyloma acuminata, Paget's disease, in situ carcinoma, invasive squamous cell carcinoma and malignant melanoma of the human vulva. *Obstet. Gynecol. 39:*346, 1972.

82. Kaufman, R. H., and Gardner, H. L. Benign mesodermal tumors. *Clin. Obstet. Gynecol. 8:*953, 1965.

83. Kaufman, R. H., and Gardner, H. L. Intraepithelial carcinoma of the vulva. *Clin. Obstet. Gynecol. 8:*1035, 1965.

84. Kaufman, R. H., Gardner, H. L., Brown, D., and Beyth, Y. Vulvar dystrophies: An evaluation. *Am. J. Obstet. Gynecol. 120:*363, 1974.

85. Kersting, D. W. Clear cell hidradenoma and hidradeno-carcinoma. *Arch. Dermatol. 87:*91, 1963.

86. King, L. S., and Sullivan, M. Effects of podophyllin and of colchicine on normal skin, on condyloma acuminatum, and on verruca vulgaris. *Arch. Pathol. 43:*374, 1947.

87. Kligman, A. M. The myth of the sebaceous cyst. *Arch. Dermatol. 89:*141, 1964.

88. Kraus, F. T., and Perez-Mesa, C. Verrucous carcinoma. *Cancer 19:*26, 1966.

89. Krupp, P. J., Lee, F. Y., Batson, H. W., Allen, P. M., and Collins, J. H. Carcinoma of the vulva. *Gynecol. Oncol. 1:*345, 1973.

90. Krupp, P. J., Lee, F. Y., Bohm, J. W., Batson, H. W., Diem, J. E., and Lemire, J. E. Prognostic parameters and clinical staging criteria in epidermoid carcinoma of the vulva. *Obstet. Gynecol. 46:*84, 1975.

91. Lash, A. F., and Zibel, M. Carcinoma of the vulva in a young woman. *Am. J. Obstet. Gynecol. 62:*216, 1951.

92. Lasser, A., Cornorg, J. L., and Morris, J. M. Adenoid squamous cell carcinoma of the vulva. *Cancer 33:*224, 1974.

93. Lenette, E. H., Spaulding, W. H., and Tuant, J. P. *Manual of Clinical Microbiology*, 2nd ed. Washington, D.C., American Society for Microbiology, 1974.

94. Lever, W. F., and Schaumburg-Lever, G. *Histopathology of the Skin*, 5th ed. Philadelphia, J. B. Lippincott, 1975.

95. Lopez de la Osa Garces, L. Etiology and pathogeny of carcinoma of the vulva, *in* Lopez de la Osa Garces, L., ed. *Aspects and Treatment of Vulvar Cancer.* Basel, S. Karger, 1972, pp. 4–15.

96. Lovelady, S. B., McDonald, J. R., and Waugh, J. M. Benign tumors of the vulva. *Am. J. Obstet. Gynecol. 42:*309, 1941.

97. Lucas, W. E., Benirschke, K., and Lebherz, T. B. Verrucous carcinoma of the female genital tract. *Am. J. Obstet. Gynecol. 119:*435, 1974.

98. Lundwall, F. Cancer of the vulva. *Acta. Radiol. Suppl. 208*, 1961.

99. Lynch, P. J., and Minkin, W. Molluscum contagiosum of the adult. *Arch. Dermatol. 98:*141, 1968.

100. Machacek, G. F., and Weakley, D. R. Giant condylomata acuminata of Buschke and Lowenstein. *Arch. Dermatol. 82:*95, 1960.

101. Mann, P. R., and Cowan, M. A. Ultrastructural changes in four cases of lichen sclerosus et atrophicus. *Br. J. Dermatol. 89:*223, 1973.

102. Marshall, F. C., Uson, A. C., and Melicow, M. M. Neoplasms and caruncles of the female urethra. *Surg. Gynecol. Obstet. 110:*723, 1960.

103. Meleiro de Sousa, L., and Lash, A. F. Hemangiopericytoma of the vulva. *Am. J. Obstet. Gynecol. 78:*295, 1959.

104. Mihm, M. C., Clark, W. H., and From, L. The clinical diagnosis, classification and histogenetic concepts of the early stages of cutaneous malignant melanomas. *N. Engl. J. Med. 284:*1078, 1971.

105. Milbrath, J. R., Wilkinson, E. J., and Friedrich, E. G. Xerographic evaluation of radical vulvectomy specimens. *Am. J. Roentgenol. Radium Ther. Nucl. Med. 125:*486, 1975.

106. Mollica, G., Palmara, D., and Campagna, A. Histochemical data on adenosine triphosphatase and alkaline phosphatase in the human vulva. *Minerva Ginecol. 18:*1111, 1966.

107. Monacelli, M., and Nazzaro, P. *Behcet's Disease.* Basel, S. Karger, 1966.

108. Monif, G. R. G. *Infectious Diseases in Obstetrics and Gynecology.* Hagerstown, Harper and Row, 1974.

109. Montgomery, H. *Dermatopathology.* New York, Harper and Row, 1967, pp. 501–505.

110. Morrow, C. P., and Rutledge, F. N. Melanoma of the vulva. *Obstet. Gynecol. 39:*745, 1972.

111. Muller, G., Jacobs, P. H., and Moore, N. E. Scraping for human scabies. *Arch. Dermatol. 107:*70, 1973.

112. Nahmias, A. M., Naib, Z. M., Josey, W. E., and Clepper, A. C. Genital herpes simplex infection. *Obstet. Gynecol. 29:*395, 1967.

113. Nahmias, A. M., and Roizman, B. Infection with herpes simplex virus 1 and 2. *N. Engl. J. Med. 289:*667, 1973.

114. Naib, M. Z., Nahmias, A. J., and Josey, W. E. Relation of cytohistopathology of genital herpes virus infection to cervical anaplasia. *Cancer Res. 33:*1452, 1973.

115. Nakao, C. Y., Nolan, J. F., DiSaia, P. J., and Futoran, R. Microinvasive epidermoid carcinoma of the vulva with an unexpected natural history. *Am. J. Obstet. Gynecol. 120:*1122, 1974.

116. Neilson, D., and Woodruff, J. D. Electron microscopy in in-situ and invasive vulvar Paget's disease. *Am. J. Obstet. Gynecol. 113:*719, 1972.

117. Niebyl, J. R., Genadry, R., Friedrich, E. G., Wilkinson, E. J., and Woodruff, J. D. Vulvar carcinoma with hypercalcemia. *Obstet. Gynecol. 45:*343, 1975.

118. Novak, E. R., and Woodruff, J. D. *Novak's Gynecologic and Obstetric Pathology*, 7th ed. Philadelphia, W. B. Saunders, 1974.

119. Oberfield, R. A. Lichen sclerosus et atrophicus and kraurosis vulvae. *Arch. Dermatol. 83:*144, 1961.

120. O'Duffy, J. D., Carney, J. A., and Deodhar, S. Behcet's disease. *Ann. Int. Med. 75:*561, 1971.

121. Olansky, S. Serodiagnosis of syphilis. *Med. Clin. N. Am. 56:*1145, 1972.

122. Oriel, J. D. Natural history of genital warts. *Br. J. Vener. Dis. 47:*1, 1971.

123. Oriel, J. D., and Almeida, J. D. Demonstration of virus particles in human genital warts. *Br. J. Vener. Dis. 46:*37, 1970.

124. Parker, R. T., Duncan, I., Rampone, J., and Creasman, W. Operative management of early invasive epidermoid carcinoma of the vulva. *Am. J. Obstet. Gynecol. 123:*349, 1975.

125. Parmley, T. H., Woodruff, J. D., and Julian, C. G. Invasive vulvar Paget's disease. *Obstet. Gynecol.* 46:341, 1975.

126. Parry-Jones, E. Lymphatics of the vulva. *J. Obstet. Gynecol. Br. Commonw.* 70:751, 1963.

127. Pinkus, H., and Mehregan, A. H. *A Guide to Dermatohistopathology,* New York, Appleton-Century-Crofts, 1969.

128. Piver, M. S., Tsukada, Y., and Barlow, J. Epithelioid sarcoma of the vulva. *Obstet. Gynecol.* 40:839, 1972.

129. Plentl, A. A., and Friedman, E. A. *Lymphatic System of the Female Genitalia,* Philadelphia, W. B. Saunders, 1971.

130. Powell, L. C. Condyloma acuminatum. *Clin. Obstet. Gynecol.* 15:948, 1972.

131. Ridley, C. M. *The Vulva.* Philadelphia, W. B. Saunders, 1975.

132. Rorat, E., Ferenczy, A., and Richart, R. M. Human Bartholin gland, duct, and duct cyst. *Arch. Pathol.* 99:367, 1975.

133. Saltzstein, S. L., Woodruff, J. D., and Novak, E. R. Postgranulomatous carcinoma of the vulva. *Obstet. Gynecol.* 7:80, 1956.

134. Sanz Esponera, J. The histopathology and degree of malignancy in invasive carcinoma of the vulva, *in* Lopez de la Osa Garces, L., ed. *Aspects and Treatment of Vulvar Cancer.* Basel, S. Karger, 1972, pp. 28–30.

135. Sarkany, I., Taplin, D., and Blank, H. The etiology and treatment of erythrasma. *J. Invest. Dermatol.* 37:283, 1961.

136. Schreiber, M. M. Vulvar von Recklinghausen's disease. *Arch. Dermatol.* 88:136, 1963.

137. Schueller, E. F. Basal cell cancer of the vulva. *Am. J. Obstet. Gynecol.* 93:199, 1965.

138. Seiji, M., and Mizuno, F. Electron microscopic study of Bowen's disease. *Arch. Dermatol.* 99:3, 1969.

139. Shane, J. M., and Naftolin, F. Aberrant hormone activity by tumors of gynecologic importance. *Am. J. Obstet. Gynecol.* 121:133, 1975.

140. Siegel, A. Malignant transformation of condyloma acuminatum. *Am. J. Surg.* 103:613, 1962.

141. Sobel, H. J., Marquet, E., and Schwarz, R. Is schwannoma related to granular cell myoblastoma? *Arch. Pathol.* 95:396, 1973.

142. Sparling, P. F. Diagnosis and treatment of syphilis. *N. Engl. J. Med.* 284:642, 1971.

143. Stegmaier, O. C. Cosmetic management of nevi. *J. Am. Med. Assoc.* 199:167, 1967.

144. Steigleder, G. K., and Raab, W. P. Lichen sclerosus et atrophicus. *Arch. Dermatol.* 84:87, 1961.

145. Stenchever, M. A., McDivitt, R. W., and Fisher, J. A. Leiomyoma of the clitoris. *J. Reprod. Med.* 10:75, 1973.

146. Suurmond, D. Lichen sclerosus et atrophicus of the vulva. *Arch. Dermatol.* 90:143, 1964.

147. Swerdlow, M. Nevi: A problem of misdiagnosis. *Am. J. Clin. Pathol.* 22:1054, 1952.

148. Szodoray, L. Histologic characteristics of the so-called precancerous processes of the skin. *Arch. Dermatol. Syph.* 36:552, 1937.

149. Taki, I., and Janovski, N. A. Paget's disease of the vulva: presentation and histochemical study of four cases. *Obstet. Gynecol.* 18:385, 1961.

150. Taylor, P. R., Stenwig, J. T., and Klausen, H. Paget's disease of the vulva. *Gynecol. Oncol.* 3:46, 1975.

151. Tchang, F., Okagaki, T., and Richart, R. Adenocarcinoma of Bartholin's gland associated with Paget's disease of vulvar area. *Cancer* 31:221, 1973.

152. Warvi, W. N., and Gates, O. Epithelial cysts and cystic tumors of the skin. *Am. J. Pathol.* 19:765, 1943.

153. Way, S. Carcinoma of the vulva. *Am. J. Obstet. Gynecol.* 79:692, 1960.

154. Wharton, J. T., Gallager, S., and Rutledge, F. N. Microinvasive carcinoma of the vulva. *Am. J. Obstet. Gynecol.* 118:159, 1974.

155. Wharton, L. R., and Everett, H. S. Primary malignant Bartholin gland tumors. *Obstet. Gynecol. Surv.* 6:1, 1951.

156. Wilkinson, E. J., and Hause, L. Probability in lymph node sectioning. *Cancer* 33:1269, 1974.

157. Wisdom, A. *Color Atlas of Venereology.* Chicago, Year Book Med. Publishers, 1973.

158. Woodruff, J. D., and Baens, J. S. Interpretation of atrophic and hypertrophic alterations in the vulvar epithelium. *Am. J. Obstet. Gynecol.* 86:713, 1963.

159. Woodruff, J. D., Borkowf, H. I., and Holzman, G. B., Arnold, E. A., and Knack, J. Metabolic activity in normal and abnormal vulvar epithelia. *Am. J. Obstet. Gynecol.* 91:809, 1965.

160. Woodruff, J. D., Davis, H. J., Jones, H. W., Recio, R. G., Salimi, R., and Park, J. Correlated investigative techniques of multiple anaplasias in the lower genital canal. *Obstet. Gynecol.* 33:609, 1969.

161. Woodruff, J. D., Julian, C. G., Puray, T., Mermut, S., and Katayama, P. The contemporary challenge of carcinoma in situ of the vulva. *Am. J. Obstet. Gynecol.* 115:677, 1973.

162. Woodruff, J. D., and Richardson, E. H. Malignant vulvar Paget's disease. *Obstet. Gynecol.* 10:10, 1957.

163. Woodruff, J. D., and Williams, T. F. The dopa reaction in Paget's disease of the vulva. *Obstet. Gynecol.* 14:86, 1959.

164. Woodworth, H., Dockerty, M. B., Wilson, R. B., and Pratt, J. H. Papillary hidradenoma of the vulva: A clinicopathologic study of 69 cases. *Am. J. Obstet. Gynecol.* 110:501, 1971.

165. Word, B. Office treatment of cyst and abscess of Bartholin's gland duct. *South. Med. J.* 61:514, 1968.

166. Yackel, D. B., Symmonds, R. E., and Kempers, R. D. Melanoma of the vulva. *Obstet. Gynecol.* 35:625, 1970.

Ancel Blaustein, M.D.

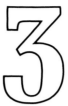

# Diseases of the Vagina

The vagina as a consequence of its relationship to the vulva, as well as similarity of its mucosa and supporting mesenchymal structures, is subject to some of the infections and tumors that affect the vulva. The upper third of the vagina is of Müllerian derivation and is at times subject to lesions that arise in particular from this tissue.

## Anatomy

The vagina extends from the vestibule to the uterus, lying dorsal to the urinary bladder and ventral to the rectum. Its axis forms an angle of over 90° with that of the uterus (Figure 3.1). It measures 6 to 7.5 cm along its ventral wall and 9 cm along its dorsal wall. In early life it is constricted at its commencement, dilated in the middle, and narrowed near its uterine extremity. The vagina surrounds the exocervix but attaches higher up on the uterine wall. The spaces formed between the cervix and the site of attachment of the vagina are called fornices. The attachment on the dorsal wall is higher up than on the ventral wall of the uterus and the posterior fornix is larger than the anterior or lateral fornices (Figure 3.2).

The ventral surface of the vagina lies in relation with the fundus of the urinary bladder and the urethra. Its dorsal surface is separated from the rectum by the recto-uterine excavation in its upper fourth and by the rectovaginal fascia in its middle two-fourths. The lower fourth is

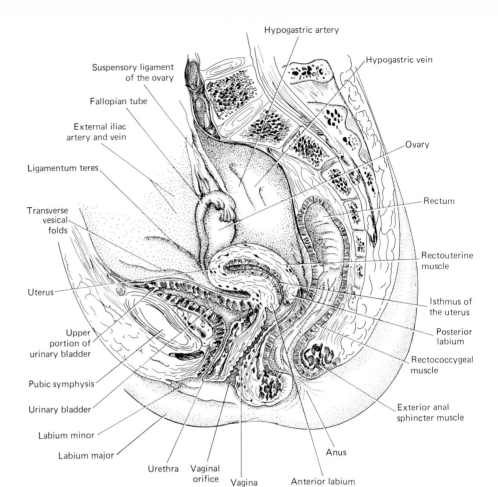

**3.1** Structural relationships of the vagina. Its axis forms an angle of over 90° with that of the uterus.

[Modified from *Gray's Anatomy*, 29th ed., 1973, courtesy of Lea & Febiger.]

Hypogastric artery

Suspensory ligament of the ovary

Hypogastric vein

Fallopian tube

External iliac artery and vein

Ovary

Ligamentum teres

Rectum

Transverse vesical folds

Rectouterine muscle

Uterus

Isthmus of the uterus

Upper portion of urinary bladder

Posterior labium

Pubic symphysis

Rectococcygeal muscle

Urinary bladder

Exterior anal sphincter muscle

Labium minor

Labium major

Anus

Urethra

Vaginal orifice

Vagina

Anterior labium

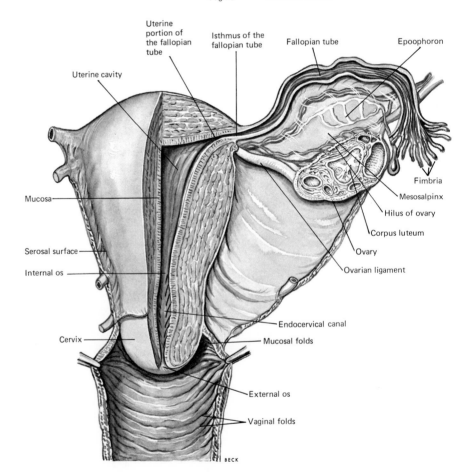

**3.2** Attachment of the vagina on the uterine wall showing lateral process (arrows).

[Modified from *Gray's Anatomy*, 29th ed., 1973, courtesy of Lea & Febiger.]

Uterine portion of the fallopian tube

Isthmus of the fallopian tube

Fallopian tube

Epoophoron

Uterine cavity

Mucosa

Fimbria

Mesosalpinx

Serosal surface

Hilus of ovary

Internal os

Corpus luteum

Ovary

Ovarian ligament

Endocervical canal

Cervix

Mucosal folds

External os

Vaginal folds

BECK

separated from the anal canal by the perineal body (Figure 3.1).

The inner surface of the vagina is covered by mucous membrane composed of stratified squamous epithelium and a muscular coat composed of an outer longitudinal layer (by far the stronger) and an inner circular layer. These are connected by decussating fasciculi that pass from one layer to another. The longitudinal layer is continuous with the superficial muscular fibers of the uterus and there are strong bands that are attached to the rectovaginal fascia on either side. Near the vestibule there is a concentration of erectile tissue and a band of striate muscular fibers called the bulbocavernosus. External to the muscle coat is a layer of connective tissue containing a large plexus of blood vessels.

## Vascular and Nerve Supply

The vaginal artery takes origin from the uterine artery or from the adjacent internal iliac artery. It supplies the mucous membrane and anastomoses with the uterine, inferior vesical, and middle rectal arteries. The branch of the uterine artery to the cervix descends on the dorsal wall, forming the azygous artery of the vagina (Figure 3.3).

The veins run along both sides, forming plexuses with the uterine, vesical, and rectal veins and ending in a vein that opens into the internal iliac vein (Figure 3.4).

The nerve supply is derived from the lumbar plexus and pudendal nerve.

## Lymph Drainage

There are three levels of lymphatics that serve the vagina.

1. Channels from the upper third of the vagina drain into the external iliac nodes.
2. Channels from the middle third drain into the internal iliac lymph nodes.
3. Channels from the lower third drain into the common iliac nodes (Figures 3.5 and 3.6).

## Mucous Membranes

There are two longitudinal ridges, one on the anterior and one on the posterior wall, and from these transverse folds extend outward. Rugae are divided by furrows of variable depth, suggesting papilla formation (Figure 3.7). These are more prominent near the vaginal orifice. The submucosa contains mucous crypts and a plexus of veins.

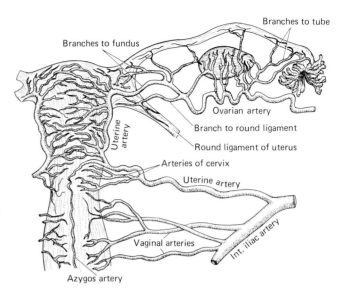

**3.3** Arterial blood supply of the vagina.

[Modified from *Gray's Anatomy*, 29th ed., 1973, courtesy of Lea & Febiger.]

### Histology of the mucous membranes

The mucous membrane consists of a wavy, stratified squamous epithelium with an underlying tunica propria of fibrous connective tissue (Figure 3.8). Epithelial folds dip down into the tunica propria, producing an undulating pattern. There is a distinctive basement membrane separating the mucosa from its underlying stroma. The epithelium consists of a single layer of basilar cells, three to four layers of parabasal cells, intermediate cells, and superficial cells. As maturation proceeds to the surface nuclei become smaller and the cytoplasm increases in volume (Figure 3.9). Scanning electron microscopy of the surface cells of the vaginal mucosa reveals the polygonal outline of the cells. The cytoplasm is flattened. The surface of the cells is roughened. Terminal bars can be seen between adjacent cells (Figure 3.10). Higher magnification shows that the surface plasma membrane contains an intricate network of microridges (Figure 3.11). The prepubertal child has a thin vaginal mucosa composed of a single layer of basal epithelium and three to seven layers of parabasal cells (Figure 3.12). At times the vaginal mucosa may show maturation caused by maternal estrogens that cross the placental circulation (Figure 3.13). The mucosa is hormonally responsive; at the time of puberty it increases in thickness under the influence of estrogens and the epithelium undergoes

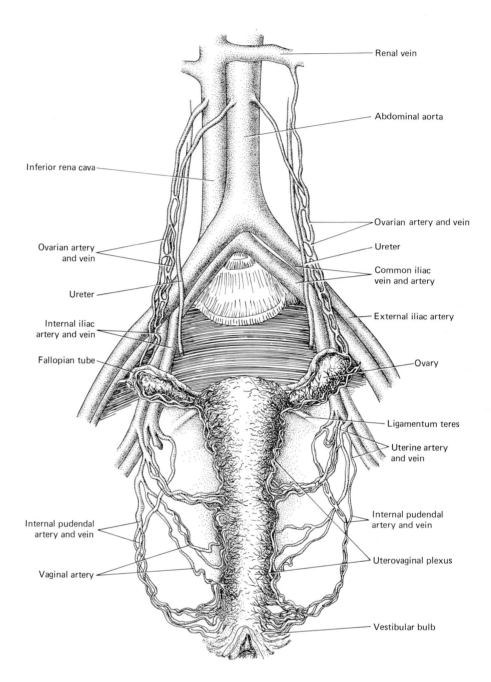

**3.4** Venous drainage of the vagina.

[Modified from *Gray's Anatomy*, 29th ed., 1973, courtesy of Lea & Febiger.]

Renal vein

Abdominal aorta

Inferior rena cava

Ovarian artery and vein

Ureter

Common iliac vein and artery

External iliac artery

Ovarian artery and vein

Ureter

Internal iliac artery and vein

Fallopian tube

Ovary

Ligamentum teres

Uterine artery and vein

Internal pudendal artery and vein

Internal pudendal artery and vein

Uterovaginal plexus

Vaginal artery

Vestibular bulb

maturation. Throughout the menarche the mucosa responds to the estrogen–progesterone cycle. Progesterone inhibits maturation of vaginal epithelium to the extent that it stops maturation at the intermediate cell level. Just prior to ovulation, when estrogen output is at its peak, superficial cells are dominant in the vaginal smear. Post-ovulation and throughout pregnancy, intermediate cells predominate. Menopause is characterized by the absence of menstrual cycling; vaginal cells undergo less maturation (Figure 3.14), and the thinned mucosa is susceptible to infection (Figure 3.15). These facts are useful in evaluating the hormonal status of women (see Chapter 36).

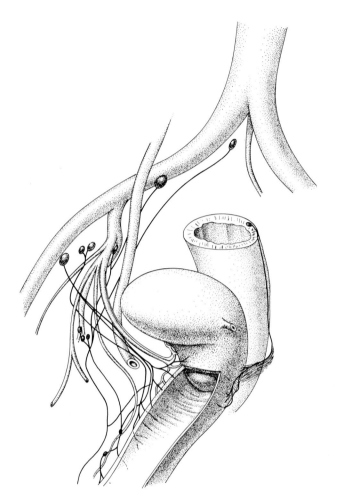

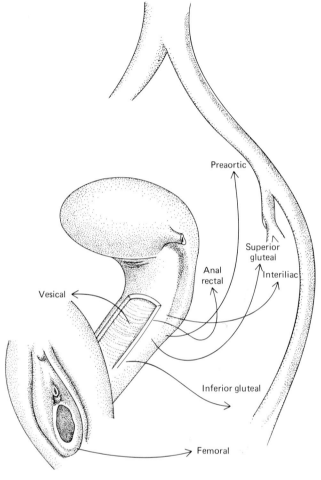

**3.5** Lymphatic drainage of the vagina.

[Modified from A. A. Plentl and E. A. Friedman, eds., *Lymphatic System of the Female Genitalia,* W.B. Saunders, 1971.]

**3.6** Lymphatic drainage of the vagina.

[Modified from A. A. Plentl and E. A. Friedman, eds., *Lymphatic System of the Female Genitalia,* W.B. Saunders, 1971.]

# Inflammatory Lesions

## Gonorrhea

The many layered vaginal mucosa of adults is resistant to *Neisseria gonococcus.* There may be some edema and hyperemia, but there is no penetration of the mucosa by organisms. In children this is not so. The vaginal mucosa is thin, less vascular, and readily penetrable by *N. gonorrhea,* which enters the submucosa. There is edema, hyperemia, and round cell infiltration, and purulent vaginitis may develop.

## *Haemophilus vaginalis*

*Haemophilus vaginalis* is probably the commonest infecting agent in the vagina (probably accounting for more than 90% of previously classified "nonspecific" infections.[12,29,37] The organism is a minute, rod-shaped,[4] gram-negative bacillus. It is essentially a venereal disease transmitted by sexual intercourse. There is a high rate of recovery of the organisms from the male partner. The infection is found primarily during the reproductive years.

Natural or exogenous estrogens stimulate the vagina to produce the nutrients that support a heavy growth of

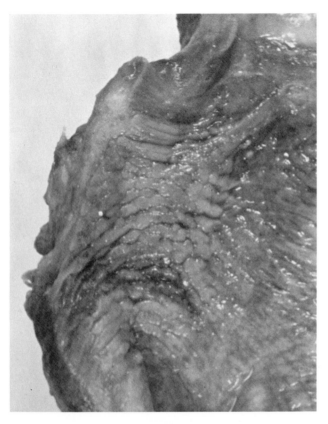

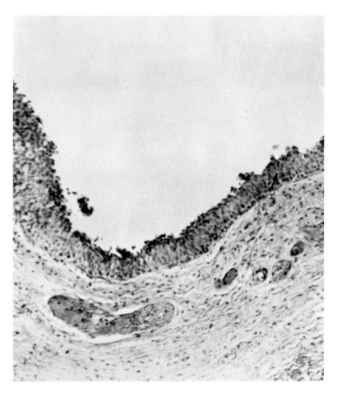

**3.8** Mucosa of the vagina. The mucosa is separated from the submucosa by a basement membrane. In the submucosa there are nerves and blood vessels.

**3.7** Rugal folds of the vaginal mucosa.

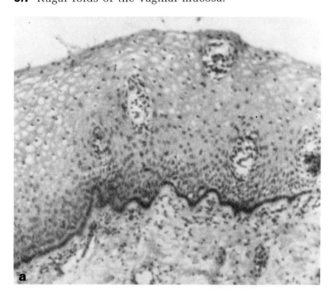

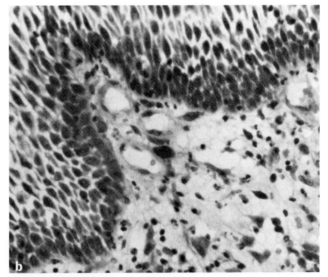

**3.9 a.** Mucosa of the adult vagina. There is a single layer of dark-staining basilar cells, three to four layers of parabasal cells, intermediate cells, and matured surface cells. **b.** Mucosa of the vagina. A high-power view of the basement membrane, basilar, and parabasal cells. Note decreasing size of the nuclei in the upper layers.

**3.10** Scanning electron microscopy of normal vaginal epithelium. The most superficial cells
have polygonal outlines and
flattened cytoplasmic substance.
Note the rough surface and
well-developed terminal bars
between adjacent superficial
squamous cells.

[Courtesy of A. Ferenczy.]

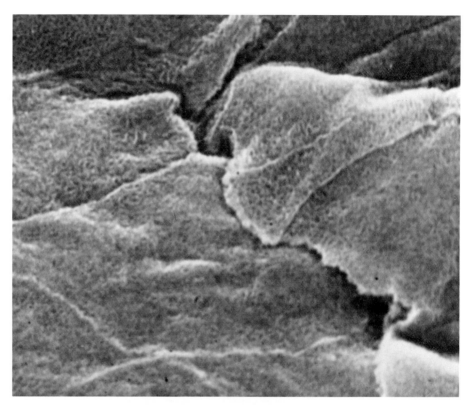

**3.11** Higher magnification of
Figure 3.10, illustrating the surface of the most superficial
squamous cells of the vaginal
epithelium. The surface plasma
membrane contains an intricate
network of microridges.

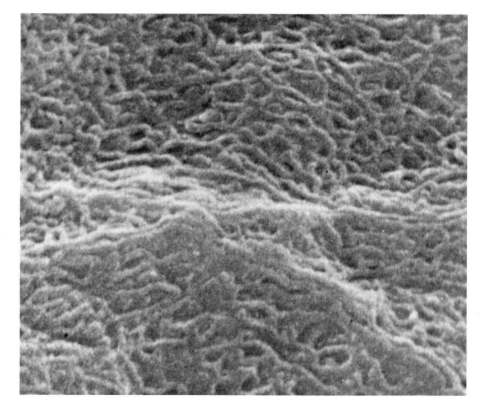

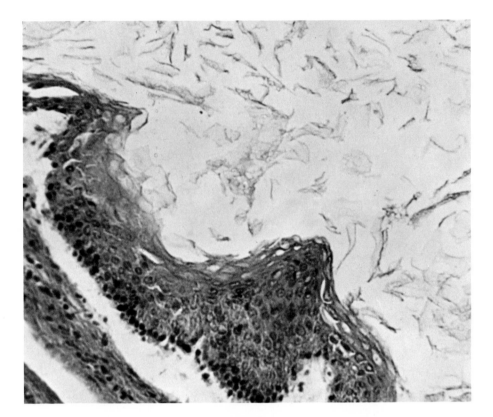

**3.12** Vaginal mucosa of a newborn. Parabasal cells are about six layers deep.

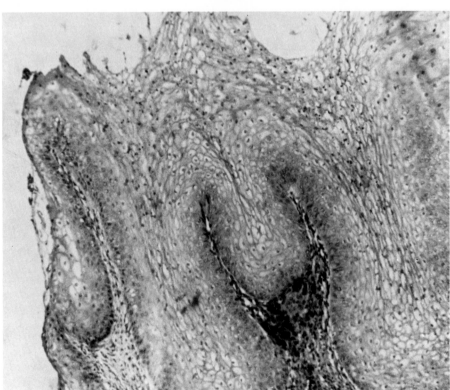

**3.13** Vaginal mucosa of newborn, showing maturation of epithelium.

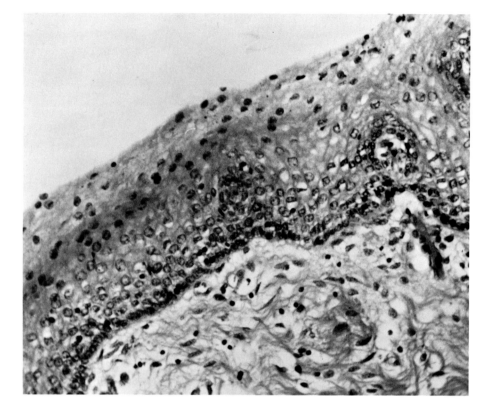

**3.14** Atrophic vagina. Many layers of parabasal cells.

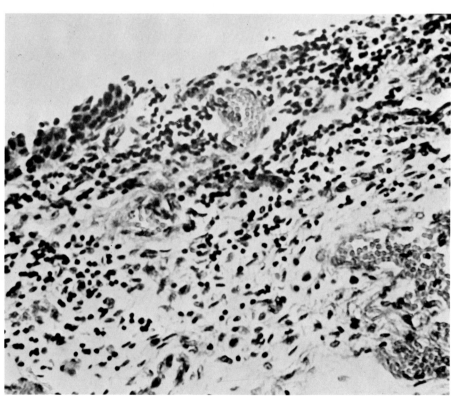

**3.15** Atrophic thinned vagina. There is ulceration of the mucosa and a dense lymphocytic infiltrate in the submucosa.

*H. vaginalis.* It is for this reason that it is more prevalent in females during the reproductive period. The organisms are less able to flourish in the postmenopausal vagina unless the patient is producing endogenous estrogens or receiving exogenous therapy.

### Histopathology

The organism does not penetrate the mucosa or invoke an inflammatory reaction. Microscopic sections appear normal.

### Diagnosis

Diagnosis is made by examining wet mount preparations of the vaginal discharge. Epithelial cells laden with organisms can be seen floating freely. These are called "clue cells." Because the organisms are very small, these "clue cells" (see Figure 36.15, Chapter 36) should not be confused with epithelial cells laden with lactobacilli. These organisms are much longer. Fluorescent antibody methods[8,22] are useful in diagnosis, as are culture techniques using Casman's blood agar base. However, wet smear examination should be adequate and is surely less expensive.

*Streptococcus pyogenes, Staphylococcus aureus,* and *Escherichia coli* may all produce vulvovaginitis. *Mycoplasma*[8,46] has been found in association with *Trichomonas* infections but, by itself, has not been incriminated as a cause of vaginitis. *Leptothrix* has never been proved to be the initiating or sole cause of vaginitis and is usually found in association with *Trichomonas* when vaginitis is present. Tuberculosis may produce vaginitis, but this is extremely rare. The appearance of the lesion is similar to that found in other sites, namely, granulomata, that may or may not show caseation. Viral infections[16] can occasionally produce vaginitis. Unless there are facilities for immediate inoculation of specimen, a high number of negatives is likely to be reported.

## Vaginal Candidiasis

The organisms of *Candida* do not penetrate the mucosa of the vagina, but they do result in an inflammatory reaction in the submucosa and mild edema. The cellular infiltrate is composed of lymphocytes, a few plasma cells, and an occasional neutrophil. On the mucosal surface there are cellular debris, neutrophils, and the buds and hyphae of *Candida*. The clinical appearance of the lesion is "thrush"-like[11,21,35] white patches that rub off freely, in contrast to leukoplakia where the white patch is more tenacious. Diagnosis is readily made from a wet preparation, a Papanicolau smear, or a preparation of vaginal material fixed in 10 to 20% potassium hydroxide.

## Trichomoniasis

These organisms were recognized as a source of vaginal infection as far back as 1836 by Donne. In fact, he recognized the venereal nature[7] of the disease when he found the organisms in purulent discharge from the genital tract of males.[50] Infection of the vulvovaginal tissue is clinically divided into three distinct states depending on the severity of the infection. The first is the "carrier" state that usually follows postacute infection. Chronic infection is characterized by increased vaginal secretions, odor, and elevated pH. Sections of the vagina show some evidence of chronic inflammation. Acute trichomoniasis is characterized by edema, erythema, and profuse vaginal discharge.[36]

The causative organism is *Trichomonas vaginalis,* which is a unicellular protozoa with prominent flagella that render it actively mobile. The organism is large, averaging 15 to 20 cm in length and is fusiform in shape (see Figure 36.16, Chapter 36). It is transmitted essentially by sexual contact; other sources, such as toilet seats, can be the source of infection but this is rare. There are some predisposing factors, such as normal or high estrogen levels and hypoacidity (vaginal). It is found most prevalent during the reproductive years.[34]

### Histopathology

Vaginal biopsy for trichomoniasis is by no means the rule, but specimens have been reviewed. There may be focal areas of edema, ulceration, and minute hemorrhages. There may be infiltration of leukocytes, lymphocytes, and plasma cells (Figure 3.16). The inflammatory exudate may extend into the epidermis and pseudoabscesses may form. If a pseudomembrane has developed, the epidermal surface becomes coated with inflammatory cells. In the chronic state the mucosa is essentially similar in appearance, with perhaps less edema being seen. In the carrier state there may simply be some hyperemia.

### Diagnosis

Hanging drop preparations reveal the mobile organisms. They can also be detected in smears stained for routine cytology, but the hanging drop is perhaps the best way to find them.

## Emphysematous Vaginitis

This condition was first described by Hugier in 1847. It has been variously called vaginitis emphysematosa, colpocervicitis cystica, emphysema vaginae, and colpocervicitis emphysematosa.[1,10,29,32] It is a self-limiting disease process.

### Incidence

The exact incidence is not known. Although numbers of published cases are not necessarily a reflection of incidence, fewer than 200 cases have been reported and one can deduce that it is not a common disorder.

### Clinical manifestations

Symptomatology may be limited to vaginal discharge caused by some organism. The occasional patient may complain of the embarrassing popping sound from the vaginal area. The sounds are caused by the release of gases from tense cystic spaces. Vaginal examination may show gas-filled blebs projecting above the mucosal surface. They vary in size from pinheads to 2 cm in diameter. There may be only a few blebs seen on the exocervix or the vagina may be extensively involved, with the blebs being clustered or diffusely scattered.

### Microscopic appearance

The mucosa is usually intact and the cystic spaces are found in the lamina propria (Figure 3.17). The cystic spaces are surrounded by lymphocytes, histiocytes, and multinucleate giant cells (Figure 3.18). They are lined by epidermoid epithelium.[23] Larger cavities may no longer have an identifiable lining epithelium.

## Desquamative Inflammatory Vaginitis

This is a rare form of vaginitis resembling the atrophic condition seen in postmenopausal patients yet occurring in females with normal estrogen levels.[24] Its rarity is underscored by Gardner's finding only eight cases in 3,000 patients with vaginitis.

The vagina appears to be thin and reddened, and smears reveal numerous pus cells and parabasal cells. The etiology and pathogenesis are not yet known. Microscopic examination of the vaginal mucosa reveals an intense inflammatory reaction consisting of edema, congestion of vessels, and infiltrates of monocytes, histiocytes, and plasma cells.

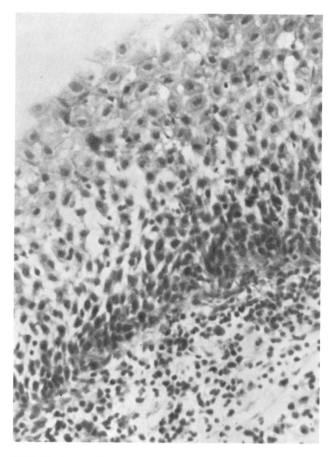

**3.16** Vagina (trichomoniasis). There is edema in the epithelial layer and leukocytic and lymphocytic infiltration in the submucosa.

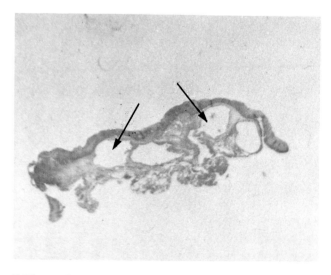

**3.17** Emphysematous vaginitis. Submucosal blebs (arrows).

69

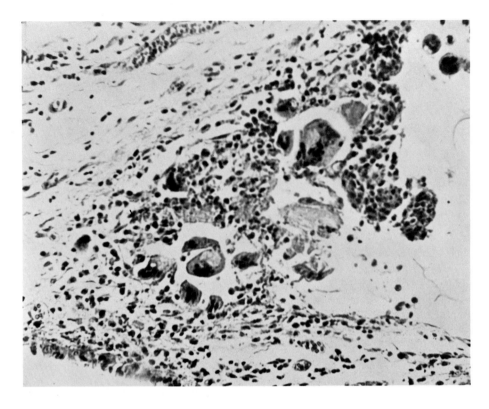

**3.18** Emphysematous vaginitis. Cystic spaces surrounded by histiocytes, multinucleate giant cells, and lymphocytes.

## Vaginitis Caused by Parasites

*Entameba histolytica* affects the colon primarily but can secondarily involve the vagina.[9,11] It is not a common disease and is most often seen in tropical countries where opportunities for good hygiene do not prevail.

Genital schistosomiasis has been reported in Egypt, Africa, the Orient, and the West Indies.[2,17] It involves the cervix and the upper third of the vagina. It occurs in patients who have infestation of the urinary bladder caused by *Schistosoma hematobium*.

## Vaginal Changes Associated with Prolapse

Prolapse of the uterus results in varying degrees of inversion of the vaginal mucosa. Exposure of the mucosa and chafing results in the hyperkeratosis of varying degrees (Figure 3.17). The mucosa may become ulcerated (Figure 3.19). Following total hysterectomy granulation tissue is seen at the site of closure of the vault (Figure 3.20).

## Cysts of the Vagina

Vestigial remnants of the Wolffian duct (Gartner's duct cyst) are quite common. They are located on the antero-lateral wall of the vagina or on the lateral wall. They vary in size and can sometimes be large and protrude through the introitus. Others are small and are simply incidental observations (Figure 3.21a). They are lined by low cuboidal epithelium that may or may not be ciliated (Figure 3.21b). Ackerman has reported finding adenocarcinoma arising in two Gartner duct cysts. He emphasizes that unlike cervical adenocarcinoma, these do not produce mucin.

"Epidermoid inclusion cysts" are common and they frequently follow manipulative surgery or trauma (most often birth trauma).

## Fibroepithelial Polyps of the Vagina

Burt, Prichard, and Kim[13] have found that vaginal polypoid lesions are uncommon. In 1966 Norris and Taylor[43] had reported a series of 24 cases. Two polyps were

**3.19** Prolapse of the vagina. Prominent cornification on the surface epithelium.

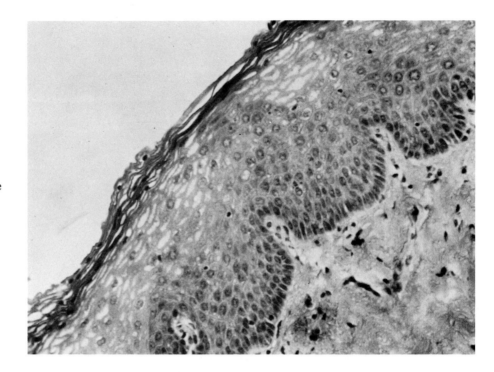

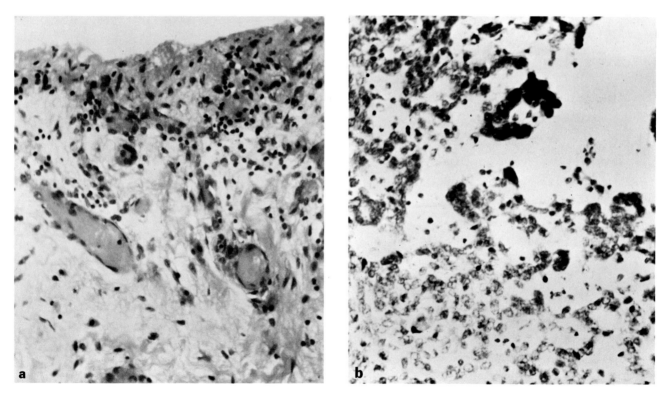

**3.20 a.** Prolapse of the vagina. Ulceration of the mucosa with formation of granulation tissue. **b.** Prolapse of the vagina. Granulation tissue at the site of vault closure following hysterectomy.

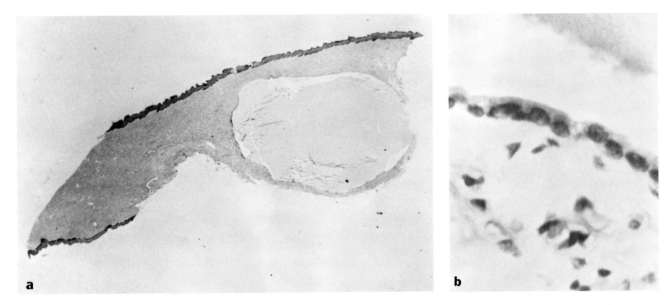

**3.21 a.** Vagina. Gartner's duct cyst. **b.** Gartner's duct cyst, lining epithelium.

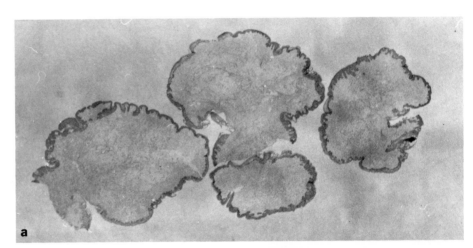

**3.22 a.** Vagina. Squamous papilloma. **b.** Squamous papilloma of the vagina. Pseudosarcomatous stromal cells.

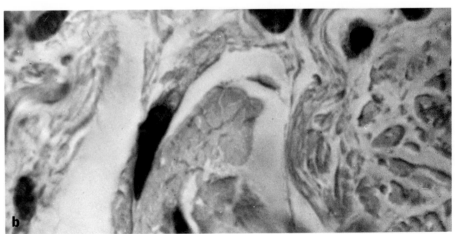

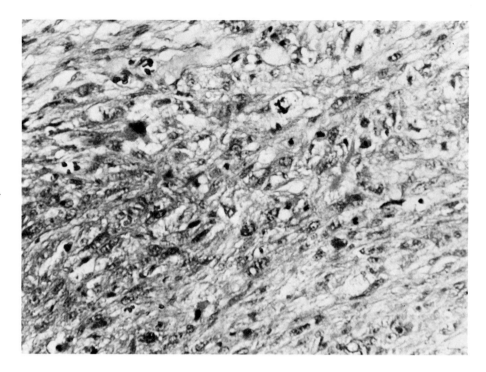

**3.23** Vagina, cellular leiomyoma. Some atypia and mitoses. Initially considered to be leiomyosarcoma, but the patient was alive and well 10 years later.

present in infants. They may be single and measure up to 1.5 cm in diameter, with only one exception being noted, in which the polyp measures 3.5 by 2 by 1.5 cm. Occasionally they may have multiple fingerlike projections. This lesion may not only be confused in the clinician's mind with sarcoma botryoides, but because there may be some bizarre cells in the stroma, pathologists have similarly regarded the lesion as malignant. These lesions are rubbery in consistency, they usually have a pedicle which may be short, they are gray-white in appearance, and they are covered by vaginal mucosa. The stroma is composed of loose fibrous connective tissue (Figure 3.22), and contains numerous dilated capillaries. Large atypical cells may be present (Figure 3.22a and b). The nuclei of the atypical cells may be single or multiple and nucleoli may be prominent. Mitotic figures are rare and usually do not exceed 2 to 3 per microscopic section. These polyps are benign and have a benign course. They merely require local excision. They lack the features of sarcoma botryoides, a neoplasm not found in the vagina of adults. Elliot and Elliot[24] have described a 0.5- to 5-mm subepithelial myxoid stromal zone which runs from endocervix to the vulva in mature females. In this stroma they find bizarre nuclei and it is their feeling that fibroepithelial polyps represent florid focal hyperplasia of this myxoid zone. Ceremsak[15] reported a case of a pedunculated rhabdomyoma in the vagina of a 34-year-old female.

# Benign Tumors of the Vagina

Leiomyoma (Figure 3.23),[6,39,45] fibromyoma, myxoma, fibroma, and neurofibroma occur in the submucosa and usually are located in the rectovaginal septum. They vary in size and on occasion can form pedunculated masses that project into the vagina or to the exterior. Endometriosis involving the rectovaginal septum can produce a large tumorlike mass that clinically resembles carcinoma. There can be rectal bleeding as well as vaginal bleeding. The history of bleeding from this site in association with menses is usually elicited. Biopsy shows endometriosis or its residue. It must be kept in mind that there are rare instances of endometrioid carcinoma developing in endometriosis at this site.

## Granular Myoblastoma (Granular Cell Tumor)

These tumors are usually small but can measure up to 5 cm in diameter. They are firm in consistency and have ill-defined borders.[4] Nests of cells can be found lying deep beneath the mucosa (Figure 3.24). They are composed of large cells that have a granular cytoplasm (Figure 3.25).[5,25] If they impinge on the epithelium, the tumor can produce a pseudoepitheliomatous hyperplasia that at

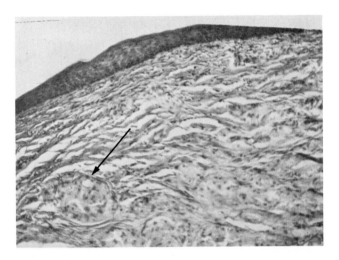

**3.24** Granular myoblastoma of vagina. Nest of tumor cells (arrow) beneath the mucosa.

times has been incorrectly interpreted as cancer. The majority of these tumors are benign, but there are several recorded instances of distant metastases. The histogenesis is not yet clear.[3] Some believe that the lesion arises from Schwann cells, whereas others believe it is of muscle origin.

# Malignant Tumors

Primary malignant neoplasms of the vagina are infrequent, representing approximately 1% of all gynecologic cancers.[1]

Primary epidermoid carcinoma of the vagina is not a common neoplasm.[38,54,55] It is important to demonstrate that there is no cancer of the cervix present, in order to regard the lesion as primary in origin. Most epidermoid carcinomas of the vagina are extensions from a cervical lesion. The upper third of the vagina and its anterior and lateral walls are sites of predilection (Figure 3.26). Primary epidermoid carcinoma of the vagina occurs most often in the fifth to seventh decade of life.[47,53]

## Microscopic Appearance

The lesion may be ulcerated and endophytic or nodular and exophytic. Microscopic examination reveals sheets and masses of epidermoid epithelium infiltrating the stroma (Figures 3.27 and 3.28). Transmission electron microscopy (Figure 3.29) reveals prominence of the intercellular bridges (curved arrow) and tonofibrils (straight arrow). Scanning electron microscopy reveals somewhat flat neoplastic squamous cells that display a lack of organization

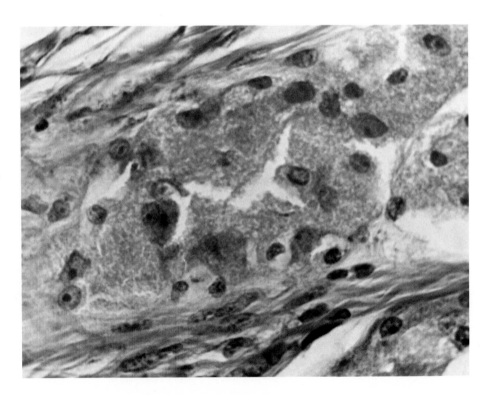

**3.25** Granular myoblastoma of vagina. High-power view of tumor cells. Note their uniformity.

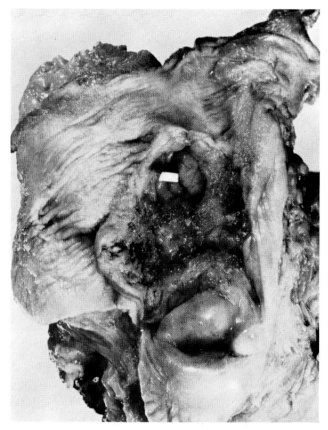

**3.26** Primary epidermoid carcinoma of the vagina. The tumor is exophytic and ulcerating.

[Reprinted by permission from L. Ackerman and A. Rosai, *Surgical Pathology*, 5th ed., C.V. Mosby, 1974.]

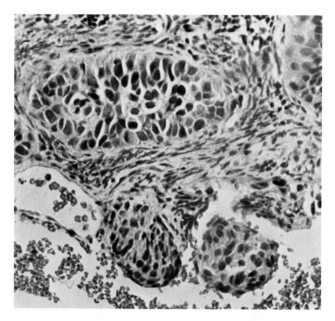

**3.27** Primary epidermoid carcinoma of the vagina. Nests of pleomorphic epidermoid cells infiltrate the submucosa.

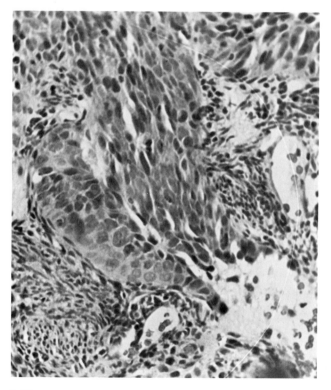

**3.28** Primary epidermoid carcinoma of the vagina showing invading tongues of moderately well-differentiated squamous epithelium.

and cellular cohesion (Figure 3.30a,b). The well-differentiated neoplastic cells contain cytoplasmic microridges, but the less mature cells are covered by microvilli.

## Metastatic Spread

Tumors may directly invade the urinary bladder or the rectum. Metastases generally are via lymphatics. A review of a total of 679 cases of epidermoid carcinoma of the vagina revealed lymph node metastases in 141 cases (20.8%). The reliability of these data is colored by the fact that not all authors have indicated whether all lymph nodes have been examined by histology or simply have been deemed positive or negative based on size and palpation. In those papers where histologic criteria were used, iliac nodes were as commonly involved as femoral nodes.

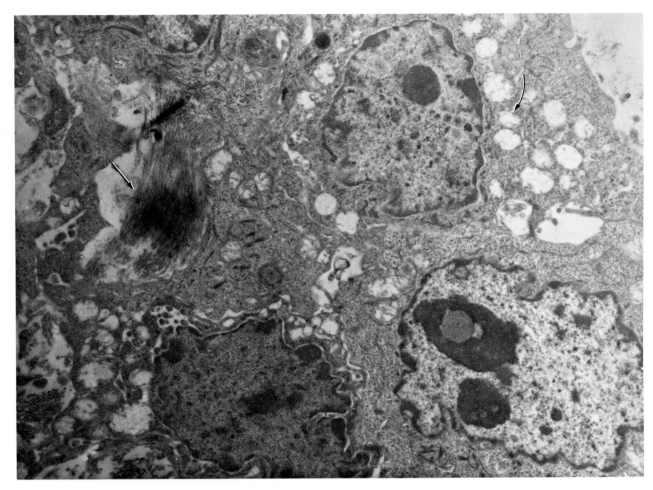

**3.29** Primary epidermoid carcinoma of the vagina. Transmission electron microscopy demonstrates intracellular bridges (curved arrow) and tonofibrils (straight arrow).

Once lymph node involvement was found, the prognoses was exceedingly poor. Only one purported cure has been reported.

## Dysplasia and Carcinoma in Situ

These lesions may arise *de novo,* coexist, or follow carcinoma of the cervix. There may be multifocal sites, including the vulva. As in the cervix, dysplasia may be mild (Figure 3.31) or severe (Figure 3.32) or may involve the full thickness (carcinoma in situ) (Figure 3.33). Carcinoma in situ has also been reported following the use of immunosuppressive therapy.[50]

## Carcinoma of the Vagina in Infancy

Sarcoma botyroides is the tumor that is usually thought of when an infant presents with vaginal bleeding or discharge associated with a tumoral mass. Vawter,[52] however, reported two cases of embryonal carcinoma of the vagina, one in an infant 16 months old and a second in an infant 14 months old. In both instances the tumors were large friable, polypoid tumor masses clinically indistinguishable from sarcoma botyroides. One case arose from the posterior vaginal wall; the other from the anterolateral vaginal wall. In one case metastases occurred 6 months later and death 11 months following the initial diagnosis. At au-

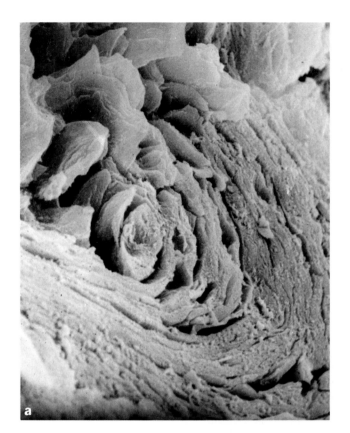
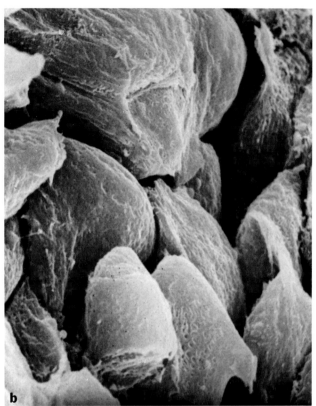

**3.30 a.** Scanning electron microscopy of moderately differentiated squamous cell carcinoma of the vagina. The somewhat flat neoplastic squamous cells display lack of organization and cellular cohesion and penetrate deep into the subjacent connective tissue stroma. **b.** Detailed view of neoplastic squamous cells. Although the well-differentiated neoplastic cells contain cytoplasmic microridges, the less mature cells are covered by microvilli.

**3.31** Vagina, mild dysplasia. Only the inner third is abnormal.

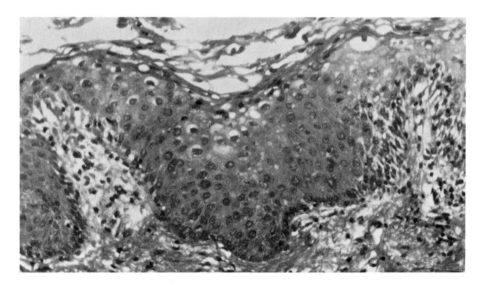

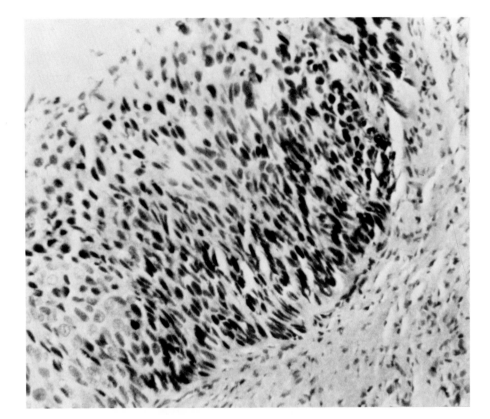

**3.32** Vagina. Severe dysplasia involving more than two-thirds of the mucosa.

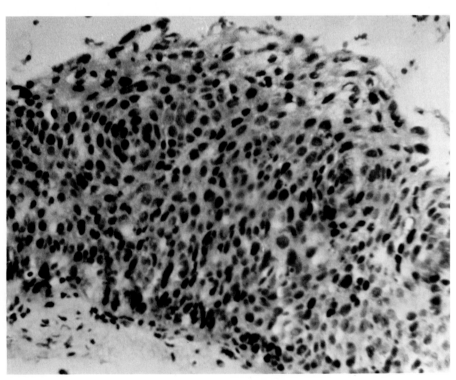

**3.33** Vagina. Carcinoma in situ showing full thickness involvement of the mucosa.

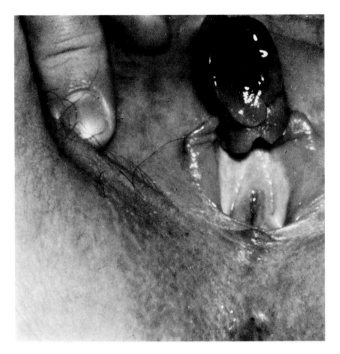

**3.34** Malignant melanoma in the outer third of the vagina showing the blue-black pigmented lesion.

topsy metastases were present in inguinal nodes, pelvic nodes, liver, and lungs. In the second case death occurred 14 months following the initial diagnosis with metastases being present in the pelvis, lung, and spinal cord transection. Both cases were treated by irradiation and actinomycin D. Itoh, Shirai, Naka, and Matsumoto[33] described four cases of endodermal sinus tumors including a case arising in the vagina of an infant.

## Malignant Melanoma

The vagina is not a common site for this lesion; however, malignant melanomas may occur as a primary vaginal tumor.[19,41,42] They usually are seen in the outer third of the vagina and are often pigmented (blue or black) (Figure 3.34). The lesions tend to ulcerate and the prognosis is poor. Microscopic examination reveals pleomorphic pigment-laden cells (Figure 3.35).

## Sarcomas of the Vagina

Sarcomas comprise less than 2% of all malignant vaginal neoplasms and of these sarcoma botyroides appears to

**3.35** Malignant melanoma, pleomorphic cellularity. Note the fine granules of pigment in cell cytoplasm.

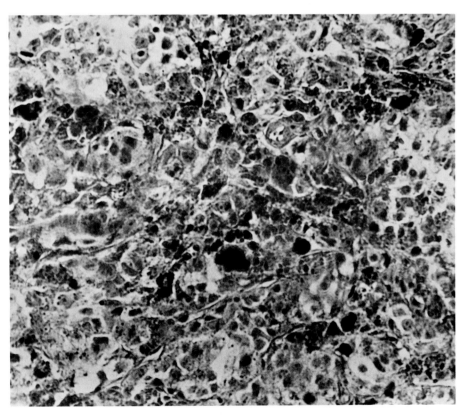

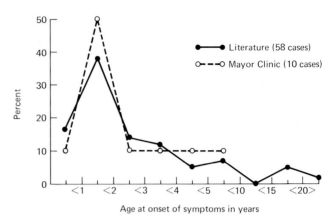

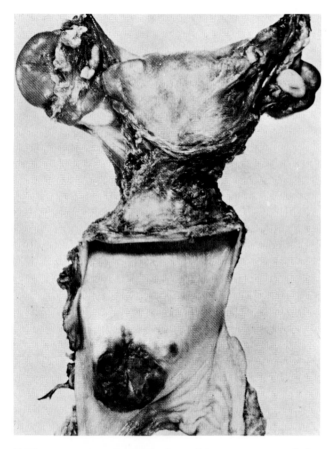

**3.36** Vagina. An ulcerating large leiomyosarcoma of the vagina in a 62-year-old patient.

[Reprinted by permission from L. Ackerman and A. Rosai, *Surgical Pathology*, 5th ed., C.V. Mosby, 1974.]

**3.37** Sarcoma botyroides of the vagina. Age distribution at onset of symptoms in years.

[Reprinted by permission from R. D. Hilgers, G. D. Malkasian, Jr., and E. H. Soule, Embryonal rhabdomyosarcoma (botyroid type) of the vagina, *Am. J. Obstet. Gynecol. 107*:484–502, 1970.]

be most common. It is almost exclusively found in infants and young girls with few exceptions in postpubertal patients. Leiomyosarcoma usually occurs in middle age and older women. It is an uncommon lesion but is the commonest one occurring in adults. In a review of 16 sarcomas of the vagina, Davos and Abell[20] found two cases of reticulum cell sarcoma, a malignant schannoma, and a Müllerian stromal sarcoma.

### Leiomyosarcoma

These are rather bulky lesions that may vary from 3 to 10 cm in diameter (Figure 3.36). They commence in the rectovaginal septum[20] and may produce ulceration in the vaginal mucosa and extend into the rectum. The microscopic appearance is similar to that of leiomyosarcoma found in other sites. The tumor carries a poor prognosis,[49]

which to some extent is reflected in the number of mitotic figures in 10 high-power fields.[51] The majority of deaths occur within 2 years. Metastases occur via the vascular route.

### Sarcoma Botyroides (Embryonal Rhabdomyosarcoma)

This is an extremely rare tumor largely found in infants and young children.[18,20,31,48] The peak incidence is between 1 and 2 years of life with 90% of cases seen in girls under 5 years of age, and almost two-thirds within the first 2 years (Figure 3.37). The tumor originates in the lamina propria, arising from the undifferentiated mesenchyme, and infiltrates the vaginal wall and pelvic structures.[20] The gross appearance is that of a confluence of polypoid masses resembling a bunch of grapes (Figure 3.38). The lesions may be extensive, and have a tendency to ulcerate (Figure 3.39). The polypoid masses may be hemorrhagic and/or myxoid in appearance (Figures 3.40 and 3.41). The microscopic appearance of the tumor usually reveals a mass of poorly differentiated, round or spindle cells (Figure 3.42). Tumor cells tend to crowd around blood vessels (Figure 3.43). The stroma is myxoid (Figure 3.44) and may contain striate muscle cells (Figure 3.45). Crowding of tumor cells beneath the vaginal epithelium results in a distinctive subepithelial dense zone referred to as the "cambium" zone of Nicholson (Figure 3.46). The prognosis is poor and Hilgers *et al.*[31] have reported death from the tumor in 5 of 10 cases studied. Davos and Abell[20] noted that 5 of

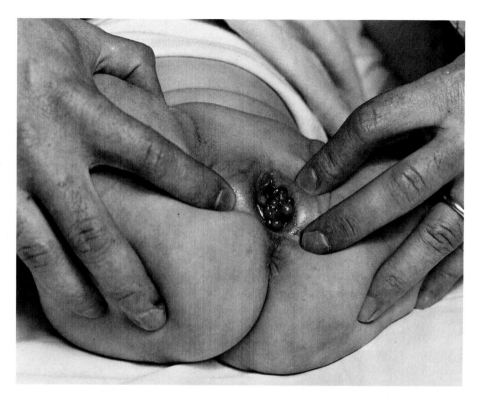

**3.38** Sarcoma botyroides of the vagina. The gross appearance is that of a confluence of polypoid mass resembling a bunch of grapes.

[Reprinted by permission from R. D. Hilgers, G. D. Malkasian, Jr., and E. H. Soule, Embryonal rhabdo-myosarcoma (botyroid type) of the vagina, *Am. J. Obstet. Gynecol.* *107*:484–502, 1970.]

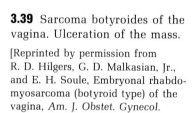

**3.39** Sarcoma botyroides of the vagina. Ulceration of the mass.

[Reprinted by permission from R. D. Hilgers, G. D. Malkasian, Jr., and E. H. Soule, Embryonal rhabdo-myosarcoma (botyroid type) of the vagina, *Am. J. Obstet. Gynecol.* *107*:484–502, 1970.]

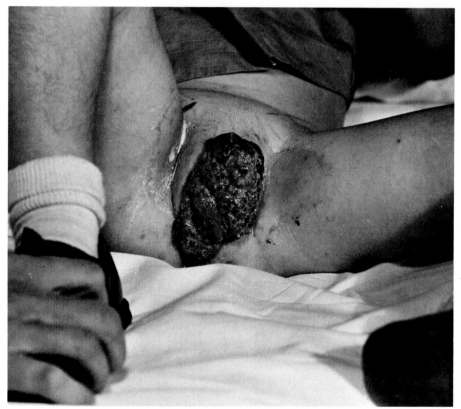

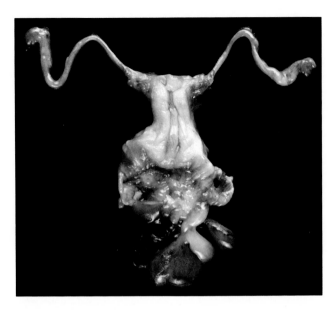

**3.40** Sarcoma botyroides. Resected lesion composed of polypoid masses; hemorrhagic and myxoid in appearance.

[Reprinted by permission from R. D. Hilgers, G. D. Malkasian, Jr., and E. H. Soule, Embryonal rhabdomyosarcoma (botyroid type) of the vagina, *Am. J. Obstet. Gynecol. 107:*484–502, 1970.]

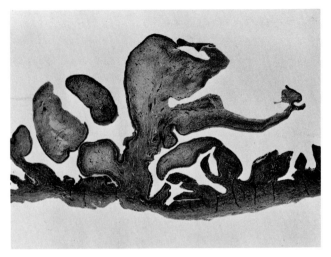

**3.41** Sarcoma botyroides. Cross section of a resected mass.

[Reprinted by permission from R. D. Hilgers, G. D. Malkasian, Jr., and E. H. Soule, Embryonal rhabdomyosarcoma (botyroid type) of the vagina, *Am. J. Obstet. Gynecol. 107:*484–502, 1970.]

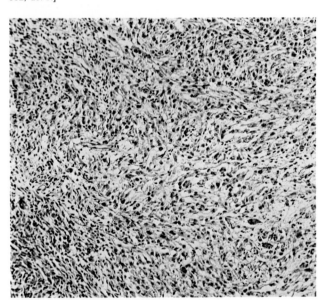

**3.42** Sarcoma botyroides. Tumor composed of poorly differentiated round or spindle cells.

[Reprinted by permission from R. D. Hilgers, G. D. Malkasian, Jr., and E. H. Soule, Embryonal rhabdomyosarcoma (botyroid type) of the vagina, *Am. J. Obstet. Gynecol. 107:*484–502, 1970.]

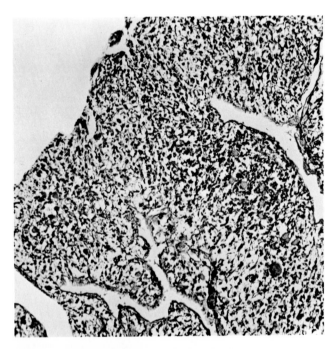

**3.43** Sarcoma botyroides. Tumor cells tend to crowd around blood vessels.

[Reprinted by permission from R. D. Hilgers, G. D. Malkasian, Jr., and E. H. Soule, Embryonal rhabdomyosarcoma (botyroid type) of the vagina, *Am. J. Obstet. Gynecol. 107:*484–502, 1970.]

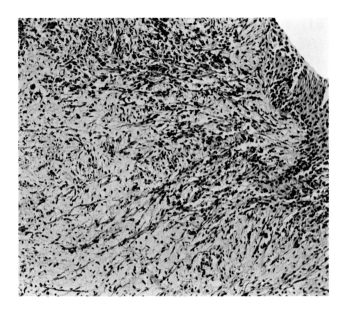

**3.44** Sarcoma botyroides. Myxoid stroma.

[Reprinted by permission from R. D. Hilgers, G. D. Malkasian, Jr., and E. H. Soule, Embryonal rhabdomyosarcoma (botyroid type) of the vagina, *Am. J. Obstet. Gynecol.* *107*:484–502, 1970.]

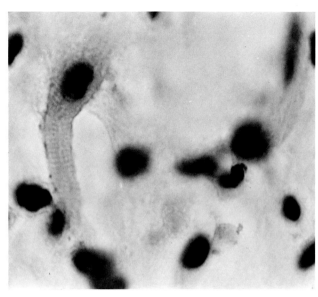

**3.45** Sarcoma botyroides. Striated muscle cells are present.

[Reprinted by permission from R. D. Hilgers, G. D. Malkasian, Jr., and E. H. Soule, Embryonal rhabdomyosarcoma (botyroid type) of the vagina, *Am. J. Obstet. Gynecol.* *107*:484–502, 1970.]

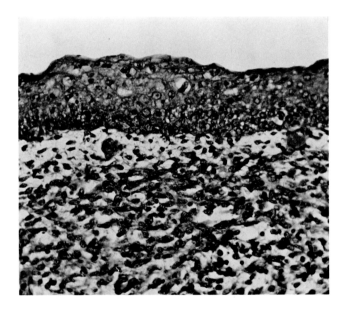

**3.46** Sarcoma botyroides. Cambium layer beneath the epithelium.

[Reprinted by permission from R. D. Hilgers, G. D. Malkasian, Jr., and E. H. Soule, Embryonal rhabdomyosarcoma (botyroid type) of the vagina, *Am. J. Obstet. Gynecol.* *107*:484–502, 1970.]

the 9 cases they studied succumbed to the disease. The cause of death is by direct extension of the tumor more often than by distant metastases. Metastases are both by the lymphogenous or hematogenous route. Hilgers *et al.*[31] found in their series that the tumor was confined to the pelvis in 50% of the cases they studied at autopsy. The 5-year survival rate has been variously estimated between 10 and 30%, but in the series reported by Hilgers *et al.*,[31] the survival rate increased to almost 50% after pelvic exenteration, regional lymphadenectomy, and partial or total vaginectomy. Radium treatment and chemotherapy have up to now yielded poor results. Radium treatment combined with surgical extirpation have resulted in improved survival.

## Metastatic Tumors to the Vagina

Tumors arising from the endometrium and the cervix are the commonest sources of metastases. Tumors of the ovary, rectum, and kidney[40] may also metastasize to the vagina but this is not as common an observation. Metastases from endometrial adenocarcinoma usually reach the vagina by submucosal lymphatics. They usually are in the

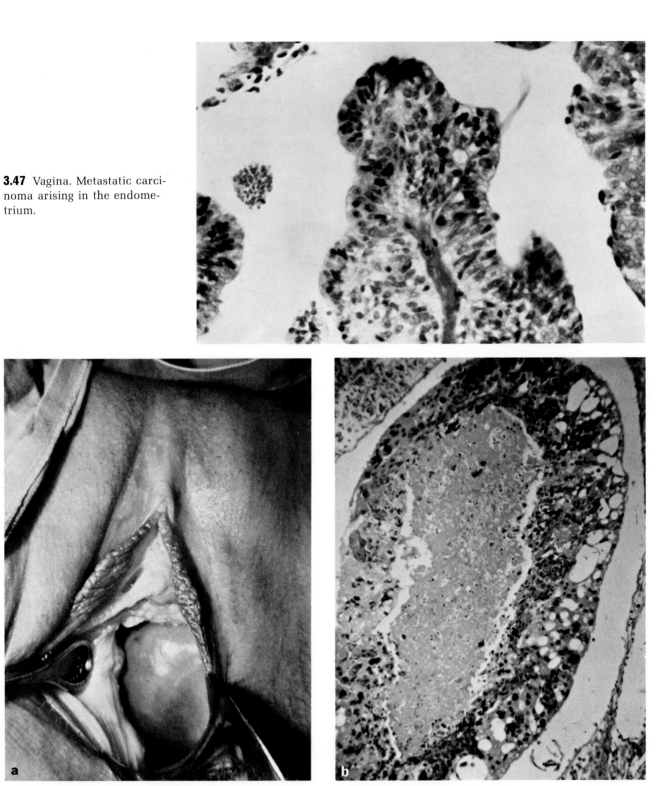

**3.47** Vagina. Metastatic carcinoma arising in the endometrium.

**3.48 a.** Vagina. Metastatic choriocarcinoma. **b.** Vagina. Microscopic pattern of metastatic choriocarcinoma shown in (**a**).

upper third and on the anterior wall. The metastases may be small and at times can resemble granulation tissue. The microscopic appearance is similar to the original tumor (Figure 3.47).

Choriocarcinoma can metastasize to the vagina (Figure 3.48a). The vagina in this case was filled with solid tumor covered over by intact mucosa. Microscopic appearance shows cyto- and syncytial trophoblastic tumoral tissue (Figure 3.48b).

# REFERENCES

1. Abell, M. R. Cervicocolpitis (vaginitis) emphysematosa. *Surg. Gynecol. Obstet.* 107:631, 1958.

2. Arean, V. M. Manson's schistosomiasis of the female genital tract. *Am. J. Obstet. Gynecol.* 72:1038, 1956.

3. Azzopardi, J. G. Histogenesis of the granular cell myoblastoma. *J. Pathol. Bacteriol.* 71:85, 1956.

4. Bangle, R. Jr. Morphological and histochemical study of the granular cell myoblastoma. *Cancer* 3:950, 1952.

5. Bangle, R. Jr. Early granular cell myoblastoma confined within a small peripheral myelinated nerve. *Cancer* 6:790, 1953.

6. Bennett, H. G., and Ehrlich, H. M. Myoma of the vagina. *Am. J. Obstet. Gynecol.* 42:314, 1941.

7. Bercovici, B., Persky, S., Rozansky, R., and Razin, S. Mycoplasma (pleuropneumonia-like organisms) in vaginitis. *Am. J. Obstet. Gynecol.* 84:687, 1962.

8. Bergman, S., Lundgren, K. M., and Lundstrom, P. Haemophilis vaginalis in vaginitis. *Acta Obstet. Gynecol. Scand.* 44:8, 1965.

9. Bhaduri, K. P. *Endamoeba histolytica* in leukorrhea and salpingitis. *Am. J. Obstet. Gynecol.* 74:4341, 1957.

10. Blaustein, A. U., and Shenker, L. Emphysematous vaginitis. *Obstet. Gynecol.* 22:295, 1963.

11. Braga, C. A., and Teoh, T. B. Amoebiasis of the cervix and vagina. *J. Obstet. Gynaecol. Br. Commonw.* 71:299, 1964.

12. Bray, G. Haemophilus vaginalis. *Acta Clin. Belg.* 18:248, 1963.

13. Burt, R. L., Prichard, R. W., and Kim, S. B. Fibroepithelial polyp of the vagina. *Obstet Gynecol.* 47(Suppl. 1):525, 1976.

14. Carter, B., Jones, C. P., Creadich, R. N., Parker, R. T., and Turner, J. The vaginal fungi. *Ann. N.Y. Acad. Sci.* 83:265, 1959.

15. Ceremsak, R. J. Benign rhabdomyoma of the vagina. *Am. J. Clin. Pathol.* 52:604, 1969.

16. Chaves, E., and Politot, P. Pelvic schistosomiasis. *Am. J. Obstet. Gynecol.* 89:1000, 1964.

17. Christian, R. T., Ludovici, P. P., Miller, N. F., and Riley, G. M. Viral studies of the female reproductive tract. *Am. J. Obstet. Gynecol.* 91:430, 1965.

18. Daniel, W. W., Koss, L. G., and Brunschwig, A. Sarcoma botyroides of the vagina. *Cancer* 12:74, 1959.

19. Das Gupta, J., and D'Urso, S. Melanoma of female genitalis. *Surg. Gynecol. Obstet.* 119:1074, 1964.

20. Davos, I., and Abell, M. R. Sarcomas of the Vagina. *Obstet. Gynecol.* 47(3):342, 1976.

21. Dawkino, S. M., Edwards, J. M. B., and Riddell, R. W. Yeasts in the vaginal flora: Their incidence and importance. *Lancet,* 2:1230, 1953.

22. Dukes, C. D., and Gardner, H. L. Identification of *Haemophilus vaginalis. J. Bacteriol.* 81:277, 1961.

23. Edmunds, P. N. The biochemical, serological and haemagglutination reactions of "Haemophilus vaginalis." *J. Pathol. Bacteriol.* 83:411, 1962.

24. Elliot, G. B., and Elliot, J. D. A. Superficial stromal reactions of lower genital tract. *Arch. Pathol.* 95:100, 1973.

25. Fisher, E. R., and Wechsler, S. Granular cell myoblastoma, a misnomer. *Cancer* 5:936, 1962.

26. Gardner, H. L. Vaginitis emphysematosa. *Am. J. Obstet. Gynecol.* 56:123, 1948.

27. Gardner, H. L. Desquamative inflammatory vaginitis; a newly-defined entity. *Am. J. Obstet. Gynecol.* 102:1102, 1968.

28. Gardner, H. L., Dampeir, T. K., and Dukes, C. D. The prevalence of vaginitis. *Am. J. Obstet. Gynecol.* 73:1080, 1957.

29. Gardner, H. L., and Dukes, C. D. *Haemophilus vaginalis* vaginitis. *Am. J. Obstet. Gynecol.* 73:1080, 1957.

30. Gray, L. A., and Christopherson, W. M. In situ and early invasive carcinoma of the vagina. *Obstet. Gynecol.* 34:226, 1969.

31. Hilgers, R., Malkasian, G. D. Jr., and Soule, E. H. Embryonal rhabdomyosarcoma (botyroid type) of the vagina; a clinico pathologic review. *Am. J. Obstet. Gynecol.* 107:484, 1970.

32. Hoffman, D. B., and Grundfest, P. Vaginitis emphysematosis. *Am. J. Obstet. Gynecol.* 78:428, 1959.

33. Itoh, T., Shirai, T., Naka, A., and Matsumoto, S. Yolk sac tumor and alpha fetoprotein: Clinico-pathological study of four cases. *Gann* 65:215, 1974.

34. Karnaky, K. J. Trichomonas vaginalis vaginitis—Pathognomonic lesion and pathologic findings in 4000 cases. *Texas J. Med.* 32:803, 1937.

35. Kearns, P. R., and Gray, J. E. Mycotic vulvovaginitis: Incidence and persistence of specific yeast species during infection. *Obstet. Gynecol.* 22:621, 1963.

36. Lamb, W. R., and Ludmir, A. A pathognomonic culposcopic sign of *Trichomonas vaginalis* vaginitis. *Acta Cytol.* 5:390, 1961.

37. Lapage, S. P. *Haemophilis vaginalis* and its role in vaginitis. *Acta Pathol. Microbiol. Scand.* 52:34, 1961.

38. Marcus, S. L. Multiple squamous cell carcinomas involving cervix, vagina and vulva: Theory of multicentric origin. *Am. J. Obstet. Gynecol.* 80:802, 1960.

39. Mochassi, K. Myoma of the vagina. *Obstet. Gynecol.* 15:235, 1960.

40. Nerdrum, T. A. Vaginal metastases of hypernephroma; report of three cases. *Acta Obstet. Gynecol. Scand.* 45:515, 1966.

41. Nigogosyan, G., DeLa Pava, S., and Pichren, J. W. Melanoblasts in the vaginal mucosa: origin for primary malignant melanoma. *Cancer* 17:912, 1964.

42. Norris, H. J., and Taylor, H. B. Melanomas of the vagina. *Am. J. Clin. Pathol.* 46:420, 1966.

43. Norris, H. J., Taylor, H. B. Polyps of the vagina: A benign lesion resembling sarcoma botyroides. *Cancer* 19:227, 1966.

44. Norris, J. W., and Cooper, J. R. Primary neurofibroma of the vagina, a case report. *J. Kansas Med. Soc.* 51:128, 1950.

45. Quan, A., and Birnbaum, S. J. Vaginal leiomyoma: Report of a case and review of the literature. *Obstet Gynecol Vol 18,* p. 360, 1961.

46. Rubin, A., and Morton, H. E. The incidence and clinical

significance of pleuro-pneumonia-like organisms in the genital tract of the human female. *Ann. N.Y. Acad. Sci. 79*:642, 1960.

47. Rutledge, F. Cancer of the vagina. *Am. J. Obstet. Gynecol. 97*:635, 1967.

48. Rutledge, F., and Sullivan, M. P. Sarcoma botyroides. *Ann. N.Y. Acad. Sci. 142*:694, 1967.

49. Schrum, M. Leiomyosarcoma of the vagina. *Obstet. Gynecol. 12*:1915, 1958.

50. Simpkins, P. B., Chir, B., and Hull, M. G. R. Intraepithelial vaginal neoplasia following immuno-suppressive therapy treated with topical 5-FU. Obstet. Gynecol. *46*(3):360, 1975.

51. Tobon, H., Murphy, A. and Salazar H. Primary leiomyo-sarcoma of the vagina. Light and electron microscopic observations. *Cancer 32*:450, 1973.

52. Vawter, G. F. Carcinoma of the vagina in infancy. *Cancer 18*:1479, 1965.

53. Watt, L., and Jennison, R. F. Incidence of *Trichomonas vaginalis* in marital partners. *Br. J. Vener. Dis. 36*:163, 1960.

54. Whelton, J., and Kottmeier, H. L. Primary carcinomas of the vagina; a study of a Radium Hamüt series of 145 cases. *Acta Obstet. Gynecol. Scand. 41*:22–40, 1962.

55. Young, E. E., and Gamdsle, C. H. Primary adenocarcinomas of the rectovaginal septum arising from endometriosis; report of a case. *Cancer 27*:596–601, 1969.

Stanley J. Robboy, M.D.,
Robert E. Scully, M.D.,
and Arthur L. Herbst, M.D.

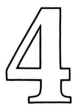

# Vaginal and Cervical Abnormalities Related to Prenatal Exposure to Diethylstilbestrol (DES)

Primary neoplasms of any type are uncommon in the vagina, with the malignant forms accounting for less than 2% of all cancers of the female genital tract. The most common type of cancer is the squamous cell carcinoma, which usually occurs in elderly women. Clear cell adenocarcinomas, which have also been called mesonephromas and mesonephric carcinomas, are much more rare. Prior to 1970 only sporadic cases were known to have occurred in older women and only four examples had been reported in young females.[12] When seven young women with clear cell adenocarcinoma of the vagina were unexpectedly encountered at the Massachusetts General Hospital between 1966 and 1969,[12] a search for a common factor in their medical histories led to the association of these tumors with exposure *in utero* to diethylstilbestrol (DES), a synthetic, nonsteroidal estrogen that had been administered to their mothers for high-risk pregnancy.[15] Later, a highly significant but less constant association of clear cell adenocarcinoma of the cervix with prenatal exposure to DES became apparent. Nonneoplastic changes of the female genital tract, including vaginal adenosis and cervical erosion, were also found not only in the great majority of the cancer patients but subsequently in a high percentage of asymptomatic young females who had been exposed prenatally to DES and the chemically related drugs, hexestrol and dienestrol.[1,3,5,8-15,25,29,32,33,36]

# Clear Cell Adenocarcinoma

Shortly after the discovery of the link between prenatal exposure to DES and the development of vaginal and cervical clear cell adenocarcinomas, the Registry of Clear Cell Adenocarcinoma of the Genital Tract in Young Females was established to centralize information about this unusual form of cancer. By June 1975 over 250 cases had been accessioned, mostly from North America but also from Europe, Australia, and Africa. The average age of the patients at the time of diagnosis has been 17 years.[11] The youngest patient was 7 years of age; although the oldest exposed patient to date has been 28 years of age at the time of diagnosis, it is possible that the average and oldest ages will increase as the exposed population grows older. Approximately two-thirds of the patients with available maternal histories have had a documented exposure to DES *in utero* and all of these women were born after 1942, several years after DES was synthesized and introduced in the United States.[20] Although the dosage and duration of maternal therapy have varied greatly, the drug had been administered prior to the eighteenth week of gestation in all the cases with accurate treatment records.[11]

The tumors have involved all portions of the vagina and cervix; two-thirds have been confined to the vagina, whereas about one-third has been classified as cervical.[1] Large tumors frequently involve much of the length and circumference of the vagina, whereas smaller ones are usually located in the upper third, most commonly in the anterior wall (Figure 4.1), and somewhat less often in the posterior wall. An occasional tumor is confined to the lateral wall or the lower third of the vagina or lies behind a ridge. Almost every cervical cancer involves the exocervix and occasionally is confined to it (Figure 4.2). In some cases the tumor is situated largely in the vagina, suggesting an origin therein, but must be classified as cervical because the external os has been involved. Only a rare tumor is confined to the endocervix.

The tumors vary greatly in size. The smallest has been 3 mm in greatest diameter and the largest more than

**4.1** Opened uterus and vagina. A polypoid carcinoma, bordered by a dark zone of adenosis, lies on the anterior vaginal wall (lower left). Another patch of adenosis occupies the posterior wall (lower right). The cervix is extensively eroded. The adenosis and erosion appeared red in the fresh state.

[Reprinted by permission from A. L. Herbst and R. E. Scully, Adenocarcinoma of the vagina in adolescence: A report of 7 cases including 6 clear-cell carcinomas (so-called mesonephromas), *Cancer* 25:745, 1970.]

10 cm. Many are polypoid or nodular (Figure 4.3) but some are flat or ulcerated with an indurated or granular surface. On occasion the tumor is confined to the lamina propria and apparently entirely covered by the squamous epithelium lining the lower genital tract.

On microscopic examination the majority of vaginal tumors are superficial, invading less than 3 mm into the vaginal wall (Figure 4.3); however, even some small neo-

---

[1] All Registry cases are classified and staged according to the criteria of the International Federation of Gynecologists and Obstetricians (FIGO). A tumor is considered primary in the vagina if it is confined to the vagina or if it involves the vagina and only a part of the cervix portio. A cancer involving the external cervical os is designated as cervical, even if the bulk of the tumor lies in the vagina. Growths extending to the vulva are designated as vulvar, but no tumors of this type have been encountered.

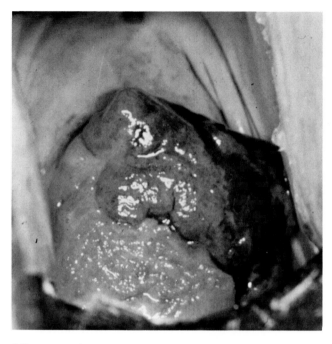

**4.2** Clear cell adenocarcinoma confined entirely to the exocervix.

[Reprinted by permission from S. J. Robboy, R. E. Scully, and A. L. Herbst, Pathology of vaginal and cervical abnormalities associated with prenatal exposure to diethylstilbestrol (DES), J. Reprod. Med. 15:13, 1975.]

plasms penetrate more deeply or extend more laterally than can be ascertained by gross palpation.

The microscopic appearance is similar to the clear cell adenocarcinoma that occurs elsewhere in the female reproductive tract, especially the ovary and endometrium.[28,30,31] The most commonly encountered patterns are sheets (Figure 4.4), tubules (Figure 4.5), and cysts (Figure 4.6), which may contain highly developed papillae (Figure 4.7). The most frequent cell types are clear cells, in which the abundant cytoplasm is filled with glycogen (Figure 4.4), and hobnail cells, characterized by bulbous nuclei protruding into the lumens of tubules and cysts (Figure 4.5). Dilated cysts, which can contain a proteinaceous or mucinous secretion, may be lined by flattened cells with a deceptively benign appearance (Figure 4.6). On occasion clear or hobnail cells are rare or absent and the tumor resembles to various degrees an endometrioid (Figure 4.8) or a poorly differentiated adenocarcinoma. In very rare cases the cells are arranged in cords (Figure 4.9). Often, several patterns are encountered in a single tumor.

The patterns and cell types of the clear cell adenocarcinoma should not be confused with those of the Arias–Stella reaction, which can be encountered in curettings of the endometrium and occasionally the endocervix during pregnancy.[29] In contrast to the clear cell carcinoma, the

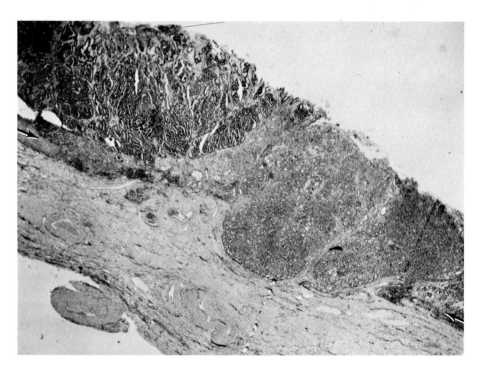

**4.3** Polypoid adenocarcinoma arising in the vagina. An imaginary line drawn between the borders of the adjacent normal mucosa (arrows) illustrates the superficial nature of many of the tumors. Hematoxylin–eosin, ×5.

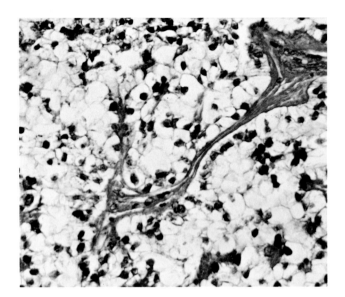

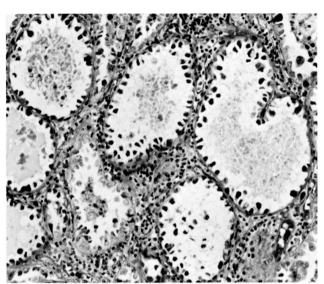

**4.4** Clear cell pattern of the tumor, which resembles the clear cell carcinoma of the ovary and endometrium. Hematoxylin–eosin ×300.

[Reprinted by permission from R. E. Scully, S. J. Robboy, and A. L. Herbst, Vaginal and cervical abnormalities including clear-cell adenocarcinoma, related to prenatal exposure to stilbestrol, *Ann. Clin. Lab. Sci.* 4:222, 1974.]

**4.5** Tubules lined by hobnail cells. Hematoxylin–eosin, ×180.

[Reprinted by permission from R. E. Scully, S. J. Robboy, and A. L. Herbst, Vaginal and cervical abnormalities including clear-cell adenocarcinoma, related to prenatal exposure to stilbestrol, *Ann. Clin. Lab. Sci.* 4:222, 1974.]

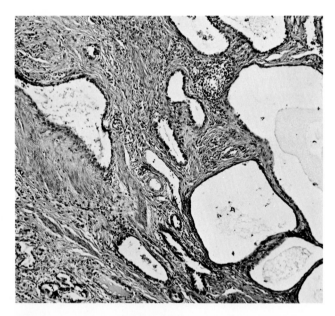

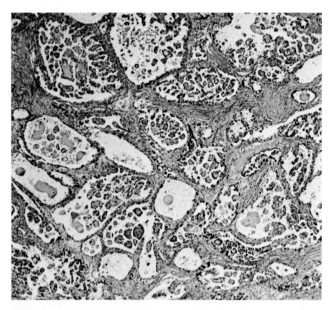

**4.6** Cystic pattern adjacent to the tubular pattern of tumor. Hematoxylin–eosin, ×80.

[Reprinted by permission from R. E. Scully, S. J. Robboy, and A. L. Herbst, Vaginal and cervical abnormalities including clear-cell adenocarcinoma, related to prenatal exposure to stilbestrol, *Ann. Clin. Lab. Sci.* 4:222, 1974.]

**4.7** Papillary pattern of the tumor. Hematoxylin–eosin, ×140.

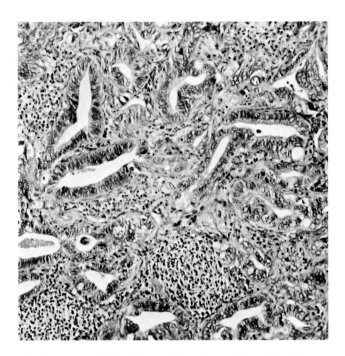

**4.8** Endometrioid pattern of the tumor. Hematoxylin-eosin, ×140.

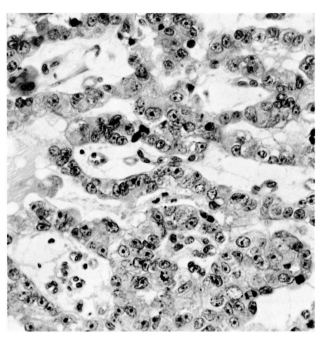

**4.9** Cords and solid tumor with unusually deeply eosinophilic cytoplasm and nuclei with prominent nucleolus and delicate chromatin. Hematoxylin-eosin, ×290.

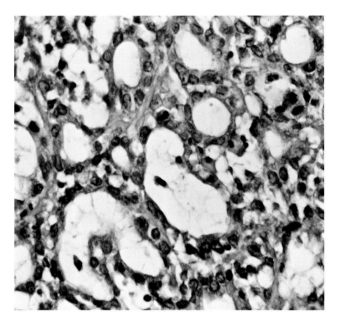

**4.10** Microglandular hyperplasia arising in vaginal adenosis. Although the glands are closely packed and are separated by little or no stroma, the nuclei are uniform and have relatively fine, evenly dispersed chromatin. Mucin is present in the glandular lumina as well as within the cytoplasm of the cells. Hematoxylin-eosin, ×490.

glands of the Arias–Stella phenomenon are arranged in an orderly fashion and are not invasive; when papillae are present they are uniform in distribution. Another source of diagnostic confusion is microglandular hyperplasia, which may appear as a granular or polypoid mass arising in an area of vaginal adenosis, sometimes as a result of ingestion of oral contraceptive.[24] Although the glands are closely packed and separated by little or no stroma, the nuclei are uniform and have relatively fine, evenly dispersed chromatin (Figure 4.10).

Most patients with clear cell adenocarcinoma of the vagina or cervix complain of abnormal bleeding or bloody intermenstrual discharge. Occasionally a suspicious or positive vaginal smear provides the first indication of an asymptomatic carcinoma.[34] In cytologic preparations the tumor cells usually resemble large endocervical cells and occur individually or in clumps (Figures 4.11 and 4.12). The large size of the nuclei, their irregular borders, and their prominent nucleoli are features more suggestive of adenocarcinoma than squamous cell carcinoma. Occasionally the cytoplasm may be delicate or clear, but it is generally impossible to differentiate the clear cell adenocarcinoma from an adenocarcinoma of ovarian, tubal, or endometrial origin. In cases in which a cytologic diagnosis

**4.11** Vaginal and cervical smears of adenocarcinoma. **a.** A clump of adenocarcinoma cells varies markedly in size; large cytoplasmic vacuoles are filled with polymorphonuclear leukocytes. **b.** A cluster of four tumor cells with prominent nucleoli. **c.** A clump of tumor cells with strikingly large nucleoli. The nuclei vary in size more than in shape. Their borders are delicate and the chromatin is granular. The cytoplasm is finely vacuolated with indefinite borders. **d.** Well-preserved adenocarcinoma cells with large nuclei, course chromatin, and multiple nucleoli. The cytoplasm is variable; several nuclei are naked. Papanicolaou stain, ×540.

[Reprinted by permission from P. D. Taft, S. J. Robboy, A. L. Herbst, and R. E. Scully, Cytology of clear-cell adenocarcinoma of the genital tract in young females. Report of 95 cases from the Registry, *Acta Cytol.* 18:279, 1974.]

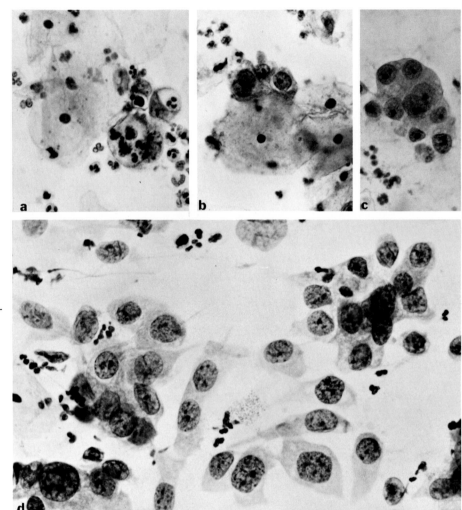

of adenoscarcinoma is made the most useful clues to its source are the age of the patient and a history of DES exposure. False-negative smears have been reported in about one-sixth of patients with clear cell carcinomas. In some cases polymorphonuclear leukocytes cover the smear. In other cases cells that are small or have a delicate chromatin pattern have not had the diagnostic features of malignant cells. The diagnosis of carcinoma may be also missed because of inadequate sampling. At present the most accurate and efficient method of sampling appears to be a direct scrape of the vagina, especially of the fornices, as well as a separate scrape of the cervix.

As in cases of squamous cell carcinoma of the cervix and vagina, the frequency of metastasis to pelvic lymph nodes can be correlated with the clinical stage of the tumor. The smallest tumor associated with a nodal metastasis in the Registry measured 1.5 cm in greatest diameter. Approximately one-sixth of the cancers that are considered clinically to be confined to the vagina (stage I vaginal) and one-third of cervical neoplasms thought to be confined to the cervix and vagina (stages I and IIa cervical) are associated with lymph node metastases. In contrast, over half of the more advanced tumors spread to the regional lymph nodes. The size of the tumor and its depth of invasion also correlate with the risk of lymph node metastasis.[23] Occasionally paraaortic lymph nodes are involved, but in such cases the pelvic lymph nodes also contain metastases, suggesting that as with most neoplasms of the cervix and upper vagina the usual route of lymphatic drainage is to the pelvic lymph nodes. Rarely,

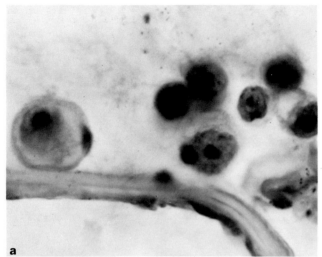

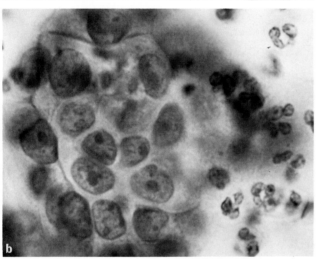

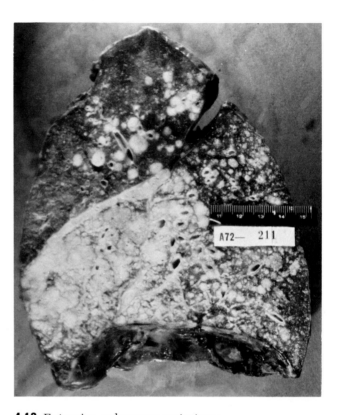

**4.13** Extensive pulmonary metastases.

[Reprinted by permission from S. J. Robboy, R. E. Scully, and A. L. Herbst, Pathology of vaginal and cervical abnormalities associated with prenatal exposure to diethylstilbestrol (DES), *J. Reprod. Med.* 15:13, 1975.]

**4.12 a.** Adenocarcinoma cells with macronucleoli and clear cytoplasm. Papanicolaou stain, ×1,000. **b.** A clump of adenocarcinoma cells with strikingly large nucleoli. Papanicolaou stain, ×1,100.

[Reprinted by permission from P. D. Taft, S. J. Robboy, A. L. Herbst, and R. E. Scully, Cytology of clear-cell adenocarcinoma of the genital tract in young females. Report of 95 cases from the Registry, *Acta Cytol.* 18:279, 1974.]

tumor also metastasizes to the inguinal lymph nodes. Radical surgery and radiation therapy have been used to treat most tumors.[11, 18, 38]

Among all of the Registry patients for whom followup data are available, about one-fourth have had tumors that have persisted or recurred after therapy. The predominant patterns and cell types of the recurrences have been similar to those of the primary tumors in most cases, although sometimes the recurrence has been less well differentiated.

Approximately half are in the pelvis but one-third are in the lungs or supraclavicular lymph nodes. This pattern of spread resembles that of adenocarcinoma of the corpus more closely than that of squamous cell carcinoma of the cervix or vagina. Postmortem examinations have confirmed the high frequency of pulmonary metastases (Figure 4.13).[23]

## Nonneoplastic DES-related Changes

Nonneoplastic alterations of the genital tract related to prenatal exposure to DES include vaginal adenosis (Figure 4.1), cervical erosion (Figure 4.1), and vaginal (Figure 4.14) and cervical ridges (Figure 4.15) (Table 4.1). Vaginal adenosis, which is defined as the presence of a glandular epithelium or its secretory products in the vagina, has been recognized since the late 1800s. The term "adenomatosis"

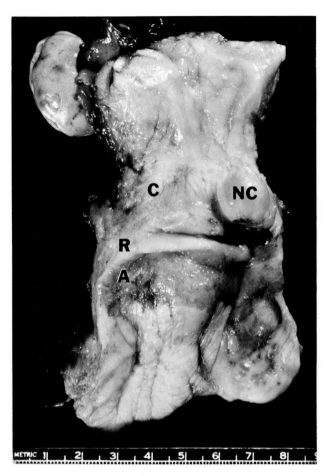

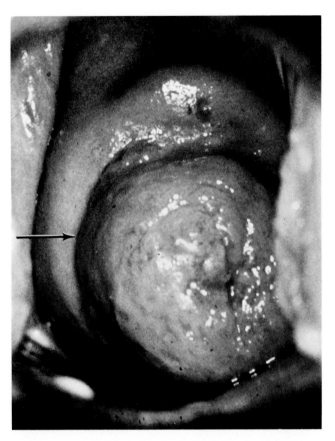

**4.14** Opened uterus and vagina with transverse vaginal ridge (R), cervix (C), and zone of adenosis (A). A Nabothian cyst (NC) of the cervix is also visible along the right margin of the specimen.

[Reprinted by permission from A. L. Herbst, R. J. Kurman, R. E. Scully, and D. C. Poskanzer, Clear-cell adenocarcinoma of the genital tract in young females: Registry report, *N. Engl. J. Med.* 287:1259, 1972.]

**4.15** Concentric ridge (arrow) in the cervix creating the appearance of a "pseudopolyp" in the center of which is the external os. A circular fold gives the appearance of a hood covering the cervix.

[Courtesy of Dr. Duane Townsend; reprinted by permission from S. J. Robboy, R. E. Scully, and A. L. Herbst, Pathology of vaginal and cervical abnormalities associated with prenatal exposure to diethylstilbestrol (DES), *J. Reprod. Med.* 15:13, 1975.]

was introduced for this disorder in 1911 and later changed to "adenosis".[21] Despite earlier views that it was acquired after puberty,[26,27] it is now recognized that it may be congenital, for it has been found in the human fetus and newborn[16] and has been produced experimentally in mice injected with estrogens during the neonatal period.[7,35]

Adenosis should be suspected clinically when the vaginal mucosa contains red or granular spots or patches (Figure 4.1), does not stain with an iodine (Schiller's or Lugol's) solution (Figure 4.16), or is colposcopically abnormal. On microscopic examination it is usually characterized by an epithelium that resembles the lining of the

endocervix (Figure 4.17), endometrium, or fallopian tube (Figure 4.18). Mucinous columnar cells of the endocervical type are encountered twice as frequently as cells of the tuboendometrial type, which may have dark (eosinophilic) or occasionally clear cytoplasm, with or without cilia, and form a single or occasionally pseudostratified layer.[1,25] Typically, the columnar epithelium lines glands in the lamina propria, is accompanied by vascular congestion, and is surrounded by a round cell infiltrate of varying degrees of severity; acute inflammatory cells are encountered less often. Sometimes mucinous epithelium lies directly on the lamina propria, completely replacing the surface squamous

**Table 4.1** Vaginal and cervical abnormalities in DES-exposed females and unexposed controls[a]

| Abnormality | Exposed (%) | Control (%) |
|---|---|---|
| Vaginal adenosis identified by biopsy specimens | 35 | 1 |
| Failure of part of the vagina to stain with iodine | 56–78 | 2 |
| Colposcopic abnormalities in the vagina | 78 | 2 |
| Cervical erosion identified in biopsy specimens | 85 | 38 |
| Failure of part of the cervix to stain with iodine | 95 | 49 |
| Vaginal or cervical ridges | 22–39 | 0 |

[a] Adapted from Refs. 3 and 9.

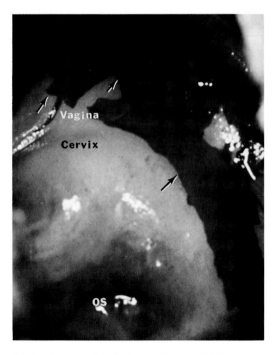

**4.16** Abnormal Schiller stain in which aglycogenated (nonstaining) areas in both the vagina and the cervix appear white in the photograph and represent the so-called transformation zone. The glycogenated vaginal epithelium stains black. Arrows demarcate the staining from the nonstaining areas.

[Reprinted by permission from S. J. Robboy, R. E. Scully, and A. L. Herbst, Pathology of vaginal and cervical abnormalities associated with prenatal exposure to diethylstilbestrol (DES), *J. Reprod. Med. 15*:13, 1975.]

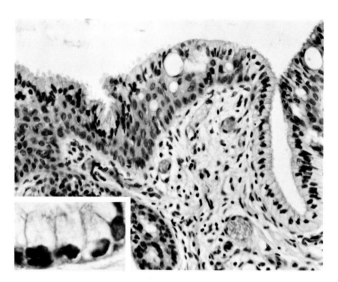

**4.17** Vaginal adenosis with mucinous columnar epithelium lying on the surface of metaplastic squamous epithelium (center and left). To the right the mucinous epithelium appears to line the neck of a gland in the lamina propria. Hematoxylin–eosin, ×250. Inset: Detail of mucinous columnar epithelium. Hematoxylin–eosin, ×780.

[Reprinted by permission from S. J. Robboy, R. E. Scully, and A. L. Herbst, Pathology of vaginal and cervical abnormalities associated with prenatal exposure to diethylstilbestrol (DES), *J. Reprod. Med. 15*:13, 1975.]

epithelium (Figure 4.17). On occasion the glands are observed to open into the vaginal lumen (Figure 4.19).

Frequently, the glandular epithelium, both on the surface and in the glands in the lamina propria, appears to have been undermined or replaced by metaplastic squamous epithelium, the low glycogen content of which accounts for the negative results on iodine staining. In biopsy specimens where the columnar epithelium in the glands has been extensively replaced, the metaplastic squamous cells may appear in the form of pegs, which sometimes are observed to be continuous with the squamous epithelium lining the vaginal lumen (Figure 4.18 and 4.19). These pegs, which may contain abortive pearls with varying degrees of keratinization, may occasionally be of such prominence as to be confused on superficial examination with dysplasia or rarely even with well-differentiated squamous cell carcinoma (Figure 4.20). The metaplastic squamous cells may eventually become highly glycogenated and appear similar to normally glycogenated (mature) squamous epithelium.[10]

In some specimens the glandular epithelium is inconspicuous or absent and the only evidence of adenosis is the

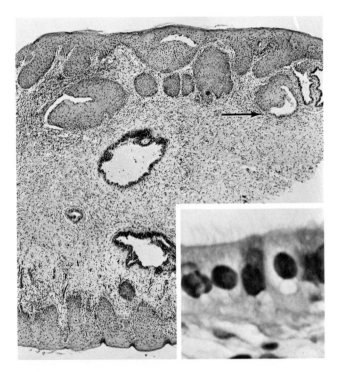

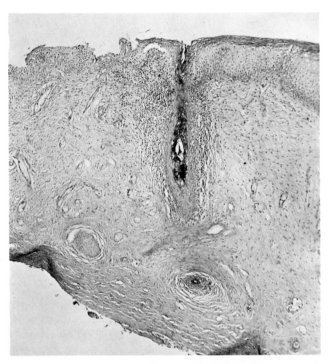

**4.18** Vaginal adenosis. Glands lined by ciliated dark cells similar to tubal or endometrial epithelium are present in the inflamed lamina propria and merge with squamous pegs (arrow). The surface epithelium is composed of glycogen-free squamous cells that account for the abnormal Schiller staining. Hematoxylin–eosin, ×41. Inset: Detail of ciliated dark cells. Hematoxylin–eosin, ×1,122.

[Reprinted by permission from A. L. Herbst, S. J. Robboy, G. J. MacDonald, and R. E. Scully, The effects of local progesterone on stilbestrol-associated vaginal adenosis, *Am. J. Obstet. Gynecol.* 118:607–615, 1974.]

**4.19** Sagittal section through a squamous peg. The central core, lined by mucinous epithelium, is the neck of a gland. Periodic acid Schiff, ×65.

[Reprinted by permission from A. L. Herbst, S. J. Robboy, G. J. MacDonald, and R. E. Scully, The effects of local progesterone on stilbestrol-associated vaginal adenosis, *Am. J. Obstet. Gynecol.* 118:607–615, 1974.]

presence of rare intercellular pools or intracellular droplets of mucin in areas of metaplastic squamous epithelium.[9] With special stains, the mucinous pools are often found to be surrounded by inconspicuous flat cells, the cytoplasm of which is filled with mucin (Figure 4.21). Small droplets of mucin within the cytoplasm of squamous cells are often difficult to identify without the use of special stains (Figure 4.22). However, mucinous droplets and pools are important to identify because they provide the only direct proof of the existence of glandular epithelium in some cases of adenosis.

Cervical erosion (ectropion) refers to the presence of glandular epithelium or its secretory products in the portio vaginalis of the cervix (exocervix). This process has been found in a typically extensive form in nearly all exposed females (Table 4.1). Although cervical erosion and vaginal adenosis are frequently indistinguishable on microscopic examination, several findings repeatedly encountered suggest that the two conditions in part may be different. The glandular epithelium in erosion almost always consists of mucinous cells; unlike vaginal adenosis, cells resembling those of the fallopian tube and endometrium are rare. The mucinous cells in cervical erosion lie on the surface of the laminia propria and form micropapillae much more frequently than in vaginal adenosis, where the glandular epithelium is usually within the laminia propria (Figure 4.23). Last, droplets and pools of mucin in metaplastic squamous epithelium and the inflammatory response tend to be more prominent in cervical erosion.

Vaginal adenosis and cervical erosion can be detected in cytologic smears.[3,19,22,37] Mucinous columnar cells resembling those of the normal endocervix and metaplastic squamous cells, with or without cytoplasmic droplets of mucin, have been identified in about one-third of vaginal

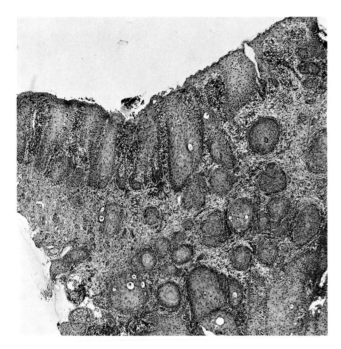

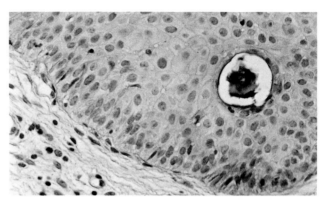

**4.21** Vaginal adenosis. A pool of mucin is surrounded by flat cells with mucinous cytoplasm obvious only with mucin stains. Mucicarmine stain, ×259.

[Reprinted by permission from S. J. Robboy, R. E. Scully, and A. L. Herbst, Pathology of vaginal and cervical abnormalities associated with prenatal exposure to diethylstilbestrol (DES), *J. Reprod. Med.* 15:13, 1975.]

**4.20** Large numbers of squamous pegs in cross section; not to be confused with invasive squamous cell cancer. The squamous epithelium of the pegs and the surface epithelium are composed of glycogen-free cells. Mucinous pools and droplets are present in many pegs. Hematoxylin–eosin, ×40.

[Reprinted by permission from A. L. Herbst, S. J. Robboy, G. J. MacDonald, and R. E. Scully, The effects of local progesterone on stilbestrol-associated vaginal adenosis, *Am. J. Obstet. Gynecol.* 118:607–615, 1974.]

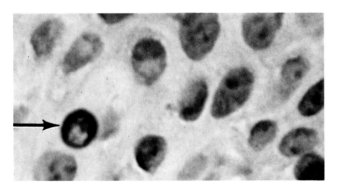

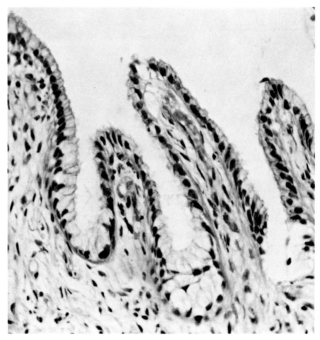

**4.22** Vaginal adenosis. The single mucin droplet (arrow) is bright red, the nuclei of the cells are brown-black, and the cytoplasm is pale yellow in the tissue slide. Mucicarmine stain, ×1,350.

[Reprinted by permission from S. J. Robboy, R. E. Scully, and A. L. Herbst, Pathology of vaginal and cervical abnormalities associated with prenatal exposure to diethylstilbestrol (DES), *J. Reprod. Med.* 15:13, 1975.]

**4.23** Cervical erosion. Mucinous columnar cells line fibrovascular papillae. This lesion appears red on macroscopic examination and does not stain with an iodine solution. Hematoxylin–eosin, ×378.

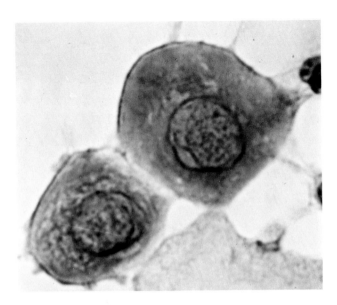

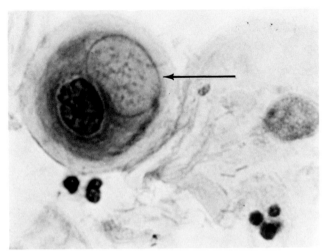

**4.25** Metaplastic squamous cell with a mucin droplet (arrow); from a vaginal scrape in a patient with vaginal adenosis. Papanicolaou stain, ×1,445.

[Reprinted by permission from S. J. Robboy, R. E. Scully, and A. L. Herbst, Pathology of vaginal and cervical abnormalities associated with prenatal exposure to diethylstilbestrol (DES), *J. Reprod. Med. 15:*13, 1975.]

**4.24** Two metaplastic squamous cells in a vaginal scrape from a patient with vaginal adenosis. Papanicolaou stain, ×1,890.

[Reprinted by permission from S. J. Robboy, R. E. Scully, and A. L. Herbst, Pathology of vaginal and cervical abnormalities associated with prenatal exposure to diethylstilbestrol (DES), *J. Reprod. Med. 15:*13, 1975.]

scrapes and two-thirds of cervical scrapes of exposed subjects (Figures 4.24 and 4.25). Ciliated cells are rarely encountered. Although the presence of the above cellular abnormalities in a vaginal scrape smear should raise a suspicion of DES exposure, they are not pathognomonic of a prenatal exposure to DES as they are encountered rarely in nonexposed individuals.

The reported incidence of adenosis in the DES-exposed population has varied from 35%[9] to 90%,[32] probably reflecting differences in terminology and variations in the composition of the population examined. For example, two factors that are known to greatly affect the incidence of adenosis are the week in pregnancy in which the DES therapy was initiated and the definition of the boundary demarcating the vagina from the cervix.[13] In one series in which accurate information was available about the exact time during pregnancy when DES was begun, the incidence of adenosis was 70% when it was given prior to the eighth week, with a progressive decline to 0% when it was begun after the eighteenth week.[9]

Transverse ridges are found in about one-fourth of young females exposed to DES (Table 4.1). Most are low, fibrous bars that involve part or all of the circumference of the upper vagina or cervix. A rare ridge may be so prominent that it must be excised before the cervix can be seen (Figure 4.14). Various descriptive terms have been applied to the ridges in the vicinity of the cervicovaginal junction, some based on the configuration they impart to the cervix: hood (Figure 4.15), cockscomb, rim, and collar. The pseudopolyp is caused by a peripheral concentric cervical band, which imparts to the portio vaginalis central to it the appearance of a protruding cervical polyp; however, the presence of the external os at its center enables it to be differentiated from a true polyp (Figure 4.15). Frequently in these patients the boundary between the cervix and the vagina is poorly delimited, especially when a ridge is present. On microscopic examination the core of the ridge is composed of fibrous connective tissue. Glands lined by mucinous epithelium are found commonly in both vaginal and cervical ridges; glands with tuboendometrial epithelium are found usually only in vaginal ridges.

## Preneoplastic Lesions

Little is known about the mechanism by which the clear cell adenocarcinoma arises and its cell of origin. Circumstantial evidence suggests that vaginal adenosis and cervical erosion may provide the bed from which the

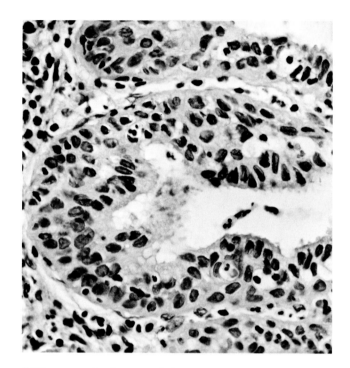

**4.26** Atypical adenosis of the vagina. The nuclei vary both in size and in shape and the cells are stratified. Hematoxylin–eosin, ×500.

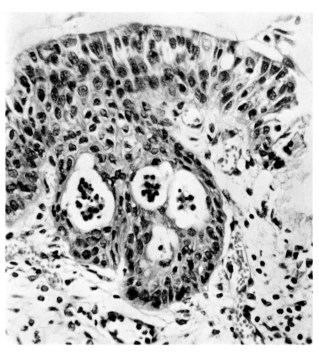

**4.27** Squamous metaplasia in vaginal adenosis. Although the immature squamous cells have large nuclei, they are uniform in size and shape and have finely dispersed chromatin and should not be misdiagnosed as dysplastic. Hematoxylin–eosin, ×310.

[Reprinted by permission from A. L. Herbst, R. E. Scully, and S. J. Robboy, Effects of maternal DES ingestion on the female genital tract, *Hosp. Prac.* 10:51, 1975.]

carcinomas arise because of the high degree of association of these benign lesions with the cancers. Several investigators have suggested that the adenocarcinoma can arise through an intermediate stage of atypical adenosis but only one reported case purports to show such a change in an exposed female.[2] The transition from atypical adenosis to cancer has also been reported once in an older female born prior to the DES era.[4] The diagnosis of atypical adenosis must be made with caution because the glands of the clear cell adenocarcinomas, especially at their periphery, can be highly differentiated and can simulate atypical and even benign glands microscopically. Among the registry cases several tumors with nearby foci of atypical adenosis have been identified, but usually the atypicality has consisted of little more than one or several glands in which few cells have displayed irregularity in the size and shape of their nuclei, prominent nucleoli, or nuclear stratification (Figure 4.26). However, similar changes have been found in biopsy specimens of asymptomatic exposed females and their relation to the clear cell adenocarcinoma is yet to be established.

The suggestion has also been made that dysplasia, squa-

mous cell carcinoma in situ (CIS), and invasive squamous cell carcinoma of the cervix and vagina are going to develop with a greatly increased frequency as the population exposed to DES reaches the ages at which the incidences of these diseases are at their peaks.[33] This concern is based on several pieces of clinical evidence extrapolated from experience with cervical abnormalities in older women who were not exposed *in utero* to DES.[32,33] In several studies based on the examinations of large numbers of DES-exposed patients, the frequency of dysplasia on histologic examination has usually ranged from 0 to 5%,[1,5,9,17,32] with the highest reported frequency being 15%.[6] In most instances the dysplasia has been of a mild degree. One potential source of confusion in the diagnosis of dysplasia is active (immature) squamous metaplasia (Figure 4.27). Although several cases of severe dysplasia and carcinoma in situ have been reported,[6,17,32] the statistical significance of these rare findings has not yet been proved.

# Summary

The story of the changes encountered in the DES-exposed female and the mechanisms by which these changes are produced is continuously unfolding. To date much data have been collected about the incidence, pathology, and clinical characteristics of adenosis and the clear cell adenocarcinoma. Major questions to be answered concern the relation between the two entities, the significance of atypical adenosis as a premalignant condition, and the cell of origin of the clear cell cancer. Much remains to be learned about the embryology of the vagina and the mechanism by which prenatal exposure to DES induces persistence of glandular tissue in the vagina. It is hoped that some of these questions can be answered through careful followup of exposed females as the population ages, new experimental approaches, and the development of an animal model in which the transplacental exposure to DES results in adenosis and adenocarcinoma.

# ACKNOWLEDGMENTS

Supported in part by Grant R01-CA13139-04 and Contract N01–CN-45157 from the National Cancer Institute.

# REFERENCES

1. Antonioli, D. A., and Burke, L. Vaginal adenosis, analysis of 325 biopsy specimens from 100 patients. *Am. J. Clin. Pathol.* 64:625, 1975.

2. Barber, H. R. K., and Sommers, S. C. Vaginal adenosis, dysplasia, and clear-cell adenocarcinoma after diethylstilbestrol treatment in pregnancy. *Obstet. Gynecol.* 43:645, 1974.

3. Bibbo, M., Al-Naqeeb, M., Baccarini, I., Gill, W., Newton, M., Sleeper, K. M., Sonek, M., and Wied, G. L. Follow-up study of male and female offspring of DES-treated mothers. A preliminary report. *J. Reprod. Med.* 15:29, 1975.

4. Blaikley, J. B., Dewhurst, D. J., Ferreira, H. P., and Lewis, T. L. T. Vaginal adenosis: Clinical and pathological features with special reference to malignant change. *J. Obstet. Gynaecol. Br. Commonw.* 78:1115, 1971.

5. Burke, L., Antonioli, D., Knapp, R. C., and Friedman, E. A. Vaginal adenosis. Correlation of colposcopic and pathologic findings. *Obstet. Gynecol.* 44:257, 1974.

6. Fetherston, W. C. Squamous neoplasia of vagina related to DES syndrome. *Am. J. Obstet. Gynecol.* 122:176, 1975.

7. Forsberg, J. G. The development of atypical epithelium in the mouse uterine cervix and vaginal fornix after neonatal oestradiol treatment. *Br. J. Exp. Pathol.* 50:157, 1969.

8. Herbst, A. L., Kurman, R. J., and Scully, R. E. Vaginal and cervical abnormalities after exposure to stilbestrol in utero. *Obstet. Gynecol.* 40:287, 1972.

9. Herbst, A. L., Poskanzer, D. C., Robboy, S. J., Friedlander, L., and Scully, R. E. Prenatal exposure to stilbestrol. A prospective comparison of exposed female offspring with unexposed controls. *N. Engl. J. Med.*, 292:334, 1975.

10. Herbst, A. L., Robboy, S. J., MacDonald, G. J., and Scully, R. E. The effects of local progesterone on stilbestrol-associated vaginal adenosis. *Am. J. Obstet. Gynecol.* 118:607, 1974.

11. Herbst, A. L., Robboy, S. J., Scully, R. E., and Poskanzer, D. C. Clear-cell adenocarcinoma of the vagina and cervix in girls: An analysis of 170 Registry cases. *Am. J. Obstet. Gynecol.* 119:713, 1974.

12. Herbst, A. L., and Scully, R. E. Adenocarcinoma of the vagina in adolescence: A report of 7 cases including 6 clear-cell carcinomas (so-called mesonephromas). *Cancer* 25:745, 1970.

13. Herbst, A. L., Scully, R. E., and Robboy, S. J. Problems in the examination of the DES-exposed female. *Obstet. Gynecol.* 46:353, 1975.

14. Herbst, A. L., Scully, R. E., and Robboy, S. J. Effects of maternal DES ingestion on the female genital tract. *Hosp. Prac.* 10:51, 1975.

15. Herbst, A. L., Ulfelder H., and Poskanzer, D. C. Adenocarcinoma of the vagina: Association of maternal stilbestrol therapy with tumor appearance in young women. *N. Engl. J. Med.* 284:878, 1971.

16. Kurman, R. J., and Scully, R. E. The incidence and histogenesis of vaginal adenosis: An autopsy study. *Hum. Pathol.* 5:265, 1974.

17. Lanier, A. P., Noller, K. L., Decker, D. G., Elveback, L. R., and Kurland, L. T. Cancer and stilbestrol: a follow-up of 1719 persons exposed to estrogen in utero and born in 1943–59. *Mayo Clin. Proc.* 48:793, 1973.

18. Morrow, C. P., and Townsend, D. E. Management of adenosis and clear-cell adenocarcinoma of vagina and cervix. *J. Reprod. Med.* 15:25, 1975.

19. Ng, A. B. P., Reagan, J. W., Hawliczek, S., and Wentz, W. B. Cellular detection of vaginal adenosis. *Obstet. Gynecol.* 46:323, 1975.

20. Noller, K. L., and Fish, C. R. Diethylstilbestrol usage: Its interesting past, important present, and questionable future. *Med. Clin. North Am.* 58:793, 1974.

21. Plaut, A., and Dreyfuss, M. L. Adenosis of vagina and its relation to primary adenocarcinoma of vagina. *Surg. Gynecol. Obstet.* 71:756, 1940.

22. Robboy, S. J., Friedlander, L., Taft, P. D., Scully, R. E., and Herbst, A. L. Vaginal and cervical cytology of 535 young females exposed prenatally to diethylstilbestrol (DES). *Obstet. Gynecol.*, in press.

23. Robboy, S. J., Herbst, A. L., and Scully, R. E. Clear-cell adenocarcinoma of the genital tract in young females. Analysis of 37 tumors that persisted or recurred after primary therapy. *Cancer* 34:606, 1974.

24. Robboy, S. J., Herbst, A. L., Welch, W. R., Keh, P., and Scully, R. E. Microglandular hyperplasia (so-called "pill lesion") arising in vaginal adenosis. Unpublished data.

25. Robboy, S. J., Scully, R. E., and Herbst, A. L. Pathology of vaginal and cervical abnormalities associated with prenatal exposure to diethylstilbestrol (DES). *J. Reprod. Med.* 15:13, 1975.

26. Sandberg, E. C. The incidence and distribution of occult vaginal adenosis. *Am. J. Obstet. Gynecol.* 101:322, 1968.

27. Sandberg, E. C., Danielson, R. W., and Prince, E. Benign vaginal adenosis. *Obstet. Gynecol.* 30:93, 1967.

28. Scully, R. E., and Barlow, J. F. "Mesonephroma" of ovary. Tumor of Müllerian nature related to the endometrioid carcinoma. *Cancer 20:*1405, 1967.

29. Scully, R. E., Robboy, S. J., and Herbst, A. L. Vaginal and cervical abnormalities including clear-cell adenocarcinoma, related to prenatal exposure to stilbestrol. *Ann. Clin. Lab. Sci. 4:*222, 1974.

30. Silberberg, S. G. Ultrastructure and histogenesis of clear-cell carcinoma of the ovary. *Am. J. Obstet. Gynecol. 115:*394, 1973.

31. Silberberg, S. G., and DeGiorgi, L. S. Clear-cell carcinoma of the endometrium. Clinical, pathologic, and ultrastructural findings. *Cancer 31:*1127, 1973.

32. Stafl, A. Colposcopy. *Clin. Obstet. Gynecol. 18:*195, 1975.

33. Stafl, A., and Mattingly, R. F. Vaginal adenosis—a precancerous lesion? *Am. J. Obstet. Gynecol. 120:*666, 1974.

34. Taft, P. D., Robboy, S. J., Herbst, A. L., and Scully, R. E. Cytology of clear-cell adenocarcinoma of the genital tract in young females. Report of 95 cases from the Registry. *Acta Cytol. 18:*279, 1974.

35. Takasugi, N. Morphogenesis of estrogen-independent proliferation and cornification of the vaginal epithelium of neonatally estrogenized mice. *Proc. Jpn. Acad. 47:*193, 1971.

36. Ulfelder, H. Stilbestrol, adenosis, and adenocarcinoma. *Am. J. Obstet. Gynecol. 117:*794, 1973.

37. Vooijs, P. G., Ng, A. B. P., and Wentz, W. B. The detection of vaginal adenosis and clear-cell carcinoma. *Acta Cytol. 17:*59, 1973.

38. Wharton, J. T., Rutledge, F. N., Gallagher, H. S., and Fletcher, G. Treatment of clear-cell adenocarcinoma in young females. *Obstet. Gynecol. 45:*365, 1975.

Alex Ferenczy, M.D.

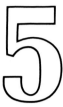

# Anatomy and Histology of the Cervix

## Gross Anatomy

Although the cervix was recognized as an organ entity as early as 4500 B.C. during the third Egyptian Dynasty, it was Soranus, in the first century A.D., who gave the first accurate description of the cervix uteri as a separate portion of the uterus.[48] The cervix (term taken from the Latin, meaning "neck") is the most inferior portion of the uterus protruding into the upper vagina. The vagina is fused circumferentially and obliquely around the distal part of the cervix, dividing it into an upper, supravaginal and lower, vaginal portion.[26] The cervix is generally cylindrical in shape, measures in the adult nulligravida 2.5 to 3.0 cm in length, and its normal position is slightly angulated downward and backward. The vaginal portion (portio vaginalis) of the cervix, also referred to as the exocervix, is delimited by the anterior and posterior fornices and has a convex elliptical surface. It is covered by a smooth, shiny squamous mucous membrane and centered by the external os, a circular (in the nulligravida) or slitlike (in the parous woman) opening (Figure 5.1). The portio may be divided into anterior and posterior lips, of which the anterior is shorter and projects lower than its posterior counterpart. The external os is interconnected with the isthmus (internal os) by the cervical canal. The canal is an elliptical, fusiform cavity, measuring in its greatest width 8 mm, and contains longitudinal mucosal ridges, the plicae palmatae (Figure 5.2). These, when hypertrophied or fused because of inflammation, may render the introduction of a uterine curette or dilator difficult because they form blind passages in the canal. The area between the endocervical and endometrial cavity is called the isthmus or lower uterine segment. The latter term is used principally for descriptive purposes during gestation and labor. The use of the terms anatomic and histologic "internal os" seems arbitrary as no convincing morphologic evidence is offered to support such a geographic subdivision of the uterus and the uterus may be divided into corpus, isthmus, and cervix. The muscular layer in the region of the isthmus is less developed than in the corpus, a feature that facilitates effacement and dilatation during labor. The blood supply of the cervix is provided by the descending branches of the uterine arteries, reaching the lateral walls along the upper margin of the paracervical ligaments (cardinal ligaments of Mackenrodt). These ligaments are the main source of fixation, support, and suspension of the organ. Another means of fixation is provided by the uterosacral ligaments, which attach the supravaginal portion of the cervix to the second through fourth sacral vertebrae. Excision of nerve fibers (denervation) within these ligaments is used to relieve intractable dysmenorrhea. The venous drainage parallels the arterial system, with communication between the cervical plexus and neck of the urinary bladder. The lymphatics of the cervix have a dual origin:[36] beneath the mucosa and deep in the fibrous stroma. Both systems collect into two lateral plexuses in the region of the isthmus and give origin to four efferent channels running toward: (1) the external iliac and obturator nodes, (2) the hypogastric and

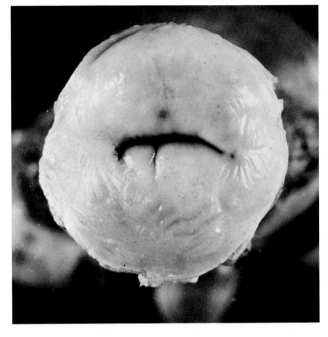

**5.1** Multiparous exocervix with slitlike external os.

common iliac nodes, (3) the sacral nodes, and (4) the nodes of the posterior wall of the urinary bladder. The innervation of the cervix is chiefly limited to the endocervix and peripheral deep portion of the exocervix.[26] This distribution is responsible for the relative insensitivity to pain of the portio vaginalis. The cervical nerves derive from the pelvic autonomic system, the superior, middle, and inferior hypogastric plexuses.

**5.2** Transected multiparous uterus. The endocervical canal is delimited by the isthmus (I) and external os (E). Note prominent mucosal folds of endocervical canal.

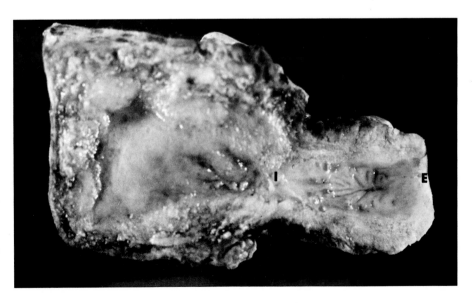

# Normal Morphology and Physiology

The cervix is made of an admixture of fibrous, muscular, and elastic tissue, of which the fibrous connective tissue is the predominant component.[6] Smooth muscle, making about 15% of the substance, is mainly located in the endocervix, the portio vaginalis being virtually devoid of smooth muscle fibers.[26] By contrast, at the isthmus 50 to 60% of the supportive tissue is made of muscular elements arranged in a concentric fashion, serving the function of sphincter.

## Squamous Epithelium

The exposed, or vaginal, portion of the cervix is generally lined by a nonkeratinizing, squamous stratified epithelium, which is referred to as "the native portio epithelium" (Figure 5.3). The portio epithelium is sensitive, although to a lesser degree than the vaginal mucosa, to ovarian sex steroid hormones and is constantly being remodeled by proliferation–maturation–desquamation during the reproductive period. The epithelium is completely replaced by a new population of cells every 4 to 5 days[25,37] and the process of squamous epithelial maturation can be accelerated to 3 days by the administration of estrogenic compounds.[25] In general, estradiol-17$\beta$ stimulates epithelial proliferation, maturation, and desquamation, whereas progesterone inhibits maturation at the upper midzone level of the epithelium. As a result, the portio epithelium during the postnatal period is fully mature and contains large amounts of glycogen from the influence of maternal estrogens. Maturation and glycogen, however, are rapidly lost as the hormones disappear from the infant's circulation and the epithelium remains atrophic until the time of menarche when, under the stimulatory effect of ovarian hormones, maturation and glycogen reappear. During pregnancy, when progesterone levels are elevated, superficial cell maturation is absent.

The mature cervical squamous epithelium is similar to the vaginal epithelium but under normal circumstances lacks the rete pegs seen in the vagina.[13,26] It contains three zones of cells:[25] (1) the basal or germinal cell layer, which is responsible for continuous epithelial renewal; (2) the midzone or stratum spinosum, the dominant portion of the epithelium; and (3) the superficial zone, made of the most mature cell population (Figure 5.3). The basal zone is composed of one or two layers of elliptical cells of about 10 $\mu$ in diameter with scant cytoplasm and oval nuclei characteristically oriented perpendicular to the underlying basal lamina (Figure 5.3). Epithelial regeneration is the

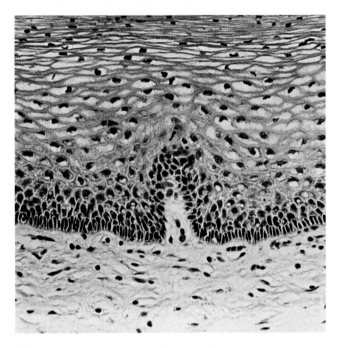

**5.3** Mature squamous epithelium of the portio of the cervix. Note gradual ascending maturation, vacuolization of midzone cells, and a single layer of basal cells in which the nuclei are perpendicularly oriented to the basal lamina. The stromoepithelial junction contains a fingerlike, fibrovascular stromal papilla penetrating the lower portion of the epithelium.

major function of the basal cells; their fine structural organization[1,12,17,18] and mitotic activity are those seen in an actively dividing cell population (Figure 5.4). The lower third of the midzone contains larger cells than the basal variety, with a comparatively more abundant cytoplasm. Because of their geographic placement they are called parabasal cells. They may occasionally exhibit mitotic divisions, and radioautographic studies[2] have demonstrated a high uptake of tritiated thymidine, a nucleoprotein precursor, into the nuclei of parabasal cells suggesting that they also contribute to epithelial growth. Ultrastructurally, the parabasal cells are attached by numerous tonofilament–desmosomal complexes and there is a beginning of intracytoplasmic glycogenization (Figure 5.5). Phosphorylase and amylo-1,6-glucosidase, enzymes essential for glycogen synthesis, are localized in this region.[14] The upper portion of the midzone is occupied by cells that are involved in a process of ascending maturation, during which there is a gradual increase in the volume of the cytoplasm. Nuclear size, however, remains

**5.4** Electron micrograph of basal cells of the native portio epithelium. The cells have prominent nuclei and nucleoli and the cytoplasm contains bundles of tonofilaments and abundant free ribosomes, mitochondria, and Golgi. Cellular integrity is maintained by desmosomal and hemidesmosomal attachments to neighboring squamous cells and basal lamina, respectively. S, Stroma ×2,720. Inset: Detailed view of cytoplasmic organelles, tonofilaments, hemidesmosomes (arrow), and basal lamina. ×6,120.

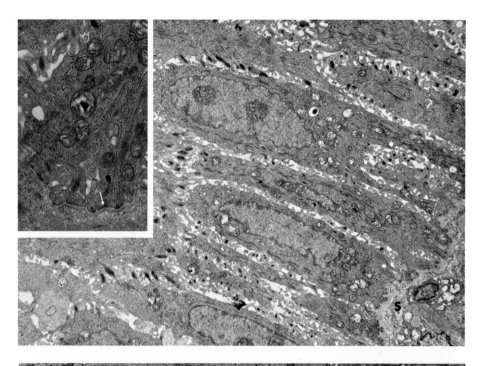

**5.5** Electron micrograph of parabasal cells, one of which is in mitosis. The organelle-rich cytoplasm contains small collections of glycogen granules (G). ×4,250.

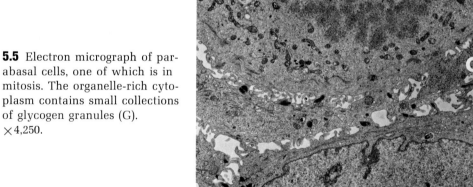

constant up to the most superficial cell level. These cells are referred to as intermediate cells when exfoliated. They do not divide.[37] Intermediate cells have abundant PAS-positive, diastase-labile intracellular glycogen (Figure 5.6), which is responsible for the clear "vacuolated" appearance of their cytoplasm (Figure 5.3). The superficial zone forms the most differentiated compartment of the squamous epithelium. Here, the cells are flattened and have a larger area of cytoplasm (50 $\mu$ in diameter) and smaller pyknotic nuclei than the underlying intermediate cells (Figure 5.7).

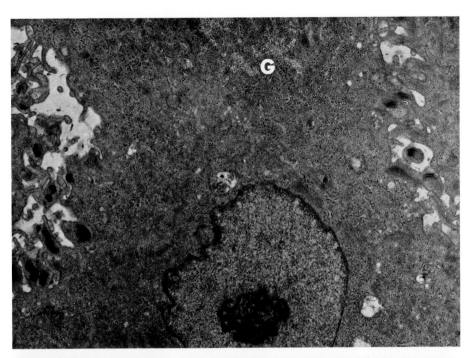

**5.6** Electron micrograph of an intermediate cell with well-preserved nucleus and abundant cytoplasm. In the latter are numerous glycogen particles (G) intermingling with bundles of tonofibrils. Tonofilament–desmosomal complexes are evident. ×6,120.

**5.7** Electron micrograph of superficial cells. The cells have pyknotic nuclei (N) and flattened cytoplasm packed with glycogen (G). The most superficial cells are rich in microfilaments and contain irregular surface membrane projections. Note the lack of desmosomal attachments between the most superficial cells, a feature facilitating desquamation. ×4,795. Inset: Higher magnification of intracytoplasmic microfilaments in the most superficial cells. ×11,370.

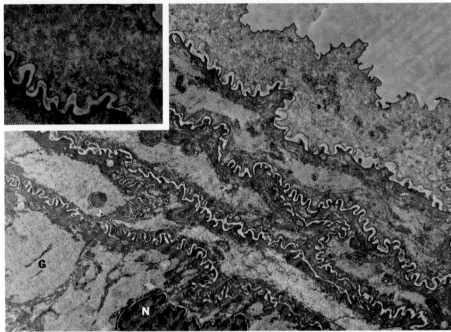

The pink, eosinophilic, and glycogen-rich cytoplasm is rich in microfilaments which provide its rigidity (Figure 5.7, inset). Superficial cells also contain occasional membrane-bound keratinosomes. These structures are the source of protein-bound disulfide keratin precursors,[1,15] which are responsible for cornification and the complex network of microridges seen on the surface of the most superficial and mature cells.[11,12,27] The function of the cornified surface is to protect the underlying epithelial cells and subepithelial vasculature from trauma and infections.

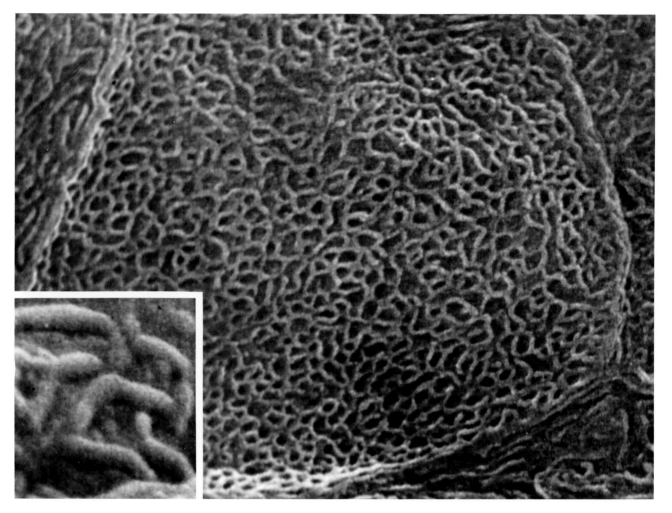

**5.8** Scanning electron micrograph of the most superficial cells of the native squamous portio epithelium. The surface contains an intricate system of microridges. ×8,240. Inset: Higher magnification of microridges representing nodular evaginations of the surface plasma membrane. ×22,660.

The microridges are believed to enhance surface adhesiveness (Figure 5.8). The virtual lack of desmosomes between the upper superficial cells explains their loose attachment and easy desquamation (Figure 5.7).

In postmenopausal women, who no longer produce ovarian hormones, the squamous epithelium is atrophic with no, or scant, intracytoplasmic glycogen and lacks surface epithelial maturation and stromal papillae (Figure 5.9). These cellular alterations should not be confused with cervical intraepithelial neoplasia. The thin epithelial covering cannot adequately protect the subepithelial vasculature against trauma, a situation that frequently leads to bleeding and inflammatory reactions. The squamous epithelium of the portio is supported by a fibrous connective tissue stroma, devoid of endocervical glands. There is a well-developed capillary network at the stromoepithelial junction with occasional fingerlike extensions into the epithelium, the stromal papillae[24] (Figure 5.3). The penetrating vessels supply the epithelial cells with nutrients and oxygen. With the colposcope, under normal conditions, the subepithelial vasculature appears as a spiderlike or hairpin capillary network.[24] In addition to connective tissue fibers and capillaries, occasional free nerve endings are seen entering the stromal papilla.[26]

## Columnar Epithelium

The mucosa of the cervical canal (endocervix) is composed of a single layer of mucus-secreting, columnar epithelium, which lines both the surface and the underlying glandular structures. The latter are traditionally called compound, tubular racemose, endocervical glands. Fluhman,[13] however, using three-dimensional plastic reconstructions from serial histologic sections, has demonstrated that the endocervical glands actually represent deep, uncrossed, cleftlike infoldings of the surface epithelium with numerous blind, tunnel-like collaterals (Figure 5.10). According to Fluhman,[13] it is in the tunnels or blind tubes that Nabothian cysts are formed. Because of the complex organization of these clefts, or grooves, including oblique, transverse, and longitudinal arrangements, in histologic sections they often appear as single glandular units (Figure 5.10). Because the epithelium lining the clefts is identical with that lining the surface, the endocervical mucus-producing apparatus is not considered glandular but a complexly infolding mucinous membrane. True glands have different epithelia in their secretory portions than in their excretory (ductal) or surface epithelial portions. The columnar epithelial cells characteristically have basally placed nuclei and tall, uniform, finely granular cytoplasm filled with mucous droplets (Figure 5.11). These have great affinity for alcian blue stains, reflecting their sulfated, sialic acid mucopolysaccharide content.[10] Cells lining the luminal surface have been termed "picket cells" because of their resemblance to a picket fence (Figure 5.11). Occasionally, nonsecretory cells with cilia are observed[12] (Figure 5.11, inset), the main function of which appears to be related to the distribution and mobilization of endocervical mucus. Although cyclic morphologic alterations in the endocervix are rather subtle, a peak of cellular growth and secretory activity is reached at the time of ovulation; in the progestational phase of the cycle,[13] these alterations progressively decrease. On the other hand, unlike the endocervical epithelium, its viscoelastic secretory product, the cervical mucus, is subject to profound cyclic changes. Under estrogenic stimulation, the endocervical secretions are profuse, watery, and alkaline, facilitating sperm penetration, whereas during the postovulatory phase they are scant, thick, and acid; contain numerous leukocytes; and so are unfavorable for sperm penetration. Biochemical[33] and fine structural analyses[3,12,46] have shown that the cervical mucus gel is made of a heterogenous micellar network of glycoproteins. The intermicellar space is occupied by cervical plasma rich in sodium chloride and potassium, the ions of which are

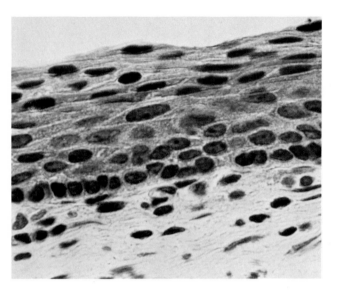

**5.9** Atrophic squamous portio epithelium. The epithelium is thin and devoid of glycogen-rich vacuolated cells. The cells in the lower half of the epithelium have prominent nuclei and nucleoli but cellular cohesion is normal and cytologic atypia is absent.

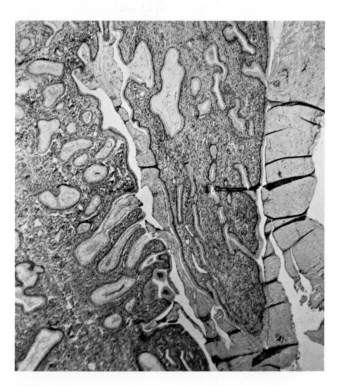

**5.10** Endocervical mucosa with cleftlike infoldings and tunnel-like collaterals. The neighboring glandlike structures represent tangentially sectioned cleft-tunnel complexes.

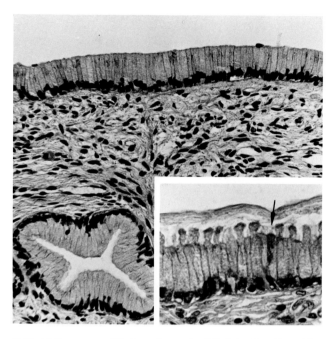

**5.11** Tall, mucus-filled endocervical "picket" cells with basal nuclei. Inset: Endocervical cells engaged in apocrine secretion whereby portions of apical cytoplasm are expelled. Ciliated cells are present (arrow).

responsible for the crystallization of mucus or ferning (arborization) reaction (Figure 5.12). Under estrogenic influence the glycoprotein micelles are arranged parallel to each other at a distance of 5 to 15 $\mu$,[46] creating a channel system that is favorable to sperm penetration. During progestogenic stimulation, the micellar channel system is replaced by a dense network composed of interlacing micellar fiber bridges that preclude sperm penetration (Figure 5.13). Ultrastructurally,[12,17,34,35] endocervical secretory activity operates by both the apocrine and the merocrine type of expulsion of secretory products. In the former type, a portion of apical cytoplasm packed with secretory granules is detached (Figure 5.14), whereas in the latter, secretory products are released from apical granules through porelike openings of the surface cytoplasmic membrane (Figure 5.15, inset). As in other mucus-secreting systems of the body,[49] in the endocervical mucinous cells synthesis of mucoproteins is initiated in the Golgi cisternae and perigolgian vesicles.[12,17,34,35] The coalescence of perigolgian vesicles leads to the formation of larger secretory units, which in turn form by further intercoalescence prominent granules with granulofilamentous content. The Golgi is associated with free ribosomes, granular endoplasmic reticulum, and mito-

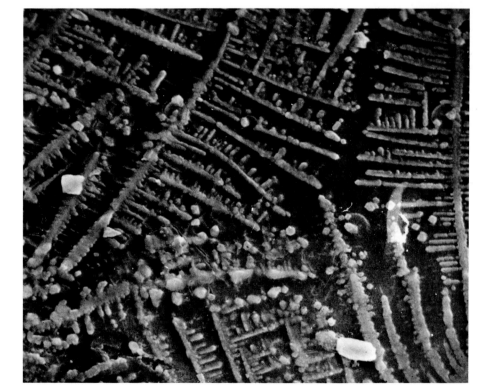

**5.12** Scanning electron photomicrograph of ferning reaction in cervical mucus during the ovulatory period. ×850.

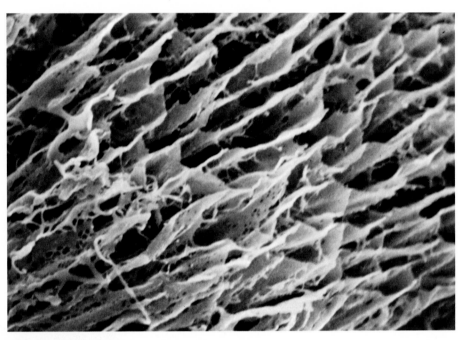

**5.13** Scanning electron microscopic appearance of unpurified cervical mucus in the secretory phase of the menstrual cycle. The mucoid material is made of interlacing filamentous micellar meshwork, unfavorable for sperm migration. ×4,000.

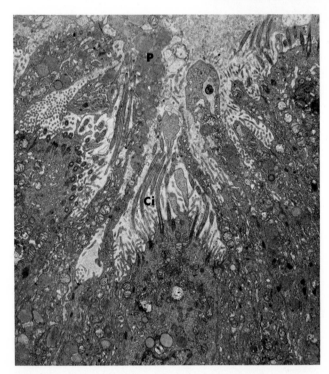

**5.14** Electron micrograph of mucus-containing endocervical cells alternating with ciliated cells (Ci). Mucous secretion is of the apocrine type, as indicated by intraluminal protrusions (P) of apical cytoplasmic substance packed with mucous droplets and various organelles. ×4,030.

chondria, providing the essential protein matrix and energy for mucoprotein synthesis (Figure 5.15). It is of interest to note that, despite the continuous desquamation of endocervical cells, mitosis in the columnar epithelium is not seen under normal conditions. Whether epithelial renewal is generated from the underlying subcolumnar reserve cells,[25] which under normal circumstances are seldom seen even at the ultrastructural level, or from the persisting mature endocervical cells is presently unknown. An uninterrupted, well-defined basal lamina produced by the endocervical cells and continuous with that of the squamous epithelium is always present and separates the endocervical cells from the underlying stroma. Unlike the attenuated vascular stromal papillae of the original squamous portio epithelium, the subepithelial capillary network in the endocervical mucosa is well developed, resembling the vessels of the intestinal villi[24] (Figure 5.16). The stroma of the endocervix is comparatively better innervated than that of the portio vaginalis. The nerve fibers are found running parallel to muscle bundles but sensory free endings have not been clearly demonstrated.[26] True lymphoid follicles, with or without germinal centers, are encountered in the subepithelial stroma of both the exo- and the endocervix. They may be numerous in association with chronic inflammatory conditions or cervical intraepithelial neoplasia and are produced by long-standing or intense antigenic stimulation (Figure 5.17).

The squamocolumnar junction of the cervix is the line

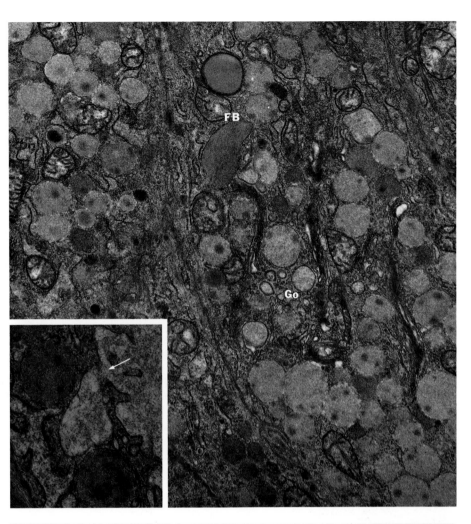

**5.15** Detail of endocervical mucinogenesis. The membrane-bound mucin-containing secretory granules derive from Golgi (Go) and mature through progressive stages of intercoalescence. The Golgi are associated with free and bound ribosomes and mitochondria, providing the protein matrix and energy for mucin synthesis. A characteristic feature of endocervical mucinous cells is the presence of fibrillar bodies (FB), presumably representing a fibrillar form of mucoprotein storage. ×19,320. Inset: Electron microscopic view of the merocrine type of secretion. Filamentous mucus is discharged through focal porelike opening (arrow) of the surface plasma membrane. ×22,080.

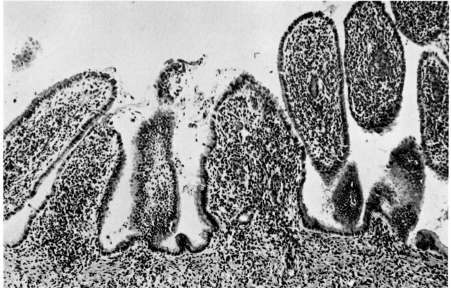

**5.16** Chronic papillary endocervicitis. The chronically inflamed lamina propria contains a prominent subepithelial capillary network.

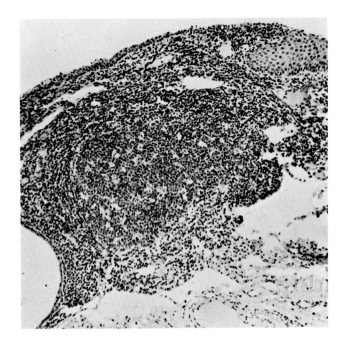

**5.17** A subepithelial lymphoid follicle with a prominent germinal center is engaged in active phagocytosis of acute inflammatory exudate. When lymphoid follicles are numerous, the condition is referred to as follicular cervicitis.

along which the stratified squamous epithelium meets the mucus-secreting columnar epithelium of the endocervix. Morphogenetically, there are two types of squamocolumnar junctions (Figure 5.18). One is termed the "original" squamocolumnar junction, where the native squamous covering of the portio vaginalis joins the columnar epithelium. The union between the two epithelia is a sharp one (Figure 5.19). The second is called the "physiologic" or "functional" squamocolumnar junction and is established between the newly formed squamous epithelium of the transformation zone and the endocervical columnar cells. In this instance the transition may be abrupt or gradual[13] (Figure 5.20).

## The Transformation Zone

In most women during the reproductive period, the mucus-secreting columnar epithelium of the endocervix extends onto the cervical portio, forming the so-called endocervical eversion (ectropion or ectopy). This occurs twice as commonly on the anterior as on the posterior lip,[38,39,50] but both lips may simultaneously be involved. The everted endocervical mucosa appears as a red velvety zone, contrasting with the neighboring pink and shiny squamous portio epithelium. Because of its gross appear-

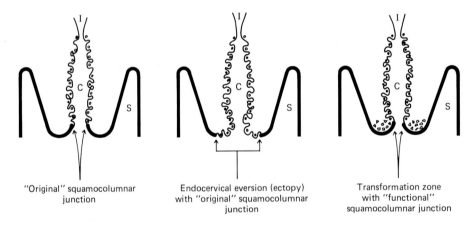

"Original" squamocolumnar junction

Endocervical eversion (ectopy) with "original" squamocolumnar junction

Transformation zone with "functional" squamocolumnar junction

**5.18** Schematic representation of "original" and "functional" squamocolumnar junctions and three basic types of portios. The left drawing diagrams a portio completely covered with native squamous epithelium. The squamocolumnar junction is at the external os. The middle drawing denotes an endocervical eversion, with the squamocolumnar junction being located on the exocervix below the external os. The right drawing indicates areas of eversion covered with squamous epithelium. This area is the cervical transformation zone. The new or "functional" squamocolumnar junction of the transformation zone is at the external os. S, Squamous epithelium; C, endocervical columnar epithelium; I, uterine isthmus.

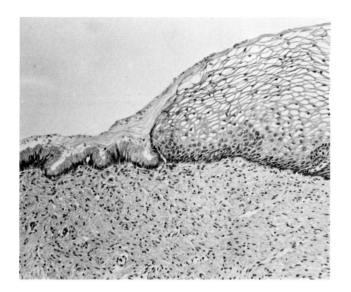

**5.19** "Original" squamocolumnar junction. Note the abrupt transition between the mature squamous epithelium of the portio and the endocervical mucosa. A similar sharp demarcation may be seen at the squamocolumnar junction of the mature transformation zone.

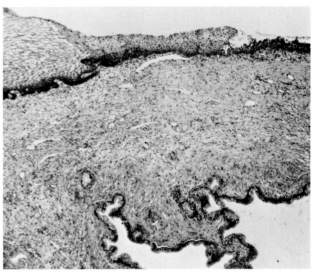

**5.20** "Functional" squamocolumnar junction of the immature transformation zone. Note the gradual transition between mature (left) and immature squamous epithelium (right). The latter is continuous with proliferating subcolumnar reserve cells. There are endocervical clefts in the subjacent area.

ance, the term cervical erosion is often used by clinicians. The term is incorrect, however, because there is no epithelial denudation (true erosion) but numerous villus or papillary excrescences of varying size, resembling a bunch of grapes when viewed with the colposcope (Figure 5.35a). Histologically, these are blunt-ended papillae lined by endocervical columnar epithelium and supported by a chronically inflamed fibrovascular stroma (Figure 5.21). The pathogenesis of endocervical eversion is not clear. Characteristically, it develops during fetal life, at the time of puberty, and during the reproductive years (especially during pregnancy) and is absent in postmenopausal women. These periods in the life of women are associated with exaggerated hormonal stimuli, which produce changes in the volume of the cervical portio and the shape of the cervical lips. Under the action of increased hormonal stimuli, the volume of the portio increases and the lips of the portio protrude.[13, 19] These observations, together with the high incidence of endocervical eversion in young girls with a history of *in utero* exposure to nonsteroidal synthetic estrogens (diethylstilbestrol, DES)[21] and experimentally induced cervical and vaginal endocervical ectopy in the rodent with large doses of DES,[16] seem to indicate that a strong estrogenic influence is primarily responsible for the development of endocervical eversion. During the postmenopausal period, when estrogenic influence is in-

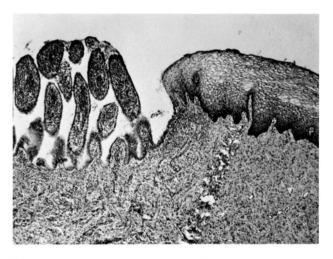

**5.21** Endocervical eversion meets the native squamous portio epithelium. The everted endocervical mucosa has a papillary configuration and the lamina propria is obscured by chronic inflammatory exudate.

conspicuous, the volume of the portio is considerably decreased. Consequently, the lips are retracted and the endocervical mucosa is brought into the endocervical canal (entropion). As a result, the squamocolumnar junction is

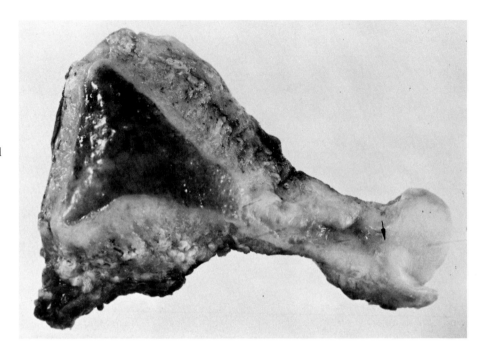

**5.22** Prolapsed, postmenopausal uterus. The cervix is atrophic and elongated and the squamocolumnar junction is visualized above the external os (arrow).

virtually always located above the external os and often within the cervical canal (Figure 5.22). The dynamics of events by which the columnar epithelium extends onto the portio are uncertain. However, it is suspected that either the columnar epithelium directly migrates from the endocervix onto the portio vaginalis or is passively carried out onto the exposed face of the cervix following protrusion[19] and/or laceration[13] of the cervical lips. The surface columnar epithelium of the everted endocervical mucosa is subsequently replaced by squamous epithelium, forming the clinical transformation or transitional zone, the direction of transformation being centripetal.[40] The squamous transformation of ectopic endocervical tissue is probably excited by the low (acid) pH of the vagina[5] and provides a protective surface for the underlying endocervical tissue. Because endocervical eversion and its squamous transformation occur in the majority of women, they are regarded as normal physiologic processes. The movements of endocervical eversion and its squamous reepithelialization are under the influence of both the women's hormonal status and local (vaginal) environmental factors. Accordingly, the physiologic squamocolumnar junction of the transformation zone is topographically fluid and follows the movements of the transformation zone. The transformation zone may be difficult to visualize with the naked eye. Its localization, however, is greatly enhanced with the use of the colposcope (see Chapter 8, Diagnostic Procedures).

The presence of squamous epithelium with circular openings and spherical "bumps" of 2 to 4 mm (which correspond to the underlying endocervical glands and Nabothian cysts, respectively) represents the outer limits of the transformation zone (Figure 5.35d). Nabothian cysts are formed when the mouths of endocervical clefts become obliterated by the proliferating surface squamous epithelium. As mucous secretion continues but excretion is blocked, the secretory products accumulate, leading to cystic glandular dilatations or Nabothian cysts. With the colposcope, the squamous mucous membrane over the cysts appears characteristically stretched, thinned out, and yellowish because of the abundant, thick intracystic mucus (Figure 5.35d). Microscopically the cystic spaces are lined by low columnar endocervical cells, supported by a distended basal lamina (Figure 5.23).

There are two histogenetic mechanisms proposed by which the cervical epithelium is replaced by squamous epithelium. The first mechanism consists in a direct ingrowth from the native portio epithelium bordering the everted columnar epithelium. Histologic, colposcopic, colpomicroscopic, and electron microscopic observations[11, 12, 41, 42] have shown that tongues of native squamous epithelium of the portio grow beneath the adjacent columnar epithelium and expand in between the mucinous epithelium and its basement membrane. As the squamous cells expand and mature, the endocervical cells

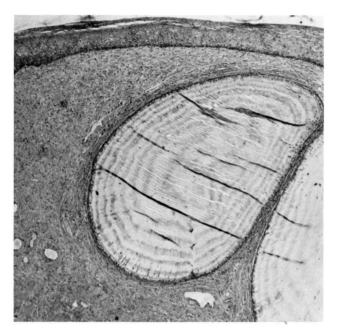

**5.23** Microscopic appearance of the outer portio limit of the transformation zone. Mature squamous epithelium covers underlying Nabothian cysts filled with laminated mucin. In this case, the cysts represent the "last glands" of previously everted endocervical mucosa.

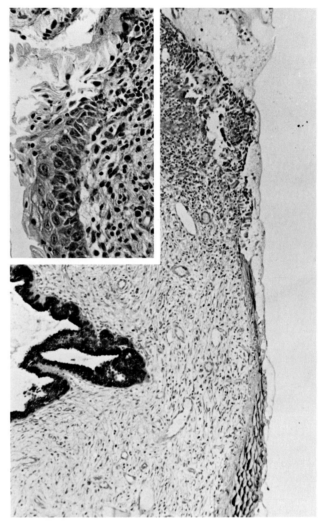

**5.24** Outer edge of the early transformation zone. A narrow tongue of glycogen-containing native squamous epithelium of the portio (right) grows onto everted and eroded endocervical mucosa. The underlying endocervical epithelium is rich in mucin (PAS stain). Inset: Detail of advancing edge of squamous cells growing beneath endocervical columnar cells, which are displaced upward. Nuclei and nucleolar enlargement in squamous cells are a reflection of epithelial hyperplasia associated with repair.

are gradually displaced upward, degenerate, and eventually are sloughed away (Figures 5.24 and 5.25). A similar process is observed in the reepithelialization of true pathologic erosion of the everted endocervix, the so-called ascending healing of Meyer[30] or squamous epithelization of the endocervix.[22] Rapid squamous reepithelialization of areas of everted columnar epithelium may also be produced artificially by electrocautery or cryosurgery. The rationale of these therapeutic techniques is to replace the often bleeding and inflamed endocervical tissue by a more protective epithelial surface. The process of squamous epithelialization is thought to be responsible for the obliteration of the peripheral portions of endocervical ectopy.

The second mechanism involved in the genesis of squamous epithelium of the transformation zone is most commonly termed squamous metaplasia, but such names as epidermidization and squamous prosoplasia[13] are also used. The latter term, derived from the Greek meaning "forward" and "to form," has been proposed by Fluhman[13] and is probably the most accurate one. It refers to a proliferation of undifferentiated subcolumnar reserve cells of the endocervical epithelium and their gradual transformation into a fully mature squamous epithelium. In contrast, squamous metaplasia implies an isolated morphologic event in which mature or adult cells are changed into another type of mature cell population that is not normal for that tissue, i.e., squamous metaplasia of the endometrium. The morphogenetic development of squamous

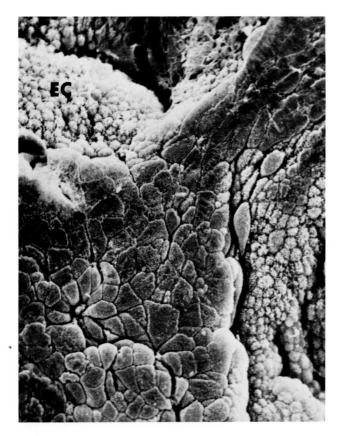

**5.25** Scanning electron microscopic appearance of the outer edge of the early transformation zone. Narrow tongues of squamous epithelium with a pavementlike surface pattern extend onto the everted endocervical mucosa (EC). ×428.

Reprinted by permission from A. Ferenczy and R. M. Richart, Scanning electron microscopy of the cervical transformation zone, *Am. J. Obstet. Gynecol. 115:*151–157, 1973.

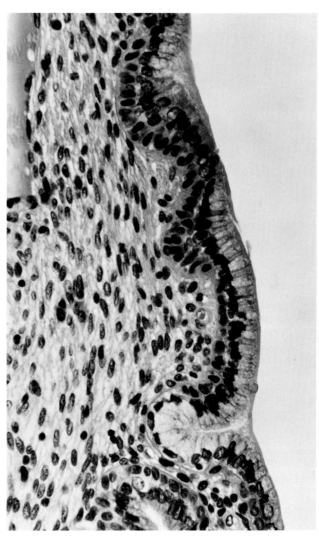

**5.26** A single layer of cuboidal to low, columnar reserve cells is seen between tall, columnar endocervical cells and basal lamina.

prosoplasia has been thoroughly documented by Fluhman[13] and others.[4,47] The first stage of prosoplasia is manifested by the appearance of small cuboidal cells beneath the columnar mucinous epithelium, the so-called subcolumnar reserve cells (Figure 5.26). Ultrastructurally, the cells have large nuclei that have an increased rate of nucleic acid synthesis when examined by radioautography.[44] The organelle-poor cytoplasm has scattered tonofilaments and the cells are attached to the overlying columnar cells and underlying basal lamina by desmosomes and hemidesmosomes, respectively (Figure 5.27). Their general fine structural characteristics are closely similar to the basal cells of the mature squamous portio epithelium.

The origin of subcolumnar reserve cells is controversial.

Some investigators suggest a direct derivation from columnar mucinous secretory cells[13] and others favor the squamous portio epithelium, squamous basal cells, embryonal rests of urogenital origin, and stromal cells as possible sources.[5] In any event, the basic feature of these cells is their bipotency and ability to evolve into either columnar or squamous epithelium. The subsequent steps are characterized by a progressive growth and stratification of reserve cells (subcolumnar reserve cell hyperplasia), followed by differentiation into immature squamous (Figure 5.28) and, ultimately, fully mature squamous epithelium indistinguishable from the native portio epithelium

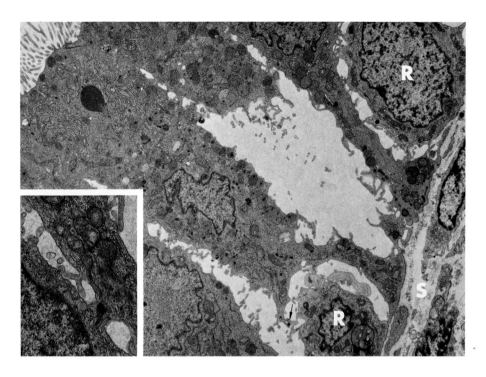

**5.27** Electron microscopy of subcolumnar reserve cells (R). The nucleocytoplasmic ratio is in favor of the nucleus and the cells are attached to neighboring endocervical cells and underlying basal lamina by desmosomes (arrow) and hemidesmosomes, respectively. The stroma (S) contains spindle-shaped fibroblasts. ×4,345. Inset: Cytoplasmic details of reserve cells containing bundles of tonofilaments, free and bound ribosomes, and mitochondria. Note the immature tonofilament–desmosome complex between two reserve cells. ×7,170.

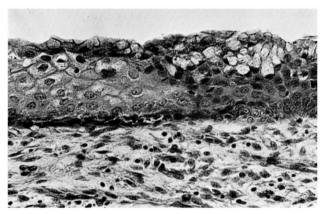

**5.28** Immature squamous prosoplastic epithelium. Note the endocervical cells on top of the proliferating squamous cells.

(Figure 5.29). The immature, squamous, prosoplastic epithelium is distinguished from its mature counterpart by lack of surface maturation and inconspicuous intracytoplasmic glycogen. It is, characteristically, sharply demarcated from the native portio epithelium by a perpendicular or oblique line to the surface (Figure 5.30). As a result, the uninitated observer may mistake immature squamous prosoplasia (metaplasia) for cervical intra-

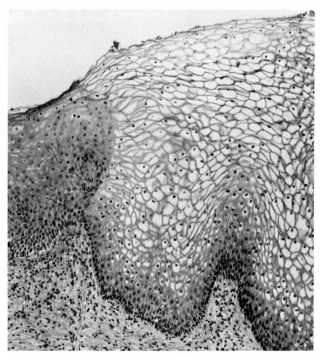

**5.29** Transformation zone epithelium. On the right, the epithelium has achieved full maturation and is identical with normal native portio epithelium, whereas on the left, squamous differentiation, including glycogenization, is incomplete.

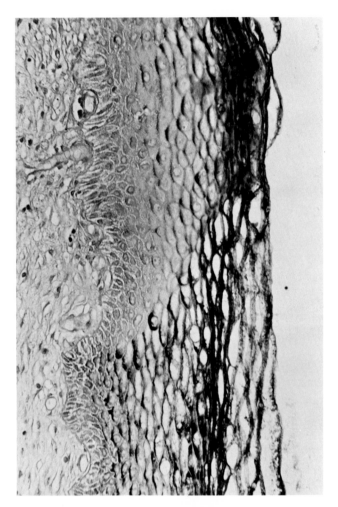

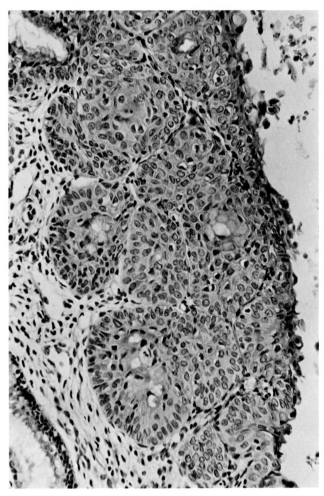

**5.30** PAS-stained squamous epithelium with a sharp demarcation between poorly glycogenized immature squamous epithelium (upper half) of the transformation zone and heavily glycogenized, mature native portio epithelium (lower half).

**5.31** Early squamous cell prosoplasia (metaplasia) involving both the surface and the deeper endocervical epithelium. Note trapped mucinous endocervical cells in the center of prosoplastic foci. Unlike cervical intraepithelial neoplasia with "gland involvement," in squamous cell prosoplasia nuclear atypia is totally lacking and cellular cohesion is normal.

epithelial neoplasia, particularly when the process also involves the underlying glands (Figure 5.31). However, in contrast to neoplastic epithelium, in the young squamous prosoplastic epithelium, cell organization and cohesion are maintained, nuclear atypia is absent, and usually a single row of endocervical cells on top of squamous cells is seen. Fine structurally, the immature, squamous, prosoplastic cells resemble the parabasal cells of the portio epithelium and have well-developed tonofilaments, abundant desmosomes, and evidence of early glycogenization (Figure 5.32). Unlike the most superficial cells of the mature squamous epithelium, the superficial cells of the young transformation zone epithelium are covered by numerous microvillus projections rather than surface microridges[11,12,27,51] (Figure 5.33). Unlike squamous epithelialization, which involves the peripheral regions of the everted endocervical tissue, squamous prosoplasia has a random distribution within the everted endocervical tissue. Indeed, with the aid of the colposcope, islands of squamous prosoplastic epithelium are seen on the summit of endocervical papillae, expanding centripetally and developing delicate epithelial bridges that fuse with neighbor-

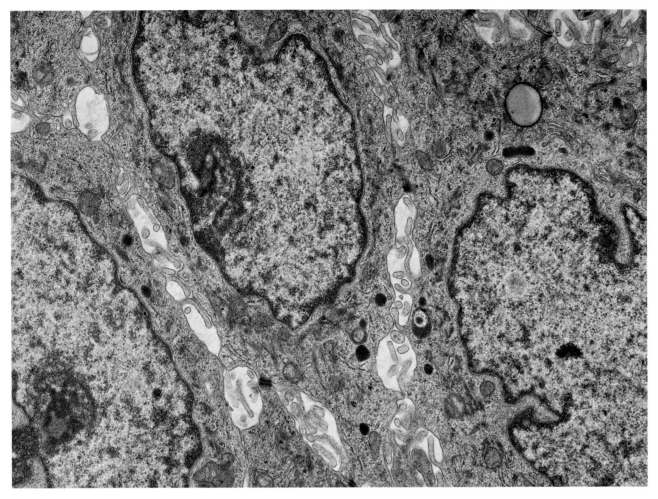

**5.32** Electron microscopy of immature squamous prosoplastic cells. Squamous differentiation is suggested by the presence of intracytoplasmic tonofilaments and abundant interdigitating microvilli. Unlike mature squamous epithelial cells, in the immature variety desmosomes are infrequent and poorly developed. ×12,750.

ing epithelial proliferations (Figure 5.35b, Plate V). Further growth, expansion, and interanastomosis between epithelial islands eventually lead to complete obliteration of the underlying everted endocervical mucosa (Figure 5.35c,d, Plate V).

The major events involved in the histogenesis of the transformation zone are summarized in Figure 5.34 and illustrated in Figure 5.35a–d, Plate V. The transformation zone epithelium originates simultaneously by ingrowth from the native portio epithelium and by squamous prosoplasia (metaplasia) from the reserve cells of everted columnar epithelium. The two epithelial proliferations by expanding merge into each other, interanastomose, and

ultimately form the so-called transformation zone of the cervix uteri. The squamous replacement of everted endocervical epithelium is designed to protect the columnar epithelium from infections and trauma.

The clinical identification of the squamocolumnar junction of the transformation zone is important because virtually all cervical squamous neoplasia begins at this junction.[42] The transformation zone is important because the extension and limits of cervical intraepithelial neoplasia coincide with the distribution of the transformation zone.[42] It is also important to remember that during the childbearing ages and pregnancy the transformation zone is located in almost all instances on the exposed portion of

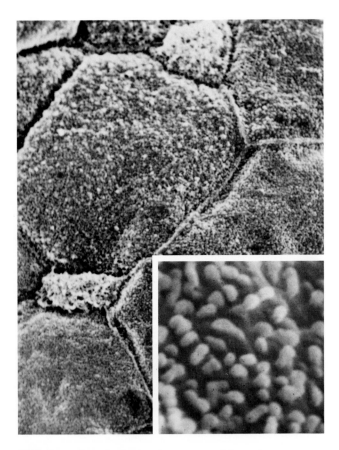

**5.33** Scanning electron microscopy of immature squamous prosoplastic cells with well-developed terminal bars. In contrast to the superficial cells of the mature squamous epithelium, which are covered by microridges, the superficial cells of the young transformation zone are covered by microvilli. Among the squamous cells is an entrapped endocervical cell (lower left). ×2,500. Inset: Higher magnification of surface microvilli. ×15,000.

the cervix. Consequently, the vast majority of cervical neoplasia can be removed for histologic diagnosis by punch biopsy.

# The Cervix during Pregnancy and Puerperium

The morphologic alterations that occur in the ante- or postpartum cervix are not pathognomonic of pregnancy or partuition but are seen more commonly at these times than in the nonpregnant postpartum state. They are corre-

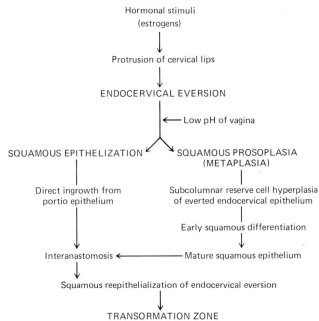

**5.34** Summary of the sequence of events in the histogenetic development of the transformation zone.

lated with the stimulatory actions of the gestational hormones. The spongy enlargement of the pregnant cervix is caused by increased vascularity and edema of the stroma accompanied by acute inflammation.[9,13,23] The massive destruction of collagen fibers and accumulation of extracellular glycoproteinic ground substance[7] prior to labor result in cervical softening and effacement, facilitating dilatation of the cervix to about 10 cm during labor. Pseudodecidualization of the stroma, either patchy or diffuse, occurs in about one-third of the cases examined histologically (Figure 5.36) and disappears by 2 months postpartum.[23] It is presumably mediated by the high levels of progesterone during pregnancy.

The most conspicuous histologic changes are observed in the endocervical mucosa. The columnar cells become tall, with the nuclei located in the middle of the cytoplasm, and mucous secretion is prominent (Figure 5.37). The gestational cervical mucus is thick, tenacious, and rich in leukocytes and forms a mucous plug that obliterates the cervical canal, sealing the endometrial cavity from the vagina and thus providing protection against bacterial invasion. Subcolumnar reserve cell hyperplasia is a common feature of pregnancy and may be found in a multifocal pattern on the tip of the endocervical papillae or deep within the endocervical clefts and tunnels. Similar changes

PLATE V

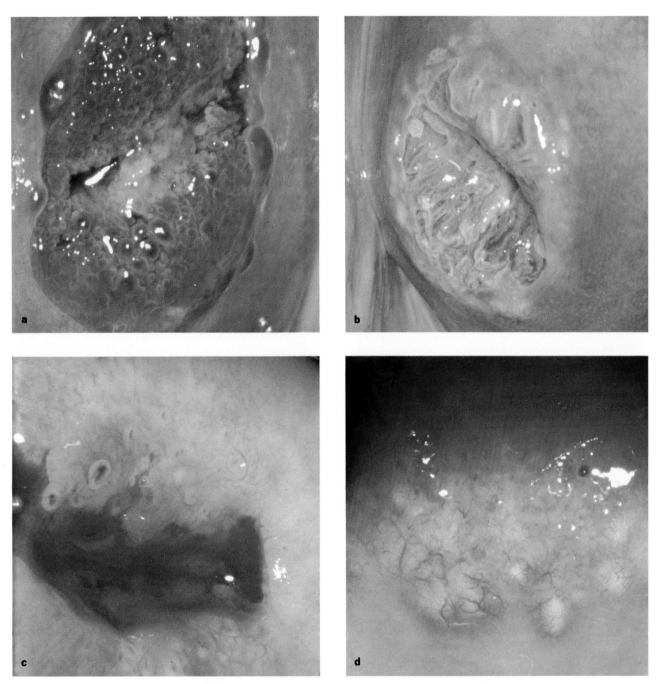

**5.35** Colpophotographs illustrating the genesis of the cervical transformation zone. **a.** Endocervical eversion. Grapelike endocervical mucosa is everted on both the anterior and the posterior lip and surrounds the anatomic external os. The "original" squamocolumnar junction is displaced below the os. **b.** Early transformation zone. Everted endocervical mucosa with tonguelike ingrowths from the native squamous portio epithelium. Some of these tongues appear to interanastomose with whitish, young squamous prosoplastic epithelium, which covers the tip of endocervical villi. Note the irregular outline of the squamocolumnar junction of the young transformation zone. **c.** Mature transformation zone with endocervical "gland" openings. The squamocolumnar junction of the transformation zone is at the os. **d.** Outer limit of the mature transformation zone, indicated by the presence of several Nabothian cysts. These appear as elevated yellowish areas with blood vessels on the surface.

PLATE VI

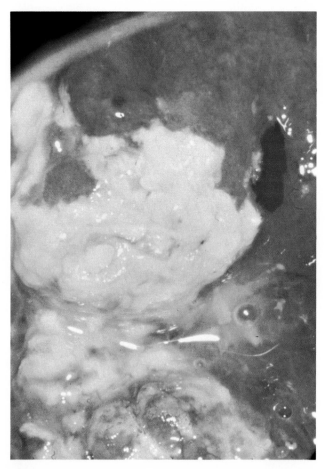

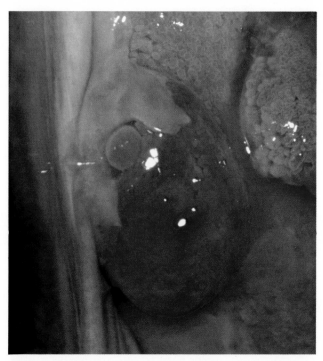

**6.12** Colpophotograph of endocervical mucous polyp. The congested surface is partially covered by whitish squamous prosoplastic epithelium. Note the villous configuration of adjacent endocervical mucosa.

**6.2** Colpophotograph of an elevated, white plaque (leukoplakia) involving the anterior lip of a prolapsed cervix.

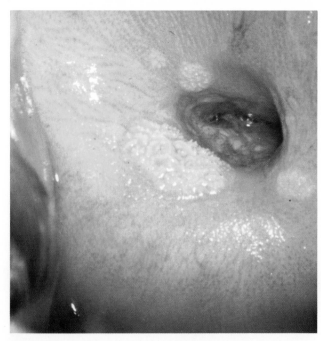

**6.24** Colpophotograph of multiple condylomata acuminata of the cervix with white verruciform surface.

PLATE VII

**7.15** Colposcopy of noninvasive and invasive cervical squamous cell carcinomas. **a.** Colpophotograph taken with green filter, illustrating punctation pattern. The abnormal white epithelium appears to be "perforated" by numerous, irregularly spaced terminal capillaries. Biopsy contained grade 3 CIN. **b.** Mosaic pattern. The neoplastic epithelium is compartmentalized into a myriad of irregular mosaics by the compressed vascular. **c.** Early invasive carcinoma of the cervix. Note the irregular horizontal vessels running parallel to the surface and greatly increased intercapillary distance. **d.** Clinically invasive squamous cell carcinoma of the cervix. Vessels display atypical branching and enlargement.
[**(c)** and **(d)** are courtesy of Dr. A. Stafl, The Medical College of Wisconsin, Milwaukee.]

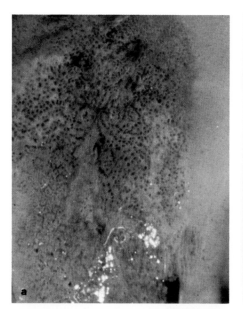
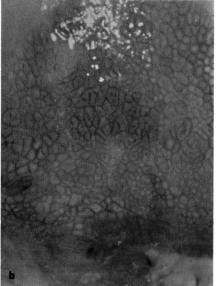
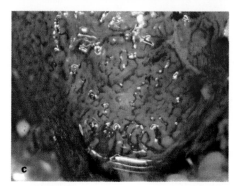
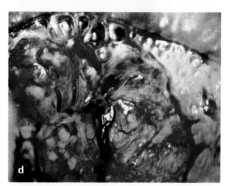

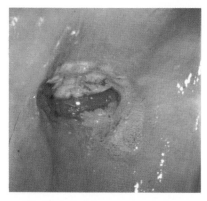

**7.20** Colpophotograph depicting the location and extent of abnormal punctated white epithelium, which histologically contained grade 3 CIN. The entire lesion is visualized at the external os with extension onto the anterior lip and minimally into the endocervical canal. Note sharp demarcation between neoplastic and adjacent normal transformation zone epithelium.

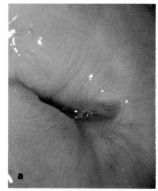
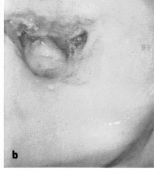

**7.23 a.** Colpophotograph of the cervix seen in Figure 7.20, 1 min after cryosurgery with nitrous oxide. The ice ball extends 4 mm beyond the outer limits of punctated lesion. **b.** Same cervix 3 months after cryosurgery, containing typical spokelike striations. No residual lesion is seen.

PLATE VIII

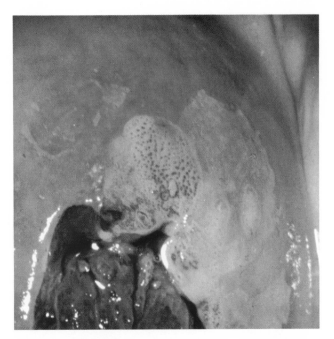

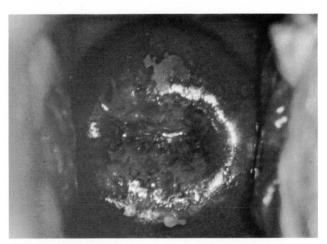

**8.3** Schiller test outlining the iodine-negative, non-glycogen-containing, light areas. Biopsy contained grade 3 cervical intraepithelial neoplasia (carcinoma in situ).

**8.2** Colpophotograph of cervix after the application of 3% acetic acid. Note white focal epithelium with focal punctation and sharp margins located at the squamo-columnar junction of the anterior lip. Colposcope-oriented punch biopsy contained grade 2 cervical intra-epithelial neoplasia (moderate dysplasia).

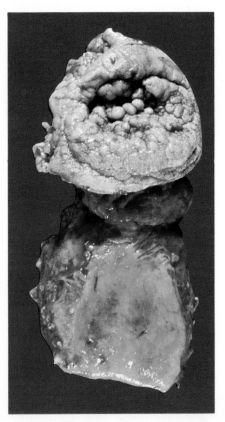

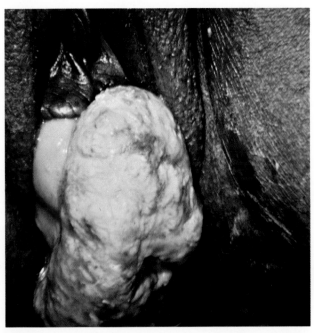

**9.13** Verrucous carcinoma of the cervix. The tumor is made of confluent, exophytic papillary masses involving both the os and the portio.

[Courtesy of Dr. A. Blaustein, New York University Medical Center, New York.]

**9.7** Polypoid, invasive squamous cell carcinoma of the cervix. A bulky friable mass projects from the external os.

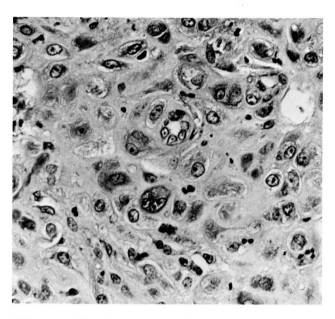

**5.36** Pseudodecidual reaction of cervical stromal cells during pregnancy. The cells are identical with gestational decidual cells of the endometrium. Pseudodecidual change in the cervix should be distinguished from poorly differentiated invasive squamous cell carcinoma or undifferentiated carcinoma.

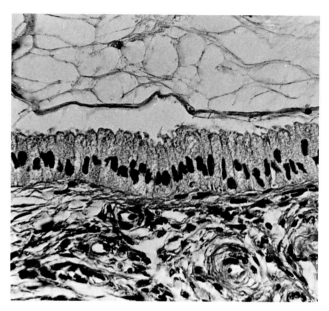

**5.37** Endocervical epithelium during pregnancy. Note palisading nuclei in the middle of the cytoplasm.

with or without squamous prosoplasia (metaplasia) may also be seen in lobules of tightly packed, small endocervical glandular units forming polypoid protrusions into the canal. The term "microglandular endocervical hyperplasia" is used for this type of lesion. A histologically identical endocervical proliferation is seen in patients using oral contraceptives (see Chapter 6, Microglandular Endocervical Hyperplasia). The intense proliferation of endocervical mucinous cells is associated with enlargement and softening of the portio during the course of gestation and leads to eversion of the endocervix onto the exposed portion of the cervix. Indeed, endocervical eversion is encountered in the majority of ante- and postpartum cervices with its maximum incidence occurring after the first pregnancy and in women under 20 years old.[5] Eversion of columnar epithelium occurs twice as commonly on the anterior as on the posterior lip of the cervix.[50] It is rapidly replaced by young, immature squamous epithelium of both native portio and subcolumnar reserve cell origin.[5,13,23] As a result, in most primigravida a young cervical transformation zone is seen, which often persists for long periods of time. The squamocolumnar junction of the transformation zone is nearly always located distal to the external os. Endocervical eversion and its squamous transformation occur to a comparatively lesser extent in subsequent pregnancies.[13] True pathologic erosion during pregnancy is observed to involve the everted endocervix next to the native portio epithelium in about 10% of biopsies.[23] Postpartum injuries, such as lacerations produced during labor, are seen in most primiparous and half of multiparous patients,[23] with a distribution of 2:1 in favor of the anterior lip.[50] The denuded areas are subsequently reepithelized by ingrowing native squamous epithelium of the portio vaginalis. In general, the squamous portio epithelium remains intact during pregnancy. It often contains basal cell hyperplasia, which is believed to occur in response to underlying severe inflammatory reaction.[22]

# Vestigial and Heterotopic Structures of the Cervix

## Mesonephric Duct Remains

The vestigial elements of the distal ends of mesonephric ducts are found in about 1% of cervices.[32] They consist of small tubules or cysts[45] and are located deep in the lateral cervical wall. Characteristically, the tubules are arranged in

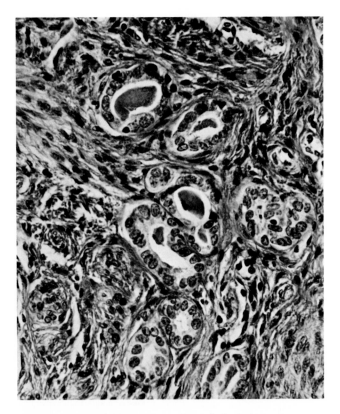

**5.38** Mesonephric tubules with pink, homogeneous intraluminal secretions.

small clusters or have an orderly, Indian-file distribution reminiscent of the ampullary portion of the fetal mesonephric duct. The tubules are lined by a nonciliated, low columnar or cuboidal epithelium.[28,29,32,45] The lining cells contain no glycogen or mucin, features which distinguish them from the endocervical epithelium.[29] The tubular lumen, however, is often filled with pink, homogeneous, PAS-positive secretions (Figure 5.38). A few cases of non-mucous-producing adenocarcinoma (mesonephric carcinoma) presumably arising in mesonephric remnants have been reported[20,28,29] (see Chapter 9, Adenocarcinoma of the Cervix).

## Heterotopic Ectodermal and Mesodermal Structures

Among the pathologic curiosities of the cervix are reports of true epidermidization of the cervical mucosa. In these instances sebaceous glands,[8,31,52] hair, and sweat glands[52] are found. The presence of these ectodermal structures, which are normally appendages of the epider-

mis, on a mucous membrane of mesodermal derivation is difficult to explain. It is conceivable, however, that squamous stratified epithelium under certain circumstances, such as long-standing chronic inflammation, can form the appendages of its epidermal analogue. Four cases of heterotopic mature cartilage in the cervix were reported by Roth and Taylor.[43] The finding of these structures alone has no clinical significance and they should not be confused with a malignant mixed mesodermal tumor.

## ACKNOWLEDGMENTS

This work was aided by grant MA5137 from the Medical Research Council of Canada.

## REFERENCES

1. Ashworth, C. T., Luibel, F., and Sanders, E. Epithelium of normal cervix uteri studied with electron microscopy and histochemistry. *Am. J. Obstet. Gynecol.* 79:1149, 1960.

2. Averette, H. E., Weinstein, G. D., and Frost, P. Autoradiographic analysis of cell proliferation kinetics in human genital tissues. I. Normal cervix and vagina. *Am. J. Obstet. Gynecol.* 108:8, 1970.

3. Chretien, F. C., Gernigon, C., David, G., and Psychoyos, A. The ultrastructure of human cervical mucus under scanning electron microscopy. *Fertil. Steril.* 24:746, 1973.

4. Coppleson, M., Pixley, E., and Reid, B. *Colposcopy. A Scientific and Practical Approach to the Cervix in Health and Disease,* 1st ed. Springfield, Ill., Charles C Thomas, 1971.

5. Coppleson, M., and Reid, B. *Preclinical Carcinoma of the Cervix Uteri,* 1st ed. Oxford, Pergamon Press, 1967.

6. Danforth, D. N. The distribution and functional activity of the cervical musculature. *Am. J. Obstet. Gynecol.* 68:1261, 1954.

7. Danforth, D. N., Veis, A., Breen, M., Weinstein, H. G., Buckingham, J. C., and Manalo, P. The effect of pregnancy and labor in the human cervix: Changes in collagen, glycoproteins, and glycosaminoglycans. *Am. J. Obstet. Gynecol.* 120:641, 1974.

8. Dougherty, C. M., Moore, W. R., and Cotten, N. Histologic diagnosis and clinical significance of benign lesions of the nonpregnant cervix. *Ann. N.Y. Acad. Sci.* 97:683, 1962.

9. Epperson, J. W. W., Hellman, L. M., Galvin, G. A., and Busby, T. The morphological changes in the cervix during pregnancy, including intraepithelial carcinoma. *Am. J. Obstet. Gynecol.* 61:50, 1951.

10. Fand, S. B. The histochemistry of human cervical epithelium, in Blandau, R. J., and Maghissi, K. S., eds.: *The Biology of the Cervix.* Chicago, University of Chicago Press, 1973, pp. 103–124.

11. Ferenczy, A., and Richart, R. M. Scanning electron microscopy of the cervical transformation zone. *Am. J. Obstet. Gynecol.* 115:151, 1973.

12. Ferenczy, A., and Richart, R. M. *Female Reproductive System. Dynamics of Scan and Transmission Microscopy,* 1st ed. New York, John Wiley & Sons, 1974.

13. Fluhman, C. F. *The Cervix Uteri and Its Diseases*, 1st ed. Philadelphia, W. B. Saunders, 1961.

14. Foraker, A. G., and Marino, G. Glycogen-synthesizing enzymes in the uterine cervix. *Obstet. Gynecol.* 17:311, 1961.

15. Foraker, A. G., and Wingo, W. J. Protein bound sulfhydryl and disulfide group in squamous carcinoma of the uterine cervix. *Am. J. Obstet. Gynecol.* 71:1182, 1956.

16. Forsberg, J. G. Estrogen, vaginal cancer, and vaginal development. *Am. J. Obstet. Gynecol.* 113:83, 1972.

17. Friedrich, E. R. The normal morphology and ultrastructure of the cervix, in Blandau, R. J., and Maghissi, K. S., eds.: *The Biology of the Cervix.* Chicago, University of Chicago Press, 1973, pp. 79–102.

18. Hackeman, M., Grubb, C., and Hill, K. R. The ultrastructure of normal squamous epithelium of the human cervix uteri. *J. Ultrastruct. Res.* 22:443, 1968.

19. Hamperl, H., and Kaufmann, C. The cervix uteri at different ages. *Obstet. Gynecol.* 14:621, 1959.

20. Hart, W. R., and Norris, H. J. Cervix adenocarcinoma of mesonephric type. *Cancer* 29:106, 1972.

21. Herbst, A. L., Poskanzer, D. C., Robboy, S. J., Friedlander, L., and Scully, R. E. Prenatal exposure to stilbestrol. *N. Engl. J. Med.* 292:334, 1975.

22. Johnson, L. D. The histopathological approach to early cervical neoplasia. *Obstet. Gynecol. Surv.* 24:735, 1969.

23. Johnson, L. D. Dysplasia and carcinoma in-situ in pregnancy, in Norris, H. J., Hertig, A. T., and Abell, M. R., eds.: *The Uterus*, Internatl. Acad. Path. Monogr. Baltimore, Williams & Wilkins, 1973, pp. 382–412.

24. Kolstad, P., and Stafl, A. *Atlas of Colposcopy*, 1st ed. Baltimore, University Park Press, 1972.

25. Koss, L. G. *Diagnostic Cytology and Its Histopathologic Bases*, 2nd ed. Philadelphia, J. B. Lippincott, 1968.

26. Krantz, K. E. The anatomy of the human cervix, gross and microscopic, in Blandau, R. J., and Moghissi, K., eds.: *The Biology of the Cervix.* Chicago, University of Chicago Press, 1973, pp. 57–69.

27. Llanes, A., Farre, C., Ferenczy, A., and Richart, R. M. Scanning electron microscopy of normal exfoliated squamous cervical cells. *Acta Cytol.* 17:507, 1973.

28. Mackles, A., Wolfe, S. A., and Neigus, I. Benign and malignant mesonephric lesions of the cervix. *Cancer* 11:292, 1958.

29. McGee, C. T., Cromer, D. W., and Greene, R. R. Mesonephric carcinoma of the cervix. Differentiation from endocervical adenocarcinoma. *Am. J. Obstet. Gynecol.* 84:358, 1962.

30. Meyer, R. The basis of the histological diagnosis of carcinoma with special reference to carcinoma of the cervix and similar lesions. *Surg. Gynecol. Obstet.* 73:14, 1941.

31. Nicholson, G. W. Sebaceous glands in the cervix uteri. *J. Pathol. Bacteriol.* 22:252, 1918.

32. Novak, E., Woodruff, J. D., and Novak, E. R. Probable mesonephric origin of certain female genital tumors. *Am. J. Obstet. Gynecol.* 68:1222, 1954.

33. Odeblad, E. The functional structure of human cervical mucus. *Acta Obstet. Gynecol. Scand.* 47(Suppl. 1):57, 1968.

34. Philipp, E. On the granulo-filamentous transformation of secretory granules in the mucous producing epithelium of the human endocervix. *Z. Zellforsch. Mikrosk. Anat.* 134:555, 1972.

35. Philipp, E., and Overbeck, L. Die Ultrastuktur des Zervixepithels. *Z. Geburtsh. Gynaek.* 171:159, 1969.

36. Reiffenstuhl, G. *The Lymphatics of the Female Genital Organs,* 1st ed. Philadelphia, J. B. Lippincott, 1964.

37. Richart, R. M. A radioautographic analysis of cellular proliferation in dysplasia and carcinoma in situ of the uterine cervix. *Am. J. Obstet. Gynecol.* 86:925, 1963.

38. Richart, R. M. The growth characteristics in vitro of normal epithelium, dysplasia and carcinoma in situ of the uterine cervix. *Cancer Res.* 24:662, 1964.

39. Richart, R. M. Colpomicroscopic studies of the distribution of dysplasia and carcinoma in situ on the exposed portion of the human uterine cervix. *Cancer* 18:950, 1965.

40. Richart, R. M. Colpomicroscopic studies of cervical intraepithelial neoplasia. *Cancer* 19:395, 1966.

41. Richart, R. M. Natural history of cervical intraepithelial neoplasia. *Clin. Obstet. Gynecol.* 10:748, 1967.

42. Richart, R. M. Cervical intraepithelial neoplasia, in Sommers, C. C., ed.: *Pathology Annual.* New York, Appleton-Century-Crofts, 1973, pp. 301–328.

43. Roth, E., and Raylor, H. B. Heterotopic cartilage in the uterus. *Obstet. Gynecol.* 27:838, 1966.

44. Schellhas, H. F., and Heath, G. Cell renewal in the human cervix uteri. A radioautographic study of DNA, RNA, and protein synthesis. *Am. J. Obstet. Gynecol.* 104:617, 1969.

45. Scherrick, J. C., and Vega, J. G. Congenital intramural cysts of the uterus. *Obstet. Gynecol.* 19:486, 1962.

46. Singer, A., and Reid, B. L. Effects of the oral contraceptive steroids on the ultrastructure of human cervical mucus. *J. Reprod. Fertil.* 23:249, 1970.

47. Stafl, A., and Mattingly, R. F. Vaginal adenosis: A precancerous lesion? *Am. J. Obstet. Gynecol.* 120:666, 1974.

48. Temkin, O. (Translator). *Soranus' Gynecology.* Baltimore, Johns Hopkins University Press, 1956.

49. Whaley, W. G., Dauwalder, M., and Kephart, J. E. Golgi apparatus: Influence on cell surface. *Science* 175:596, 1972.

50. Wilbanks, G. D., and Richart, R. M. The puerperal cervix, injuries and healing: A colposcopic study. *Am. J. Obstet. Gynecol.* 97:1105, 1967.

51. Williams, A. E., Jordan, J. A., Allen, J. M., and Murphy, J. F. The surface ultrastructure of normal and metaplastic cervical epithelia and of carcinoma in situ. *Cancer Res.* 33:504, 1973.

52. Willis, R. A. *The Borderland of Embryology and Pathology,* 2nd ed. Washington, D.C., Butterworth, 1962.

Alex Ferenczy, M.D.

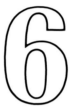

# Benign Lesions
# of the Cervix

## Inflammatory Diseases

### Nonspecific Acute Cervicitis

Acute inflammation of the cervix results from direct infection by nonspecific microorganisms or by secondary invaders. The former group includes streptococci, staphylococci, and enterococci, and infections with these organisms are prone to occur in puerperal infections. Among the most common secondary invaders are the gram-negative diplococci, *Neisseria gonorrhoea, Trichomonas vaginalis,* and *Candida albicans*. Foreign bodies introduced into the vagina, namely, fragments of residual tampons and pesseries, may also lead to acute cervical inflammation. Clinically, acute cervicitis is manifested by purulent vaginal discharge, which is yellowish green when the infection is caused by *Trichomonas* and whitish with white flakes when *Candida* is the causative agent. Backache, vulvar pruritus, and painful urination, when the urethra is involved, are often accompanied by vaginal discharge. An acutely inflamed cervix is swollen and reddened because of an increase in stromal edema and terminal vasculature of the cervix. Histologically, there is extensive stromal edema with polymorphonuclear leukocytic infiltration and often focal loss of mucous membrane.

## Nonspecific Chronic Cervicitis

Chronic cervicitis occurs principally in women of child-bearing age, being infrequent after the menopause and virtually nonexistent before the menarche. Clinically, the chief complaint is whitish, greenish, or yellowish discharge. On gross and colposcopic examination, the cervical mucosa is hyperemic because of an increased number of terminal vessels, often contains patchy areas of endocervical eversion, and rarely contains true epithelial erosions or lacerations. The microorganisms most often identified in chronic cervicitis are *Streptococcus, Staphylococcus,* and *Enterococcus.* The condition is so common that its histologic diagnosis seems meaningless. Microscopically there is a variable degree of submucosal accumulation of lymphocytes and plasma cells. Occasionally lymphoid follicles with germinal centers are found beneath the epithelium (see Figure 5.17). The inflammatory exudate may be confined to the transformation zone but may also involve the portio and endocervical glandular mucosa. Squamous prosoplasia (metaplasia) and endocervical polyps are often seen in association with chronic cervicitis.

## Atypia of Repair (Anaplasia of Repair)

In cases of severe acute or long-standing chronic inflammation, especially those associated with *Trichomonas vaginalis* or epithelial injury of any kind—true erosion, biopsy, or conization—the squamous epithelium, and occasionally the endocervical epithelium, undergoes considerable epithelial disorganization and nuclear atypia may be present (Figure 6.1a–c). The lower half of the squamous epithelium may not mature normally and may be occupied by atypical cells of the basal type. These changes are often confused in both histology[60] and cytology[41] with intraepithelial neoplasia. However, they are distinct from the undifferentiated cells that are found in intraepithelial neoplasia for the cytoplasmic membrane is better defined, the nuclei are uniform in shape and size, and the chromatin is aggregated in prominent chromocenters. The epithelium is often studded with migrating inflammatory cells. Mitotic figures are normal in architecture and are confined to the proliferating basal and parabasal cell population. Characteristically, the cells in the upper half of the epithelium are not abnormal and maturation occurs in a normal fashion. In the endocervical columnar cells, the abnormal morphologic alterations include nuclear enlargement and hyperchromasia, cytoplasmic eosinophilia, and loss of mucous

droplets (Figure 6.1c). Although this type of glandular epithelium appears highly atypical, the changes are focal, alternating with normal mucous-secreting columnar cells, and are confined to areas with massive inflammation or mucosal injury. In addition, the deep cytoplasmic eosinophilia (which is caused by an increase in ribosomes and mitochondria) and the absence of abnormal mitoses, are features that distinguish the inflammatory lesions from an in situ adenocarcinoma of the endocervix. The atypical cellular changes accompany the increased DNA and RNA synthesis that occurs during the repair of the damaged or inflamed epithelial membrane.

## Hyperkeratosis and Parakeratosis

Cervical hyperkeratosis or parakeratosis usually involves the portio vaginalis and clinical appearance of a whitish or greasy plaque (leukoplakia) (Figure 6.2, Plate VI). When cervical hyperkeratosis is diffuse, the portio is covered by a thickened, white, and wrinkled epithelial membrane. Most patients with diffuse hyperkeratosis have prolapsed uteri. Microscopically, the whitish plaque corresponds to the presence of a thick keratin layer, which is referred to as hyperkeratosis (Figure 6.3). When pyknotic nuclei are found within the keratin layer, the term parakeratosis is used (Figure 6.4). The epithelium is often acanthotic with a well-developed granular layer, prominent intercellular bridges, and elongated rete pegs. Characteristically, the epithelial cells contain sparse glycogen but cytologic atypicality is absent, whether associated with chronic cervicitis or not. There is neither morphologic nor clinical indication that either hyperkeratosis or parakeratosis represents precursor lesions to cervical neoplasia. However, it should be emphasized that hyperkeratosis or parakeratosis may be a feature of cervical intraepithelial neoplasia or invasive carcinoma, and so all clinical white plaques on the portio vaginalis or vaginal epithelium, should be biopsied. The precise mechanism of hyperkeratosis is not well understood. The fine structural organization of the keratin layer and underlying epithelial cells is normal. There is no evidence of defective formation of desmosomal attachments, which would lead to precocious or accelerated desquamation. Increased mitotic activity and double-nucleated epithelial cells are not observed, suggesting that hyperkeratosis occurs in response to exaggerated keratin formation and that there is a relative decrease in its desquamation instead of an increase in the turnover rate of epithelial cells.[24]

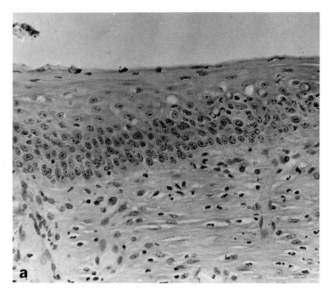

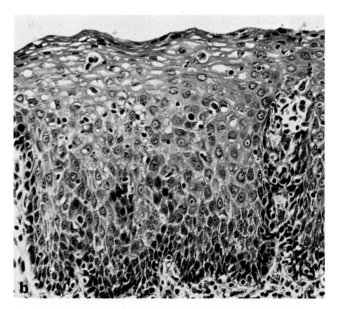

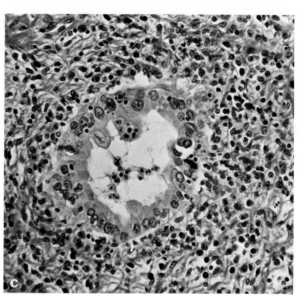

**6.1** Atypia (anaplasia) of repair. **a.** Basal cell hyperplasia involving the lower one-third of the squamous epithelium of the cervix. The nuclei contain prominent chromocenters but lack nuclear abnormalities associated with neoplasia. The epithelial cells above the enlarged basal zone display normal maturation. These alterations are often associated with mucosal denudation caused either by trauma or by severe inflammation. **b.** Trichomonas cervicitis. The epithelium exhibits intercellular edema, elongation of rete pegs, and poor glycogenization. The lower half is occupied by parabasal-type cells with prominent nucleoli and intercellular bridges. Both the epithelium and the stromal papillae are infiltrated by acute inflammatory cells. **c.** Trichomonas cervicitis. Endocervical epithelium exhibiting nuclear enlargement, mitosis, microabscesses, and inconspicuous intracellular mucus. Note the diffuse distribution of nuclear chromatin, the cytoplasmic eosinophilia, and the absence of abnormal mitoses, features distinguishing endocervical atypia of inflammation from in situ adenocarcinoma of the cervix.

## Specific Inflammations

### Herpesvirus infection

Although the precise incidence of cervical *Herpes simplex* virus infection (herpes genitalis) is not known, it is far greater than generally recognized.[5,6,49] This is because a large number of patients experience mild symptoms or no symptoms at all. It has been shown, however, that 9% of patients seen in private gynecologic practice and 22% of those seen in hospital's out-patient gynecologic clinics have positive serology for *Herpes simplex* virus type 2 (HSV-2) infection.[5,6] Genital herpesvirus infections are caused most commonly by the type 2 strain, but approximately 13% are caused by herpesvirus type 1 (HSV-1).[50] Both have several common features, including architecture, size, envelope, mode of multiplication, and double-stranded DNA genetic content. However, type 1 is chiefly found in the oropharyngeal region (herpes buccalis) and has different biologic and epidemiologic properties from type 2 virus.[50] HSV-2 has been identified as a human,

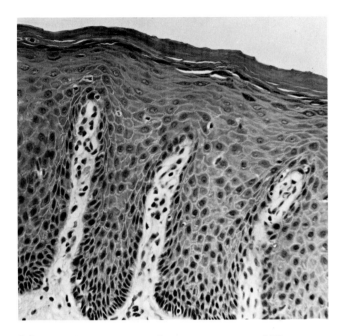

**6.3** Hyperkeratosis. Histologic appearance of Figure 6.2. A prominent keratin layer covers the epithelium of the portio.

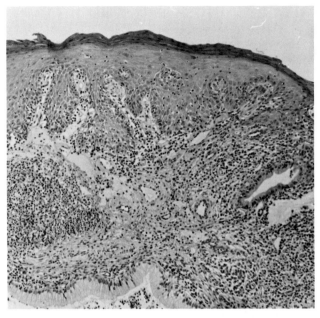

**6.4** Parakeratosis. Within the keratin layer are pyknotic nuclei. The epithelium and the subjacent stroma are infiltrated by chronic inflammatory cells.

DNA-containing virus, a member of the poxvirus group. The virus can be demonstrated by neutralizing antibodies, serologic techniques,[5,6] and viral growth in monkey kidney and human amnionic cells. It can also be grown on the chorioallantoic membrane of chick embryos. Ultrastructurally,[50,72] the *Herpes simplex* virions measure 150 nm (1 nm = $10^{-9}$ m) in diameter. They are surrounded by a protein-containing, hexagonal capsid of about 100 nm in diameter. The capsid, in turn, is enveloped by an inner glycoprotein-rich and an outer lipid-rich membrane of about 150 to 200 nm (Figure 6.5). Viral particles are thought to replicate within the host cell nuclei, where they interfere with normal biosynthetic activity and membrane functions and modify the host cell to synthesize viral proteins that are necessary for replication of viral DNA.[72] HSV-2 is acquired through sexual contact and most patients are teenage or unmarried women. Primary herpetic infections produce symptoms within 3 to 7 days after exposure, principally severe vulvar pain, tenderness and painful urination, and profuse watery vaginal discharge.[38] The symptoms of recurrent herpes genitalis are comparatively less severe than those experienced during the primary infection. The disease is characterized by the development of multiple, painful vesicles involving the vulva, perineum, vagina, and cervix. These are rapidly trans-

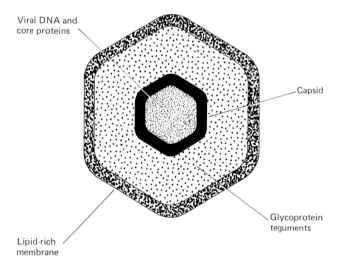

Viral DNA and core proteins

Capsid

Glycoprotein teguments

Lipid-rich membrane

**6.5** Drawing of a virion of *Herpes simplex* virus, type 2.

formed into shallow and painful ulcerations. Occasionally, the ulceronecrotic process is so extensive as to produce a fungating, necrotic mass on the cervical portio, which can be mistaken for carcinoma.[68] Herpesvirus infection may be diagnosed by cervical cultures, by neutralizing antibodies serology, and in Papanicolaou smears.[51] In the latter, large multinucleated cells with the characteristic intranuclear "ground-glass" viral inclusions are observed. Occasionally, during the vesicular phase, a biopsy may reveal the presence of suprabasal intraepidermal vesicles filled with serum, degenerated epidermal cells, and multinucleated giant cells, some of them containing eosinophilic, intranuclear inclusions surrounded by a clear halo (Figure 6.6). Herpes genitalis has two important implications for the clinician. First, it may result in spontaneous abortion, fetal morbidity, and mortality. Second, evidence is now accumulating that suggests a close association between HSV type 2 infections of the female genital tract and the genesis of cervical carcinoma (see Chapter 7).

### Tuberculous cervicitis

Tuberculosis of the cervix[18,55,65,67] is almost invariably secondary to tuberculous salpingitis and endometritis, with and occasionally without[18,55] accompanying pulmonary tuberculosis. The incidence of cervical tuberculosis in a population with genital tuberculosis varies between 2 and 60% with an incidence rate of 5% in the United States.[65] There are no macroscopic alterations in the cervix that are specific for tuberculous infection. The cervix may appear normal or inflamed or may resemble invasive carcinoma. Histologically tuberculous infection of the cervix is recognized by the presence of multiple granulomata or tubercles. These are characterized by central caseous necrosis surrounded by epithelioid histiocytes and multinucleated giant cells of Langhans, in which the nuclei are distinctively distributed at the periphery of the cytoplasm. The periphery of the tubercle is made of a heavy lymphoplasmocytic infiltrate (Figure 6.7). It should be emphasized that tuberculous cervicitis often presents as a non-caseating granulomatous lesion and that caseating-like granulomata other than tuberculosis (lymphogranuloma venerum, sarcoidosis) may be encountered in the cervix. Therefore, the unequivocal diagnosis requires demonstration of acid-fast *Mycobacterium tuberculosis,* a straight, rod-shaped bacillus either in sections stained with the Ziehl–Neelsen technique or by culture or animal inoculation of cervical tissue. Because culture or inoculation yields far better results than staining of tissue sections, unfixed biopsy material should be obtained for microbiology whenever tuberculosis is suspected. The most common granulomatous lesions that are to be distinguished from tuberculous cervicitis include foreign body giant cell granulomata to suture, crystal, or cotton; lymphogranuloma venerum; schistosomiasis; and sarcoidosis.

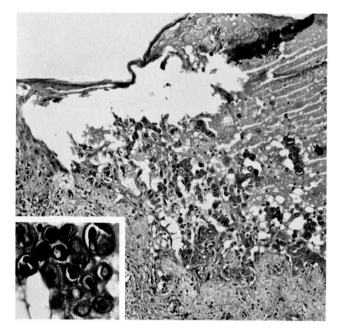

**6.6** Suprabasal herpetic vesicle in squamous epithelium of the portio. Inset: High-power view of acantholytic intravesicular epithelial cells with "ground-glass" intranuclear viral inclusions.

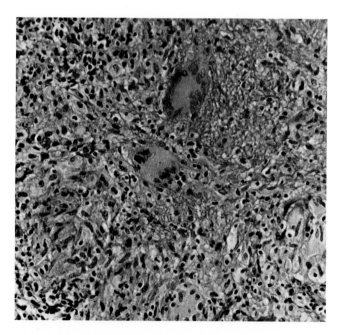

**6.7** Tuberculous cervicitis. Typical granuloma with palisading epithelioid cells, multinucleated Langhans giant cells, and central caseous necrosis. Acid-fast stain for *Mycobacterium tuberculosis* was positive.

OTHER GRANULOMATOUS INFECTIONS. Certain venereally transmitted diseases that are commonly encountered in the vulva may also involve the cervix. These include syphilis, either as the primary chancre, secondary mucous patches, or tertiary gumma[16,18,26]; lymphogranuloma venerum[18]; granuloma inguinale[7,18,59]; and chancroid.[26] All of these conditions may resemble carcinoma clinically. In addition to characteristic morphologic features, there are specific bacteriologic and immunologic techniques available for identifying each of these diseases (see Chapter 2).

### Diphtheritic cervicitis

Diphtheritic cervicitis, caused by *Corynebacterium diphtheriae,* has been recorded in association with vaginal diphtheria.[8,26] Characteristically, the portio is covered with a firmly adherent frosty white membrane.

### Parasitic infections

Rare instances of parasitic infestations, such as echinococcis or hydatid cysts[43,48] and ulceronecrotic amebiasis[15] (Figure 6.8), have been encountered in the cervix. However, schistosomiasis (bilharziasis) of the cervix,[9,22] generally caused by *Schistosoma haematobium* and occasionally by *S. mansoni,* is prevalent in Africa (Egypt), South America, Puerto Rico, and several Asian countries. A large number of cases of cervical schistosomiasis are associated with urinary schistosomiasis and sterility. The latter condition is presumably related to increased *Schistosoma*-stimulated antispermatozoal antibodies.[22] Microscopically, noncaseating granulomata (pseudotubercles) with ova surrounded by multinucleated giant cells are seen (Figure 6.9), and the ova are often calcified. The *S. mansoni* type has a long lateral spine, whereas the *S. haematobium* has a short spine extending from one of its poles. Cervical schistosomiasis may be associated with extensive pseudoepitheliomatous hyperplasia of the covering cervical squamous mucous membrane, masquerading both clinically and histologically as verrucous carcinoma.

### Actinomycosis

Actinomycosis infection of the female genital organs, including the cervix[26,61] is caused by *Actinomycosis israelii* (*bovis*) and results from surgical instrumentation, clinical abortion, intrauterine contraceptive devices, and direct extension from parametrial and appendiceal lesions, or from the anus. Until 1972 there were approximately 300

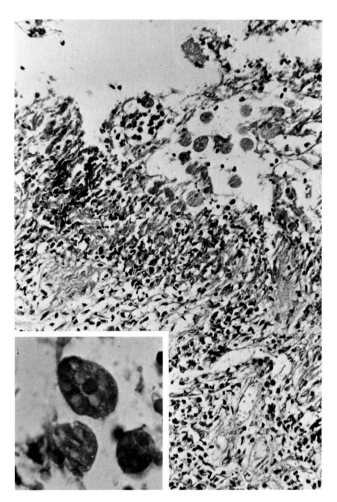

**6.8** Ulceronecrotic amebiasis of cervix with numerous amebae in the superficial exudate. Inset: Detail view of *Entamoeba histolytica* with vacuolated cytoplasm.

cases of genital actinomycosis reported in the literature.[61] The diagnosis is made by demonstrating the fungus granules in the center of large abscesses. The granules are composed of branching, gram-positive filaments with peripheral palisading clubs (Figure 6.10). The granules appear yellow to the naked eye; hence the term "sulfur granules."

### Cervicovaginitis emphysematosa

This unusual disease is characterized by multiple blue-gray subepithelial cysts of the portio vaginalis and vagina.[2,28,73] The cause of this condition is unknown but it is often associated with trichomoniasis.[28,73] Gas-forming

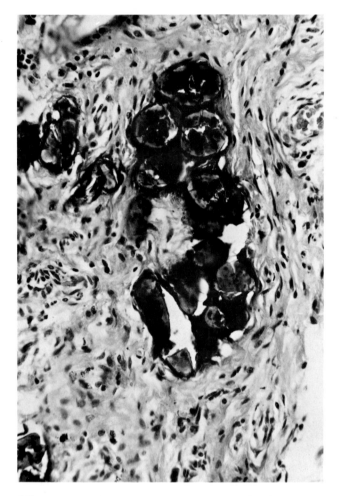

**6.9** Cervical schistosomiasis. Note calcified *Schistosoma hematobium* ova.

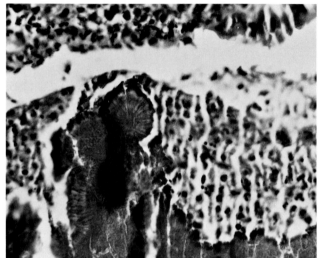

**6.10** Actinomycosis in endocervix. Portion of actinomycotic "sulfur" granules in pus with felted mycelium and peripheral palisading clubs.

[Courtesy of Dr. J. Haddad, St. Clare's Hospital, New York.]

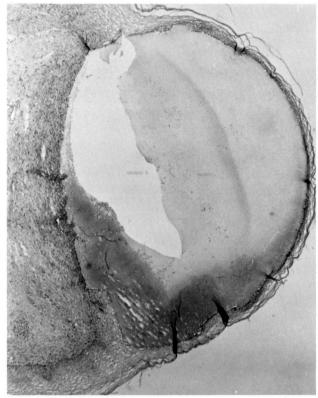

**6.11** Suprabasal, intraepithelial vesicle with blood in the portio epithelium.

bacteria have never been identified. The cysts are dilated connective tissue spaces without a lining epithelium and contain air and carbon dioxide.[28] Some of the cysts are surrounded by multinucleated foreign body giant cells and the subepithelial veins and lymphatics are often dilated. The disappearance of the disease following eradication of trichomoniasis suggests an etiologic relationship. This contention is supported by the experimental production of gas by *Trichomona vaginalis* in subcutaneous tissue of guinea pigs.[52] The high incidence of cardiovascular and pulmonary disease associated with cervicovaginitis emphysematosa may result from the high percentage of cases found at autopsy rather than an etiologic relationship.

*Herpes-like lesions*

Vesicular and bullous lesions of the cervical squamous mucous membrane, other than herpetic cervicitis, have been reported. Small, intra- and subepithelial vesicles containing blood and inflammatory exudate, but not mucus, are found in approximately 1% of cervices examined histologically[10] (Figure 6.11). The significance and pathogenesis of these vesicles are unknown, although severe inflammation associated with intracellular edema followed by focal epithelial degeneration by lytic enzymes of leukocytic origin may lead to the formation of such vesicles. Pemphigus vulgaris of the cervical squamous epithelium[39] is a rather common finding in women with generalized disease. Microscopically, there are multiple intraepithelial bullae in a suprabasal location containing the characteristic acantholytic Tzank's cells.

# Pseudotumors

*Endocervical polyps*

*Endocervical polyps*[1,18,23,26] constitute the most common newgrowths of the uterine cervix. Cervical polyps are composed of mature endocervical epithelium and are considered as focal, hyperplastic protrusions of endocervical folds, including the epithelium and substantia propria, rather than true neoplasms. The stimulus for the polypoid outgrowths is presently unknown. Cervical polyps are most often found during the fourth to sixth decades and in multigravidas.[1,23] Although many of them are symptomless, they may be a cause of profuse leukorrhea, or abnormal bleeding.[1,23] These symptoms are caused by hypersecretion of mucus by severely inflamed endocervical epithelium and ulceration of the surface epithelium, respectively. Clinically, cervical polyps are rounded or elongated structures with a smooth or lobulated surface that is often reddened because of increased vascularity (Figure 6.12, Plate VI). They are attached to the endocervical mucosa or uterine isthmus by a narrow stalk, but occasionally they have a broad base. Most polyps occur singly and measure from a few millimeters to 2 to 3 cm. In rare instances they may reach gigantic dimensions, protruding beyond the introitus and resembling carcinoma.[44,64] Various cervical lesions with a polypoid gross appearance are presented in Table 6.1. Microscopically, cervical polyps contain a variety of structural patterns that vary according to the preponderance of one or another tissue component normally found in all cervical polyps (Table 6.2). The

most common type is the endocervical mucosal or mucous polyp. It is composed of mucous-secreting epithelial infoldings and crypts, with or without cystic or adenomatous glandular changes (Figure 6.13). Occasionally they may be mainly fibrous, representing an overgrowth of the connective tissue stroma of the portio. This type of lesion is referred to as cervical fibrous polyp. When vascular structures predominate, the lesion is called vascular polyp. Squamous prosoplasia (metaplasia) involving the surface or glandular epithelium of polyps is frequently observed. These changes are not difficult to differentiate from carcinoma arising in a polyp. The supporting connective tissue of polyps is generally loose, with centrally placed "feeding" vessels, and is almost always infiltrated by chronic inflammatory exudate. Occasionally, such infiltration may be so extensive as to be the principal tissue constituent of the polyp. In these cases, a polypoid granulation tissue devoid of surface epithelium is observed (Figure 6.14). Polyps originating in the isthmus often have an admixture of endocervical- and endometrial-type epithelial components and are referred to as mixed polyps (Figure 6.15). During gestation, cervical polyps may contain focal stromal pseudodecidual changes. Rarely, massive pseudodecidualization of endocervical stroma produces a polypoid protrusion from the endocervix, the so-called true decidual polyp (Figure 6.16). In addition to decidua-like

**Table 6.1** Differential diagnosis of polypoid lesions of the cervix—macroscopy

| | |
|---|---|
| Polyps | Squamous papilloma, |
| Microglandular endocervical hyperplasia | Condylomata acuminata |
| | Papillary adenofibroma |
| Leiomyoma | Squamous cell carcinoma |
| Adenomyoma | Adenocarcinoma |
| Fibroadenoma | Sarcomas, primary or secondary |

**Table 6.2** Histologic patterns of cervical polyps

| | |
|---|---|
| Endocervical mucosal type (cervical mucous polyp) | Inflammatory type (polypoid granulation tissue) |
| Fibrous type | |
| Vascular type | Pseudodecidual type |
| Mixed endocervical-endometrial type | Pseudosarcomatous type |

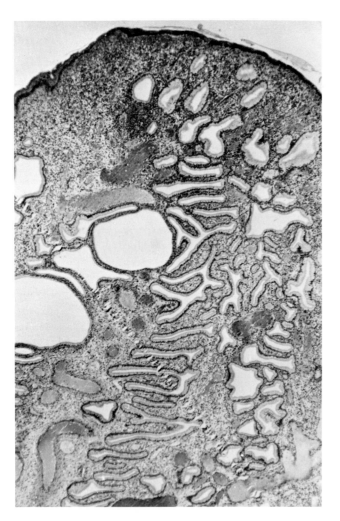

**6.13** Tip of endocervical mucous polyp.

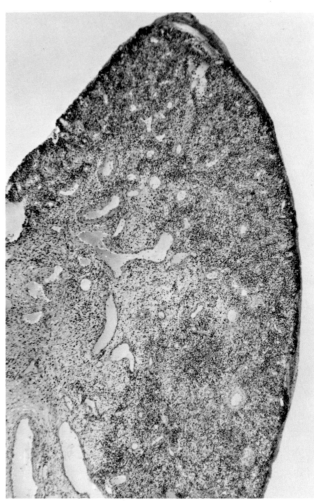

**6.14** Endocervical polyp with extensive inflammation resembling polypoid granulation tissue. This type of lesion often leads to bleeding.

cystoplasmic changes, focal areas of bizarre stromal cell reaction with irregular, hyperchromatic nuclei resembling radiation fibroblasts are seen which may simulate the subepithelial cambium layer seen in sarcoma botryoides[20,21] (Figure 6.17). Similar morphologic alterations are encountered in pseudosarcomatous botryoid polyps of the cervix[21] and vagina[56] as well as in the subepithelial myxoid stromal zone, which is often seen running from the endocervix to the vulva in adult women.[20] All these conditions are benign, most likely representing a peculiar form of stromal cell hyperplasia. Carcinoma, either *in situ* or invasive (adeno- or squamous), arising in cervical polyps is extremely rare, with an incidence of 0.2%[23] to 0.4%.[1] Endocervical polyps with adenocarcinomatous changes (Figure 6.18) must be differentiated from polypoid adenocarcinoma of the endocervix and

from endocervical polyps that are secondarily involved by adjacent adenocarcinoma. The most useful criterion for differentiating between the two conditions is to determine whether or not the base of the pedicle of the polyp is involved by carcinoma. The base of a polyp that harbors primary malignancy is free of disease and the carcinoma usually has a focal distribution within an otherwise benign polyp. In a polypoid carcinoma, the entire mass is malignant, including its base and neighboring areas. A focus of carcinoma in a cervical polyp without involvement of its base but associated with similar carcinoma in the adjacent regions should be regarded as a secondary rather than a primary focus. Adenocarcinoma confined to a polyp has an excellent prognosis.[4]

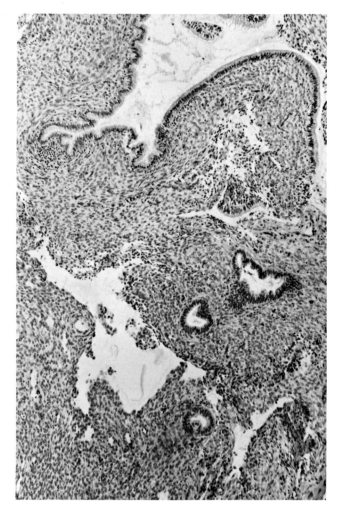

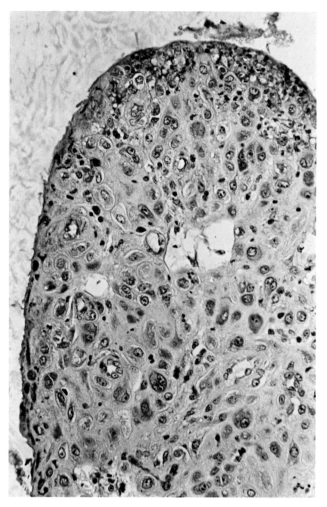

**6.15** Mixed endocervical–endometrial polyp of uterine isthmus origin. Note dense endometrial stroma with endometrial glands admixed with mucinous endocervical epithelium (top).

**6.16** True decidual polyp of cervix in pregnancy. Note typical decidual cells.

### Microglandular endocervical hyperplasia (MEH)

Among the various benign cervical lesions occurring in women receiving oral contraceptive agents,[42,45a] such as glandular hypersecretion, squamous prosoplasia (metaplasia), basal cell hyperplasia, stromal edema, and pseudodecidual reaction, MEH is considered the most important because of its possible confusion with endocervical adenocarcinoma.[70] Clinically, this benign condition most often resembles a cervical polyp measuring 1 to 2 cm in size. Some patients complain of postcoital bleeding or spotting. This distinctive endocervical lesion occurs almost without exception in women with history of oral progestin use or in pregnant or postpartum patients.[12,31,42,53,70] It is therefore considered that MEH is a reflection of progestogenic stimulation.[53] Persistence of the condition for long periods of time following discontinuation of pills or termination of pregnancy suggests that increased levels of progestogens are needed for inducing but not for maintaining the lesion.[53] Histologically, MEH may be single, polypoid, or distributed in multiple foci. It may involve the surface and/or deeper portions of endocervical clefts. Two histologic types of MEH are recognized. The most common form, termed "microglandular hyperplasia,"[12] consists of tightly packed, varying-sized glandular or tubular units lined by flattened to cuboidal cells with eosinophilic granular cytoplasm, which is generally poor in

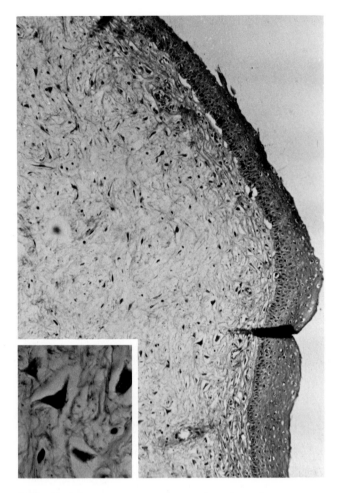

**6.17** Pseudosarcomatous "botryoid" polyp of cervix. Spindle-shaped and stellate fibroblasts are embedded in a loose myxoid stroma simulating sarcoma botryoides. Note absence of subepithelial cambium layer. Inset: High magnification of stellate atypical fibroblasts.

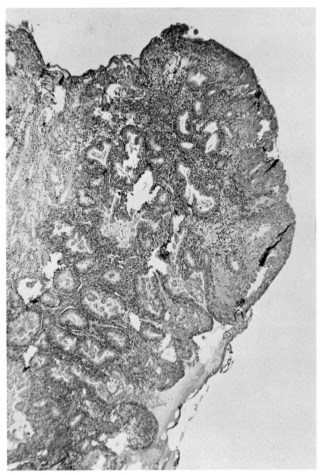

**6.18** Adenocarcinoma *in situ* within endocervical polyp. The neoplastic growth is confined to the superficial area of the polyp.

mucous content (Figure 6.19). The nuclei are uniform, with occasional pleomorphism and hyperchromasia. Associated squamous prosoplasia (metaplasia) and subcolumnar reserve cell hyperplasia are seen in a large number of cases. The second form was described by Taylor and associates[70] under the term of "atypical endocervical hyperplasia." It is this type of florid microglandular proliferation that can be mistaken for adenocarcinoma. In these lesions the glandular elements are arranged in a reticulated or solid pattern with areas of nuclear hyperchromasia and pleomorphism, features that may cause concern as to whether the lesion is malignant (Figure 6.20). However, the benign nature of

the lesion is supported by lack of stromal invasion, scant mitotic activity, and the consistently irregular nuclear morphology as compared to the inconsistently irregular nuclear pattern of endocervical adenocarcinoma. Other evidence in favor of the benign nature of atypical microglandular hyperplasia is that no patients are yet reported to have developed malignancies subsequent to the diagnosis.

*Epithelial inclusion cysts*

Epithelial inclusion cysts[26] are solitary, unilocular cystic structures measuring 1 to 2 cm in diameter and lined by nonkeratinizing squamous epithelium. Because they are found beneath the native portio epithelium, at a distance from the transformation zone, they are believed to result

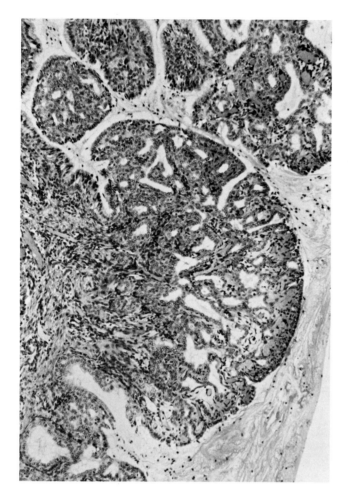

**6.19** Polypoid microglandular hyperplasia in women taking oral contraceptive. Adenomatous pattern with cuboidal lining cells and focal squamous prosoplasia.

from misplaced portio epithelium following surgical or obstetric trauma rather than from squamous prosoplasia (metaplasia) of a dilated endocervical gland.

There are 15 recorded cases in which neuroglial tissue was found in the cervix and endometrium.[54] Although the term "glioma" is used for this condition, the high degree of differentiation of the glial tissue, the absence of mitoses, and the absence of recurrence are against its being neoplastic (Figure 6.21). The lesion should not be confused with a pure heterologous sarcoma. The neural tissue is believed to represent either implantation of fetal cerebral glia at the time of instrumentation of the gravid uterus[54] or heterotopic maldevelopment during embryogenesis. When the cervix is involved, the lesion usually presents as a polyp that bleeds readily.

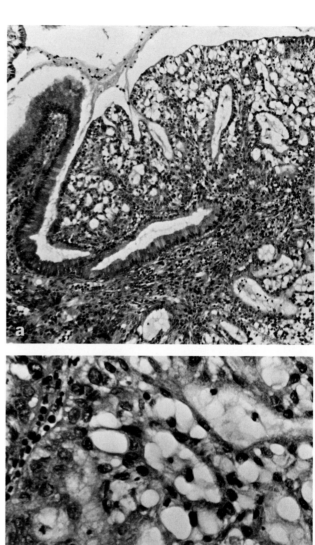

**6.20 a.** Polypoid atypical microglandular hyperplasia in women taking oral contraceptives. The lesion is made of a myriad of glandular units. The hyperplastic cells sharply contrast with adjacent normal endocervical picket cells. **b.** High magnification illustrating the reticulated pattern of atypical microglandular hyperplasia. Note extensive vacuolization, which is caused by cystic dilatation of intercellular spaces. The cells are poor in intracellular mucin.

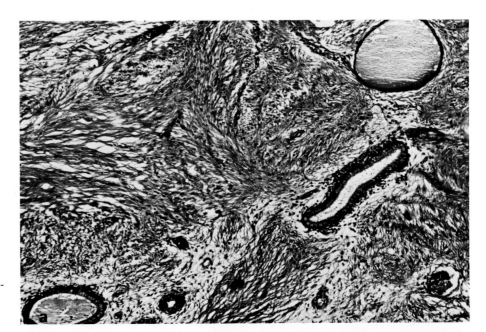

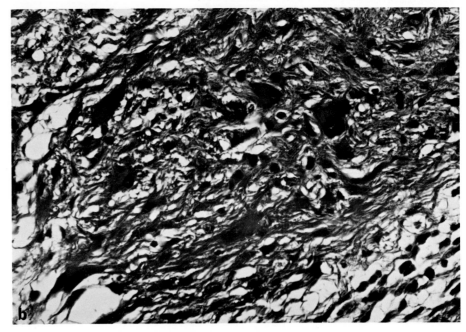

**6.21 a.** "Glioma" of the endo-cervix. Bundles of well-differentiated neuroglial tissue intermingle with normal endocervical epithelium. **b.** Detail of glial tissue with astrocytic elements.

[Courtesy of Dr. Y. Boivin, Hotel-Dieu Hospital, Montreal.]

# Benign Neoplasms

## Leiomyomas

Cervical leiomyomas, composed of interlacing bundles of smooth muscle fibers, represent about 8% of all uterine myomas.[26] They usually occur singly and produce unilateral enlargement of the cervical portio. As a result, the external os and cervical canal are markedly distorted. At times the lesion may protrude from the canal, resembling an endocervical polyp, and in pregnancy it may produce dystocia. The usual therapeutic approach to leiomyoma of the cervix is hysterectomy because they are often associated with fundal leiomyomata, but a myomectomy may be effective in isolated lesions. Cervical leiomyomata are simi-

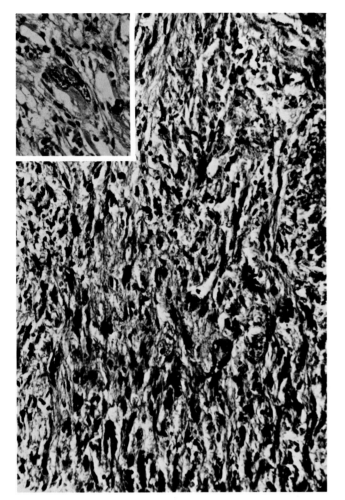

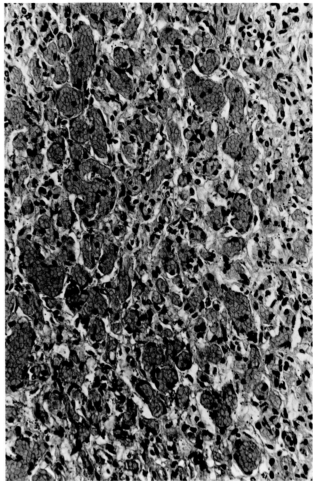

**6.22** Cellular (atypical) leiomyoma of the cervix in a pregnant woman with atypical giant cells and pleomorphism but no mitotic figures. Such neoplasms should not be interpreted as sarcoma. Inset: Detail of atypical neoplastic smooth muscle cells.

[Courtesy of Dr. B. Bigelow, Bellevue Hospital, New York.]

lar grossly, microscopically, and ultrastructurally to those observed in the myometrium, and bizarre histologic patterns, including nuclear palisading, hyalinization, and giant nuclei, may be encountered (Figure 6.22). They arise from the muscular tissue of the cervical stroma or the muscular wall of stromal blood vessels. A variant of cervical as well as myometrial leiomyomas is the so-called vascular leiomyoma. In these lesions, the muscular growth is associated with an abundance of varying-sized, thick-walled, and many times hyalinized blood vessels. Histologic continuity between the smooth muscle fibers and the muscular wall of blood vessels is often demonstrated,

**6.23** Capillary hemangioma of the cervix.

suggesting that the latter represents the source of the neoplastic growth.

### Hemangiomas

Hemangiomas are rarely found in the cervix[23,26,34,58] and may be of capillary or cavernous type. They consist of proliferating capillaries and large distended vascular channels, respectively. They are lined by endothelial cells and the lumen is filled with red blood cells (Figure 6.23). A variant of the capillary hemangioma is the so-called granuloma pyogenicum. One such case was reported in the cervix.[47] The lesion consists of a submucosal, dull red, polypoid capillary hemangioma. Because it is often inflamed it has been widely assumed to be caused by a pyogenic infection. Histologically the lesion is composed of lobules of proliferating capillaries embedded in a loose, edematous stroma. Granuloma pyogenicum occurs in the gums during pregnancy, where it is termed pregnancy tumor or granuloma gravidarum. A single instance of cervical lymphangioma was reported by Stout[69] and several cases of lipoma of the cervix are on record.[35,63] Neoplasms of neurogenic derivation arising in the cervix are extremely rare and include neurofibroma[11] and ganglioneuroma.[25] Fourteen cases of benign blue nevus of the endocervix have been reported.[37] Histologically, these lesions are indistinguishable from those arising in the dermis. They are composed of melanin-containing fusiform cells with dendritic cytoplasmic processes, located in the stroma of the endocervix. Blue nevus of the cervix is thought to be derived from the endocervical Schwann cells, which presumably may be transformed into melanocytes.[37]

### Papillomas

Papillomas of the cervix[23,29,30,32,40,46,74,76] are focal papillary outgrowths of the cervical squamous mucous membrane supported on projecting cores of fibrovascular tissue. Their growth and clinical course are benign. Papillomas constitute 0.24%[23] of all benign tumors of the uterine cervix, with the majority occurring during the childbearing ages. The high incidence of papillomas reported during pregnancy is only relative and is a reflection of the fact that pregnant patients receive comparatively more vaginal examinations than their nonpregnant counterparts. According to their number and distribution,[23,46] as opposed to their histologic appearance,[30,76] papillomas of the cervix are divided into two groups: When they are solitary, the term squamous papilloma is used; when they are multiple, either on the cervix alone or in association with similar lesions in the vulva and vagina, they are referred to as condylomata acuminata. The precise etiology of the squamous papilloma remains to be determined. Condylomata acuminata, however, are generally considered viral induced, and viral particles of the human papilloma virus type have been demonstrated by electron microscopy.[19] Although the exact mechanism of transmission is unclear, the venereal route is the most likely possibility. Grossly, condylomata are polypoid, with reddish to whitish verruciform surface and a broad base (Figure 6.24, Plate VI). Individual lesions seldom exceed 1 to 2 cm. Most large papillary growths represent locally invasive exophytic verrucous carcinomas of the cervix rather than papillomas.[29] Condylomata acuminata during pregnancy often undergo rapid enlargement with occasional occlusion of the vagina. Using microscopy, Godforth[30] and

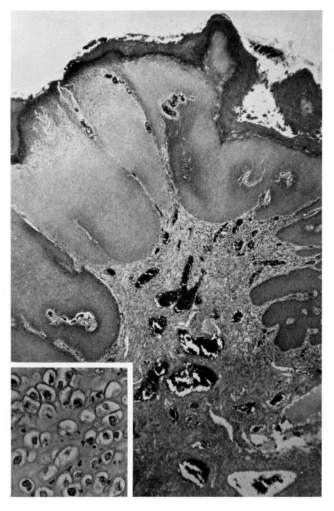

**6.25** Condyloma accuminatum of the cervix in the late stage of development. Acanthotic rete pegs converge toward the vascular base and are separated from each other by stromal papillae. Note the surface hyperkeratosis. Inset: Higher-power view of vacuolated cells with atypical nuclei in the upper strata.

Woodruff, and Peterson[76] presented histologic criteria for distinguishing condylomata acuminata from the solitary squamous papilloma. Condylomata are characterized by parakeratosis and little or no hyperkeratosis, whereas in the squamous papilloma hyperkeratosis and a well-developed granular layer are the predominant findings. Most morphologists feel, however, that there is a considerable degree of overlapping of these features, precluding accurate differentiation between the two lesions on a morphologic basis.[23,32,46] In general, in the early phase of cervical papillomas, hyperkeratosis is minimal or absent. There is evidence of extensive squamous cell hyperplasia (acantho-

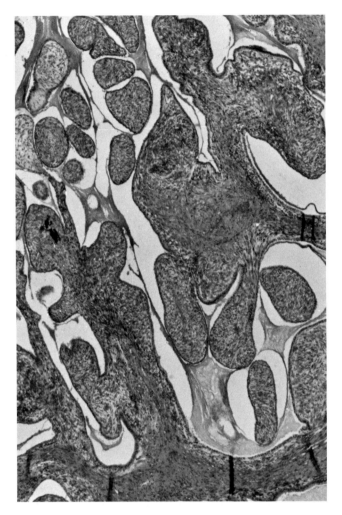

**6.26** Papillary adenofibroma of the endocervix. Fibro-epithelial papillae project into cystic spaces. The endocervical lining epithelium produces abundant mucus.

sis) with elongation and clubbing of the rete ridges, which are divided by ascending connective tissue cores (papillomatosis). The underlying connective tissue stroma is uniformly infiltrated by chronic inflammatory exudate. Characteristically, the rete ridges converge toward the vascular base of the lesion and the upper strata contain cells with mitotic figures, nuclear atypia, and intracytoplasmic vacuoles (Figure 6.25). The vacuoles result from the accumulation of large amounts of intracytoplasmic glycogen associated with central vacuolar degeneration.[24] The older lesions are usually covered by a hyperkeratotic layer associated with a thickened granular cell layer. Despite the cytonuclear atypia observed in many of these lesions, it is felt that most cervical papillomas of limited size (1 to 2 cm) are benign and should not be regarded as premalig-

nant neoplasms. The relatively high incidence of malignant transformation (5%)[40] of the larger squamous papillomas is believed to result from erroneous diagnosis. Indeed, retrospective examination of such lesions demonstrated that most of them were malignant from their inception,[23,29] most being well-differentiated verrucous carcinomas. Similarly, the danger of overdiagnosing podophyllin-treated condylomata acuminata is well known. Podophyllin-treated cells become swollen with pale cytoplasm, the nuclei appear hyperchromatic and pyknotic, and mitotic activity is increased. These changes result from podophyllin effects that include cytoplasmic edema and an arrest of mitosis in metaphase. Occasionally, larger condylomatous lesions contain surface ulceration and secondary infection associated with such severe cytologic atypia as to be indistinguishable from well-differentiated squamous cell carcinoma with a hyperkeratotic papillary surface or verrucous carcinoma. In these instances, response to therapy rather than histologic appearance seems to be the best diagnostic guide (see Chapter 9, Verrucous Carcinoma of the Cervix). Lesions reported in the past as "giant condylomata acuminata of Buschke and Lowenstein" are currently considered to be verrucous carcinomas[45] and to be unrelated to benign condylomata acuminata.

### Papillary adenofibroma

In 1971, Abell[3] described three polypoid lesions of endocervical origin that contained histologic features which were distinct from the classic endocervical polyp and its variants. The tumors consist of branching clefts and papillary excrescences lined by mucous-secreting epithelium with foci of squamous prosoplasia (metaplasia) (Figure 6.26). The epithelium is supported by a compact cellular fibrous tissue composed of spindle-shaped and stellate fibroblasts, with an occasional storiform pattern. The stroma is devoid of smooth muscle fibers and mitoses are rare. Because of their resemblance to adenofibroma of the ovary, the term papillary adenofibroma of the cervix was suggested.[3] The lesions are regarded as true benign neoplasms. Similar papillary growths have since been reported in the endometrium[33,71] and fallopian tube. The hypercellular stromal component of papillary adenofibroma may resemble cervical stromal sarcoma. However, the latter is usually not papillary, and in it the nuclei are pleomorphic and mitoses are frequent. Although a focus of adenocarcinoma has been found[71] in one case of papillary adenofibroma of the endometrium, to date all the patients are alive and well. Papillary adenofibroma of the female reproductive tract including the cervix occurs ex-

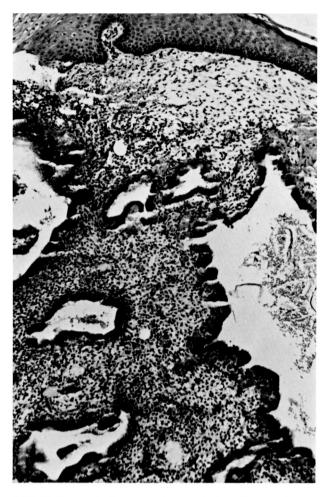

**6.27** Endometriosis containing typical endometrial glands and stroma subjacent to the squamous portio epithelium.

[Courtesy of A. Blaustein, New York University Medical Center, New York.]

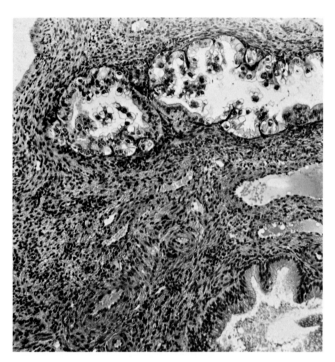

**6.28** Arias–Stella reaction in the gestational endocervix. Such cellular changes should not be confused with clear cell adenocarcinoma of the cervix.

clusively in menopausal and postmenopausal women. Papillary adenofibroma must also be distinguished from its malignant counterpart, the so-called Müllerian adenosarcoma.[14] In this lesion, there is increased mitotic activity in the stromal elements.

### Adenomyoma and fibroadenoma

These neoplasms are composed of an admixture of fibroconnective tissue and smooth muscle elements intermingling with mucous-secreting endocervical epithelium.[23] Depending on the predominance of the fibrous or muscular tissue component, they are classified as fibroade-

noma or adenomyoma. These lesions are rare and probably represent variants of cervical leiomyoma. Because of their large size (up to 6 cm) and polypoid configuration, they must be distinguished from polypoid endocervical stromal sarcoma or malignant mixed mesodermal tumor.

### Mesonephric papilloma of children

Rare instances of benign, papillary growths of the cervix in children have been described.[36,66] They are composed of complex papillary projections lined by flat cuboidal epithelium with cores of loose fibrovascular tissue. Cytologic atypia and mitoses are absent. The lesions are thought to be of mesonephric duct origin, although they have not been encountered in association with mesonephric remnants.

### Endometriosis

The term endometriosis refers to lesions that are composed of aberrant endometrial glands and stroma. Endometriosis of the cervix is not as uncommon as originally believed[57,62,75] and may occur on the portio or in the endocervical canal.[23,27,57,62,75] Endometriotic lesions of the endocervix are incidental findings in hysterectomy or cervicectomy specimens. Most areas of endometriosis of the exocervix appear as one or more small blue or red nodules, measuring a few millimeters in diameter. Occasionally, however, the lesion may be larger or cystic and may produce abnormal vaginal bleeding. Histologically, the glands and stroma are identical with the endometrium. The glands as well as the stroma usually have a proliferative pattern (Figure 6.27) but may contain pools of extravasated red blood cells, or respond to hormonal stimuli with differentiation into secretory glands and pseudodecidua.

During pregnancy, the ectopic glands occasionally exhibit gestational Arias–Stella reaction (Figure 6.28). The development of cervical endometriosis is best explained by Samson's implantation theory.[62] According to this theory, endometrial tissue is implanted into the cervical mucosa or submucosa following postmenstrual cauterization[57,62] or during delivery. Clinically, bleeding endometriosis of the portio may be confused with primary carcinoma or metastatic choriocarcinoma. A biopsy, however, will establish the benign nature of the lesion. Hemorrhagic Nabothian cysts and inflamed gestational pseudodecidua may also masquerade as endometriosis. A case of adenocarcinoma arising within cervical endometriosis has been reported.[13]

# ACKNOWLEDGMENT

This work was aided by Grant MA5137 from the Medical Research Council of Canada.

# REFERENCES

1. Aaro, L. A., Jacobson, L. J., and Soule, E. H. Endocervical polyps. *Obstet. Gynecol. 21*:659, 1963.

2. Abell, M. R. Cervicocolpitis (vaginitis) emphysematosa. *Surg. Gynecol. Obstet. 107*:631, 1958.

3. Abell, M. R. Papillary adenofibroma of the uterine cervix. *Am. J. Obstet. Gynecol. 110*:990, 1971.

4. Abell, M. R., and Gosling, J. R. G. Gland cell carcinoma (adenocarcinoma) of the uterine cervix. *Am. J. Obstet. Gynecol. 83*:729, 1962.

5. Adam, E., Kaufman, R. H., Melnick, J. L., Levy, A. H., and Rawls, W. E. Seroepidemiologic studies of herpesvirus type 2 and carcinoma of the cervix. III. Houston, Texas, *Am. J. Epidemiol., 96*:427, 1972.

6. Adam, E., Kaufman, R. H., Melnick, J. L., Levy, A. H., and Rawls, W. E. Seroepidemiologic studies of herpesvirus type 2 and carcinoma of the cervix. IV. Dysplasia and carcinoma in situ. *Am. J. Epidemiol., 98*:77, 1973.

7. Adams, J. Q., and Packer, H. Granuloma inguinale of the cervix. *South. Med. J. 48*:27, 1955.

8. Beacham, W. D., and Rice, M. Diphtheria of the uterine cervix. *Am. J. Obstet. Gynecol. 47*:417, 1944.

9. Berry, A. A cytopathological and histopathological study of bilharziasis of the female genital tract. *J. Pathol. Bacteriol. 91*:325, 1966.

10. Burd, L. I., and Esterly, J. R. Vesicular lesions of the uterine cervix. *Am. J. Obstet. Gynecol. 110*:887, 1971.

11. Busby, J. G. Neurofibromatosis of the cervix. *Am. J. Obstet. Gynecol. 63*:674, 1952.

12. Candy, J., and Abell, M. R. Progestogen-induced adenomatous hyperplasia of the uterine cervix. *JAMA 203*:323, 1968.

13. Chang, S. H. and Maddox, W. A. Adenocarcinoma arising within cervical endometriosis and invading the adjacent vagina. *Am. J. Obstet. Gynecol. 110*:1015, 1971.

14. Clement, P. B., and Scully, R. E. Müllerian adenosarcoma of the uterus. *Cancer 34*:1138, 1974.

15. Cohen, C. Three cases of amoebiasis of the cervix uteri. *J. Obstet. Gynaecol. Brit. Commonw. 80*:476, 1973.

16. Crossen, R. J. A case of gumma of cervix. *Am. J. Obstet. Gynecol. 19*:708, 1930.

17. Danforth, D. N., Veis, A., Breen, M., Weinstein, H. G., Buckingham, J. C., and Manalo, P. The effect of pregnancy and labor in the human cervix: Changes in collagen, glycoproteins, and glycosaminoglycans. *Am. J. Obstet. Gynecol. 120*:641, 1974.

18. Dougherty, C. M., Moore, W. R., and Cotten, N. Histologic diagnosis and clinical significance of benign lesions of the nonpregnant cervix. *Ann. N.Y. Acad. Sci. 97*:683, 1962.

19. Dun, A. E. G., and Ogilvie, M. M. Intranuclear virus particles in human genital wart tissue: Observation on the ultrastructure of the epidermal layer. *J. Ultrastruct. Res. 22*:282, 1968.

20. Elliott, G. B., and Elliott, J. D. A. Superficial stromal reactions of lower genital tract. *Arch. Pathol. 95*:100, 1973.

21. Elliott, G. B., Reynolds, H. A., and Fidler, H. K. Pseudosarcoma botryoides of cervix and vagina in pregnancy. *J. Obstet. Gynaecol. Brit. Commonw. 74*:728, 1967.

22. El-Mahgoub, S. Antispermatozoal antibodies in infertile women with cervicovaginal schistosomiasis. *Am. J. Obstet. Gynecol. 112*:781, 1972.

23. Farrar, H. K. Jr., and Nedoss, B. R. Benign tumors of the uterine cervix. *Am. J. Obstet. Gynecol. 81*:124, 1961.

24. Ferenczy, A., and Richart, R. M. *Female Reproductive System. Dynamics of Scan and Transmission Electron Microscopy,* 1st ed. New York, John Wiley & Sons, 1974.

25. Fingerland, A., and Sikl, H. Ganglioneuroma of cervix uteri. *J. Pathol. Bacteriol. 47*:631, 1938.

26. Fluhman, C. F. *The Cervix Uteri and Its Diseases,* 1st ed. Philadelphia, W. B. Saunders, 1961.

27. Gardner, H. L. Cervical and vaginal endometriosis. *Clin. Obstet. Gynecol. 9*:358, 1966.

28. Gardner, H. L., and Fernet, P. Etiology of vaginitis emphysematosa. *Am. J. Obstet. Gynecol. 88*:680, 1964.

29. Gilbert, E. F., and Palladino, A. Squamous papillomas of the uterine cervix: review of the literature and report of a giant papillary carcinoma. *Am. J. Clin. Pathol. 46*:115, 1966.

30. Godforth, J. L. Polyps and papillomas of the cervix uteri. *Texas State J. Med. 49*:81, 1953.

31. Govan, A. D. T., Black, W. P., and Sharp, J. L. Aberrant glandular polypi of the uterine cervix associated with contraceptive pills: pathology and pathogenesis. *J. Clin. Pathol. 22*:84, 1969.

32. Greene, R. R., and Peckham, B. M. Squamous papillomas of the cervix. *Am. J. Obstet. Gynecol.* 67:883, 1954.

33. Grimalt, M., Argueles, M., and Ferenczy, A. Papillary cystadenofibroma of endometrium. A histochemical and ultrastructural study. *Cancer* 36:137, 1975.

34. Gusdon, J. T. Hemangioma of the cervix. *Am. J. Obstet. Gynecol.* 91:204, 1965.

35. Henriksen, E. Lipoma of the uterus. Report of 3 cases. *West. J. Surg.* 60:609, 1952.

36. Janovski, M. S., and Kasdon, E. J. Benign mesonephric papillary and polypoid tumors of the cervix in childhood. *J. Pediatr.* 63:211, 1963.

37. Jiji, V. Blue nevus of the endocervix. Review of literature. *Arch. Pathol.* 92:203, 1971.

38. Kaufman, R. H., Gardner, H. L., Rawls, W. E., Dixon, R. E., and Young, R. L. Clinical features of herpes genitalis. *Cancer Res.* 33:1446, 1973.

39. Kaufman, R. H., and Watts, J. M., and Gardner, H. L. Pemphigus vulgaris genital involvement. *Obstet. Gynecol.* 33:264, 1969.

40. Kistner, R. W., and Hertig, A. T. Papillomas of the uterine cervix—their malignant potentiality. *Obstet. Gynecol.* 6:147, 1955.

41. Koss, L. G., and Wolinska, W. H. Trichomonas vaginalis cervicitis and its relationship to cervical cancer; a histocytological study. *Cancer* 12:1171, 1959.

42. Kyriakos, M., Kempson, R. L., and Konikor, N. F. A clinical and pathologic study of endocervical lesions associated with oral contraceptives. *Cancer* 22:99, 1968.

43. Langley, G. F. Primary echinococcal cyst of the uterus. *Br. J. Surg.* 30:278, 1943.

44. Lippert, L. J., Richart, R. M., and Ferenczy, A. Giant benign endocervical polyp: Report of a case. *Am. J. Obstet. Gynecol.* 118:1140, 1974.

45. Lucas, W. E., Benirschke, K., and Lebherz, T. B. Verrucous carcinoma of the female genital tract. *Am. J. Obstet. Gynecol.* 119:435, 1974.

45a. Maqueo, M., Azuela, J. C., Calderon, J. J., and Goldzieher, J. W. Morphology of the cervix in women treated with synthetic progestins. *Am. J. Obstet. Gynecol.* 96:994, 1966.

46. Marsh, M. R. Papilloma of the cervix. *Am. J. Obstet. Gynecol.* 64:281, 1952.

47. Morehead, R. P., Woodruff, W. D., Thomas, W. C., and Winston-Salem, N. C. Granuloma pyogenicum of the cervix. *Am. J. Obstet. Gynecol.* 47:546, 1944.

48. Murray, H. L. Hydatid cyst of the cervix uteri. *Lancet* 1:911, 1926.

49. Nahmias, A. J., Dowdle, W. R., Naib, Z., Josey, W., McClone, D., and Domescik, G. Genital infection with type 2 herpes virus hominis. A commonly occurring venereal disease. *Br. J. Vener. Dis.* 45:294, 1969.

50. Nahmias, A. J., and Roizman, B. Infection with *Herpes-simplex* viruses 1 and 2. *N. Engl. J. Med.* 289:667, 719, 781, 1973.

51. Naib, Z. M., Nahmias, A. J., and Josey, W. E. Cytology and histopathology of cervical *Herpes simplex* infection. *Cancer* 19:1026, 1966.

52. Newton, W. L., Reardon, L. V., and DeLeva, A. M. A comparative study of the subcutaneous innoculation of germ free and conventional guinea pigs with two strains of *Trichomonas vaginalis. Am. J. Trop. Med. Hyg.* 9:56, 1960.

53. Nichols, T. M., and Fidler, H. K. Microglandular hyperplasia in cervical cone biopsies taken for suspicious and positive cytology. *Am. J. Clin. Pathol.* 56:424, 1971.

54. Niven, P. A. R., and Stansfeld, A. G. "Glioma" of the uterus. A fetal homograft. *Am. J. Obstet. Gynecol.* 115:534, 1973.

55. Nogales, F., and Vilar, E. Etude chimique et thérapeutique de la tuberculose du col utérin. (Travail basé sur l'étude de 102 cas). *Rev. Franç. Gynecol.* 52:275, 1957.

56. Norris, H. J., and Taylor, H. B. Polyps of the vagina: A benign lesion resembling sarcoma botryoides. *Cancer* 19:226, 1966.

57. Overton, D. H., Wilson, R. B., and Dockerty, M. B. Primary endometriosis of the cervix. *Am. J. Obstet. Gynecol.* 79:768, 1960.

58. Pedowitz, P. Vascular tumors of the uterus. *Am. J. Obstet. Gynecol.* 69:1291, 1955.

59. Pund, E. R., and Greenblatt, R. B. Granuloma venerum of cervix uteri (granuloma inguinale) simulating carcinoma. *JAMA* 108:1401, 1937.

60. Richart, R. M. Cervical intraepithelial neoplasia, in Sommers, C. C. ed.: *Pathology Annual.* New York, Appleton-Century-Crofts, 1973, pp. 301–328.

61. Richter, G. A., Pratt, J. H., Nichols, D. R., and Coulam, C. B. Actinomycosis of the female genital organs. *Minn. Med.* 55:1003, 1972.

62. Ridley, J. H. The histogenesis of endometriosis. A review of facts and fancies. *Obstet. Gynecol. Surv.* 23:1, 1968.

63. Rilke, F., and Cantaboni, A. Lipomas of the uterus. Presentation of 2 cases and review of the recent literature. *Ann. Ostet. Gynecol.* 86:645, 1964.

64. Saier, F. L., Hovadhanakul, P., and Ostapowicz, F. Giant cervical polyp. *Obstet. Gynecol.* 41:94, 1973.

65. Schaefer, C. Tuberculosis of female genital tract. *Clin. Obstet. Gynecol.* 13:965, 1970.

66. Selzer, F., and Nelson, H. M. Benign papilloma (polypoid tumor) of the cervix uteri in children; report of two cases. *Am. J. Obstet. Gynecol.* 84:165, 1962.

67. Sered, H., Falls, F. H., and Zummo, F. H. Recent trends in management of tuberculosis of the cervix. *J. Int. Coll. Surg.* 20:409, 1953.

68. Stein, B. J., and Siciliano, A. Necrotizing *Herpes simplex* viral infection of the cervix during pregnancy: Mimic of squamous cell carcinoma. *Am. J. Obstet. Gynecol.* 94:249, 1966.

69. Stout, A. P. Hemangio-endothelioma: A tumor of blood vessels featuring vascular endothelial cells. *Ann. Surg.* 118:445, 1943.

70. Taylor, H. B., Irey, N. S., and Norris, H. J. Atypical endocervical hyperplasia in women taking oral contraceptives. *JAMA* 202:637, 1967.

71. Vellios, F., Ng, A. B. P., and Reagan, J. W. Papillary adenofibroma of the uterus. A benign mesodermal mixed tumor of Müllerian origin. *Am. J. Clin. Pathol.* 60:543, 1973.

72. Wagner, E. K. The replication of herpesvirus. *Am. Sci.* 62:584, 1974.

73. Wilbanks, G. D., and Carter, B. Vaginitis emphysematosa. *Obstet. Gynecol.* 22:301, 1963.

74. Wolfe, S. A. Papilloma of the cervix. *Am. J. Obstet. Gynecol.* 60:448, 1950.

75. Wolfe, S. A., Mackles, A., and Greene, H. J. Endometriosis of the cervix. *Am. J. Obstet. Gynecol.* 81:111, 1961.

76. Woodruff, J. D., and Peterson, W. F. Condylomata acuminata of the cervix. *Am. J. Obstet. Gynecol.* 75:1354, 1958.

Alex Ferenczy, M.D.

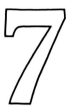

# Cervical Intraepithelial Neoplasia

## Terminology and Definitions

The precursors to invasive squamous cell (epidermoid) carcinoma of the cervix are among the most extensively studied lesions occurring in women. The studies have been facilitated by the anatomic location of the organ, which is readily accessible to both clinical and morphologic investigations without significant danger to the patient, and by the high rate of cervical cancer precursors, providing a generous source of supply of study material. Despite such advantages for investigations, there are considerable differences of opinion regarding the natural history of preinvasive cervical neoplasia. Most of these controversies are attributable to differences in definitions and terminology of the disease as well as to differences in techniques of investigation and methods of data analysis.

Traditionally, among the various forms of epithelial abnormalities of the cervix, lesions designated as "carcinoma in situ" (CIS) were regarded as representing the precursor stage of invasive cervical carcinoma. In 1961, at the First International Congress on Exfoliative Cytology, the Committee on Histological Terminology for Lesions of the Uterine Cervix[74] defined carcinoma *in situ* as follows: "Only those cases should be classified as carcinoma in situ which, in the absence of invasion, show as surface lining epithelium in which, throughout its whole thickness, no differentiation takes place. The process may involve the lining of the cervical glands without thereby creating a new group. It is recognized that the cells of uppermost layers may show some slight flattening. The very rare case of an otherwise characteristic carcinoma in situ which shows a greater degree of differentiation belongs to the exceptions for which no classification can provide." Although most practicing pathologists adhere to the above definition, others, who also have vast experience in the field,[33,51,53] firmly believe that it is "too narrow and excludes from this category of lesions many that deserve to be placed there."[33] A similar opinion was expressed by the late and distinguished pathologist, Dr. Arthur Purdy Stout who wrote:[70] "In the cervix the diagnosis of carcinoma in situ is generally not made if the surface is covered by a single layer of flattened cells that are not obviously anaplastic. This has always seemed to me to be a very arbitrary decision. If the anaplastic cells are in fact cancer cells, then a cancerous process is present whether or not it has involved the full thickness of the mucus membrane."

Largely because of the strict morphologic standards used for the definition of CIS cytologically atypical lesions that failed to meet the full thickness dedifferentiation of the cervical epithelium remained an issue of great controversy. Some considered these lesions as precursors to CIS, whereas others were uncertain of their clinical significance; still others regarded them as harmless epithelial alterations. Accordingly, such lesions were variously being treated, followed, or ignored depending on the concepts at the institution in which they were detected. Uncertainty regarding the precise nature of these lesions is also reflected by their terminology, which includes atypical hyperplasia, basal cell hyperactivity, anaplasia, metaplasia, precanceroses, benign dysplasia, premalignant dysplasia, borderline lesions, and dysplasia. Of these names, dysplasia is currently the most widely used term. Dysplasia, from the Greek, can literally be translated as "bad molding" (dys, bad; plasia, molding), and in the context of the uterine cervix it refers to an abnormal epithelial growth without further indicating the biologic characteristics of the lesion. Later, the so-called dysplastic lesions were subdivided into very mild, mild, moderate, and severe categories, according to the extent to which undifferentiated cells occupied the full thickness of the epithelium. The 1961 Committee on Terminology[74] defined dysplasia of the cervix as: "All other (than CIS) disturbances of differentiation of the squamous epithelial lining of surface and glands are to be classified as dysplasia. They may be characterized as of high or low degree, terms which are preferable to suspicious and non-suspicious, as the proposed terms describe the histological appearance and do not express an opinion."

This definition is so broad as to encompass anything but an entirely normal cervical epithelium. As a result, diagnostic uncertainties and disagreements continued to be perpetuated among pathologists concerning the histologic distinction between the various types of intraepithelial abnormalities.

Despite the serious drawbacks of the international definitions of CIS and dysplasia, the concept of a two-disease system—carcinoma in situ and dysplasia—has become anchored in the literature. The concept that underlies the more than often fanatic diagnostic separation of dysplasia from CIS is that the latter has been established to be an intraepithelial neoplasm, which if untreated progresses to invasive cancer in 60%[6] to 70%[36] of cases. In contrast, dysplasia has not been established as the precursor of CIS. It has been claimed that dysplasias if left undisturbed either[8,33] persist or regress and seldom progress to the CIS stage.[31]

The evidence on which the separation of dysplasia from CIS is based largely derives from histologic observations and, to a lesser degree, from retro- and prospective studies, recently reviewed in detail by Patten[42] and Burghart.[8] However, most of the earlier studies suffer from several pitfalls pertaining to the histologic and cytologic criteria used for diagnosing dysplasia and CIS as well as to the diagnostic techniques employed in the followup of patients.[8,51,53] Indeed, should a review be made of published photomicrographs shown as being representative of CIS that progressed to invasive carcinoma, a surprisingly large number of these would currently be classified as dysplasia. Similarly, a good number of illustrated cases designated as mild, moderate, or severe dysplasia and reported to regress spontaneously would now be regarded as reparative epithelial atypia occurring in response to severe inflammation or injury, both of which are unrelated to cervical neoplasia. Most studies employed diagnostic cervical punch or conization biopsies in the followup of patients. The use of these techniques is of special importance, for lesions measuring less than 40 mm$^2$ can completely be excised by a single punch biopsy[71] and up to 95% of lesions may be eradicated by diagnostic conization. In addition, it has been reported that a certain proportion of lesions, even if not completely removed, may be destroyed during the process of wound healing after the punch biopsy.[35,50] When these factors are considered, it is estimated that 50% of lesions followed by surgical means have been in fact removed and presumably cured by the first or subsequent diagnostic procedures. Unfortunately, this situation was not recognized by the earlier investigators and consequently the results were erroneously interpreted as a reflection of spontaneous regression. This contention is reinforced by the strikingly lower spontaneous regression rates reported in studies in which biopsy was excluded in both the initial diagnosis and the followup observations.[54] The validity of retrospective and prospective studies in the followup of patients with cervical dysplasia and CIS can also be argued. The number of patients studied is relatively small, the precise histology of each biopsy is often not published, and the followup period of patients with dysplasia is generally too short to provide evidence of progression to CIS. Finally, the statistical analyses in interpreting long-term followup studies are inappropriate if no consideration is given to the multiple entries of patients during the period of followup observation; there is, in general, a lack of rigid morphologic ascertainment in admitting the patients to the study; and progression rates are reported as single percentages instead of by an actuarial statistical analysis.

The major clinical implication of separating carcinoma in situ from dysplasia lies in the vastly different management of the two lesions. If a patient receives a diagnosis of CIS, she is classically treated by hysterectomy. In contrast, if undifferentiated cells do not reach the surface but have one or several layers of cells exhibiting some degree of differentiation, then the patient is either treated by conization or simply followed with cervical cytology, or in some cases entirely disregarded. The decision to remove a woman's uterus in one case or leave it intact in another is therefore essentially based on a difference in the histologic appearance of two to five layers of surface cells.

In more recent years, a variety of sophisticated clinical[23,27,54] and laboratory[32,46,55,56,60,76] experiments have appeared in the literature concerning the natural history of cervical cancer precursors and the relationship between dysplasia and carcinoma in situ. The results of the data obtained seem to be in disagreement with the traditional concepts of dysplasia and CIS of the uterine cervix. Convincing evidence has been presented for regarding lesions currently named dysplasia and CIS as part of a disease continuum or a single disease system.[51,53] It has been suggested that the continuous nature of the process be designated by a generic term, cervical intraepithelial neoplasia (CIN),[51] because the use of a compound term (dysplasia–CIS) implies a two-disease system. *CIN is defined as a spectrum of intraepithelial changes that begins as a generally well-differentiated intraepithelial neoplasm, which has traditionally been classified as very mild dysplasia, and ends with invasive carcinoma.* The CIN may or may not pass through the full spectrum of intraepithelial change, including the lesion traditionally referred to as carcinoma

in situ. The very end stage of CIN is identified when a clone (or clones) of cells is selected that breaks through the epithelial basement membrane and invades the underlying stroma (Figure 7.1). In support of the lesional continuum concept are the foregoing morphologic, laboratory, and clinical observations accumulated over the past 15 years. Light and transmission electron microscopy[60] as well as cytogenetics[32] and DNA microspectrophotometry[76] coupled with tissue culture[55,56] and radioautography[46] have shown that changes occurring in cells of dysplasia and CIS are qualitatively similar and remain constant throughout the disease spectrum. The abnormal changes observed vary quantitatively, however, depending on the stage of epithelial differentiation (Figure 7.1). Histologically, the lesions have in common cytonuclear pleomorphism, loss of cellular cohesion and maturation, and a large number of mitotic accidents. Many of the alterations in CIN cells may be related to the generation of an abnormal number of chromosomes, which corresponds to abnormal or aneuploid nuclear DNA values as determined by chromosomal examination using the direct squash technique[32] and DNA microspectrophotometry.[76] An aneuploid chromosomal content is a specific feature of non-endocrine-dependent invasive cancer cells in general and is absent in benign neoplasms. The finding of a pattern that is similar to invasive carcinoma in even the earliest form of CIN (very mild dysplasia)[76] is the strongest available evidence supporting the view that dysplastic lesions of the cervix are in fact preinvasive neoplasms. The aneuploid nuclear changes can be recognized histologically by the "irregularly irregular" nuclear configuration of CIN cells, which is associated with hyperchromasia and coarse, granular, or filamentous chromatin patterns. Radiautographic studies[46] using short-term, *in vitro* incubation techniques with tritiated thymidine, a nucleoprotein precursor, have shown a logarithmic increase in the labeling index and, presumably, in mitotic rates paralleling histologic dedifferentiation without evidence of two distinct diseases—dysplasia and CIS. The generation time (the time between two successive cell divisions) and renewal time (time necessary for the replacement of the entire cell population by new cells) are approximately 12 times greater in advanced CIN than in early CIN. The epithelium with carcinoma in situ therefore may be totally replaced every 12 hr, a finding that explains the abundance of exfoliated, undifferentiated cells in the smears obtained from patients with high-grade lesions as compared to better differentiated CIN. Fine structurally,[60] both the nuclear and cytoplasmic alterations are consistent with a progressive lack of normal differenti-

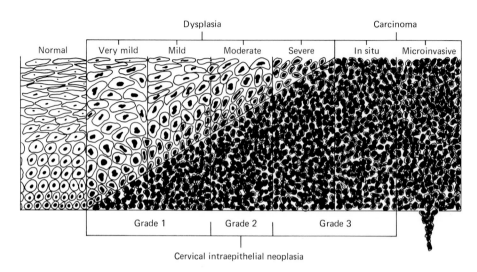

**7.1** Drawing representing cervical cancer precursors. There is a logarithmic increase in the number of malignant basal cells with increasing severity of disease. Note that the basal cells of carcinoma *in situ* are morphologically identical with those of very mild dysplasia. According to the disease continuum concept, grade 1 cervical intraepithelial neoplasia (CIN) corresponds to very mild–mild dysplasia, grade 2 to moderate dysplasia, and grade 3 to severe dysplasia–carcinoma in situ. The precursor stage ends when clones of malignant cells invade the stroma; this is microinvasive carcinoma.

ation (Figures 7.2 and 7.3). The nucleus becomes larger, resulting in a reversed nucleocytoplasmic ratio, and the nuclear chromatin undergoes segregation. The most striking ultrastructural changes are observed in free and membrane-bound ribosomes, in mitochondria, and in a decrease in glycogen and tonofilaments with increasing severity of the lesion. A gradual decrease in the number of desmosomes and specialized junctional units or nexuses (see Chapter 9, Invasive Carcinomas, Ultrastructure) is observed with increasing histologic dedifferentiation and is correlated with a progressive decrease in cellular adhesions and cell contact inhibition demonstrated by time-lapse cinematography in cells grown *in vitro*.[55,56] The surface ultrastructure of cervical cancer precursors also differs from the normal architecture,[19,77] the most outstanding feature being the absence of surface microridges and the presence of abundant microvilli (Figure 7.4). The microridges have been shown to interdigitate in apposed normal superficial cell surfaces and presumably contribute to maintain cellular integrity.[19]

Evidence that dysplasia is a neoplasm representing the early part of the disease continuum between normal cervical epithelium and invasive cervical cancer is also supported by long-term prospective clinical followup studies of patients with dysplasia.[23,27,54] The studies were based on the generally accepted concept that CIS was a precursor to invasive carinoma.[8,21,22,29,33,53] If dysplasia progresses to classical CIS, which in turn progresses to invasive carcinoma, then the original dysplastic lesion may be regarded as preinvasive carcinoma itself. In contrast to the earlier prospective analyses, the most recent investigations contain a large number of women with dysplasia ascertained initially by two or three consecutive abnormal smears and followed without biopsy, using only cytology[23,27,54] and colpomicroscopy[54] at 1- to 4-month intervals for 6[54] to 9[23] years. The major advantage of this type of approach is that patients with dysplasia can accurately be diagnosed and followed without altering the natural course of the disease. The results of these followup studies were analyzed by actuarial life-table methods[3,54] and showed that about 50% of patients with various forms of dysplasia progressed to CIS. A substantial proportion of cases that did not progress to CIS remained in the stage in which they were detected (28%), whereas the remainder progressed to a higher stage of dysplasia.[54] Although spontaneous regressions did occur, they were confined to patients with very mild dysplasia and their number was negligible (6%) compared to the progression rate values.[54]

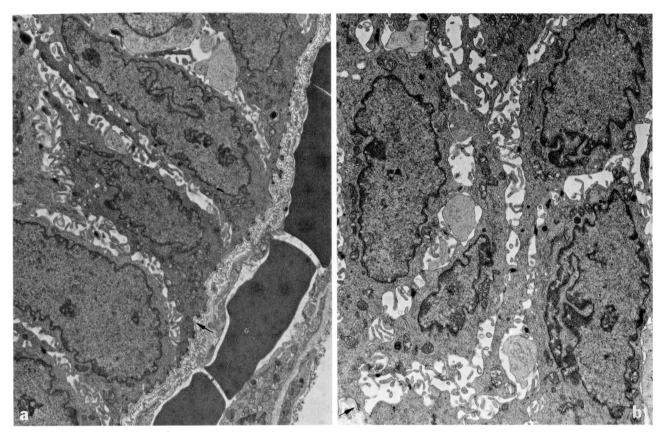

**7.2** Electron microscopic appearance of the basal cells in (**a**) grade 1 CIN (mild dysplasia) and (**b**) grade 3 CIN (carcinoma in situ). The cells contain identical ultrastructural features, including nuclear pleomorphism, convoluted nuclear membranes, and spare desmosomal attachments. The arrows point the basal lamina. A subepithelial capillary with red blood cells is seen in (**a**). **a**, ×3,973; **b**, ×5,160.

Barron and Richart[3] noted that "The results of this study indicate that dysplasia represents a subcritical process and there is, therefore, a small probability that a given clone, once established, can spontaneously vanish, die, or disappear. This probability estimated from these data appears to be very small and for the CIS (carcinoma in situ) lesion is effectively zero." The followup examinations have also shown that the rate of progression increases with increasing severity of dysplasia and that the transit time to carcinoma in situ becomes gradually shorter with increasing dedifferentiation. Therefore the probability that dysplasia progresses to CIS is directly dependent on the severity of the atypia. These observations indicate, furthermore, that lesions develop progressively from a better to a lesser differentiated state. The median transit time to CIS was approximately 7 years for very mild dysplasia, 5 years

for mild dysplasia, 3 years for moderate dysplasia, 1 year for severe dysplasia, and 4 years for all the dysplastic lesions taken together.[54] The gradual decrease in progression rates and transit time with increased severity of lesions is consistent with the clinical findings of comparatively more cases of early than advanced intraepithelial neoplasia. The data are also in agreement with epidemiologic investigations of patients with dysplasia and CIS. The prevalence (rate of disease in a population when first examined) of dysplasia proportionally decreases with advancing age, whereas that of CIS increases with age[8,29,69]; new lesions arise in the form of dysplasia instead of CIS as determined by calculations of the incidence rate[29,69] (development of new lesions in a previously screened disease-free population); and there is a thousand times higher annual incidence of CIS in women with dysplasia compared to those

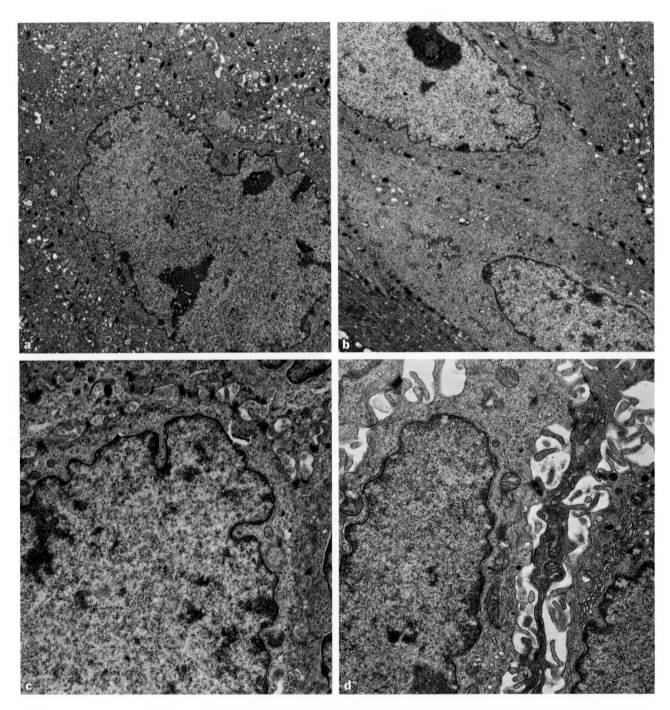

**7.3** Electron micrographs of neoplastic cells from the middle third of the epithelium in (**a**) grade 1 CIN (mild dysplasia), (**b**) grade 2 CIN (moderate dysplasia), (**c**) grade 3 CIN (severe dysplasia), and (**d**) grade 3 CIN (carcinoma in situ). The common features include increased nucleocytoplasmic ratio, irregular nuclear contour, prominent nucleoli, and abundant free and bound ribosomes. Note the gradual decrease in the number of desmosomes, tonofilaments, and glycogen particles from (**a**) to (**d**). **a**, ×5,000; **b**, ×5,000; **c**, ×10,200; **d**, ×10,200.

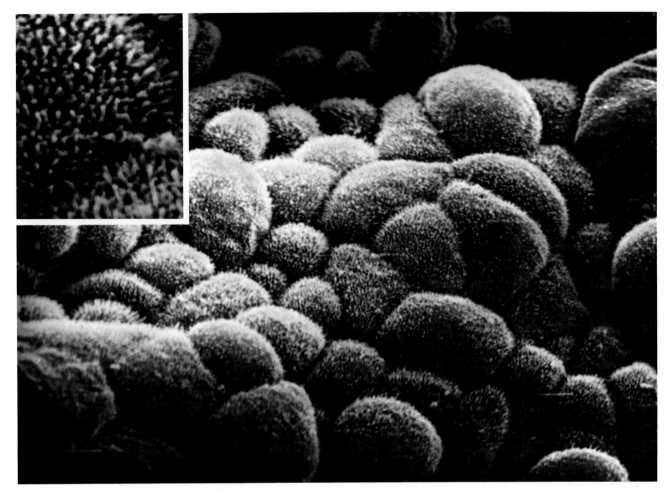

**7.4** Scanning electron microscopy of the surface of grade 3 CIN (carcinoma in situ). Note the cellular disorganization, pleomorphism, and bulging microvillous surface membranes and the lack of intercellular terminal bars. Compare this photomicrograph with Figures 5.8 and 5.36. ×2,280. Inset: Higher magnification of tightly packed surface microvilli. ×9,120.

with normal cytologic findings.[68] Animal models of chemically induced carcinogenesis of the cervix provide additional credence to the spectrum of progression of cervical neoplasia in humans. In animals, cervical lesions also develop through progressive stages of dysplasia, carcinoma in situ, and invasive carcinoma.[59]

In conclusion, the current objective data indicate that dysplasia and CIS are parts of a continuous process that precedes invasive cervical carcinoma rather than a two-stage, two-disease system. It is felt, therefore, that treatment of preinvasive cervical disease should not be based on arbitrary histologic division (dysplasia–CIS) but instead should be individualized and based on both the histologic appearance and anatomic distribution of the lesions. The implications of the disease continuum concept for the pathologist are in deciding whether the patient has normal cervical epithelium, intraepithelial neoplasia, or invasive carcinoma. If the disease is noninvasive, the clinician should determine its geographic distribution and apply the appropriate therapeutic approach that is most consistent with the wellbeing of the patient.

## Epidemiology

Cervical intraepithelial neoplasia is a disease of young women. The overall age-adjusted annual incidence rates (newly diagnosed cases) for *in situ* carcinoma in the

United States of America according to the 1969–1970 Third National Cancer Survey[14] are 32.5 per 100,000 white and 62.5 per 100,000 black women. The peak in the age-adjusted incidence rate of CIS is in the decade from 30 to 34 years of age which is 120 per 100,000 white and 230 per 100,000 black women. The difference in incidence rates between white and nonwhite disappears when economic status is controlled by studying low-income women exclusively.[10] The mean age of patients with CIS is 35 years, 15 years younger than that for patients with invasive disease.[14] The incidence progressively increases from age 15 to 19 years (12 per 100,000) through 34 years and decreases rapidly thereafter, with an incidence rate of 86 per 100,000 at ages 35 to 39 years and 8.2 per 100,000 in women aged 85 years and over.[14] The incidence of *in situ* cervical cancer has doubled among both whites and nonwhites in the United States since 1950. This increase is largely caused by an increase in cytologic screening and earlier disease detection. Although accurate figures are not available, the average incidence rates of dysplasia appear comparatively higher than that of CIS, and the peak incidence occurs several years earlier.[68,69] Most epidemiologic studies have shown that the presence or absence of cervical neoplasia is primarily related to coitus and that a major determining factor appears to be the age at which that event is initiated.[4,11] Consequently, it has recently been recommended that cytologic screening be initiated when the patient begins sexual intercourse[34] rather than by age 20 as previously practiced. Several large epidemiologic surveys[4,11] found an early age at first intercourse, an early age at first pregnancy, a large total number of pregnancies, a short mean time interval between pregnancies to be the most significant and distinctive associated factors in the population of women with abnormal cytologic smears compared to those with normal cytology. It must be emphasized that because of the complex interrelationship between these variables, accurate prediction of the relative risk of developing cervical neoplasia can only be made in a population and not in the individual case. There are, in addition, a large number of covariables[4,11] that are believed to be only secondarily related to the incidence of cervical carcinoma because they are a common feature of the population who have early sexual contacts. These include frequent coitus, many sexual partners, low socioeconomic level, poor hygiene, race, and religion. Similarly, certain venereally transmitted diseases, such as syphilis, gonorrhea, and trichomonas vaginalis, that are reported in association with cervical neoplasia seem to characterize the sexual history of the population at risk rather than play an etiologic role themselves. Data on the occurence of cervical neoplasia and methods of contraception have been published. No statistically significant differences were found in the incidence rates of CIN in oral contraceptive, diaphragm, and IUD users.[37] In 1936, it was suggested that circumcision of the spouse reduces the risk of cervical neoplasia in Jews.[26] Since then, numerous epidemiologic studies have been undertaken to confirm this hypothesis. However, the findings are controversial and most recently the hypothesis has been totally rejected.[72]

## Etiology

Because the factors associated with a high risk of cervical cancer are related to sexual events and the disease is absent in virgins, it seems clear that cervical cancer is a venereal disease and that the causative agent(s) is transmitted by intercourse. The epidemiology and natural history of the disease suggest, furthermore, that the patient must be exposed to this agent (or agents) at an early age and that the exposure must be sustained over a long period of time in order to develop cervical neoplasia. Because cervical cancer is a venereally transmitted disease, it has been postulated that cervical cancer may be caused by a venereally transmitted virus. The suspected virus is *Herpes simplex* virus type 2 (HSV-2), which can be cultured from the genitalia. There has been a vast amount of research into the role of HSV-2 infection as an etiologic agent of cervical cancer.

Although irrefutable evidence establishing a causal relationship has not been presented to date, the combined weight of accumulated data suggests a positive association between the virus and cervical malignancy. Seroepidemiologic studies have shown that patients with invasive and noninvasive cancers of the cervix have a higher incidence of neutralizing antibodies against HSV-2 than among controls, matched for race, age, and socioeconomic status.[38] Herpesvirus antigens have been detected by immunofluorescence in exfoliated cervical squamous carcinoma cells[58] and the virus has been identified at the ultrastructural level in cervical carcinoma cells grown in tissue culture[2] (Figure 7.5). Herpesvirus oncogenecity was demonstrated by its ability to transform hamster embryo cells into cell lines that produced malignant tumors when injected into newborn hamsters.[18] Patients with antibodies to HSV-2 are 10, 7, and 6 times more likely to develop invasive cervical carcinoma, CIS, and dysplasia, respectively, than are women without antibodies to the virus.[39] Antibodies to HSV-2 virus were found in 36% of women who subsequently developed CIS and in only 7% of

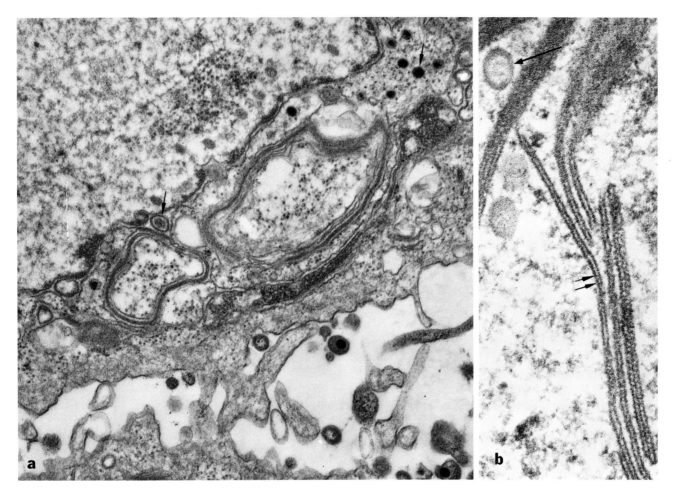

**7.5** Electron micrographs of two areas from HEp-2 cells infected with HSV-2 isolated from cervical carcinoma cells *in vitro*. **a.** Most of the infected HEp-2 cells have an obviously productive infection and contain viral components in all stages of maturation (arrows). ×27,000. **b.** A smaller percentage of cells contains intranuclear arrays of capsomeres (double arrow) and empty viral capsids (long arrow). In these cells complete virion formation is not observed.

[Courtesy of L. Aurelian, Johns Hopkins University, Laboratory of Animal Medicine, Baltimore.]

matched controls who did not develop CIS during the same period of observation[9]; and after conization and presumptive cure of CIS, type 2 antibodies were present in only 9% of patients compared to 32% of matched controls.[9] In a prospective study of women with herpes genitalis, cervical dysplasia developed twice as often and CIS eight times as often compared to controls.[24] The results of these studies and the age-specific incidence rates of cervical neoplasia suggest that infection by the virus precedes neoplastic changes in the cervix.

If HSV-2 is a human oncogenic virus, the mechanism by which it initiates the neoplastic process in human cervical epithelium is not known at the present time. However, it is known that, experimentally,[18] neoplastic transformation of virus-infected cells requires (1) maintenance of viral genes in a persistently or latent infected state and (2) partial or incomplete expression of the latent viral genome. In these conditions, the synthesis of viral proteins (cancer proteins) is triggered and these alter cell contacts and cellular functions and eventually lead to the malignant state. In support of this concept, Aurelian[1] has demonstrated that human cervical tumor cells contain HSV-2 genome in a partially repressed state characterized by the expression of only some viral functions. This is in contrast to the complete expression of viral genome, which is characterized by inhibition of host cell DNA and RNA synthesis, during which the cell is modified to produce HSV-2-specific RNA, required for viral replication and formation of infectious "noncancerogenic" virions.

The hypothesis of HSV-2 oncogenicity also seems to fit the previous postulates[4] that cervical neoplasia develops through a sequence of initiating events and promoting factors. The initiating factor might be the type 2 herpes genitalis gaining access to cervical cells at an early age, during which period cells involved in active generation of the transformation zone would be particularly sensitive to an initiating agent,[4,66] i.e., *Herpes simplex* virus type 2. Promotion could occur by repeated exposure to the original initiating agent during multiple pregnancies, when healing of the transformation zone epithelium is activated. A similar promotion-like effect is observed in the wound-healing, regenerating epithelium in the classic initiation–promotion chemical carcinogenesis experiments of the cervix.[59] Direct colpomicroscopic[49] and histologic observations add plausibility to the theory of viral-induced cervical carcinogenesis because early cervical neoplasia begins virtually without exception in the squamous epithelium of the transformation zone.[49]

An alternate hypothesis regarding the etiologic agent of cervical carcinoma has been proposed by Coppleson,[12] who has suggested that the nuclear DNA of spermatozoa, rather than HSV-2, is the initiating agent in cervical oncogenesis. Sperm heads were found to be incorporated in the cytoplasm and later in the nuclei of subcolumnar reserve cells, from which cervical neoplasia presumably arises. The intracellular presence of spermatozoa, however, may be a reflection of the phagocytic properties of reserve cells and there are no experimental facts to date indicating that sperm DNA has a carcinogenic potential for the human cervix.

## Microscopic Morphology

A histologic diagnosis of CIN implies that the lesion so diagnosed is capable of progressing to invasive carcinoma. The morphologic evaluation of these lesions is based on the histologic organization and cytologic characteristics of the epithelium.[8,25,33,42] The accurate assessment of these features is considerably enhanced by proper orientation

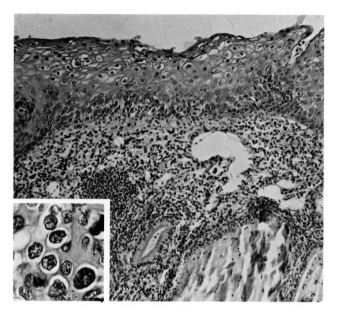

**7.6** Cervical intraepithelial neoplasia (CIN) grade 1 (very mild dysplasia). The entire epithelium is occupied by neoplastic cells, with only the two or three lowermost layers being replaced by undifferentiated, basal-type cells. However, disturbed maturation is observed in the upper strata, in which nuclei are prominent, vary in shape and size, and are often binucleated. These changes are associated with disturbed cellular orientation and cohesion. Inset: Characteristically, the nuclei of malignant basal cells are hyperchromatic and have irregular membranous or coarse chromatin.

and fixation of tissues, as well as by appropriate staining of tissue sections (see Chapter 8, Tissue Examination). The spectrum of epithelial alterations that comprises CIN has been quantitatively classified, according to the number of undifferentiated malignant cells occupying the cervical epithelium, into three categories: CIN grade 1, grade 2, and grade 3[53] (Figure 7.1). CIN grade 1 corresponds to the classic very mild to mild dysplasia (Figures 7.6 and 7.7), CIN grade 2 to moderate dysplasia (Figure 7.8), and CIN grade 3 to severe dysplasia (Figure 7.9) to carcinoma in situ (Figure 7.10). In order to achieve a high degree of diagnostic reproducibility, grading of CIN should be based on the greatest degree to which the epithelium is replaced by undifferentiated cells. It is of great importance to keep in mind that because CIN represents a single disease process, grading of CIN serves only to provide diagnostic references for statistical analysis of (1) the incidence and prevalence rates of the disease in its early, middle, and late stages and (2) progression with transit

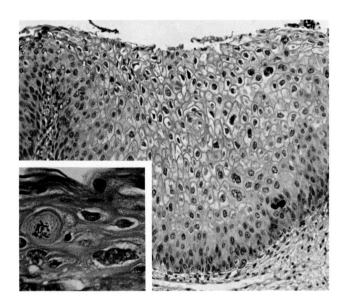

**7.7** Grade 1 CIN (mild dysplasia). This lesion is similar to that of Figure 7.6 but the neoplastic cells may occupy more than the lower third of the epithelium. Characteristically, the cells have atypical large nuclei and lack maturation and organization. Inset: Neoplastic (dyskaryotic) cells of the upper layer, demonstrating abnormal mitosis, binucleation, and chromatin aggregation.

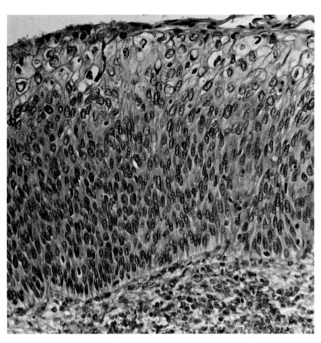

**7.8** Grade 2 CIN (moderate dysplasia). Undifferentiated neoplastic cells replace 50 to 70% of the epithelium. The nucleocytoplasmic ratio is in favor of the nucleus and the cytoplasmic membranes are indistinct.

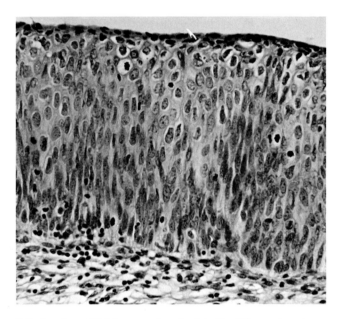

**7.9** Grade 3 CIN (severe dysplasia). Undifferentiated basal-type cells involve approximately two-thirds of the full thickness of the epithelium. There is a large number of mitoses in prometaphase. Note absence of intracytoplasmic glycogenization.

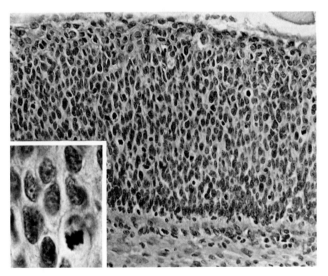

**7.10** Grade 3 CIN (carcinoma in situ). The full thickness of the epithelium is composed of small, undifferentiated neoplastic cells. This is the classic "small-cell carcinoma in situ." Note numerous mitotic figures and a complete loss of cellular maturation and organization. Inset: Detail of aggregated nuclear chromatin and mitosis in metaphase. Characteristically, cell membranes are ill defined.

times of one category of disease into another. Therefore, subclassification of CIN into grades 1, 2, and 3 should not be used as an indicator of the choice of the therapeutic approach. The critical decision to be made from a clinical point of view is whether the lesion is intraepithelial or invasive. CIN, regardless of its grade, is characterized by an abnormal epithelium in which cellular organization and maturation are disturbed and the cells display nuclear and cytoplasmic abnormalities consistent with malignant neoplastic cells (Figures 7.2 through 7.10). The malignant cells may be recognized by their hyperchromatic and irregular nuclei, in which the chromatin is coarse, granular, or filamentous throughout the nuclear mass (Figures 7.7 through 7.10). The abnormal chromatin patterns are perhaps the most important factors in the histologic identification of CIN and serve to distinguish it from lesions that mimic intraepithelial neoplasia. These nuclear alterations are found at all levels of the epithelium regardless of the degree of cytoplasmic maturation. In the early forms of CIN (CIN grades 1 and 2), cells of the middle and upper strata demonstrate evidence of cytoplasmic differentiation but their nuclei contain all the features that are commonly associated with malignancy, such as marked hyperchromasia, variation in nuclear size and shape, nucleomegaly, and abnormal chromatin organization. These cells are commonly referred to by cytopathologists as dyskaryotic cells.[33] Dyskaryotic cells are therefore capable of cytoplasmic maturation, but the nucleus retains the multiplication potential of a younger cell. The proliferative abilities of cells of the upper epithelial layers are demonstrated in both cytologic smears and tissue sections in which they may be found in mitotic division. Proliferation of cells in the upper and lower strata results in disorganization of the normal cellular cohesion, with cells being chaotically arranged throughout the entire thickness of the epithelium (Figures 7.6 and 7.7). The cytoplasmic membranes and intercellular bridges become indistinct. With an increasing degree of atypia the cells progressively lose cytoplasmic maturation and consequently, the nucleocytoplasmic ratio is in favor of the nucleus. Eventually the epithelium is completely replaced by undifferentiated neoplastic cells. The progressive dedifferentiation is accompanied by a progressive decrease in intracytoplasmic glycogen, loss of stratification, and an increase in mitotic figures at all levels of the epithelium.

Advanced, grade 3 CIN lesions (carcinoma in situ) are classified by some investigators into three main cytologic subtypes:[33,42,44] small-cell anaplastic carcinoma in situ, large-cell keratinizing or squamous cell carcinoma in situ, and large-cell nonkeratinizing or moderately differentiated

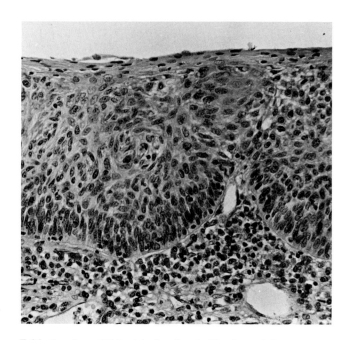

**7.11** Grade 2 CIN with focal spindle-shaped features.

carcinoma in situ. They are believed to be the precursor of small-cell, well-differentiated, and moderately differentiated invasive carcinomas, respectively. The small-cell variety is usually found within the external os or endocervical canal, is composed of small undifferentiated malignant cells of the basal cell type, and contains no surface maturation or keratinization (Figure 7.10). Occasionally the small tumor cells appear spindle shaped (Figure 7.11). The large-cell keratinizing lesion originates on the exposed portion of the cervix, away from the external os, and displays prominent intercellular bridges, macronucleoli, and extensive surface keratinization (Figure 7.12). The latter phenomenon appears clinically as a white patch (leukoplakia). Because cervical neoplasia may be associated with hyperkeratosis or clinical leukoplakia, all lesions with a white surface must be biopsied to rule out the presence of an underlying intraepithelial carcinoma. Large-cell nonkeratinizing lesions are by far the most frequent of all intraepithelial carcinomas of the cervix and are found within the cervical transformation zone. The epithelium is composed of undifferentiated cells the size of normal parabasal cells. Individual cell keratinization may be encountered (Figure 7.13). Because accurate studies concerning the invasive potential of each of these subtypes are lacking, it is felt that prediction as to the likelihood of progression to invasive carcinoma should not be based on the above subclassification.

Parallel to the epithelial abnormalities observed in CIN,

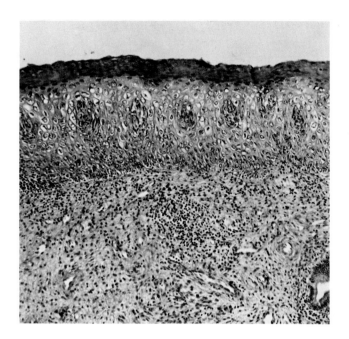

**7.12** Large-cell keratinizing CIN grade 3. Note cellular prominence, well-defined cytoplasmic membranes, and extensive surface keratinization. Clinically the lesion appeared as a white plaque or leukoplakia of the cervix.

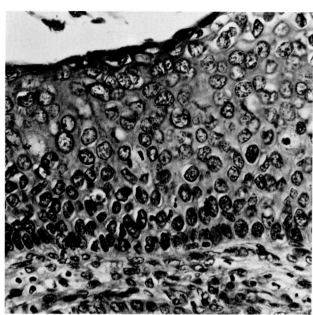

**7.13** Large-cell nonkeratinizing CIN grade 3. The neoplastic cells have hyperchromatic nuclei with clumping of chromatin. There is a high degree of cellular disorderliness and cytoplasmic membranes are indistinct.

the subepithelial vascular network undergoes profound alterations as determined by histochemical vascular preparations and colposcopic observations.[67] These presumably occur to provide an adequate supply of oxygen and nutrients that are necessary for neoplastic growth. The flat capillary network, which is found beneath the normal cervical epithelium, becomes tortuous and compressed vertically by the neoplastic epithelium, with extension close to the surface (Figure 7.14a–d), producing a colposcopic pattern of punctation (Figure 7.15a, Plate VII). Further proliferation and interconnection of proliferating masses of neoplastic tissue results in compression of the vascular network into basketlike structures around the neoplastic epithelium, producing a colposcopic mosaic (Figure 7.15b, Plate VII). Because of severe compression some of the capillaries eventually disappear, which results in an increase in the intercapillary distance. In early invasive carcinoma, a system of new capillaries is generated from capillaries of punctation or mosaic structures and is observed to run parallel to and beneath the surface of neoplastic epithelium (Figure 7.14c); this is the so-called horizontal capillary network (Figure 7.15c, Plate VII). These vascular changes and variation in the intercapillary dis-

tance are the most important diagnostic criterion of colposcopy and serve to distinguish noninvasive from invasive cervical squamous cell carcinoma (Figure 7.15c, d, Plate VII).

Lesions that are commonly confused with CIN include atypia of repair (Figures 6.1 and 7.16), squamous prosoplasia (metaplasia) (Figures 5.28, 5.31, and 7.17), immature transformation zone epithelium (Figure 5.29), and atrophic cervical epithelium (Figure 5.22). Although these lesions lack the normal maturation process, they are devoid of the cytonuclear pleomorphism that is seen in intraepithelial cervical neoplasia.

## Origin

Opinions vary as to whether the multicellular as opposed to the single-cell origin of CIN is most appropriate. The proponents of the multicellular theory[13,28,63] suggest that CIN arises in a predetermined (preneoplastic) field or fields in the transformation zone epithelium containing an abnormal cell population. This primary lesion, originating from either prosoplastic (metaplastic) epithelium[13,45] or

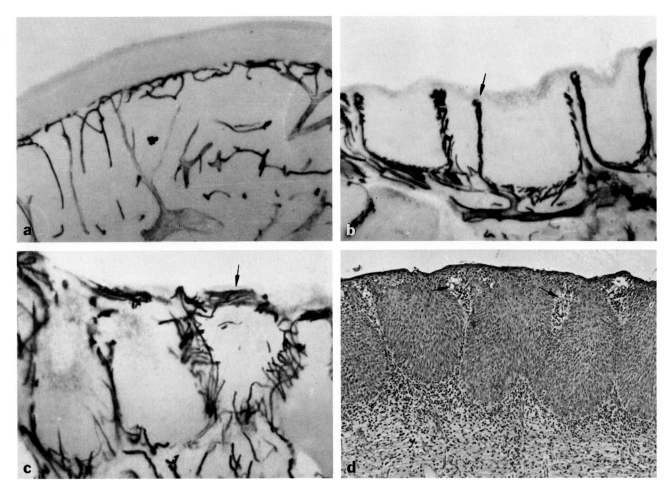

**7.14** Histochemical preparations of the terminal vascular network of the cervix. **a.** Flat capillary network beneath normal squamous epithelium. **b.** Abnormal vascular growth (arrow) in advanced CIN, producing colposcopic mosaic pattern. **c.** Abnormal horizontal vascular pattern (arrow) in early invasive carcinoma of cervix. **d.** Histology of grade 3 CIN, in which the vascular stromal papillae are compressed vertically by masses of neoplastic epithelium, with extension near the surface (arrows) producing a colposcopic pattern of punctation.

[Courtesy of Dr. A. Stafl, The Medical College of Wisconsin, Milwaukee.]

subcylindrical cells of the endocervix,[28,45] eventually progresses in a vertical fashion by transforming the adjacent normal epithelium into neoplastic epithelium or by coalescence of multiple predetermined neoplastic fields, producing a larger lesion. This theory of the multicellular origin of CIN and its vertical proliferation is based primarily on histologic[28] and colposcopic[13,63] observations of the distribution and changes in the distribution of presumed preinvasive cervical lesions.

The unicellular theory proposed that CIN began in a single cell or at most in an extremely circumscribed group of cells. Support for the unicentric single-cell origin theory has been offered by direct colpomicroscopic[49] and histologic[43] observations, as well as by cytogenetic chromosomal preparations[62] and glucose-6-phosphate dehydrogenase X-linked chromosome marker studies.[41,61] Using colpomicroscopy, Richart[49] showed that 95% of early CIN grade 1 lesions were confined to a single focus. Although he was not able to trace these lesions back to a single-cell origin, some of them were as small as 10 cells in diameter. Multifocal lesions or coalescence of multiple lesions were only rarely observed. Colpomicroscopic followup of pa-

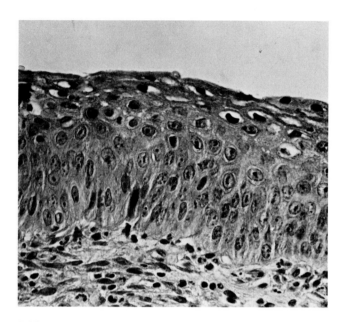

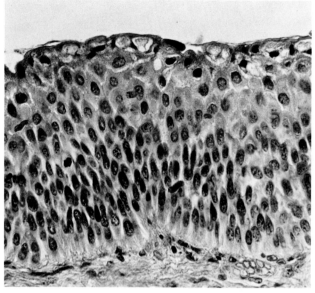

**7.16** Atypia (anaplasia) of repair. Note the disorganization in normal maturation. Atypical basal cells occupy the lower half of the epithelium, simulating CIN grade 2 lesion. Unlike CIN, however, the basal cells in atypia of repair have regular nuclear outline, prominent chromocenters, and distinct cell membranes. Additionally, cells in the upper half of the epithelium are not atypical and demonstrate normal maturation.

**7.17** Immature squamous prosoplastic epithelium of the clinical transformation zone. The newly formed cells proliferate beneath the mucinous endocervical cells, which are degenerating as a result of their separation from the basal lamina. Note the basal cell hyperplasia with occasional mitotic divisions and the attempt at maturation in the upper half of the epithelium. The cells in the upper strata of the epithelium are regularly orientated, with uniformly disposed nuclear chromatin and cellular borders. Intercellular bridges are well defined.

tients with minute CIN lesions has shown that they expand centrifugally by mechanically displacing and eventually replacing the adjacent benign squamous and/or endocervical epithelium. Histologically, CIN lesions were demonstrated to be unifocal and confluent in nearly 95% of serially step-sectioned conization specimens.[43] In direct chromosomal preparations,[62] dysplasia, carcinoma *in situ,* and microinvasive carcinoma were shown to contain the same neoplastic clone, which presumably derived from a single cell. The evidence consisted of finding similar abnormal modal number and marker chromosomes in dysplasia and CIS as well as microinvasive carcinoma.

Recently, the electrophoretic variants of the X-linked enzyme glucose-6-phosphate dyhydrogenase (G-6-PD) have been applied to determine the single versus multicellular origin of cervical neoplasia.[41,61] The G-6-PD system relies on the Lyon hypothesis; one X chromosome in each somatic cell is inactivated during early embryogenesis and subsequently all cells deriving from this cell have the same X chromosome active. The G-6-PDase enzyme is an X-linked enzyme that, in about one-third of American Negro

women, has two electrophoretic variants, the slow and fast or A and B. These women are heterozygous for G-6-PDase electrophoretic variants and so have two types of cells, those with only type A enzyme and those with only type B enzyme. If neoplastic cells arising in a heterozygous woman contain only one electrophoretic variant, either A or B, they can be assumed to be of single-cell origin, providing that the Lyon hypothesis operates in tumorigenesis. However, if tumor cells have a double-enzyme phenotype, both A and B enzymes, the lesion has a multiple-cell origin. Therefore, this system can be used to trace the cellular origin of neoplasms. The results with CIN lesions were, in most cases, consistent with a single-cell origin,[41,61] suggesting that the initial tumorigenic event affects one rather than a large number of cells simultaneously.

At the present time, there is no unanimous opinion on the cellular origin of CIN. Three cellular sites of origin have been proposed: basal cells of the squamous epithe-

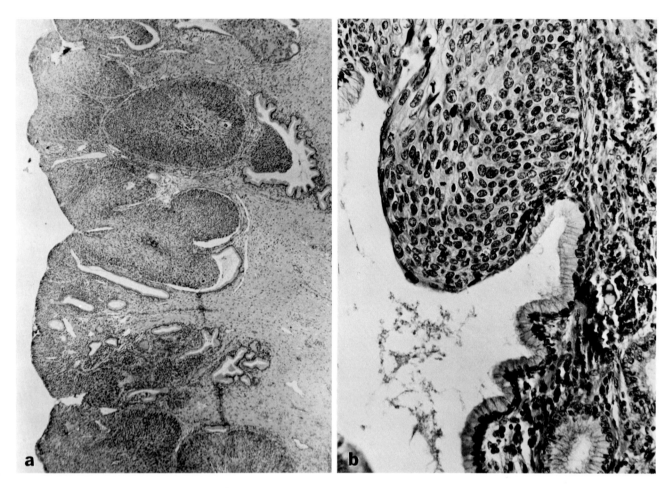

**7.18** Endocervical "gland" involvement by CIN. **a.** Masses of neoplastic epithelium grow into and distend endocervical clefts. Note the smooth margins of ingrowing neoplastic epithelium retaining the normal configuration of endocervical mucosa. **b.** The neoplastic cells grow in between the endocervical epithelium and its basal lamina.

lium of the portio, basal cells of the transformation zone epithelium, and subcylindrical reserve cells of the endocervix.[28] Colposcopic, colpomicroscopic, and histologic observations have shown that virtually all CIN begins at the squamocolumnar junction of the transformation zone, with one edge of the lesion bordering the endocervical columnar epithelium[49] (Figure 7.18a). The line of demarcation between the squamous epithelium of the native portio or transformation zone and CIN is sharp and perpendicular to the surface (Figure 7.18b). Early, well-differentiated preinvasive disease is usually found in the squamous epithelium at the squamocolumnar junction and is seldom seen in the endocervix. In general, the exposed portion of CIN is well differentiated and of the CIN grade 1 type, whereas the endocervical involvement is less well differentiated and of the CIN grade 3 type. From

these observations it is now proposed that most CIN arises in the basal cells of the transformation zone epithelium, which is formed by the coalescence of squamous prosoplastic (metaplastic) epithelium and native squamous epithelium. In the squamous prosoplastic and native portio epithelium, the cell of origin is the subcylindrical reserve cells of the everted endocervix and basal cells of the native portio epithelium, respectively.

## Distribution

Colpomicroscopic studies[48] have shown that CIN occurs on the anterior lip of the cervix twice as commonly as on the posterior lip and is rarely seen at the lateral cervical angles. The distribution of CIN was similar to the distri-

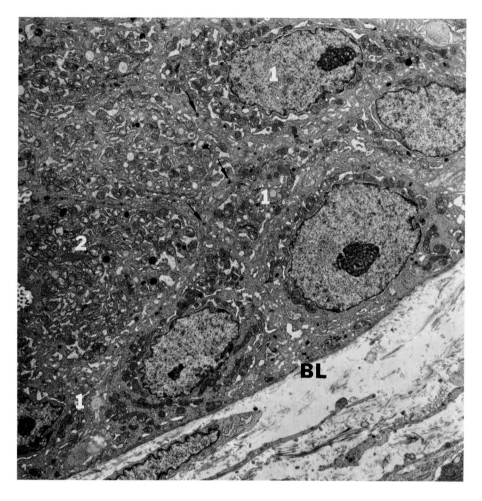

**7.19** Electron micrograph of the advancing edge of grade 3 CIN cells (1) extending along the basal lamina (BL) of the endocervical epithelium (2). The neoplastic squamous cells are attached by small desmosomes (arrows) to subjacent endocervical cells. ×4,550.

bution of both the everted endocervical epithelium and transformation zone during the postpartum period.[75] CIN has been seen to expand progressively and horizontally and may involve the entire area of transformation zone, but it stops abruptly at the junction with native portio epithelium. The area of the transformation zone therefore predetermines the distribution and extent of CIN on the exposed portion of the cervix. In view of these observations the traditional and standardized four–quadrant–punch biopsy technique, in which tissue is removed at positions 12, 3, 6, and 9 o'clock from the exposed portion of the cervix, is no longer recommended. Instead, the area to be biopsied should be determined according to the location of the squamocolumnar junction of the transformation zone.

The mechanism through which CIN is able to extend into normal squamous epithelium and into the columnar epithelium of the endocervix is also a matter of contention. Some believe that CIN spreads by transformation of cells from normal to malignant in a vertical direction.[13,28,45] Others on the basis of colpomicroscopy,[48] tissue culture studies,[47] and light and electron microscopy[19] have suggested that CIN spreads horizontally along the basement membrane by mechanically lifting up the adjacent normal squamous and endocervical columnar cells (Figure 7.18a,b). Ultrastructural observations[60] of the junction of CIN and the endocervical epithelium have failed to demonstrate subcylindrical reserve cells or prosoplastic squamous cells at the interface of these lesions and normal tissues (Figure 7.19), suggesting that the expansion is not through transformation of prosoplastic cells. Moreover, because endocervical involvement is seldom seen in CIN grade 1 lesions and the vast majority of patients with CIN grade 3 lesions have endocervical involvement, it is reasonable to believe that such extension occurs during the progression of the disease. The mechanical replacement of the normal epithelium by neoplastic cells is not confined to the endocervix, as cases have been described in which CIN has extended along the entire endocervical canal up to the endometrial cavity.[20] However, CIN stops at the junction of the transformation zone and the normal native portio epithelium, the line of demarcation being sharp. CIN rarely extends onto the portio past the junction of the transformation zone with the native portio mucosa.[48] Although the precise significance of this phenomenon is obscure, it has been suggested that a tissue-specific antimitotic substance, such as the epidermal chalone,[7] may be responsible for the geographic distribution and growth pattern of CIN.[52] According to this theory a diffusable substance (chalone) is produced by normal squamous epithelium of the cervix, which keeps mitosis in check and allows physiologic maturation to proceed. This factor is presumably specific only for normal squamous portio epithelium. The production of cervical chalone offers an explanation for the near universality of CIN arising at the squamocolumnar junction, because the columnar epithelium produces a chalone that is specific for mucus-secreting epithelium only and so does not affect the squamous epithelium of the portio. Hence, the squamocolumnar junction would represent a unique site for the origin of cervical carcinogenesis because one epithelial border would not produce antimitotic substance and the concentration of squamous epithelial chalone would be expected to be lower at the squamocolumnar junction than at any other region. The concept might also explain the frequent endocervical involvement by CIN for squamous neoplastic cells would not be influenced by endocervical chalone, whereas the relative large quantity of chalone produced by the native squamous portio epithelium would provide resistance against the expanding squamous neoplastic cells onto the portio.

## Management

Many different therapeutic modalities have been advocated for noninvasive cervical neoplasia, including electrocauterization,[57] conization, simple hysterectomy, and radical hysterectomy. The most widely used therapeutic protocol advocates conization for patients with dysplasia and simple vaginal or abdominal hysterectomy for patients with CIS who no longer desire to conceive.[15] Patients with CIS who wish to preserve their ability to bear children are treated with conization followed by cervical cytology. Patients during pregnancy are either followed by cytology or punch biopsies or receive conization and are treated by hysterectomy after delivery.[15] One of the major arguments against conization as an adequate

therapeutic means for preinvasive cervical neoplasia is the seemingly high frequency of residual disease found in postconization hysterectomy specimens, reported by some to be as high as 22[15] to 35%.[40] This high incidence of residual disease, however, does not seem to be a strong argument, because the recurrence rates in patients treated by conization are only 5 to 7%[15] compared to less than 3% in those treated by hysterectomy.[15] The discrepancy between the high-residual and low-recurrence rates is presently explained by the histologic overdiagnosis of atypical epithelium at the healing site, destruction of a certain proportion of residual lesions during the process of healing, and incomplete conization. It is therefore believed that therapeutic conization when properly performed in carefully evaluated cases, especially with regard to the extent of the disease, is a highly reliable method for managing cervical cancer precursors.

With current knowledge and understanding of the natural history of preinvasive cervical lesions and the improved precision of evaluating their extent in the cervix by colposcopic examination, a trend toward a more conservative and highly individualized treatment of CIN has developed in more recent years.[16, 17, 30, 57, 64, 65, 73] In contrast to the traditional and rather radical two-disease, dysplasia–carcinoma in situ approach, the modern approach to a patient with cytologic evidence of preinvasive neoplasia is based on the concept that dysplasia and CIS are a part of a disease continuum, cervical intraepithelial neoplasia, that may lead to invasive cancer of the cervix. The concept of CIN as a disease continuum has been accepted and recommended at the 1973 National Conference on Cancer Prevention and Detection, which was held in Bethesda, Maryland.[34] With this concept of the disease, the question of whether a given lesion is mild, moderate, or severe dysplasia or carcinoma in situ becomes meaningless and artificial. The important features for the clinicians are (1) to rule out invasive carcinoma; (2) if the lesion is noninvasive, to determine its distribution; and (3) to remove the lesion in the easiest, most reliable, and least costly way possible, and if appropriate, to preserve the patient's reproductive functions. In the majority of cases with abnormal cytology, colposcopy can accurately determine the precise location and extent of the disease (Figure 7.20, Plate VII), and colposcopically directed punch biopsies (Figure 7.21) coupled with endocervical curettage (see Chapter 8, Tissue Examination) can provide histologic confirmation of the existence of either invasive or noninvasive neoplasia. With these techniques, it is possible to eliminate the need for diagnostic conization and its inherent complications (bleeding and infection) in 95% of

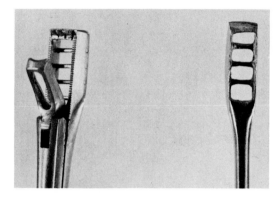

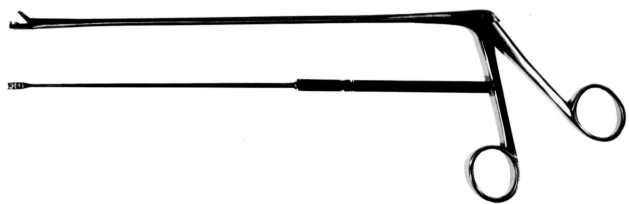

**7.21** Kevorkian cervical biopsy punch and endocervical curette. Inset: The slightly rectangular jawed biopsy punch has shallow penetration into the cervical stroma, resulting in little discomfort for the patient, and the tissue removed has straight edges, facilitating orientation. The curette is rectangular with sharp edges.

nonpregnant[65] and 99% of pregnant[17] patients. The clinical–pathologic diagnosis and treatment and followup of patients with abnormal cytology are outlined in Figure 7.22. According to the colposcopic findings, the patients are divided into three major groups:[64] (1) patients with abnormal colposcopic findings, (2) patients with normal colposcopic findings, and (3) patients with unsatisfactory colposcopic findings.

### Patients with abnormal colposcopic findings

If the process is noninvasive and confined to the exposed portion of the cervix, the patient may be managed on an out-patient basis using electrocauterization[57] or cryocauterization[16,30,73] and followed with cervical cytology for possible recurrence. Cryocautery is now the most frequently used technique for large lesions limited to the portio and, although a longer term of followup is still required, the failure rate in experienced hands does not exceed that of therapeutic conization.[16,30,73] On the other hand, complications and costs of cryosurgery are negligible compared to conization. Cryosurgery is also preferred to electrocautery because it is less painful and does not inter-

fere with fertility. The mechanism of cryoinjury on cervical tissue is not well known. However, it is believed that damage is caused during freezing and thawing when the tissue is exposed to excess thermal stress.[16] The temperature delivered through the cryoprobe to the cervix varies from $-90°C$ to $-160°C$, depending on the refrigerant used ($CO_2$, $N_2O$, or liquid nitrogen). Minute ice crystals are formed, both within the cells and in the extracellular spaces, which presumably produce mechanical disruption leading to fragmentation of cell membranes and cytoplasmic organelles. In addition, crystallization dehydrates cells so that high electrolyte concentrations produce biochemical injury associated with lysosomal enzyme release, which results in cell destruction. Although double freeze–thaw cycles with timed freezes were initially used, it has become clear that the only significant end point for the cryosurgical management of CIN is that the margins of the ice ball extend 3 to 4 mm beyond the limits of the lesion (Figure 7.23a, Plate VII).

Postcryotherapy, the cervix becomes edematous and the epithelium sloughs. Reepithelialization begins within 24 hr of the procedure and healing is generally completed within approximately 12 weeks (Figure 7.23b, Plate VII).

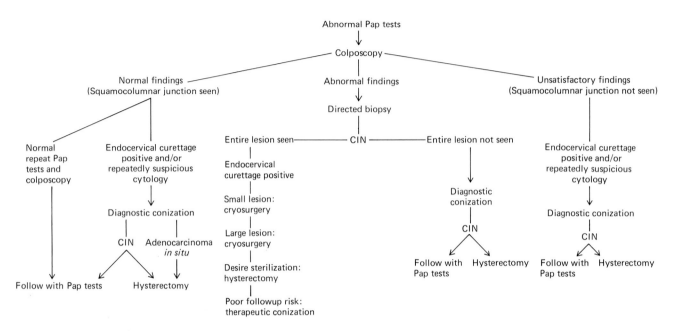

**7.22** Diagnostic evaluation, treatment, and followup of patients with abnormal cytology when colposcopy and an experienced colposcopist are available.

If the patient has colposcopic evidence of an exocervical lesion that extends into the endocervical canal and the limits of the lesion cannot be visualized with the colposcope, a diagnostic conization should be performed. If the disease in the conization specimen is not invasive, the patient may be followed cytologically every 3 months for the first year and once a year thereafter, so long as the smears remain negative.

*Patients with normal colposcopic findings*

These patients have a fully visible squamocolumnar junction and no colposcopic evidence of lesional tissue on the portio. There is no evidence of neoplasia either in the endocervical curettage or on repeat smears and colposcopy. They are followed as described in the previous paragraph. A diagnostic conization is indicated only if the endocervical curettage contains strips of neoplastic epithelium or repeated cytology remains or becomes positive.

*Patients with unsatisfactory colposcopy*

These are patients in whom the squamocolumnar junction is not fully visible and in whom one cannot exclude colposcopically the possibility of a lesion higher in the endocervical canal. In these patients, a diagnostic conization is indicated. If the diagnostic cone obtained from patients with either normal or unsatisfactory colposcopic findings contain CIN, they may be followed with repeated Pap smears or treated by hysterectomy. In patients with a histologic diagnosis of invasive carcinoma, the treatment must depend on the stage of the disease, including hysterectomy, radical surgery, radiotherapy, and chemotherapy.

It should be emphasized that the above outlined approach to patients with abnormal cytology requires a highly skilled and experienced team of cytopathologist, histopathologist, and colposcopist working in consultation. Those clinicians who have less experience with outpatient diagnosis and management or who do not have access to highly accurate cytology and pathology laboratories should either rely on conization as the major diagnostic and therapeutic modality or refer the patient for colposcopic consultation.

# Summary

In summary, the modern concept of the natural history of cervical cancer precursors may be outlined as follows: (1) Current evidence indicates that lesions traditionally termed dysplasia and carcinoma in situ are a part of the same neoplastic process, cervical intraepithelial neoplasia (CIN), and represent the transition from normal cervical epithelium to invasive carcinoma. (2) Cervical intraepithelial neoplasia begins at the squamocolumnar junction, is usually unifocal, and has a predilection for the anterior lip in a ratio of 2:1 over the posterior lip. (3) In the process of continuous growth, the lesion progressively becomes less differentiated and spreads into the transformation zone on the exposed portion of the cervix and into the endocervical canal by replacement of adjacent normal epithelium. (4) The distribution and maximum extent of CIN on the portio coincides with the distribution of the transformation zone. (5) There is a logarithmic increase in the tritiated thymidine labeling index and presumably in the mitotic rate and loss of desmosomes, cell contact inhibition, and intracellular glycogen with increased severity of the lesion. (6) In CIN lesions, regardless of degree of differentiation, the majority of cells contain abnormal chromosomal constitutions similar to those which characterize cancer and their precursors in other non-endocrine-dependent epithelium. (7) In the majority of untreated CIN lesions, one or more clones of cells are finally selected that are capable of penetrating the basement membrane and producing invasive carcinoma. (8) The major clinical implication of the disease continuum concept is that once the diagnosis of CIN is established, management be based on the lesion's distribution rather than on its arbitrary division into dysplasia and carcinoma in situ.

## ACKNOWLEDGMENTS

This work was aided by Grant MA5137 from the Medical Research Council of Canada.

## REFERENCES

1. Aurelian, L. Persistence and expression of the herpes simplex virus type 2 genome in cervical tumor cells. *Cancer Res.* 34:1126, 1974.

2. Aurelian, L., Strandberg, J. D., Melendez, L. V., and Johnson, L. A. Herpesvirus type 2 isolated from cervical tumor cells grown in tissue culture. *Science* 74:704, 1971.

3. Barron, B. A., and Richart, R. M. A statistical model of the natural history of cervical carcinoma based on a prospective study of 557 cases. *J. Natl. Cancer Inst.* 41:1343, 1968.

4. Barron, B. A., and Richart, R. M. An epidemiologic study of cervical neoplastic disease. *Cancer* 27:978, 1971.

5. Beacham, W. D., and Rice, M. Diphteria of the uterine cervix. *Am. J. Obstet. Gynecol.* 47:417, 1944.

6. Boyes, D. A., Fidler, H. K., and Lock, D. R. *The Significance of In Situ Carcinoma of the Uterine Cervix.* Proceedings of the First International Congress of Exfoliative Cytology. Philadelphia, J. B. Lippincott, 1963.

7. Bullough, W. S., and Laurence, E. B. Epigenetic mitotic control, in Tier, H., and Rytomaa, T., eds.: *Control of Cellular Growth in Adult Organisms.* New York, Academic Press, 1967, pp. 28–40.

8. Burghart, E. *Early Histological Diagnosis of Cervical Cancer,* 1st ed. Philadelphia, W. B. Saunders, 1973.

9. Catalano, L. W., and Johnson, L. D. Herpesvirus antibody and carcinoma in situ of the cervix. *JAMA* 217:447, 1971.

10. Christopherson, W. M., and Parker, J. E. A study of the relative frequency of carcinoma of the cervix in the Negro. *Cancer* 13:711, 1960.

11. Christopherson, W. M., and Parker, J. E. Relation of cervical cancer to early marriage and child bearing. *N. Engl. J. Med.* 273:235, 1965.

12. Coppleson, M. The origin and nature of premalignant lesions of the cervix uteri. *Int. J. Gynecol. Obstet.* 8:539, 1970.

13. Coppleson, M., and Reid, B. *Preclinical Carcinoma of the Cervix Uteri,* 1st ed. Oxford, Pergamon Press, 1967.

14. Cramer, D. W., Cutler, S. J. Incidence and histopathology of malignancies of the female genital organs in the United States. *Am. J. Obstet. Gynecol.* 118:443, 1974.

15. Creasman, W. T., and Rutledge, F. Carcinoma in situ of the cervix. *Obstet. Gynecol.* 39:373, 1972.

16. Creasman, W. T., Weed, J. C., Jr., Curry, S. L., Johnston, W. W., and Parker, R. T. Efficiency of cryosurgical treatment of severe intraepithelial neoplasia. *Obstet. Gynecol.* 41:501, 1973.

17. De Petrillo, A. D., Townsend, D. E., Morrow, C. P., Lickrish, G. M., Di Saia, P. J., and Roy, M. Colposcopic evaluation of the abnormal Papanicolaou test in pregnancy. *Am. J. Obstet. Gynecol.* 121:441, 1975.

18. Duff, R., and Rapp, F. Properties of hamster embryo fibroblasts transformed *in vitro* after exposure to ultraviolet-irradiated herpes simplex virus type 2. *J. Virol.* 8:469, 1971.

19. Ferenczy, A., and Richart, R. M. *Female Reproductive System. Dynamics of Scan and Transmission Electron Microscopy,* 1st ed. New York, John Wiley & Sons, 1974.

20. Ferenczy, A., Richart, R. M., and Okagaki, T. Endometrial involvement by cervical carcinoma in situ. *Am. J. Obstet. Gynecol.* 110:590, 1971.

21. Fidler, H. K., Boyes, D. A., and Worth, A. J. Cervical cancer detection in British Columbia. *J. Obstet. Gynaecol. Br. Commonw.* 75:392, 1968.

22. Fidler, H. K., Boyes, D. A., Nichols, T. M., and Worth, A. J. Cervical cytology in the control of cancer of the cervix. *Modern Medicine of Canada* 25:9, 1970.

23. Fox, C. H. Biologic behavior of dysplasia and carcinoma in situ. *Am. J. Obstet. Gynecol.* 99:960, 1967.

24. Franklin, E., and Jenkins, R. Prospective studies of the association of genital herpes simplex infection and cervical anaplasia. *Cancer Res.* 33:1491, 1973.

25. Friedell, G. H., Hertig, A. T., and Younge, P. A. *Carcinoma In Situ of the Uterine Cervix,* 1st ed. Springfield, Ill., Charles C Thomas, 1960, pp. 108–109.

26. Handley, W. S. The prevention of cancer. *Lancet* 1:987, 1936.

27. Hulka, B. S. Cytological and histological outcome following an atypical cervical smear. *Am. J. Obstet. Gynecol.* 101:190, 1968.

28. Johnson, L. D. The histopathological approach to early cervical neoplasia. *Obstet. Gynecol. Surv.* 24:735, 1969.

29. Johnson, L. D., Nickerson, R. J., Easterday, C. L., Stuart, R. S., and Hertig, A. T. Epidemiologic evidence for the spectrum of change from dysplasia through carcinoma in situ to invasive cancer. *Cancer* 22:901, 1968.

30. Kaufman, R. H., Strama, T., Norton, P. K., and Conner, S. J. Cryosurgical treatment of cervical intraepithelial neoplasia. *Obstet. Gynecol.* 42:881, 1973.

31. Kirkland, J. A. Atypical epithelial changes in the uterine cervix. *J. Clin. Pathol.* 16:150, 1963.

32. Kirkland, J. A., Stanley, M. A., and Cellier, K. M. Comparative study of histologic and chromosomal abnormalities in cervical neoplasia. *Cancer* 20:1934, 1967.

33. Koss, L. G. *Diagnostic Cytology and Its Histopathologic Bases,* 2nd ed. Philadelphia, J. B. Lippincott, 1968.

34. Koss, L. G., and Phillips, A. Summary and recommendations of the workshop on uterine cervical cancer. *Cancer* 33:1753, 1974.

35. Koss, L. G., Stewart, F. W., Foote, F. W., Jordan, M. J., Bader, G. M., and Day, E. Some histological aspects of behavior of epidermoid carcinoma in situ and related lesions of the uterine cervix. A long-term prospective study. *Cancer* 16:1160, 1963.

36. Kottmeier, H. L. Evolution et traitement des épithéliomas. *Rev. Franç. Gynécol.* 56:821, 1961.

37. Melamed, M. R., and Flehinger, B. J. Early incidence rates of precancerous cervical lesions in women using contraceptives. *Gynecol. Oncol.* 1:290, 1973.

38. Melnick, J. L., Adam, E., and Rawls, W. E. The causative role of herpes virus type 2 in cervical cancer. *Cancer* 34:1375, 1974.

39. Nahmias, A. J., and Roizman, B. Infection with herpes-simplex viruses 1 and 2. *N. Engl. J. Med.* 289:667, 719, 781, 1973.

40. Nelson, J. H., Jr., and Hall, J. E. Detection, diagnostic evaluation, and treatment of dysplasia and early carcinoma of the cervix. *Cancer J. for Clinicians* 20:150, 1970.

41. Park, I. J., and Jones, H. W., Jr. Glucose-6-phosphate dehydrogenase and the histogenesis of epidermoid carcinoma of the cervix. *Am. J. Obstet. Gynecol.* 102:106, 1968.

42. Patten, S. F., Jr. *Diagnostic Cytology of the Uterine Cervix,* 1st ed. Baltimore, Williams & Wilkins, 1969.

43. Przybora, L. A., and Plutowa, A. Histological topography of carcinoma in situ of the cervix uteri. *Cancer* 12:263, 1959.

44. Reagan, J. W., and Hamonic, M. J. The cellular pathology in carcinoma in situ; a cytohistopathological correlation. *Cancer* 9:385, 1956.

45. Reagan, J. W., Ng, A. B. P., and Wentz, W. B. Concepts of genesis and development in early cervical neoplasia. *Obstet. Gynecol. Surv.* 24:860, 1969.

46. Richart, R. M. A radioautographic analysis of cellular proliferation in dysplasia and carcinoma in situ of the uterine cervix. *Am. J. Obstet. Gynecol.* 86:925, 1963.

47. Richart, R. M. The growth characteristics *in vitro* of normal epithelium, dysplasia and carcinoma in situ of the uterine cervix. *Cancer Res.* 24:662, 1964.

48. Richart, R. M. Colpomicroscopic studies of the distribution of dysplasia and carcinoma in situ on the exposed portion of the human uterine cervix. *Cancer* 18:950, 1965.

49. Richart, R. M. Colpomicroscopic studies of cervical intraepithelial neoplasia. *Cancer* 19:395, 1966.

50. Richart, R. M. The influence of diagnostic and therapeutic procedures on the distribution of cervical intraepithelial neoplasia. *Cancer* 19:1635, 1966.

51. Richart, R. M. Natural history of cervical intraepithelial neoplasia. *Clin. Obstet. Gynecol.* 10:748, 1967.

52. Richart, R. M. A theory of cervical carcinogenesis. *Obstet. Gynecol. Surv.* 24:874, 1969.

53. Richart, R. M. Cervical intraepithelial neoplasia, in Sommers, C. C. ed.: *Pathology Annual.* New York, Appleton-Century-Crofts, 1973, pp. 301–328.

54. Richart, R. M., Barron, B. A. A follow-up study of patients with cervical dysplasia. *Am. J. Obstet. Gynecol.* 105:386, 1969.

55. Richart, R. M., Lerch, V. Time-lapse cinematographic observations of normal human cervical epithelium, dysplasia and carcinoma in situ. *J. Natl. Cancer Inst.* 37:317, 1966.

56. Richart, R. M., Lerch, V., and Barron, B. A. A time-lapse cinematographic study *in vitro* of mitosis in normal human cervical epithelium, dysplasia and carcinoma in situ. *J. Natl. Cancer Inst.* 39:571, 1967.

57. Richart, R. M., Sciarra, J. J. Treatment of cervical dysplasia by out-patient electrocauterization. *Am. J. Obstet. Gynecol.* 101:200, 1968.

58. Royston, I., and Aurelian, L. Immunofluorescent detection of herpes virus antigens in exfoliated cells from human cervical carcinoma. *Proc. Natl. Acad. Sci. USA* 67:204, 1970.

59. Rubio, C. A., and Lagerlöf, B. Studies on the histogenesis of experimentally induced cervical carcinoma. *Acta Pathol. Microbiol. Scand.* 82:153, 1974.

60. Shingleton, H. M., Richart, R. M., Wiener, J., and Spiro, D. Human cervical intraepithelial neoplasia. Fine structure of dysplasia and carcinoma in situ. *Cancer Res.* 28:695, 1968.

61. Smith, J. W., Townsend, D. E., and Sparks, R. S. Genetic variants of glucose-6-phosphate dehydrogenase in the study of carcinoma of the cervix. *Cancer* 28:529, 1971.

62. Spriggs, A. I., Bowey, C. E., and Cowdell, R. H. Chromosomes of precancerous lesions of the cervix uteri. *Cancer* 27:1239, 1971.

63. Stafl, A. The clinical diagnosis of early cervical cancer. *Obstet. Gynecol. Surv.* 24:976, 1969.

64. Stafl, A., Friedrich, E. G., Jr., and Mattingly, R. F. Detection of cervical neoplasia. Reducing the risk of error. *Clin. Obstet. Gynecol.* 16:238, 1973.

65. Stafl, A., and Mattingly, R. F. Colposcopic diagnosis of cervical neoplasia. *Obstet. Gynecol.* 41:168, 1973.

66. Stafl, A., and Mattingly, R. F. Vaginal adenosis: A precancerous lesion? *Am. J. Obstet. Gynecol.* 120:666, 1974.

67. Stafl, A., and Mattingly, R. F. Angiogenesis of cervical neoplasia. *Am. J. Obstet. Gynecol.* 121:845, 1975.

68. Stern, E. Epidemiology of dysplasia. *Obstet. Gynecol. Surv.* 24:711, 1969.

69. Stern, E., Neely, P. M. Carcinoma and dysplasia of the cervix: A comparison of rates for new and returning populations. *Acta Cytol.* 7:357, 1963.

70. Stout, A. P. Observations on biopsy diagnosis of tumors. *Cancer* 10:912, 1957.

70a. Sugimori, H., and Gusberg, S. B. Quantitative measurement of DNA content of cervical cancer cells before and after test dose radiation. *Am. J. Obstet. Gynecol.* 104:829, 1969.

71. Takeuchi, A., and McKay, D. B. The area of the cervix

involved by carcinoma in situ and anaplasia (atypical hyperplasia). *Obstet. Gynecol. 15*:134, 1960.

72. Terris, M., Wilson, F., and Nelson, J. H., Jr. Relation of circumcision to cancer of the cervix. *Am. J. Obstet. Gynecol. 117*:1056, 1973.

73. Townsend, D. E., and Ostergard, D. R. Cryocauterization for preinvasive cervical neoplasia. *J. Reprod. Med. 6*:171, 1971.

74. Weid, G. L. *Proceedings of the First International Congress on Exfoliative Cytology,* 1st ed. Philadelphia, J. B. Lippincott, 1961.

75. Wilbanks, G. D., and Richart, R. M. The puerperal cervix, injuries and healing: A colposcopic study. *Am. J. Obstet. Gynecol. 97*:1105, 1967.

76. Wilbanks, G. D., Terner, J. Y., and Richart, R. M. The DNA content of cervical intraepithelial neoplasia studied by two-wave length Feulgen cytophotometry. *Am. J. Obstet. Gynecol. 98*:792, 1967.

77. Williams, A. E., Jordan, J. A., Allen, J. M., and Murphy, J. F. The surface ultrastructure of normal and metaplastic cervical epithelia and of carcinoma in situ. *Cancer Res. 33*:504, 1973.

Alex Ferenczy, M.D.

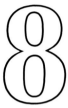

# Diagnostic Procedures for Lesions of the Cervix

## Colposcopy

In the United States for a number of years colposcopy[8] and exfoliative cytology were regarded as competitive methods in the early detection of cervical neoplasia. In the last decade, however, colposcopy became accepted and used as a complementary technique to cytology.[4] Cytology is a laboratory method of detection, based on the evaluation of the morphologic alterations of the exfoliated cells. Colposcopy is a clinical method designed for the early diagnosis of noninvasive, preclinical invasive, and frank invasive cervical cancers. Colposcopy evaluates the modifications in the surface vascular system of cervical epithelium, which occur in response to biochemical and metabolic alterations in neoplastic tissues. When colposcopy and cytology are combined their diagnostic accuracy is near 100%.[1,8] The colposcope (Figure 8.1) is a stereoscopic microscope with focused illumination that provides a three-dimensional image of tissue surfaces. It is particularly useful in the cervix, vagina, and vulva. When the instrument is positioned 6 to 7 cm from the introitus, the image is magnified from 10 to 40 times. The technique of colposcopic examination includes the application of a 3 to 4% solution of acetic acid over the exposed portion of the cervix uteri. Acetic acid serves (1) to coagulate the mucus, facilitating its removal, and (2) to dehydrate cells. In areas of nuclear crowding, as occurs in cervical neoplasia, the dehydrated, abnormal mucous membrane has de-

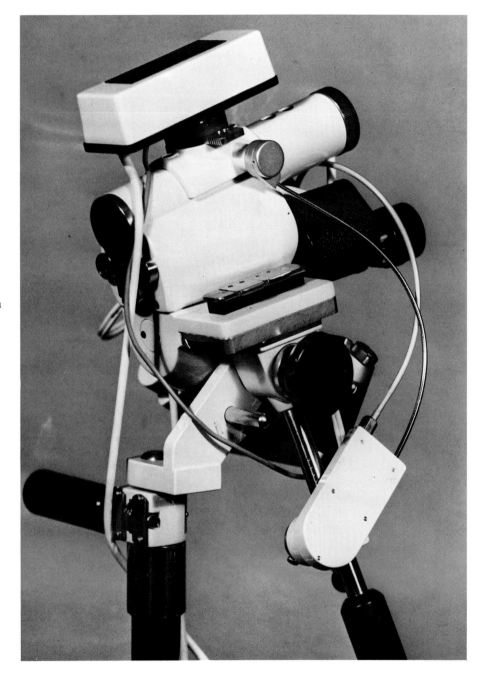

**8.1** Photograph of a Leisegang colposcope with a Leica camera attachment for colpophotographs. The basic principle of colposcopy is that of stereoscopic visualization of tissue surfaces with bright illumination.

creased transparency and appears white. Colposcopists refer to this phenomenon as the "acetic acid or Hinselmann test"[2] (Figure 8.2, Plate VIII). Colposcopic examination of the cervix is limited to the portio and outer third of the endocervical canal. Colposcopic diagnosis is based on evaluating the vascular pattern, intercapillary distance, surface contour, color tone, and clarity of demarcation of lesions.

Detailed observations and descriptions of the colposcopic appearance of normal and neoplastic cervical epithelium have appeared[1,3] and are illustrated in Chapters 5 through 9. It should be emphasized that colposcopy is neither a practical nor an economic means for cervical cancer screening. Its main role lies in the clinical evaluation of patients with abnormal cytologic smears. Because of the high-resolution capability of the colposcope, the distribution and extension of cervical neoplasia, either intraepithelial or invasive, can accurately be determined and selection of areas for punch biopsy is facilitated. As a result, the traditional diagnostic conization of relatively high morbidity (10%) may be considerably reduced. A diagnostic conization is indicated only if (1) cytology remains repeatedly positive with normal colposcopic findings; (2) cytology is repeatedly positive and the squamocolumnar junction is not visible because of its localization higher in the endocervical canal (unsatisfactory colposcopy); and (3) the colposcopic lesion extends into the endocervical canal and its limits are beyond the reach of colposcopic visualization. In all these instances a diagnostic conization can provide histologic diagnosis of whether the lesion is invasive or not.

## Staining Tests

Examination of the cervix with the naked eye generally reveals no significant differences between the cervix with cervical intraepithelial neoplasia (dysplasia and carcinoma in situ) and one without lesional tissue. When a weak aqueous iodine solution is applied to the exposed portion of a normal cervix the entire mucous membrane stains a deep mahogany brown (iodine-positive or Schiller dark areas) caused by the presence of intracellular glycogen. Areas of clinically normal appearing squamous epithelium, which fail to stain (iodine-negative or Schiller light areas), may be composed of neoplastic epithelium, devoid of glycogen (Figure 8.3, Plate VIII). The staining reaction is known as the Schiller test or iodine test and is widely used as a tool to aid in the delineation of suspicious areas for biopsy. There are several drawbacks, however, in the application of the Schiller test. These are, on one hand, that not all areas of the cervix which fail to take the iodine represent foci of neoplasia as columnar epithelium, inflammatory regions, and prosoplastic (metaplastic) regions also fail to stain with iodine and, on the other hand, a certain number of cases with cervical neoplasia remain iodine positive. Indeed, Richart[6] found that 28% of patients with advanced cervical intraepithelial neoplasia (carcinoma in situ) were iodine positive and 72% were iodine negative. In patients with cervical neoplasia of lesser severity (dysplasia) the iodine test failed to detect 48% of lesions. In addition, the test failed to detect the actual distribution of cervical neoplasia in a high proportion of cases. In view of the relatively high false-negative rate of the Schiller test, its use must be combined with considerable clinical expe-

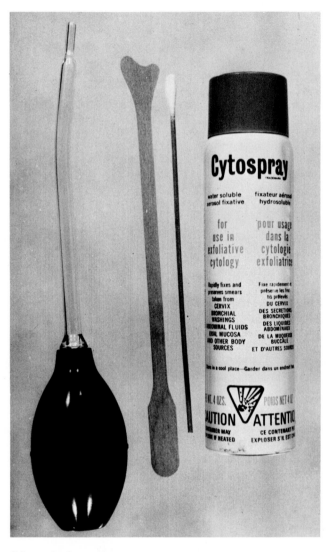

**8.4** Tools for exfoliative cervical cytology: endocervical cytopipette, wooden spatula, cotton tipped applicator, and cytospray fixative.

rience focusing on the delineation of the limits of the transformation zone, because the limits of cervical neoplasia will be within the limits of that zone. Toluidine blue dye has also been used as a clinical staining procedure, staining dark blue in regions of high nuclear concentration.[5] Although the test yields a comparatively lower false-negative rate than the Schiller test, it suffers from many of the pitfalls of any clinical staining procedure. Other staining tests that have been suggested but not proved to be of substantial value include acridine orange fluorescence and tetracycline fluorescence.[9]

**8.5** Drawing illustrating orientation, fixation, and microtome sectioning of a specimen obtained by cervical punch biopsy.

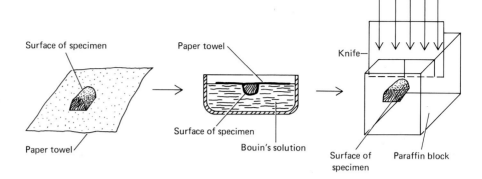

Surface of specimen

Paper towel

Direction of cut

Knife

Paper towel

Surface of specimen

Bouin's solution

Surface of specimen

Paraffin block

# Cytologic Examination

The cytology of the cervix is described in detail in Chapter 36, but certain aspects with regard to cell collection techniques deserve special mention in this chapter. The major goal of cervical cytology is to achieve a high detection rate and a high degree of diagnostic predictability. When these criteria are met, cytology can be utilized as an important tool in the clinical management of patients with abnormal Papanicolaou smears. Previous experience[7] has shown that the most accurate sampling technique combines the use of an aspirator for recovering a specimen from the external os and a wooden spatula for obtaining a sample from the exposed portion of the cervix (Figure 8.4). It should be emphasized that a large (25 ml) rubber bulb must be used to provide adequate suction force and that the glass pipette must have a narrowed tip. The tip of the aspirator is placed at the os, the canal contents are aspirated, and the material obtained is then placed on a glass slide. This is done by placing the tip of the pipette against the glass slide at a 90° angle and then pressing on the rubber bulb one or more times until the sample is fully recovered. In cases of severe cervical stenosis or "dry cervical os" a cotton tipped applicator can be used instead of a cytopipette. Os aspiration is immediately followed by circumferential scraping of the exposed portion of the cervix with the aid of a wooden spatula. The specimen obtained is then gently mixed with the aspiration sample and the two are evenly smeared on the same glass slide and fixed immediately. When a combination of aspiration and scraping is employed and two or more specimens are obtained over a period of time, the diagnostic accuracy of cytology can reach 98%.[7] When cellular samplings are performed by os aspiration or cervical scraping alone, the diagnostic accuracy is reduced to 93% and 85%, respectively.[7]

# Tissue Examination

The pathologist may receive punch biopsies, conization biopsies, or endocervical curettings from the cervix. To achieve diagnostic accuracy and reproducibility, a mutual understanding between the pathologist and clinician must be established regarding orientation, fixation, and preparation of surgical specimens.

## Punch Biopsy

The clinician should be instructed to place the tissue samples on end on a piece of paper towel, so that the mucosal surface faces upward. The specimen, with its adhesive blood, should then immediately be placed in Bouin's fixative upside down, the specimen facing the bottom of the container (Figure 8.5). In this manner, the tissue will be fixed undistorted and will be easy to orient in the paraffin block. The clinician should instruct the technician or the pathologist of the orientation of the specimen, which is then to be reoriented on edge in the paraffin block to obtain sections perpendicular to the surface (Figure 8.5). In this way, tangential sections of the epithelium will be eliminated, facilitating histologic interpretation. All tissue received must be submitted *in toto*.

## Endocervical Curettage

Endocervical curettage of the endocervical canal is performed chiefly to determine whether the canal harbors invasive or noninvasive carcinoma. The specimen obtained consists of endocervical tissue fragments, blood, and mucus. In order to avoid loss of tiny tissue fragments (one or several of which may be neoplastic) during laboratory processing, the clinician should collect and place the sample, including mucus and blood, on a piece of paper towel.

The specimen is then placed in Bouin's solution in the fashion described for cervical biopsy punches (Figure 8.5). By this method, even the smallest fragments can easily be recovered for pathologic evaluation. All tissue submitted must be embedded and sectioned.

## Conization Biopsy

Conization biopsy consists of a conical structure of varying size according to whether the operator has performed a shallow conization for an exocervical lesion or a deep cone, for an endocervical lesion. The apex and base of the sample represent the endocervical and exocervical portion, respectively. The specimen should preferably be received fresh, opened in the middle of either the anterior or posterior lip, pinned out on a cork board, and fixed in Bouin's solution. Following fixation, 2-mm thick step sections of the entire cone taken perpendicular to the surface should be prepared. Similar sectioning should be made in prefixed cone specimens. For the study of all biopsy material, the use of cytologic fixative, such as Bouin's solution, and a light hematoxylin and eosin stain is preferred because of the importance of cytologic features in the histologic diagnosis of cervical neoplasia. The use of noncytologic fixatives, such as 10% formalin, or the heavy hematoxylin and eosin stain precludes the observation of fine nuclear details that are essential for accurate diagnosis and grading of lesions.

# ACKNOWLEDGMENT

This work was aided by Grant MA5137 from the Medical Research Council of Canada.

# REFERENCES

1. Coppleson, M., Pixley, E., and Reid, B. *Colposcopy. A Scientific and Practical Approach to the Cervix in Health and Disease,* 1st ed. Springfield, Ill., Charles C Thomas, 1971.

2. Hinselmann, H. *Colposcopy,* 1st ed. Trans. by Lang, W. R. Girardet, Wuppertal-Elberfeld, 1955.

3. Kolstad, P., and Stafl, A. *Atlas of Colposcopy,* 1st ed. Baltimore, University Park Press, 1972.

4. Navratil, E., Burghardt, E., Bajardi, F., and Nash, W. Simultaneous colposcopy and cytology used in screening for carcinoma of the cervix. *Am. J. Obstet. Gynecol. 75:*1292, 1958.

5. Richart, R. M. A clinical staining test for the *in vivo* delineation of dysplasia and carcinoma in situ. *Am. J. Obstet. Gynecol. 86:*703, 1963.

6. Richart, R. M. The correlation of Schiller-positive areas on the exposed portion of the cervix with intraepithelial neoplasia. *Am. J. Obstet. Gynecol. 90:*697, 1964.

7. Richart, R. M., and Vaillant, H. W. Influence of cell collection technic upon cytologic diagnosis. *Cancer 18:*1474, 1965.

8. Stafl, A., and Mattingly, R. F. Colposcopic diagnosis of cervical neoplasia. *Obstet. Gynecol. 41:*168, 1973.

9. Wilbanks, G. D., and Carter, B. Fluorescence of cervical intraepithelial neoplasia induced by tetracycline and acridine orange. *Am. J. Obstet. Gynecol. 106:*726, 1970.

Alex Ferenczy, M.D.

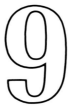

# Carcinoma and Other Malignant Tumors of the Cervix

## Invasive Carcinomas

### Preclinical Microinvasive and Occult Invasive Squamous Cell Carcinomas

#### Terminology and definitions

The concept of microinvasive carcinoma of the cervix was first introduced in 1947 by Mestwerdt.[78] The almost infinite number of descriptive terms used to designate preclinical invasive disease of the cervix include microcarcinoma, incipient invasion, very small carcinoma, overt invasive carcinoma, and intraepithelial carcinoma with microinvasive foci.[102] To date the most widely accepted term is microinvasive carcinoma. The term implies the earliest stromal extension of cervical intraepithelial neoplasia and signifies its growth potential. Microinvasive carcinoma is considered a preclinical stage in the progressive spectrum of cervical intraepithelial neoplasia and frank clinical invasive carcinoma of the cervix uteri. It is classified as clinical stage Ia according to the 1974 FIGO (International Federation of Gynecologists and Obstetricians) staging of carcinoma of the cervix (Table 9.1). Because the lesion cannot be visualized on gross inspection, the diagnosis is based on histologic examination of cervical tissue removed by punch biopsy, conization, or hysterectomy.

The definition of microinvasive carcinoma is one of the most confused and controversial issues in the pathology of

**Table 9.1**  1974 modification of FIGO staging of carcinoma of the cervix uteri

| Stage | Description |
| --- | --- |
| 0 | Preinvasive carcinoma (intraepithelial carcinoma, carcinoma in situ) |
| I[a] | Carcinoma strictly confined to the cervix (extension to the corpus should be disregarded) |
| Ia | Carcinoma in situ with early stromal invasion (microinvasive carcinoma) diagnosed on tissue removed by biopsy, conization, or portio amputation or on the removed uterus |
| Ib | Clinically invasive carcinoma confined to the cervix |
| Ib occ | Histologic invasive carcinoma of the cervix that could not be detected at routine clinical examination but that was diagnosed on a large biopsy, a cone, or the amputated portio |
| II | Invasive carcinoma that extends beyond the cervix but has not reached either lateral pelvic wall; involvement of the vagina is limited to the upper two-thirds |
| III | Invasive carcinoma that extends to either lateral pelvic wall and/or the lower third of the vagina |
| IV | Invasive carcinoma that involves urinary bladder and/or rectum or extends beyond the true pelvis |

[a] Notes to the Staging: Stage Ia (microinvasive carcinoma) represents those cases of epithelial abnormalities in which histologic evidence of early stromal invasion is unambiguous. The diagnosis is based on microscopic examination of tissue removed by biopsy, conization, or portio amputation or of the removed uterus. Cases of early stromal invasion should therefore be allotted to stage Ia. The remainder of stage I cases should be allotted to stage Ib. As a rule, these cases can be diagnosed by routine clinical examination. Occult cancer is an evidently invasive cancer that cannot be diagnosed by routine clinical examination. They are as a rule diagnosed on a cone or on the amputated portio. They should be included in stage Ib and should be marked "stage Ib, occ."

the cervix.[12,61] The main subjects of contention concern the exact depth of stromal invasion, vascular invasion, and confluence between invasive tongues of neoplastic epithelium. The maximal permissible depth of stromal invasion reported in the literature varies from 1 mm[8,12] and 3 mm[41,114] to 5 mm.[13,15,73,78,81,83,84,92,101] Some characterize microinvasion by the absence of confluency of invasion foci[12,15,73,102] and/or by absence of vascular permeation,[12,73,102] whereas for others, lymphatic in-

volvement[13,81,83,99,101] and confluency[99] do not exclude the diagnosis of microinvasive disease. The lack of a uniform definition is reflected in the conflicting reports regarding the incidence of pelvic node metastasis complicating microinvasion, which varies from 0[13,83,92,99] to 5%,[12] with a composite incidence of 3.6%.[12] These figures are difficult to interpret, as in most studies no information is given regarding the methods used to measure the depth of stromal invasion. In other series, the depth of stromal penetration is not even stated.[102] Similarly, precise data on the incidence of recurrences and survival rates are not available because of the different definitions and methods of treatment employed (cone biopsy, hysterectomy, radical hysterectomy, irradiation) for early invasive lesions[61] and because of limited followup information.[92] Despite these pitfalls, analysis of the literature indicates that lymph node metastases,[12,81] recurrences,[13,15,101] and deaths[101] tend to occur in lesions that contain lymphatic penetration, confluency, and more than 1-mm deep stromal penetration. Recently, Rubio, Soderberg, and Einhorn[101] reported that 4% of 210 patients with 1- to 5-mm microinvasive carcinomas died of disseminated cervical cancer an average of 7 years after diagnosis, and about 3% experienced recurrences. In contrast, there is convincing evidence presented that no metastases or recurrences occur in lesions that are not confluent, contain no vascular invasion, and do not exceed 1-mm deep stromal penetration.[12] In the opinion of the author and of others,[12] a meaningful definition of the early invasive stage must reflect its biologic malignancy with relation to management and survival. In other words, a stage should be defined at which there is stromal invasion but there are no metastases. Such a lesion can be treated differently than the invasive lesions with the potential of metastasis. In the light of presently available data, *microinvasive carcinoma is best defined as one or several tongues of neoplastic epithelium extending into the stroma through the plane of the basement membrane that do not exceed 1 mm in depth from the point of origin, do not invade vessels, and are not confluent.* This type of lesion can be treated conservatively by simple hysterectomy. All other preclinical carcinoma with more than 1-mm stromal invasion, vascular invasion, and/or confluence should be considered as occult invasive carcinoma and managed accordingly.

*Incidence and age distribution*

According to various investigators, the incidence rates of microinvasion in patients with cervical intraepithelial neoplasia varies from 4[15] to over 50%.[68] The significant variations in incidence rates reflect wide differences in the definition of microinvasive carcinoma and methods of

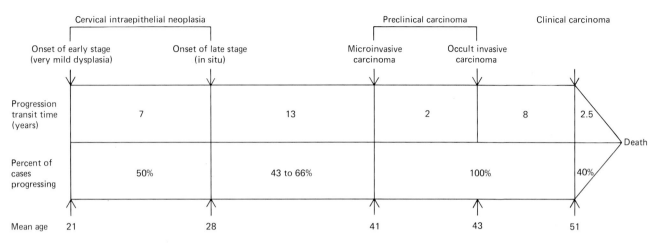

**9.1** Diagram of the progression, transit time and proportion of cases of CIN progressing to invasive squamous carcinoma estimated according to the mean age of the patients.

[Adapted from H. K. Fidler, D. A. Boyes, T. M. Nichols, and A. J. Worth. Cervical cytology in the control of cancer of the cervix, *Modern Medicine of Canada* 25:9, 1970.]

sampling of cervical specimens. A 4% frequency rate was demonstrated by serial step sections in specimens with cervical intraepithelial neoplasia by Boyes and associates[15] and is the incidence figure that has gained general acceptance. As a result of improved cytologic diagnosis in recent years, about 10% of squamous cell carcinomas of the cervix are demonstrated in a microinvasive stage.[83] The mean age of patients at the time of histologic detection of microinvasion with up to 5-mm stromal penetration is 41 years.[38] From an age standpoint, microinvasive carcinoma is observed, on the average, 13 years later than the onset of the advanced stage of CIN or carcinoma *in situ*—mean age at onset 28 years—and 2 years earlier than preclinical occult invasive carcinoma of the cervix—mean age 43 years[38] (Figure 9.1).

### Symptoms and signs

The majority of patients with stage Ia microinvasive disease are asymptomatic and are seen for routine pelvic examination. The cervix demonstrates a grossly normal appearance or nonspecific findings, such as chronic cervicitis or true erosion.[13,61]

### Diagnosis

As has been mentioned earlier, a definite diagnosis of microinvasion is made on histologic evaluation of cervical tissue removed by various surgical means. These surgical procedures are performed because cervical smears obtained during routine examination suggest the presence of cervical intraepithelial neoplasia or invasive carcinoma. However, cytopathologists and colposcopists with wide experience are able to detect early stromal invasion with a high degree of accuracy. Ng and associates,[84] on the basis of cellular characteristics, correctly predicted 27 of 31 patients with proved microinvasive carcinoma, an accuracy of 87%. According to these authors, the major cytologic features diagnostic of microinvasion are coarse, irregular chromatin distribution; micro- and macronucleoli; background of exudates and cellular debris (tumor diathesis); and syncytial arrangement of neoplastic cells. The colposcopic diagnosis[12,109] of early invasive lesion is based on abnormal vascular patterns of the cervical epithelium. Characteristically, the epithelium displays a marked degree of whiteness consistent with cervical intraepithelial neoplasia in which one or more foci contain bizarre surface branching of vessels (Figure 7.15c). The recommended approach in diagnosing microinvasion is colposcope-oriented punch biopsy of the area suspicious for microinvasion, followed by conization in order to exclude the possibility of a more advanced disease.

### Histology

According to the definition of microinvasive carcinoma of the cervix, one or more tongues of malignant cells are seen to break through the plane of the basement mem-

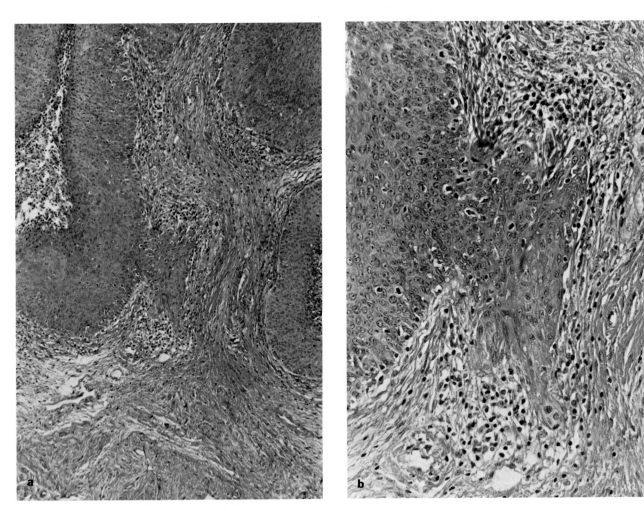

**9.2** Microinvasive squamous cell carcinoma of the cervix. **a.** Minute tongue of neoplastic epithelium projecting into the stroma from an area of grade 3 CIN that has replaced a preexisting endocervical cleft. Stromal extension is less than 1 mm in depth. **b.** Higher magnification of the microinvasive focus, which characteristically displays irregular margin and better differentiated neoplastic cells than those confined above the basal lamina. The stromoepithelial junction of the invasive focus is typically infiltrated by chronic inflammatory cells.

brane of the epithelium (Figure 9.2a). The latter invariably demonstrates intraepithelial neoplasia of varying severity and in most instances the underlying endocervical "glands" are extensively replaced by the advancing intraepithelial disease. Typically in the microinvasion foci, the cells are usually better differentiated than those in the associated CIN, with abundant cytoplasm and prominent nucleoli. Occasionally, small centers of keratinization are seen. Because of focal disruption of the basement membrane, the margin of the invading nests is ragged, flanked by intact basement membrane on either side (Figure 9.2b).

This irregular contour pattern is probably the most reliable criterion in the diagnosis of microinvasive carcinoma. It is easily distinguished from the smooth and regular contour of masses of neoplastic cells that represent endocervical "gland" involvement by intraepithelial carcinoma. At the site of initial stromal invasion, disruption of the basement membrane is confirmed by electron microscopy. The neoplastic cells are seen encroaching directly onto the collagen fibers of the stroma, and their cytoplasmic membrane is markedly convoluted with numerous microvilli. The factors that initiate a clone or clones of cells to invade

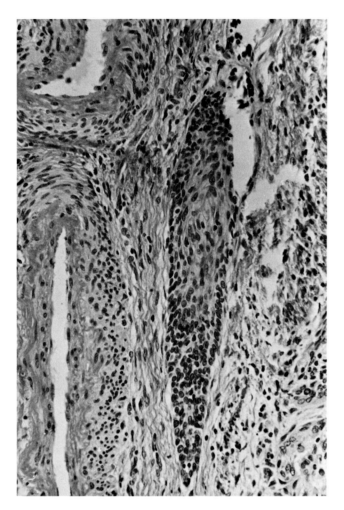

**9.3** Lymphatic invasion by tumor cells. Neoplastic cells tightly adhere to the endothelial lining of a lymphatic capillary space. Although the lesion contained non-confluent, less than 2 mm deep microinvasive sprouts, because of vascular invasion the lesion was interpreted as preclinical, occult invasive carcinoma. Two of 28 pelvic lymph nodes contained metastasis.

within the basement membrane, as evidenced by the often conspicuous lymphoplasmacytic infiltrates surrounding the tips of invasive epithelial prongs. The presence of lymphatic or venous involvement by the tumor or confluency of invading tongues regardless of the size of the lesion should exclude the disease from the microinvasive category (Figure 9.3). Early invasion of lymphatic spaces is difficult to identify, however. Roche and Norris[99] define lymphatic space invasion when endothelial-lined spaces contain tumor cells that are contiguous with the stroma. The authors note, however, that "there is no evidence that the capillary-like spaces in question are, in fact, lymphatic spaces."[99] The extent of neoplastic projections should not exceed 1 mm from the initial site of invasion either from the surface epithelium or from endocervical "glands" replaced by intraepithelial neoplasia. The most accurate method to measure the depth of stromal penetration is with a calibrated slide of occular microscale,[83,99] although such devices are seldom used in routine practice. A more convenient but perhaps less accurate means of establishing the size of penetrating foci consists of using a microscopic field that corresponds to a diameter of 1 mm. This may be determined by direct microscopic visualization of a transparent metric ruler. Although variation in microscopic objectives and occulars exists, in general a microscopic field of $\times 160$ measures a little more than 1 mm in diameter. The depth of penetration also depends on the angle at which sections are prepared, and efforts should be made to secure vertically sectioned tissue samples. Special attention should be paid to the interpretation of recently biopsied conization specimens. These often harbor individual nests of neoplastic epithelium scattered within the cervical stroma at the site of a previous punch biopsy (Figure 9.4). Such nests represent clusters of intraepithelial carcinoma that may be disrupted and incorporated into the stroma by the punch biopsy and masquerade as microinvasive carcinoma. Therefore, a diagnosis of microinvasion should be carefully evaluated when such a phenomenon is seen at or near a recent biopsy site.

*Treatment*

Many methods of treatment for early invasion are used, ranging from cervical conization to radical hysterectomy with pelvic node dissection and from radium insertion to total pelvic irradiation. The trend in the more recent literature, however, appears to be in the direction of more conservative management, with attempts at individualization of treatment based on the definition of the lesion.[12] The general consensus is that microinvasive carcinoma

the stroma are obscure. Morphologically, invasive squamous cells have fewer cellular attachments and presumably elaborate more lysosomal lytic substances than their intraepithelial counterparts. It is conceivable that these morphophysiologic changes, when acquired in a small group of intraepithelial neoplastic cells, can lead to a decrease in cellular adhesiveness, loss of contact inhibition, and presumably disruption of the basement membrane, respectively, and thus enable them to penetrate the underlying connective tissue stroma. Host factors probably also play an important role in restraining the neoplastic cells

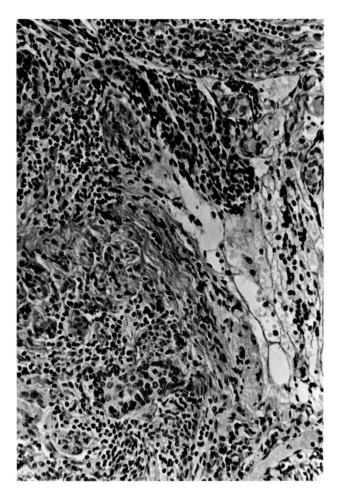

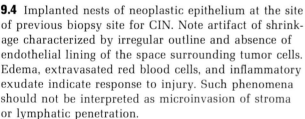

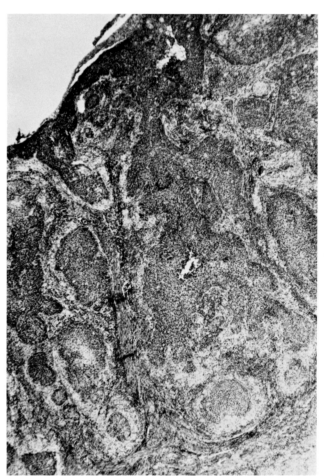

**9.4** Implanted nests of neoplastic epithelium at the site of previous biopsy site for CIN. Note artifact of shrinkage characterized by irregular outline and absence of endothelial lining of the space surrounding tumor cells. Edema, extravasated red blood cells, and inflammatory exudate indicate response to injury. Such phenomena should not be interpreted as microinvasion of stroma or lymphatic penetration.

**9.5** Unifocal, preclinical, occult invasive squamous cell carcinoma of the cervix. The lesion was not visible to the naked eye. The entire lesion measured 4 mm in diameter and maximum penetration. In contrast to microinvasive carcinoma, in this lesion invasive tongues are confluent. Note the extensive inflammatory cell infiltration at the interface between tumor cells and stroma.

with less than 1-mm stromal extension devoid of vascular invasion and confluency can safely be treated by simple hysterectomy.[12]

## Occult Invasive Carcinoma

Occult invasive carcinoma bridges microinvasive carcinoma and frank clinical invasive carcinoma of the uterine cervix. In the currently modified 1974 FIGO staging of carcinoma of the cervix, it is classified as stage Ib, "occult" carcinoma (Table 9.1). The stage Ib acknowledges its more serious potential than stage Ia microinvasive neoplasia and the term "occult" refers to a frank invasive growth that cannot be detected on gross examination and that is discovered on histologic sections of surgical specimens. *Such occult invasive carcinoma is defined as invasive tongues that are greater than 1 mm in depth and/or are confluent, regardless of size, with or without involvement of vascular spaces* (Figures 9.3 and 9.5). This type of lesion is usually unifocal and measures in depth from a few millimeters to over 1.5 cm.[15] The mean age of patients with occult invasive carcinoma is 43 years,[38] as compared to 51 years for those with clinical visible stage Ib–IV disease[24] (Figure 9.1). Several large series of patients with preclinical malignant cervical neoplasms with more than 1-mm stromal extension demonstrated a close relationship between the extent of stromal extension and lymphatic permeation as well as lymph node involvement and death rate.[12,15,61,101] Vascular invasion occurred in 2% of lesions measuring up to 3 mm in depth compared to 26% in those with 3- to 5-mm stromal extension.[101] Boyes, Worth, and Fidler[15] found lymphatic vessel invasion in one-third of 218 cases of occult confluent lesions. Pelvic node metastasis was observed in 5% of 40 patients with 1- to 3-mm microinvasion.[12] The mortality rate is 4[101] to 7%.[15] Patients who die of disseminated carcinoma in general have lymphatic channel involvement[15,61] and tumors measuring more than 5 mm in greatest extent.[15,41] In view of these data, the pathologist should specify the extent of the disease and the presence or absence of vascular penetration in order to predict the prognosis of the patient. The better 5-year survival rate (96%)[15,101] of patients with occult invasive carcinoma as compared to stage Ib frank invasive carcinoma (5-year survival rate, 86%) justifies the former being distinguished from the latter variety. At the present state of knowledge, radical hysterectomy with pelvic lymphadenectomy is considered to be the most appropriate therapeutic approach to occult invasive carcinoma of the cervix.

## Clinical Invasive Squamous Cell Carcinoma

### Incidence and age distribution

According to the 1969–1970 Third National Cancer Survey,[24] invasive squamous cell carcinoma of the uterine cervix represents the most common malignancy in the female reproductive system in American women, both white and black, aged younger than 50. In black women, cancer of the cervix is the most common genital malignancy throughout life, followed by cancer of the fundus and ovary. In white women over 50, cancer of the cervix represents only the third most common malignant lesion of the genital organs, preceded by cancer of the endometrium and ovary. The differences in the incidence of cervical carcinoma according to age and race are attributed primarily to the declining occurrence of squamous cell carcinoma among Caucasian women and the observation that in black women cancer of the endometrium develops significantly less frequently than in white women.[25] Geographic factors are also significant in the incidence of invasive cervical carcinoma, the Southern United States

with its low socioeconomic background having the highest rates for both black and white women.[24] The age-adjusted incidence rates per 100,000 women for invasive cervical cancer fell from 34 in 1947 (Second National Cancer Survey) to 15.3 in 1970, an approximately 58% decrease. This spectacular decline is thought to result from the increased use of mass screening by cervical cytology, which significantly contributes to the early detection and eventual removal of invasive cervical cancer precursors.[23] The primary role of cytology in reducing cervical cancers is also supported by the different incidence rates reported in screened population (4.5 cases per 100,000) and unscreened population (29 cases per 100,000), both cohorts exhibiting similar epidemiologic characteristics.[37] The decline of cervical carcinoma accounts for a decrease in all female genital malignancies, which fell from 118 cases per 100,000 women aged 20 and over in 1947 to 88 cases per 100,000 in 1970.[24] Whereas the cervix comprised over 50% of the invasive cancers in the 1947 survey, today it accounts for less than a third of the cases.[24] Most investigators feel that the gradual reduction in cervical cancer morbidity is the primary factor responsible for the progressive decrease in mortality rates[23,94] observed over the past two decades. The average reduction in the crude mortality rate is estimated to be about 30%,[23] ranging from 1.1 to 57.4% in various parts of the United States.[23,94] A positive correlation between the rate of effective cancer detection programs used in each state of the United States and a decrease in mortality rate can be demonstrated.[23,94] In areas with high-quality mass screening cytologic programs, there has been over 50% reduction in the death rate for cervical carcinoma.[94] Despite the success so far achieved in mortality rate cut, only half of the United States women aged 20 or over have ever received a Pap test. As a result, cervical malignancy remains a common and highly lethal disease, amounting to the third most frequent cause of death from malignancy (after breast and lung) in women 35 to 54 years old according to the 1975 Cancer statistics from the American Cancer Society.[105] An estimated 19,000 new cases of invasive cervical carcinoma are discovered annually in the United States, and 7,800 women died of cancer of the cervix in 1975.[105] The average age of patients with invasive squamous cell carcinoma is 51.4 years, 15 to 23 years older than patients with advanced cervical intraepithelial neoplasia (carcinoma *in situ*).[24] Cervical cancer occurs, however, at almost any age between 17 and 90 years. In young women, aged 30 or less, it accounts for 7% of all invasive lesions of the cervix.[66] The epidemiologic characteristics, including socioeconomic status and sexual history, of these patients are similar to those of the older age group.[66] Contrary to earlier studies, indicating a less favorable prognosis for young women with invasive cervical neoplasia, recent data[66] showed no significant differences in the histologic differentiation, stage of disease, and survival rates between young women and patients in the perimenopausal and menopausal periods. Patients aged 70 years and older have the lowest risk of developing invasive squamous cell carcinoma, as only 4.5% of all invasive cervical cancers are observed in this age group.[2]

*Etiology and pathogenesis*

A considerable body of evidence has been accumulated in the past decade suggesting that invasive squamous cell carcinoma develops from cervical intraepithelial neoplasia (CIN). Patients with invasive disease have similar environmental variables and seroimmunologic characteristics to those with preinvasive precursor lesions (see Chapter 7). The majority of women with invasive cancer of the cervix classically are from lower socioeconomic groups, have begun heterosexual activity early in life, marry early, are multiparous, and have usually many sexual partners. Most of these attributes are interrelated, having for a common basis intercourse. Although the precise etiologic agent in the development of cervical cancer has not yet been convincingly identified, data derived from seroimmunologic studies on herpesvirus type 2 and cervical cancer patients support the concept of a cause–effect relationship.[59]

The usual pathogenetic sequence of events of cervical carcinomas is cervical intraepithelial neoplasia (mild to moderate to severe dysplasia to carcinoma in situ), microinvasive carcinoma, preclinical occult invasive carcinoma, and frank clinical invasive carcinoma.[14,19,37,38] The mean progression transit time of early CIN (very mild dysplasia) to advanced CIN (carcinoma in situ) as determined by cytology and colpomicroscopy is approximately 7 years.[97] The average duration of the *"in situ"* phase is estimated to be in between 13[38] and 15 years.[24] It is known, however, that a certain number of cases progress more quickly and others more slowly. It has been estimated that only 43 to 66% of untreated intraepithelial lesions eventually progress to microinvasive carcinoma.[37,38] The estimated average duration of preclinical microinvasive disease to occult invasive carcinoma is 2 years and that of occult carcinoma to overt clinical carcinoma is about 8 to 9 years[38] (Figure 9.1). It is believed that all cases of microinvasive and occult invasive carcinomas, if untreated, progress to frank invasive carcinoma. About 10% of invasive squamous cell carcinomas of the cervix are thought to arise *de novo,* not

preceded by intraepithelial precursor lesions.[2,5] This form of invasive cancer, referred to as "monophasic carcinoma"[2] or "spray carcinoma of Schiller,"[103] usually occurs later in life and is rapidly progressing.[5] It presumably develops from the basal cells of the normal native squamous epithelium of the portio. Whether such a pathogenetic form of cervical neoplasia really exists is debatable. Histologic sampling alone does not necessarily provide accurate data on the precise geographic distribution of associated intraepithelial alterations, particularly if the changes represent a minute focus. Such a small focus may therefore easily be missed in 3- to 5-mm thick step sections. In addition, in "monophasic cervical carcinomas," epithelial atypia, consistent with early CIN, has invariably been demonstrated in the squamous mucous membrane of the transformation zone adjacent to the invasive lesion.[10,55] It is therefore highly unlikely that invasive carcinoma of the cervix ever arises in normal squamous epithelium.

*Symptoms and signs*

Nearly all patients (99%) with clinically visible invasive carcinoma of the cervix complain of abnormal vaginal bleeding. The most significant and common feature is bleeding following intercourse or douching. Intermittent spotting, serosanguinous discharge, or frank hemorrhage are also frequently encountered. Ten to 20% of patients complain of bloody malodorous discharge and pain, often radiating to the sacral region. Weakness, pallor, weight loss, edema of extremities, rectal pain, and hematuria are symptoms and signs of either locally advanced or metastatic disease.

*Diagnosis*

Means for accurate detection and diagnosis of frank invasive carcinoma include cytology, colposcopy, and colposcope-oriented punch biopsy. Although the high degree of diagnostic accuracy of cytology (95% of cases)[94] and colposcopy[12,107,108] (Figure 7.15d) is no longer questioned, a tissue diagnosis is required for a definitive histologic confirmation. A diagnosis of invasive cervical carcinoma obtained by punch biopsy need not be followed by dilatation and curettage, because the latter often complicates therapy by producing pelvic infection and because involvement of the fundus by the tumor does not influence the clinical stage (Table 9.1). Thorough rectovaginal examination, intravenous pyelography, cystoscopy, proctosigmoidoscopy, and skeletal survey are required to assess the exact clinical stage of the disease.

**Table 9.2** Distribution of carcinomas (squamous and adenocarcinomas) of the uterine cervix by clinical stage

| Series | Stage | | | |
|---|---|---|---|---|
| | I | II | III | IV |
| Campos[16] (311 patients) | 37% | 34% | 27% | 2% |
| Abell[2][a] (3,694 patients) | 30% | 35% | 23% | 6.5% |
| Total | 33.5% | 34.5% | 30% | 4.2% |

[a] In Abell's series the clinical stage was not available in 5.5% of patients.

### Clinical stage

The rationale in determining the clinical stage or extent of cervical carcinoma is that a definite relationship exists between survival rate and staging. The histologic grade or degree of differentiation of the neoplasm influences the prognosis only by its possible effect on the stage. Therefore, the most critical factor in predicting the eventual outcome of cervical malignancy is the clinical extent of the disease. The International Federation of Gynecologists and Obstetricians (FIGO), after several modifications of its original 1961 classification, has adopted in 1974 the clinical staging system for both squamous and adenocarcinoma of the cervix given in Table 9.1. Although the FIGO classification is the one generally used, it has a major drawback. With the exception of stage Ia microinvasive and Ib occult invasive cancers, it is limited to the clinical findings based on pelvic examination. As a result, a large proportion of patients treated by radical surgery are found to have more advanced stage than originally has been determined. Metastatic node involvement was reported[60,85] in 8 to 25% of stage I, 21 to 38% of stage II, and 32 to 46% of stage III lesions. The distribution of cervical carcinomas according to clinical stages is shown in Table 9.2. Two-thirds of all lesions are stage I and II, nearly one-third are stage III, and fewer than 5% are stage IV.[2,16]

### Gross morphology

The appearance of invasive cervical carcinoma on gross inspection depends on the extent of involvement. The early lesions may produce focal induration, shallow ulcera-

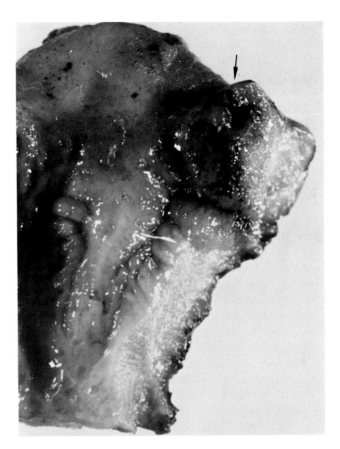

**9.6** Noduloinvasive squamous cell carcinoma of the cervix. Note the circumscribed margin of the tumor elevating the squamous portio epithelium (arrow), which is devoid of ulceration.

tions, or a slightly elevated granular area that bleeds readily on touch. Approximately 98% of early carcinomas are localized within the transformation zone, with variable degree of encroachment onto the neighboring native portio. The more advanced growths have two major types of gross appearance: endophytic and exophytic. Endophytic carcinomas are either ulceroinvasive or noduloinvasive, whereas the exophytic variety may be polypoid or papillary (verrucous carcinoma).[2]

The ulceroinvasive lesion presents a craterlike excavation with necrotic base and indurated, elevated margins. This type of lesion produces extensive tissue destruction and parametrial fixation associated with fistulas into the urinary bladder, rectum, and peritoneal cavity.

The noduloinvasive type is characterized by stoney-hard, irregular, nodular masses with elevation of the squamous and endocervical epithelium, both of which often appear normal but eventually ulcerate (Figure 9.6).

Polypoid carcinoma consists of a bulky, friable, often bleeding and necrotic exophytic growth with granular or papillary surface. The lesion protrudes through the cervical os and may fill the vaginal apex (Figure 9.7, Plate VIII). The rare exophytic papillary or verrucous carcinoma is described in detail on page 188. The vagaries of growth patterns have generally no relationship to the microscopic appearance of the tumor.

### Microscopic morphology

The majority (94%) of malignant epithelial neoplasms of the cervix used to be classified microscopically as squamous cell (epidermoid) carcinomas. However, a recent analysis of large series of cervical cancers[2,95] revealed that when rigid histologic criteria are used in the histologic classification of cervical carcinomas, only 75 to 77% are of the squamous cell type. The remainder, 23 to 25%, include various types of adenocarcinomas, subcolumnar reserve cell carcinomas, double primary carcinomas, and collision carcinomas (Table 9.3). Several attempts have been made to classify cervical squamous cell carcinomas according to the predominant cell type or degree of differentiation. Reagan and Ng[95] proposed to classify squamous cell lesions into large-cell keratinizing, large-cell nonkeratinizing, and small-cell nonkeratinizing carcinomas. When considered in relation to prognosis, the best 5-year survival rate is associated with large-cell nonkeratinizing carcinomas (68.3%), followed by the large-cell keratinizing type (41.7%), whereas small-cell carcinomas have 20% 5-year survival rate. Others[74] prefer such terms as spinal, transitional, and spindle or basal cell types. To date, the most accepted and widely used histologic classification is based on the degree of differentiation. The lesions are divided into well-differentiated (grade 1), moderately differentiated (grade 2), and poorly differentiated (grade 3) carcinomas. The largest proportion of squamous cell carcinomas is moderately differentiated (grade 2), followed by poorly differentiated (grade 3) and well-differentiated lesions (grade 1).

In general, invasive squamous cell carcinomas are char-

**Table 9.3** Histologic classification of invasive carcinomas of the cervix

| | |
|---|---|
| Squamous cell (epidermoid) carcinoma | Subcolumnar reserve cell carcinoma |
| Adenocarcinoma | Double primary carcinomas |

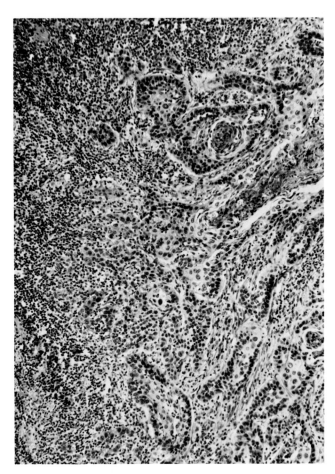

**9.8** Invasive squamous cell carcinoma of the cervix. Note the irregular contour of infiltrative nests. There is evidence of neoplastic cell degeneration and conspicuous inflammatory exudate at the epitheliostromal junction.

acterized by interanastomosing tongues or solid masses of neoplastic epithelium infiltrating the fibrous stroma of the cervix (Figure 9.8). Characteristically, the contour of the infiltrating nests and clusters is irregular and ragged. Stromal reactions of the cervix to invasive carcinoma are variable. In most cases, there is a moderate lymphoplasmocytic infiltration of the invaded connective tissue. There are cases, however, with marked inflammatory reaction, especially at the interface of neoplastic tumor cells and stroma, suggesting a cellular immunologic response to tumoral antigens. The existence of a cellular immune mechanism in the host response to cervical carcinoma is supported by the comparatively better survival rates and fewer regional node metastases reported for patients with intense stromal reaction than those without.[2,49] Further

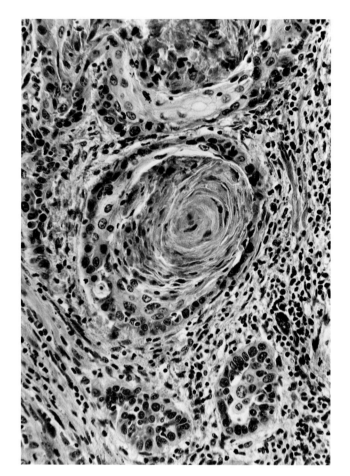

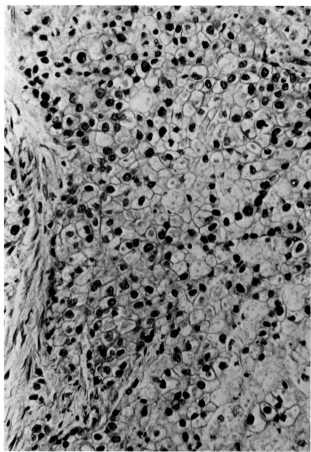

**9.9** Well-differentiated, grade 1 invasive squamous cell carcinoma of the cervix. Keratin pearl formation is evident.

**9.10** Invasive squamous cell carcinoma of the cervix with clear cell features. The cells are rich in glycogen, which results in their floculent, clear cytoplasmic appearance. The cellular borders are well defined.

support is provided by the inhibition of immuno-competent leukocyte migration by extracts of patients' autochthonous cervical squamous carcinoma cells.[47] Although extensive inflammatory reaction may be seen in polypoid carcinomas, it cannot be correlated with survival rates, presumably because inflammation occurs secondarily to trauma and necrosis in this type of cervical neoplasm.

In the well-differentiated type, the most striking feature is the abundance of keratin formation, which is deposited as concentric whorls (keratin pearls) in the centers of neoplastic epithelial nests (Figure 9.9). The cells appear mature with voluminous, eosinophilic cytoplasm. Individual cell keratinization (dyskeratosis) is recognized by intense cytoplasmic eosinophilia. Occasionally, the cells assume a clear appearance which is caused by the accumulation of intracytoplasmic glycogen (Figure 9.10).

The cells are tightly packed together and produce well-developed intercellular bridges. The nuclei are large, irregular, and hyperchromatic, with numerous chromocenters. Mitotic divisions are present with maximum concentration at the periphery of the advancing epithelial nests. The stroma is often infiltrated by chronic inflammatory cells and, occasionally, a foreign body giant cell reaction is observed (Figure 9.11).

In moderately differentiated carcinomas, the neoplastic cells are more pleomorphic than in grade 1 lesions, are characterized by large irregular nuclei, and have less abundant cytoplasmic matrix. The cellular borders, as well as intercellular bridges, appear indistinct. Keratin pearl formation is virtually nonexistent, but individual cell kera-

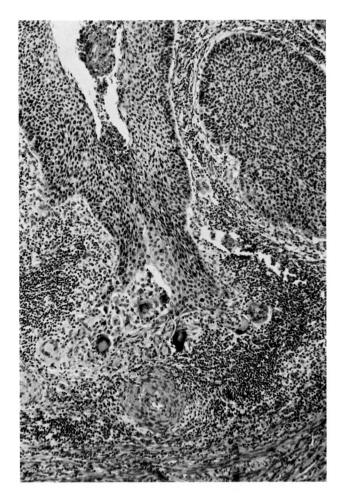

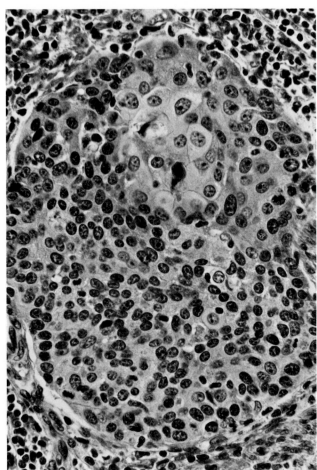

**9.11** Moderately differentiated, grade 2 squamous cell carcinoma of the cervix. Note foreign body giant cell reaction to infiltrating tumor cells. Such host response is associated with good prognosis.

**9.12** Moderately differentiated, grade 2 squamous cell carcinoma of the cervix. Note attempt at keratinization.

tinization is seen in the center of cancer nests. Mitotic figures are more numerous than in the better differentiated lesions (Figure 9.12).

Poorly differentiated squamous cell carcinomas are generally composed of small cells with hyperchromatic oval nuclei and scant indistinct cytoplasm, resembling the malignant basal cells of grade 3 intraepithelial neoplasia or carcinoma in situ (Figures 9.13 and 9.14). Search for squamous differentiation reveals rare foci of abortive dyskeratosis. Mitoses and areas of necrosis are abundant. Poorly differentiated lesions are occasionally made of large, pleomorphic cells with giant, bizarre nuclei and abnormal mitotic figures. In rare instances, the neoplastic cells assume a spindle-shaped configuration resembling a sarcoma

(Figure 9.15). In these instances, reticulin stain demonstrates the epithelial nature of the spindle-shaped growth (reticulin fibers encircle nests of cells rather than individual cells), and in most instances histologic continuity between the fibroblastoid neoplastic cells and the usual squamous epithelial cells can be demonstrated.

### Ultrastructure

Ultrastructurally, the neoplastic cells of invasive squamous cell carcinoma of the cervix display nuclear, cytoplasmic, and plasma membrane abnormalities that are more severe in high-grade than in low-grade, well-differentiated neoplasms.[36] The neoplastic squamous cells have large nuclei with indented nuclear membrane and promi-

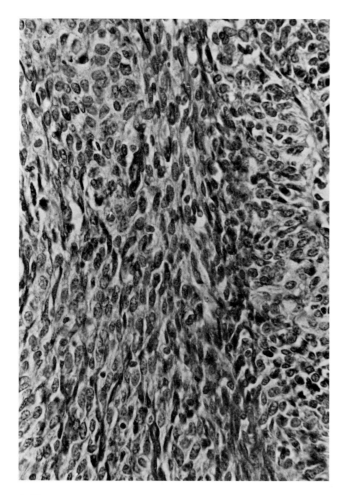

**9.13** Poorly differentiated, grade 3 squamous cell carcinoma of the cervix. The cells have hyperchromatic, oval nuclei; scant cytoplasm; and indistinct cell membranes.

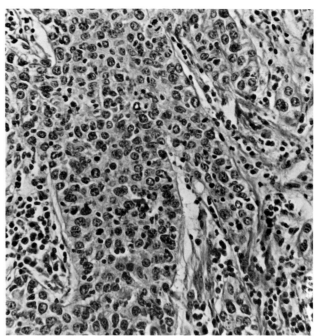

**9.14** Poorly differentiated, grade 3 squamous cell carcinoma. Note anisonucleosis associated with numerous mitotic divisions.

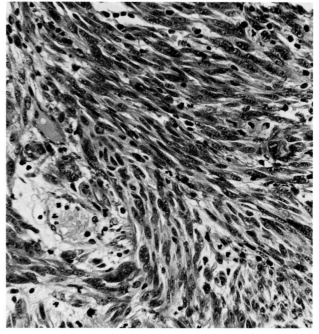

**9.15** Invasive squamous cell carcinoma with spindle shape features. Note fusiform configuration of cells, resembling a sarcoma. This area was continuous with moderately differentiated squamous cell carcinoma.

nent nucleoli associated with segregation of nuclear DNA and nucleolar RNA. In contrast to normal squamous cells, in the malignant variety, there is a decrease in polyribosomes and tonofilaments[119] and an increase in pleomorphic mitochondria and autophagocytic activity (Figure 9.16). The granular endoplasmic reticulum is dilated and fragmented. These morphologic alterations are associated with higher anaerobic glycolytic rates than are observed in normal cervical squamous cells. These changes in metabolic characteristics reflect adaptation to a new form of cellular function by which malignant cells rely on anaerobic glycolysis as an energy source.[6] By doing so, the neoplastic cells become independent of the normal controls of extracellular energy supply, which is required for

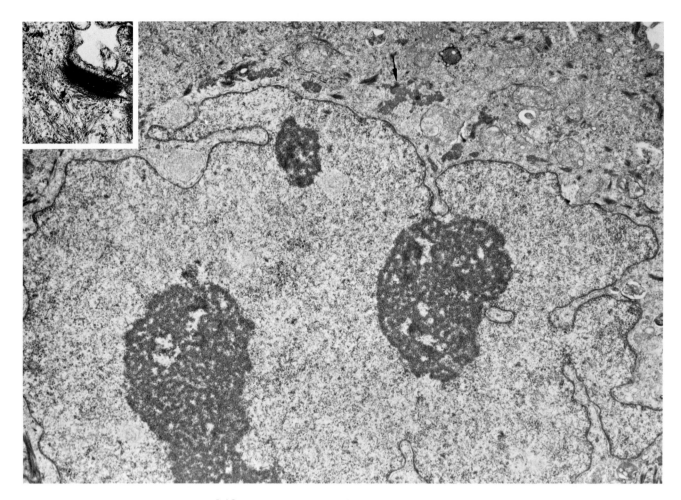

**9.16** Electron micrograph of moderately differentiated squamous carcinoma cell of the cervix. Intracytoplasmic bundles of tonofilaments (arrow) and well-developed desmosome–tonofilament intercellular attachment complexes are characteristic features of malignant cells of squamous origin. Note irregular nuclear membrane and prominent nucleoli. ×5,550; Inset, ×17,760.

cellular growth. The tonofilaments are aggregated and often form large globular masses, resulting in intense cytologic eosinophilia of neoplastic cells that are engaged in individual cell keratinization (Figure 9.17). Aggregation of tonofilaments is caused by separation and retraction of desmosomal–tonofilament attachments. In the lesser differentiated lesions, tonofilaments and desmosomal plates are reduced and poorly developed. Loss of desmosomal attachments and separation of desmosomal–tonofilament complexes lead to loss of cellular cohesion. Another characteristic feature of squamous cell carcinoma cells is the profound decrease in gap-junction nexuses compared to normal cervical squamous epithelium.[77] Nexuses are specialized junctional units, where adjacent cell membranes

are very closely apposed, with an intercellular space of about 20 Å in diameter. The nexus consists of closely packed, hollow, hexagonal tubules arranged in a honeycomb pattern and forming an open-channel system between adjacent cells. The system facilitates the passage of electrolytes and proteins from one cell to another without traversing the intercellular space. It has been suggested that nexuses play a role in cell contact inhibition and in the formation of low-resistance electrical coupling sites between normal cells.[77] A deficiency of nexuses in invasive cervical carcinoma may therefore be responsible for the reduced cellular adhesiveness, cell contact inhibition, and the altered electrical coupling that have been observed in malignant neoplastic cells[77] and perhaps the invasive char-

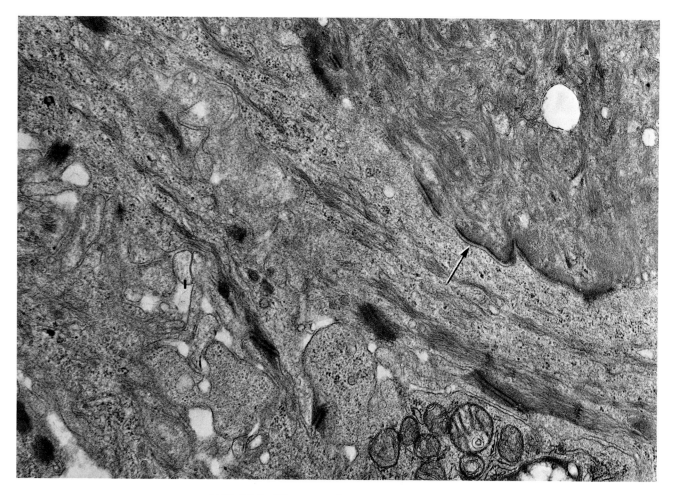

**9.17** Well-differentiated invasive squamous cell carcinoma of the cervix. Electron microscopic appearance of individual cell keratinization (dyskeratosis). Lobular masses of tonofilaments are responsible for intense eosinophilia on light microscopy. Aggregation of tonofilament is caused by separation and retraction of desmosomal–tonofilament attachments (arrow). The intercellular space (I) contains interdigitating microvilli. ×7,438.

acter of malignant neoplasms. The plasma membrane is complexly convoluted, with numerous interdigitating microvilli. A well-developed basement membrane is produced by the invading neoplastic cells, although it often appears fragmented.

### Differential diagnosis

Histologically, the lesions most commonly confused with invasive squamous cell carcinomas are squamous prosoplasia (metaplasia) with extensive endocervical "gland" involvement, pseudodecidual reaction, squamous papilloma, condylomata acuminata, and pseudoepithelio-

matous hyperplasia associated with chronic granulomatous diseases, such as lymphogranuloma venerum and granuloma inguinale. Careful evaluation of the cytonuclear appearance of these lesions, however, reveals their benign nature.

### Modes of spread

Squamous cell carcinoma of the cervix spreads principally by direct local invasion to the adjacent tissues and by lymphatics, and less commonly through blood vessels. Initially, the tumor grows by direct continuity along tissue spaces of least resistance, the perineural and perivascular tissues, into the paracervical and parametrial areas and into the cardinal and uterosacral ligaments. Ultimately, lateral spread may reach the bony pelvis and so encompasses and obstructs one or both ureters as they traverse the paracervical region. Direct extension may also involve the uterine cavity and vagina, with extension into the urinary bladder and rectum resulting in vesicovaginal and rectovaginal fistulas.

The spread of cervical cancer via lymphatics occurs relatively early in the course of the disease and is found in 25 to 50% of patients with stage Ib and II carcinomas.[17,60] The preferential course of dissemination is via the paracervical, hypogastric, and external iliac lymph nodes[91] and then extension to lateral sacral, common iliac, paraaortic, and inguinal nodes. Isolated invasion of the sacral, external iliac, and hypogastric nodes is occasionally observed. Distant lymph node metastases above the diaphragm including the supraclavicular lymph nodes are uncommon[32] and are a feature of widespread disease. In these cases, cancer cells are transported from the paraaortic nodes into the mediastinum and then into the thoracic duct.

Hematogenous dissemination is the least common metastatic pathway of cervical carcinoma, although nearly 50% of surgically removed specimens may contain histologic evidence of blood vessel invasion.[42] Blood-borne metastases are generally seen in stage IV lesions or when the local growth has previously been irradiated. They are produced in the lung, liver, bone, heart, skin, and brain.

## Therapy

The three basic modalities in the curative treatment of invasive carcinoma of the cervix are surgery, radiation, and combination of both radiation and surgery. In selected early stage Ib and IIa cases, radical hysterectomy and bilateral pelvic lymphadenectomy or intracavitary radiation followed by radical surgery may be carried out. Because metastatic lymph node involvement remains one of the most important prognostic factors, the use of preoperative and peroperative lymphography has been recommended in recent years as an aid during the dissection and excision of the pelvic lymphatic system.[62] Advanced lesions with involvement of the bladder or rectum or both may be treated by pelvic exenteration. The preferred treatment for most stage II and III cases is combined external and intracavitary radiotherapy. Modern techniques of radiotherapy use a variety of intracavitary radium applicators and low-intensity needles.

External megavoltage with cobalt-60 is required for adequate radiation of the pelvis. The total cancericidal dose of both radium and x rays to control squamous cell carcinoma of the cervix is in the order of 6,000 to 7,000 rads. The incidence of serious morbidity and mortality from irradiation is 30% and 2.4%, respectively.[115] The most common complications in decreasing frequency are: proctitis; vault necrosis; hemorrhagic cystitis; peritonitis resulting from obstruction, perforation, and necrosis of the bowel; vesicovaginal fistula; and profuse hemorrhage. The incidence of major complications associated with radical surgery is about 9% and includes bladder atony, thrombophlebitis, cuff abscesses, and hematoma. The operative death rate is 0.6%.[89] Chemotherapy, using methotrexate and 5-fluorouracil, is employed in carcinomas with widespread distribution or recurrent neoplasms, but the results are disappointing. Immunotherapy with DNA from patient's tumor plus Freund's adjuvant and autogenous vaccine made from patient's tumor was tried without significant success.[48]

## Prognosis and causes of death

The results of treatment of invasive cervical carcinoma are primarily related to the extent of the tumor at the time of initial diagnosis. The general 5-year survival rates for adequately treated cases of all stages are 60%. Local recurrences of invasive disease are principally located in the vaginal vault, pelvis, bladder, and rectum and occur in about 15% of patients. Typically, the majority of recurrences appear within 2 years after the initial therapy. The 5-year survival rate after treatment of recurrent disease by means of irradiation, exenteration, and radical hysterectomy is 20 to 35%.[51] The significantly lower incidence of recurrence (6%) in patients treated by surgery is presumably because of the less advanced stage of the malignancy selected for operation. Results of radical surgery and radiation therapy are essentially similar. The actuarial 5-year salvage rates according to the FIGO clinical stages are: stage I, 85 to 90%; stage II, 70 to 75%; stage III, 30 to 35%; and stage IV, 10%.[60,71] In general, the survival rates are reduced to 30 to 50%, even in the early stages (Ib), when metastatic lymph nodes are discovered compared to those patients without node involvement.[51,60]

A good correlation between immunocompetence and prognosis of cervical cancer patients has recently been demonstrated.[82] Patients with adequate cutaneous delayed hypersensitivity reaction to standard skin antigens and to contact allergen (difluorobenzene) have a better prognosis than those with impaired or no reactivity. The role of immunology in assessing prognosis was also demonstrated by Davidsohn and associates.[28] By using the mixed-cell agglutination reaction they have shown that isoantigens A, B, and H, which are present in normal squamous epithelium and red blood cells, are absent in nearly all primary and metastatic cervical squamous cell carcinomas. According to the investigators, the findings indicate that the loss of demonstrable antigens precedes the formation of distant metastases. Failure to demonstrate antigens in squamous cell carcinoma of the cervix is therefore regarded as an indicator of the probability of metastases.[28] Elevated levels of plasma carcinoembryonic antigen (CEA), a tumor associated antigen, were reported in 50% of patients with invasive squamous cell carcinoma of the cervix and 84% of the patients with recurrent carcinoma.[33] Carcinoembryonic antigen determinations may be used as an adjunctive help in the early detection of recurrent disease or metastasis. A tumor-specific complement-fixing antibody, induced by HSV-2, has recently been detected in 91% of untreated invasive carcinomas, 68% of *in situ* lesions, and 5% of control patients studied.[7] The antibody (AG-4) was absent in all 22 women treated by ionizing radiation or surgery for invasive disease. These findings, if confirmed, would be of considerable prognostic value in evaluating the clinical course as well as the therapeutic response of patients with cervical neoplasia.

Other factors that influence prognosis are the gross characteristics of invasive cervical carcinomas; polypoid lesions are less aggressive than nodulo- or ulceroinvasive cancers. In general, histologic grading has no direct influence on survival rate. Although well-differentiated neoplasms progress slower than poorly differentiated lesions, the latter has a better response to ionizing irradiation therapy than the former and so the overall end results are similar for carcinomas of different grades.[2] However, neoplasms with marked lymphoplasmocytic stromal infiltration have a more favorable course than those without significant stromal inflammatory reaction.[2]

Ureteral compression caused by both ureteral wall compression and periureteral lymphatic obstruction by the tumor leads to hydroureter, hydronephrosis, hydronephrotic renal atrophy, pyelonephritis, and loss of renal function. Obstruction of both ureters results in uremia and is the leading cause of death, being found in about 40 to 50% of patients with cervical carcinoma.[106] Peritonitis caused by obstruction and perforation of large or small bowel, respiratory failure associated with pulmonary metastasis, or massive edema are the other major causes of death. Hemorrhage, cardiac failure, massive venous thrombosis, pulmonary embolism, and complications of radiation therapy represent the less common causes of death.

## Carcinoma of the Cervical Stump

Invasive carcinoma either of the squamous or glandular type may develop in the cervical stump that remains following subtotal hysterectomy, with an incidence of 0.2 to 3% of patients.[121] According to various series, patients with cervical stump cancer represents 0.5 to 10% of all cancers of the cervix uteri. In a study of 173 women with carcinoma of the cervical stump, Wolff and associates[121] divided their patients into those in whom the neoplasm was found within 2 years of the subtotal hysterectomy and those in whom the lesion appeared more than 2 years after the operation. The 5-year survival rate of patients of the first subgroup was found worse (30%) than either those of the second subgroup (49%) or those with cancer of the cervix in general. The prognosis for patients of the second subgroup was comparable to that for patients with cancer of the cervix in general. Similarly, metastatic disease developed more frequently (17%) in the first subgroup than in the second group of patients. On the basis of these observations, the authors[121] postulated that cervical stump cancers occurring within the first 2 years following surgery represent "left behind" or residual malignancy, whereas those discovered after 2 years are "true" cancers arising *de novo* from the cervical stump. The existence of two such distinct groups of patients, however, remains speculative as no morphologic data were available either on the subtotal hysterectomy specimens or on the cervix prior or after removal of the fundus. The fact that carcinoma may arise in cervical stumps indicates that subtotal hysterectomy has no place in contemporary gynecologic practice.

## Carcinoma in Pregnancy

Invasive carcinoma of the cervix is uncommon during gestation, occurring approximately once in 3,500 pregnancies in a high-risk population for cervical cancer.[35] In average, pregnant women, the incidence is about one in 6,000 pregnancies or fewer. Nonetheless, routine cervical cytology should be part of the initial prenatal examination. Suspicious cytology should be repeated and if the findings are confirmed colposcope-oriented cervical punch biopsy obtained. Cone biopsy should be avoided because of the danger to induce massive bleeding. The treatment of pregnant patients with invasive cervical cancer depends essentially on the clinical stage of the disease. Patients with stage Ia microinvasive carcinoma (with less than 1-mm stromal invasion) are allowed to progress to term under careful and frequent colposcopic examinations and then treated either by vaginal hysterectomy following vaginal

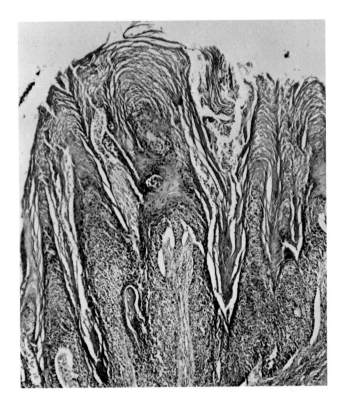

**9.19** Verrucous carcinoma of the cervix. Note frondlike papillae with extensive surface keratinization. The circumscribed, cone-shaped edges of neoplastic fronds expand into the underlying stroma.

[Courtesy of Dr. A. Blaustein, New York University Medical Center, New York.]

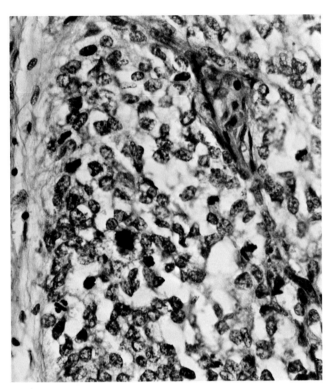

**9.20** Verrucous carcinoma of the cervix. High-power view illustrating the edge of advancing epithelial fronds. Note marked nuclear pleomorphism, hyperchromasia, loss of cellular cohesion, and numerous mitotic figures, consistent with malignant growth.

[Courtesy of Dr. A. Blaustein, New York University Medical Center, New York.]

delivery or by cesarean section hysterectomy.[31] Stages Ib or more are immediately treated without regard to the fetus. Exceptions are made, however, during the last trimester when treatment may be delayed to carry the infant to viability. The management of stage Ib and IIa lesions is radical hysterectomy and bilateral pelvic lymphadenectomy[35] or combined radiation therapy.[26] Irradiation is the therapeutic choice for more advanced disease or for patients who have medical contraindication or refuse radical surgery. External radiation usually causes abortion in about 6 weeks and intracavitary radium is applied to the cervix to complete therapy. Pregnancy per se does not influence the prognosis of cancer of the cervix.[35,45a]

## Verrucous Carcinoma

Verrucous carcinoma is a variant of well-differentiated squamous cell carcinoma. In the female genital tract, the most commonly involved region is the vulva, but at least

eight well-documented cases have been described in the cervix.[30,45,65,69] Clinically, the lesion is a slow growing but a potentially lethal locally invasive verrucous neoplasm (Figure 9.18, Plate VIII). Five of eight patients with verrucous carcinoma of the cervix died of tumor shortly after the diagnosis.[69] In the past, this distinctive growth has often been reported under the term "giant condylomata acuminata of Buschke and Lowenstein."[69] Histologically, the neoplasm is composed of well-differentiated squamous cells arranged in frondlike papillae (Figures 9.19 and 9.20) with or without surface keratinization. The epithelium often lacks significant cytologic atypia, although in several cases cytonuclear pleomorphism and numerous mitoses are found in the upper layers. The edge of neoplastic tongues is expanding instead of infiltrating the underlying stroma and there is a conspicuous inflammatory reaction at the epitheliostromal junction.

Certain investigators[65] have suggested that verrucous carcinoma may be distinguished histologically from the well-differentiated squamous cell carcinoma with a keratinized papillary surface and from condylomata acuminata. Verrucous carcinoma lacks the small infiltrating clusters of anaplastic cells and central fibroconnective tissue cores in the epithelial papillae, which are seen in the warty squamous cell carcinoma and condylomata, respectively.[65] However, the general contention is that verrucous carcinoma in the absence of metastasis is not possible to distinguish histologically from well-differentiated squamous cell carcinoma or large condylomata acuminata of the cervix.[69] In view of this difficulty, the most accurate diagnosis in differentiating these lesions lies in their prospective behavior following surgical removal. The most common complication associated with verrucous carcinoma is local recurrence, particularly when irradiation is used as a sole therapeutic means. Another, as yet unexplained, complication of verrucous carcinoma is its high rate (30%)[30] of anaplastic transformation with accelerated growth following radiation therapy. Because of these features, together with the relative resistance to radiation, roentgen therapy is contraindicated in the treatment of verrucous carcinoma. The most appropriate therapeutic approach of the disease is early wide local excision. Regional lymph nodes are rarely involved and distant metastases are exceedingly rare.[69]

# Adenocarcinoma of the Cervix

## Incidence and age distribution

The incidence of primary adenocarcinoma has been variously assessed as 5 to 8% of all epithelial malignancies of the cervix, with an incidence rate from 0.42 to 11.7%.[2,3,50,79,112] However, in recent years the average incidence has doubled[2,94] and rates as high as 34% are reported in certain series.[29] It seems, however, that the increased frequency is not absolute but only relative to an improved cytologic detection and a decreasing number of cases of cervical squamous cell carcinoma observed in current years.[24,37,94] The mean age of patients with invasive adenocarcinoma is 56 years, 5 years older than those with squamous cell carcinoma.[24]

## Symptoms and signs

The presenting symptom is abnormal vaginal bleeding in about 75% of patients, and 80% have their disease confined to the cervix (stage I) or advanced into the parametrium or vagina (stage II) at the time of discovery.[2,3,29,50,79,112]

## Diagnosis

The diagnostic accuracy of cytopathology in the detection of cervical adenocarcinoma varies according to the cytologic experience of the pathologist and the techniques used for material sampling. When the sampling technique includes aspiration of the endocervical canal with an endocervical pipette, the diagnostic accuracy can reach 95%.[95] The definitive diagnosis of either invasive or in situ adenocarcinoma is achieved by microscopic examination of tissue recovered by punch biopsy or conization biopsy.

## Etiology and pathogenesis

At present, there is little information on the etiology and pathogenesis of endocervical adenocarcinoma. This lack of knowledge is attributable to the relatively low incidence and distant location of the lesion, precluding early detection and meaningful prospective followup studies of a large number of cases. It is believed, however, that unlike squamous cell carcinoma of the cervix, adenocarcinoma is not associated with venereal etiologic factors. The finding of in situ endocervical columnar cell adenocarcinomas with[3] and without[116] invasive disease suggests that the most common type of cervical adenocarcinoma originates in the epithelium of the endocervix. The occurrence of adenocarcinoma in situ 5 to 6 years earlier[116] than the invasive form indicates that the former is the precursor of invasive carcinoma of the endocervix. The development of clear cell adenocarcinoma of the cervix and vagina in young patients who were exposed in utero to abnormal estrogenic (diethylstilbestrol) stimulation is histogenetically unrelated to the conventional adenocarcinoma of the cervix.

## Gross morphology

On gross examination, 50% of the patients have a fungating, polypoid, or papillary mass, whereas nearly 15% have no gross lesion as the carcinoma is located within the canal or deep within the endocervical clefts.

## Microscopic morphology and ultrastructure

Histologically, there are many variations in both the cell types and growth patterns.[2,3] The diagnosis is not always obvious, particularly in lesions with lesser differentiation. In assessing whether the malignancy is of primary endocervical origin or metastatic in the cervix, the pathologist should evaluate the following morphologic features: (1) neoplastic growth pattern, (2) coexistent in situ

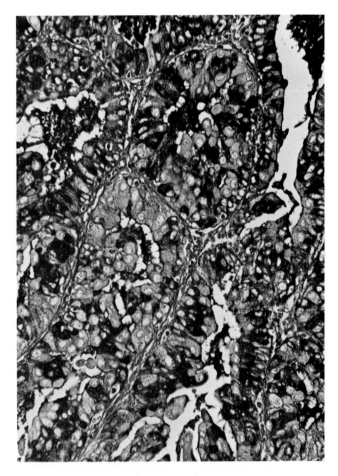

**9.21** Moderately differentiated adenocarcinoma of the cervix. The endocervical origin of the lesion is confirmed by finding of abundant intracytoplasmic acid mucin in neoplastic gland cells (alcian blue stain at pH 2.5).

changes, (3) cell type, and (4) histochemical characteristics. The majority of cervical adenocarcinomas are well to moderately differentiated,[2,3,50,79,112] arranged in a complex racemose of glandular pattern reproducing the cleft–tunnel configuration of the normal endocervical mucosa. Transition between *in situ* and invasive carcinoma provides the strongest evidence for a primary origin and is found in certain series up to 43% of the cases.[3] Most cervical adenocarcinomas contain well-differentiated cells that closely resemble the normal columnar endocervical epithelium. Histochemistry, especially the alcian blue stain, is a useful adjunct in differentiating between adenocarcinoma of the cervix and metastatic adenocarcinoma of endometrial origin.[29] The former contains variable amounts of intracellular alcian blue- positive acid mucin, which may be diffuse or spotty within the neoplastic growth (Figure 9.21), whereas the latter lacks mucin within the cytoplasmic substance. In endometrial adenocarcinoma cells, the alcian blue staining reaction is faint and is confined to the apex and luminal cytoplasmic membrane. Alcian blue stain, however, is of no diagnostic aid in poorly differentiated endocervical adenocarcinoma as mucinogenesis is generally minimal or absent. Cervical adenocarcinomas may be divided into two histogenetic groups: (1) neoplasms of endocervical mucinous cell origin and (2) neoplasms of presumable subcolumnar reserve cell derivation (Table 9.4). Those arising from endocervical mucinous epithelium are classified according to the predominant histologic growth patterns because they can be correlated with clinical course and survival rate.[112] Histologic classification of the second group can be debated as this group has a poor prognosis, regardless of histologic type.

Adenocarcinoma of endocervical columnar cell type

**Table 9.4**  Adenocarcinoma of the uterine cervix: histogenetic and histologic classification

| Endocervical columnar cell origin | Endocervical subcolumnar origin | Mesonephric duct remnants origin |
| --- | --- | --- |
| Adenocarcinoma, endocervical columnar cell type | Undifferentiated reserve cell carcinoma | Mesonephric adenocarcinoma |
| Clear cell adenocarcinoma | Adenosquamous carcinoma | |
| Medullary adenocarcinoma | Mucoepidermoid carcinoma | |
| Papillary adenocarcinoma, serous type | Adenoid cystic carcinoma (cylindroma) | |
| Mucinous (colloid) adenocarcinoma, intestinal type | | |
| Endometrioid carcinoma | | |
| Carcinoma with stromal fibroplasia (scirrhous carcinoma) | | |

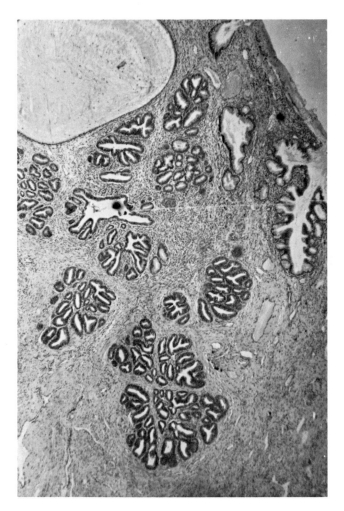

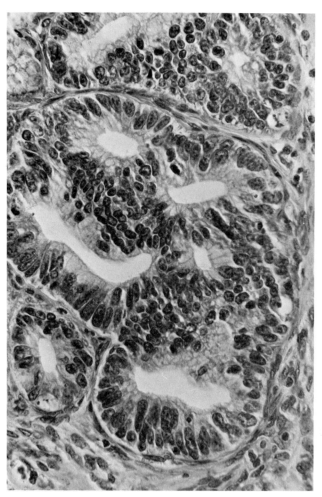

**9.22** *In situ* adenocarcinoma of the cervix. The neoplastic glands contrast in the arrangement and staining characteristics from those of normal endocervical epithelium.

**9.23** *In situ* adenocarcinoma of the endocervix. Note the nuclear enlargement and pseudostratification with coarse chromatin, mitoses, and reduced intracytoplasmic mucin.

represents the most common variety of cervical glandular malignancies. Histologically, it varies from well-differentiated *in situ* carcinoma,[116] in which most of the general characteristics of endocervical epithelium are retained except the nuclei are enlarged and hyperchromatic and mitoses are present (Figures 9.22 and 9.23), to poorly differentiated adenocarcinoma without an easily recognizable glandular pattern. The most common type is moderately differentiated with interbranching glands and variable amount of intracytoplasmic mucin (Figures 9.21, 9.24, and 9.25). Transmission electron microscopy (Figure 9.26) confirms the light microscopic and histochemical observations of a gradual decrease and an eventual loss of mucin production in increasingly dedifferentiated adenocarci-

noma of the cervix.[36] In occasional instances, lesions under the term "adenoma malignum"[76] have been reported. This peculiar type of lesion is currently regarded as an extremely well-differentiated adenocarcinoma with minimal deviation from that of the normal endocervical columnar epithelium (Figure 9.27). The cytoplasm remains tall columnar, with abundant mucin, and nuclear atypia is inconspicuous. In addition, the lesion may exhibit a similar branching arrangement to that of the normal endocervical grooves and tunnels.

When the pathologist is confronted with such a well-differentiated growth, it is difficult to determine whether it represents an *in situ* or an invasive carcinoma. The most reliable criterion in assessing the true nature of the disease

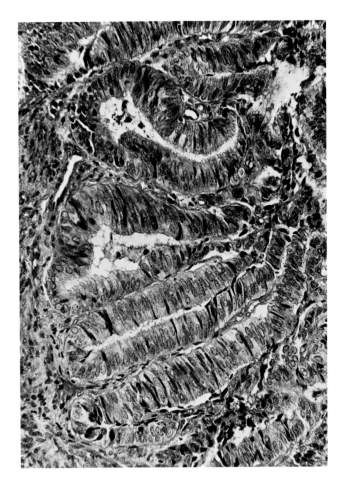

**9.24** Moderately differentiated invasive adenocarcinoma of the cervix.

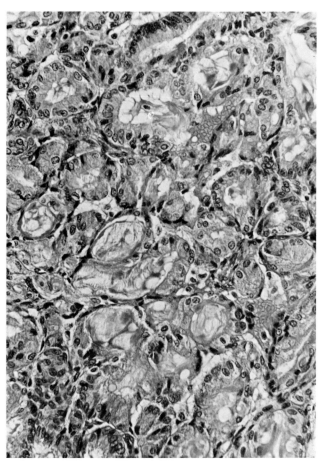

**9.25** Moderately differentiated invasive adenocarcinoma of the cervix. Note the conspicuous mucin production and finely granular pale cytoplasm of the neoplastic cells.

is to carefully evaluate its depth within the endocervix. If the lesion involves more than two-thirds of the cervical stroma, the neoplasm may be regarded invasive, for endocervical crypts and tunnels do not extend beyond that level under normal circumstances. A condition likely to be confused with invasive adenocarcinoma of the cervix is atypical microglandular hyperplasia of the endocervical epithelium (see Chapter 6, Microglandular Endocervical Hyperplasia), but providing that the pathologist is well informed of this disease entity, mistakes are not likely to be made. Similarly, endocervical epithelial atypia associated with trauma or severe inflammation (Figure 6.1c) should be distinguished from *in situ* adenocarcinoma.

The less frequent histologic varieties of endocervical adenocarcinoma of columnar cell origin include medullary adenocarcinoma[2] with abortive gland formation; papillary carcinoma,[2,79] which arises from the surface epithelium of

the endocervix, resembling well-differentiated papillary serous carcinoma of the ovary including psammoma bodies[79] (Figure 9.28); mucinous (colloid) carcinoma with conspicuous mucus production, identical with adenocarcinoma of large bowel with occasional argentaffin and Paneth cells[9] (Figure 9.29); endometrioid carcinoma[2] with or without foci of squamous metaplasia, in all respects similar to endometrial adenocarcinoma; carcinoma with stromal fibroplasia[2] (scirrhous carcinoma), a rare lesion resembling that seen in the female mammary gland (Figure 9.42); and clear cell adenocarcinoma. The latter type of neoplasm is of particular interest as about 170 cases (100 in the vagina and 70 in the cervix) have recently been reported in young women with a history of prenatal exposure to diethylstilbestrol (DES).[54] In the cervix, the lesion

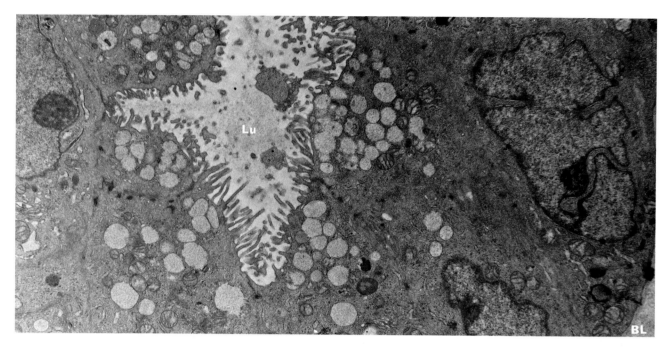

**9.26** Electron micrograph of neoplastic endocervical gland cells with apical, mucin-containing secretory granules. Mucinogenesis is reduced in neoplastic as compared to normal endocervical epithelium. Lu, Lumen; BL, basal lamina. ×6,810.

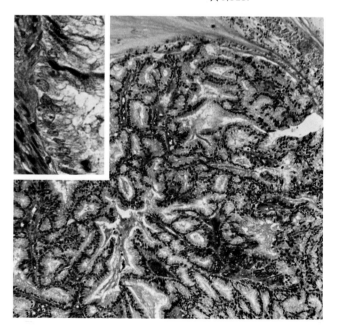

**9.27** Well-differentiated adenocarcinoma of the cervix (adenoma malignum). Note the complex branching pattern and abundant mucin production. The lining cells closely resemble normal endocervical epithelium. Inset: Detail of lining cells with minimal nuclear atypia.

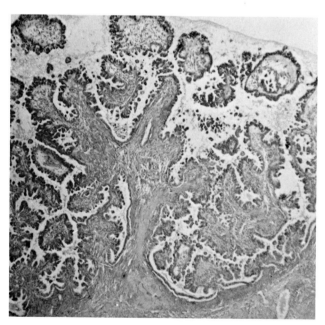

**9.28** Papillary adenocarcinoma of the cervix. Note the branching papillae lined by atypical villous epithelium and supported by connective tissue stroma resembling well-differentiated papillary serous carcinoma of the ovary.

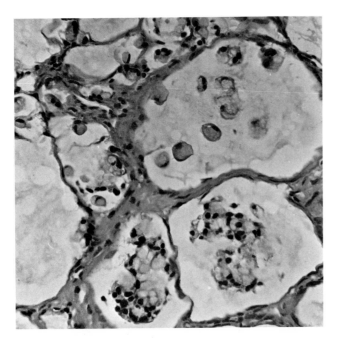

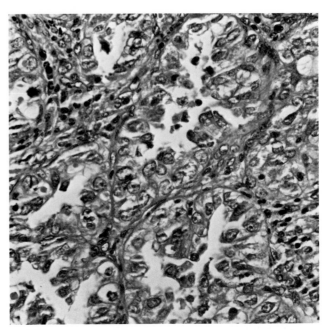

**9.29** Mucinous, colloid carcinoma of the cervix. Note the malignant signet-ring cells in lakes of extracellular mucin.

**9.30** Clear cell carcinoma of the cervix in a young woman with a history of prenatal exposure to diethylstilbestrol. The neoplastic gland cells have clear cytoplasm and hobnail nuclear architecture.

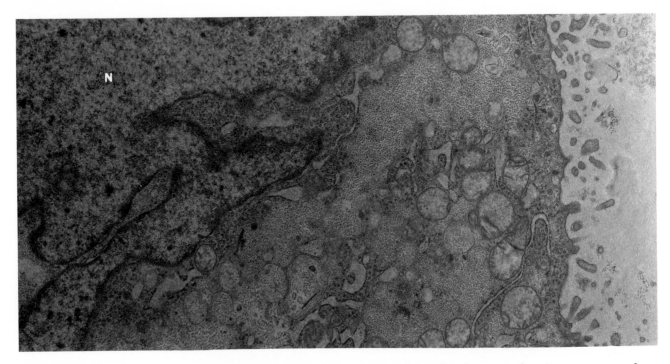

**9.31** Electron microscopy of Figure 9.30. The clear cytoplasmic appearance of neoplastic cells is caused by a massive accumulation of glycogen granules. The nucleus (N) has an irregular membrane. ×12,750.

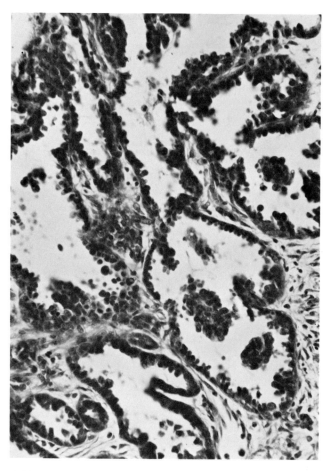

**9.32** Mesonephric carcinoma of the cervix. The gland lining cells demonstrate hobnail nuclear pattern and scant cytoplasm that is not clear and contains an inconspicuous amount of glycogen. The lesion was continuous with mesonephric remnants in the cervix.

[Courtesy of Dr. A. Blaustein, New York University Medical Center, New York.]

arises within the endocervical mucosa and is arranged in glands, tubules, and solid nests (Figure 9.30). The neoplastic cells have a large clear cytoplasm and hyperchromatic pleomorphic nuclei, which often are in an atypical position resulting in a hobnail cytonuclear pattern. Ultrastructurally, (Figure 9.31) there is abundant intracytoplasmic PAS-positive diastase-labile glycogen, which is thought to be responsible for the clear cytoplasmic appearance of the neoplastic cells. The presently available morphologic[36,54] and experimental[40] data favor a Müllerian rather than a mesonephric[52] origin for clear cell adenocarcinomas of the cervix and vagina. This contention

is supported by the frequent coexistence of clear cell adenocarcinoma of the cervix and normal endocervical epithelium[100] and the observation of histologically and ultrastructurally similar neoplasms in the endometrium and ovary.[36] In the vagina, clear cell carcinoma is associated with Müllerian-derived vaginal adenosis.[54] In view of these observations, the term mesonephric carcinoma[52] should not be used for clear cell adenocarcinoma of the female genital tract. Arias–Stella reaction occurs on occasion in endocervical epithelium with intrauterine or ectopic pregnancy and may be mistaken for clear cell adenocarcinoma. Arias–Stella cells are distinctive by their cytonucleomegaly, they contain no mitosis, and their clear cytoplasmic appearance is not caused by glycogen but by increased cytoplasmic matrix in which the organelles are dispersed.

In contrast to the superficial location of cervical clear cell adenocarcinomas, true mesonephric adenocarcinomas are found deep in the lateral wall of the cervix, in a site corresponding to the general location of mesonephric duct remnants. Histologic transitions between mesonephric duct remains and carcinomas have rarely been demonstrated[53]; the cells of mesonephric adenocarcinoma are not clear and have negligible amount of intracytoplasmic glycogen (Figure 9.32).

### Modes of spread and prognosis

Endocervical adenocarcinoma follows similar pathways of progression, including lymphatic metastasis, to that of squamous carcinoma. However, local extension[2] as well as lymph node metastases[85] occur comparatively earlier in adeno- than squamous carcinoma. As a result, the general 5-year survival rates are lower for adenocarcinoma (56%) than for squamous carcinoma patients (68%)[2,50,79,112] and recurrences are a common feature (25%).[112]

### Therapy

The two most widely used therapeutic modalities for stages I and II adenocarcinoma are radiation alone and radiation followed by conservative hysterectomy. Although not generally agreed on,[112] the latter approach seems to yield better results: 80% 5-year survival compared to the former 66% 5-year survival rate.[57] For patients with adenocarcinoma in situ, hysterectomy is considered to be the treatment of choice.[116] In general, the degree of differentiation has no significant influence on survival for adenocarcinoma patients.[112] However, survival rate may be correlated with histologic types of growth. Papillary and clear cell adenocarcinomas[98] are associated with the best survival rates, whereas medullary carcinoma, endometrioid carcinoma, and carcinoma with fibroplasia (scirrhous carcinoma) have the poorest prognoses.[2]

## Carcinomas of Subcolumnar Reserve Cell Origin

Lesions with mixed patterns of differentiation or no differentiation at all constitute about 10% of all cervical carcinomas. They are believed to arise from subcolumnar reserve cells of the endocervical mucous membrane.[2]

Undifferentiated subcolumnar reserve cell carcinoma is made of compact, uniform, small cells with dark nuclei resembling basal cells. Mitoses are common and neither squamous nor glandular differentiation is seen (Figure 9.33). According to Abell,[2] subcolumnar reserve cell carcinoma has a comparatively worse prognosis than poorly differentiated small-cell squamous cell carcinoma.

Adenosquamous carcinomas[34,104,118] contain an admixture of histologically malignant squamous and gland cells (Figure 9.34). Both cell types are thought to arise from undifferentiated subcolumnar reserve cells. This type of lesion is more aggressive and has a less favorable prognosis than squamous cell carcinoma of similar clinical stage.[118]

Mucoepidermoid carcinomas[34,88] consist preponderantly of malignant squamous cells disposed in sheets, clumps, and ribbons in which are scattered mucous-secreting cells (Figure 9.35). The mucin from these cells is extruded into the intercellular spaces or fibrous stroma where it may collect in small or large lakes. The mucinous cellular elements most often are of the goblet or signet-ring cell type and contain mucinocarminophilic, PAS-positive, diastase-resistant mucopolysaccharides. They presumably derive from neoplastic squamous cells or cells intermediate between squamous and mucinus cells. Mucoepidermoid carcinoma is separated from the squamous cell carcinoma group because the distribution of this lesion in other parts of the body is chiefly confined to glandular tissues, such as the salivary glands, and because subcolumnar reserve cells of the endocervix are capable of differentiating into both squamous and glandular cell lines. The prognosis of mucoepidermoid carcinoma of the cervix is extremely poor.

Adenoid cystic carcinoma (cylindroma) of the cervix[43,75,80] is distinguished by its stroma, particularly by the presence of characteristic cylindrical hyalin bodies that lie within solid nests or between interanastomosing cords of uniform basaloid tumor cells. In cross section, hyalin

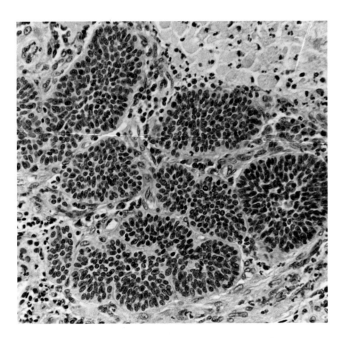

**9.33** Undifferentiated subcolumnar reserve cell carcinoma of the cervix. The cells have small, hyperchromatic nuclei and scant, indistinct cytoplasm, resembling subcolumnar reserve cells. The neoplasm was located in the endocervical canal with deep penetration into the cervical wall. Note the lobular configuration of the tumor, reminiscent of endocervical "glandular" units.

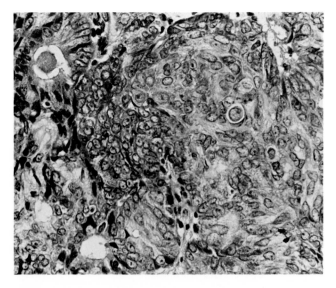

**9.34** Adenosquamous carcinoma of the cervix. Both the glandular and the squamous components contain malignant morphologic features. In this case the endometrium was free of disease.

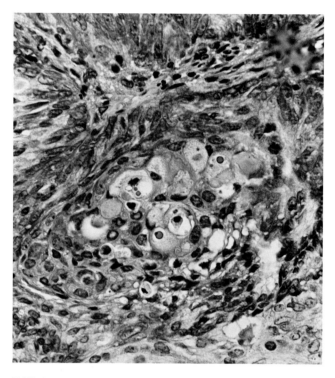

**9.35** Mucoepidermoid carcinoma of the cervix. Note the pale, mucin-containing cells within masses of neoplastic squamous cells.

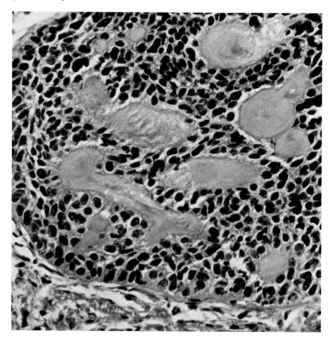

**9.36** Adenoid cystic carcinoma (cylindroma) of the cervix. Within solid nests of basaloid tumor cells are cylindrical hyalin bodies.

cylinders appear round or ovoid, giving the neoplasm a sievelike appearance (Figure 9.36). Curiously, the hyalin material at the electron microscopic level was shown to be partly made of coalesced masses of basal lamina produced by the epithelial tumor cells[63] and partly by fine procollagen and collagen fibers of fibroblastic origin. Inconspicuous glandular lumina are sometimes seen filled with amorphous material, representing partly digested cellular debris. Adenoid cystic carcinoma may be associated with squamous and adenocarcinoma as well as carcinosarcoma of the cervix.[2] The lesion is most often seen in between the sixth and seventh decades and it has similar aggressive behavior to that of most cervical adenocarcinomas.

## Multiple Primary Carcinoma

Examples of synchronous adeno- and squamous cell carcinomas occurring independently in the cervix have been reported.[2,3,34,116] They may be either invasive[3] or *in situ*.[116] In the invasive form, one carcinoma often invades the other, resulting in a collision tumor. Although such lesions closely resemble adenosquamous carcinomas, the different neoplastic components remain histologically distinct, separated from each other by narrow stroma or their respective basal lamina. Direct transition from one cell type into another, such as seen in adenosquamous carcinoma, is not seen.

## Morphology of the Uterine Cervix Following Ionizing Irradiation

In general, electromagnetic irradiation in the form of either x rays or γ rays produces cellular injury that affects especially the nucleus.[11] Characteristic cytologic changes are observed in the nucleus during different phases of mitotic division, such as chromosome breaks (scission), bridge formation between chromosomes at anaphase, and chromosomal fragmentation. Cells in early $G_1$ and $G_2$ phases of mitosis are the least sensitive and cells in $M_1$, late $G_1$, or early S phases are the most sensitive to ionizing radiation. These alterations are a result of profound biochemical changes that occur in the nuclear DNA and that in turn are caused by the interaction of x rays or γ rays with atoms in the target cells. Appropriate doses of radiation ultimately lead to vacuolization of nuclei and nuclear dissolution. In the cytoplasm of irradiated cells are swollen mitochondria with disrupted cristae. The cytoplasmic vacuolization seen by light microscopy corresponds to dilated Golgi and granular and agranular endoplasmic reticulum.[44] An increase in lysosomes and lysosomal enzyme activity, such as alkaline phosphatase, contributes to accelerated cell death.[96]

The morphologic effects of radiation on the cervix are well described by Krauss.[64] The normal cervical squamous cells immediately after intracavitary radiation for cervical carcinoma demonstrate cytoplasmic swelling and vacuolization. The nuclei are enlarged and contain one or two prominent nucleoli. The intercellular spaces are dilated (spongiosis) because of the accumulation of intercellular edema with concomitant loss of desmosomal attachments. The underlying supportive connective tissue is necrotic and contains numerous inflammatory cells. By the sixth postirradiation week there is severe atrophy of the squamous epithelium, and nuclear enlargement associated with a decrease in mucin content is seen in the endocervical epithelial cells. The cervical fibrous stroma is obscured by chronic inflammatory cells and macrophages and contains foci of partly necrotic, partly hyalinized collagen tissue scattered with a few atypical fibroblasts. These have abundant fibrillar cytoplasm and voluminous dark nuclei with several enlarged nucleoli (Figure 9.37). Characteristically the small arteries near the surface are obliterated by hyalin tissue, whereas others have intimal thickening (Figure 9.37). The endothelial cells lining capillaries are often enlarged, with hyperchromatic nuclei. In the following years, radiation changes are recognized by extensive hyalinization of the cervical fibrous tissue, which results in severe contraction. Most vessels are transformed into circular fibrohyalin masses surrounded by fragmented, wrinkled elastic fibers. Giant atypical fibroblasts with bizarre nuclear architecture can be found even 10 years after radiation. The squamous mucous membrane of the cervix remains atrophic and poor in intracytoplasmic glycogen.

Radiation of invasive squamous cell carcinoma of the cervix produces decrease in tumor size and eventual regression.[72] Although tumor regression is generally faster in neoplasms of small size and in those confined to the cervix (stage I) than in larger lesions with advanced stages, 90% of 493 patients with all stages had no gross tumor 12 weeks after termination of combined external radiation ([60]Co, 5,000 R) and intracavitary radium (4,000 R) therapy.[72] The rapidity of tumor regression is apparently unrelated to histologic patterns and degree of differentiation.[72] Morphologic changes in cervical squamous carcinoma cells that are considered evidence of response to ionizing radiation are cellular differentiation with keratinization, cell degeneration with cytoplasmic vacuolization, pyknosis, and nucleomegaly[46] with polyploid DNA content. Nuclear polyploidy, i.e., generation of multiple double sets of

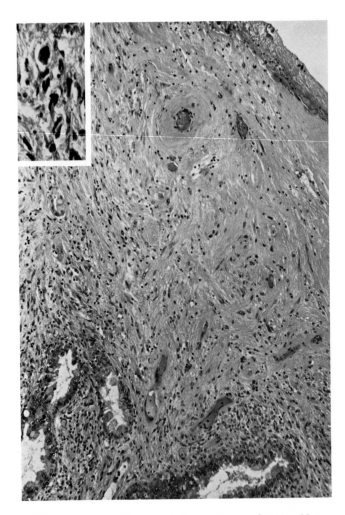

**9.37** Cervix 6 weeks after intracavitary radiation. Note the amorphous, hyalinized appearance of stroma; decreased mucin in endocervical epithelium; fibroblasts with atypical nuclei; and hyalin obliteration of vessels. Inset: Atypical giant fibroblasts are a typical feature of radiated connective tissue.

DNA, is the result of arrest of mitotic activity caused by radiation. Radiation-induced changes in adenocarcinoma of the cervix include nuclear shrinkage and pyknosis, cytoplasmic vacuolization, decrease in mucin synthesis, and a striking abundance of intracytoplasmic cytophagosomes (Figure 9.38).

The incidence of a second squamous cell carcinoma of the cervix or vagina or adenocarcinoma of the endometrium after irradiation for antecedent cervical malignancy is not greater than in the general population.[87] Only 1% of 1,297 patients treated with radiation for invasive carci-

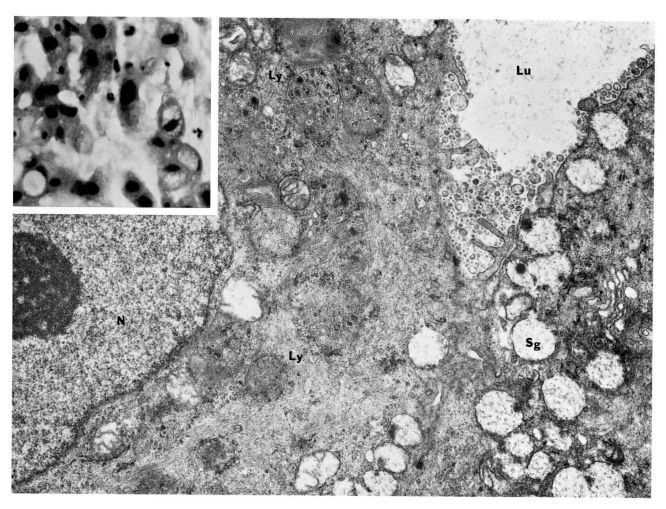

**9.38** Ultrastructural appearance of invasive adenocarcinoma of the cervix 6 weeks postirradiation. The cells are rich in membrane-bound autophagosomes (Ly), in which are incorporated cytoplasmic vesicles and membranes. The number of secretory granules (Sg) is considerably reduced as compared to normal or moderately differentiated neoplastic endocervical cells without radiation effect. N, Nucleus; Lu, glandular lumen. ×19,435. Inset: Histologic appearance of heavily irradiated adenocarcinoma of the cervix. Note shrunken pyknotic nuclei, vacuolization, and inconspicuous intracytoplasmic mucin.

noma of the cervix subsequently developed independent vaginal carcinomas.[58] It is not certain whether the second vaginal malignancy is initiated by radiation or represents a delayed multicentric development in the lower female genital tract. Morphologic alterations of the squamous epithelium of the uterine cervix and vagina of women who successfully have been treated with irradiation for cervical carcinoma occur in approximately 23% of cases.[117] The condition, termed "postirradiation dysplasia"[90] (PRD), is thought to be specifically induced by ionizing

radiation and to be histogenetically unrelated to spontaneously occurring cervical intraepithelial neoplasia. The abnormal epithelial cells, both in smears and in histologic sections, have large nuclei and a variable degree of cytoplasmic differentiation. Histologically, the lesion resembles early cervical intraepithelial neoplasia (mild dysplasia) (Figure 9.39). The clinical significance of PRD according to Wentz and Reagan[117] lies in the positive correlation between the early appearance of PRD and the subsequent recurrence of cervical carcinoma. Indeed, if PRD is de-

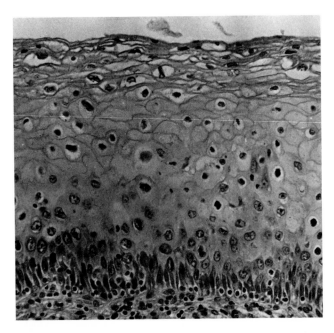

**9.39** Postirradiation dysplasia of the cervix observed 26 months after irradiation of invasive squamous cell carcinoma of the cervix.

tected within 3 years of irradiation for carcinoma of the cervix, the likelihood of recurrence is considerably increased and there is only a 34% 5-year survival rate. In contrast, if PRD occurs after 3 years, a 100% 5-year survival rate is observed and in many instances the abnormal changes revert to normal without therapy. Recently attempts were made with the aid of microspectrophotometry to separate PRD with nuclear diploidy (normal DNA content) and polyploidy (multiple normal DNA content) from those with aneuploidy (abnormal DNA content, interclass values).[86] Understandably, patients with PRD of the aneuploid type, in which the nuclei contain all the characteristic changes of malignancy, had significantly higher recurrence and death rates than those with nuclear diploidy or polyploidy. In view of these observations, careful evaluation of the cytonuclear changes of PRD is recommended because it may provide useful information for the early detection and treatment of recurrences and contribute to the improvement in patient survival.

## Rare Carcinomas

Primary malignant melanoma is among the least common of the malignancies that arise in the cervix. Nine patients with such disease have been reported in the litera-

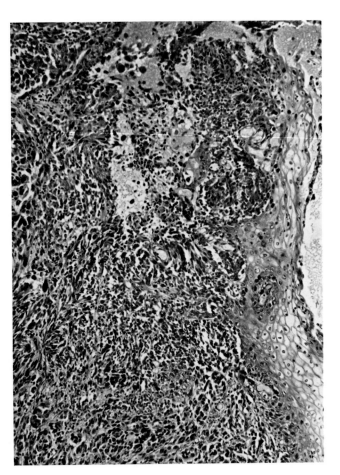

**9.40** Invasive malignant melanoma of the cervix. Note junctional changes in squamous epithelium and spindle-shaped configuration of neoplastic cells. Fontana stain was strongly positive for melanin. Patient died of dissiminated disease 2 years following the original diagnosis.

ture.[56] All the patients in whom followup was available died with widespread metastases from 6 months to 14 years[56] after diagnosis. In most instances, the lesion is pigmented and dark brown. The diagnosis of primary melanoma of the cervix uteri is based on the histologic demonstration of junctional changes in the cervical squamous epithelium and the absence of similar lesions elsewhere in the body (Figure 9.40). Morphologically, melanoma of the cervix is identical with those arising in the skin and extragenital mucous membranes and frequently contains intracytoplasmic melanin pigment granules.

The histogenesis of malignant melanoma of the cervix is unclear, although its origin may be ascribed to the melanin-containing cells of the Schwannian sheath of the normal cervix.[20] Choriocarcinoma, primary in the cervix, is a rare occurrence, and presumably results from a preexisting cervical pregnancy or displaced intrauterine molar tissue. About a dozen such cases are recorded in the English literature.[93] The gross and microscopic appearance as well as the clinical course are identical with those found in the uterine corpus.[93]

## Sarcomas of the Cervix

Sarcomas of the uterine cervix are exceedingly rare. They include endocervical stromal sarcoma, leiomyosarcoma, malignant mixed mesodermal tumors (carcinosarcoma),[4,39] embryonal rhabdomyosarcoma of infancy and childhood (sarcoma botryoides),[120] and malignant lymphoma.[18,21,111] With the exception of the botryoid sarcoma, which is exclusively a disease of infancy and childhood, sarcomas of the cervix generally occur between the fourth and sixth decades. They are usually discovered as projecting polypoid masses arising from the cervix and have as the dominant clinical complaint abnormal vaginal bleeding. According to Abell and Ramirez,[4] only those cervical sarcomas should be considered primary that are centered in the cervix of a uterus in which the endomyometrium is free of disease.

Leiomyosarcoma, endocervical stromal cell sarcoma, and malignant mixed mesodermal tumors, with either homologous or heterologous components, have a histologic pattern and clinical behavior similar to those of their more common counterparts of the uterine corpus.[4] Except for the low-grade endocervical stromal sarcomas, most patients succumb to their disease within 2 years after the original diagnosis.[4] The pathogenesis of cervical sarcomas and that of malignant mixed mesodermal tumors is obscure. In general, pure homologous and pure heterologous sarcomas are believed to be derived from a single mesenchymal stem cell, the endocervical fibroblast, whereas the mixed mesodermal variety, containing an admixture of carcinoma and sarcoma(s), probably has two separate cellular origins (composite tumors), the cervical epithelium and stromal fibroblasts.[4]

Sarcoma botryoides is a variant of embryonal rhabdomyosarcoma. It usually originates in the supportive stroma of the vagina and rarely in the cervix of infants and young children.[120] Sarcomas with botryoid elements are occasionally encountered in the corpus or cervix in the adult. These lesions also contain other heterologous tissues, such as chondrosarcoma, and so should be regarded as malignant mixed mesodermal sarcoma rather than pure botryoid sarcoma.

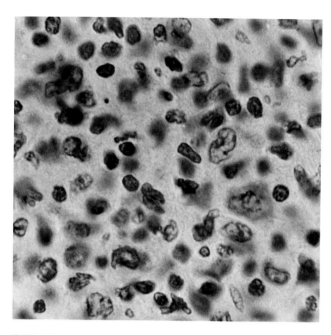

**9.41** Histiocytic lymphoma (reticulum cell sarcoma), presumably primary in cervix from a 52-year-old woman. Note deeply indented nuclear membranes, prominent nucleoli, and lack of cellular adherence. The patient is free of disease 3 years following hysterectomy, bilateral salpingo-oophorectomy, and irradiation.

Primary malignant lymphomas of the uterine cervix are considerably less common than metastatic systemic lymphoma.[67] Until 1974, a total of 28 cases had been reported, of which 14 were histiocytic lymphomas (reticulum cell sarcomas), six were Hodgkin's disease, six were lymphocytic lymphomas, and two were cases of granulocytic leukemia.[18,21,111] Malignant lymphomas appear as sessile or polypoid masses with a "fish-flesh" appearance. Histologically, some cases of histiocytic lymphoma may mimic pseudosarcomas or pseudodecidual reaction of gestation, poorly differentiated squamous cell carcinoma, undifferentiated epithelial carcinoma, and endocervical stromal sarcoma. Histiocytic lymphoma is characterized by a diffuse infiltrate of large mononuclear cells, replacing the stroma without destroying the endocervical epithelial elements. The latter feature is characteristic of all malignant lymphomas and differs from that of primary or metastatic epithelial carcinoma, which tends to obliterate the architecture of the cervix. In addition, histiocytic lymphoma is devoid of the cellular adherence that characterizes epithelial carcinomas and contains numerous mitotic figures and prominent nucleoli. A centrally folded nuclear membrane giving a "kidneybean" appearance to the nuclei is present in many neoplastic cells (Figure 9.41).

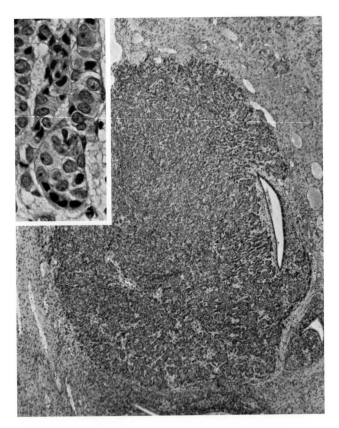

**9.42** Metastatic carcinoma in the cervix following carcinoma of female mammary gland. Inset: Cellular detail of neoplastic cells arranged in typical narrow cords.

Whether lymphomas are truly derived from the cervix or represent a localized, initial manifestation of a systemic process cannot be established at the present time because most patients have not been adequately evaluated as to the possibility of associated node involvement. Nonetheless, the overall survival of patients with lymphoma initially limited to the corpus or cervix is considerably better than that of patients with metastatic lymphomatous involvement of the cervix or patients with other extranodal lymphomas of similar histologic type. This comparatively favorable prognosis presumably results from the earlier clinical signs and the greater ease of radiation and surgical therapy because of the cervix's accessibility.

## Metastatic Disease

The most common metastatic lesion in the cervix is endometrial adenocarcinoma, although some cases may be direct extensions from the corpus instead of metastases.

Another lesion that has a relatively high incidence of cervical metastasis is choriocarcinoma. Rarely, carcinoma of the urinary bladder directly invades, rather than metastasizes, to the adjacent cervix. Sarcomas of the corpus uteri may also involve the cervix. Metastases in the cervix from distant primary foci are rare, the two most frequent sources being the female mammary gland (Figure 9.42) and stomach. Instances of metastatic carcinoma of ovary, gallbladder, rectosigmoid, pancreas, thyroid,[113] and malignant melanoma have been described. Leukemic infiltration of the cervix, especially of the granulocytic type, is a rather common occurrence in women with leukemia at autopsy.[70] Secondary lymphomatous involvement of the cervix is reported in 6% of women dying with generalized disease.[67]

## ACKNOWLEDGMENT

This work was aided by Grant MA5137 from the Medical Research Council of Canada.

## REFERENCES

1. Abell, M. R. Papillary adenofibroma of the uterine cervix. *Am. J. Obstet. Gynecol. 110:*990, 1971.

2. Abell, M. R. Invasive carcinomas of uterine cervix, *in* Norris, H. J., Hertig, A. T., and Abell, M. R., eds. *The Uterus,* Internatl. Acad. Path. Monogr. Baltimore, The Williams and Wilkins Co., 1973, pp. 413–456.

3. Abell, M. R., and Gosling, J. R. G. Gland cell carcinoma (adenocarcinoma) of the uterine cervix. *Am. J. Obstet. Gynecol. 83:*729, 1962.

4. Abell, M. R., and Ramirez, J. A. Sarcomas and carcinosarcomas of the uterine cervix. *Cancer 31:*1176, 1973.

5. Ashley, D. J. B. Evidence for the existence of two forms of cervical carcinoma. *J. Obstet. Gynaecol. Brit. Commonw. 73:*372, 1966.

6. Auersperg, N. Histogenetic behavior of tumors. III. Possible relationships to patterns of glycolysis. *J. Natl. Cancer Inst. 48:*1589, 1972.

7. Aurelian, L., Schumann, B., Marcus, R. L., and Davis, H. J. Antibody to HSV-2 induced tumor specific antigens in serums from patients with cervical carcinoma. *Science 181:*161, 1973.

8. Averette, H. E. Indications for radical hysterectomy. *Medical Opinion and Review 7:*73, 1971.

9. Azzopardi, J. G., and Tsun, H. L. Intestinal metaplasia with argentaffin cells in cervical adenocarcinoma. *J. Path. Bacteriol. 90:*686, 1965.

10. Bangle, R. Jr., Berger, M., and Levin, M. Variations in the morphogenesis of squamous cell carcinoma of the cervix. *Cancer 16:*1151, 1963.

11. Berdjis, C. C. *Pathology of Irradiation,* 1st ed. Baltimore, Williams and Wilkins Co., 1971.

12. Boronow, R. C., Averette, H. E., Nelson, J. H. Jr., Richart, R. M., and Townsend, D. E. Defining cervical microinvasive carcinoma. *Contemp. Obstet. Gynecol.* 5:121, 1975.

13. Boutselis, J. G., Ullery, J. C., and Charme, L. Diagnosis and management of stage Ia (microinvasive) carcinoma of the cervix. *Am. J. Obstet. Gynecol.* 110:984, 1971.

14. Boyes, D. A., Fidler, H. K., and Lock, D. R. *The Significance of in situ Carcinoma of the Uterine Cervix.* Proceedings of the First International Congress of Exfoliative Cytology. Philadelphia, J. B. Lippincott Co., 1963.

15. Boyes, D. A., Worth, A. J., and Fidler, H. K. The results of treatment of 4389 cases of preclinical cervical squamous carcinoma. *J. Obstet. Gynaecol. Brit. Commonw.* 77:769, 1970.

16. Campos, J. L. Mortality trends in carcinoma of the cervix uteri. *J. Chronic Dis.* 24:701, 1971.

17. Cherry, C. P., and Glücksmann, A. Lymphatic embolism and lymph node metastasis in cancers of vulva and of uterine cervix. *Cancer* 8:564, 1955.

18. Chorlton, I., Karnei, R. F. Jr., King, F. M., and Norris, H. J. Primary malignant reticuloendothelial disease involving the vagina, cervix, and corpus uteri. *Obstet. Gynecol.* 44:735, 1974.

19. Christopherson, W. M., and Parker, J. E. Microinvasive carcinoma of the uterine cervix; a clinical-pathological study. *Cancer* 17:1123, 1964.

20. Cid, J. M. La pigmentation mélanique de l'endocervix. Un argument viscéral "neurogénique." *Ann. Anat. Pathol.* 4:617, 1959.

21. Cihak, R. W., and Hamada, J. Primary reticulum cell sarcoma of the uterus. *Cancer* 33:1039, 1974.

22. Coppleson, M. The origin and nature of premalignant lesions of the cervix uteri. *Int. J. Gynecol. Obstet.* 8:539, 1970.

23. Cramer, D. W. The role of cervical cytology in the declining morbidity and mortality of cervical cancer. *Cancer* 34:2018, 1974.

24. Cramer, D. W., and Cutler, S. J. Incidence and histopathology of malignancies of the female genital organs in the United States. *Am. J. Obstet. Gynecol.* 118:443, 1974.

25. Cramer, D. W., and Cutler, S. J., and Christine, B. Trends in the incidence of endometrial cancer in the United States. *Gynecol. Oncol.* 2:130, 1974.

26. Creasman, W. T., Rutledge, F., and Fletcher, G. H. Carcinoma of the cervix associated with pregnancy. *Obstet. Gynecol.* 36:495, 1970.

27. Danforth, D. N. The distribution and functional activity of the cervical musculature. *Am. J. Obstet. Gynecol.* 68:1261, 1954.

28. Davidshon, I., Norris, H. J., Stejskal, R., and Lill, P. Metastatic squamous cell carcinoma of the cervix. The role of immunology in its pathogenesis. *Arch. Pathol.* 95:132, 1973.

29. Davis, J. R., and Moon, L. B. Increased incidence of adenocarcinoma of uterine cervix. *Obstet. Gynecol.* 45:79, 1975.

30. Demian, S. D. E., Bushkin, F. L., and Echevarria, R. A. Perineural invasion and anaplastic transformation of verrucous carcinoma. *Cancer* 32:395, 1973.

31. De Petrillo, A. D., Townsend, D. E., Morrow, C. P., Lickrish, G. M., Di Saia, P. J., and Roy, M. Colposcopic evaluation of the abnormal Papanicolaou test in pregnancy. *Am. J. Obstet. Gynecol.* 121:441, 1975.

32. Diddle, A. W. Carcinoma of the cervix uteri with metastases to the neck. *Cancer* 29:453, 1972.

33. Di Saia, P. J., Haverbeck, B. J., Dyce, B. J., and Morrow, C. P. Carcinoembryonic antigen in patients with gynecologic malignancies. *Am. J. Obstet. Gynecol.* 121:159, 1975.

34. Dougherty, C. M., and Cotten, N. Mixed squamous-cell and adenocarcinoma of the cervix; combined, adenosquamous, and mucoepidermoid types. *Cancer* 17:1132, 1964.

35. Dudan, R. C., Yon, J. L., Ford, J. H., and Averette, H. E. Carcinoma of the cervix and pregnancy. *Gynecol. Oncol.* 1:283, 1973.

36. Ferenczy, A., and Richart, R. M. *Female Reproductive System. Dynamics of Scan and Transmission Electron Microscopy*, 1st ed. New York, John Wiley & Sons, 1974.

37. Fidler, H. K., Boyes, D. A., and Worth, A. J. Cervical cancer detection in British Columbia. *J. Obstet. Gynaecol. Brit. Commonw.* 75:392, 1968.

38. Fidler, H. K., Boyes, D. A., Nichols, T. M., and Worth, A. J. Cervical cytology in the control of cancer of the cervix. *Modern Medicine of Canada* 25:9, 1970.

39. Fluhman, C. F. *The Cervix Uteri and Its Diseases*, 1st ed. Philadelphia, W. B. Saunders Co., 1961.

40. Forsberg, J. G. Estrogen, vaginal cancer, and vaginal development. *Am. J. Obstet. Gynecol.* 113:83, 1972.

41. Frick, H. C., Janovski, N. A., Gusberg, S. B., and Taylor, H. C. Early invasive cancer of the cervix. *Am. J. Obstet. Gynecol.* 85:926, 1963.

42. Gardner, H. L., and Parsons, L. Blood vessel invasion in cancer of the cervix. *Cancer* 15:1269, 1962.

43. Gallager, H. S., Simpson, C. B., and Ayala, A. G. Adenoid cystic carcinoma of the uterine cervix: Report of 4 cases. *Cancer* 27:1398, 1971.

44. Ghidoni, J. J. Light and electron microscopic study of primate liver 36 to 48 hours after high doses of 32 million electron volt protons. *Lab. Invest.* 16:268, 1967.

45. Gilbert, E. F., and Palladino, A. Squamous papillomas of the uterine cervix: review of the literature and report of a giant papillary carcinoma. *Am. J. Clin. Pathol.* 46:115, 1966.

45a. Glücksmann, A. Relationships between hormonal changes in pregnancy and the development of "mixed carcinoma" of the uterine cervix. *Cancer* 10:831, 1957.

46. Glücksmann, A., and Spear, F. G. The qualitative and quantitative histological examination of biopsy material from patients treated by radiation for carcinoma of the cervix uteri. *Brit. J. Radiol.* 18:313, 1945.

47. Goldstein, M. S., Shore, B., and Gusberg, S. B. Cellular immunity as a host response to squamous carcinoma of the cervix. *Am. J. Obstet. Gynecol.* 111:751, 1971.

48. Graham, J., Graham, R., and Hirabayaski, K. Recurrent cancer of the cervix uteri. *Surg. Gynecol. Obstet.* 126:799, 1968.

49. Gusberg, S. B., Yannopoulos, K., and Cohen, C. J. Virulence indices and lymph nodes in cancer of the cervix. *Am. J. Roentgenol.* 111:273, 1971.

50. Haggard, J. L., Cotten, N., Dougherty, C. M., and Mickal, A. Primary adenocarcinoma of the cervix. *Obstet. Gynecol.* 24:183, 1964.

51. Halpin, T. F., Frick, H. C., and Munnell, E. W. Critical points of failure in the therapy of cancer of the cervix: a reappraisal. *Am. J. Obstet. Gynecol.* 114:755, 1972.

52. Hameed, K. Clear cell "mesonephric" carcinoma of uterine cervix. *Obstet. Gynecol.* 32:564, 1968.

53. Hart, W. R., and Norris, H. J. Cervix adenocarcinoma of mesonephric type. *Cancer* 29:106, 1972.

53a. Hepler, T. K., Dockerty, M. B., and Randall, L. M. Primary adenocarcinoma of cervix. *Am. J. Obstet. Gynecol.* 63:800, 1952.

54. Herbst, A. L., Robboy, S. J., Scully, R. E., and Poskanzer, D. C. Clear-cell adenocarcinoma of the genital tract in young

females. Analysis of 170 Registry cases. *Am. J. Obstet. Gynecol.* 19:713, 1974.

55. Johnson, L. D. The histopathological approach to early cervical neoplasia. *Obstet. Gynecol. Surv.* 24:735, 1969.

56. Jones, H. W., Droegemueller, W., and Makowski, E. L. A primary melanocarcinoma of the cervix. *Am. J. Obstet. Gynecol.* 111:959, 1971.

57. Kagan, A. R., Nussbaum, H., Chan, P., and Ziel, H. K. Adenocarcinoma of the uterine cervix. *Am. J. Obstet. Gynecol.* 117:464, 1973.

58. Kanbour, A. I., Klionsky, B., and Murphy, A. I. Carcinoma of the vagina following cervical cancer. *Cancer* 34:1838, 1974.

59. Kaufman, R. H., and Rawls, W. E. Herpes genitalis and its relationship to cervical cancer. *Cancer J. Clinicians, Am. Cancer Soc.* 24:258, 1974.

60. Ketcham, A. S., Hoye, R. C., Taylor, P. T., Deckers, P. J., Thomas, L. B. and Chretien, P. B. Radical hysterectomy and pelvic lymphadenectomy for carcinoma of the uterine cervix. *Cancer* 28:1272, 1971.

61. Kirk, M. E. Carcinoma of the cervix, stage Ia. *Human Pathol.* 5:253, 1974.

62. Kolbenstvedt, A., and Kolstad, P. Pelvic lymph node dissection under peroperative lymphographic control. *Gynecol. Oncol.* 2:39, 1974.

63. Koss, L. G., Brannan, C. D., and Ashikari, R. Histologic and ultrastructural features of adenoid cystic carcinoma of the breast. *Cancer* 26:1271, 1970.

64. Krauss, F. T. Irradiation changes in the uterus, *in* Norris, H. J., Hertig, A. T., and Abell, M. R., eds.: *The Uterus,* Internatl. Acad. Pathol. Monograph. Baltimore, Williams and Wilkins Co., 1973, pp. 457–488.

65. Krauss, F. T., and Perez-Mesa, C. Verrucous carcinoma. *Cancer* 19:26, 1966.

66. Kyriakos, M., Kempson, R. L., and Perez, C. A. Carcinoma of the cervix in young women. *Obstet. Gynecol.* 38:930, 1971.

67. Lathrop, J. C. Views and reviews: Malignant pelvic lymphomas. *Obstet. Gynecol.* 30:137, 1967.

68. Latour, J. P. A. Results in the management of preclinical carcinoma of the cervix. *Am. J. Obstet. Gynecol.* 81:511, 1961.

69. Lucas, W. E., Benirschke, K., and Lebherz, T. B. Verrucous carcinoma of the female genital tract. *Am. J. Obstet. Gynecol.* 119:435, 1974.

70. Lucia, S. P., Mills, H., Lowenhaupt, E., and Hunt, M. L. Visceral involvement in primary neoplastic diseases of the reticuloendothelial system. *Cancer* 5:1193, 1952.

71. Marchant, D. J. Cancer of the cervix. *New Engl. J. Med.* 281:602, 1969.

72. Marcial, V. A., and Bosch, A. Radiation-induced tumor regression in carcinoma of the uterine cervix: Prognostic significance. *Am. J. Roentgenol.* 108:113, 1970.

73. Marcuse, P. M. Incipient microinvasive carcinoma of the cervix. Morphology and clinical data of 22 cases. *Obstet. Gynecol.* 37:360, 1971.

74. Martzloff, K. H. Carcinoma of the cervix uteri: A pathological and clinical study with particular reference to the relative malignancy of the neoplastic process as indicated by the predominant cell type of cancer cell. *Bull. Johns Hopkins Hospital.* 34:141, 184, 1923.

75. Maza, L. M., Thayer, B. A., and Naeim, F. Cylindroma of the uterine cervix with peritoneal metastases: Report of a case and review of the literature. *Am. J. Obstet. Gynecol.* 112:121, 1972.

76. McKelvey, J. L., and Goodlin, R. R. Adenoma malignum of the cervix: A cancer of deceptively innocent histological pattern. *Cancer* 16:549, 1963.

77. McNutt, N. S., and Weinstein, R. S. Carcinoma of the cervix: Deficiency of nexus intercellular junctions. *Science* 165:597, 1969.

78. Mestwerdt, G. Probeexzision und Kolposkopie in des Frühdiagnose des Portiokarcinoms. *Zentr. Gynäk.* 4:326, 1947.

79. Mikuta, J. J., and Celebre, J. A. Adenocarcinoma of the cervix. *Obstet. Gynecol.* 33:753, 1969.

80. Miles, P. A., and Norris, H. J. Adenoid cystic carcinoma of the cervix: An analysis of 12 cases. *Obstet. Gynecol.* 38:103, 1971.

81. Mussey, E., Soule, E. H., and Welch, J. S. Microinvasive carcinoma of the cervix. Late results of operative treatment in 91 cases. *Am. J. Obstet. Gynecol.* 104:738, 1969.

82. Nalick, R. H., Di Saia, P. J., Rea, T. H., and Morrow, C. P. Immunocompetence and prognosis in patients with gynecologic cancer. *Gynecol. Oncol.* 2:81, 1974.

83. Ng, A. B. P., and Reagan, J. W. Microinvasive carcinoma of the uterine cervix. *Am. J. Clin. Pathol.* 52:511, 1969.

84. Ng, A. B. P., Reagan, J. W., and Lindner, E. A. The cellular manifestations of microinvasive squamous cell carcinoma of the uterine cervix. *Acta Cytol.* 16:5, 1972.

85. Nogales, F., and Bottela-Llusia, J. The frequency of invasion of the lymph nodes in cancer of the uteri cervix: A study of the degree of extension in relation to the histological type of tumor. *Am. J. Obstet. Gynecol.* 93:91, 1965.

86. Okagaki, T., Meyer, A. A., and Sciarra, J. J. Prognosis of irradiated carcinoma of cervix uteri and nuclear DNA in cytologic post-irradiation dysplasia. *Cancer* 33:647, 1974.

87. Palmer, J. P., and Spratt, D. W. Pelvic carcinoma following irradiation for benign gynecological diseases. *Am. J. Obstet. Gynecol.* 72:497, 1956.

88. Papadia, S. Mucinous patterns in epidermoid carcinomas. *Gynecologia* 153:337, 1962.

89. Park, R. C., Patow, W. E., Rogers, R. E., and Zimmerman, E. A. Treatment of stage I carcinoma of the cervix. *Obstet. Gynecol.* 41:117, 1973.

90. Patten, S. F. Jr., Reagan, J. W., Obenauf, M., and Ballard, L. Post-irradiation dysplasia of uterine cervix and vagina. An analytical study of cells. *Cancer* 16:173, 1963.

91. Pilleron, J. P., Durand, J. C., and Hamelin, J. P. Location of lymph node invasion in cancer of the uterine cervix: Study of 140 cases treated at the Curie Foundation. *Am. J. Obstet. Gynecol.* 119:453, 1974.

92. Przybora, L. A. Incipient invasion of cervical cancer: Morphological aspects of carcinogenesis in 74 cases. *Gynaecologia* 160:69, 1965.

92a. Rampone, J. F., Klem, W., and Kolstad, P. Combined treatment of stage Ib carcinoma of the cervix. *Obstet. Gynecol.* 41:163, 1973.

93. Rashbaum, M., Daub, W. W., and Lisa, J. R. Primary cervical choriocarcinoma. *Am. J. Obstet. Gynecol.* 64:451, 1952.

94. Reagan, J. W. Cellular pathology and uterine cancer. *Am. J. Clin. Pathol.* 62:150, 1974.

95. Reagan, J. W., and Ng, A. B. P. The cellular manifestations of uterine carcinogenesis, *in* Norris, J. J., Hertig, A. T., and Abell, M. R., eds.: *The Uterus,* Internatl. Acad. Path. Monograph. Baltimore, Williams and Wilkins Co., 1973, pp. 320–347.

96. Rene, A. A., Darden, J. H., and Parker, J. L. Radiation induced ultrastructural and biochemical changes in lysosomes. *Lab. Invest. 25*:230, 1971.

97. Richart, R. M., and Barron, B. A. A follow-up study of patients with cervical dysplasia. *Am. J. Obstet. Gynecol. 105*:386, 1969.

98. Robboy, S. J., Herbst, A. L., and Scully, R. E. Clear-cell adenocarcinoma of the vagina and cervix in young females: Analysis of 37 tumors that persisted or recurred after primary therapy. *Cancer 34*:606, 1974.

99. Roche, W. D., and Norris, H. J. Microinvasive carcinoma of the cervix. The significance of lymphatic invasion and confluent patterns of stromal growth. *Cancer 36*:180, 1975.

100. Roth, L. M., and Hornback, N. B. Clear-cell adenocarcinoma of the cervix in young women. *Cancer 34*:1761, 1974.

101. Rubio, C. A., Söderberg, G., and Einhorn, N. Histological and follow-up studies in cases of microinvasive carcinoma of the uterine cervix. *Acta Pathol. Microbiol. Scand. 82*:397, 1974.

102. Savage, E. W. Microinvasive carcinoma of the cervix. *Am. J. Obstet. Gynecol. 113*:708, 1972.

103. Schiller, W., Daro, A. F., Collin, H. A., and Primiano, N. P. Small preulcerative invasive carcinoma of the cervix: The spray carcinoma. *Am. J. Obstet. Gynecol. 65*:1088, 1953.

104. Sidhu, G. S., Koss, L. G., and Barber, H. R. K. Relation of histologic factors to the response of stage I epidermoid carcinoma of the cervix to surgical treatment: Analysis of 115 patients. *Obstet. Gynecol. 35*:329, 1970.

105. Silverberg, E., and Holleb, A. I. Major trends in cancer: 25 year survey. *Cancer J. Clinicians 25*:2, 1975.

106. Sotto, L. S. J., Graham, J. B., and Pickren, J. W. Postmortem findings in cancer of the cervix. *Am. J. Obstet. Gynecol. 80*:791, 1960.

107. Stafl, A. The clinical diagnosis of early cervical cancer. *Obstet. Gynecol. Surv. 24*:976, 1969.

108. Stafl, A., Friedrich, E. G. Jr., and Mattingly, R. F. Detection of cervical neoplasia. Reducing the risk of error. *Clin. Obstet. Gynecol. 16*:238, 1973.

109. Stafl, A., and Mattingly, R. F. Angiogenesis of cervical neoplasia. *Am. J. Obstet. Gynecol. 121*:845, 1975.

110. Stern, E. Epidemiology of dysplasia. *Obstet. Gynecol. Surv. 24*:711, 1969.

111. Stransky, G. C., Acosta, A. A., Kaplan, A. L., and Friedman, J. A. Reticulum cell sarcoma of the cervix. *Obstet. Gynecol. 41*:183, 1973.

112. Tasker, J. T., and Collins, J. A. Adenocarcinoma of the uterine cervix. *Am. J. Obstet. Gynecol. 118*:344, 1974.

113. Twombley, G. H., and Di Palma, S. Growth and spread of cancer of cervix uteri. *Am. J. Roentgenol. 65*:691, 1951.

114. Ullery, J. C., Boutselis, J. G., and Botschner, A. C. Microinvasive carcinoma of the cervix. *Obstet. Gynecol. 26*:866, 1965.

115. Villasanta, U. Complications of radiotherapy for carcinoma of the uterine cervix. *Am. J. Obstet. Gynecol. 114*:717, 1972.

116. Weisbrot, I. M., Stabinsky, C., and Davis, A. M. Adenocarcinoma in situ of the uterine cervix. *Cancer 29*:1179, 1972.

117. Wentz, W. B., and Reagan, J. W. Clinical significance of post-irradiation dysplasia of the uterine cervix. *Am. J. Obstet. Gynecol. 106*:812, 1970.

118. Wheeless, C. R., Graham, R., and Graham, J. B. Prognosis and treatment of adenoepidermoid carcinoma of the cervix. *Obstet. Gynecol. 35*:928, 1970.

119. Wiernik, G., Bradbury, S., Plant, M., Cowdell, R. H., and Williams, E. A. A quantitative comparison between normal and carcinomatous squamous epithelia of the uterine cervix. *Brit. J. Cancer 28*:488, 1973.

120. Williamson, H. O., and McIver, F. A. Sarcoma botryoides of the cervix treated by vaginal hysterectomy and subtotal vaginectomy. *Obstet. Gynecol. 31*:689, 1968.

121. Wolff, J. P., Lacour, J., Chassagne, D., and Berend, M. Cancer of the cervical stump. *Obstet. Gynecol. 39*:10, 1972.

Lila Nachtigall, M.D.

# 10

# Hormones of the Menstrual Cycle

The ovary has as its functions the production of mature ova for reproduction and the elaboration of sex steroid hormones. These are interdependent functions. For example, before menarche ever commences, estrogens are produced that are essential for genital and somatic development, i.e., linear growth, breast development, genital maturation, and the growth of axillary and pubic hair.[2]

Sex steroids can be separated into three main groups based on the number of carbon atoms within the steroid (Figure 10.1). The C-21 series includes progestins and corticoids, in which the basic structure is the "pregnane" nucleus. The C-19 series includes all androgens with androstane as the basic structure. The C-18 series incorporates the estrogens, with estrane being the basic nucleus. Since the nomenclature of steroids can be confusing to non-endocrinologists, these are clearly outlined in Table 10.1.

## Hormonal Activity during the Menstrual Cycle

### Estrogens

In the initial phase of follicle development, estradiol levels are low. Then there is a slow rise followed by a sharp rise that reaches its peak, coincident with the peak elevation of luteinizing hormone (LH) (Figure 10.2). The subsequent sharp drop in LH is paralleled by a similar drop

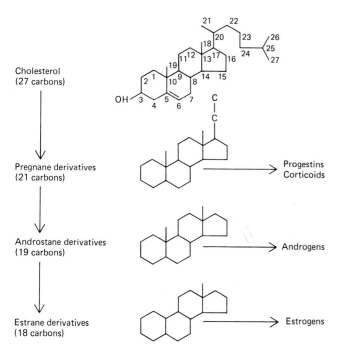

**10.1** The main groups of sex steroids according to their numbers of carbon atoms.

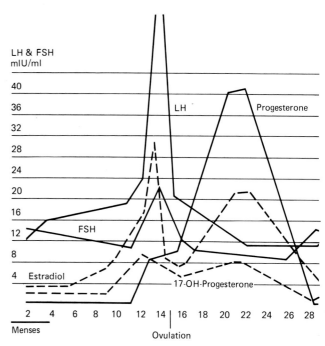

**10.2** Hormonal activities during the menstrual cycle.

**Table 10.1**  Nomenclature of steroids

| Suffix or prefix | Significance |
| --- | --- |
| -Ene, -diene, -triene | One, two, or three double bonds |
| -Ol, -diol, -triol | One, two, or three hydroxyl groups |
| -One, -dione, -trione | One, two, or three ketones |
| Dihydro- | Elimination of two hydrogens |
| Dioxy- | Elimination of oxygen |
| Nor- | Elimination of carbon |
| Delta- | Location of double bond |

Pregnenolone → Progesterone

**10.3** Conversion of pregnenolone to progesterone.

of androstanedione to estrone.[3] The estrone produced by this conversion is available to the target organ and does exert biologic activity.

## Progesterone and 17-O,H-Progesterone

The changes in progesterone and 17-O,H-progesterone are also illustrated in Figure 10.2. Progesterone was always believed to be secreted in the ovary only by the corpus luteum, but analyses of normal ovarian follicles have demonstrated its presence, and it is probably produced in small quantities during the follicular phase of the cycle.[4] Plasma progesterone assays are not useful in determining follicular production because the major portion of circulating progesterone results from conversion of adrenal pregnenolone and pregnenolone sulfate to progesterone[5] (Figure 10.3).

in estradiol. This change corresponds to between the fourteenth and sixteenth day in the cycle and the time of ovulation. Estradiol then rises again, reaching its second peak between the twentieth and twenty-fourth day. The vast majority of estradiol produced is from the ovary,[1] with less than 0.2% of testosterone converted to estradiol.[1] Estrone is also secreted by the ovary and the changes are similar to those of estradiol; however, most of the estrone in the circulation is derived from the peripheral conversion

There is a small elevation in progesterone at the beginning of the rise in circulating LH (Figure 10.2) and a second major rise from day 16 to day 20. At that time progesterone peaks. This rise in progesterone parallels that of estradiol in the luteal phase of the cycle. The first preovulatory rise in progesterone levels probably is the consequence of the high levels of LH stimulating the follicle.[6]

The mechanism by which estrogen secretion is turned off and progesterone secretion rises has not yet been elucidated.[10] There are a number of intriguing studies and one recently reported is appealing. Radioactive labeled estrogen has been found to bind to nuclei in cells in the hypothalamus and anterior lobe of the pituitary. It is postulated that when these nuclei are saturated by estrogen, follicle-stimulating hormone (FSH) releasing factor is turned off and estrogen production by the follicle diminishes markedly.

$17\alpha$-O,H-Progesterone shows two clear-cut peaks during the menstrual cycle[7] (Figure 10.2), one during the late stage of follicle maturation and the second during the latter half or luteal part of the cycle. $\Delta_5$-Pregnenolone and $17\alpha$-O,H-$\Delta_5$-pregnenolone are found in the follicular phase of the cycle as well as in the luteal phase. It is more prominent in the latter.[8]

## Androgens

Lloyd et al.[4] measured the secretion of testosterone, dehydroepiandrosterone, and $\Delta_4$-androstenedione both in the ovarian and peripheral blood. $\Delta_4$-Androstenedione is the major androgen secreted by the ovary, but testosterone is secreted in small amounts throughout the menstrual cycle. The adrenal gland produces the majority of dehydroepiandrosterone and dehydroepiandrosterone sulfate; only a small amount is produced by the ovary.

## Hypothalamic–Pituitary–Ovarian Relationship

It was long known that there were hypothalamic influences on the pituitary. In recent years gonadotropin releasing factors have both been isolated and synthesized.[16] Dhariwal and his co-workers[3] achieved separation of luteinizing hormone releasing factor and follicle stimulating hormone releasing factor. It now appears that the hypothalamus plays an important intermediary role between the central nervous and the endocrine systems in the area of reproduction as well as in other bodily functions.[13] It appears that a humoral agent is secreted by neuroendocrine cells, which then passes through the hypothalamic–hypo-

physial portal blood vessels to act on the pituitary cells.[13] It is not known at this time whether this acts as a releasing mechanism or whether these factors are directly involved in the biosynthesis of FSH and LH.

## Feedback Mechanisms

Circulating estrogen is the key factor in increasing or decreasing release of FSH and LH from the pituitary gland.[15] The negative feedback is well understood as it functions in menopause. Cessation or diminution of estrogen production and circulation results in high circulating levels of FSH and LH.

The positive-feedback system is the key factor in the regulation of the menstrual cycle. As estrogen levels rise in the blood, LH levels also rise, reaching a peak at the time of ovulation. Estrogens do not have this positive feedback effect on FSH. Positive and negative feedback are obviously occurring simultaneously and the result and net change in the secretion of gonadotropins represent the algebraic sum of the positive- and negative-feedback inputs.[11]

# Follicle Growth, Maturation, and Atresia

Follicle growth commences in the latter half of the luteal phase of the menstrual cycle. Estrogen levels are on the rise during this period. A significant increase in estrogen is detectable 6 to 7 days before the LH surge and examination of ovaries at this time reveals follicular growth. The increase in estrogens is triggered by a rise in FSH levels that follows diminished estrogen production by the involuting corpus luteum. There is also a corresponding rise in LH.[1]

Follicle maturation is dependent on the stimulatory effect of FSH and LH in appropriate ratios.[1,9] By their feedback effect on the hypothalamic–pituitary axis the gonadal hormones indirectly influence follicle maturation but they also appear to modulate follicle growth by a direct intraovarian mechanism.[1,10] Intraovarian estrogen contributes to stimulating follicle maturation and rendering the follicle more susceptible to gonadotropin stimulation. Androgens produced within the ovary exert an inhibitory effect on follicle maturation.[4] It is therefore necessary to take into account the stimulation not only of FSH and LH but also of the ratio of the stimulatory and inhibitory effects of the intraovarian concentrations of estrogens and androgens.[11] During the phase of maturation of the follicle,[12] estrogens rise at first gradually and then more rapidly, reaching a peak just before ovulation.[9] As estrogens rise, FSH decreases because of a negative-feedback effect of estrogens. At the same time LH increases slowly but steadily. Only one follicle each month normally grows to full maturity and others become atretic. The mechanism resulting in atresia is not known. Atresia may be caused by decreasing levels of FSH that are unable to influence the mature follicle or possibly may be caused by intraovarian androgens, which can inhibit their growth and development.

## Ovulation

Just before ovulation there is a rapid rise in the secretion of LH. Rupture and the release of the ovum follow this rise. Recent evidence suggests that the variations and rising titer of estrogens trigger the LH surge.[13] At the same time that this surge occurs, there is a less dramatic FSH rise. The factors that play a role in terminating the LH surge are not known. Just prior to rupture of the follicle, plasma estrogen levels drop, probably representing morphologic alterations in the follicle induced by LH, namely, luteinization of granulosa cells. The abrupt fall in estrogen levels prior to ovulation may have a structural effect on the follicle; certainly LH exerts its effects as well, probably mediated through progesterone produced in the follicle.

## Corpus Luteum, Maturation and Regression

The luteal phase of the cycle is marked by an increase in the plasma levels of progesterone, estradiol, estrone, and 17α-hydroxyprogesterone.[14] Luteinizing hormone and FSH levels are lower than in the preovulatory period and are lowest when progesterone secretion is maximum. The corpus luteum reaches full maturity 8 or 9 days postovulation, and this is followed by regression if pregnancy has not occurred. The normal length of the luteal phase is dependent on complete follicle maturation prior to ovulation and adequate LH levels during the luteal phase.

It has been shown[9] that short luteal phases result from the lack of complete maturation of the follicle prior to rupture. In patients with short luteal phases, the LH surge was normal. Once corpus lutein maturation is achieved and if pregnancy does not occur, progesterone and estrogen levels drop and menstruation occurs. The drop in

estrogens triggers a rise in FSH and LH and the commencement of a new cycle.

The alterations in endometrium during the menstrual cycle are a reflection of the interaction of hypothalamic, pituitary, and ovarian functions and are described in Chapter 11.

## Receptor Sites in Endometrium and Steroid Interaction

Radioimmunoassay has contributed to accurately following blood levels of steroid hormones, LH, FSH, and hypothalamic releasing factors during the menstrual cycle. Molecular endocrinology has recently contributed to understanding what happens when a given hormone reaches a specific tissue and initiates changes in its structural and functional characteristics.[16] It seems unlikely that any hormone has a single primary effect on its target cells. Each probably operates via several, perhaps many, different sites of action, even within a single cell. Hormones in low concentrations can exert marked cellular responses both in structure and function and it is believed that there must be a mechanism of biologic amplification in order to have so profound a response.[15] It appears that during the process of cellular differentiation certain cells develop specific protein receptors, which bind to specific hormones and form specific hormone–receptor complexes.[17] Specifically there have been found estrogen receptors in the uterus. It has not yet been determined whether these receptors represent a mechanism for accumulating an effective concentration of the hormone in the cells or whether they represent a first step in the action of the hormone. The estrogen receptor has been studied in the rat uterus.[18] The receptor is present in the cytoplasm and may serve to move estradiol through the cytoplasm to the nucleus. The estradiol comes in contact with DNA in the chromosomes and initiates the synthesis of messinger RNA on the DNA template. Some studies suggest that estradiol stimulates RNA synthesis only when it is bound to a receptor protein. Estrogen receptors are similarly found in other target sites, such as breast, vagina, hypothalamus, and anterior pituitary lobe, suggesting tissue specificity for hormone action.

Experimental evidence[7] shows that the cellular response to estrogens is increased synthesis of ribosomal, transfer, and messenger RNA, not simply the latter. This synthesis corresponds to the proliferation of glands, stroma, and blood vessels in the endometrium during the preovulatory phase of the cycle.

Progesterone exerts equally marked effects on the endometrium but, as is well known, only after the cells have responded to estrogen. As yet there is no molecular explanation for this requirement of prior exposure to estrogen. It is possible that a prior production of RNA and the subsequent alterations induced by them is a prerequisite for further protein synthesis, such as the intraluminal secretions present on day 21 in the menstrual cycle.

# REFERENCES

1. Baird, D. T., and Guevara, A. Concentration of unconjugated estrone and estradiol in peripheral plasma in non-pregnant women throughout the menstrual cycle, castrate and post menopausal women and in men. *J. Clin. Endocrinol. 29:149, 1969.*

2. Baird, D. T., Horton, R., Longcope, C., et al. Steroid dynamics under steady state conditions. *Recent Prog. Horm. Res. 25:611, 1969.*

3. Dhariwal, A. D. S., Nallar, R., Batt, M., and McCann, S. M. Separation of follicle stimulating hormone releasing factor from luteinizing hormone releasing factor. *Endocrinology 76:291, 1965.*

4. Lloyd, C. W., Lobotsky, J., Baird, D. T., et al. Concentration of unconjugated estrogens, androgens and gestagens in ovarian and peripheral venous plasma of women. The normal menstrual cycle. *J. Clin. Endocrinol. Metab. 32:155, 1971.*

5. Midgley, A. R. Jr., and Jaffe, R. B. Regulation of human gonadotropins. X. Episodic fluctuation of L.H. during the menstrual cycle. *J. Clin. Endocrinol. 33:962, 1971.*

6. Musliner, T. A., Chader, G. J., and Villee, C. A. Studies on estradiol receptors of the rat uterus: Nuclear uptake in vitro. *Biochemistry 9:4448, 1970.*

7. O'Malley, B. W., McGuire, W. L., Kohler, P., and Korenman, S. Studies on the mechanism of steroid hormone synthesis of specific proteins. *Recent Prog. Horm. Res. 29:105, 1969.*

8. Ross, G. T., Cargille, C. M., et al. Pituitary and gonadal hormones in women during spontaneous and induced ovulatory cycles. *Recent Prog. Horm. Res. 26:1, 1970.*

9. Ross, G. T., Vaiturastis, J. L., et al. Pituitary gonadotropins and pre-antral follicular maturation in women. Amsterdam, *in* Excerpta Medica, Intern. Congress Ser. 273, 1973.

10. Ross, G. T., and Vande Wiele, R. L., eds. The ovaries *In Textbook of Endocrinology,* 5th ed. Baltimore, Williams and Wilkins, 1974, p. 368.

11. Speroff, L., and Vande Wiele, R. L. Regulation of the human menstrual cycle. *Am. J. Obstet Gynecol. 109:234, 1971.*

12. Strott, C. A., and Lipsett, M. B. Measurement of 17-hydroxy-progesterone in human plasma. *J. Clin. Endocrinol. 28:1426, 1968.*

13. Taymor, M. *Advances in Endocrinology—A Ten Year Review.* Special Article in Gynecology of the Woman Over 65. New York, Hoeber Medical Division, Harper & Row, 1967.

14. Toft, D., and Gorski, J. A Receptor molecule for estrogens: Isolation from the rat uterus and preliminary characterization. *Proc. Natl. Acad. Sci. USA 55:1574, 1966.*

15. Vande Wiele, R. L., Bogumil, R. J., and Dyrenfurth, I. Mechanisms regulating the menstrual cycle in women. *Recent Prog. Horm. Res. 26:63, 1970.*

16. Vande Wiele, R. L., and Dyrenfurth, I. Gonadotropin-steroid interrelationships. *Pharmacol. Res. 25:2, 1973.*

17. Villee, C. A. *Pharmacologic Physiology of the Endometrium and Steroid Interactions.* In M. Abell, ed., *The Uterus.* Baltimore, Williams & Wilkins, 1973.

18. Yoshimi, T., and Lipsett, M. B. The measurements of plasma progesterone. *Steroids 11:527, 1968.*

Rita Iovine Demopoulos, M.D.

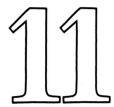

# Normal Endometrium*

Endometrium, the lining mucosa of the uterus, is a labile tissue hormonally responsive to sex steroids elaborated in the ovary. In the first half of the menstrual cycle all its elements undergo proliferation under the influence of estrogens, and in the latter half, it responds to progesterone by the production of secretions and stromal alterations necessary for implantation of a fertilized ovum. The factors in the hypothalamus and anterior lobe of the pituitary gland that control and regulate hormone production in the ovary are discussed in Chapter 10.

## Development of the Uterus

### Neonatal Uterus

At birth the corpus and cervix together measure 3 to 4 cm in length; however, the length of the cervix is greater than that of the uterus roughly in a ratio of 2:1 to 4:1 (Figure 11.1). Over the next 9 years the combined length remains quite stationary, and the cervix is considerably longer than the uterine corpus. Between 9 and 13 years, the cervix grows in length from approximately 2 cm to over 3 cm. The uterus enlarges much more dramatically in this period, so that at about 13 years it measures over 3 cm and is about equal in length to the cervix.

\* Contributions on scanning electron microscopy of the normal endometrium are by A. J. White and H. J. Buchsbaum.

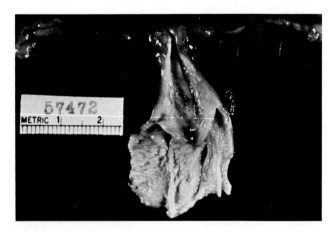

**11.1** Gross anatomy of newborn vagina, cervix, corpus uteri, and fallopian tubes.

The endometrium at birth is characteristically thin and consists of a continuous surface of cuboidal epithelium which occasionally dips down to line a few small sparse tubular glands (Figure 11.2). The endometrial stroma at this time is just developing as a definitive layer, separate from the myometrium. In a study of the endometria of 169 neonatal infants, Ober[13] found inactive endometrium in 52%, proliferative endometrium in 16%, and secretory changes in 27% (Figure 11.3). Predecidual changes or menstrual endometrium were seen in 5%. Ober attributed these hormonal responses to maternal hormones that crossed the placental barrier. In these cases the endometrium becomes inactive following delivery. There is a slow steady growth of the uterus, including the endometrium, in childhood. Estrogens are elaborated before menarche commences and this leads to the development of secondary sexual characteristics before and at the time of puberty. It is the premenarchal production of estrogens that promotes the growth of endometrial glands and stroma. At puberty, the nulliparous uterus weighs between 40 and 50 gm. The ratio of cervix to corpus is 1:1. The overall dimensions are: length, 5.5 to 8 cm; width, 4.5 to 6.0 cm; and anterior–posterior diameter, 2.5 to 3.5 cm.

## Menarche

The menarche normally occurs between 9 and 16 years of age, after other secondary sex characteristics have begun to develop. Breast development and pubic and axillary hair generally precede the onset of the first menstrual period. It is common for the first few cycles to be anovulatory and irregular in their occurrence, with intervals as long as 2 to 3 months, until a more regular ovulatory pattern is established. The usual cycle lasts from 3 to 6 weeks, with the mean occurring at 4 weeks. The onset of bleeding corresponds to day 1. Because the interval of time between ovulation and the subsequent onset of bleeding is fairly fixed at 2 weeks, most of the variation in the duration of the menstrual cycle results from variations in the duration of the preovulatory portion of the cycle. The average duration of bleeding is from 2 to 7 days.

Menstrual blood does not usually clot because it con-

**11.2** Newborn endometrium at term shows resting endometrium characterized by sparse simple glands lined by flat epithelium and ill-defined stroma.

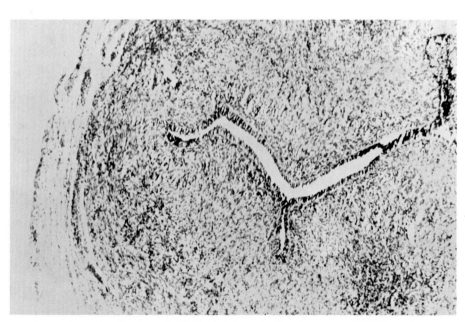

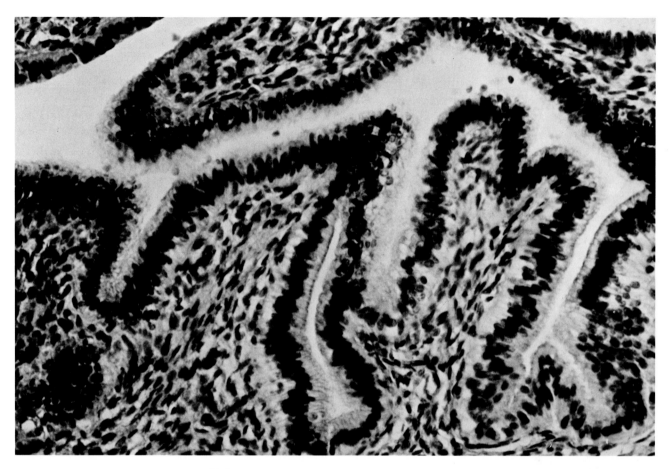

**11.3** Newborn endometrium showing secretory changes from stimulation by maternal estrogens and progesterone.

tains fibrinolysin in sufficient concentration to inhibit clot formation. Occasionally, if bleeding is heavy, however, the ability of fibrinolysin to lyse fibrin may be overcome and clots may form in the vagina.[2]

## The Adult Uterus

The parous uterus is considerably larger than the nulliparous and weighs from 50 to 80 gm. It measures as follows: length, 7 to 9 cm; width, 4.5 to 6 cm; and anterior–posterior diameter, 2.5 to 3.5 cm. The ratio of corpus to cervix reverses so that the corpus is now considerably larger than the cervix, averaging 2:1. The corpus is symmetrical about a vertical axis and roughly triangular in shape with the apex at the bottom. The endometrial cavity is similarly symmetrical. The endometrium varies from 1 to 8 mm in thickness and the myometrium averages 1.5 to 2.5 cm in thickness.

## Blood Supply

### Arterial

Blood is delivered to the endomyometrium via branches of uterine and ovarian arteries. These form arcuate branches that penetrate the lateral wall of the uterus and traverse the uterus between the outer and middle third of the myometrium. They divide into two sets of vessels; one supplies the myometrium, and the other sends branches which enter the basilar endometrium (Figures 11.4 and 11.5) and give rise to spiral arterioles that supply the upper two-thirds of the endometrium. The basal arteries are not as responsive to ovarian steroid hormones as are the spiral arterioles. During the proliferative phase of the menstrual cycle, the spiral arterioles grow in height and in number; it is in the latter half of the cycle that they are near the surface of the endometrium. Spiral arterioles

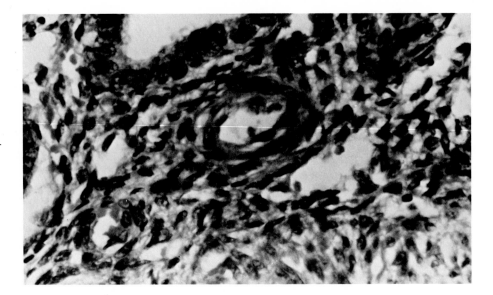

**11.4** Basilar artery at the endomyometrial junction.

have smooth muscle and adventitia in their walls. When they reach the upper third of the endometrium, they lose the smooth muscle and adventitia and terminate as capillaries. Elastic tissue stains demonstrate elastic fibers between the media and adventitia in spiral arterioles, and it is this tissue that facilitates changes in length and diameter of the vessels. As they course through the endometrium they give rise to numerous perpendicular vessels that supply the stroma and glands. Routine hematoxylin and eosin stains do not outline the structure of blood vessels very

well, and Fanger and Barker[5] have used alkaline phosphatase stains to visualize detail in vessel walls. They described variations in the caliber of vessels in the endometrium during the menstrual cycle. In the latter half of the cycle the capillaries were of larger dimension and the spiral arterioles were markedly increased in number. The hormonal responsiveness of the arterioles and capillaries was demonstrated by Markee,[8] by transplanting homologous endometrium into the eyes of rhesus monkeys.

## Venous Drainage

The venous drainage of endometrium was studied by Farrer-Brown[6] using injections of a radio-opaque medium followed by microradiography. They found that venous capillaries originated just under surface endometrium. They intercommunicate like the rungs of a ladder. In the basal endometrium they join to form large collecting veins, which run through the inner one-third of the myometrium. The inner one-half of the myometrium is considerably less vascular than the endometrium. The veins increase in size as they travel outward to join the arcuate veins.

## Normal Histologic Response of Endometrium to Sex Steroids

The dating system that the majority of clinicians and pathologists are familiar with is based upon a 28-day normal cycle. However, the 28-day cycle is quite elusive

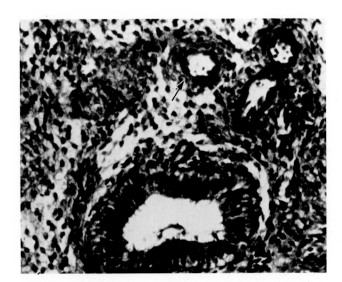

**11.5** Spiral arteriole showing smooth muscle in its walls (arrow).

and the range varies from 23 to 34 days. The old dating system is based on a 28-day cycle. Day 1 is the first day of menses and ovulation is day 14 in the cycle. The first few days are menstrual; the rest of the preovulatory period is designated as early, mid, and late proliferative. In the postovulatory phase, the changes are sufficiently specific as to permit dating to within 24 hr. Noyes et al.[12] found that the dating of endometrium correlated with the expected day of menstruation 60% of the time within ±1 day. Gynecologists have recommended that endometrial dating be done according to days after ovulation because the sequence of events in the secretory phase are more uniform from patient to patient and cycle to cycle. Because ovulation occurs on the fourteenth day, day 16 in the first system of dating would be considered in this new dating system as day 2. In illustrating the day-to-day changes in the postovulatory phase, we give the dating as determined by both systems.

## Menstrual Endometrium

On the first day of bleeding, the endometrium grossly appears congested and hemorrhagic (Figure 11.6). Hemorrhage, dissecting through the stroma, fragments and disrupts endometrial glands. Microscopically, despite vascular congestion and focal hemorrhage, it is possible to evaluate whether ovulation has occurred since the glands and stroma show evidence of progestational stimulation. There is extensive leukocytic stromal infiltration (Figure 11.7). Fibrin thrombi are noted and glands appear exhausted. On the second and third days of bleeding, degenerative changes become pronounced. The glands are fragmented

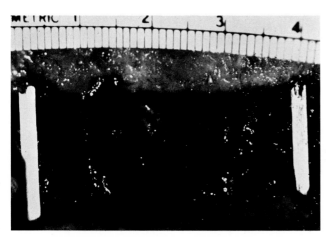

**11.6** Gross view of endometrium, first day of menses. The surface is hemorrhagic.

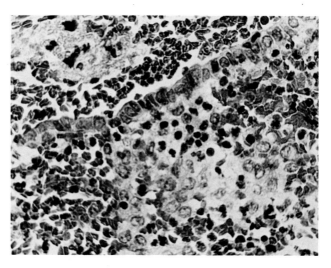

**11.7** Endometrium, first day of menses. High-power view showing hemorrhage and leukocytic infiltration in stroma.

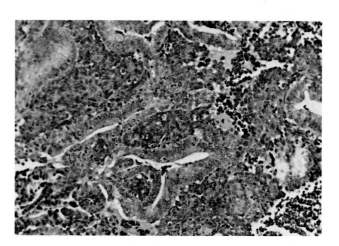

**11.8** Endometrium, third day of menses. Glands are collapsed and fragmented. There is necrosis and condensation of stroma.

and collapsed. The stroma is condensed and varies in its staining properties. The nuclei become pyknotic and plasma membranes indistinct (Figure 11.8). At this time there is too much architectural and cytologic disruption to determine whether ovulation occurred.

## Preovulatory Phase of the Cycle

Following about 4 days of menses, the endometrium regenerates from the basilar glands. There is evidence to suggest that regeneration begins before menses are com-

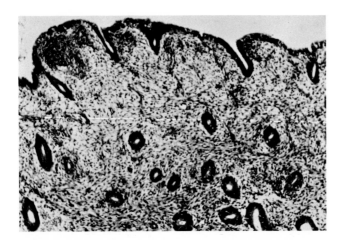

**11.9** Early proliferative endometrium. Glands are small and tubular and on cross section appear spherical.

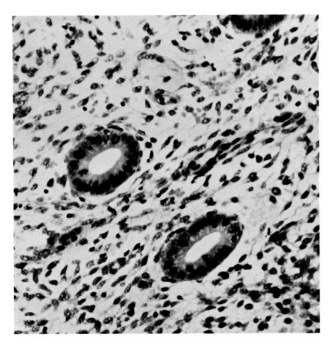

**11.10** Early proliferative endometrium showing mitoses in gland epithelium.

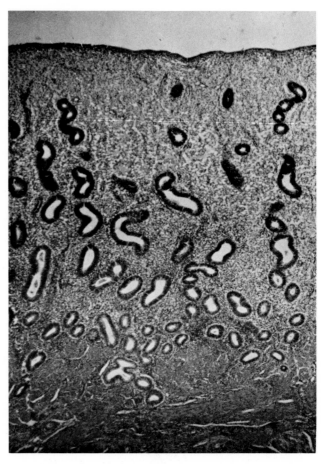

**11.11** Midproliferative endometrium. Glands become elongated and slightly tortuous.

pleted. In the proliferative phase, the endometrium grows rapidly in response to circulating estrogens. It triples in thickness from approximately 1 to 3 mm. In the early stages (days 4 to 7 old system), the glands are small, tubular, and short and on cross section appear spherical (Figure 11.9).

The lining epithelium is cuboidal to columnar and the nuclei are ovoid and basally or centrally located. Mitoses increase as proliferation proceeds (Figure 11.10). These may be seen both in the glands and in the stroma. In the midproliferative phase the glands become elongated and somewhat tortuous (Figure 11.11). The lining cells are tall columnar and pseudostratification of nuclei is seen. Mitoses continue to be abundant (Figure 11.12). The nucleus in a dividing cell moves to the luminal side of the cell and therefore can be detected by the density of its chromatin. About 8 to 10 days into the preovulatory phase there is a transient period of mild edema in the stroma (Figure 11.13). Blood vessels are not as conspicuous as in the postovulatory phase. Some scattered lymphocytes may be present and occasionally lymphoid follicles with germinal centers are seen. They are probably a normal component of the tissue as in other organ sites. In late proliferative endometrium, the glands are maximally elongated, per-

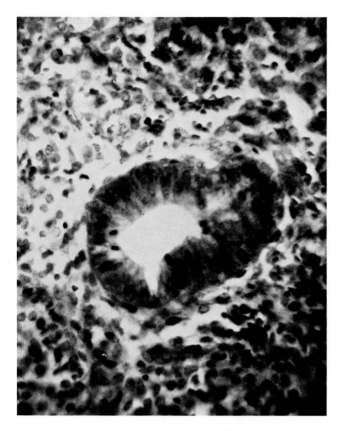

**11.12** Midproliferative endometrium showing mitoses in gland epithelium. There is loose stroma, in which nuclei are fusiform and oval, and there is scant cytoplasm.

pendicular to the surface, and markedly convoluted (Figure 11.14a). The nuclei are large and pseudostratified (Figure 11.14b). The stroma is dense and abundant and the nuclei are oval with scant cytoplasm (Figure 11.15). Spiral arterioles are thin walled and inconspicuous.

## Postovulatory Phase

The endometrium, which up until now has been estrogen-primed, shows changes due to the additional stimulation by progesterone, which is secreted by the corpus luteum. Gross examination of secretory endometrium reveals it to be thick (3 to 5 mm) and to have a creamy yellow appearance (Figure 11.16). It is soft in consistency and at curettage is so abundant that in premenopausal patients it is often erroneously regarded as hyperplastic by the gynecologist, merely because of the volume obtained. Assuming that day 14 represents the day of ovulation (day 1 in the new system of dating), the first evidence of it is seen 48 hr later (day 16 in the old dating system, or day 3 in the new dating system). On day 16 small subnuclear vacuoles begin to appear in some of the glands (Figure 11.17). By day 17, these vacuoles are conspicuous and uniformly seen in virtually all the endometrial glands (Figure 11.18). They are clear vacuoles, rich in glycogen and lipid, and are located beneath the nucleus, displacing the nucleus to a midzonal position. By day 18, the secretory vacuoles have largely migrated to a supranuclear or luminal position (Figure 11.19). Mitoses are not seen

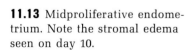

**11.13** Midproliferative endometrium. Note the stromal edema seen on day 10.

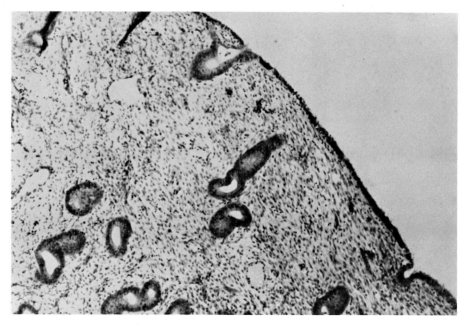

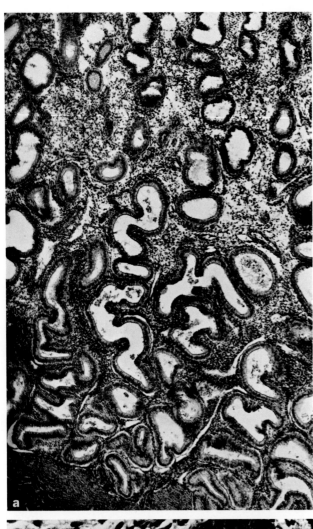

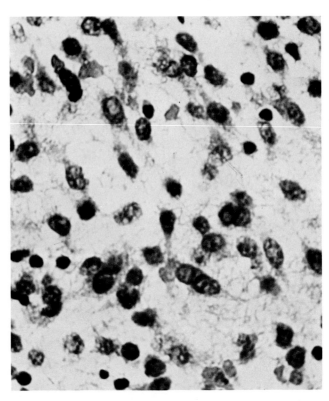

**11.15** Late proliferative endometrium. Stromal cells have plump nuclei and scant cytoplasm.

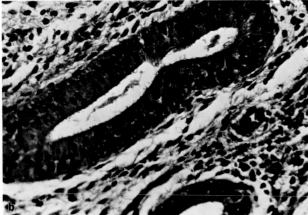

**11.14 a.** Late proliferative phase. Glands are maximally elongated and are convoluted. **b.** Late proliferative endometrium. There is pseudostratification and nuclei are large.

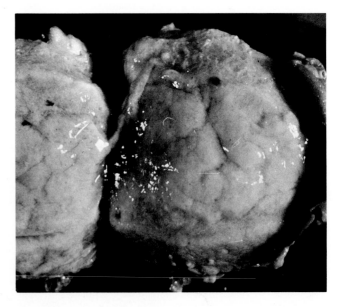

**11.16** Gross appearance of secretory endometrium. It is thick and pseudopolypoid.

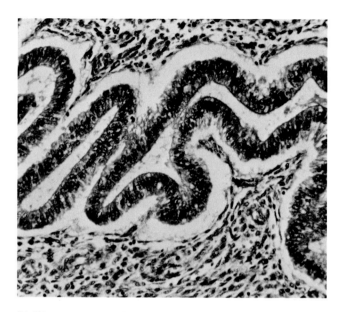

**11.17** Secretory endometrium, day 16. There is focal subnuclear vacuolation.

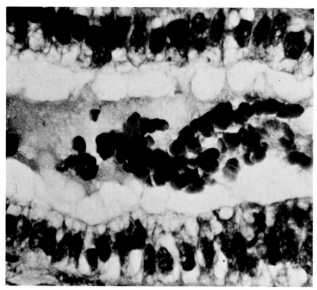

**11.19** Secretory endometrium, days 18 to 19. Vacuoles can be seen on the sides of the nuclei as well as above them.

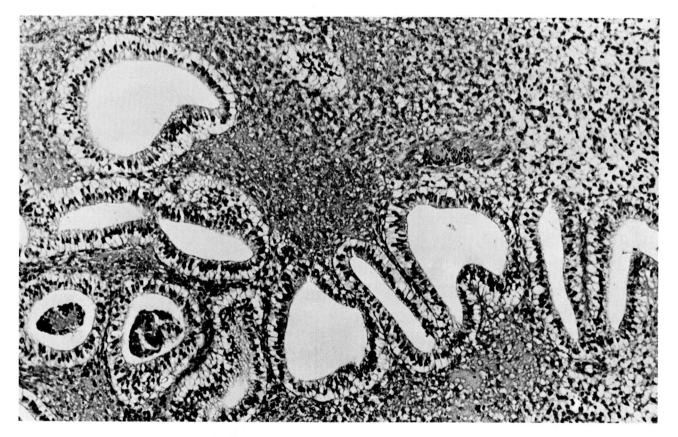

**11.18** Secretory endometrium, day 17. High-power view of subnuclear vacuoles.

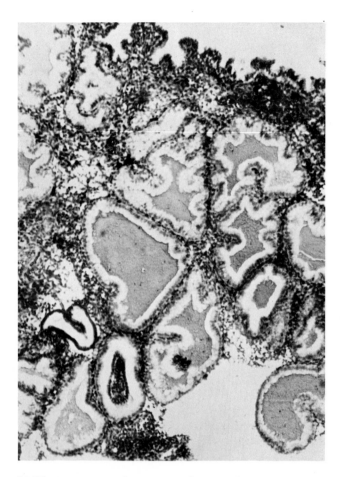

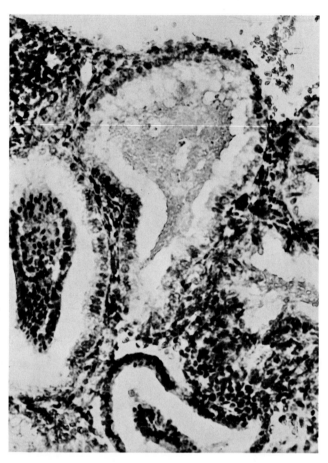

**11.20** Secretory endometrium, day 20. The secretions now fill the lumen of the glands.

**11.21** Secretory endometrium, day 20. Epithelial lining cells are low cuboidal and the luminal borders are frayed.

either in the glands or stroma in this phase of the cycle. By day 20 the secretions are released into the lumina of the glands (Figure 11.20). The lining cells now become cuboidal in shape and the luminal border of the epithelial cells is no longer sharply defined; it becomes frayed and irregular (Figure 11.21). The stromal changes now become dramatic. On day 20 the stromal cell nuclei are spindle shaped and the cytoplasm and cell borders are poorly defined. Stromal edema begins on day 21, focally, causing the nuclei to spread apart. This is clearly seen on day 22, when stromal edema reaches its peak (Figure 11.22). Some of the glands appear dilated and the epithelium lining them appears exhausted. The blood vessels, which have been inconspicuous and have appeared singly during the proliferative and early secretory stages, have proliferated, elongated, and become coiled so that by day 23 they are seen in clusters of two to five on cross section (Figure

11.23). The earliest predecidual changes are perivascular. The stromal cells surrounding the spiral arterioles no longer have bare nuclei; there is a distinct cytoplasm. The cytoplasm increases and stains deeper than usual and on day 24 has the appearance of predecidua (Figure 11.24). The nuclei become round and are centrally located. The change in the stromal cells extends beyond the spiral arterioles and by day 25 (Figure 11.25) predecidua can be seen about the glands as well as beneath the surface endometrium. The cell borders become distinct, forming a mosaic-like pattern (Figure 11.26). Glycogen stains, such as Best's carmine or periodic acid Schiff, reveal glycogen to be present in the cytoplasm. The terms, predecidua or pseudodecidua are reserved for nonpregnancy states, and the term, decidua, for gestational stroma. The predecidual change may be less well developed in women approaching the menopause, and in patients who have poor corpus

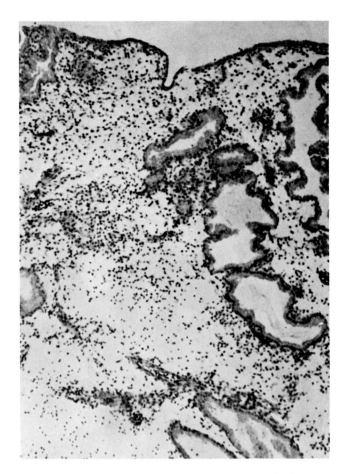

**11.22** Secretory endometrium, day 22. Stromal edema is at its peak. Glands are dilated and tortuous and the epithelium is exhausted.

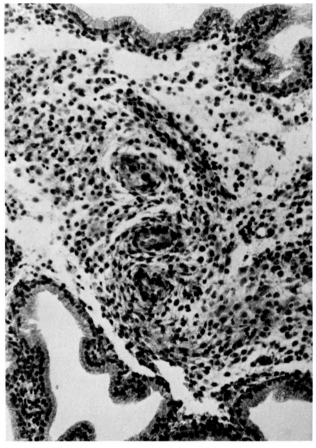

**11.23** Secretory endometrium, day 23. Spiral arterioles are prominent and appear clustered.

luteum development. After day 24, secretions in the glands diminish and become inspissated. The glands take on a sawtooth appearance and this is prominent on day 26. Other glands appear dilated and exhausted. Spiral arterioles are prominent and dilated. On day 27 polynuclear leukocytes appear in the stroma (Figures 11.27 and 11.28). Just prior to the onset of menstruation, nuclear debris often appears at the base of the endometrial glands (Figure 11.29). This debris consists of fragmented bits of nuclear chromatin, often sequestered in vacuoles beneath the nucleus of the endometrial lining cell. The origin of this nuclear debris is not clear. It resembles degenerating polymorphonuclear leukocytes; however intact leukocytes are not seen in this location.

The origin of the polymorphonuclear leukocytes seen in the stroma is disputed. They have in the past generally been thought to be derived from the circulation by diapedesis across the wall of the dilated spiral arterioles. However, Dallenbach-Hellweg[4] suggests that they are derived from stromal cells and refers to them as endometrial granulocytes. She demonstrated paranuclear phloxinophilic granules in stromal appearing cells around spiral arterioles on day 24, and postulated that these developed into "endometrial granulocytes." She believed that polymorphonuclear leukocytes only appeared in a menstrual endometrium in association with frank hemorrhage and necrosis.

According to Noyes et al.,[12] two pathologists independently evaluating 1,007 endometria dated them identically 30% of the time, agreed to within ±1 day 60% of the time, and agreed within ±2 days 80% of the time. The correlation between histologic dating and patients' basal body temperatures concurred within ±2 days 75% of the time.

221

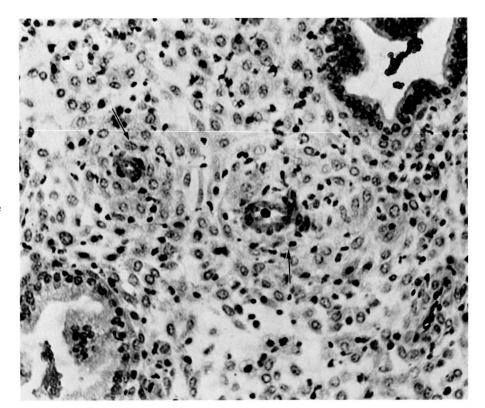

**11.24** Secretory endometrium, day 24. Spiral arterioles. The stromal cells (arrows) now have prominent cytoplasm and are predecidual.

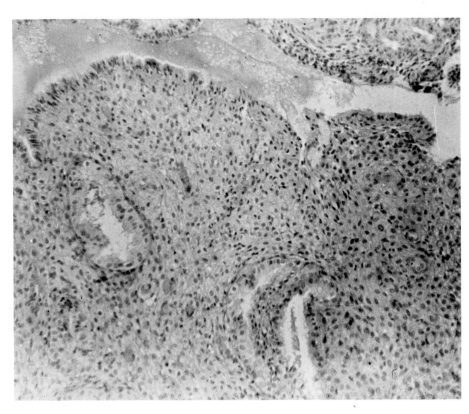

**11.25** Secretory endometrium, day 25. Pseudodecidua in broad sheets, surrounding glands and beneath the surface epithelium.

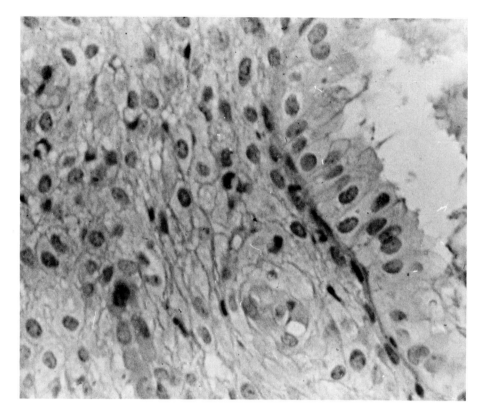

**11.26** Secretory endometrium, day 26. Pseudodecidua has a mosaic pattern.

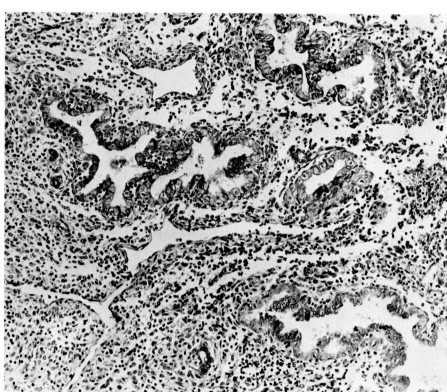

**11.27** Secretory endometrium, day 27. Glands are tortuous and there is a stromal infiltrate composed of lymphocytes and polymorphonuclear leukocytes.

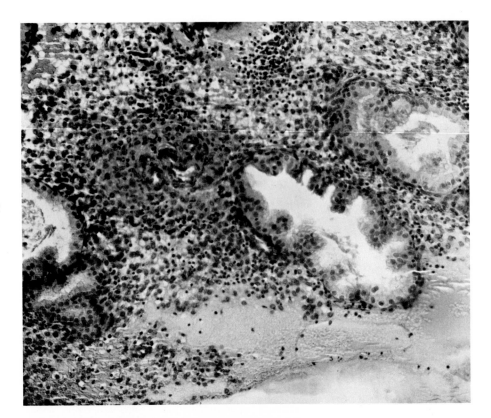

**11.28** Secretory endometrium, day 27. Glands are sawtoothed, and secretions are minimal and inspissated. There is leukocytic infiltration, and beginning stromal dissolution.

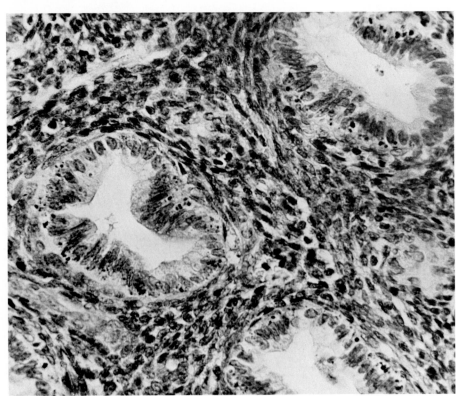

**11.29** Premenstrual secretory endometrium. Nuclear debris at the base of nuclei in the glands.

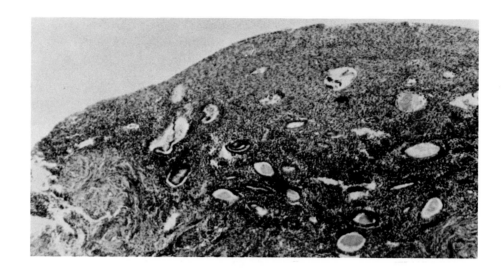

**11.30** Inactive endometrium, postmenopause. Stroma is dense; glands are small and lined by cuboidal epithelium.

## The Endometrium at Menopause

Menopause is defined as 6 months of amenorrhea occurring usually in the fourth and fifth decades of life and is characterized by cessation or marked diminution of estrogen production by the ovary. The age at which menopause occurs is to some extent genetically determined. Menopause occurring prior to age 35 is considered to be premature ovarian failure. This is discussed in greater detail in Chapter 35. There is some evidence to suggest that over the past several decades, the average duration of fertility has been increased somewhat.[14] It appears that girls are experiencing menarche at slightly younger ages than their grandmothers did. There is also an impression that some women continue to have regular menstrual cycles into their late fifties. This observation is supported by a comparison of histologic patterns of sequential endometrial curettage performed at Booth Memorial Medical Center in 1961 and 1973 in women of different age groups (Table 11.1). This demonstrated that 9% of secretory endometria occurred in women over 50 in 1973 as compared to 1.5% in 1961. Proper nutrition and freedom from chronic systemic illness may favor prolongation of ovulation. Physiologically, the menopause is caused by failure of the ovary to respond to gonadotropic hormones. This failure may be abrupt and the patient may go from regular cycles to complete permanent cessation of menstruation. In the absence of estrogen stimulation, the endometrium becomes thinned and inactive. It is better to use the term "inactive" instead of "atrophic" because it can be subsequently stimulated by exogenously administered estrogens at any age. Inactive endometrium becomes thin and may measure 1 mm in thickness. Microscopic examination may show few small glands that are simple, tubular, and lined by cuboidal epithelium. The nuclei are centrally placed and do not show pseudostratification (Figure 11.30). Mitoses are not seen. The glands are indistinguishable from the basilar glands. Thinned endometrium in which blood vessels are scant may become readily infected and so it is not unusual to see mild degrees of endometritis in postmenopausal endometrium. Occasionally in examining inactive endometrium from postmenopausal patients, squamous metaplasia may be present, and when it is extensive it is referred to as ichthyosis uteri. It is not uncommon for ovulation in the perimenopausal period to be irregular and there may be a number of episodes of anovulation prior to menopause. The longer the period of unopposed estrogen stimulation, the more likely there is to be glandular and stromal hyperplasia. The subject of hyperplasia is more fully discussed in a later chapter.

**Table 11.1** Secretory endometrium in curettage specimens

| | Age (years) | | | | |
|---|---|---|---|---|---|
| | <40 | >40 | >45 | >50 | >55 |
| N = 216 1961 | 74% | 26% | 9% | 1% | 0.5% |
| N = 204 1973 | 62% | 38% | 21% | 8% | 1% |

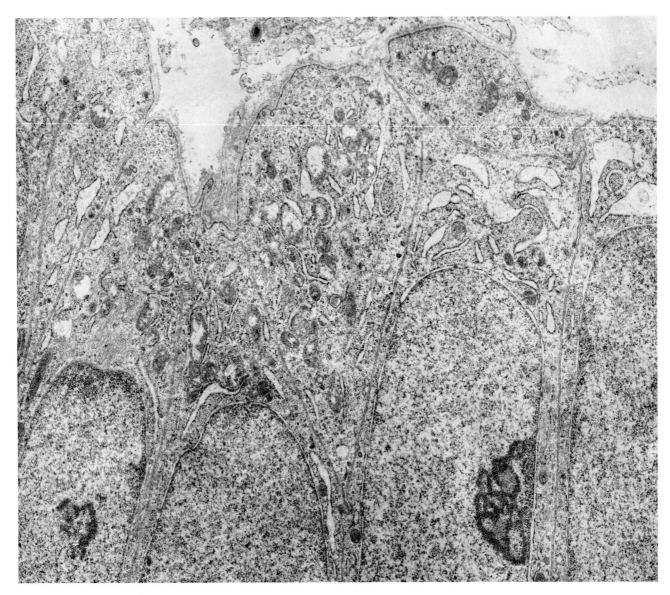

**11.31** Proliferative endometrium, TEM. Pseudostratification is seen. Microvilli are present at the cell surface. Pinocytic vesicles are present.

# The Fine Structure of the Endometrium

## Glandular Epithelium

### *Preovulatory*

The fine structure of early (day 8) proliferative glandular epithelial cells is shown in Figures 11.31, 11.32, and 11.33. The lining cells are columnar and the nuclei are centrally located with some pseudostratification. The nuclei are ovoid and not indented; the chromatin is diffusely distributed with very little condensed on the nuclear membrane. The nucleoli are prominent, large, and complex. The cell membrane at the luminal surface shows differentiation into microvilli. Pinocytic vesicles are present. In addition, the luminal surface has a "fuzzy" layer (Figure 11.31) which represents surface glycoproteins. The lateral cell boundaries show typical differentiations of columnar gland-forming cells. Near the luminal surface

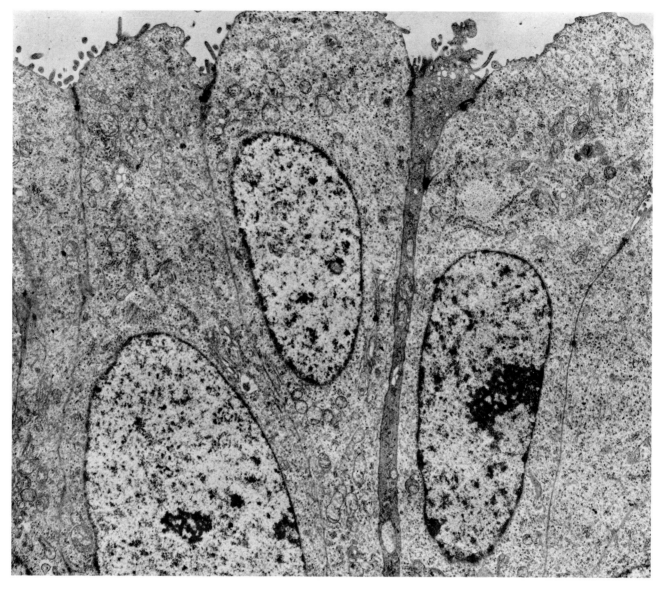

**11.32** Proliferative endometrium, TEM. Tight junctions and desmosomes connect the cells.

the lateral cell borders show tight junctions and desmosomes (Figure 11.32). The majority of the lateral cell boundaries are simple; however, as the base of the columnar cell is approached they exhibit extensive interdigitations (Figure 11.33). The basilar attachment of the columnar cell to the basement membrane is relatively simple (Figure 11.34).

The Golgi apparatus is located between the nucleus and the luminal surface (Figure 11.32). It is generally prominent and composed of vesicles, vacuoles, and lamellae. The endoplasmic reticulum (ER) is present in rough and smooth forms and is generally abundant. Large numbers of free ribosomes are present in the cytoplasm. This reflects the production of proteins for intracellular utilization. The mitochondria are distributed throughout the cytoplasm and are generally elongated.

Occasional cells contain abundant large bundles of microtubules in juxtaposition to the nuclei. The microtubules in this location may represent remnants of the mitotic spindle.

227

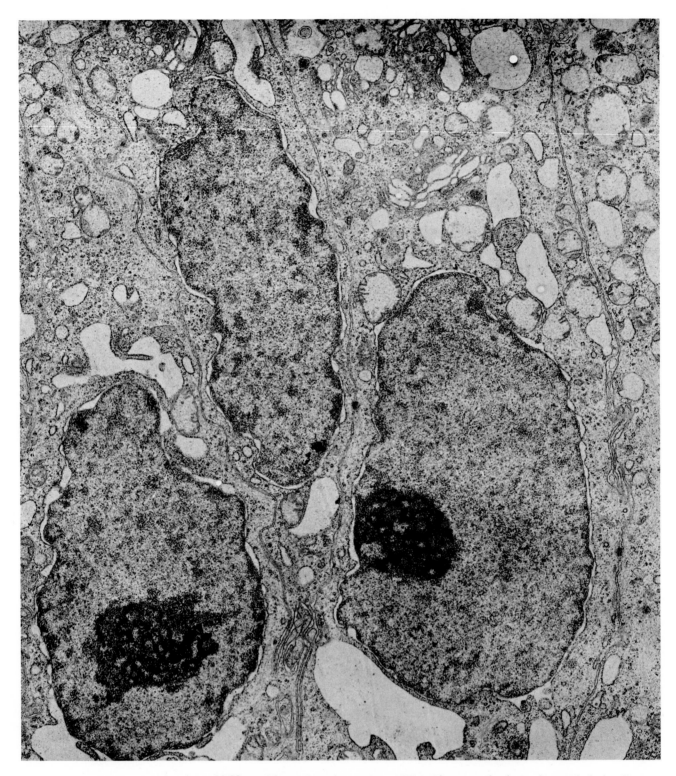

**11.33** Proliferative endometrium, TEM. Closer to the base the epithelial cells exhibit extensive interdigitations.

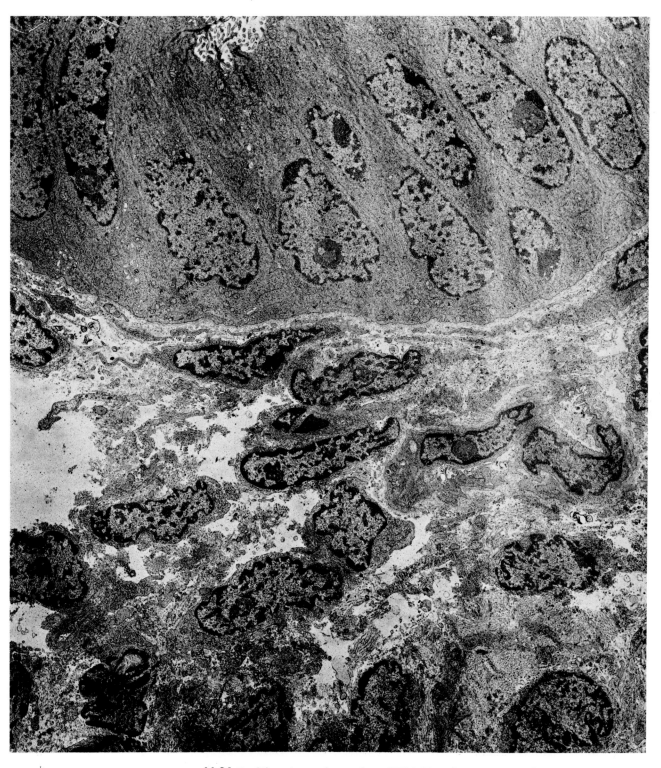

**11.34** Proliferative endometrium, TEM. Note basement membrane separating glandular epithelium from stroma. Stromal cells have prominent nuclei and cytoplasm that is electron dense.

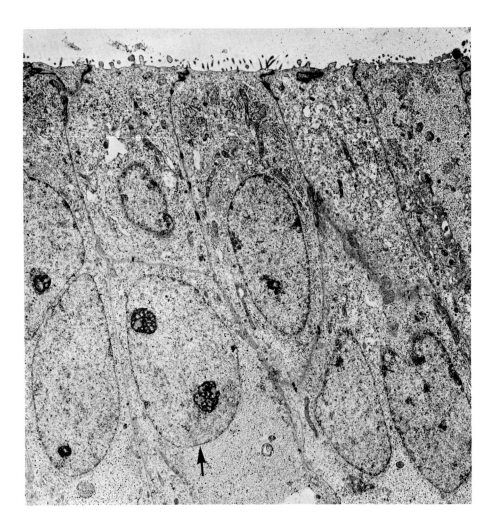

**11.35** Secretory endometrium, day 17, TEM. Nucleus pushed up by subnuclear glycogen (arrow).

At the time of ovulation, a distinctive ultrastructural feature involving mitochondria is seen. A small proportion of them, in almost all epithelial cells, enlarge and become "giant" mitochondria.[1] This is due to a true increase in the amount of material that comprises the outer and inner membranes. Accordingly, there is an increase in the number of cristae in the usual lamellar configuration. Although these "giant" structures do not differ from most other mitochondria, in ultrastructural terms, they do have an unusual association with a circumferential loop of rough ER.[1] The nature of this subcellular complex is not understood but may be related to the synthesis of membrane phospholipids and proteins by the ER, which can then be easily transported to the mitochondrion. There are active lipid exchanges between the ER and the mitochondria, facilitated by phospholipid exchange proteins. The giant mitochondria, surrounded by a loop of ER, may be a manifestation of some phase of such an exchange.

*Postovulatory*

Secretory glandular epithelium is depicted in Figures 11.35 and 11.36. The principal change from the proliferative stage is an accumulation of glycogen in the cell cytoplasm. In Figure 11.35 the glycogen occupies the basilar portions of some cells and the mid and apical portions of others. The glycogen accumulations are sufficiently massive to push aside virtually all other organelles. The mechanism of releasing glycogen into the lumen includes the formation of blebs off the cell surface (Figure 11.36). The cell membrane shows no other striking changes except for the presence of electron dense homogeneous material in the intercellular spaces near the apex. This could represent part of the secretory mechanism of the cell. Complex lysosomes appear in small numbers, some of which are in proximity to the glycogen (Figure 11.35).

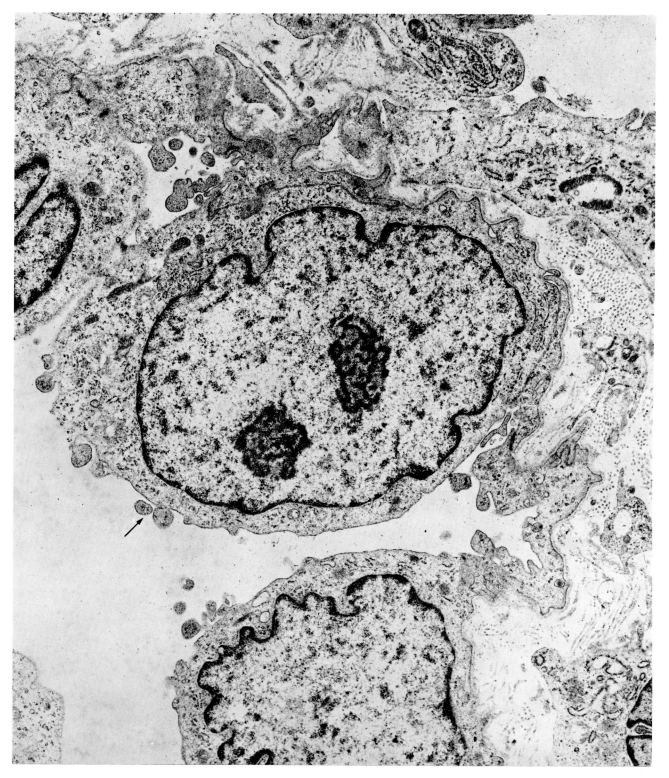

**11.36** Secretory endometrium, day 21, TEM. Cytoplasmic blebs (arrow) contain secreted glycogen.

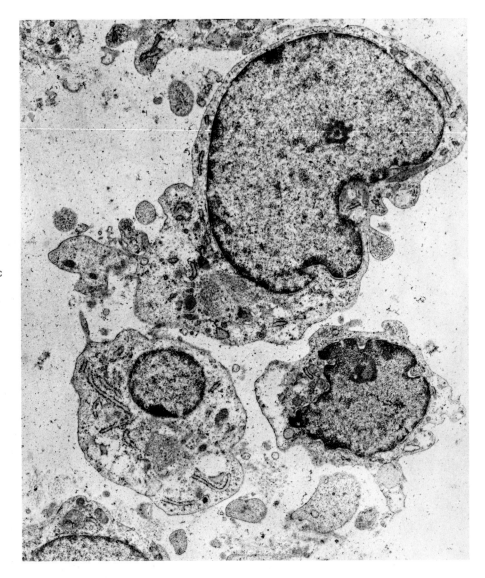

**11.37** Secretory endometrium, TEM. Stromal cells at day 21. Rough and smooth endoplasmic reticulum, and glycogen are present. The stromal cell is more complex and larger than in the proliferative phase.

The nucleus shows several modifications when compared to the proliferative phase. The nuclear envelope contains multiple convolutions. The chromatin is relatively more coarsely aggregated along the nuclear envelope as well as in the nucleoplasm (Figure 11.36). This is consistent with the cessation of mitoses, and the production of specialized proteins and other secretory products. The aggregation of chromatin represents a cell biologic mechanism for turning off gene sites. This chromatin is termed heterochromatin. The active chromatin is finely dispersed and termed euchromatin. In the proliferative phase, all of the chromatin appears active because the cells are replicating and all of the DNA must be duplicated. The nonmitosing, secreting cell in the latter half of the menstrual cycle has no need for large segments of chromatin and shuts down part of the machinery.

## Ultrastructure of Stromal Cells

Several recent papers[7,10,11,20,21] have illustrated the sequential changes in stromal cells throughout the cycle.

The stromal cells display cell biologic changes that are similar to those observed in epithelial cells. The proliferative phase is marked by ultrastructural simplicity, with biosynthesis of substances for use by the cell in division. As the proliferative phase progresses, the nucleus develops a dispersed chromatin pattern (euchromatin); because DNA is being replicated frequently, there is little or no

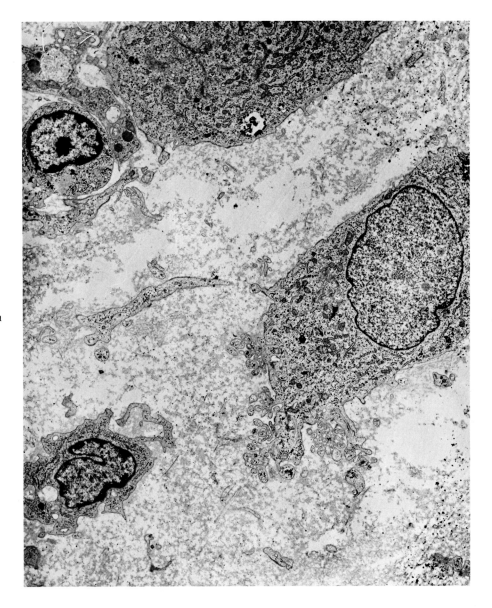

**11.38** Stromal cell, TEM, pseudodecidua. The cell is more complex. Glycogen (dark granules) is abundant. Mitochondria are prominent.

clumping (heterochromatin). The cytoplasm in this phase is relatively less complex, compared with the secretory phase. The Golgi and smooth ER are scanty; however, the rough ER progressively increases during the proliferative phase. Mitochondria remain undistinguished through this phase, as well as the secretory part, and therefore are in contrast to the giant mitochondria that form at ovulation in the adjacent glandular epithelial cells. Lysosomes, although present in the early proliferative stages, become less prominent in the late proliferative phase. There are few cell-to-cell contacts, and the intercellular spaces are sparse in collagen content.

During the secretory phase, the halt in cell division is marked by differentiation and the elaboration of materials that are destined for extracellular use (Figure 11.37). The secretory part of the cycle is accompanied by a gradual shift of euchromatin to heterochromatin. By the late secretory phase, there is extensive clumping. The amount of rough ER increases considerably and in the later secretory phase, the Golgi and smooth ER become prominent (Figure 11.38). Vesicles from the ER and Golgi are seen to contain granular material that is discharged into the extracellular matrix as a result of fusion of vesicle and plasma membranes. This material is apparently tropocollagen, and

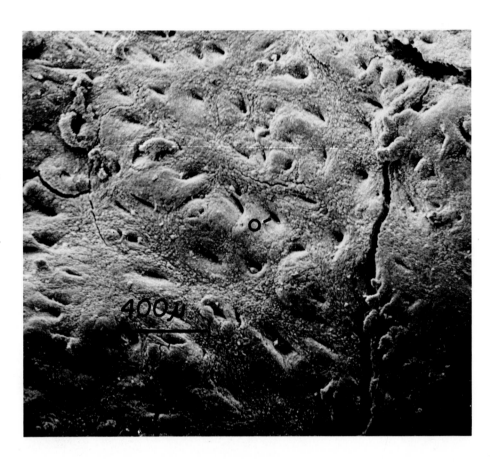

**11.39** Early proliferative endometrium showing elliptical gland ostia (O). Vertical fissure is an artifact. ×52, SEM.

[Reprinted by permission from A. J. White and H. J. Buchsbaum, Scanning electron microscopy of the human endometrium, *Gynecol. Oncol.* 1:333, 1973.]

collagen fibrils are seen to develop in the matrix. Glycogen is synthesized in increasing amounts throughout the secretory phase, and large autophagic lysosomes become prominent in the premenstrual part of the secretory phase. Cell-to-cell contacts increase as the predecidual cells enlarge, but these areas are not marked by any specializations of the plasma membrane.

## Scanning Electron Microscopy of the Normal Endometrium

The surface of the human endometrium viewed with the scanning electron microscope (SEM) shows changes throughout the ovarian cycle.[7,18,19] The surface changes are more subtle than those seen in the glands with conventional light microscopy. Variations exist in adjacent areas in a specimen at any point in the cycle, and the SEM has not proved useful in dating of the endometrium.

Under low magnification the surface appears relatively flat with gland ostia randomly dispersed (Figure 11.39). Two types of cells can be seen under higher magnification,

ciliated and secretory (Figure 11.40). Approximately 1 in 20 cells has cilia and these are found in increased numbers around gland ostia (Figure 11.41).

The cells vary in shape from round to ovoid and polyhedral, and the cell size varies from approximately 5 by 5 $\mu$ during the proliferative phase to approximately 6 by 11 $\mu$ during the menstrual phase (Table 11.2). The luminal surface of both types of cells is convex and covered with microvilli, 150 to 200 per cell. The ciliated cells have 60 to 70 cilia per cell and the cilia measure 3.0 $\mu$ in length and 2,500 Å in diameter. The ratio of ciliated to nonciliated cells varies with the phase of the endometrium. White and Buchsbaum[19] could find no difference in the number of ciliated cells at different anatomic sites in the uterus, the anterior, posterior, or lateral walls. Takeguchi, Tanaka, and Sawaragi[18] report a greater number of ciliated cells in the endometrium of the fundus and cornual regions.

### Proliferative Phase

The surface appearance of the endometrium during the proliferative phase is shown in Figure 11.39. In some areas

**11.40** Proliferative phase of endometrium. A ciliated cell is seen surrounded by secreting cells with microvilli. Secretory droplets are seen on the surface of these cells.

[Reprinted by permission from A. J. White and H. J. Buchsbaum, Scanning electron microscopy of the human endometrium, *Gynecol. Oncol.* 1:333, 1973.]

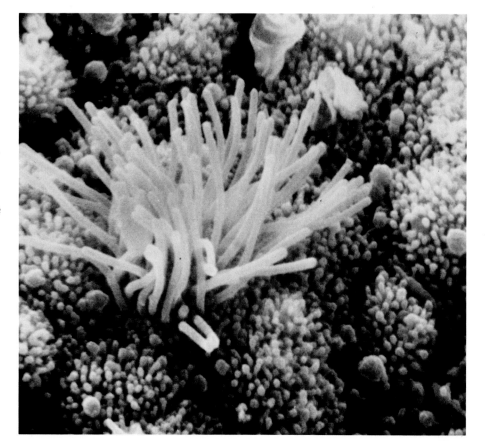

the surface may be raised because of variations in the height of the endometrium. The surface is generally flat with elliptical gland ostia. The gland ostia measure 20 to 30 $\mu$ in diameter and the interglandular distance is approximately 125 $\mu$.

During the proliferative phase the gland ostia appear

rolled as a result of cell proliferation, as shown in Figure 11.42. Ferenczy and Richart[7] suggest progressive dilatation of the gland ostia through the proliferative phase and continuing into the secretory phase. Cell size and shape remain relatively constant throughout the proliferative phase.

**Table 11.2**  Microstructural variations during the normal ovarian cycle[a]

| Phase | Number of patients | Cell size ($\mu$) | Percent ciliated cells | Number per cell | Cilia Length ($\mu$) | Cilia Width (Å) | Number per cell | Microvilli Length (Å) | Microvilli Width (Å) | Gland ostia ($\mu$) |
|---|---|---|---|---|---|---|---|---|---|---|
| Menstrual | 4 | 6.6 × 11.3 | 5 | 71 | 3.1 | 2,850 | 200 | 6,000 | 2,100 | 20 × 26 |
| Proliferative | 2 | 4.9 × 5.4 | 16 | 70 | 3.4 | 2,150 | 160 | 3,000 | 1,400 | 27 × 25 |
| Secretory | 5 | 5.9 × 5.5 | 15 | 83 | 2.2 | 2,500 | 180 | 4,800 | 1,950 | 52 × 25 |

[a] Representative measurements from over 150 photographs. $\mu$ = micron (1 $\mu$ = $10^{-3}$ mm); Å = Ångstrom (1 Å = $10^{-7}$ mm). From White and Buchsbaum.[4]

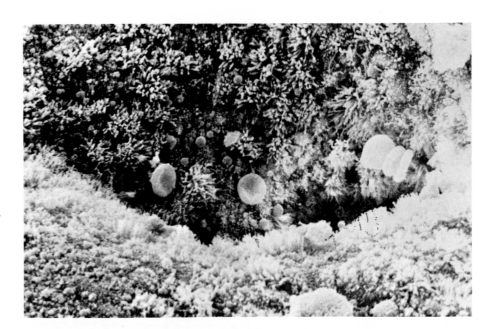

**11.41** Gland ostium with a great number of ciliated cells. Red blood corpuscles can be seen in the gland lumen. ×1,056, SEM.

[Reprinted by permission from A. J. White and H. J. Buchsbaum, Scanning electron microscopy of the human endometrium, *Gynecol. Oncol.* 1:333, 1973.]

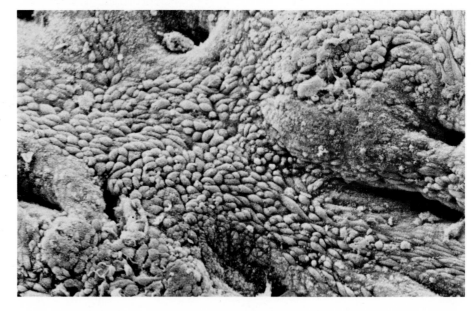

**11.42** Gland ostia appear rolled as a result of cell proliferation— proliferative phase. ×220, SEM.

[Reprinted by permission from A. J. White and H. J. Buchsbaum, Scanning electron microscopy of the human endometrium, *Gynecol. Oncol.* 1:333, 1973.]

## Secretory Phase

The endometrial surface during the secretory phase shows marked changes from the proliferative phase. The surface is convoluted, giving the appearance of ridges and clefts (Figure 11.43). Gland ostia are not obvious on the surface.

There is a relative increase in the number of ciliated cells during this phase. The cells appear uniform in size during the luteal phase. The microvilli are dense with approximately 180 microvilli per cell. The cilia appear slightly shorter, measuring 2.2 $\mu$ in length. Secretory droplets are prominent in the gland ostia and on the surface of the endometrium (Figure 11.44). By day 24 of the normal ovarian cycle, the secretory cells become distended and portions of the surface bulge into the endometrial cavity (Figure 11.45). The microvilli have bulbous dilatations at their terminal portions. These expansions of the distal

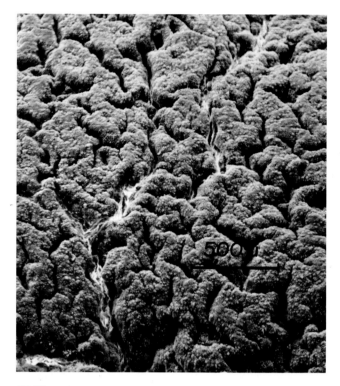

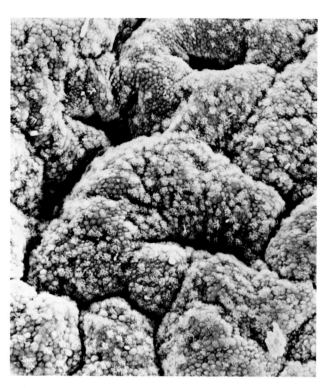

**11.43** Endometrial surface during the secretory phase. Surface appears convoluted, obscuring the gland ostia. ×80.

[Reprinted by permission from A. J. White and H. J. Buchsbaum, Scanning electron microscopy of the human endometrium, *Gynecol. Oncol. 1:*333, 1973.]

**11.44** At greater magnification cellular detail can be seen, allowing identification of ciliated and secretory cells. ×232, SEM.

[Reprinted by permission from A. J. White and H. J. Buchsbaum, Scanning electron microscopy of the human endometrium, *Gynecol. Oncol. 1:*333, 1973.]

**11.45** Late secretory endometrium. The microvilli (S) on the secretory cells show bulbous dilatations. ×6,826, SEM.

[Reprinted by permission from A. J. White and H. J. Buchsbaum, Scanning electron microscopy of the human endometrium, *Gynecol. Oncol. 1:*333, 1973.]

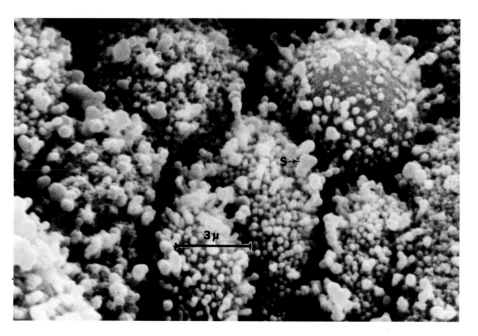

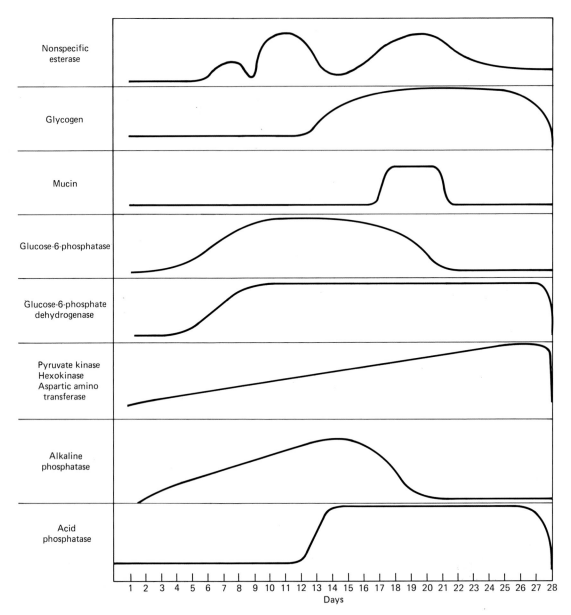

**11.46** Relative enzyme activities in endometrial glandular epithelium in the menstrual cycle.

portion of the microvilli may be the site of emission of secretory material from the cell. Individual cells maintain their configuration, but the cell margins are more sharply defined as a result of the increasing surface convexity.

## Menstrual Phase

The surface appearance of the endometrium during the menstrual phase is irregular and shaggy as a result of shedding. There is a relative decrease in the number of

ciliated cells; the secretory cells are large, with prominent microvilli.

## Cell Physiology of Endometrium

### Histochemistry and Biochemistry

Although knowledge of the distribution and concentration of enzymes in normal endometrium throughout

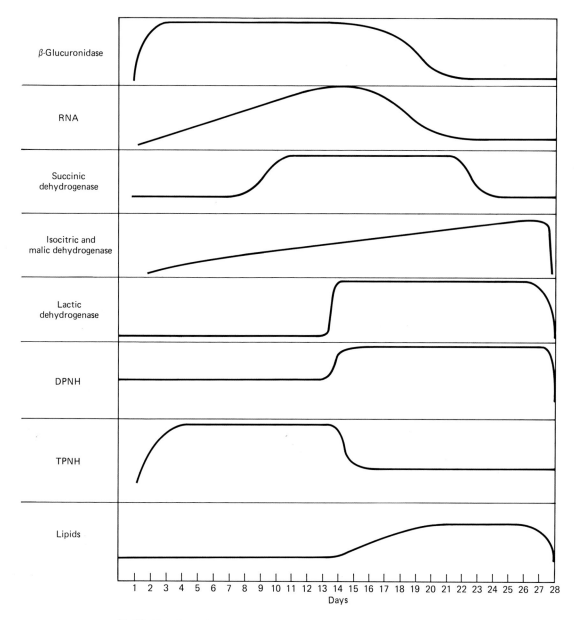

**11.46** Continued

the menstrual cycle has been available for many years, only recently has this information been correlated with normal and abnormal uterine function.

Analysis of enzyme concentrations by histochemical staining of freshly frozen endometrial tissue was carried out by Boutselis *et al.*[3] The women were from 22 to 35 years of age and had an intact pituitary–ovarian–endometrial axis. Based on his findings and those of Spellman[16] and other investigators,[17] the localization of various enzymes in glandular epithelium throughout the menstrual

cycle is schematically represented in the following chart (Figure 11.46). The curves have no quantitative significance and merely represent in a diagrammatic way the histochemical descriptions of "increases" or "decreases" of enzyme activities during the cycle.

Biochemical quantitations of these enzymes in endometrial homogenates yield data that may vary from those depicted in Figure 11.46. The reason for this is that homogenates include stroma, blood vessels, and glands. Enzyme concentrations in blood vessel endothelium parallels the concentration of enzymes in epithelium for DPNH. Alkaline phosphatase concentration in endothelium remains high throughout the secretory cycle, in contrast to its activity in glandular epithelium. Isocitric, succinic, and malic dehydrogenase are not present in significant amounts in the endothelium. The stroma contains low levels of lactic dehydrogenase and β-glucuronidase throughout the cycle and minimal DPNH, alkaline phosphatase, acid phosphatase, and succinic dehydrogenase. Lipids are seen in the postovulatory period. Nonspecific esterase is contained in stromal macrophages throughout the cycle.

In the proliferative part of the cycle (Figure 11.46) during estrogenic stimulation, the most active enzymes in glandular epithelium are alkaline phosphatase, β-glucuronidase, and glucose-6-phosphatase. These are accompanied by elevations of NADPH (TPNH) and RNA.

Although the true significance of these elevations in terms of cell physiology cannot be easily determined, some limited interpretations can be made. Stuermer and Stein[17] and McKay[9] have pointed out that the rapid growth rate of glandular epithelium and stromal cells during the proliferative phase proceeds at a time when the vasculature is poorly developed. Therefore, the proliferating tissues are relatively hypoxic and consequently anaerobic glycolytic pathways are utilized.

An essential feature of glycolysis is the initial phosphorylation of glucose by hexokinases. These are widely distributed and used by most cells for this purpose. This enzyme activity is rapidly inhibited by its own product, glucose 6-phosphate. The presence of high levels of glucose-6-phosphatase in the proliferative cycle may serve as a modulating mechanism. It may stand by, ready to dephosphorylate excessive amounts of glucose 6-phosphate, and thus allow steady rather than intermittent, hexokinase activity. The overall glycolytic pathway would then have an even input of phosphorylated glucose, the production of which would be a key regulatory step in glycolysis.

The elevated levels of TPNH (NADPH, nicotinamide adenine dinucleotide phosphate) in its reduced form are significant and suggest the presence of an active hexose monophosphate shunt (phosphogluconate pathway or pentose phosphate pathway). In this multistep pathway glucose 6-phosphate is dehydrogenated and eventually converted to D-ribose 5-phosphate. TPNH (NADPH) is a product of the dehydrogenation. The ribose 5-phosphate is essential for the synthesis of RNA, which is active in the proliferative phase.

In the postovulatory phase, there are elevations in the activities of the following enzymes: acid phosphatase, glucose 6-phosphate dehydrogenase, lactic acid dehydrogenase, succinic acid dehydrogenase, cytochrome oxidase, malic acid dehydrogenase, isocitric acid dehydrogenase, and others. In addition, the content of DPNH (NADH), mucin (glycoproteins), glycogen, and lipids is increased.

The combined effects of estrogen plus progesterone in this phase result in a cessation of cell proliferation and a stimulation of differentiation. This generally is accompanied by greater oxidative metabolism, facilitated by the better vascular supply of the endometrium in this part of the cycle, and is manifested by elevations of enzymes in the tricarboxylic acid (Krebs citric acid) cycle and in electron transport.

A shift to greater oxidative respiration (Krebs citric acid cycle and electron transport) as a function of differentiation is observed in other types of tissues and is an expected correlation. In addition, the increased content of glycoproteins, glycogen, and lipids is a further indication that the ATP produced by the nonproliferating epithelial cells is now being used for the synthesis of differentiated cellular product, instead of for replication, as was the case in the proliferative stage.

The increased content of NADH (DPNH) is related to the enhanced activity of lactic acid dehydrogenase (LDH). NADH is requisite for converting pyruvic acid to lactic acid. Increased LDH is usually associated with tissues that are proliferating and glycolyzing and, therefore, may not be expected in differentiated states. However, in differentiated tissues such as secretory endometrium, LDH serves a vital role in consuming NADH (DPNH) and converting it to NAD. The striking increases in the various dehydrogenases requires molecules that can receive hydrogen removed from malic and isocitric acids. NAD picks up the hydrogen and is reduced to NADH; eventually the "excess" hydrogen is transferred to pyruvic acid, converting it to lactic acid.

The changes in enzyme activities and content of various substances are the result of the influence of estrogens, progesterone, and possibly other factors as well.

## Mechanism of Action of Steroid Hormones

All of the target cells of the steroidal hormones respond in similar ways. Steroids, because of their hydrophobic or amphipathic nature, can readily cross the lipoidal plasma membrane of any cell and enter the cytosol (cytoplasm). In the specific target cell, however, there are proteins that can bind with the hormone. These cytosol receptors are present only in target cells. The subsequent fate of the bound hormone includes transport to the nucleus and then binding to the chromatin. Presumably the latter binding results in the production of messenger RNAs to direct the syntheses of the many proteins that characterize the target cell's response to a particular steroid hormone. Cells that do not normally respond to specific steroid hormones lack the particular cytosol receptor and, therefore, are not affected.

From the point of view of pathologic and physiopathologic conditions that involve a lack of response by a target cell to a specific hormone, the molecular pathologic "lesion" may be the loss of the particular cytosol receptor, or a lack of stability of the hormone–receptor complex; e.g., a change in pH is known to influence the stability of the estradiol–receptor complex. If stability is lost, then transport to the nucleus and chromatin binding may be compromised, resulting in an altered, or no response. Intracellular pH fluctuations can be brought about by changes in the activities of certain enzymes and metabolic pathways, such as increased activity of LDH, resulting in greater production of lactic acid. In the secretory phase of the cycle, estrogen levels are high but no proliferation takes place. Clearly, the glandular and stromal cells have had their DNA sites for proliferation silenced. Although highly speculative, the following explanation serves as an example of the possible complex interrelationships. The arrival of progesterone in the endometrial cells may result in increasing the activity of LDH and yield more lactic acid. If the pH drops, then the estrogen–receptor complexes may destabilize (progesterone–receptor complex may not destabilize or may be more stable at lower pH) and not bind to chromatin. Therefore, some or all of the DNA sequences that have been activated by estrogens are silenced, particularly those concerned with replication.

The dysfunction or absence of these specific cytosol receptors may play a role in the observed overall clinical response of a target tissue to hormones. In some malignant tumors these cytosol receptors may be absent. In some endometrial cancers, progesterone-binding proteins have been shown to be lacking, and such cells as this are therefore exposed to virtually unbroken stimulation by estrogens; theoretically, because progesterone cannot bind, LDH does not increase and the pH does not drop to destabilize the estrogen–receptor complex.

The opportunity for more involved interactions rises considerably when the cyclic nucleotides, cAMP and cGMP, are introjected together with the prostaglandins. Many humoral agents, e.g., pituitary hormones, epinephrine, and so forth, have been shown to act on their target cells by a series of "second messengers." The target cell has a receptor site on the surface of its membrane and can bind the specific humoral agent. The hormone does not enter the cell but instead a chain of events is started. Within the plasma membrane, specific prostaglandins (PG) will respond to the perturbation induced by the surface receptor,

which has bound a nonsteroidal hormone. The PG then, in turn, activates adenyl cyclase or guanosyl cyclase, resulting in cAMP or cGMP production. In general, the E class of PGs activates adenyl cyclase, whereas the F class stimulates guanosyl cyclase. The cAMP and cGMP are produced from ATP, by their respective enzymes located on the inner side of the plasma membrane. The ratio of cAMP/cGMP influences cell division. Alteration of the latter ratio is possible by agents that affect the enzymes that form cAMP and cGMP, as well as by drugs that affect phosphodiesterases, which specifically inactivate the cyclic nucleotides. The cAMP or cGMP acts on a cell by activating a broad range of kinases. These are enzymes that become phosphorylated and, when thus activated, specifically stimulate the synthesis of RNA, DNA, proteins, lipids, carbohydrates, and so forth. In this way, the cyclic nucleotides can have very broad cellular effects, including an influence on replication. High levels of cGMP and/or low cAMP are generally associated with rapid replicative rates in most normal tissues and in some malignant neoplasms.

Specificity of action by a humoral agent on a target cell is therefore brought about by the presence or absence of *surface receptors,* in the case of those mediated by the PG–cyclic nucleotide–kinase axis, or by *cytosol receptors,* in the case of the steroids.

In human endometrium $PGE_2$ and $PGF_2$ have been studied and correlated with the menstrual cycle. In normal endometrium, $PGE_2$ in the early proliferative phase is 110 ng per 1 gm wet weight; in late proliferative, 150; in early secretory, 125; in late secretory, 185; and during menstruation, 345; the corresponding levels of $PGF_2$ are 125, 165, 210, 400, and 545.[15] The relative increase in $PGF_2$ is much greater and in the secretory phase the PGF : PGE ratio is high.

In rat endometrium, estradiol stimulates the appearance of adenyl cyclase activity on the plasma membrane of the epithelial cells, at their free apical surface. This was demonstrated in ovariectomized rats. The capillary endothelial cells demonstrate a baseline level of adenyl cyclase activity, which is not cycle dependent. The administration of progesterone to ovariectomized rats blunts the estradiol-induced increase of adenyl cyclase activity, apparently by affecting the estrogen-binding receptors. Whether the steroid hormones exert any of their effects through prostaglandins is not known. The rise in adenyl cyclase following estradiol administration may be similar to the elevations in other enzyme activities with estrogens and simply represent newly synthesized enzyme molecules following the estrogen binding to DNA. It is important to distinguish between the *activation* of preexisting molecules of enzymes, as in the case of PGE activation of adenyl cyclase, and the synthesis of new enzyme molecules, as in the case of steroid hormones.

At present, most of the interest in the PG–cyclic nucleotide–kinase axis lies in the physiology and pathophysiology of the uterine smooth muscle; however, there appears to be a growing body of literature with respect to endometrium, with attempts to relate this axis to the steroid hormones.

# REFERENCES

1. Armstrong, E. M., Moore, I. A. R., McSeveney, D., and Carty, M. The giant mitochondrion–endoplasmic reticulum unit of the human endometrial glandular cell. *J. Anat.* 116:375, 1973.

2. Beller, F. Personal communication, 1970.

3. Boutselis, J. G., DeNeef, J. C., Ullery, J. C., and George, O. T. Histochemical and cytologic observations in the normal human endometrium. *Obstet. Gynecol.* 21:423, 1963.

4. Dallenbach-Hellweg, G. *Histopathology of the Endometrium.* New York, Springer-Verlag, 1971, p. 24.

5. Fanger, H., and Barker, B. E. Capillaries and arterioles in normal endometrium. *Am. J. Obstet. Gynecol.* 17:543, 1961.

6. Farrer-Brown, G. G., Beilby, J. O. W., and Tarbit, M. H. The blood supply of the uterus, venous pattern. *J. Obstet. Gynaecol. Br. Commun.* 77:682, 1970.

7. Ferenczy, A., and Richart, R. M. *Female Reproductive System: Dynamics of Scan and Transmission Electron Microscopy.* New York, John Wiley & Sons, 1974.

8. Markee, J. E. Menstruation in intraoccular endometrial transplant in the rhesus monkey. Carnegie Inst. Wash. Publ. 518, *Contrib. Embryol.* 28:219, 1940.

9. McKay, D. G., Hertig, A. T., Bardawil, W. A., and Velardo, J. T. Histochemical observations in the endometrium. *Obstet. Gynecol.* 8:22, 1956.

10. More, I. A. R., Armstrong, E. M., Carty, M., and McSeveney, D. Cyclical changes in the ultrastructure of the normal human endometrial stromal cell. *J. Obstet. Gynaecol. Br. Commun.* 81:337, 1974.

11. Nilssen, O., Kottmeier, H. L., and Tillenger, K. G. Some differences in the ultrastructure of normal and cancerous human uterine epithelium. *Acta Obstet. Gynecol. Scand.* 42:73, 1963.

12. Noyes, R. W., Hertig, A. T., and Rock, J. Dating the endometrial biopsy. *Fertil. Steril.* 1:3, 1950.

13. Ober, W. B., and Bernstein, J. Observations on the endometrium and ovary in the new born. *Pediatrics* 16:445, 1955.

14. Shenker, L. Booth Memorial Medical Center. Unpublished data, 1976.

15. Singh, E. J., Baccarini, I. M., and Zuspan, F. P. Levels of prostaglandins $F_2\alpha$ and $E_2$ in human endometrium during the menstrual cycle. *Am. J. Obstet. Gynecol.* 121:1003, 1975.

16. Spellman, C. M., Fottrell, P. F., Baynes, S., O'Dwyer, E. M., and Clinch, J. D. A study of some enzymes and isoenzymes of carbohydrate metabolism in human endometrium during the menstrual cycle. *Clin. Chim. Acta* 48:259, 1973.

17. Stuermer, V. M., and Stein, R. J. Cytodynamic properties of the human endometrium. V. Metabolism and enzymatic activity in the human endometrium during the menstrual cycle. *Am. J. Obstet. Gynecol.* 63:359, 1952.

18. Takeguchi, H., Tanaka, M., and Sawaragi, I. A scanning electron microscopic study on the ultrastructure of the surface of the human endometrium and endocervix. *J. Clin. Electr. Microsc.* 7:3, 1974.

19. White, A. J., and Buchsbaum, H. J. Scanning electron microscopy of the human endometrium. I. Normal. *Gynecol. Oncol.* 1:330, 1973.

20. White, A. J., and Buchsbaum, H. J. Scanning electron microscopy of the human endometrium. II. Hyperplasia and adenocarcinoma. *Gynecol. Oncol.* 2:1, 1974.

21. Wienke, E. C., Cavazos, F., Hall, D. G., and Lucas, F. V. Ultrastructural effects of norethynodrel and mestranol on human endometrial stromal cell. *Am. J. Obstet. Gynecol.* 102:111, 1969.

L. Shenker, M.D., F.A.C.O.G.

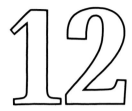

# Clinical Considerations of Gynecologic Pathology

## Suggestions for Fruitful Cooperation

The level of gynecologic care can directly be related to the degree of cooperation between the clinician and the pathologist. Inadequate communication or understanding of details on the part of either physician will seriously mar any cooperative effort. For communication to be realistic the practicing gynecologist must have a working understanding of gynecologic pathology and the pathologist must learn of the specific clinical problems facing the gynecologist if he or she is to be ideally helpful.

Training in pathology for the gynecologist usually begins in medical school, where most clerkships in obstetrics and gynecology devote time to specific areas of gynecologic pathology. The most important phase of the training of the gynecologist in pathology takes place during the residency program. A block of time should be set aside during residency for an intensive experience under the supervision of a pathologist. This time should allow the resident to study and describe gross surgical specimens and to be responsible for their microscopic diagnosis. He or she should have training in cytology with an opportunity to review pertinent biopsy specimens from outpatient services. A 3- or 4-month assignment to GYN pathology on an active service should serve as a reasonable orientation to the subject. Most important is the subsequent opportunity for training during the residency and especially in practice. The usual mechanism for this type of training is a weekly gynecologic pathology conference. All cases from the preceding week are reviewed, with detailed presentation of clinical data and active participation of residents in both specialties. At regular staff conferences, the gynecologic pathologist should be present for discussion of relevant material.

Whatever skills obtained as a result of a program described above, even if supplemented with formal postgraduate courses, require that a clinician review with the pathologist all slides on his or her own patients for the rest of the clinician's professional life if he or she is to remain proficient in pathology.

Unless such review of his or her own clinical material occurs, communication between clinician and pathologist becomes faulty. It is not in the patient's best interest for a gynecologist to plan therapy based on biopsy material reported formally but not studied independently by the doctor responsible for the patient's care.

There are many areas of diagnosis in which proper communication between surgeon and pathologist is important. One constant source of inaccuracies is the failure of the gynecologist to provide the laboratory with a concise clinical history of the patient and an indication of what pathologic information would be helpful. Unless the date of the patient's last menstrual period is known to the pathologist, his or her interpretation of the endometrial biopsy or curettage specimen loses its significance. This is especially true when the patient's problem is infertility. Many subtleties in endometrial morphology take on added significance if the pathologist is aware of when in the cycle the endometrium is biopsied. The diagnosis of luteal phase deficiency, for example, can be rulled in or out more accurately when all the clinical data are available to the pathologist. The same statement is true for irregular shedding of the endometrium. Accurate dating of the endometrium and, of equal importance, the clinician's knowledge of the limitations of accuracy of dating, become meaningful only when both clinician and pathologist know the patient's menstrual history.

If the pathologist is to provide accurate diagnosis in malignant tumors of the uterus, his or her communication with the gynecologist must be intimate. The clinician has the responsibility of providing a detailed history, performing a meticulous fractional curettage of the uterus with special attention to the separate preservation of the tissues removed, with their accurate labeling as to the part of the uterus from which they originated. Only under these conditions can the pathologist provide a diagnosis which may be the most important part, in determining the type and extent of therapy. The pathologist must share with the clinician the staging of all endometrial carcinomas and, because therapy is very often dictated by stage of disease, cooperation here is essential.

Another area where the team concept is much more than a cliche is in the diagnosis of early cervical neoplasia. Cytologic reporting among pathologists has been very variable and each gynecologist must know exactly what the laboratory report specifies. Moreover, the gynecologist must know his or her laboratory's limitations. Does the cytology lab diagnose definitively "invasive cervical carcinoma" as well as "positive for noninvasive cervical carcinoma"? More important, is the laboratory accurate in its diagnosis? Although cytology may never be, and should not be, accepted as definitive diagnosis, the more accurate the cytologic detection, the easier becomes the subsequent workup. Colposcopy with directed biopsy has become an integral second step in patients with abnormal cytology. The pathologist should be aware of whether biopsies are directed or random. Directed biopsies theoretically should be from the most advanced change in the cervix and this knowledge aids the pathologist in making a diagnosis. The need for fewer cervical conizations as a result of expert colposcopy will put even more responsibility for accurate diagnosis on the pathologist. He or she will probably require more sections of the biopsy specimen, more time for deliberation and study of multiple sections, and more understanding of the clinical problem facing the colposcopist.

The recognition of gross pathology in the operating room is so fundamentally a major responsibility of the operating gynecologist that he or she is likely to frequently call the pathologist to consult in the decision making process. The surgeon must be able to recognize and distinguish between the commonly occuring ovarian tumors. Unless he or she has this capability, therapy will all too often be inadequate or, perhaps worse, too radical. The use of frozen section to confirm the presence of ovarian carcinoma will permit better planning of therapy at the time of laparotomy. Well-understood dialogue between gynecologist and pathologist should make for optimal therapy in such clinical situations.

In summary, the excellence of gynecologic care is heavily dependent on an intelligent working relationship between clinician and pathologist. This relationship, in turn, depends on mutual comprehension of each specialty's problems and attention to details clearly communicated between responsible physicians. Some examples of the importance of this relationship have been presented and explored in detail. Many more examples can have been cited but the details can be mastered if the relationship between specialists is ideal.

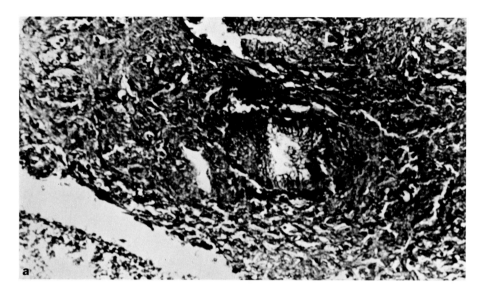

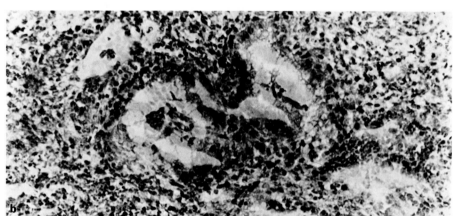

**12.1 a.** Irregular shedding. Exhausted secretory gland surrounded by dense compact stroma. **b.** Irregular shedding; a high-power view of Figure 12.1a. Glands are exhausted; the stroma shows no evidence of pseudodecidual change.

# Dysfunctional Uterine Bleeding

The most common indication for dilatation and curettage of the uterus is dysfunctional (functional) uterine bleeding. It may be defined as an abnormal bleeding pattern occurring in the absence of organic disease of the uterus and its endometrium. It is almost always related to anovulation and the resultant unopposed estrogen effect on the endometrium. Dysfunctional uterine bleeding often is a diagnosis made by exclusion of organic causes for abnormal bleeding and therefore requires diagnostic dilatation and curettage.

In patients with dysfunctional uterine bleeding, the most common histologic finding is proliferative endometrium. If the exposure to unopposed estrogens is prolonged, endometrial hyperplasia is found. Mixtures of proliferative endometrium with focal areas of hyperplasia may be present.

Although most patients with dysfunctional uterine bleeding have not ovulated, there is a very small group in which the endometrium shows some evidence of progestational activity (however, not normal secretory endometrium).

# Irregular Shedding of the Endometrium

A rare condition, usually manifested by prolonged menstruation, is irregular shedding of the endometrium. It results from persistence of corpus luteum function beyond 14 days after ovulation in the absence of pregnancy. The endometrium obtained at curettage performed by design after the seventh day of bleeding will show characteristic dense, dehydrated stroma surrounding collapsed star-shaped endometrial glands retaining evidence of hypersecretion (Figures 12.1a and 12.1b). Confirmatory elevated

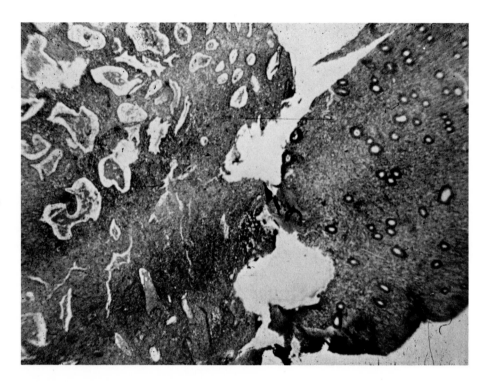

**12.2** Mixed endometrium. Proliferative endometrium on the left and secretory endometrium on the right.

levels of plasma progesterone or urinary pregnanediol measured at the time of diagnostic curettage will confirm the persistent corpus luteum activity.

## Short Luteal Phase

Inadequate corpus luteum function (short luteal phase) may manifest itself by abnormal bleeding, usually metrorrhagia, but more frequently results only in infertility. The endometrium obtained at the time of bleeding or as a part of infertility workup will show stromal glandular asynchrony or a mixed endometrium. The term stromal glandular asynchrony is used to describe an endometrium in which glands and stroma are out of phase with one another by more than a week. The term "mixed endometrium" refers to the occurrence of glands and stroma that are consistent in appearance with one date; another portion of the curettings contain glands and stroma that suggest greater or lesser degrees of maturation (Figure 12.2).

The anovulatory patient who is bleeding abnormally and has been treated with progestational agents prior to endometrial sampling, or who has spontaneously ovulated and produced her own progesterone after several months of anovulation, has an endometrium that shows a combi-

nation of hyperplastic and secretory changes. This might be referred to as "secretory hyperplasia" (Figure 12.3).

In patients whose symptoms suggest dysfunctional uterine bleeding but in whom endometrial sampling reveals only a normal secretory endometrium, the gynecologist must be aware that he or she is dealing with one of two situations. Either an organic cause for the bleeding exists (e.g., myomata, polyps) or the timing of the endometrial sampling has been inappropriately delayed, allowing for return of normal ovulatory function.

## Indications for Endometrial Biopsy

1. Determination of the etiology of abnormal bleeding
   a. Menorrhagia (hypermenorrhea): abnormally heavy periods or periods lasting more than 7 days
   b. Metrorrhagia (intermenstrual bleeding): bleeding between periods
   c. Polymenorrhea: periods occurring more frequently than every 21 days
   d. Postmenopausal bleeding: bleeding after 1 year of amenorrhea
2. To remove products of conception
   a. After incomplete abortion or missed abortion
   b. Voluntary interruption of pregnancy

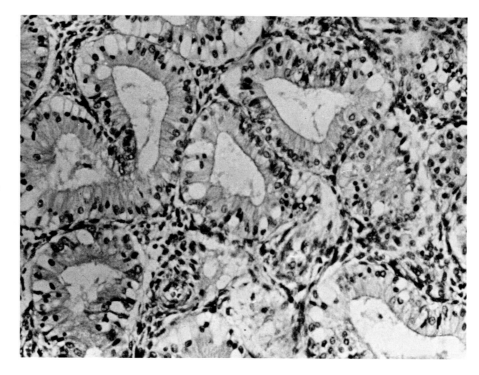

**12.3** Secretory hyperplasia. Closely packed glands show secretory changes.

3. As part of an infertility study (see Chapter 35)
4. As followup for patients who have had atypical adenomatous hyperplasia of the endometrium and are being treated medically
5. Routine procedure in patients at high risk for development of endometrial carcinoma: this should be performed annually

## Techniques for Endometrial Sampling

Endometrium may be obtained for study by several different methods. These are:

1. *Fractional dilatation and curettage of the uterus.* This is a hospital procedure performed in the operating room, most commonly requiring general anesthesia. It is the most thorough diagnostic procedure. Its main advantage is the capability of separately curetting the endocervical canal and endometrial cavity, submitting the specimens individually. This is of critical importance in the diagnosis and staging of endometrial carcinoma. Selection of appropriate therapy is entirely dependent on the accurate interpretation of fractional curettings. A second advantage of dilatation and curettage is the capability of exploring the uterine cavity for polyps with a special polyp forceps. If only a curette is used, polyps may be entirely overlooked. Hospitalization for dilatation and curettage allows the gynecologist the opportunity to perform a pelvic examination under anesthesia, often necessary to delineate and identify pelvic masses and accurately measure their size. The dilatation of the cervix and the patient's freedom from pain permits a much more complete sampling of the endometrium than other methods.

2. *Endometrial biopsy.* This is an office procedure performed either without anesthesia or occasionally with paracervical block. The endometrium is either mechanically removed with a narrow instrument with a collecting basket at its tip (such as a Meig's curette), or by hollow biopsy curettes (Novak or Randall), in which a syringe provides negative pressure to withdraw endometrium removed by scraping with the sharp edge of the instrument. The advantages of this technique are the speed and convenience and the lack of need for hospitalization and anesthesia. The disadvantage is the relatively incomplete sampling of the endometrium and incomplete removal of polyps.

3. *Suction curettage* (Vabra). The newest method for the collection of endometrial tissue for diagnostic purposes uses a very narrow metal cannula attached to a plastic

247

collection chamber containing a filter. This, in turn, is attached to a negative pressure source provided by a vacuum pump. The diameter of the curette is smaller than that of other office biopsy instruments, allowing a more thorough endometrial sampling; however, polyps may be entirely missed. The correlation of diagnoses for tissue removed by office suction curettage and that removed by subsequent dilatation and curettage is excellent.

In patients with postmenopausal bleeding, metrorrhagia, or any abnormal bleeding occuring at any age, if the tissue diagnosis on samples removed by office endometrial biopsy do not explain the abnormal bleeding, hospitalization for a diagnostic dilatation and curettage is mandatory.

# REFERENCES

1. Holmstrom, E. G., and McLennan, C. E. Menorrhagia associated with irregular shedding of the endometrium. A clinical and experimental study. *Am. J. Obstet. Gynecol.,* 53:727, 1947.

2. Jones, G. E. S., and Madrigal-Castro, V. Hormonal findings in association with abnormal corpus luteum function in the human. The luteal phase defect. *Fertil. Steril.* 21:1, 1970.

3. Jones, G. E. S. Luteal phase Insufficiency. *Clin. Obstet. Gynecol.* 16:255, 1973.

4. McKelvey, J. C., and Samuels, L. T. Irregular shedding of the endometrium. *Am. J. Obstet. Gynecol.* 53:627, 1947.

5. McLennan, C. E. Current concepts of prolonged or irregular endometrial shedding. *Am. J. Obstet. Gynecol.* 64:988, 1952.

6. O'Toole, R. V. Education in obstetric-gynecologic pathology. *Clin. Obstet. Gynecol.* 17:121, 1974.

Rita Iovine Demopoulos, M.D.

# 13

# Benign Diseases of the Endometrium

Benign diseases of the endometrium can be subdivided into three general categories: inflammatory, neoplastic, and functional abnormalities that may result in disturbances in the maturation pattern of the endometrium. The commonest symptoms are abnormal uterine bleeding, pelvic discomfort, and at times infertility.

## Inflammatory Endometrial Lesions

Inflammatory lesions of the endometrium are uncommon when compared with the occurrence of other pelvic inflammatory disease such as salpingitis and cervicitis. The reason is twofold. First, the endometrium is positioned so as to drain well by gravity, and second, the periodic shedding is protective against infection to some extent.

### Acute Endometritis

Grossly, an acutely inflamed endometrium appears congested, edematous, and boggy. If severe, a purulent surface exudate may be visible as well as focal ulceration. In very severe cases the infection may spread to the myometrium and parametrium and pelvic thrombophlebitis may ensue. Septic emboli can cause multiple pelvic abscesses, or cul de sac, or subdiaphragmatic abscesses. However, these complications are rare since the advent of antibiotics.

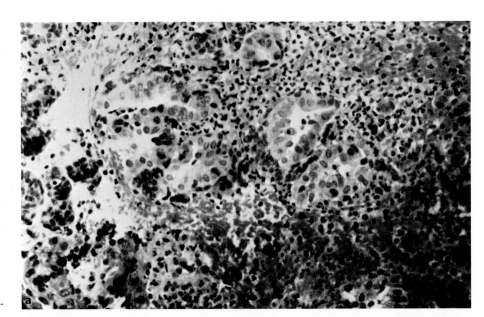

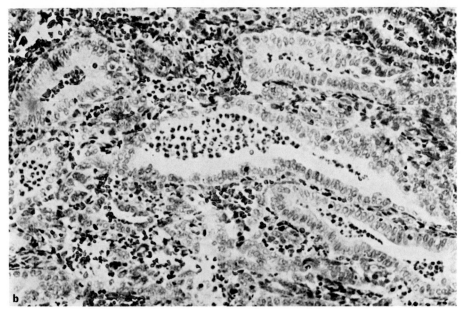

**13.1 a.** Acute endometritis. There is hemorrhage and leukocytic infiltration in the stroma. **b.** Acute endometritis. Polynuclear leukocytes in gland lumina.

Acute endometritis is less prevalent than chronic. It is characterized histologically by multiple foci, or by diffuse infiltration of endometrial stroma by polymorphonuclear leukocytes. Frequently, collections of polymorphonuclear leukocytes fill some of the gland lumina (Figure 13.1a,b). There is associated vascular congestion and varying degrees of stromal edema. The endometrium frequently shows abnormalities in the maturation pattern and may be difficult or impossible to date.

*Etiology*

Acute endometritis is most often seen following abortion or full term delivery, particularly deliveries in which there has been prolonged or difficult labor. The organisms commonly responsible for puerperal endometritis are anaerobic streptococci, *Escherichia coli, Bacteroides, Pseudomonas,* and rarely *Clostridium perfringens.* Before the days of legalized abortion, it was not uncommon for criminally

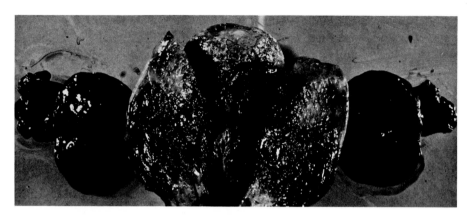

**13.2** Uterus with marked endometritis and myometritis secondary to intrauterine lavage with green soap. The fallopian tubes and ovaries are infarcted.

induced abortion to be followed by severe diffuse endometritis, physically or chemically induced. In some cases, infection spreads to involve myometrium and parametrial tissues. This is illustrated in Figures 13.2 and 13.3 in which there are marked necrotizing vasculitis and myometrial muscle necrosis. This patient used green soap installation into the uterus to induce abortion. A transient acute endometritis almost invariably succeeds insertion of intrauterine contraceptive devices. After about 72 hr the acute inflammatory cells tend to diminish in number as lymphocytes and plasma cells increase. The presence of devitalized tissue in the endometrial cavity predisposes to the development of infection. Occasionally, twisted endometrial polyps, pedunculated ischemic submucosal leiomyomata, uterine malignancies, or surgical wounds may serve as a nidus for infection. Following an abortion or delivery, fragments of retained decidua or placental tissue undergoing degeneration may become infected. Gonorrheal endometritis is rarely a clinical problem. *Neisseria gonorrhea,* a gram-negative diplococcus, causes an ascending infection; the vaginitis, cervicitis, and urethritis, as well as salpingitis, are most often symptomatic. The endometritis is transient and usually asymptomatic. Thayer-Martin cultures can be used to detect gonorrheal endometritis, and positive cultures have been reported in asymptomatic patients.

Since granulocytes are present normally at the end of the secretory phase of the menstrual cycle, their presence at this time is not indicative of infection. However, these granulocytes are present only in the stroma, whereas in true inflammatory states they are most prominently seen in gland lumina. Granulocytes physiologically present are not related to foci of stromal dissolution. In inflammatory states, polymorphonuclear leukocytes are often surrounded by areas of stromal edema, vascular congestion, and tissue necrosis. This may produce dissolution of stromal reticu-

lum, and destruction of glandular epithelium with focal abscess formation. Microabscesses may become confluent causing grossly visible ulcers. When extension into myometrium occurs, this usually begins as a perivascular cuffing by polymorphonuclear leukocytes. Vasculitis and thrombosis may lead to myometrial necrosis.

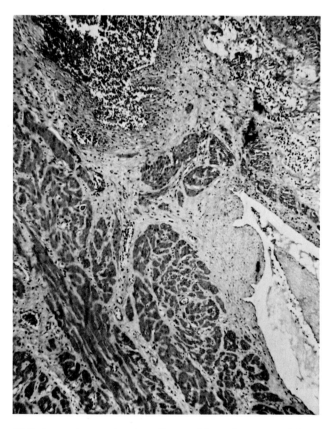

**13.3** Acute hemorrhagic endometritis and myometritis. Same case as Figure 13.2.

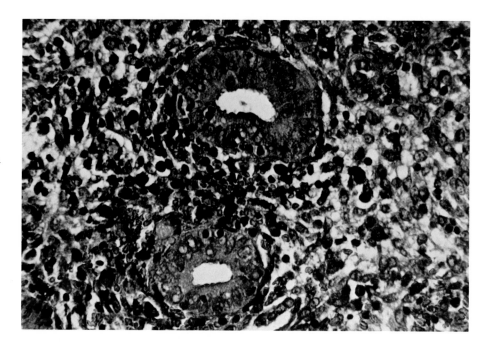

**13.4** Chronic endometritis with foci of plasma cells and lymphocytes in the stroma.

## Chronic Endometritis

### Nonspecific chronic endometritis

Chronic endometritis is diagnosed far more commonly than acute endometritis, probably because acute endometritis can rapidly progress to a chronic state if inadequately treated or not responsive to therapy. Grossly the endometrium is pale and swollen. Since scattered lymphocytes and lymphoid follicles may normally be present in endometrium, the diagnosis of chronic inflammation requires the presence of plasma cells as well as lymphocytes (Figure 13.4). Histiocytes may also be present and the inflammatory infiltrate may be diffuse or multifocal, but is often limited to the interstitial tissues. Varying degrees of stromal edema and vascular congestion are concomitant. There may be vascular and fibroblastic proliferation, causing the stroma to be converted into granulation tissue. At times the fibrous proliferation is so striking as to form large confluent areas of stromal fibrosis. If infection is severe, there are associated disturbances in the maturation pattern. In mild infections the glands are uninvolved. In a study of chronic nonspecific endometritis, Vasudeva et al.[15] found a plasma cell infiltration to be present in 2.8% of endometrial specimens including curettings, biopsies, and hysterectomy specimens. In other studies[5] the incidence is as high as 19.2%. Eighty-three percent of the patients in the former study presented with irregular vaginal bleeding; two-thirds were between the ages of 20 and 40 years. At the end of 1 year 89% were asymptomatic. The authors therefore concluded that the disease is self-limiting and therapy should be individualized according to the patients' symptoms. In a review by Cadena et al.[3] of 152 patients with chronic endometritis, they found a specific etiologic factor in 84% (pelvic inflammatory disease in 25%, intrauterine contraceptive device in 14%, postpartum factors in 12%, and postabortal factors in 41%—some individuals had more than one condition).

ETIOLOGY. Chronic endometritis is generally present to some extent in patients with an intrauterine contraceptive device.[11,12] The endometrium occasionally grows over the device. The inflammation is usually limited to the endometrium present in the region of the foreign body. There may be focal squamous metaplasia of surface epithelium (Figure 13.5). It is postulated that the endometritis may be a necessary requisite for the contraceptive effect. Occasionally, an intrauterine device may penetrate into or through the myometrium to the peritoneal cavity.

### Puerperal endometritis

Endometritis following spontaneous or induced abortion or spontaneous delivery, usually begins with acute inflammation and may become chronic. This is particularly true if fragments of decidua are retained or if segments of placenta are adherent. Such foci of retained secundines may

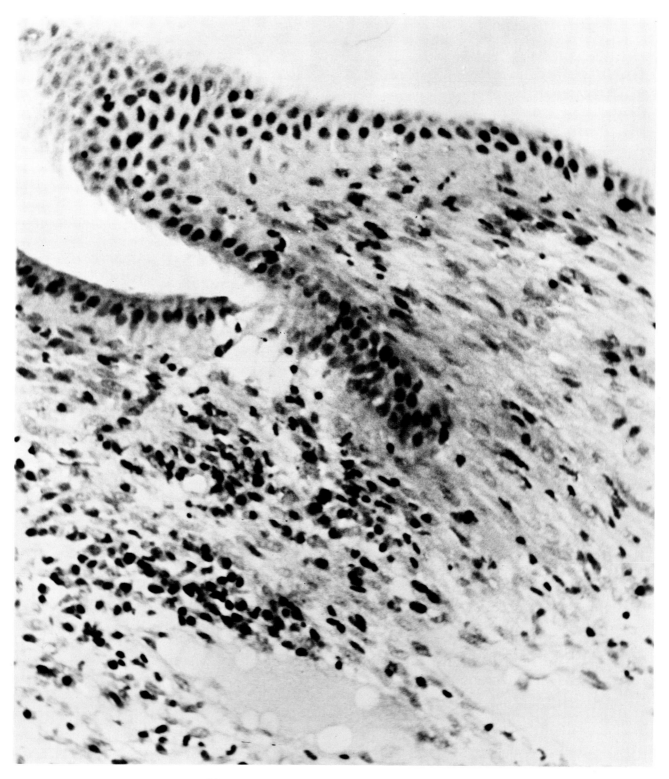

**13.5** Endometrium with chronic inflammation and squamous metaplasia, due to an intrauterine device.

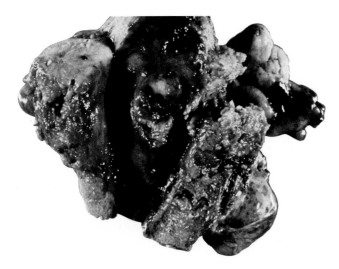

**13.6** Uterus containing placental polyp. It is an adherent, hemorrhagic polypoid mass showing degenerative changes.

appear as polypoid hemorrhagic masses which undergo degenerative changes (Figure 13.6). Histologically, the decidua becomes hyalinized, the plasma membrane disappears, the nuclei are pale or undergo dissolution, and the amorphous hyaline mass may be difficult to recognize as decidua (Figure 13.7). If the retained secundines contain chorionic villi as well as degenerating decidua, this is known as a placental polyp. The chorionic villi frequently lose their peripheral trophoblastic cells, the mesenchyme becomes fibrotic and ultimately shadowy "ghost" villi

remain (Figure 13.8). Patients with retained degenerating decidua or with a placental polyp, usually present with bleeding. The treatment is dilatation and curettage (D and C).

### Senile endometritis

Postmenopausal women develop a thin inactive endometrium. The blood vessels are frequently thick-walled, sclerotic, and calcified. There is occasionally stromal infiltration by lymphocytes and plasma cells, and focal squamous metaplasia of surface epithelium may also be present (Figure 13.9). If the squamous metaplasia is extensive, this condition is known as icthyosis. Patients with senile endometritis are subject to uterine bleeding. This may be related to the inflammation which may lead to focal congestion or ulceration. However, the causes of bleeding from senile endometritis are not wholly understood. If cervical stenosis is also present, this may result in pyometra. In 49% of patients with atrophic endometrium studied by Meyer,[10] no organic causes were found to explain bleeding. He found three factors to be of some significance in explaining the bleeding, namely, myometrial arteriosclerosis, uterine prolapse, and endometrial glandular cyst rupture.

### Asherman's syndrome

Following menstruation the mucosa regenerates from the basal glands. No fibrosis or adhesions normally occur.

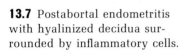

**13.7** Postabortal endometritis with hyalinized decidua surrounded by inflammatory cells.

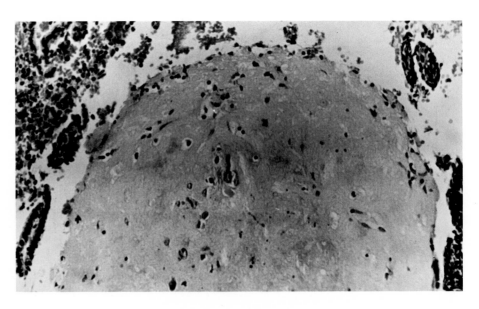

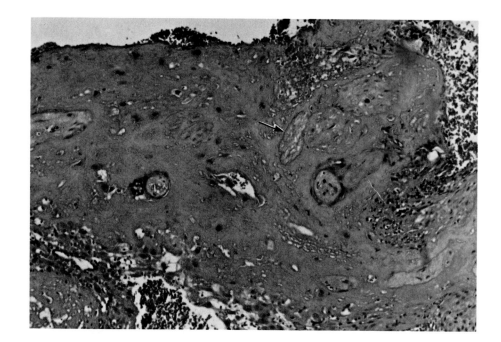

**13.8** Placental polyp showing ghost villi amidst hyalinized decidua (arrow).

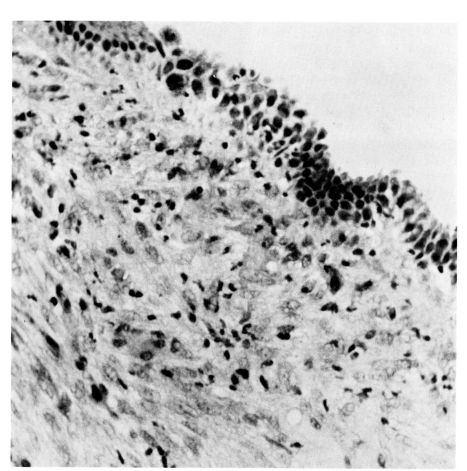

**13.9** Senile endometrium showing inflammation and squamous metaplasia.

If however, during a D and C, curettage is too vigorous, and significant basal endometrium is removed, reconstitution of surface epithelium may be difficult. If in addition, chronic inflammation follows, the glandular epithelium may not regenerate properly and stromal fibrosis may occur with the development of uterine synecchiae.[8] These patients usually develop amenorrhea. This entity is known as Asherman's syndrome. Treatment consists of surgical lysis of the uterine adhesions and the insertion of an intrauterine device to inhibit their return.

### Specific endometritis (chronic)

TUBERCULOUS ENDOMETRITIS. Tuberculous endometritis is uncommon in the United States. In 1963 Israel *et al.*[7] reported an incidence of 0.28% of unsuspected endometrial tuberculosis found on curettage, or biopsy. In a review of 132 patients with pelvic tuberculosis Henderson and co-workers[6] found that the diagnosis was made at laporatomy in 80, by curettage in 49, and in only 3 cases clinically. Pelvic tuberculosis should be suspected in any patient having pulmonary tuberculosis, particularly if amenorrhea or infertility is associated. Pelvic tuberculosis develops in about 5% of patients with pulmonary tuberculosis and usually occurs during the childbearing years. The finding of tuberculous endometritis is presumptive evidence for the presence of tuberculous salpingitis. The commonest form of menstrual disturbance found in these women is hypomenorrhea or amenorrhea. They also frequently have a history of sterility owing to the concomitant tubal disease. Of course, it should be kept in mind that amenorrhea and infertility are common complications of pulmonary tuberculosis, even in the absence of pelvic tuberculosis. The endometrial involvement is usually not extensive and very often the diagnosis is made on finding only one or two granulomata. The lesions resemble typical tuberculous granulomata of the lung except that they show little or no central caseation. Periodic sloughing of the granulomata during the menstrual cycle probably accounts for the lesions being small and young, and showing little or no caseation. The best time to do a curettage if pelvic tuberculosis is suspected is premenstrually (Figure 13.10a). Several histiocytes and giant cells often of the Langhan's type are surrounded by lymphocytes and plasma cells (Figure 13.10b). Needless to say, acid-fast stains often fail to reveal acid-fast bacilli, and the diagnosis of "granulomatous endometritis consistent with tuberculous endometritis" is made based upon the histologic pattern of the granulomatous lesion. The diagnosis must be confirmed by culture of endometrial curettings or menstrual blood. In

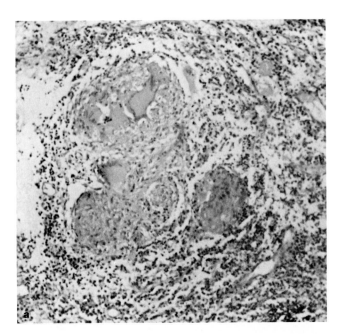

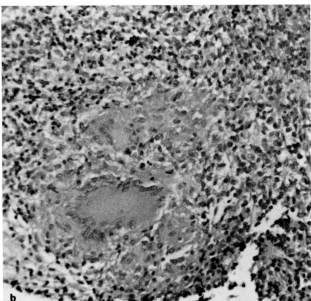

**13.10 a.** Tuberculous endometritis. Note small confluent granulomata. **b.** Tuberculous endometritis. High-power view of tubercle.

more severe infections, the granulomata are numerous and even confluent. They may involve gland epithelium and ulcerate into the lumena. Rarely, large confluent areas of caseation necrosis are present. Pelvic tuberculosis is usually treated surgically after preoperative antituberculous drugs are used, and then the therapy is continued postoperatively for a period of 2 years.

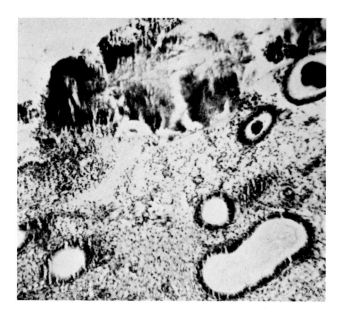

**13.11** Actinomycosis of the endometrium.

ACTINOMYCOSIS. Actinomycosis of the endometrium can occur by hematogenous dissemination from another focus or by ascending infection from the vagina. The "sulfur-granules" are found in a pool of pus surrounded by chronic inflammatory cells. On occasion these granules have been found incidently in the endometria of women having intrauterine devices removed. The "sulfur granules" show little or no surrounding inflammation (Figure 13.11). These patients are generally asymptomatic. Rarely other fungi, namely, *Blastomyces, Cryptococcus,* and *Aspergillus,* may cause infection in the endometrium. Fungal stains such as Gridley, Grocott, and periodic-acid Schiff are helpful in making the diagnosis.

SCHISTOSOMIASIS. Schistosomiasis is endemic in Africa, the Far East, and Central America. Rarely, residents of the United States who have lived in any of these areas are found to have *Schistosoma* eggs on a pap smear or on endometrial curettings. The ova elicit a granulomatous reaction and may cause uterine bleeding and fertility problems.

# Endometrial Polyps

Endometrial polyps consist of projections of endometrial glands and stroma into the uterine cavity. They are quite commonly found incidentally in uteri removed for

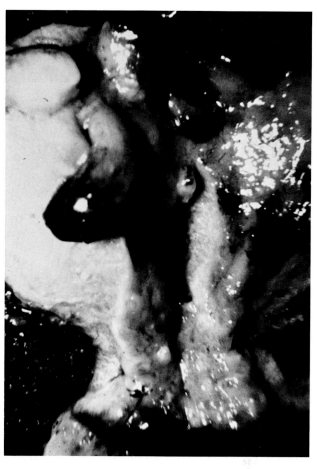

**13.12** Uterus showing multiple endometrial polyps; the largest is fingerlike and partly hemorrhagic.

fibroids or other causes. They can occur at any age but are most common between the ages of 30 and 60 years. They are also often symptomatic and may cause metrorrhagia, or menorrhagia, or both. In postmenopausal women they may similarly be asymptomatic, or be responsible for irregular spotting in which the discharge may be brown or mucoid. Grossly, polyps appear singly or in multiples and in an infinite variety of shapes and sizes. They can consist of tiny protruberances 1 to 2 mm in diameter, or fill the endometrial cavity and, at times, protrude through a dilated cervix into the vagina. They can be broad based and sessile or long and fingerlike with a narrow pedicle. They may be covered by smooth velvety mucosa, or they may show extensive hemorrhage or necrosis (Figure 13.12). During the process of curettage, the gynecologist may feel the presence of a polyp, remove it at its base, and submit it intact to the pathology laboratory, and the diagnosis of a polyp can then be made on gross examination. More often however, polyps will be curetted piecemeal and submitted

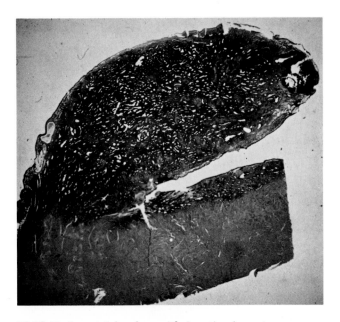

**13.13** Endometrial polyp with inactive immature glands.

admixed with fragments of endometrium. In this case the pathologist cannot rely on the finding of a polypoid structure covered on three sides by surface epithelium, but may have to rely on other criteria such as fibrosis of the stroma and a thick core of blood vessels. Most polyps are nonfunctional or inactive, which means that the glands and stroma within the polyp are not responsive to circulating hormones. Such polyps do not undergo cyclic changes, or slough each month, and therefore, will not resemble the remainder of the endometrium. The glands in such a polyp are askew, rather than being oriented linearly, perpendicular to the surface as are normal glands. They may appear inactive (Figure 13.13) and often are cystically dilated. The lining epithelium is cuboidal or columnar and nonsecretory. Mitoses are lacking or are few in number. The stroma is usually dense and fibrotic, and the blood supply to the polyp is usually via a central core of vessels which run from the base to the tip; these are often thick walled and sclerotic (Figure 13.14a,b). About 20% of endometrial polyps are functional. This means that the glands in the stroma are responsive to circulating hor-

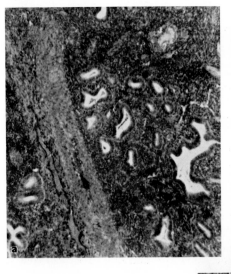

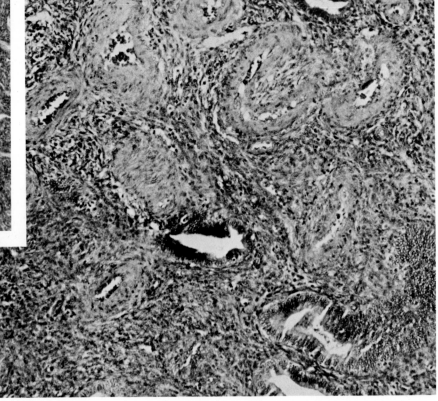

**13.14 a.** Endometrial polyp with a vascular core extending the length of the polyp.
**b.** Endometrial polyp with thick-walled vessels in the base.

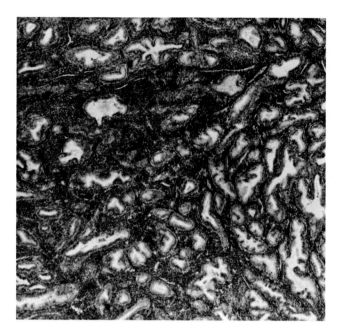

**13.15** Endometrial polyp. The glands are askew and show secretory activity.

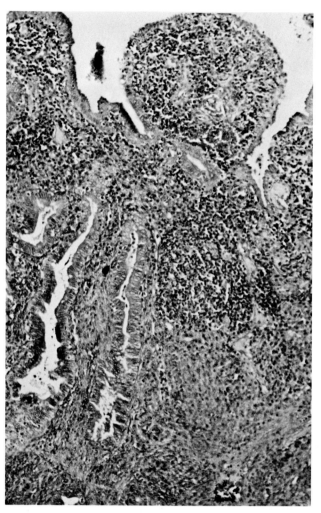

**13.16** Endometrial polyp, microscopic, showing leukocytic infiltration.

mones and they can usually be dated similarly to the remainder of the endometrium (Figure 13.15). However, it is not recommended, of course, that endometrial dating be done from polypoid structures. Functional polyps tend to be smaller than nonfunctional polyps and they probably do slough at each menstrual period. Polyps can undergo a variety of pathologic changes. The surfaces are frequently hemorrhagic, may be ulcerated, or covered by granulation tissue (Figure 13.16). This is probably due to trauma and pressure necrosis. Infection is very commonly seen within polyps, and it may be acute or chronic, or a mixture of both. Pedunculated polyps occasionally undergo torsion at the base, resulting in ischemia or infarction. Although most polyps are benign, they can be the site of glandular, or adenomatous hyperplasia, or carcinoma. A small proportion of polyps show hyperplastic changes.

## Malignancy in Endometrial Polyps

While atypical epithelium may be found in 3 to 5% of polyps, the incidence of carcinoma is lower. Peterson and Novak[14] found malignant change in only 4 of 1,100 endometrial polyps they reviewed. There have been other studies, such as those by Bianchi *et al.*,[1] in which they reported 32 cases of carcinoma within a polyp, out of a total of 1,165 polyps reviewed. The overall incidence of

malignancy (adenocarcinoma arising in a benign endometrial polyp) ranges in different series from 0.45 to 3.7%. The basic prerequisites for the designation of malignancy originating in an antecedant, benign endometrial polyp are[2,16]: (1) a preserved segment of the benign polyp, (2) limitation of malignant disease to the polyp, and (3) exclusion of malignant disease in the adjoining endometrium. In general, if all these requirements are fulfilled, the diagnosis can be made and the prognosis is excellent.

There are, however, exceptions to the rule and this we observed in a female, age 68. She had a vaginal hysterectomy performed for repair of cystocele and rectocele. A small polyp less than 1.5 cm was present in the uterine cavity (Figure 13.17). Microscopic examination showed

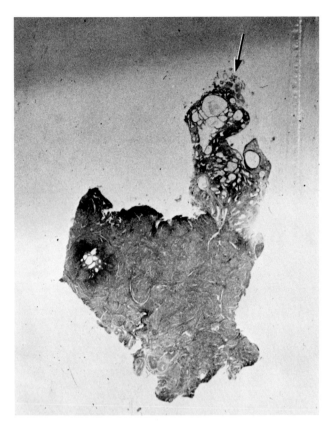

**13.17** Endometrial polyp with malignant change near the tip (arrow).

cystic glands lying in a fibrous stroma but on one surface there was distinct carcinoma (Figure 13.18). The uterus was otherwise free of tumor. Four years later she developed a lesion about the umbilicus, which on microscopic examination was metastatic carcinoma (Figure 13.19) resembling the malignant change seen in the polyp. One year later she died with widespread metastasis involving the lungs (Figure 13.20) and liver (Figure 13.21).

# Abnormal Patterns of Endometrial Maturation

A wide variety of pathophysiologic states can result in abnormal bleeding patterns. Careful documentation of the nature of the abnormal bleeding pattern, including interval between bleeding episodes, duration, and amount of bleeding is of assistance to the gynecologist and to the pathologist in determining the cause. Examination of endometrial biopsy or curettage specimens can often shed some light on the causes of dysfunctional uterine bleeding. If these problems occur in women during the childbearing years, the gynecologist should wait at least 25 days after the last bleeding episode to do a curettage, or even until the onset of the next bleeding episode. This will enable the pathologist to determine whether or not ovulation has occurred. If taken on day 1 of bleeding, it will minimize

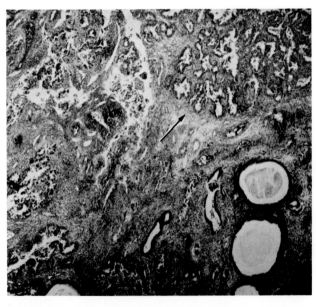

**13.18** High-power view of the focal malignant change (arrow) in polyp in Figure 13.17.

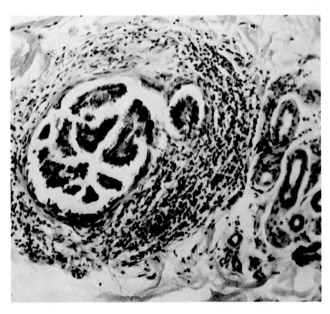

**13.19** Metastases to the umbilical region from the polyp in Figure 13.17.

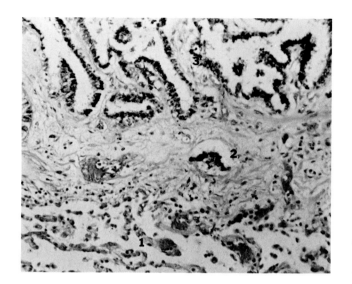

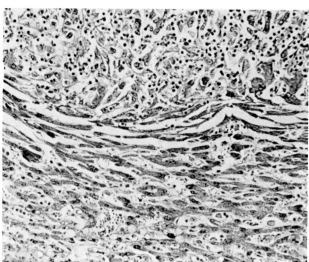

**13.20** Metastases to lung: (1) alveolar tissue, (2) lymph channel with tumor plug, (3) tumor.

**13.21** Metastases to liver.

chances of interfering with an intrauterine gestation, in those cases in which an abnormal bleeding pattern is coupled with problems of infertility, as may often be the case. In postmenopausal females with abnormal bleeding, curettage should be performed promptly. The term, menstrual endometrium, refers to sloughing tissues in which there is evidence that ovulation has occurred and progesta-

tional stimulation has been present. This is opposed to sloughing endometrium in which there are degenerative changes in the absence of progestational stimulation, i.e., in which ovulation has not occurred (Figure 13.22). This is the commonest pathologic picture found in cases of dysfunctional uterine bleeding. When anovulation is persistent for several months, varying degrees of hyperplasia

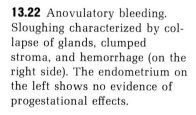

**13.22** Anovulatory bleeding. Sloughing characterized by collapse of glands, clumped stroma, and hemorrhage (on the right side). The endometrium on the left shows no evidence of progestational effects.

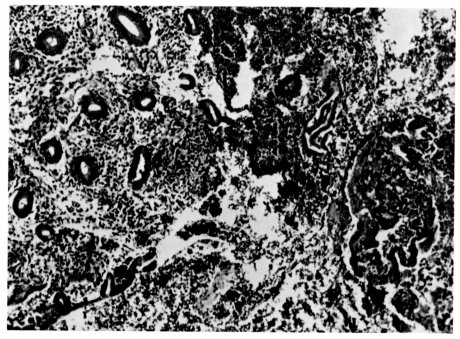

are seen in curettage specimens. The subject of endometrial hyperplasia is discussed in a later chapter.

Less common causes of dysfunctional uterine bleeding, such as persistent corpus luteum cysts and inadequate luteal phase have been previously described. The remainder of this chapter will be devoted to changes produced iatrogenically.

## Iatrogenic Abnormalities in Maturation

### Effects of combined oral contraceptives

In the combined regimen, contraceptive pills containing estrogen and progesterone are taken for 21 consecutive days, beginning on day 5 after the onset of menses. Since progesterone stimulation is begun on day 5, we see secretory changes taking place in glands that have not been fully estrogen primed. Precocious secretion begins on about day 8 and subnuclear vacuoles are seen up to day 12. However, the glands are simple and tubular, rather than elongated and tortuous, as occurs normally (Figure 13.23). The stroma is dense and compact. Secretory activity subsides and later the glands become atrophic and the stroma shows decidual changes. Venules become prominent near the surface endometrium and there is a sparse scattering of lymphocytes and polymorphonuclear leukocytes in the stroma. Bleeding commences about 3 days after cessation of the pill, and is characterized by thrombi in the dis-

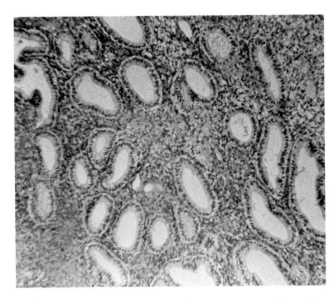

**13.23** Patient on combined oral contraceptives. D & C was performed on day 10. The glands are simple tubular in type, but show secretory changes in the form of subnuclear vacuoles.

tended venules. Stromal necrosis and hemorrhage may be seen. A small percentage of patients on oral contraceptives appear to develop idiosyncratic reactions characterized by increased responsiveness to progesterone (Figure 13.24). They usually do not reestablish their normal menstrual

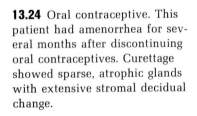

**13.24** Oral contraceptive. This patient had amenorrhea for several months after discontinuing oral contraceptives. Curettage showed sparse, atrophic glands with extensive stromal decidual change.

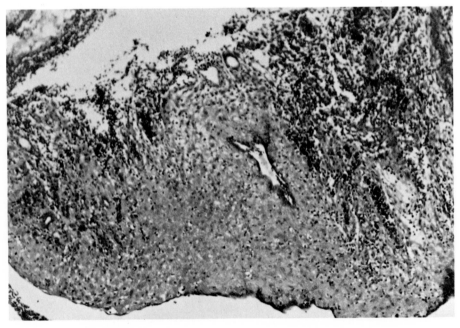

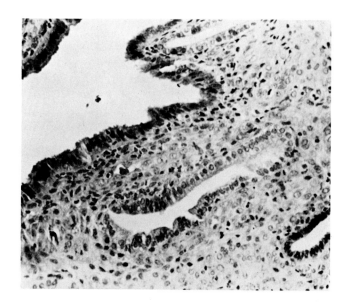

**13.25** Synthetic progestins. Note gland atrophy with marked stromal decidual change and inflammatory infiltrate.

periods after discontinuing medication, and develop amenorrhea for variable periods of time. The endometria histologically show sparse, small, atrophic glands surrounded by sheets of decidua.

### Effect of sequential oral contraceptives

In the sequential regimen, estrogen is given for 14 days (beginning on day 5 after the onset of menses) followed by a combination of estrogen and progestin in a single pill for 6 days. The estrogen component inhibits ovulation by blocking hypothalamic releasing factors.[9] On day 25, the hormones are discontinued. The endometrium shows the usual proliferative changes through day 19. Two or three days after progesterone is introduced secretory changes occur (about day 22). At this time subnuclear vacuoles form. Although progestational stimulation is evident in the endometrium through day 25, the response lags behind the normal by 5 to 7 days. On day 25, scanty predecidual changes may be seen and the development of spiral arterioles is abortive.

### Effects of synthetic progestins on the endometrium

The morphologic changes induced by synthetic progestins are related to their marked antiestrogenic properties. Initially, they produce secretions in glands, which then become exhausted and atrophic; a striking decidual

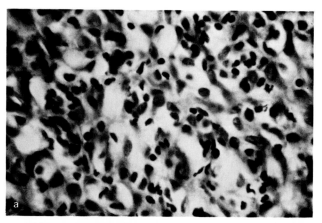
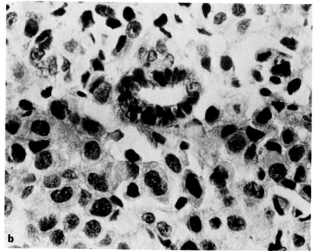

**13.26 a.** and **b.** Pseudosarcomatous alteration in decidua induced by Delalutin.

transformation of the stroma occurs (Figure 13.25) together with a vascular pattern characterized by prominent, dilated venules.[13] The response in the endometrium of a given patient may vary, and is not necessarily uniform throughout the biopsy.[9] Histologic responses vary from compound to compound. The effects depend upon the degree of estrogen exposure of the endometrium prior to initiation of progestin therapy. Individuals who have regular cycles will respond more uniformly than those who have anovulatory cycles. Because of the capacity of progestins to induce exhaustion and atrophy of endometrial glands, they have been used to treat cases of endometriosis, hyperplasia, and even carcinoma of the endometrium. Delalutin has on occasion produced a pseudosarcomatous pattern (Figures 13.26a,b). This has been described with potent progestins given for long periods of time.[4]

# REFERENCES

1. Bianchi, F., Grechi, G., and Alamanni, V. Studio sulla frequenza e le espressioni istopatologiche della degenerazione maligna nei polipi del corpo uterino e comparativamente nei polipi della cervice. *Arch. De Vecchi Anat. Pat. 48:*475, 1966.

2. Bosselman, K., and Schwarz, H. Cervical and endometrial polyps and carcinoma of female genital tract. *Geburtshilfe Frauenheilkunde 32:*687, 1972.

3. Cadena, D., Cavanzo, F. J., Leone, C. L., and Taylor, H. B. Chronic endometritis. *Obstet. Gynecol. 41:*733, 1973.

4. Dockerty, M. B., Smith, R. A. and Symmonds, R. E. Pseudomalignant endometrial changes induced by administration of new synthetic progestins. *Mayo Clin. Proc. 34:*321, 1959.

5. Farooki, M. A. Epidemiology and pathology of chronic endometritis. *Int. Surg. 48:*566, 1967.

6. Henderson, D. N., Hawkins, J. L., and Sitt, J. F. Pelvic tuberculosis. *Am. J. Obstet. Gynecol. 94:*630, 1966.

7. Israel, S. L., Roitman, H. B., and Clancy, C. Infrequency of unsuspected endometrial tuberculosis. *JAMA 183:*63, 1963.

8. Jones, W. E. Traumatic intrauterine adhesions. *Am. J. Obstet. Gynecol. 89:*304, 1964.

9. Kistner, R. W. *Endometrial Alterations in the Uterus.* Int. Acad. Pathol. Monograph. Williams & Wilkins, Baltimore, 1973.

10. Meyer, W. C., Malkasian, G. D., Dockerty, M. B., and Decker, D. G. Postmenopausal bleeding from atrophic endometrium. *Obstet. Gynecol. 38:*731, 1971.

11. Mishell, D. R., Jr., Bell, J. H., Good, R. G., and Moyer, D. L. The intrauterine device: Bacteriologic study of the intrauterine cavity. *Am. J. Obstet. Gynecol. 96:*119, 1966.

12. Moyer, D. L., Mishell, D. R., Jr. Reaction of the human endometrium to the intrauterine foreign body. II Long term effects on the endometrial histology and cytology. *Am. J. Obstet. Gynecol. 111:*66, 1971.

13. Ober, W. B. Synthetic progestagen-estrogen preparations and endometrial morphology. *J. Clin. Pathol. 19:*138, 1966.

14. Peterson, W. F., and Novak, E. R. Endometrial polyps. *Obstet. Gynecol. 8:*40, 1956.

15. Vasudeva, K., Thrasher, T. V., Richart, R. M. Chronic endometritis. A clinical and electron microscopic study. *Am. J. Obstet. Gynecol. 112:*749, 1972.

16. Wolf, S. A., and Mackles, A. Malignant lesions arising from benign endometrial polyps. *Obstet. Gynecol. 20:*542, 1962.

Rita Iovine Demopoulos, M.D.

# 14

# Endometrial Hyperplasia*

Endometrial hyperplasia is the result of persistent, prolonged estrogenic stimulation of the endometrium. The commonest cause is a succession of anovulatory cycles, but hyperplasia may also result from excessive endogenously produced, or exogenously administered estrogens.

One of the difficulties in discussing hyperplasia is the confusion in existing nomenclature. The terms simple hyperplasia, glandular hyperplasia, cystic glandular hyperplasia, and endometrial hyperplasia are synonymous. Adenomatous hyperplasia can occur with and without cytologic atypia and can be difficult to distinguish from well-differentiated adenocarcinoma. Swiss-cheese hyperplasia is an outdated term which describes inactive endometrium with cystic change. The term carcinoma in situ, as interpreted by some, is synonymous with severe atypical adenomatous hyperplasia, and is used by others to describe a specific histologic change known as pink cell anaplasia. The clinical and histologic features of each of these lesions are discussed separately.

Patients with hyperplasia have, in general, some constitutional features commonly seen in women with endometrial carcinoma. These consist of obesity, hypertension, low parity, irregular menses, and abnormal glucose tolerance curves. Obviously, individual cases may vary from these generally observed characteristics and show only

*Contributions on scanning electron microscopy of endometrial hyperplasia are by A. J. White and H. J. Buchsbaum.

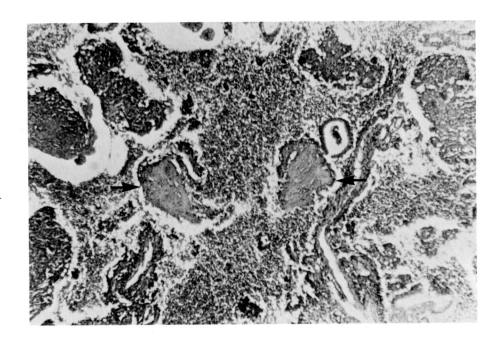

**14.1** Endometrial hyperplasia, sloughing of surface. Note thrombi in surface vessels (arrows).

some or none of these features. Hyperplasia occurs with greater frequency in women of Jewish extraction, as does endometrial carcinoma.

# Endometrial or Glandular Hyperplasia

## Clinical Observations

Endometrial hyperplasia occurs most often in young girls just after the menarche, and in older women in the climacteric, since at these times anovulation is quite common. At the commencement of the menarche, anovulation is often associated with a follicle cyst and the condition is self-limiting. In the older perimenopausal women, failure of ovulation is also common and may be associated with glandular hyperplasia of the endometrium. If hyperplasia is seen during the second and third decades, estrogen-producing ovarian tumors and Stein–Leventhal syndrome should be kept in mind as possible etiologies. The incidence of endometrial hyperplasia in patients with granulosa–theca cell tumors is variously reported as between 10 and 25%. Similar figures are given for the occurrence of hyperplasia in patients with untreated Stein–Leventhal syndrome. Once hyperplasia is present, the relatively high estrogen levels necessary to maintain it, may at times, be lacking and bleeding occurs. The amount of bleeding

bears no relationship to the degree of hyperplasia. Bleeding may be profuse when the hyperplasia is mild or may result in only spotting when the curettings are abundant. When bleeding occurs, the endometrium shows thick-walled blood vessels, fibrin thrombi in surface vessels, sloughing, and necrosis (Figure 14.1).

## Gross and Histologic Appearance

Endometrial hyperplasia is characterized by proliferation of both glands and stroma. The resulting endometrium is grossly thick, velvety, creamy-yellow, often measuring greater than 5 mm in thickness and appearing lobulated or pseudopolypoid (Figure 14.2). Curettings are abundant. Microscopically, the glands often lose their perpendicular orientation to the surface and are askew, i.e., they show a loss of polarity. Since both glands and stroma proliferate, there is little or only focal crowding of the glands. They are tubular or slightly convoluted and vary considerably in size and shape. Occasional glands may be cystically dilated (Figure 14.3). The lining cells are columnar and the nuclei are large, vesicular, and stratified. There is absent or focal, sporadic secretory activity. Mitoses are present, but oddly enough are not more numerous than in a proliferative endometrium. Nucleoli are prominent. There is little or no budding of gland epithelium into the lumen, or into stroma in this type of hyperplasia. The stroma is dense; the stromal nuclei are closely packed and surrounded by sparse,

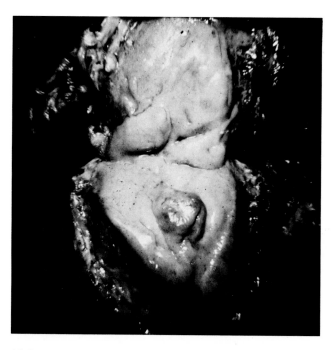

**14.2** Endometrial hyperplasia. The endometrium is thick and creamy-yellow in appearance.

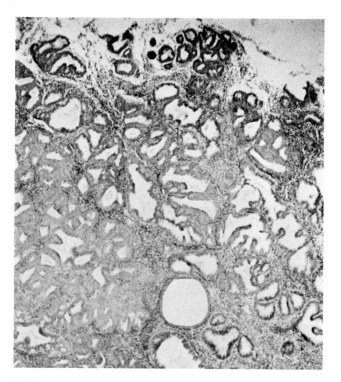

**14.3** Endometrial hyperplasia. Note the abundance of glands and stroma. The glands show a loss of polarity and vary in size and shape.

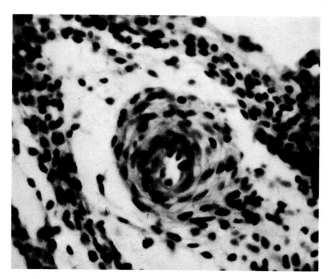

**14.4** Endometrial hyperplasia. Hypertrophy of smooth muscle in the wall of spiral arterioles.

[Reprinted by permission from A. U. Blaustein and L. Shenker, Responsiveness of endothelium in spiral arterioles of endometrium, *Obstet. Gynecol.* 35(1): January, 1970.]

poorly defined cytoplasm. Spiral arterioles often show hyperplasia of the smooth muscle layer[1] (Figures 14.4 and 14.5). The majority of patients who have endometrial hyperplasia follow a benign course. McBride[16] has reported that only 0.4% of patients with this type of hyperplasia subsequently develop carcinoma, compared to a risk of 0.1% among the general female population.[20]

## "Swiss Cheese Hyperplasia"

Cystic change can be seen in virtually any endometrium to a limited extent. It is a prominent feature, however, in the endometrium of some postmenopausal women. The combination of inactive glands with extensive cystic change has in the past been referred to as "swiss cheese hyperplasia." Since the endometrium in these cases is not hyperplastic but rather thin and atrophic, this term is a misnomer. A preferable designation would be inactive endometrium with cystic change (Figure 14.6a,b). Such endometria almost invariably follow a benign course.

## Adenomatous Hyperplasia

Adenomatous hyperplasia is viewed with much greater concern by gynecologists and pathologists than is glandular hyperplasia. It has come to be generally accepted as a precursor of endometrial carcinoma.

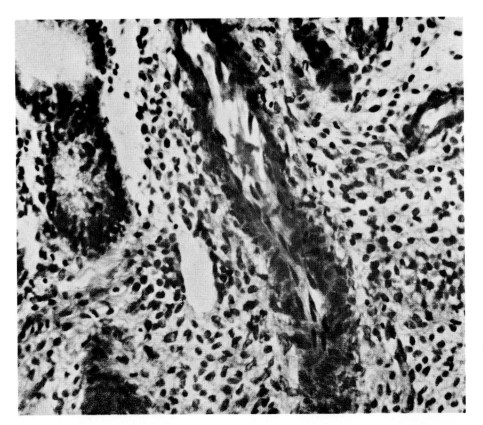

**14.5** Endometrial hyperplasia—spiral arteriole showing smooth muscle hyperplasia and desquamation of endothelium.

[Reprinted by permission from A. U. Blaustein and L. Shenker, Responsiveness of endothelium in spiral arterioles of endometrium, *Obstet. Gynecol. 35*(1): January, 1970.]

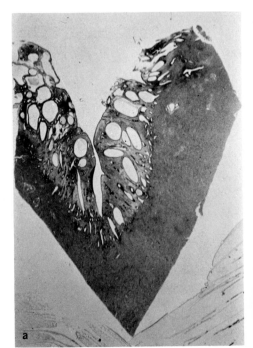

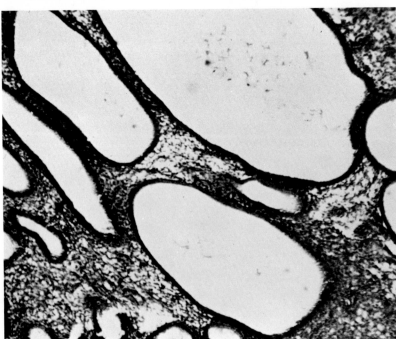

**14.6 a.** Low-power view of inactive endometrium with cystic change (menopausal patient). **b.** High-power view of Figure 14.6a.

## Gross and Microscopic Appearance

Grossly, the endometrium of adenomatous hyperplasia cannot usually be distinguished from that of glandular hyperplasia. Occasionally, adenomatous hyperplasia may be more polypoid or show microinfarcts. The distinction is histologic and consists mainly of the fact that the endometrial glands in adenomatous hyperplasia proliferate at the expense of the stroma. The glands, therefore, are crowded; they increase in number and complexity and the intervening stroma diminishes in amount. This change may be focal (Figure 14.7) or diffuse (Figure 14.8a,b). The crowding of the glands may progress to the point where they are "back to back" or separated from one another by only a very delicate band of fibrous stroma. Another feature which is often conspicuous in adenomatous hyperplasia is epithelial budding. This refers to an infolding of the gland epithelium either into the lumen or into the stroma (Figure 14.9). The lining epithelium is tall columnar, the nuclei are vesicular and stratified. Mitoses are common.

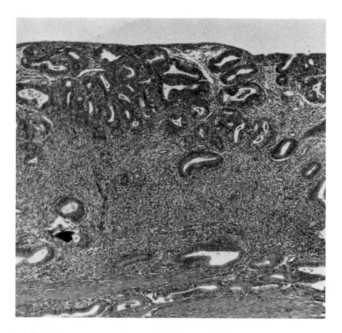

**14.7** Adenomatous hyperplasia, focal in type.

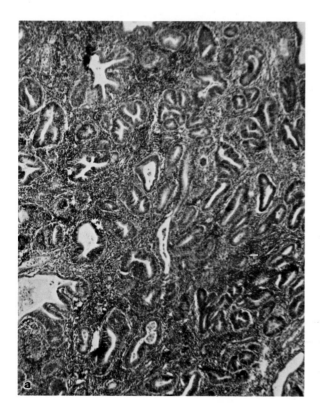

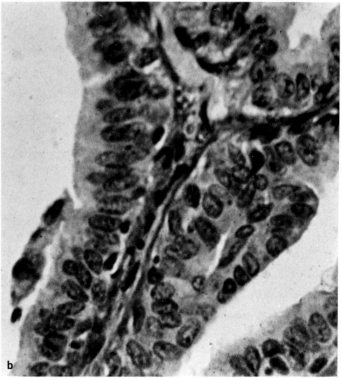

**14.8 a.** Adenomatous hyperplasia. The glands are crowded and separated by scant stroma. **b.** High-power view shows tall epithelium with stratified vesicular nuclei. Glands are virtually back to back.

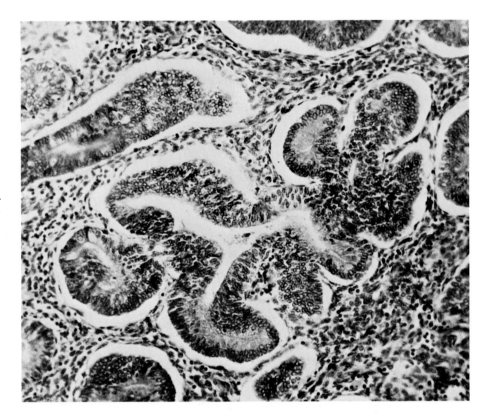

**14.9** Adenomatous hyperplasia. budding of hyperplastic epithelium.

## Scanning Electron Microscopy

The surface appearance of adenomatous hyperplasia, as viewed with scanning electron microscopy, is not very different from the surface during the proliferative phase. It is somewhat more undulated with an increase in number of gland ostia (Figure 14.10a). Under a higher magnification, only minimal changes are evident. Occasionally, there may be large secretory cells. Some fields may show a proliferation of ciliated cells with variations in the length of the cilia (Figure 14.10b).

## Atypical Adenomatous Hyperplasia

If cytologic atypia occurs in adenomatous hyperplasia, consisting of nuclear enlargement, hyperchromasia, or irregularity in shape, the term atypical adenomatous hyperplasia is appropriate (Figure 14.11). This lesion is commonly treated as if it were adenocarcinoma. A rare type of atypical adenomatous hyperplasia occurs with scattered circumscribed nodules of clustered cells called "morules" (Figure 14.12a,b). These morules are seen within the endometrial glands as well as bridging the stroma between the endometrial glands. They frequently are spheroidal but may be irregularly shaped. The constituent cells resemble squamous epithelium but do not show intercellular bridges, or intracellular keratin production. Histochemical stains fail to clarify the origin of these morules, whether epithelial, or reserve cell, or stromal cells.

Dutra[5] described several cases of adenomatous hyperplasia with morules and believed that the morules are derived from glandular epithelium. All of his cases were benign. We have seen four cases in our laboratory; all were associated with atypical adenomatous hyperplasia. They all occurred in women between 30 and 40 years of age, and all complained of infertility. One patient initially refused surgery until 10 years later. At that time, the lesion persisted unchanged. Two patients were treated immediately with hysterectomy and no malignant change was found. The last patient had deferred surgery for 16 months. Her uterus showed a focal area of well-differentiated adenocarcinoma. It is important to evaluate these cases on the basis of the glandular pattern exclusive of the morules. Electron microscopy would probably be very useful in defining the cell of origin of the morules.

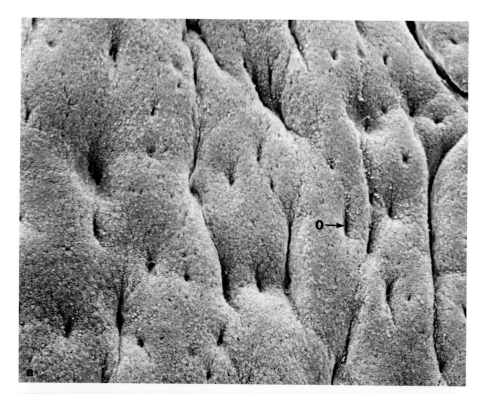

**14.10 a.** Adenomatous hyperplasia. The surface appearance of adenomatous hyperplasia is similar to normal proliferative endometrium. Multiple gland ostia (O) can be seen (×84).
**b.** Adenomatous hyperplasia. Note differences in the length of cilia in adjacent cells, probably representing differing growth rates. Secretory droplets visible in right upper and right lower corners (×6082).

[**a** and **b** reprinted by permission from A. J. White and H. J. Buchsbaum, Scanning electron microscopy of the human endometrium, *Gynecol. Oncol.* 2:1, 1974.]

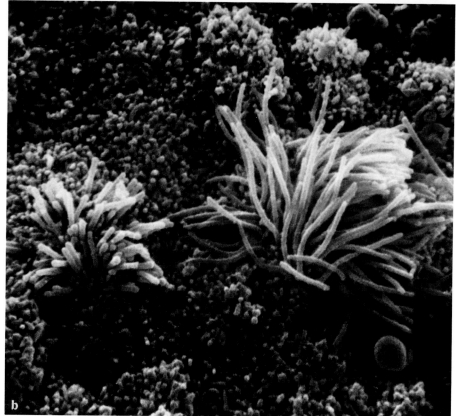

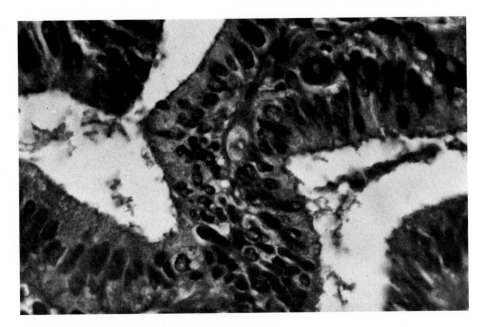

**14.11** Atypical adenomatous hyperplasia showing back to back glands lined by epithelium with large, irregular hyperchromatic nuclei.

## Carcinoma in Situ

Most pathologists agree that adenocarcinoma of the endometrium begins as a focal change in the endometrial glandular epithelium. Philosophically, there is undoubtedly a stage that precedes endometrial stromal invasion, and in which changes are limited to the endometrial glands. Just what constitutes the architectural and cytologic features of such an endometrium is not entirely clear. Sommers, Hertig, and Bengloff[22] originally described carcinoma in situ of the endometrium in 1949, as a precursor to the development of endometrial carcinoma. The gross appearance of the endometrium in in situ carcinoma is normal, thin, or focally polypoid. The microscopic pattern consists of a focus of crowded endometrial glands, composed of large cells with abundant, pale eosinophilic cytoplasm and nuclei arranged in irregular palisades, having fine granular chromatin. The adjacent stroma and surrounding endometrial glands are normal (Figure 14.13a,b). Later Buehl and Vellios et al.[2] described carcinoma in situ as a focal change in endometrial glands characterized by a piling up of epithelium, the formation of intraluminal bridges (commonly referred to as a cribriform pattern), and evidence of cytologic atypia in the form of clumping of chromatin and nuclear pleomorphism (Figure 14.14). Many pathologists and clinicians do not use the term carcinoma in situ but consider the changes described by Hertig and those described by Buehl to be examples of severe atypical adenomatous hyperplasia.

Because these lesions are customarily treated identically to carcinoma, the nomenclature is only of academic importance.

Although it is generally agreed that persistent, unopposed estrogens will produce glandular hyperplasia in all women, the development of adenomatous or atypical adenomatous hyperplasia, or carcinoma in situ implies something unusual about the host's response. There are many questions still remaining concerning the relationship of estrogens to both. At this point it seems appropriate to review the information available regarding these interrelationships.

## Estrogens, Hyperplasia, and Carcinoma of the Endometrium

In animal experiments there is good documentation of a time–dose relationship between estrogen administration and subsequent development of hyperplasia and carcinoma. Meissner, Sommers, and Sherman[17] reported production of hyperplasia and adenocarcinoma in rabbits by administration of stilbesterol. Merriam et al.[18] produced endometrial carcinoma in rabbits using methyl cholanthrene and demonstrated, by several endometrial biopsies, sequential changes in endometrium from hyperplasia, to carcinoma in situ, to invasive carcinoma. In 1947 Gusberg[7] morphologically defined adenomatous hyperplasia and suggested that it is a precursor of endometrial carci-

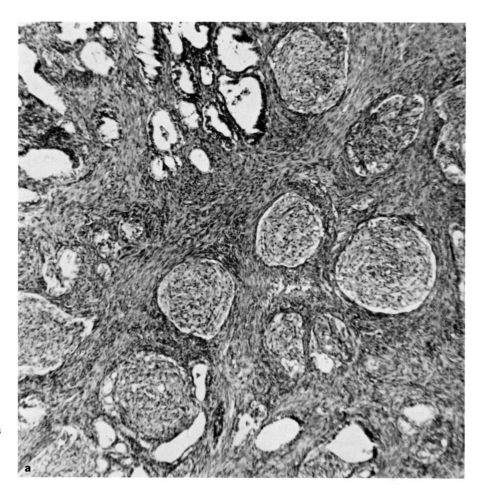

**14.12 a.** Atypical hyperplasia characterized by the presence of morules. **b.** High-power view of a morule which is contiguous with an endometrial gland.

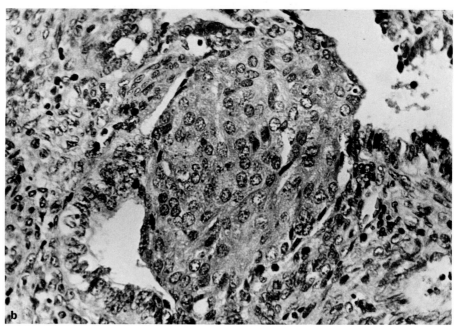

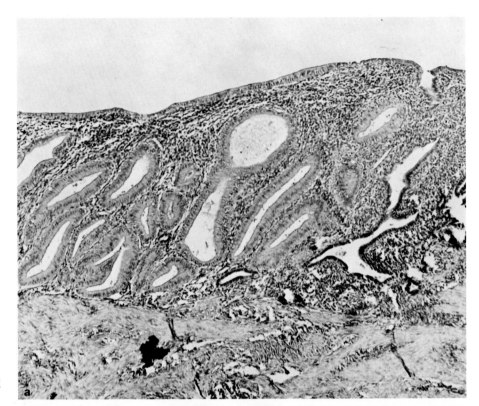

**14.13 a.** Atypical adenomatous hyperplasia, similar in appearance to Gusberg's Grade IV and Hertig's carcinoma in situ.
**b.** High-power view of Figure 14.13a. The cells have abundant pink granular cytoplasm, sometimes referred to as pink-cell anaplasia.

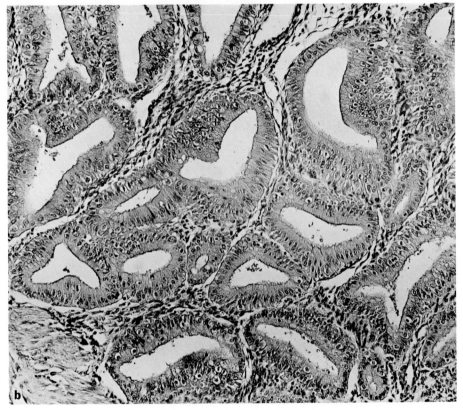

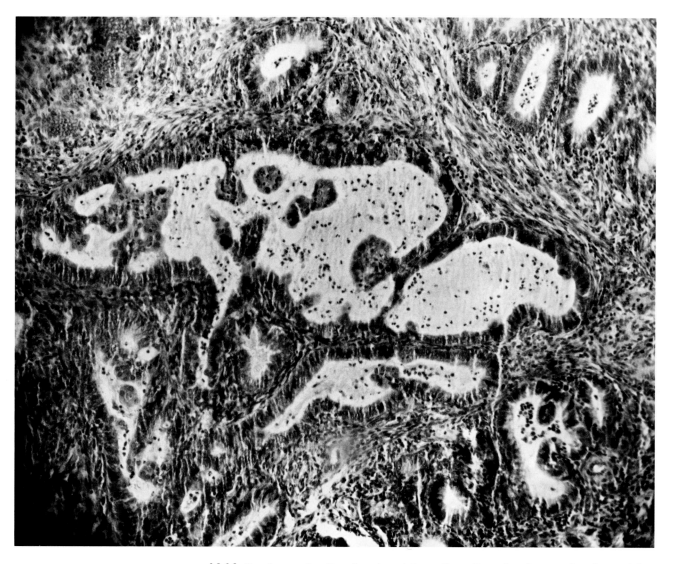

**14.14** Carcinoma in situ of endometrium. Crowding of a cluster of endometrial glands showing a cribriform pattern. All the glands surrounding this focus were proliferative in type. Hysterectomy specimen revealed no residual atypia.

noma. Later, Gusberg and Kaplan[9] did prospective follow-up studies on 191 patients with adenomatous hyperplasia diagnosed from 1934 to 1954. Of these, 90 were treated immediately by hysterectomy, and 20% were found to have coexisting carcinoma, and 13% had borderline lesions. This left 101 patients to be followed. In this group, eight patients (11.8%) went on to develop endometrial cancer (mean followup, 5.3 years). In the control groups consisting of 202 patients (all of whom presented with postmenopausal bleeding and none of whom were shown to have hyperplasia or carcinoma on initial curett-

age), only one went on to develop endometrial carcinoma. Gusberg concludes that the cumulative risk for a patient with adenomatous hyperplasia followed for 9 to 10 years is significantly higher than for women without hyperplasia.

In 1961 Gusberg and Hall[8] studied the endometria of women who had been treated with estrogen for menopausal symptoms and who had developed endometrial carcinoma. Despite the absence of controls, he concluded that the type of carcinoma developed by these patients was characteristically an "estrogen carcinoma" in that they strongly resembled atypical adenomatous hyperplasia with just enough anaplasia to call them well-differentiated adenocarcinoma. He concluded that estrogens played a role in the development of these tumors. Smith et al.[21] retrospectively compared 317 patients with adenocarcinoma of the endometrium with 317 matched controls having other gynecologic neoplasms. One hundred and fifty-two patients used estrogens in the study group, as compared to 54 in the control group. The authors found the risk of endometrial cancer was 4.5 *times* greater among women exposed to estrogen therapy. The risk is increased as the duration of estrogen therapy is prolonged.[24] Sommers, Hertig, and Bengloff[22] studied endometrial carcinoma occurring in young women, age 16 to 35 years. They found that the women gave a long history of menorrhagia alternating with periods of amenorrhea, interpreted as indicative of failure to establish normal ovulatory cycles. Sterility was also a common complaint. Multiple biopsies rarely revealed progestational change. Examination of the ovaries of 16 of these women revealed little evidence of ovulation. Sommers *et. al.* concluded that these women had evidence of endocrine dysfunction considered to be of significance in the genesis of endometrial carcinoma. Another source of support for the contention that prolonged, unopposed estrogens play a role in the development of endometrial carcinoma is the high incidence of endometrail cancer encountered in women with feminizing tumors of the ovaries. Norris and Taylor[19] found, in a group of patients with granulosa–theca cell tumors, that 22% had adenomatous hyperplasia, and 9% had endometrial carcinoma. Mansell and Hertig,[15] in a similar group, found 40% with various forms of endometrial hyperplasia and 15% with endometrial carcinoma. They found that ovarian tumors histologically suggesting hormonal activity were twice as often associated with abnormally active endometria, as those which did not. This, they felt, suggested a role of estrogens in the pathogenesis of hyperplasia and carcinoma of the endometrium. Dockerty and Mussey[4] and Ingram and Novak[11] found that approximately 15% of feminizing tumors of the ovary (granulosa and theca cell tumors) have coexisting endometrial carcinoma.

Adenocarcinoma of the endometrium is rare during the childbearing years. When it does occur, a significant number is associated with Stein–Leventhal syndrome. In a study by Jackson and Dockerty[12] of 43 patients with Stein–Leventhal syndrome, 16 (37.2%) had carcinoma of the endometrium. In another study by Chamlian and Taylor,[3] consisting of 97 women under 36 years of age who had endometrial hyperplasia, 25% had Stein–Leventhal syndrome and 14% later developed carcinoma in situ 1 to 14 years later. A study by Emge[6] challenges these

figures. He collected data from numerous medical centers throughout the country and found the incidence of coexisting carcinoma of the endometrium to be 3.1 for granulosa tumors and 3.3 for thecomas. He concludes that these figures are close to the predictable incidence for ovarian tumors and uterine cancer occurring simultaneously, by chance. An obvious limitation of all of these studies regarding the possible role of estrogen in the production of endometrial cancer is the fact that not all granulosa-theca cell tumors produce estrogens. No attempt was made to correlate the findings of endometrial carcinoma with biochemical evidence of estrogen production by the ovarian tumors.

Another argument against the case for estrogens being related to the development of endometrial carcinoma is that women who have received sterilizing doses of radiation or have had bilateral oophorectomies have occasionally developed cancer many years later. Jones and Brewer[13] reported this in 1941 and Hofmeister and Vondrak[10] in 1970 reported on 9 patients who had surgical bilateral oophorectomy and subsequently developed endometrial carcinoma. The average age at which the uterine malignancy was discovered was 56.4 years. This represented an average interval of 16.6 years after oophorectomy. Two of these patients, however, were taking estrogens for 2 to 5 years prior to the development of cancer. They discovered an additional eight women who developed endometrial carcinoma at an average of 16.1 years after having irradiation castration. This suggests that endometrial carcinoma can develop in patients deprived of their main source of estrogens, and therefore there are other factors, such as individual susceptibility, probably genetically determined. The role of adrenal estrogen production was not evaluated in these patients.

Several investigators have found beneficial effects from treating hyperplasia and carcinoma with progestins. Kistner[14] and Steiner et al.[23] treated 23 patients with atypical hyperplasia and 8 patients with carcinoma in situ with progesterone. None advanced to invasive carcinoma. They have concluded that these lesions are reversible.

In summary, it seems that evidence exists to support the view that prolonged, unopposed, endogenous or exogenous estrogen can stimulate the development of endometrial hyperplasia. Some women, because of genetically or environmentally determined individual host responses, will develop adenomatous or atypical hyperplasia and patients with these lesions are at greater risk to develop endometrial carcinoma than those with normal endometria. The problem is not simple, however. Undoubtedly, many patients develop carcinoma without ever developing any type of hyperplasia. What constitutes high circulating estrogen levels for one patient may elicit a normal response in another. Further study is necessary for a final clarification of this problem.

# REFERENCES

1. Blaustein, A. U., and Shenker, L. Responsiveness of endothelium in spiral arterioles of endometrium. *Obstet. Gynecol.* 35(1):January 1970.

2. Buehl, I. A., Vellios, F., Corten, J. E., and Huber, C. P. Carcinoma in-situ of the endometrium. *Am. J. Clin. Pathol.* 42:594, 1964.

3. Chamlian, D. L., and Taylor, H. B. Endometrial hyperplasia in young women. *Obstet. Gynecol.* 36:659, 1970.

4. Dockerty, M. B., and Mussey, E. Malignant lesion of the uterus associated with estrogen producing ovarian tumors. *Am. J. Obstet. Gynecol.* 61:147, 1951.

5. Dutra, F. R. Intraglandular morules of the endometrium. *Am. J. Clin. Pathol.* 31:60, 1959.

6. Emge, L. A. Endometrial cancer and feminizing tumors of the ovary. *Obstet. Gynecol.* 1:511, 1953

7. Gusberg, S. B. Precursors of corpus carcinoma. Estrogens and adenomatous hyperplasia. *Am. J. Obstet. Gynecol.* 54:905, 1947.

8. Gusberg, S. B., and Hall, R. I. Precursors of endometrial carcinoma. *Obstet. Gynecol.* 17:397, 1961.

9. Gusberg, S. B., and Kaplan, A. L. Precursors of corpus cancer. *Am. J. Obstet Gynecol.* 87:662, 1963.

10. Hofmeister, F. J., and Vondrak, B. F. Endometrial carcinoma in patients with bilateral oophorectomy or irradiation castration. *Am. J. Obstet. Gynecol.* 107:1099, 1970.

11. Ingram, J. M., Jr., and Novak, E. Endometrial carcinoma associated with feminizing ovarian tumors. *Am. J. Obstet. Gynecol.* 61:774, 1951.

12. Jackson, R. L., and Dockerty, M. B. The Stein–Leventhal syndrome analysis of 43 cases with special reference to association with endometrial carcinoma. *Am. J. Obstet. Gynecol.* 73:161, 1957.

13. Jones, H. D., and Brewer, J. L. Studies of ovaries and endometrium of patients with fundal adenocarcinoma. *Am. J. Obstet. Gynecol.* 42:207, 1941.

14. Kistner, R. W. Histological effects of progestins on hyperplasia and carcinoma in-situ of the endometrium. *Cancer* 12:1106, 1959.

15. Mansell, H., and Hertig, A. T. Granulosa theca cell tumors and endometrial cancer. A study of their relationship and a survey of 80 cases. *Obstet. Gynecol.* 6:385, 1955.

16. McBride, J. M. Pre-menopausal cystic hyperplasia and endometrial carcinoma. *J. Obstet. Gynaecol. Br. Emp.* 66:288, 1959.

17. Meissner, W. A., Sommers, S. C., and Sherman, G. Endometrial hyperplasia, endometrial carcinoma and endometriosis produced experimentally by estrogen. *Cancer* 10:500, 1957.

18. Merriam, J. C., Jr., Easterday, C. L., McKay, D. G., and Hertig, A. T. Experimental production of endometrial cancer in the rabbit. *Obstet. Gynecol.* 16:253, 1960.

19. Norris, H. J., and Taylor, H. B. Prognosis of granulosa theca tumors of the ovary. *Cancer* 21:255, 1968.

20. Sheehan, E. G., and Tucker, A. W. Carcinoma of the endometrium. *J.S.C. Med. Assoc.* 45:239, 1949.

21. Smith, D. C., Prentice, R., Thompson, D. J., and Herrmann, W. L. Association of exogenous estrogen and endometrial carcinoma. *New Engl. J. Med.* 293:1164, 1975.

22. Sommers, S. C., Hertig, A. T., and Bengloff, H. Genesis of endometrial carcinoma. *Cancer* 2:957, 1949.

23. Steiner, G. J., Kistner, R. W., and Craig, J. M. Histological effects of progestins on hyperplasia and carcinoma in-situ of the endometrium—further observations. *Metabolism* 14:356, 1965.

24. Ziel, H. K., and Finkle, W. D. Increased risk of endometrial carcinoma among users of conjugated estrogens. *New Engl. J. Med.* 293:1167, 1975.

Rita Iovine Demopoulos, M.D.

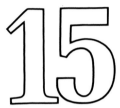

# Carcinoma of the Endometrium*

## Adenocarcinoma of the Endometrium

### Incidence

Endometrial carcinoma has been steadily increasing in incidence over the past few decades so that currently the incidence of endometrial adenocarcinoma is approximately the same as the occurrence of invasive squamous cell carcinoma of the cervix. The California Tumor Registry reported an incidence of 27.2 cases per 100,000 population in 1969 and 41.4 cases per 100,000 in 1973. This increase is in part caused by an increasing longevity of the female population. The age of the population at greatest risk for the development of endometrial carcinoma is 50 to 60 years, which is the immediate postmenopausal period. Only about 5% of cases occur in women under 40 years of age.

### Epidemiology

The prototype of the patient with endometrial carcinoma would be an obese 55-year-old woman, diabetic[9,11] and hypertensive, who has married late in life, gives a history of irregular menses and infertility, has few, if any

---

* Contributions on scanning and transmission electron microscopy of carcinoma of the endometrium are by A. J. White and H. J. Buchsbaum.

children, and has had a late menopause. The common denominator would seem be to hormone imbalance. In a study performed by Sommers and Meissner[41] on 38 women with endometrial carcinoma who were autopsied, 63% were obese, 30% were diabetic, and 53% were hypertensive. Of 136 controls, 28% were obese, 5% were diabetic, and 51% were hypertensive. They also reported ovarian cortical stromal hyperplasia to be present in 73% of patients with cancer as compared to 36% in controls. From concomitant studies of the pituitary in these women, they concluded that overproduction of hormones produced by basophils, namely; FSH, LH, and TSH, and adrenocortical hyperplasia probably play a role in the etiology of endometrial carcinoma. They studied the adrenal glands in these women and found evidence to suggest increased hormone production in the form of adrenal cortical hyperplasia in those women with cancer. The relationship between estrogen and endometrial carcinoma is discussed in Chapter 14. Recent studies by Smith et al.[40] indicate that the risk of endometrial carcinoma is 4.5 times greater among women who are on estrogen therapy. Recently, techniques for assaying the production and secretion rates of steroid hormones have been perfected. Plotz et al.[32] found that the ovaries of postmenopausal women retain steroidogenic capabilities and produce androgens that may be converted to estrogens elsewhere in the body. In a provocative study by Hausnecht and Gusberg,[18] patients with endometrial carcinoma and a control group were given radioactive androstenedione. Patients with endometrial carcinoma converted a significantly greater proportion of the androstenedione to estrone than did the controls. In a previous study these investigators[17] had shown that patients with endometrial carcinoma excreted more estrone glucosiduronate than estriol glucosiduronate. Such studies suggest that in women who develop endometrial carcinoma there may be specific metabolic pathways that differ from the normal. These observations are significant and further biochemical studies of this nature may contribute to an understanding of the pathogenesis of endometrial carcinoma.

## Diagnosis

A routine Pap smear on asymptomatic patients is only about 50% effective in detecting cases of endometrial carcinoma. When positive cervical and vaginal pool smears are compared, there is usually a greater concentration of malignant cells in the exfoliated cells of the vaginal pool, which facilitates the diagnosis by screening cytotechnologists.

Since uterine bleeding tends to be an early sign of endometrial carcinoma, all patients with this symptom should be investigated to find its cause. In a study by Hark and Sommers[15] of 500 consecutive curettages, only 2% were found to have endometrial carcinoma, 18.2% had hyperplasia, 6.2% had inactive endometrium, 3% had endometritis, 1.8% had endometrial polyps, and two-thirds had normal endometrium. This study included women of all ages, which accounts for the low proportion of patients with malignant tumors. All patients who develop postmenopausal bleeding should have a fractional diagnostic dilatation and curettage performed. Consecutive curettages in this age group disclose about 10% with malignant tumor. Fractionation of the curettage specimen, with separation of uterine from endocervical curettings, enables the pathologist to assess whether the malignant tumor has extended downward to involve the cervix. If tumor is found within segments of endocervical tissue, this modifies both the treatment and prognosis. Care should be taken not to conclude from isolated fragments of malignant tissue among the endocervical curettings, that this necessarily implies extension of tumor to endocervix, since bits of sloughing tumor from the uterus may be loose in the endocervix.

## Gross Appearance

Endometrial carcinoma tends to be a slow growing tumor and since many patients develop bleeding early in the course of the disease, most tumors are limited to endometrium or superficial myometrium when discovered.

Since the endometrium and lower uterine segment have usually been scraped, there is often little or no remaining tumor to be seen in the gross specimen. Occasionally a focal area will appear somewhat raised and granular and have a firm consistency and on sectioning will prove to be a small amount of residual tumor which was missed on curettage. The right and left cornual areas should be carefully examined for residual tumor since these areas are difficult to scrape completely. If the gross specimen is received following the administration of intracavity radium, the endometrium appears hemorrhagic and necrotic and rarely does any vestige of tumor remain in the cavity. However, numerous random sections of the entire cavity may demonstrate nests of malignant glands in the myometrium.

The uterus may be small, normal in size, or enlarged. The majority of carcinomas arise in the fundus, and more often on the posterior rather than the anterior wall. The tumors may be small and focal, or they may be diffuse and

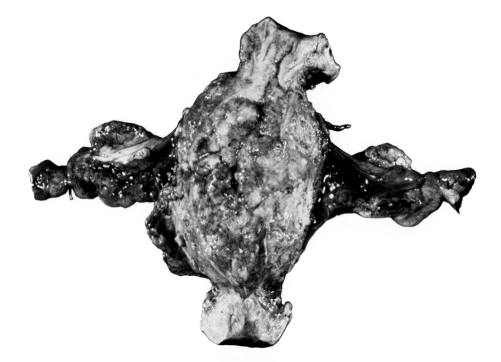

**15.1** Endometrial carcinoma that has grown extensively to involve the entire cavity.

involve much of the cavity (Figure 15.1). Diffuse lesions often show extensive hemorrhage and necrosis. The growth of the tumor may be both exophytic and infiltrative. Many sections should be taken to determine the extent of myometrial invasion. Extension into muscle appears as pale, white, irregular zones, surrounded by normal myometrium (Figure 15.2). Occasionally perforation is seen. This may be due to tumor growth through the entire thickness of the myometrium, or perforation may have occurred during curettage due to thinning of the myometrium by tumor.

Many endometrial tumors are polypoid and exophytic occupying much of the uterine cavity (Figure 15.3). Such a mass may interfere with drainage resulting in secondary infection. Pyometra usually manifests itself clinically as a purulent discharge from the uterus. Pyometra may also be a sequela of cervical stenosis, a condition which is sometimes seen in patients in this age group.

Fewer than 1% of endometrial carcinomas arise in benign polyps. It is sometimes difficult to recognize the presence of carcinoma in a polyp, but at times the mucosa at the site of malignant change appears granular, ulcerated, and hemorrhagic (Figure 15.4). Since endometrial carcinoma often arises *de novo* as a polypoid structure, the diagnosis of malignant change in a polyp can only be made when a portion of benign polyp remains microscopically.

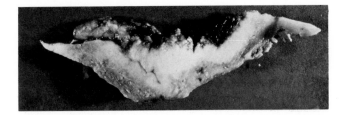

**15.2** Uterus has been longitudinally sectioned to show endometrial carcinoma deeply invading the underlying muscle. Muscle bundles are replaced by white homogeneous tumor tissue.

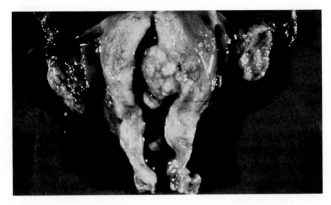

**15.3** Polypoid or exophytic endometrial carcinoma. Tumor fills the cavity and also invades underlying myometrium.

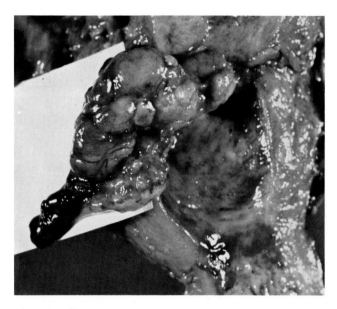

**15.4** Large endometrial polyp showing extensive hemorrhage. Although the tip was benign, malignant change occurred at the base. This area is solid and granular.

## Microscopic Appearance

Histologically, most endometrial malignancies are adenocarcinomas. There are varieties of histologic patterns and grades of differentiation seen. The use of Ewing's method of grading (1, 2, 3, and 4) is useful in establishing prognostic information.

Well-differentiated tumors composed of glands showing minimal alterations are classified as grade I (Figure 15.5a). The glands are orderly and regular and look very much like hyperplastic glands but show increased complexity and tortuosity. High-power views usually show few mitoses and little atypia in the glands (Figure 15.5b). Grade II tumors are moderately differentiated and form somewhat atypical glands (Figure 15.6) with more pronounced cytologic changes. Inflammatory changes and necrosis are frequently seen. Grade III tumors are poorly differentiated; gland formation is abortive and bizarre, if present at all (Figure 15.7). There are solid sheets of tumor with occasional areas of desmoplastic stroma. The nuclei are enlarged, hyperchromatic, irregular, and show frequent mitoses. Inflammation, necrosis, and hemorrhage are often more prominent than in the other grades. At times one can find in a given tumor, areas that are well differentiated and poorly differentiated. In such cases the lesion is likely to behave as would be expected of the poorest differenti-

ated areas, and should be graded accordingly. Grade IV tumors are undifferentiated and not gland forming. Anaplastic cells are seen in sheets, with some nesting suggesting that the lesion is a carcinoma rather than a sarcoma (Figure 15.8).

The grading of adenocarcinoma correlates quite well with tumor behavior. Keller et al.[21] report the actuarial 5-year survival for grade I to be 88%; grade II, 89%; grade III, 69%; and grade IV, 34%.

There are a vast number of variations possible in other parameters of histologic appearance in addition to the degree of differentiation. Although the majority of carcinomas are composed of glands, a smaller number are papillary. The cellular characteristics of papillary tumors frequently resemble those of serous cystadenocarcinoma of the ovary and, in fact, psammoma bodies may be present[13] (Figure 15.9). Factor[6] describes three such cases unassociated with ovarian tumors.

Approximately 5% of endometrial carcinomas are mucin-producing and these vary from scattered foci of mucin-containing cells to tumors composed almost exclusively of mucin-producing cells. Mucin can be demonstrated using a mucicarmine or periodic acid-Schiff stain. The histochemical stains are not useful in distinguishing mucinous endometrial from endocervical carcinoma.[42]

Another 5% of endometrial carcinomas have focal or extensive clear cell differentiation. These are usually well-differentiated tumors. The cytoplasm of the clear cells is foamy or vacuolated and glycogen rich.

Squamous metaplasia is perhaps one of the commonest findings in endometrial cancer. The more sections one takes of any given tumor, the more likely one is to find squamous changes. There may be only small scattered foci or large prominent masses of polygonal cells with pink-staining keratinizing cytoplasm. If the squamous epithelium is well differentiated and benign in appearance, the lesion is designated as adenoacanthoma. In those instances in which the squamous component appears histologically malignant, the term adenosquamous carcinoma is used. Rarely, pure squamous cell carcinomas of the endometrium occur. The behavior of each of these tumors will be separately discussed.

The stromal component of adenocarcinoma may be delicate and sparse or dense and fibrotic. Acute and chronic inflammatory cells are invariably present to a greater or lesser extent. Occasionally one sees clusters of lipid-laden macrophages, usually adjacent to areas of necrosis in the tumor (Figure 15.10). These histiocytes may phagocytose lipid released by the tumor cells. They are also seen occasionally in endometrial hyperplasia, polyps, and normal

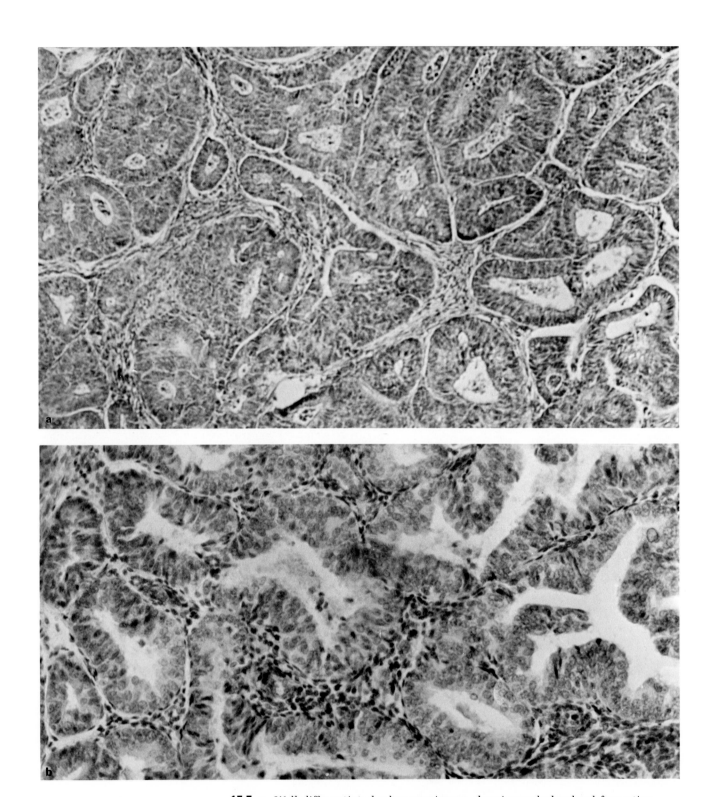

**15.5 a.** Well-differentiated adenocarcinoma showing orderly gland formation with back to back configuration very much like that seen in adenomatous hyperplasia. **b.** High-power view of a well-differentiated adenocarcinoma showing little cellular atypia and few mitoses.

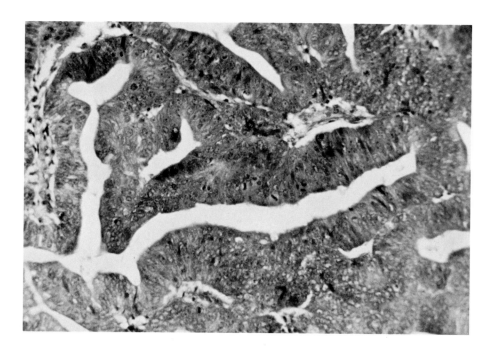

**15.6** Grade II adenocarcinoma showing stratification of nuclei and scattered mitoses.

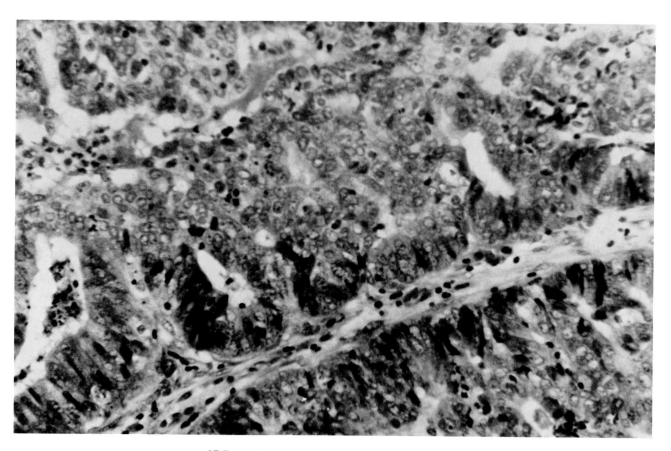

**15.7** Grade III adenocarcinoma showing abortive gland formation and stromal infiltration by polymorphonuclear leukocytes.

283

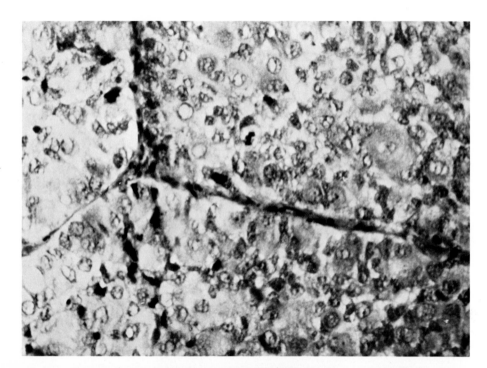

**15.8** High-power of undifferentiated carcinoma showing sheets of anaplastic cells with numerous mitoses.

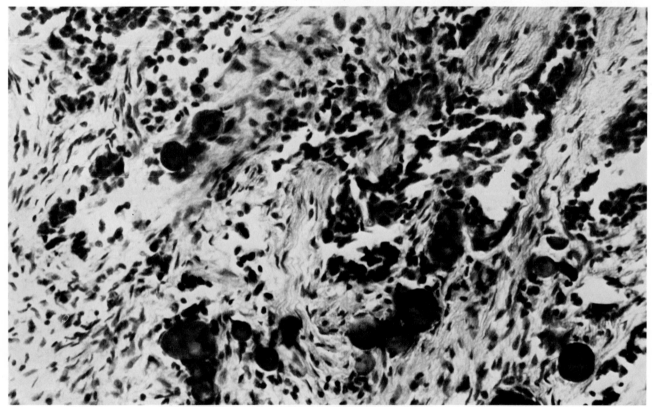

**15.9** Adenocarcinoma of the endometrium containing psammoma bodies. This is a rare finding in endometrial lesions.

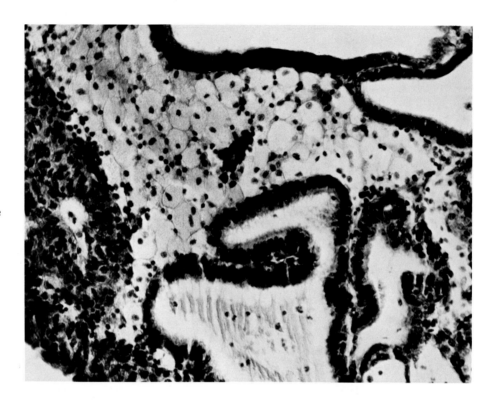

**15.10** Adenocarcinoma of the endometrium with abundant lipid-laden macrophages in the stroma.

endometrium, but to a much lesser extent than in carcinoma.[16]

Myometrial invasion usually occurs by direct downward growth of surface malignant epithelium. Tongues of tumor, often along a broad front, invade the underlying muscle bundles (Figures 15.11 and 15.12). The junction between tumor and muscle often shows a dense band of chronic inflammatory cells (Figure 15.13). Blood vessel and lymphatic invasion is uncommonly seen, but when present, is usually associated with poorly differentiated tumors.

## Ultrastructure of Adenocarcinoma of Endometrium (Transmission Electron Microscopy)

The light microscopic criteria for malignancy stress the architectural relationships of the tissue components. In a somewhat analogous manner at the ultrastructural level, the intracellular relationships and profiles of the various subcellular organelles reflect the disorder of cancer. There are no general rules to diagnose malignancy from a study of a cell's ultrastructure; however, electron microscopy is of value in providing a deeper understanding of the pathologic changes in cancer.

In most malignant tumors, there is a loss of some of the ordered subcellular relationships. In *normal* endometrial epithelium, the Golgi is located on the lumenal side of the nucleus, positioned logically to produce and efficiently deliver secretory vacuoles, and only the lumenal surface of the cell has microvilli. In most *malignant* cells the Golgi apparatus, if present at all, is not in its usual location but is in a position relative to the lumen of the dysplastic glands. Quite often, the lateral borders of the malignant cells that have formed a glandular structure tend to be separated, instead of closely apposed and have many microvilli (Figure 15.14). There are resultant intercellular spaces, and possibly this is all a reflection of the striking biochemical changes that occur on the surface of most cancer cells, that is, a greater density of negative charges as a result of altered surface glycolipids and glycoproteins.[14] It has been well demonstrated that viral transformation of cells is accompanied, within several hours, by marked changes in the complex surface carbohydrates, and the ability of cancer cells to spread and metastasize is closely tied to the surface properties. Although some endometrial cancer cells may be well ordered, as in a case of clear cell adenocarcinoma reported by Rorat, Ferenczy, and Richart,[34] even they generally show some surface abnormality. In this particular case, the cells were usually closely

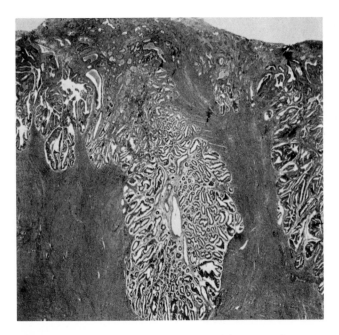

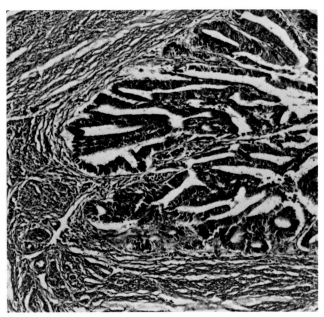

**15.11** Tongues of malignant glands with minimal stroma growing downward into myometrium.

**15.12** High-power view of well-differentiated adenocarcinoma in muscle.

apposed, had desmosomes, and had tight junctions but their lateral borders displayed microvilli projecting into slightly expanded intercellular spaces.

Other general features of malignancy are also seen in most endometrial cancers, and these include unusual nuclear outlines, with multiple infoldings and projections; more prominent nucleoli, with alterations in the pattern of condensed nucleic acids and proteins that comprise the nucleoli (Figure 15.15); a more frequent appearance of complex lysosomes, including myelin figures (Figure 15.16)[43]; and a greater proportion of free ribosomes in the cytoplasm. In addition to these features, many endometrial cancers contain large quantities of glycogen as well as lipid droplets. Both are features of endometrial epithelium in the secretory part of the normal menstrual cycle. However, surface blebs or projections of cytoplasm containing glycogen, a feature seen in normal secretory phase epithelium, is not generally seen in endometrial cancer cells. Although there is abundant rough-surfaced endoplasmic reticulum, sometimes arranged in stacks, there is generally poor development of the Golgi apparatus for packaging of secretions into vacuoles for export.[43]

In summary, the picture that emerges is that of cells, the surfaces and intracellular organelles of which are variously disordered in structure and presumably, therefore, in function. A factor that may be involved in providing an

intracellular "skeleton," and that is thought to lend subcellular order, is the presence of bundles of microtubules. These were described in normal endometrial epithelium and play a major role, in many cell types, in directing the intracellular organization of organelles, as well as attaching to the inside of the cells' plasma membranes. In endometrial cancer cells examined so far, such microtubules have not been seen. This may be a particular loss or deletion in a cancer cell that, in part, may be responsible for some of the disarray that is observed.

## Scanning Electron Microscopy of Endometrial Carcinoma

Surface characteristics of adenocarcinoma of the endometrium vary with the degree of tumor differentiation. Well-differentiated carcinomas may show focal areas of abnormal cells, whereas other fields vary only slightly from adenomatous hyperplasia. With increasing loss of differentiation, surface changes become more marked.

In well-differentiated carcinoma the surface is flat with an increased number of gland ostia. There may be considerable variation in cell size and appearance in adjoining areas as well as in the number of ciliated cells (Figures 15.17 and 15.18). The surface of the enlarged cells shows

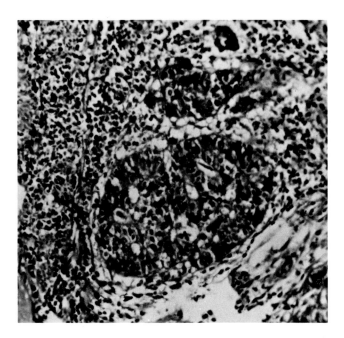

**15.13** High-power view of nests of carcinoma in muscle with surrounding chronic inflammatory infiltrate.

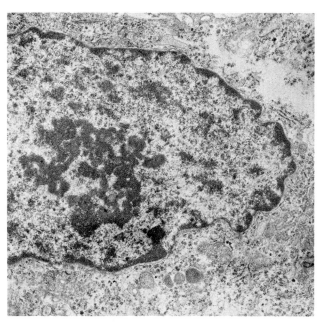

**15.15** Malignant nucleus in an endometrial adenocarcinoma containing a bizarre nucleolus. The cytoplasm contains abundant glycogen.

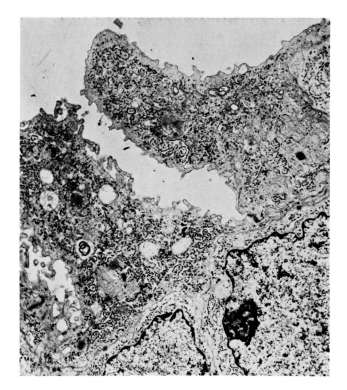

**15.14** Fine structure of endometrial carcinoma cells showing villi extending into widened intercellular spaces between the lateral borders of the cells.

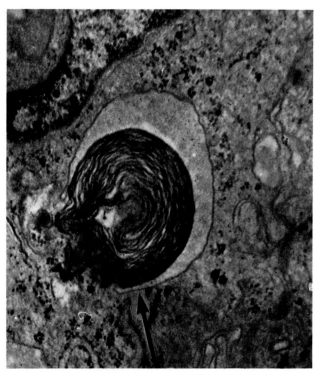

**15.16** A myelin figure (arrow) contained within the cytoplasm of a malignant epithelial cell.

**15.17** Well-differentiated adeno-carcinoma (SEM). Abnormal cells are seen in clusters. Note the absence of microvilli on the cell surface and the bulging of the luminal surface. Large cells measure up to 21 nm. in greatest dimension. ×1,029.

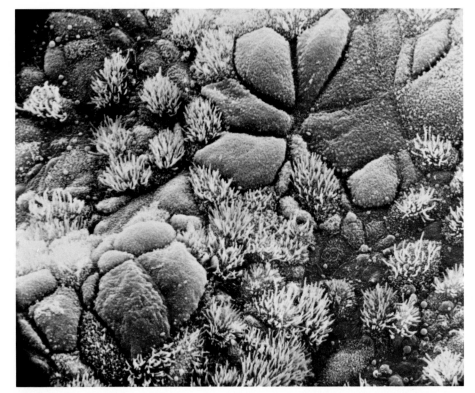

**15.18** Well-differentiated adeno-carcinoma (SEM). Marked pleomorphism of cells and marked variation in the appearance of the microvilli. ×1,936.

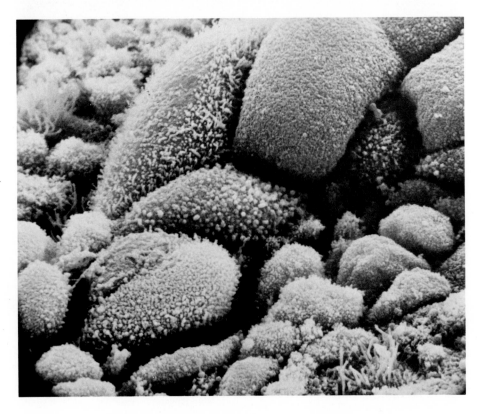

loss of surface architecture. The cells are markedly enlarged, measuring 11 by 27 $\mu$ in size. The lumenal surface appears to bulge into the endometrial cavity.

With loss of histologic differentiation, surface changes become more striking. The loss of cellular surface architecture is evident in Figure 15.19. In poorly differentiated adenocarcinoma, ciliated cells may be completely absent. Microvilli may be absent from secretory and ciliated cells, suggesting a loss of normal cell function. At greater magnification abnormalities of the cell membrane can be seen. Wrinkles may be found on the cell surface, and in some extreme cases the cell membrane may be thrown into folds or flaps (Figure 15.20). This reduplication of the cell membrane may represent a greater surface area for increased metabolic function of the tumor cells. Nilsson, Kottmeier, and Tillinger[29] noted variations and irregularities of the cell surface in adenocarcinoma cells studied with transmission election microscopy (TEM). These irregularities may correspond to the wrinkles seen on the cell surface with the scanning election microscopy (SEM). Similar changes have been described in other malignant tissues.

## Staging

Endometrial carcinoma was staged by the International Federation of Obstetricians and Gynecologists (FIGO)[8] at the Sixth World Congress in 1970,[8] as follows:

Stage I      The carcinoma is confined to the corpus.

Stage IA      The length of the uterine cavity is 8 cm or less.

Stage IB      The length of the uterine cavity is more than 8 cm.

Stage II      The carcinoma has involved the corpus and the cervix.

Stage III      The carcinoma has extended outside the uterus but not outside the true pelvis.

Stage IV      The carcinoma has extended outside the true pelvis or has obviously involved the mucosa of the bladder or rectum. A bullous edema as such does not permit allotment of a case to stage IV.

The Stage I cases should be subgrouped with regard to the histologic type of the adenocarcinoma as follows:

Grade I      Highly differentiated adenomatous carcinomas.

Grade II      Differentiated adenomatous carcinoma with partly solid areas.

Grade III      Predominantly solid or entirely undifferentiated carcinoma.

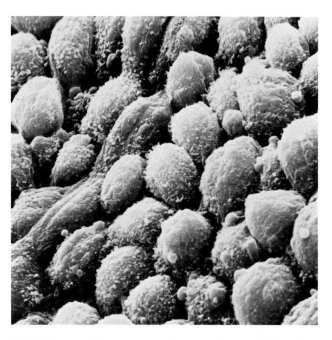

**15.19** Poorly differentiated adenocarcinoma (SEM). Although there is apparent uniformity in cell size, ciliated cells are absent and abnormal microvilli are seen on the cell surface. ×1,728.

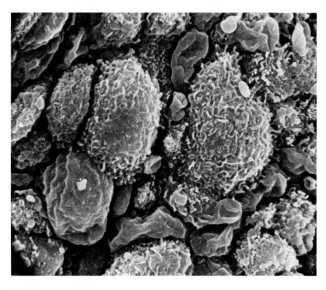

**15.20** Adenocarcinoma (SEM). Great variations in cell size and shape are apparent. Microvilli are sparse and many are fused. Note reduplication of cell membranes, giving a wrinkled appearance to the cell surface. ×2,124.

[Reprinted by permission from A. J. White, H. J. Buchsbaum, and M. A. Macasaet, Primary squamous cell carcinoma of the endometrium, *Obstet. Gynecol.* 41:912, 1973.]

An obvious fault with the above staging is that it does not take into account the depth of myometrial penetration by tumor. A patient with a lesion restricted to the endometrium has a much greater chance of surviving 5 years than a patient with deep myometrial extension. Yet both these patients would be similarly designated as stage I according to the above classification.

## Mode of Spread of Adenocarcinoma

Carcinoma of the endometrium spreads by direct extension, via lymphatics to regional nodes and through both blood vessels and lymphatics to distant sites.

Local extension can occur downward to cervix and vagina, outward to fallopian tubes and to ovaries and other peritoneal structures.[4]

Plentl and Friedman[31] reviewed patterns of lymph node metastases and found the aortic nodes to be involved most often (37.2% of patients with positive nodes). The obturator nodes were positive in 17.3% and the external and common iliac groups were the next most often involved (13.3% each). Only 9.2% had parametrial node involvement.

When extraabdominal metastases are found the lung is the commonest site, 8.3%; followed by liver in 5.9%; and bone, 3.4%.[31]

Vaginal metastases are found in 8.2% of patients and usually suggest that widespread dissemination has occurred.[31] Involvement of the lower vagina is usually hematogenous. Vaginal vault recurrence, on the other hand, probably represents local extension or implantation at the time of surgery.

## Prognosis

The management of 348 cases of adenocarcinoma and adenoacanthoma of the corpus at Presbyterian and Francis Delafield Hospitals between 1956 and 1965 was reviewed by Frick et al.[10] They found an overall relative survival of 66.1%. The correlation of 5-year survival with stage of disease was as follows: Stage Ia, 81.5%; stage Ib, 71.2%; stage II, 36.4%; stage III, 44.1%; stage IV, 3.2%. These cases were treated with surgery alone, or surgery plus radiation if the uterus was enlarged, the tumor poorly differentiated, or myometrial penetration was found.

The relationship between myometrial penetration and survival in this study was as follows: When no residual tumor was found in the uterus, the 5-year survival was 91.6%; when disease was confined to the endometrium, 79.3% survived 5 years. If superficial myometrial invasion

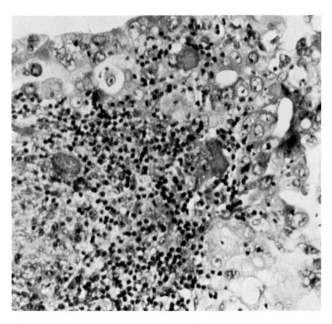

**15.21** Endometrial carcinoma following radiation therapy showing nuclear anaplasia and perinuclear cytoplasmic vacuolization.

was found, 77.2% survived 5 years. When deeper penetration, up to two-thirds of the myometrium was present, the 5-year survival was 73.3%. When deep penetration was present, involving the outer one-third of the myometrium, the 5-year survival fell to 45.2%.

Although several studies[30,33] have shown that combined preoperative radiation followed by total hysterectomy is associated with a lower incidence of vaginal vault recurrence, other investigators[24,45] report no difference in vault recurrences when compared with the results of surgical treatment alone.

Uteri examined following the administration of intracavity radium or external radiation, often show radiation effects. Surface tumor is often completely destroyed or so necrotic as to be unrecognizable. The endometrial cavity contains fibrin and necrotic debris and inflammatory cells. Nests of residual tumor, when present, frequently show evidence of mitotic arrest, with scattered cells appearing enlarged and multinucleated. The malignant glands as well as the benign, may show cytoplasmic vacuolization, often perinuclear (Figures 15.21 and 15.22). The tumor cell nuclei may be enlarged and more irregular than on the initial curettage specimen. Necrosis and inflammation are usually widespread. The stromal as well as tumor vessels show thickening and fibrosis of their walls and often endothelial proliferation.

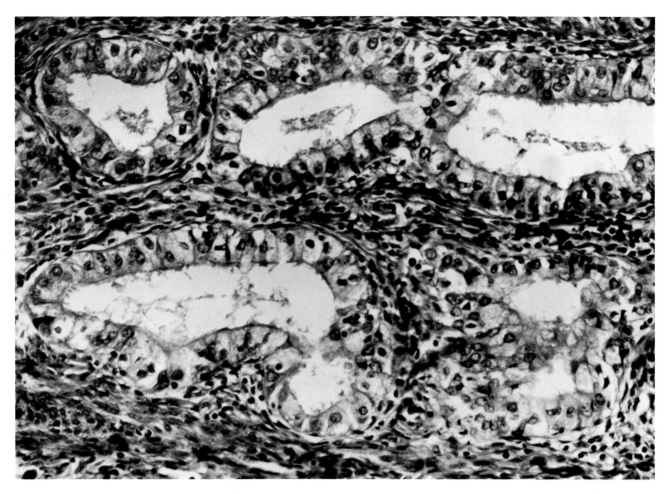

**15.22** Normal endometrial glands also show effects of radiation.

## Treatment

A simple total hysterectomy is the treatment of choice for well-differentiated endometrial carcinoma in cases in which the uterus is of normal size, and the endocervix is not involved. Enlargement of the corpus (greater than 8 cm) and the presence of a tumor whose histology suggests a poor prognosis, and endocervical extension, are generally considered indications for preoperative radiation. This serves a twofold purpose. The tumor decreases in size and so does the uterus, thus technically facilitating the surgery. It also causes thrombosis of vessels and perhaps decreases chances of spreading the tumor during surgery. Two to six weeks later total hysterectomy is performed. Bilateral salpingo-oophorectomy is mandatory because of the hormonal relationship between estrogens and endometrial carcinoma.

In those instances in which carcinoma has extended to cervix, it has been found that the disease frequently spreads as does cervical carcinoma to involve pelvic lymph nodes. Morrow[27] found in reviewing the literature that 10.6% of stage I carcinomas had pelvic node metastases as compared to 36.5% in stage II. Therefore *radical* hysterectomy is usually performed for stage II disease, including en bloc removal of cervix and corpus and a cuff of vagina, both tubes and ovaries, and bilateral pelvic lymph nodes. Kottmeier[24] reported finding endocervical involvement in 20% of 1,860 cases, whereas Davis[5] found endocervical involvement in 10.4% of his cases.

Following surgery, if examination of the uterus reveals significant myometrial penetration by tumor (usually 50% or more) or if pelvic lymph nodes contain tumor, adjuvant radiation therapy is recommended.

Patients who develop pulmonary metastases are frequently treated with progestational agents with evidence of temporary remission in some.[21,22,23] Progesterone therapy can be administered in high doses for prolonged periods with few, if any, undesirable side effects.

## Adenocanthoma of the Endometrium

### Occurrence

This morphologic variant of endometrial carcinoma consists of an adenocarcinoma with foci of benign squamous metaplasia. Liu[25] reports finding that adenocanthomas account for 10.8% of endometrial carcinomas. Silverberg et al.[38] reported a much higher figure of 29.7%, but in his review he specified that even if only a single focus of benign squamous metaplasia was found, the lesion was termed adenocathoma.

### Epidemiology

The mean age for the occurrence of adenocanthoma is 57 and similar to that for adenocarcinoma. However, Silverberg et al.[38] found that patients with adenocanthoma had a later menopause than patients with adenocarcinoma and half of the women with adenocanthoma between 50 and 59 were still menstruating.

### Gross Appearance

Grossly adenocanthomas are frequently exophytic lesions (Figure 15.23). The areas of focal squamous change are occasionally sufficiently large to be seen with the naked eye as a punctate white granular focus on the surface of the tumor. Small lesions show little necrosis or hemorrhage.

### Microscopic Appearance

Histologically acanthomas are usually well differentiated, clearly gland forming and often papillary. There is usually little cellular atypia (Figure 15.24). The nodules of squamous metaplasia appear well differentiated, with evidence of intracellular keratin production, well-defined plasma membranes, and occasionally with intercellular bridges and pearl formation (Figure 15.25).

### Prognosis

These lesions have a better 5-year survival than adenocarcinoma, probably because the associated glandular ele-

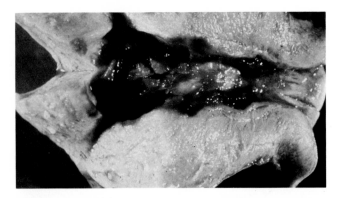

**15.23** Gross view of adenoacanthoma of the endometrium. It is exophytic and fills the endometrial cavity.

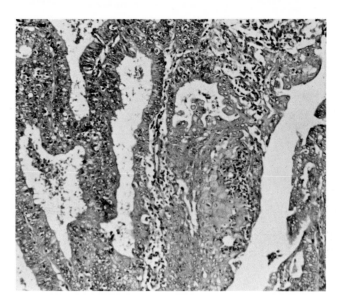

**15.24** Adenoacanthoma showing well-differentiated adenocarcinoma with focal squamous metaplasia.

ment is usually well differentiated. Silverberg et al. found, despite similar treatment regimens, the patients with adenocanthoma had a 5-year survival of 82.9% compared with 56.3% for adenocarcinoma.[38]

## Adenosquamous Carcinoma

### Occurrence

Adenosquamous carcinoma of the endometrium refers to lesions in which both the glandular and squamous elements are malignant. The term "mixed carcinoma" was

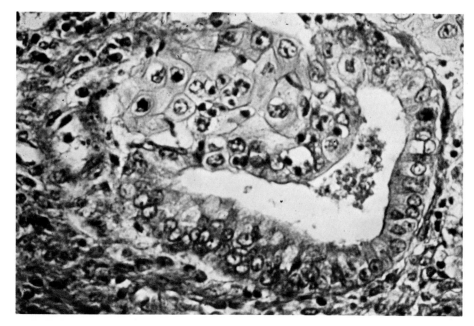

**15.25** High-power view of benign focal squamous metaplasia showing polygonal squamous cells, clearly defined plasma membranes, and intracellular keratin.

originally coined by Glucksmann and Cherry[12] to describe these lesions. These tumors have increased in frequency over the past 30 years, until currently they account for 12.6% of endometrial carcinomas.[28] These mixed malignant tumors occur in an older age group than endometrial carcinomas. In Ng's study, the mean age at detection was 65.5 years.[28]

## Gross Appearance

These lesions are often quite extensive at the time of discovery which suggests a more aggressive behavior than adenocarcinomas. Even when focal they are often associated with deep myometrial penetration (Figure 15.26). Ulceration and necrosis are common.

## Microscopic Appearance

An explanation for the aggressive biologic behavior of these tumors may be the fact that histologically the glandular component is often poorly differentiated (Figure 15.27). The glands are abortive and the lining cells show large anaplastic nuclei. Often solid sheets of undifferentiated carcinoma are present. The areas of squamous carcinoma may be scattered, small, and focal, or may be larger and confluent. The squamous cells are large and polygonal and although often showing evidence of intracellular keratin formation, rarely show intercellular bridges (Figure

15.28). Epithelial pearl formation is rare. Occasionally, sheets of large cells are so undifferentiated as to appear nonkeratinizing under light microscopy. It can then be almost impossible to determine whether such areas represent glandular or squamous cells. Electron microscopic examination of these areas is often useful in demonstrating their squamous nature. Aikawa[1] describes three such cases in which the squamous component appeared to be large cell nonkeratinizing. The fine structure revealed keratohyalin-like granules and abundant filaments which, on occasion, aggregated to form tonofilaments. Desmosomes were also present. These findings confirmed the squamous nature of the cells in question. Most of these tumors show a predominant glandular component. In one case, myo-

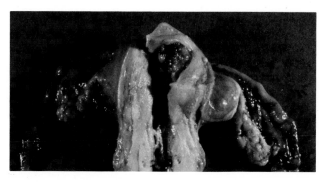

**15.26** Gross appearance of adenosquamous carcinoma showing deep myometrial invasion.

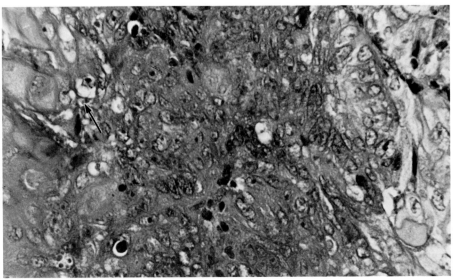

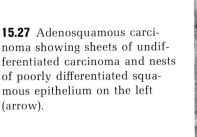

**15.27** Adenosquamous carcinoma showing sheets of undifferentiated carcinoma and nests of poorly differentiated squamous epithelium on the left (arrow).

metrial penetration was due to nests of pure squamous differentiation (Figure 15.29), although usually both elements are present. Metastases, although usually mixed, can be pure adenocarcinoma or pure squamous carcinoma.

## Prognosis

The 5-year survival is less than 20%. The finding of an adenosquamous carcinoma is considered an indication for adjuvant radiation therapy in addition to surgery because of the poor survival rates.

## Primary Squamous Cell Carcinoma of the Endometrium

Primary pure squamous cell carcinoma of the endometrium is a rare entity. Only about 16 cases have been reported in the world literature.[46] They occur in an older age group than adenocarcinoma, and squamous carcinomas are often preceded by extensive benign squamous metaplasia known as icthyosis.[19] The prognosis for these tumors is very poor. Although a history of pelvic irradiation is elicited in some of these women, an etiologic relationship has not been demonstrated. Some authors[30] find an increased incidence of fundal carcinoma following an irradiation-induced menopause, and others[3] report a low incidence. One of the problems is that long follow-up periods are required to evaluate whether radiated patients develop malignant lesions more often than controls. These data are not yet available.

## Clear Cell Carcinoma

### Occurrence

Clear cell carcinoma of the endometrium occurs as a focal change in adenocarcinoma or occasionally in pure form. They account for approximately 5% of endometrial carcinomas.

### Clinical Picture

The clinical profile of patients with clear cell carcinoma according to Silverberg and DeGiorgi[39] resembles that of patients with adenocarcinoma in that they are usually postmenopausal, have low gravidity, and tend to be hypertensive, obese, and diabetic. The clinical stage at the time of detection is somewhat more advanced than for adenocarcinoma.

### Gross and Microscopic Appearance

The gross appearance of the clear cell endometrial tumor is not distinguishable from adenocarcinoma. Histologically four basic patterns are seen; tubular, papillary, solid, and secretory. These are often admixed in a single tumor. Foci of Arias–Stella changes are often seen. Most of our cases have shown combinations of tubular or papillary with solid patterns. The tubular pattern consists of glands which are separated by a thin fibrous stroma. The lining cells have clear vacuolated cytoplasm. Some of the cells have a hobnail pattern; that is, the nucleus, which is large

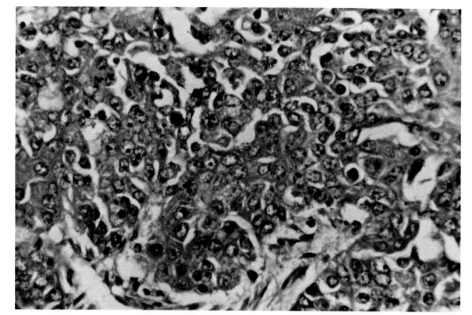

**15.28** Squamous component of adenosquamous carcinoma shows polygonal cells producing keratin. Intercellular bridges and pearl formation are lacking.

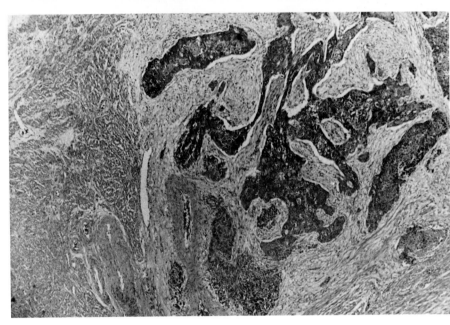

**15.29** Adenosquamous carcinoma in which the myometrium has been penetrated by nests of tumor showing pure squamous differentiation.

and hyperchromatic, is at the lumenal border of the cell, jutting prominently into the gland lumen (Figure 15.30). In the papillary form the epithelial cells line arborizing papillae of connective tissue. These cells have clear cytoplasm occasionally also showing a hobnail pattern. In the solid variety sheets of clear cells with distinct cell borders and central nuclei are present (Figure 15.31). The secretory variety is least common, consists of regular back to back

glands lined by clear cells with vesicular nuclei, and so cytologically may closely resemble secretory endometrium.

## Prognosis

In Silverberg and DeGiorgi's[39] study of 12 cases, they found the actuarial 5-year survival to be extremely poor (20.6%).[39]

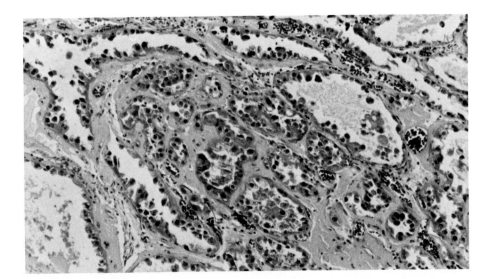

**15.30** Clear cell carcinoma, tubular variety, showing hobnail nuclei.

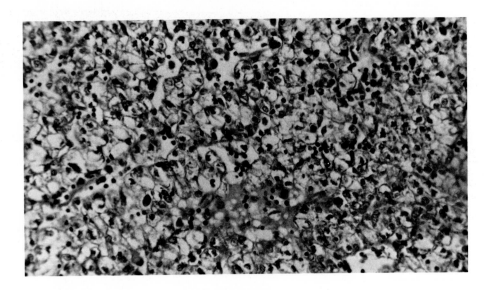

**15.31** Clear cell carcinoma. Diffuse sheets of cells with clear cytoplasm and central or eccentric nuclei, characteristic of the solid variety.

## Histochemistry

Although earlier case reports indicated that the clear cells are lipid-rich and glycogen negative,[26] more recent studies by Fechner[7] indicate occasional clear cells are alcian blue and mucicarmine positive, suggesting mucin production. Rorat *et al.*[34] found that the clear cells contain abundant intracytoplasmic and intraluminal PAS-positive material which is removed after diastase digestion. They confirmed their belief that this material is glycogen with a Best's carmine stain. They found mucicarmine and alcian blue stains to be negative.

The origin of clear cell carcinomas has long been disputed—whether of mesonephric origin as described by Schiller[36] or of Müllerian origin. Electron microscopic examination by several investigators[34,35,39] reveals the fine structure to be similar to clear cell carcinomas of ovary, vagina, and cervix, and to Arias–Stella cells. Clear cells have large nuclei with deeply indented nuclear membranes and prominent nucleoli. The plasma membranes contain microvilli projecting into slightly dilated intercellular spaces. The cytoplasmic matrix contains pools of glycogen, usually supranuclear. There is abundant granular endoplasmic reticulum appearing as parallel membranes in stacks. Golgi complexes are near the collections of glycogen. Mitochondria and free ribosomes are numerous. Based on such electron microscopic findings, these tumors are now widely accepted as derived from Müllerian anlage.

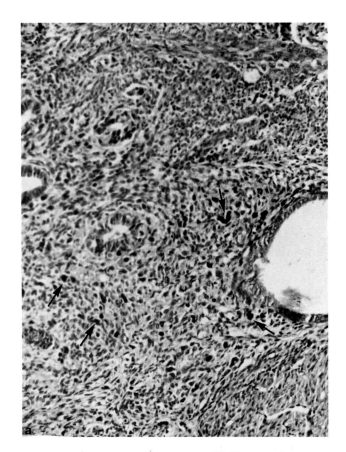
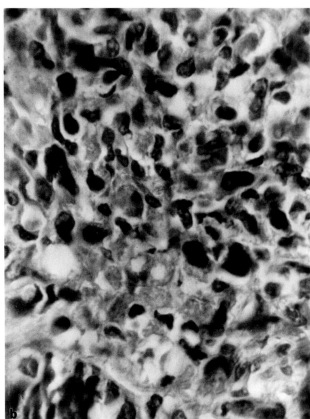

**15.32 a.** Endometrium. Metastatic cancer from breast. Tumor infiltrates seen scattered in the stroma (arrows). **b.** High-power view of tumor cells in Figure 15.31.

## Tumors Metastatic to Endometrium

Occasionally, metastatic or secondary carcinoma involves the endometrium. Carcinoma of the cervix may extend to the endometrium. When endometrioid carcinoma is present in the ovaries, and adenocarcinoma of the uterus is also found, it is difficult to determine which is primary. Scully[37] has found that one-third of patients with endometrioid carcinoma of the ovary have small adenocarcinomas of the endometrium. He believes these represent an independent primary tumor. Breast carcinoma that has metastasized to ovaries can also spread to endometrium (Figure 15.32a,b). This is not a common observation. Other tumors, such as those arising from the sigmoid colon, can involve the uterus by contiguity and infiltrate to endometrial surface. Ovarian tumors can adhere to the uterus and invade myometrium and endometrium. Lymphosarcoma (Figure 15.33), Hodgkin's disease, and leukemia can be present in endometrial stroma.[2,20,44]

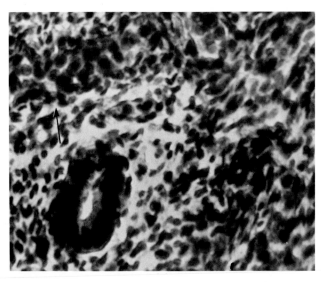

**15.33** Infiltrates of cells of lymphocytic leukemia (arrow) in the stroma of the endometrium.

# REFERENCES

1. Aikawa, M., and Ng, A. B. P. Mixed (adenosquamous) carcinoma of the endometrium. *Cancer* 31:385, 1973.

2. Blaustein, A. U., Payan, H. M., and Kish, M.: Genital stromal changes induced by malignant lymphomata and leukemia. *Obstet. Gynecol.* 20(1):112, 1962.

3. Crossen, R. J., and Crossen, H. S. Radiation therapy of uterine myoma. *JAMA* 133:593, 1947.

4. Dahle, T.: Transtubal spread of tumor cells in carcinoma of the body of the uterus. *Surg. Gynecol. Obstet.* 103:332, 1956.

5. Davis, E. W. Jr. Carcinoma of the corpus uteri. *Am. J. Obstet. Gynecol.* 88:163, 1964.

6. Factor, S. M. Papillary adenocarcinoma of the endometrium with psammoma bodies. *Arch. Pathol.* 98:201–205, 1974.

7. Fechner, R. E. Endometrium with pattern of mesonephroma. Report of a case. *Obstet. Gynecol.* 31:485, 1968.

8. F.I.G.O. News: Definitions of the different clinical stages of carcinoma of the corpus uteri to be used from January 1, 1971. Report presented by the Cancer Committee to the General Assembly of F.I.G.O. p. 176, New York, April 1, 1970.

9. Fox, H., and Sen, D. K. A controlled study of constitutional stigmata of endometrial adenocarcinoma. *Br. J. Cancer* 24:30, 1970.

10. Frick, H. C., Munnell, E. W., Richart, R. M., Berger, A. P., and Lawry, M. F. Carcinoma of the endometrium. *Am. J. Obstet. Gynecol.* 115:663, 1973.

11. Garnet, J. D. Constitutional stigmas associated with endometrial carcinoma. *Am. J. Obstet. Gynecol.* 76:11, 1958.

12. Glucksmann, A., and Cherry, C. P. Incidence, histology, and response to radiation of mixed carcinomas (adenoacanthomas) of the uterine cervix. *Cancer* 9:971, 1956.

13. Hameed, K., and Morgan, D. A. Papillary adenocarcinoma of endometrium with psammoma bodies. *Cancer* 29:1326, 1972.

14. Hakamori, S. *Tumor Lipids: Biochemistry and Metabolism.* Randell Wood, Champagne, Illinois, 1973, Vol. 18, pp. 269–284.

15. Hark, B., and Sommers, S. C. Endometrial curettage in diagnosis and therapy. *Obstet. Gynecol.* 21:636, 1963.

16. Harris, H. R. Foam cells in the stroma of carcinoma of the body of the uterus and uterine cervical polyps. *J. Clin. Pathol.* 11:19, 1958.

17. Hausknecht, R. U., and Gusberg, S. B. Estrogen metabolism in patients at high risk for endometrial carcinoma. *Am. J. Obstet. Gynecol.* 105:1161, 1969.

18. Hausknecht, R. U., and Gusberg, S. B. Estrogen metabolism in patients at high risk for endometrial carcinoma. *Am. J. Obstet. Gynecol.* 116:981, 1973.

19. Hopkin, I. D., Harlow, R. A., and Stevens, P. J. Squamous carcinoma of the body of the uterus. *Br. J. Cancer* 24:71, 1970.

20. Johnson, C. E., and Sonle, E. H. Malignant lymphoma as a gynecologic problem. *Obstet. Gynecol.* 9:149, 1957.

21. Keller, D., Kempson, R. L., Levine, G., and McLennan, C. Management of the patient with early endometrial carcinoma. *Cancer* 33:1108, 1974.

22. Kelly, R. M., and Baker, W. H. Progesterone for endometrial cancer. *New Engl. J. Med.* 264:216, 1961.

23. Kennedy, B. J. A progesterone for treatment of advanced endometrial cancer. *JAMA* 184:102, 1963.

24. Kottmeier, H. L. Carcinoma of the corpus uteri. Diagnosis and therapy. *Am. J. Obstet. Gynecol.* 78:1127, 1959.

25. Liu, C. T. A study of endometrial adenocarcinoma with emphasis on morphologically variant types. *Am. J. Clin. Pathol.* 57:562, 1972.

26. Marza, V. D., and Dobresco, D. Épithélioma de l'utérus á cellules claires. *Ann. Anat. Pathol.* 16:1023, 1940.

27. Morrow, C. P., Di Saia, P. J., and Townsend, D. E. Current management of endometrial carcinoma. *Obstet. Gynecol.* 42:399, 1973.

28. Ng, A. B. P., Reagan, J. W., Storaasli, J. P., and Wentz, W. B. Mixed adenosquamous carcinoma of the endometrium. *Am. J. Clin. Pathol.* 59:765, 1973.

29. Nilsson, O., Kottmeier, H. C., and Tillinger, K. G. Some differences in the ultrastructure of normal and cancerous human epithelium. *Acta Obstet. Gynecol. Scand.* 42:73, 1963.

30. Palmer, J. P., and Spratt, D. W. Uterus cancer after x-ray irradiation. *Obstet. Gynecol.* 72:497, 1956.

31. Plentl, A. A., Friedman, A. E. *Lymphatic System of the Female Genitalia.* Philadelphia, W. B. Saunders, p. 135, 1971.

32. Plotz, E. J., Wiener, M., Stein, A. A., and Hahn, B. D. Enzymatic activities related to steroidogenesis in postmenopausal ovaries of patients with and without endometrial carcinoma. *Am. J. Obstet. Gynecol.* 99:182, 1967.

33. Renning, E. L., and Javert, C. T. Analysis of a series of cases of carcinoma of the endometrium treated by radium and operation. *Am. J. Obstet. Gynecol.* 88:171, 1964.

34. Rorat, E., Ferenczy, A., and Richart, R. M. The ultrastructure of clear cell adenocarcinoma of endometrium. *Cancer* 33:880, 1974.

35. Roth, L. M. Clear cell adenocarcinoma of the endometrium. *Cancer* 33:990, 1974.

36. Schiller, W. Mesonephroma ovarii. *Am. J. Cancer* 35:1, 1939.

37. Scully, R. E. Recent progress in ovarian cancer. *Hum. Pathol.* 1:73, 1970.

38. Silverberg, S. G., Bolin, M. G., and DeGiorgi, L. S. Adeno-acanthoma and mixed adenosquamous carcinoma of the endometrium. *Cancer* 30:1307, 1972.

39. Silverberg, S. G., and DeGiorgi, L. S. Clear cell carcinoma of the endometrium. *Cancer* 31:1127, 1973.

40. Smith, D. C., Prentice, R., Thompson, D. J., and Herrmann, W. L. Association of exogenous estrogen and endometrial carcinoma. *New Engl. J. Med.* 293:1164, 1975.

41. Sommers, S. C., and Meissner, W. A. Endocrine abnormalities accompanying human endometrial cancer. *Cancer* 50:516, 1956.

42. Sorvani, T. E. A histochemical study of epithelial mucosubstances in endometrial and cervical adenocarcinomas with reference to normal endometrium and cervical mucosa. *Acta Pathol. Microbiol. Scand. (Suppl.)* 207:183, 1969.

43. Thrasher, T. U., and Richart, R. M. An ultrastructural comparison of endometrial adenocarcinoma and normal endometrium. *Cancer* 29:1713, 1972.

44. Walton, L. I. Lymphosarcoma of the uterus. Report of two cases. *Conn. Med. J.* 17:819, 1953.

45. Whetham, J. C. G., and Bean, J. L. M. Carcinoma of the endometrium. *Am. J. Obstet. Gynecol.* 112:339, 1972.

46. White, A. J., Buschsbaum, H. J., and Macasaet, M. A. Primary squamous cell carcinoma of the endometrium. *Obstet. Gynecol.* 41:912, 1973.

Rita Iovine Demopoulos, M.D.

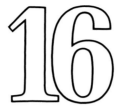

# Benign Lesions
# of the Myometrium

## Introduction

The myometrium is uniquely structured to efficiently modify its size, capacity, and contractility throughout gestation and labor. It is shaped like an upside down pear and is thick, the wall measuring approximately 2 cm on cross section, in the sexually mature female. The myometrial fibers, arranged in three layers, undergo massive hypertrophy characterized by elongation and increased diameter during pregnancy, in response to increased hormone levels. The uterus can increase its weight 10 to 20 times as it enlarges to accommodate the growing fetus. The dramatic response in terms of uterine contractility to prostaglandins $E_1$ and $F_2 \alpha$ is consistent with the presence of specific binding sites for prostaglandins in human muscle tissues[51] and is essential to its function during labor. A variety of benign pathologic conditions affect the uterine musculature and these are separately discussed.

## Leiomyomata

Leiomyomata are benign smooth muscle tumors and are by far the commonest visceral tumors in the body. Originally believed to be fibromas, the misnomer "fibroid" has come to be so widely employed that it is generally accepted as synonymous with leiomyoma.

## Epidemiology

Leiomyomata can occur at virtually any age; however, they are most common during the childbearing years and have a peak incidence from 35 to 45. They occur more often in nulliparous than multiparous females and, therefore, are more common in single than in married women. They are much more common in Blacks than in Caucasians. They are responsive to estrogen stimulation and grow rapidly during pregnancy. At times a leiomyoma not palpable before pregnancy may grow so rapidly during gestation as to be suspected of being a sarcoma.

## Clinical Picture

The signs and symptoms caused by leiomyomata depend on their number, size, and location. Myomata may be single or multiple. If they are single or small, the patient is often entirely asymptomatic. It should be kept in mind that leiomyomata are so common that they often coexist with other abnormalities and need not necessarily be responsible for the patient's symptoms. Leiomyomata can cause a wide spectrum of signs and symptoms, including abnormal bleeding, pelvic discomfort characterized by heaviness or a mass, pain, urinary frequency, stress incontinence, infertility or decreased fertility, abortion, dystocia, and pelvic inflammatory disease. In a study of 101 consecutive cases of uterine fibroids occurring in urban Blacks, Rubin and Ford[41] found that the average age of these patients was 41.8 years; 58% had menorrhagia, 26.8% had dysmenorrhea, and 63% had abdominal pain. They found no significant difference in parity between patients with or without fibroids. However, the effect of fibroids on fertility may have been obscured by the presence of chronic healed salpingitis in these patients, a variable which was not separately investigated.

Leiomyomata are found in one of three locations—submucosal, intramural, or subserosal. When they are large they may involve the whole myometrial wall. Submucosal lesions protrude into the endometrial cavity. They are often covered by thin atrophic endometrium. The increase in endometrial surface may produce menorrhagia. Compression atrophy of overlying mucosa and surface ulceration may cause metrorrhagia. Submucosal myomas may be responsible for spontaneous abortion because the anchoring site of the placenta may be too shallow. Myomata present in the lower uterine segment may interfere with the progress of labor by producing dystocia and therefore necessitate delivery by Caesarian section. Sometimes myomata are large enough to be seen protruding

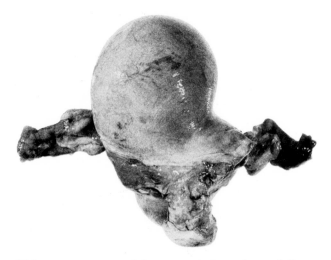

**16.1** Outer contour of the uterus is irregular and distorted by fundal and lower uterine segment myomata.

through the cervical os, which may be partially effaced and dilated. Surface ulceration and infection is common in these tumors. On occasion, submucosal leiomyomata can be diagnosed from fragments of muscle included on curettage specimens.

Intramural myomata may be asymptomatic or may produce symptoms referable to the presence of a mass, that is, pelvic discomfort or a sensation of heaviness, or bladder compression with frequency of urination. Subserosal myomata on bimanual palpation may be mistaken for ovarian tumors or other pelvic tumors. Pedunculated leiomyomata are attached by a stalk or pedicle to the myometrium. They are subject to torsion, subsequent ischemia, and infarction. Occasionally pedunculated subserosal myomata become completely separated from the uterus and are referred to as parasitic leiomyomata. These are most often found in the broad ligaments or in the cul de sac. On physical examination it may be impossible to distinguish them from ovarian tumors, bladder tumors, retroperitoneal masses, or bowel lesions.

## Gross and Microscopic Appearance

Leiomyomata often produce marked distortion and irregularity of the outer contour of the uterus (Figure 16.1). Occasionally a single myoma can produce uniform globular enlargement of the uterus and resemble adenomyosis or an intrauterine gestation (Figure 16.2). The sectioned uterus shows encapsulation of the myomata and often the presence of other myomata that may not have been previously detected (Figure 16.3). Submucosal myo-

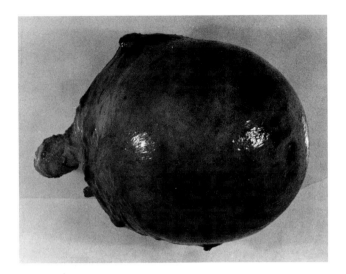

**16.2** Occasionally a single myoma may cause symmetrical globular uterine enlargement and may be mistaken for an intrauterine gestation or adenomyosis on physical examination.

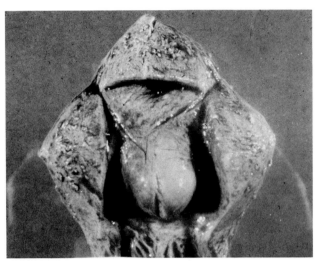

**16.4** A large submucosal leiomyoma fills the uterine cavity.

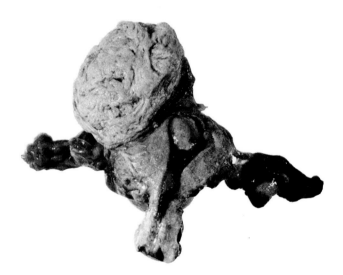

**16.3** A large fundal myoma is present in addition to intramural and submucosal myomata.

mata are covered by thin endometrium. They are usually easily distinguished from polyps because the central muscle core of myomata makes them firm and inflexible, whereas polyps are soft and pliable (Figure 16.4).

The cut surface of a leiomyoma reveals it to be a roughly spherical, solid, firm, encapsulated mass, which projects above the surrounding tissue (Figure 16.5a). On close examination, the interlacing bundles of smooth muscle form a characteristic whorled pattern. Compression of the adjacent myometrium is often evident.

Microscopic examination usually shows bundles of smooth muscle cells with delicate, spindly nuclei in wavy interlacing fascicles, with a small amount of intervening connective tissue (Figure 16.5b). Blood vessels enter through the capsule. One or several arteries derived from adjacent myometrium enter the myoma from different poles. They branch and penetrate toward the center of the myoma. The veins are located beneath the capsule and few, if any, are seen in the center of the lesion.[16]

Mast cells are relatively numerous in myometrium as compared to other viscera, and are almost as numerous in leiomyomata.[19] They can be identified only if special stains, such as alcian blue, are used.

Occasionally focal areas in a myoma show a pattern of nuclear palisading (Figure 16.6). This feature is reminiscent of neural tissue, but occasionally smooth muscle nuclei also palisade. These areas are probably not of neural origin.

Degenerative changes are often seen and are largely caused by ischemia. The tumor grows relatively faster than vessel proliferation can keep pace. Most ischemic changes tend to be centrally located in myomas because the central portions are farthest away from the arterial supply, which enters from the periphery.

Persaud and Arjoon[40] reported in a series of 298 leiomyomata that 65% of the specimens showed degenerative changes. They found hyaline degeneration to be present in 63%, myxomatous degeneration in 13%, calcification in

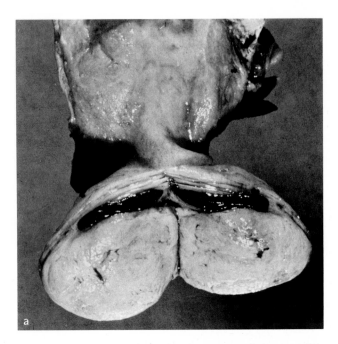
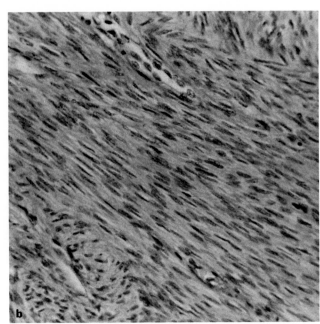

**16.5 a.** Cut section of encapsulated, submucosal leiomyoma shows interlacing bundles of smooth muscle, producing a characteristic whorled pattern and bulging on its cut surface. There is hemorrhage into the capsule. **b.** Leiomyoma showing interlacing bundles of smooth muscle with spindle nuclei without degeneration.

**16.6** Leiomyoma showing palisading of nuclei resembling neural tissue.

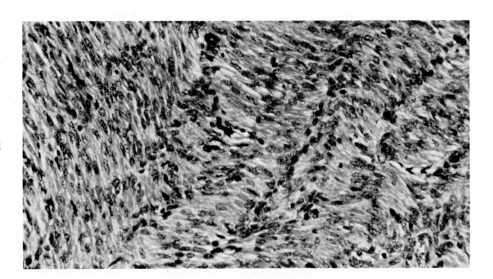

8%, mucoid degeneration in 6%, cystic degeneration in 4%, red degeneration in 3%, fatty degeneration in 3%, and sarcomatous change in 0.7%. There was no correlation between the presenting symptom and the type of degeneration present. Hyaline change causes the myoma to appear pale and homogeneous, and to be particularly firm (Figure 16.7a). Hyalinized muscle fibers are refractile, acellular, and amorphous (Figure 16.7b). Myxomatous degeneration is characterized grossly by yellowish discoloration and softening. Microscopically, areas of myxomatous change show a loose fibrillar matrix separated by pale basophilic extracellular material resembling Wharton's jelly of the umbili-

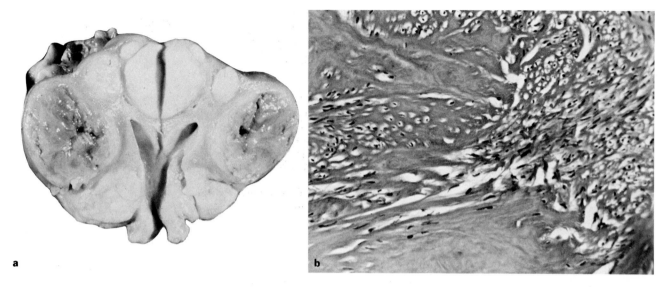

**16.7 a.** The small fundal myoma is white and homogeneous and microscopically reveals hyaline change. The lateral intramural myoma shows central necrosis and discoloration. **b.** Leiomyoma with hyalinization of muscle fibers.

**16.8** Myxomatous degeneration of a leiomyoma showing separation of muscle fibers by pale basophilic material.

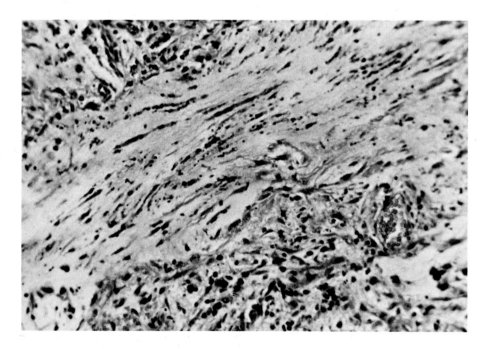

cal cord (Figure 16.8). Calcium is frequently deposited in areas of degeneration and histologically appears as irregular, dark blue granular masses (Figure 16.9). Areas of mucinous degeneration grossly appear as pale, clear mucoid foci (Figure 16.10) and, microscopically, homogeneous lakes of mucin separate muscle fibers (Figure 16.11).

Liquefaction necrosis leaves holes or spaces, where the necrotic muscle has been dissolved and removed (Figure 16.12). Such changes are singularly unimpressive microscopically, for they simply consist of clear spaces containing homogeneous pink fluid separating muscle bundles.

Red degeneration refers to the uniformly red, beefy

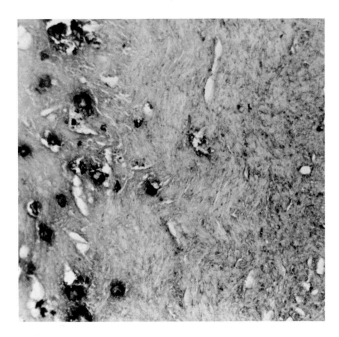

**16.9** Degenerating leiomyoma showing granular deposits of calcium.

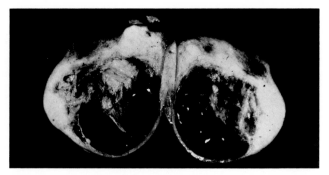

**16.10** A leiomyoma showing extensive mucinous degeneration.

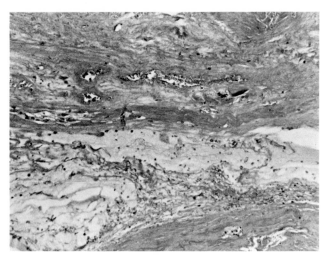

**16.11** Leiomyoma with focal mucinous degeneration.

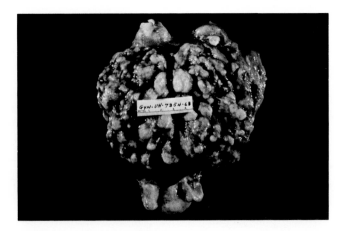

**16.12** Liquefaction necrosis involves dissolution of smooth muscle, leaving spaces between remaining muscle bundles; this is also known as cystic degeneration.

appearance of some myomas (Figure 16.13). It has been reported most often in pregnant women. However, red degeneration is by no means exclusively found in association with pregnancy. Boyd[3] describes 38 cases of red degeneration, of which 29% were associated with pregnancy. The symptomatology seems to be more severe in pregnant than in nonpregnant females. Red degeneration of a myoma may produce severe pain, often associated with fever, nausea, and vomiting. The etiology has been a source of interest since they were first described by Gebhard[20] in 1899. Faulkner[17] finds that tumors undergoing early changes of red degeneration show thin-walled arteries to be engorged with blood. Many vessels are ruptured and extravasated red blood cells are numerous throughout the muscle fibers. Swelling and edema are prominent features. He also finds that some hyaline change is always present before red degeneration occurs. He concludes, therefore, that red degeneration is caused by hemorrhagic infarction of a previously hyalinized myoma. Indeed, it seems reasonable that rapid growth of preexisting myomata during pregnancy may cause peripheral compression of veins which are located beneath the capsule. This, in turn, produces swelling, edema, engorgement, rupture of arteries, and hemolysis of red blood cells. Microscopically, the picture seen is somewhat variable, depending on the time interval between the development of

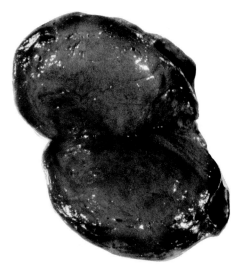

**16.13** Red degeneration is characterized by a "raw beef" color and consistency, which usually involves the entire myoma.

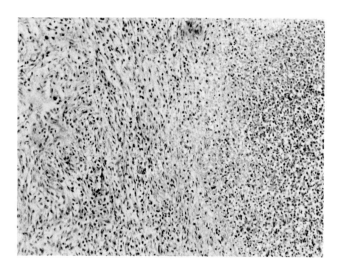

**16.14** A leiomyoma with degeneration and abscess formation.

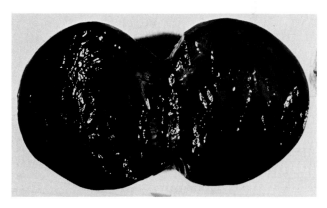

**16.15** A pedunculated subserosal leiomyoma twisted on its pedicle, resulting in massive infarction and gangrene.

symptoms and the examination of tissue. Usually there is evidence of edema, hemorrhage with extravasation and hemolysis of red cells, coagulation necrosis of muscle, and foci of hyaline change. Venous thrombosis may be present.

Fatty degeneration refers to the finding of scattered small round cells with vacuolated cytoplasm that contain stainable lipid. This fatty change is almost always co-existent with other forms of degeneration, such as hyaline and myxomatous, and this feature is useful in distinguishing fatty degeneration from benign mixed mesenchymal tumors and lipomas of the uterus.

Occasionally, foci of degeneration in leiomyomata undergo secondary infection, and abscess formation may result (Figure 16.14). We have seen one patient who presented with an abdominal fistula. On exploratory laparotomy an infected myoma was found that had become adherent to the abdominal wall, the abscessed contents of which were draining through the fistulous tract. Secondarily infected myomata can be responsible for fever, elevated white blood cell count, elevated sedimentation rate, and even septicemia.[30]

Although all the forms of degeneration so far discussed have been caused by ischemia, massive acute infarction resulting from arterial occlusion is seen most often in pedunculated leiomyomas that have undergone torsion. This may produce sudden and severe pain, often accompanied by vomiting, an elevated sedimentation rate, and in rare instances manifestations of shock. The myoma is deeply hemorrhagic, almost black in color (Figure 16.15).

It is soft and no architectural pattern can be discerned grossly. Microscopically there is marked necrosis of muscle, karyorrhexis and lysis of nuclei, and a deeply eosinophilic cytoplasm. Hemorrhage and congestion are marked.

Neoplastic change occurs rarely in leiomyomata. Leiomyosarcomas can occur as single or multifocal changes in leiomyomata, or can arise from normal myometrium unassociated with leiomyomata. This entity is described with uterine sarcomas in Chapter 17.

## Treatment

Asymptomatic myomata require no treatment as the incidence of malignant change is less than 1% and the operative mortality for hysterectomy is about the same.

These patients should be regularly examined. Myomata usually diminish in size and pose no problems following menopause.

The therapy for symptomatic leiomyomata is simple hysterectomy in women who have completed their families. This can be performed abdominally or vaginally. For women desiring children, myomectomy may be considered. However, because myomata are so often multiple, myomectomy is indicated only when preservation of the uterus for childbearing is extremely important to the patient. Myomectomy is never indicated in women over 40 years old. It should be kept in mind that the operative mortality for myomectomy is greater than hysterectomy and was reported by Te Linde et al. to be 1.9%.[49]

## Vascular Leiomyomata

These uncommon lesions are also referred to as angiomyomas. They are characterized by an increased number of blood vessels relative to the amount of smooth muscle. It is not clear whether the vessels in these lesions are proliferating as part of a neoplastic process or whether they simply represent a hyperplastic change. Vascular leiomyomata are usually submucosal in location, although they may be intramural or subserosal. The cut surface of the tumor shows increased vascularity (Figure 16.16a). Microscopic examination shows numerous small, thin-walled, well-formed blood vessels (Figure 16.16b,c). Occasionally the endothelial cells lining the vascular channels are prominent and plump.

## Clear Cell Leiomyomata

This is a rare microscopic variation in the appearance of the smooth muscle fibers of a leiomyoma that may involve

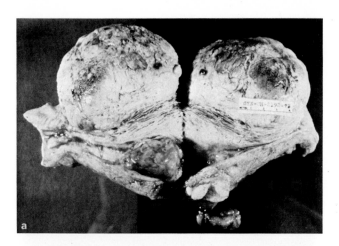

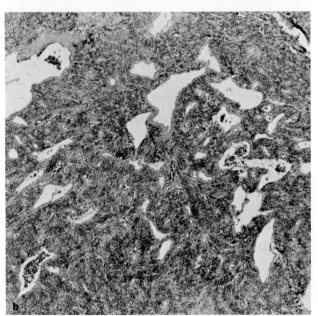
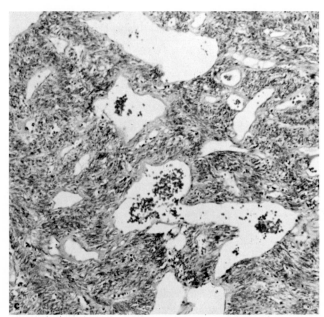

**16.16 a.** Uterus showing the cut surface of a subserosal vascular leiomyoma. It is congested and vascular. **b.** Numerous thin-walled blood vessels are seen in the parenchyma of a vascular leiomyoma. **c.** High-power view of Figure 16.16b.

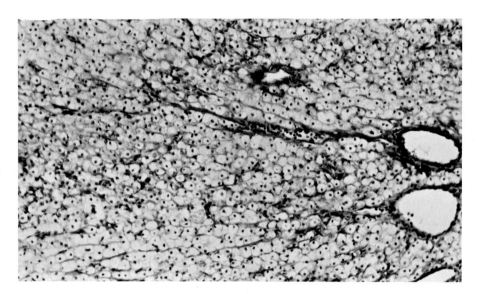

**16.17** Clear cell leiomyoma in which the muscle cells are round with central nuclei; they are epithelioid in appearance. The characteristic feature is the clarity of the cytoplasm.

the entire myoma or be a focal change. The muscle cells lose their spindle appearance and become round, with spherical central nuclei. They resemble epithelial cells. The cytoplasm is characteristically clear and vacuolated (Figure 16.17). These tumors have been referred to as leiomyoblastomata in the French literature, implying a derivation from leiomyoblasts.[9]

## Cellular Leiomyomata

This tumor is a variant of a leiomyoma characterized by increased cellularity. The spindle nuclei are closely apposed; however, they are elongated rather than plump as in many leiomyosarcomas (Figure 16.18a). The mitotic count is low [below 4 per 10 HPF (high-power field)], and little or no anaplasia is noted. The term cellular myoma should be used only descriptively and not to imply a malignant potential. These tumors have been observed to enlarge rapidly in pregnant women.

## Bizarre Leiomyomata

These smooth muscle tumors contain enlarged, bizarre hyperchromatic nuclei as well as multinucleated giant cells scattered among otherwise unremarkable smooth muscle cells. The anaplastic nuclei may appear singly and be diffusely scattered throughout the tumor (Figure 16.18b). More often, however, they aggregate focally in areas showing degenerative changes, such as hyalinization, or myxomatous change (Figure 16.18c). The intervening smooth muscle shows no increase in cellularity and has a low mitotic count. On occasion, a single tumor will show both increased cellularity and bizarre nuclei (Figure 16.18d). Such tumors can be difficult to distinguish from leiomyosarcomas. The most useful differentiating characteristic is the low mitotic count.

## Adenomyoma or Adenofibroma

This term refers to the presence of epithelial-lined glandular spaces scattered among the muscle fibers of a leiomyoma (Figure 16.19a). There may be an increase in the amount of interstitial connective tissue, in which case the term adenofibromyoma is appropriate. The glands are lined by cuboidal or columnar epithelium (Figure 16.19b). The glands may or may not be sheathed by endometrial stroma. Cullen[8] described adenomyomas in many sites other than the uterus. These include the rectovaginal septum, fallopian tube, round ligament, ovary, utero-ovarian ligament, uretosacral ligament, sigmoid flexure, rectus muscle, and umbilicus. He postulated that these benign tumors are derived from Müllerian rests.

## Intravenous Leiomyomatosis

"Intravenous leiomyomatosis" refers to the presence of well-differentiated smooth muscle in the lumina of uterine and pelvic veins. In a review of the literature prior to 1958, Marshall and Morris[35] found 17 acceptable cases of this rare lesion.

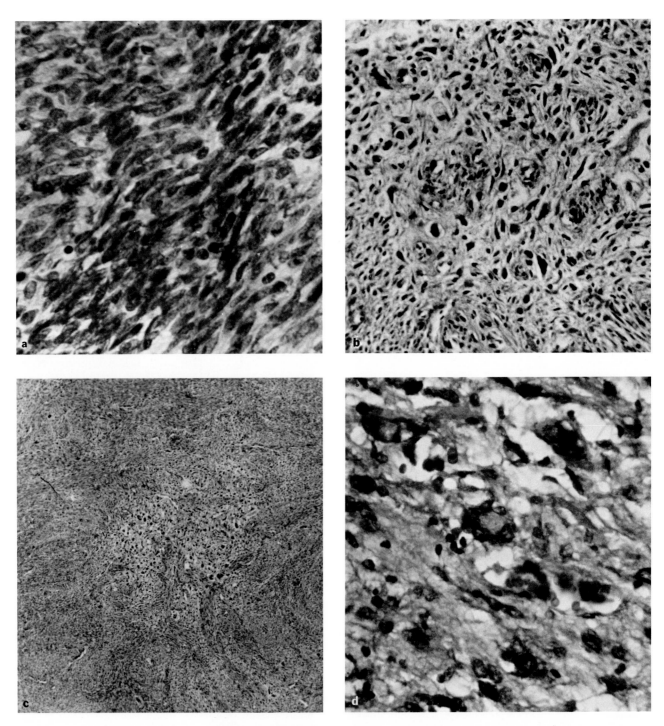

**16.18 a.** High-power view of a cellular leiomyoma. **b.** This bizarre leiomyoma from a 23-year-old pregnant female shows diffusely scattered, enlarged hyperchromatic nuclei. **c.** A bizarre leiomyoma showing central degeneration in which are clustered atypical nuclei. **d.** High-power view of a cellular bizarre leiomyoma which grew rapidly during pregnancy. The large numbers of atypical nuclei and giant cells could be worrisome; however, the mitotic count is low.

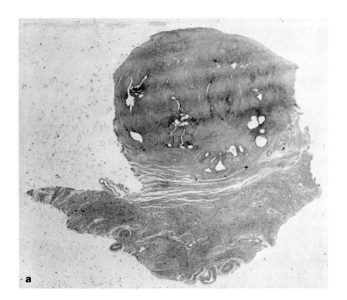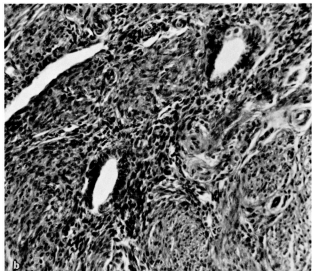

**16.19 a.** Adenomyomata are circumscribed tumors that compress the adjacent myometrium. Endometrial glands and stroma are an integral part of the tumor. **b.** Histologically, adenomyomata demonstrate endometrial glands interspersed among the fibers of a leiomyoma.

Grossly, wormlike cords of tumor can sometimes be seen extending from the myometrium into veins in the broad ligament (Figure 16.20a). Microscopically, bundles of benign appearing smooth muscle invade and distend vein walls (Figure 16.20b). There are two commonly associated histologic features; one is large plugs of lobulated smooth muscle (Figure 16.20b) and the other is the presence of thick-walled muscular vessels within the tumor (Figure 16.20c). The presence of thrombus or blood in some of the vascular channels confirms that the tumor occupies venous rather than lymphatic vessels. The presence of leiomyoma in the inferior vena cava and right atrium strengthens this view. Intravenous leiomyomatosis is almost invariably associated with uterine leiomyomas of the usual variety; only one case has failed to show coexisting extravascular leiomyomas. Harper and Scully[26] reported four cases involving vessels of the myometrium and broad ligament. They concluded that there was a continuous spectrum of cases, ranging from leiomyomas with minor intravascular extension to widespread intravenous leiomyomatosis without extravascular tumor formation. They observed that intravenous leiomyomatosis might not always be conspicuous and suggested that a careful search be made for it in cases of uterine leiomyomas; particular attention being paid to cellular and vascular leiomyomas or those that exhibit vascular thrombosis.

The two leading theories of the pathogenesis of intravenous leiomyomatosis have been those of Knauer[31] and Sitzenfrey.[45] Knauer thought that the intravascular masses arose *in situ* from the smooth muscle of the vein walls. Sitzenfrey believed they resulted from the intravenous growth of adjacent extravascular myomatous tissue. Marshall and Morris[35] offered convincing evidence supporting Knauer's view by demonstrating intravenous masses arising from vein walls and having no association with adjacent tumor tissue. Borland and Wotring similarly favored an origin from smooth muscle of vein walls,[2] despite the presence of an adjacent leiomyoma.

The differential diagnosis of intravenous leiomyomatosis includes endolymphatic stromal myosis, leiomyosarcoma, and metastasizing leiomyoma. Intravenous leiomyomatosis may not be distinguished from endolymphatic stromal myosis grossly, but microscopic examination demonstrates that the tumor cells in the former are of the smooth muscle cell type. Wilder's reticulum stain is also useful in distinguishing smooth muscle masses from endometrial stromal tissue.[18] Intravenous leiomyomatosis lacks the nuclear pleomorphism, hyperchromatism, and mitotic activity found in leiomyosarcoma, nor does it exhibit extravascular invasive properties. It is distinguished from benign metastasizing leiomyoma in that in the latter there are extravascular sites of metastasis, such as the lungs. The

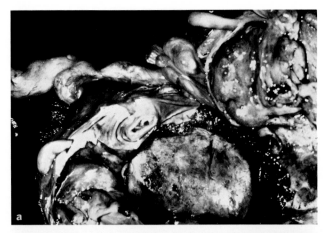

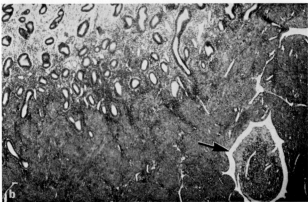

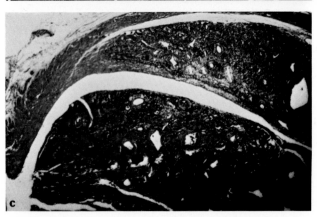

**16.20 a.** Intravenous leiomyomatosis. Cords and tongues of smooth muscle tissue are seen to invade parametrial veins. **b.** A low-power view of the endomyometrial junction, showing a vein filled with smooth muscle tissue (arrow) in a case of intravenous leiomyomatosis. The surface of the plug is covered by endothelium. **c.** High-power view of intravenous leiomyomatosis, showing vein wall distended by smooth muscle tumor. Note the lobular pattern and the numerous blood vessels within the tumor.

clinical symptoms include vaginal bleeding and, occasionally, abdominal enlargement.

## Benign Metastasizing Leiomyoma

In 1939 Steiner[46] described a fatal case of what he termed "benign metastasizing leiomyoma." He observed a patient with multiple fibroleiomyomata of the uterus with invasion of smooth muscle cells through the wall of a uterine vein forming a sessile mass projecting into the circulating blood. Pulmonary metastases consisting of well-differentiated smooth muscle nodules were present at autopsy. Additional cases have been described[1] in which patients with uterine leiomyomata have been found to have pulmonary metastases (Figure 16.21), characterized by nodules of well-differentiated, histologically benign smooth muscle (Figure 16.22). It is generally felt that this entity is closely related to intravenous leiomyomatosis. Thompson, Symmonds, and Dockerty[50] in their case report offered embolization from intravenous leiomyomatosis as the explanation for pulmonary metastases. Ariel and Trinidad[1] entertained the possibility of the primary tumor of the uterus being a leiomyosarcoma and not a benign leiomyoma. They buttress their view by referring to similar instances in which histologically benign leiomyomata have been found in the stomach wall, metastases being found at a later date that have ultimately killed the patient. They conclude that the term "benign metastasizing leiomyoma" should be abandoned and the tumor regarded as a low-grade leiomyosarcoma.

## Hemangiopericytoma

This tumor was first described by Stout and Murray[48] in 1942 as a vascular tumor composed of patent or collapsed capillaries surrounded by proliferating cells derived from the outer wall of capillaries. The cells are termed pericytes. These are not common tumors, but they have been reported in many locations in the body, including the uterus.

Grossly, the tumor has no characteristics that distinguish it. They tend to be fleshy and gray, tan, or yellow, often with blends of all three. They range in size from 1 to 10 cm in diameter and they may be submucosal, intramural, or subserosal, just as the common leiomyoma. They have been found in the cervix and in the broad ligament. Microscopically (Figure 16.23a,b), they are made up of inconspicuous capillaries and venules and most of the cells are of the pericytic type. They are uniform and monotonous in appearance. Reticulum defines the capillaries (Fig-

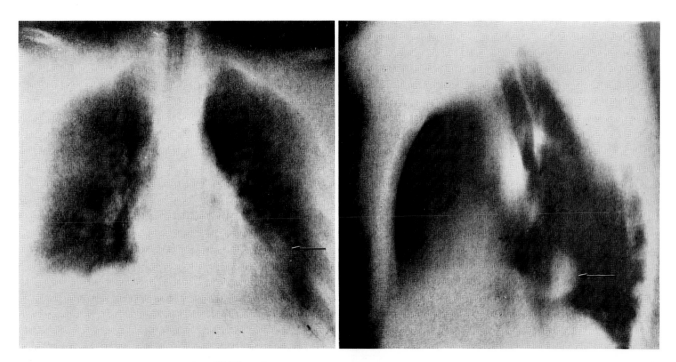

**16.21** Pulmonary metastases (arrows) from benign metastasizing leiomyoma.
[Reprinted by permission from I. M. Ariel, *Amer. J. Obstet. Gynecol.*]

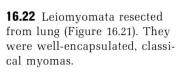

**16.22** Leiomyomata resected from lung (Figure 16.21). They were well-encapsulated, classical myomas.

[Reprinted by permission from I. M. Ariel and S. Trinidad, Pulmonary metastases from a uterine "leiomyoma," *Amer. J. Obstet. Gynecol. 94:*110, 1966.]

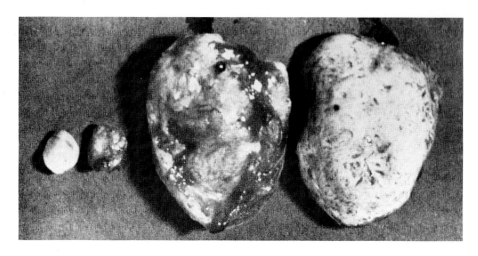

ure 16.23c), surrounds clusters of cells, and forms a mosaic pattern by surrounding individual cells.[21] They should be distinguished from cellular leiomyoma, endometrial stromal sarcoma, leiomyosarcoma, and angiosarcoma. Although the tumor does not disencapsulate as a myoma does, it has well-defined borders. This is usually not the case with the sarcomas. The relationship of the tumor cells to capillary endothelium distinguishes it from endometrial

stromal sarcoma and cellular leiomyoma. Stout[47] reviewed 25 cases and found that six had recurred or metastasized. None of these cases had arisen in the uterus and, to date, there is no known case of malignant hemangiopericytoma of the uterus. Greene *et al.*[25] and Greene and Gerbie[24] followed 12 cases of hemangiopericytoma of the uterus from 2 to 18 years postsurgery, and none showed any evidence of recurrence. A thirteenth case in his series died

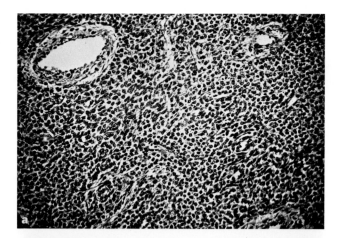

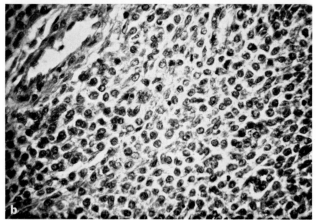

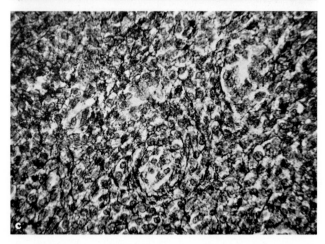

**16.23 a.** Low-power view of a hemangiopericytoma. Inconspicuous capillaries are surrounded by a uniform mass of pericytes. **b.** High-power view of a hemangiopericytoma, showing monotonous pericytes having well-defined nuclei and less well-defined cytoplasm. **c.** Hemangiopericytoma. Reticulum stain showing nests of tumor cells surrounded by reticulum.

of an unrelated malignancy. Enzinger and Smith[14] found recurrence in cases in which there were four mitoses per 10 HPF, foci of necrosis, and hemorrhage.

The clinical presentation is usually one of an abdominal mass or abnormal uterine bleeding. The diagnosis is only made following microscopic study.

# Adenomyosis

This lesion is also referred to as endometriosis interna and refers to the presence of endometrial glands and stroma lying within the myometrium. Because there is no basement membrane separating the endometrium and the myometrium and because glands may dip into the myometrium, there is a need to define what constitutes adenomyosis. It has been variously defined as the presence of endometrial mucosa, one lower power field or more beneath the endomyometrial junction,[4,38,44] or greater than one high power field beneath this junction. The former has become widely adopted and corresponds to a depth of at least 2 to 3 mm below the level of the endomyometrium.

## Clinical Data

Adenomyosis was first described by Rokitansky in 1860 and was correlated with clinical symptomatology by Cullen[7] in 1908. There have been through the years, conflicting reports concerning the clinical significance of adenomyosis. It is a common incidental finding at autopsy. Molitor[36] found adenomyosis in only 8.8% of 281 consecutive hysterectomies. He felt that adenomyosis entirely explained or contributed to the patients' symptoms in 71% of cases and was only considered in the preoperative diagnosis in 23% of cases. Hunter *et al.*[28] reported an incidence of 27.8% in the surgical specimens they studied.

The symptom triad suggesting adenomyosis is progressive, uniform enlargement of the uterus, accompanied by dysfunctional uterine bleeding, and dysmenorrhea. Emge[13] stressed that the uterine bleeding was chronic and unresponsive to hormone therapy or curettage. It usually begins in the late thirties or early forties and persists, often increasing in severity, up to the climacteric. The explanations offered for the abnormal bleeding include increasing size of the uterine cavity and endometrial surface caused by myometrial hyperplasia, coexisting endometrial hyperplasia, and loss of myometrial contractility associated with venous engorgement. The dysmenorrhea has been explained on the basis of an endocrine response of the

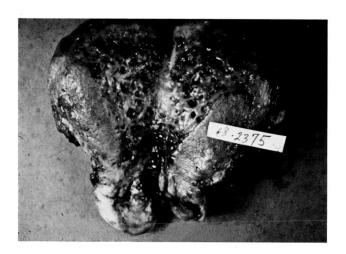

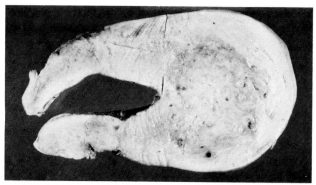

**16.25** Fundal adenomyosis showing smooth muscle hyperplasia.

**16.24** Extensive diffuse adenomyosis causing symmetrical globular enlargement of the uterine fundus, as well as thickening of the uterine walls. The dark-staining, spherical areas represent ectopic endometrium.

ectopic islands of mucosa producing congestion, bleeding, pressure, and rigidity of the myometrium. Because only about one-third of cases show hormonal responsiveness in the adenomyosis, only a minority of patients would be expected to develop dysmenorrhea. Pressure symptoms on the urinary bladder and rectum are caused by the uterine enlargement and compression of adjacent viscera. Emge[13] reported that 60 to 70% of patients with adenomyosis developed menorrhagia; 25 to 40% had dysmenorrhea, and 30% were found on curettage to have endometrial hyperplasia.

## Gross Appearance

Adenomyosis usually causes diffuse, symmetrical, globular enlargement of the fundus of the uterus (Figure 16.24). Less often, adenomyosis is focal and the uterine enlargement is then asymmetrical. On sectioning, areas of adenomyosis are diffuse and nonencapsulated and blend with adjacent myometrium (Figure 16.25). This distinguishes adenomyosis from adenomyomata, which are discrete and encapsulated tumor masses that compress adjacent tissues. The presence of endometrial mucosa in the myometrium is invariably associated with hyperplasia of adjacent smooth muscle, causing focal thickening of the uterine wall. A distinguishing gross feature is the spongy appearance of the muscle in adenomyosis caused by the cystlike spaces lined by endometrial glandular epithelium (Figure 16.26).

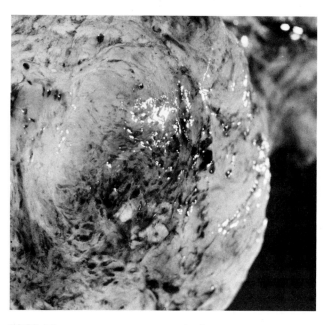

**16.26** The spongy appearance of adenomyosis is caused by cyst-like spaces consisting of endometrial glands scattered among the myometrial muscle. Concomitant smooth muscle hyperplasia is striking.

## Microscopic Appearance

Endometrial glands and stroma are found in the myometrium. The foci of displaced mucosa may be single or numerous and may be superficial or deep, or extend through the myometrium to the serosa. Usually, the glands are inactive and the stroma is quite dense, showing no evidence of functional response (Figure 16.27). Hypertrophy of adjacent smooth muscle is evident (Figure 16.28). Molitor[36] found that 33% of his cases showed

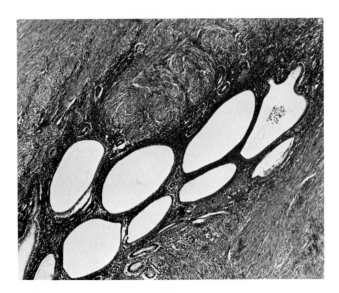

**16.27** Adenomyosis showing inactive glands and dense stroma without evidence of functional activity.

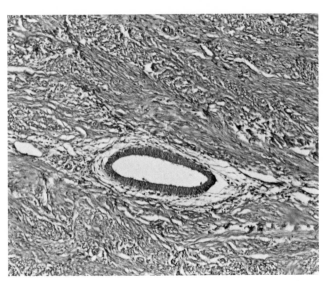

**16.28** Smooth muscle hyperplasia always accompanies, to a greater or lesser degree, areas of adenomyosis.

functional activity. In this group the mucosa may be proliferative, secretory, or menstrual, and is often consistent in appearance with surface endometrium. Decidual change may be present in adenomyosis if pregnancy exists or, on occasion, in response to progestins. We have, on occasion, found menstrual changes in adenomyosis of young patients complaining of severe dysmenorrhea (Figure 16.29). In patients with adenomyosis and endometrial hyperplasia, 44% were found to have hyperplastic changes in the ectopic endometrium[34] (Figure 16.30).

## Histogenesis

Cullen's[7] original postulate that adenomyosis represents a downward growth of basal endometrium has become generally accepted. In 1927 von Burg demonstrated the continuity between adenomyosis and surface endometrium by examining multiple serial sections. Although the mechanism is agreed upon, the underlying cause remains speculative. One of the theories postulated includes a hereditary predisposition and is supported by several cases of adenomyosis occurring in mothers and daughters, twins, and triplets. It is further supported by the finding of cases of adenomyosis in infants and children. Pappas[39] and Eckert[12] support the idea that trauma and repeated deep curettage are responsible. Prolonged unopposed estrogen may be related to the development of adenomyosis, but convincing experimental evidence has yet to be presented.

The invasion of myometrium by endometrial glands and stroma fulfills one of the criteria for malignancy. Yet the behavior of this lesion is almost invariably benign. This suggests that our understanding of factors regulating the growth potential of normal tissues is poor, and future studies in this area may shed light on the underlying etiology of adenomyosis.

## Adenomyosis and Associated Conditions

It is of some importance to determine the spectrum of conditions associated with adenomyosis as a clue to understanding its pathophysiology.

### Pregnancy

Sandberg and Cohn[43] studied the occurrence of adenomyosis in pregnancy. They examined 151 consecutive Caesarian hysterectomy specimens from clinic and private patients. They defined adenomyosis as the presence of uterine mucosa greater than one low-power field below the endomyometrial junction. Of 151 uteri examined, 27 were found to have adenomyosis, an incidence of 17%. Of the 27 uteri with adenomyosis, seven showed evidence of hormonal response in the form of decidual change.

Adenomyosis is more often found in the uteri of multiparous than nulliparous women. There are case reports of uterine rupture, postpartum hemorrhage, and uterine

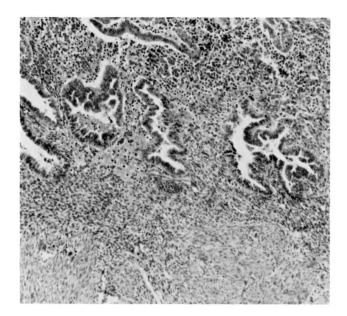

**16.29** Adenomyosis showing changes of premenstrual endometrium, as did the surface endometrium, namely, stromal hemorrhage, diffuse infiltration by granulocytes, and exhausted secretory glands.

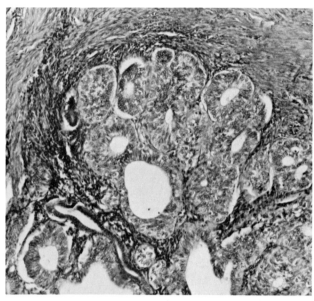

**16.30** Adenomyosis showing severe atypical adenomatous hyperplasia, as did a portion of the surface endometrium.

atony associated with adenomyosis, but it is difficult to be certain how significant adenomyosis has been in these cases.

### Adenomyosis, endometriosis, and hyperplasia

Adenomyosis may coexist with pelvic endometriosis, endometrial hyperplasia, or both. The endometrium in adenomyosis may be hyperplastic (Figure 16.30). Novak and DeLima[37] studied the relationship between adenomyosis, pelvic endometriosis, and uterine hyperplasia. In 243 cases of adenomyosis and endometriosis, they found adenomyosis alone in 92 cases, endometriosis alone in 102, and 42 cases with both lesions. Therefore, 23% had coexisting adenomyosis and endometriosis. This high figure suggests a possible common etiology, perhaps hormonal. They found that of 92 patients with adenomyosis, 36% also had endometrial hyperplasia; none of the patients with endometrial hyperplasia had evidence of functioning ectopic endometrium. Eighteen cases of adenomyosis without endometrial hyperplasia (surface) showed hyperplasia in the ectopic endometrium. It is suggested in Novak's paper that adenomyosis is due to downgrowth of basal endometrium and as such is composed of immature cells which respond only to estrogen and not to progester-

one. Since overgrowth of the basalis is a feature of endometrial hyperplasia, as well as of adenomyosis, an association between the two might be expected.

### Adenomyosis and endometrial carcinoma

Giammalvo and Kaplan[22] found that of 120 cases of endometrial carcinoma, 40 (33%) had coexisting adenomyosis, whereas only 18% of a control group, matched for age but without carcinoma, were found to have adenomyosis, a statistically significant difference. Marcus[34] also showed not only that adenomyosis is more likely to be present in association with endometrial carcinoma (60%), than without (39%), but that the adenomyosis is more extensive in uteri with carcinoma. He concurs that the common denominator may be hormonal.

Adenocarcinoma arising in adenomyosis has been reported.[6,11,23] The criteria for making this diagnosis are that the surface endometrium be free of tumor and the carcinoma confined to the area of adenomyosis.

In summary, there is evidence suggesting that adenomyosis and related conditions, including endometriosis, endometrial hyperplasia, and endometrial carcinoma, may have a related etiology and that hormones, particularly estrogen, may be involved.

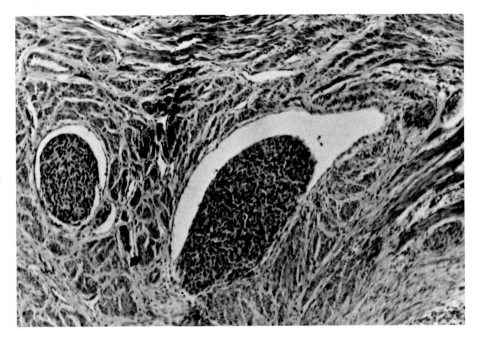

**16.31** Endolymphatic stromal meiosis depicts clumps of endometrial stroma within lymphatic channels of the myometrium.

## Endolymphatic Stromal Myosis

This uncommon entity, also known as benign stromatosis, refers to the presence of endometrial stroma within the myometrium, unassociated with endometrial glands. The downgrowth of endometrial stroma often occurs along and within lymphatic channels. This lesion can cause an area of diffuse, poorly defined thickening of the wall of the uterus or can produce a discrete tumor known as a stromal nodule. There is no associated myometrial hypertrophy, as there is in adenomyosis. Microscopically, small, closely packed clumps of endometrial stroma are seen within lymphatic channels of the myometrium (Figure 16.31). Few or no mitoses are present. Endometrial stromal myosis is the benign counterpart of a continuous spectrum of lesions, which at the other extreme is represented by the highly malignant stromal sarcoma; this entity is discussed in Chapter 17.

## Benign Mesodermal Tumors

These uncommon myometrial tumors contain a variety of tissues derived from mesoderm, including adipose tissue, smooth muscle, connective tissue, and blood vessels in varying proportions. These lesions can be named according to the predominant tissues present, such as myolipoma, fibromyolipoma, or angiomyolipoma, and so forth, or can more simply be designated as benign mixed mesodermal tumors. When these tumors are composed almost purely of adipose tissue they are termed lipomas. The presence of fat, a tissue not indigenous to the uterus, has led to considerable speculation concerning its origin in these tumors. Some of the theories include misplaced embryonic fat cells,[27] metaplasia of muscle cells to fat cells,[29] metaplasia of connective tissue into fat,[33] and fatty infiltration or degeneration.[5] The finding of proliferating dysplastic blood vessels in a significant proportion of these tumors[10] suggests that they represent a form of hamartoma, derived from an undifferentiated mesenchymal cell. Such a cell could differentiate into adipose tissue, as well as muscle, connective tissue, and blood vessels, and could well explain the various components of these tumors.

Clinically, these tumors occur over a wide age range, 20 to 80 years, but the average age is in the fifth decade. Pure lipomas usually occur in the sixth or seventh decades. The commonest presenting symptom is abnormal uterine bleeding; the patient may be otherwise asymptomatic or may have signs and symptoms associated with leiomyomata. Because these tumors are often coexistent with leiomyomata, it may be difficult or impossible to determine which tumor is causing symptoms.

Mesodermal tumors vary in size from a few millimeters to many centimeters in diameter. They can be submucosal,

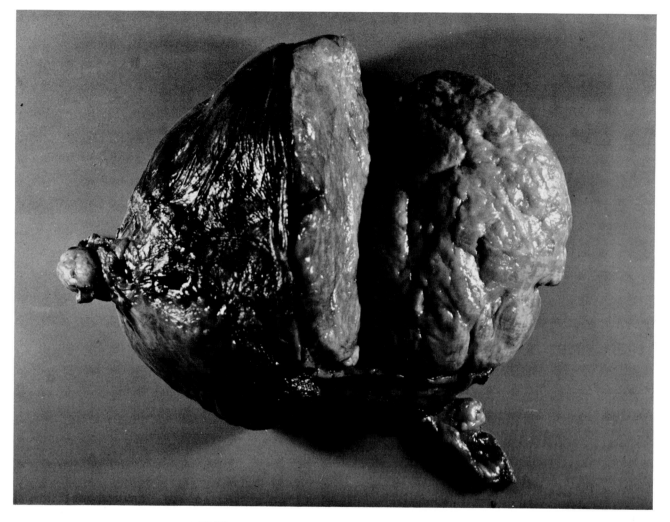

**16.32** Gross view of a lipomatous tumor of the uterus, whose pale, tan-yellow, greasy appearance suggests the presence of adipose tissue.

intramural, subserosal, or parasitic. These tumors resemble leiomyomas in that they are discrete and encapsulated. However, on section, depending upon the amount of adipose tissue, they vary from pale tan to yellow; they may be quite soft and greasy if much fat is present, and may project above the capsule (Figure 16.32). Microscopically, these tumors vary greatly from one tumor to another as well as in different portions of a given tumor. They may consist largely of mature adipose tissue and connective tissue in one area, as in Figure 16.33, whorls of smooth muscle in another (Figure 16.34), and closely packed atypical blood vessels in still others (Figure 16.35).

The clinical importance of these tumors lies in the fact

that because of their soft, yellow, sometimes rather homogeneous appearance, they can be mistaken grossly for leiomyosarcoma.

## Lymphangioma

These rare, small, asymptomatic tumors are found in various parts of the male and female genital tract in proximity to the pelvic peritoneum. They have been called by a variety of names, including adenofibroma, endothelioma, adenomatoid tumor, and mesothelioma. Evans[15] described such a tumor, demonstrated continuity with

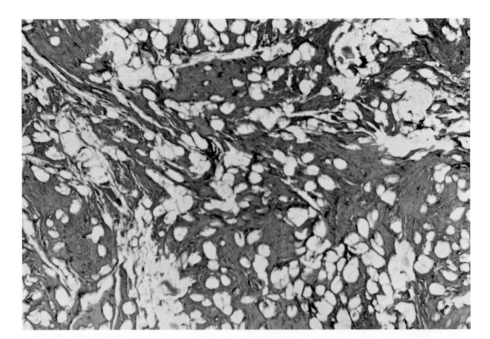

**16.33** Benign mixed mesodermal tumor showing a predominance of adipose tissue and connective tissue in this area.

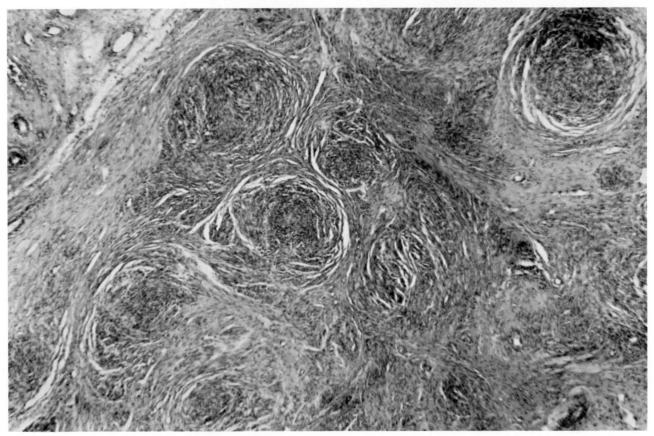

**16.34** Benign mixed mesodermal tumor containing whorls of smooth muscle in a focal area.

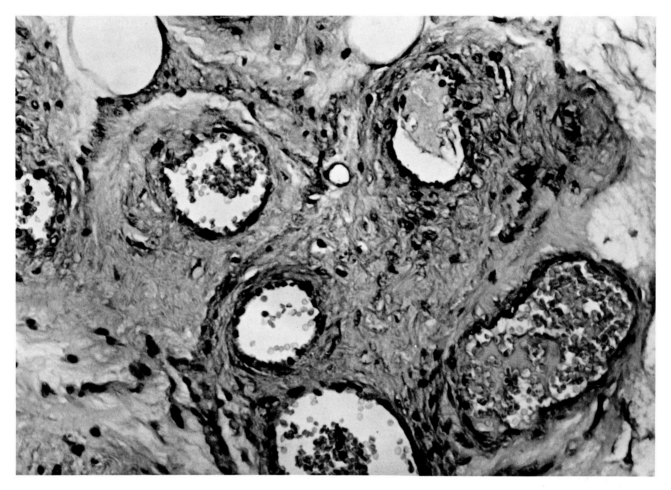

**16.35** Atypical blood vessels in a benign mixed mesodermal tumor of the uterus. The vessels have prominent endothelium and thick, fibrous, partially hyalinized walls.

serosal mesothelium, and called it a mesothelioma. The origin of these tumors remains in dispute, whether mesothelial, epithelial, or endothelial. Laufe[32] described a tumor histologically resembling those previously called mesotheliomas, but because this tumor was located largely within the wall of the fallopian tube and showed no continuity with peritoneal mesothelium, he proposes these tumors be considered lymphangiomas and postulates that they arise from submesothelial lymphatics.

Recently an electron microscopic study of these tumors has shown a resemblance to the fine structure of normal peritoneal mesothelium, favoring an origin from this structure.[42]

The tumors are small, nonencapsulated nodules usually found incidentally at surgery. They may be located on the serosal surface of the uterus or elsewhere in the pelvis. Microscopically they consist of small, closely packed, or large, widely dilated channels, lined by prominent cells separated by a small amount of intervening connective tissue (Figure 16.36a,b). They are invariably benign.

## Plexiform Tumorlets

These rare benign tumors are usually found just beneath the endomyometrial junction. Histologically, they consist of a nodule of interlacing cords of cells, having round central nuclei and foamy cytoplasm separated by a small amount of delicate connective tissue. They are usually multicentric and the cell of origin is not known.

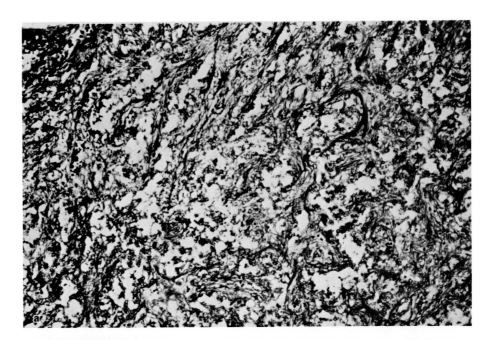

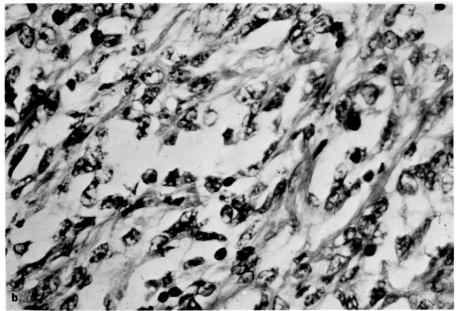

**16.36** Low- (**a**) and (**b**) high-power views of a lymphangioma or mesothelioma, characterized by dilated channels, lined by prominent cells, and separated by delicate connective tissue.

# REFERENCES

1. Ariel, I. M., and Trinidad, S. Pulmonary metastases from a uterine "leiomyoma." *Am. J. Obstet. Gynecol.* 94:110, 1966.

2. Borland, D. S., and Wotring, J. W. Intravenous leiomyomatosis of uterine and broad ligament. *Am. J. Clin. Pathol.* 42:182, 1964.

3. Boyd, W. *Textbook of Pathology, The Female Reproductive System.* Philadelphia, Lea & Febiger, 1961, Ch. 33, p. 906.

4. Brewer, J. I. *Textbook of Gynecology. Adenomyosis.* Baltimore, Williams & Wilkins, 1953, p. 200.

5. Bride, J. W. A large fatty tumor of the uterus. *J. Obstet. Gynaecol. Br. Emp.* 36:83, 1929.

6. Coleman, H. I., and Rosenthal, A. H. Carcinoma developing in areas of adenomyosis. *Obstet. Gynecol.* 14:342, 1959.

7. Cullen, T. S. *Adenomyoma of the Uterus*. Philadelphia, W. B. Saunders, 1908.

8. Cullen, T. S. The distribution of adenomyomas containing uterine mucosa. *Arch. Surg. 1*:215, 1920.

9. DeBrux, J., Ancla, M., and Bonnenfant, J. L. Leiomyoblastomes uterins (tumeurs myoides de l'uterus). *Ann. d'Anat. Pathol. 14*:107, 1969.

10. Demopoulos, R. I., Denarvaez, F., and Kaji, V. Benign mixed mesodermal tumors of the uterus. *Am. J. Clin. Pathol. 60*:377, 1973.

11. Dockerty, M. B. Malignancy complicating endometriosis—pathologic features in 9 cases. *Am. J. Obstet. Gynecol. 83*:175, 1962.

12. Eckert, J. Clinical problems of endometriosis. *Zentralbl. Gynekol. 79*:468, 1957.

13. Emge, L. A. The elusive adenomyosis of the uterus. *Am. J. Obstet. Gynecol. 83*:1541, 1962.

14. Enzinger, F. M., and Smith, B. H. Hemangiopericytoma: Analysis of 106 cases. *Hum. Pathol. 7*:61, 1976.

15. Evans, N. J. Mesothelioma of the epididymis and tunica vaginalis. *J. Urol. 50*:249, 1943.

16. Faulkner, R. L. The blood vessels of the myomatous uterus. *Am. J. Obstet. Gynecol. 47*:185, 1944.

17. Faulkner, R. L. Red degeneration of uterine myomas. *Am. J. Obstet. Gynecol. 53*:474, 1947.

18. Fienberg, R. Endometrial sarcoma. *Arch. Pathol. 29*:800, 1940.

19. Fox, J. E., and Abell, M. R. Mast cells in uterine myometrium and leiomyomatous neoplasms. *Am. J. Obstet. Gynecol. 91*:413, 1965.

20. Gebhard, C. *Veit's Handbuch der Gynakol. 2*:439, 1899.

21. Gerbie, A. B., Hirsch, M. R., and Greene, R. R. Vascular tumors of the female genital tract. *Obstet. Gynecol. 6*:499, 1955.

22. Giammalvo, J. T., and Kaplan, K. The incidence of endometriosis interna in 120 cases of carcinoma of the endometrium. *Am. J. Obstet. Gynecol. 75*:161, 1958.

23. Greene, J. W., Jr. Carcinoma arising in adenomyosis associated with a feminizing mesenchymoma of the broad ligament—a case report. *Am. J. Obstet. Gynecol. 81*:272, 1961.

24. Greene, R. R., and Gerbie, A. B. Hemangiopericytoma of the uterus. *Obstet. Gynecol. 3*:150, 1954.

25. Greene, R. R., Gerbie, A. B., Gerbie, M. V., and Eckman, T. R. Hemangiopericytomas of the uterus. *Am. J. Obstet. Gynecol. 106*:1020, 1970.

26. Harper, R. S., and Scully, R. E. Intravenous leiomyomatosis of the uterus. *Obstet. Gynecol. 18*:519, 1961.

27. Henriksen, E. Lipoma of the uterus. Report of three cases. *West. J. Surg. 60*:609, 1952.

28. Hunter, W. C., Smith, L. L., and Reiner, W. C. Uterine adenomyosis. *Am. J. Obstet. Gynecol. 53*:663, 1947.

29. Jacobson. Examen anatomique d'un lipo-fibrome de l'uterus. *Ann. Gynecol. Obstet. 58*:259, 1902.

30. Kaufmann, B. M., Cooper, J. M., and Cookson, P. *Clostridium perfringens* septicemia complicating degenerating uterine leiomyomas. *Am. J. Obstet. Gynecol. 118*:877, 1974.

31. Knauer, E. *Beitr. Geburtshilfe u. Gynakol. 1*:695, 1903; Cited by Marshall and Morris, reference 35.

32. Laufe, L. E. Lymphangiomas of the genital tract. *Am. J. Obstet. Gynecol. 68*:722, 1954.

33. Ley, G. Lipomatosis of a fibromyoma of the corpus uteri. *J. Obstet. Gynaecol. Br. Emp. 25*:42, 1914.

34. Marcus, C. C. Relationship of adenomyosis uteri to endometrial hyperplasia and endometrial carcinoma. *Am. J. Obstet. Gynecol. 82*:408, 1961.

35. Marshall, J. F., and Morris, D. S. Intravenous leiomyomatosis of the uterus and pelvis. *Ann. Surg. 149*:126, 1959.

36. Molitor, J. J. Adenomyosis: A clinical and pathologic appraisal. *Am. J. Obstet. Gynecol. 110*:275, 1971.

37. Novak, E. and DeLima, O. A. A correlative study of adenomyosis and pelvic endometriosis with special reference to the hormonal reaction of ectopic endometrium. *Am. J. Obstet. Gynecol. 56*:634, 1948.

38. Novak, E. R., and Woodruff, J. D. *Gynecologic and Obstetric Pathology*. 7th ed. Philadelphia, London and Toronto, W. B. Saunders, 1974, pp. 261–271.

39. Pappas, H. J. Endometrial adhesions and endometriosis. *Obstet. Gynecol. 13*:714, 1959.

40. Persaud, V., and Arjoon, P. D. Uterine leiomyoma. *Obstet. Gynecol. 35*:432, 1970.

41. Rubin, A., and Ford, J. A. Uterine fibromyomata in urban blacks. *S. Afr. Med. J. 48*:2060, 1974.

42. Salazar, H., Kanbour, A., and Burgess, F. Ultrastructure and observations on the histogenesis of mesotheliomas "adenomatoid tumors" of the female genital tract. *Cancer 29*:141, 1972.

43. Sandberg, E. C., and Cohn, F. Adenomyosis in the gravid uterus at term. *Am. J. Obstet. Gynecol. 84*:1457, 1962.

44. Scott, R. B. Uterine adenomyoma in adenomyosis. *Clin. Obstet. Gynecol. 1*:413, 1958.

45. Sitzenfrey, A. Ueber venenmyome des uterus mit intravaskularem wachstum. ztschr. *Geburtsch u. Gynakol. 68*:1, 1911.

46. Steiner, P. E. Metastasizing fibroleiomyoma of the uterus. *Am. J. Pathol. 15*:89, 1939.

47. Stout, A. P. Hemangiopericytoma. A study of twenty-five new cases. *Cancer 2*:1027, 1949.

48. Stout, A. P., and Murray, M. R. Hemangiopericytoma; a vascular tumor featuring Zimmermann's pericytes. *Ann. Surg. 116*:26, 1942.

49. Te Linde, R. W., and Mattingly, R. F. Operative Gynecology. 4th ed. Philadelphia and Toronto, J. B. Lippincott, 1970, Ch. 8, pp. 143–191.

50. Thompson, J. W. III, Symmonds, R. E., and Dockerty, M. B. Benign uterine Leiomyoma with vascular involvement. *Am. J. Obstet. Gynecol. 84*:182, 1962.

51. Wakeling, A. E., and Wyngarden, L. J. Prostaglandin receptors in the human, monkey, and hamster uterus. *Endocrinology 95*:55, 1974.

Rita Iovine Demopoulos, M.D.

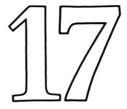

# Uterine Sarcomas

## Introduction

Sarcomas of the uterus are much less common than carcinomas, and all types of sarcomas combined account for approximately 4% of malignant uterine tumors. An analysis by Crawford[9] of all cases of cervix and corpus malignancies revealed that sarcomas accounted for 2.6% of these uterine malignancies. Fenton[11] and Novak and Anderson[25] report slightly higher figures of 5.5 and 4.5%, respectively.

In recent years, considerable data have been accumulated regarding uterine sarcomas, which has been helpful in determining incidence rates, in refining diagnostic criteria, as well as in predicting the behavior of these lesions.

## Classification

The nomenclature for sarcomas has been somewhat ambiguous in the past and this, too, has been recently clarified. Ober's classification of uterine sarcomas[26] has been simplified by Kempson[14] and this practical schema which appears in Table 17.1 is now widely used.

The homologous tissues are those normally present in the uterus, and sarcomas derived from these tissues are considered homologous sarcomas. The tissues included are smooth muscle, endometrial stromal tissue, blood vessels, and fibrous connective tissue; pure tumors derived from

**Table 17.1** Classification of uterine sarcomas

---

I. Pure sarcomas
   A. Pure homologous
      1. Leiomyosarcoma
      2. Stromal sarcoma
      3. Angiosarcoma
      4. Fibrosarcoma
   B. Pure heterologous
      1. Rhabdomyosarcoma
      2. Chondrosarcoma
      3. Osteogenic sarcoma
      4. Liposarcoma
II. Mixed sarcomas
   A. Mixed homologous
   B. Mixed heterologous
   C. Mixed homologous and heterologous
III. Malignant mixed Müllerian tumors
   A. Malignant mixed Müllerian tumor, homologous type; carcinoma plus one or more of the homologous sarcomas listed under IA above
   B. Malignant mixed Müllerian tumor, heterologous type; carcinoma plus one or more of the heterologous sarcomas listed under IB; homologous sarcoma(s) may also be present
IV. Sarcoma, unclassified
V. Malignant lymphoma

---

these elements are named, respectively, leiomyosarcomas, endometrial stromal sarcomas, hemangiosarcomas, and fibrosarcomas. The heterologous tissues most often seen in uterine sarcomas include striated muscle, cartilage, bone, and fat, and pure tumors derived from these are designated rhabdomyosarcomas, chondrosarcomas, osteogenic sarcomas, and liposarcomas. Combinations of two or more homologous malignant tissues comprise mixed homologous sarcomas. If homologous and heterologous sarcomas are mixed, or two or more heterologous tissues are present, the tumor is referred to as mixed heterologous.

The presence of carcinoma, whether it be adenocarcinoma, squamous cell carcinoma, or undifferentiated carcinoma, in addition to sarcoma, whether it be homologous or heterologous, are the components of mixed Müllerian tumors. At times more than one carcinoma and more than one type of sarcoma is present in mixed Müllerian tumors. The terms mixed mesodermal sarcomas, mixed mesenchymal sarcoma, and carcinosarcoma are often used synonymously with mixed Müllerian tumor. However, the expression carcinosarcoma should be reserved for carcinoma

plus homologous sarcoma, whereas mixed Müllerian tumor implies the presence of at least one heterologous element.

Sarcoma botryoides refers to a rare and highly malignant tumor usually occurring in the vagina of infant girls or the cervix of adolescent girls. It has a characteristic bulky, loose, soft, gross appearance. Microscopically, it usually contains myxoid elements and rhabdomyosarcoma. This tumor is discussed in Chapter 3 and is mentioned here because histogenetically it is probably related to the mixed Müllerian tumor.

# Leiomyosarcoma

## Occurrence

These malignant smooth muscle uterine tumors can arise in preexisting leiomyomas or in normal uterine musculature. Crawford[9] found that of 26 leiomyosarcomas studied, six arose in myometrium and 20 arose in a leiomyoma. According to Bartsich,[2] who analyzed 1,562 uterine malignancies, leiomyosarcomas account for 1.28% of all uterine malignancies and 16% of all uterine sarcomas. Spiro[29] similarly found that myosarcomas account for 1.3% of uterine malignancies. Christopherson[5] found the average incidence rate for leiomyosarcoma for Jefferson County residents to be 0.67 per 100,000 women 20 years of age and older.

Since leiomyomas are so common, the incidence of malignant change is of considerable importance. In a study of over 15,000 cases of clinically diagnosed leiomyomata, there were 19 cases of lethal sarcomatous change, an incidence of 0.13% or 1:800 cases.[7] Since this figure does not take into account leiomyomata not clinically diagnosed, the true incidence of sarcomatous change is even lower.

## Clinical Findings

The average age at the time of diagnosis of leiomyosarcoma is about 55 and includes a wide age span from the second to the eighth decade. Invasive leiomyosarcomas occur slightly more often in Blacks than Caucasians, according to Bartsich[2] but less often in a study by Spiro.[29] There is not good evidence to support any racial predilection for myosarcomas. These tumors occur in nulliparous women as often as multiparous, and the incidence is not affected by parity.[29]

The most common presenting symptom is vaginal bleeding. Less often, patients develop abdominal pain or an abdominal mass. Curettage is not a useful technique in the diagnosis of myosarcoma. If a uterine leiomyoma which has been observed to be relatively stationary in size, enlarges rapidly, this might suggest to the physician that malignant change has occurred. Of course, pregnancy or the occurrence of hemorrhage or edema into a leiomyoma can also produce rapid enlargement.

A history of prior irradiation has not been shown to be related to the subsequent development of myosarcoma.

## Gross Appearance

Leiomyosarcomas may be indistinguishable grossly from leiomyomas, particularly when extensive degenerative changes are present (Figure 17.1), or when sarcomatous change has occurred focally in a leiomyoma. At times, especially when the leiomyosarcomas arise from myometrium, the gross appearance of a sarcoma differs from its benign counterpart in that it is a nonencapsulated mass which merges with adjacent normal myometrium. The cut surface often demonstrates a bulging homogeneous, grayish-white soft mass, in which the whorled pattern of muscle bundles is no longer evident (Figure 17.2). Necrosis and hemorrhage are very common. Christopherson[5] found most of his cases to be intramural in location; submucosal and subserosal locations followed in that order. The tumors averaged 9 cm in diameter, with a range from 4 to 40 cm. Malignant smooth muscle tumors have a larger average diameter than benign, although there is considerable overlap. In contrast to Crawford's findings,[9] Christopherson's series did not reveal any sarcomas arising in a leiomyoma, although many patients had coexisting leiomyomas. He also did not demonstrate multiple sarcomas in any case.

## Histologic Appearance

The microscopic features distinguishing leiomyosarcoma from leiomyoma have not been well defined in the past, and the histologic criteria have not been consistently applied. In laboratories requiring evidence of vascular, myometrial, or extrauterine invasion as a prerequisite for the diagnosis of sarcoma, the 5-year survivals have been as low as zero.[25] If the diagnosis was made on histologic appearance, not requiring that invasive properties be demonstrated, the survival figures have been as high as 75%. This disparity highlights the need for additional parameters to be used to correlate histopathology and behavior.

The histologic characteristics of leiomyosarcoma, in contrast to leiomyoma, include increased cellularity, a

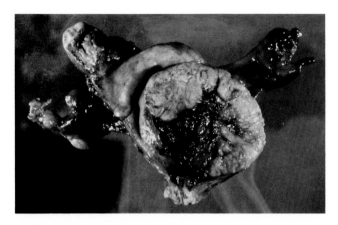

**17.1** Gross view of a leiomyoma with sarcomatous change showing myometrial invasion and extensive hemorrhage and necrosis.

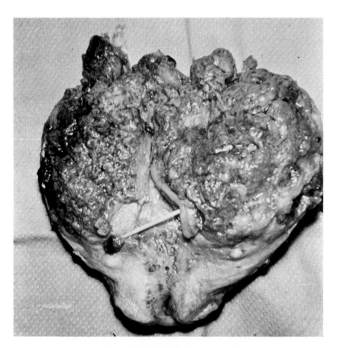

**17.2** Gross view of a leiomyosarcoma, which is nonencapsulated, has replaced most of the myometrium and shows extensive degeneration.

change in the appearance of the nuclei from thin elongated structures to plump spindle-shaped nuclei, greater nuclear variability in size and staining properties, prominent nucleoli (Figure 17.3) and increased mitotic figures (Figure 17.4). The cytoplasm is eosinophilic and poorly defined. Marked anaplasia and tumor giant cells may be present (Figures 17.5 and 17.6).

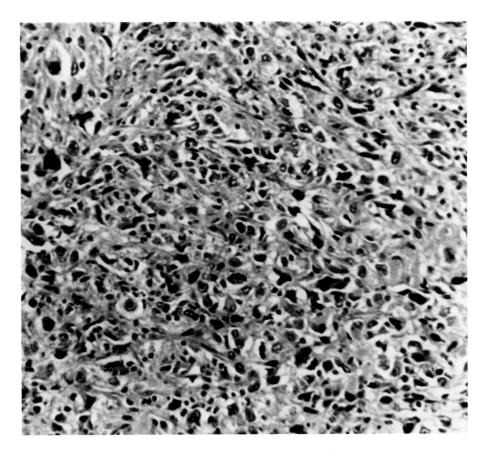

**17.3** Leiomyosarcoma which arose in a leiomyoma. The smooth muscle nuclei are closely packed, plump, and pleomorphic.

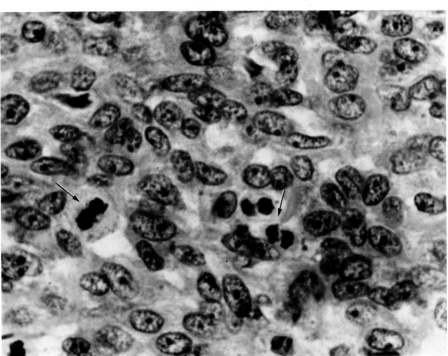

**17.4** Leiomyosarcoma showing multiple mitoses (arrows).

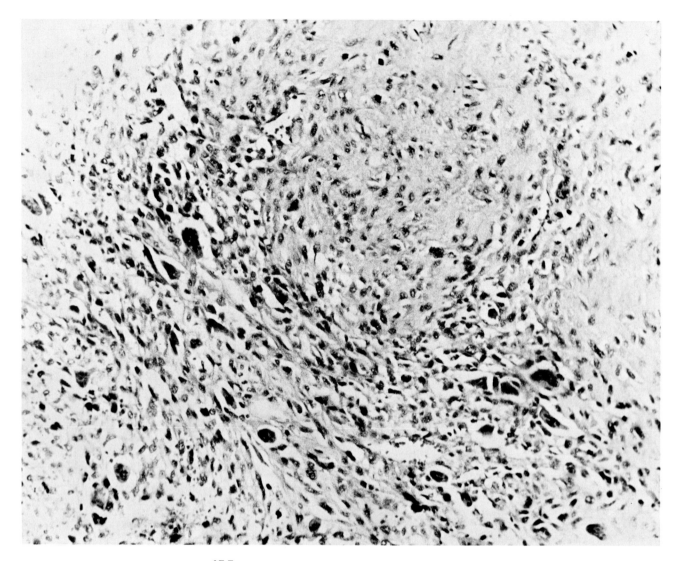

**17.5** Leiomyosarcoma showing marked anaplasia with scattered tumor giant cells.

A study by Taylor and Norris,[31] in which mitotic rate was correlated with tumor behavior, has proved to be an extremely useful adjunct in the diagnosis of uterine sarcomas. It has been especially helpful in distinguishing cellular and bizarre leiomyomas from sarcomas, for this can be extremely difficult. Subsequent studies have also carefully documented the mitotic rate in a variety of smooth muscle tumors, including cellular and bizarre leiomyomas, as well as sarcomas. A low mitotic count has consistently been correlated with a good prognosis. Kempson[14] found that smooth muscle tumors averaging less than 5 mitoses per 10 high-power fields (HPF) are benign. Those with higher mitotic counts are malignant. The prognosis for leiomyosarcomas with more than 10 mitoses per 10 HPF is poor and metastases are frequent. Christopherson,[5] in a study including 32 leiomyosarcomas, 31 cellular leiomyomas, 17 bizarre leiomyomas, and one intravascular leiomyoma, found that no patient with a tumor showing fewer than 5 mitoses per 10 HPF died of the disease. The average length of follow-up of his sarcoma cases was 12 years. The number of mitoses in 10 HPF of greatest mitotic activity should be noted in all smooth muscle tumors showing any degree of increased cellularity or atypia as a routine diagnostic procedure. Factors which might affect the mitotic

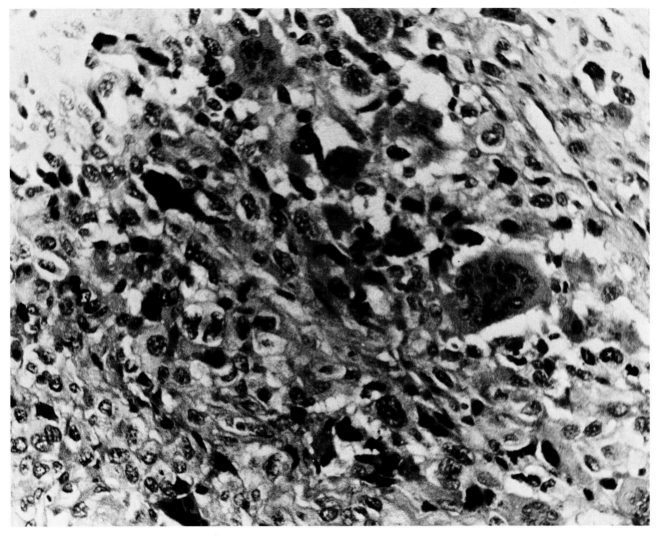

**17.6** High-power view of leiomyosarcoma showing nuclear pleomorphism and normal as well as tumor giant cells.

count such as the interval between surgery and the fixation and sectioning of the gross specimen, as well as the temperature at which the specimen is kept, must be evaluated. Variation in these conditions may modify the results of mitotic counts, perhaps causing them to be lower if the sections are taken several hours after surgery, even if the specimen is properly refrigerated.

## Therapy and Prognosis

It is obvious that numerous features must be evaluated for a smooth muscle tumor suspected of being malignant,

in order to arrive at the proper diagnosis. If evidence of invasion of contiguous extrauterine structures is present, the tumor should be designated a leiomyosarcoma. If vascular invasion is seen (except for intravenous leiomyomatosis), or if the tumor invades myometrium, endometrium, or endocervix, it should also be considered a sarcoma. If the mitotic count is 10 per 10 HPF, or more, the tumor will probably behave aggressively and should be diagnosed as malignant. Tumors showing no invasive properties and having less than 1 mitosis per 10 HPF, should be designated benign, even if pleomorphic. Also, tumors having 1 to 4 mitoses per 10 HPF with little or no cellular pleomorphism are probably benign. Kempson[13] describes two groups of smooth muscle tumors of uncertain malignant potential. The first group has 5 to 9 mitoses per 10 HPF without cellular pleomorphism, and the second group has 1 to 4 mitoses per 10 HPF with significant cellular pleomorphism. These must be individually evaluated and classified depending upon the degree of pleomorphism. Care must be taken to count mitoses in four different areas of 10 HPF each. The areas chosen should be those showing the greatest cellularity. The occurrence of giant cell forms should be disregarded since they are as likely to be present in benign lesions as in malignant.

Since the use of mitotic counts to assist in distinguishing benign from malignant smooth muscle tumors has become widespread, the range for 5-year survival figures for leiomyosarcoma has narrowed considerably. Christophersen[5] reports the 5-year survival of 32 patients with leiomyosarcomas to be 20.7%. Twenty-four of these patients were treated by hysterectomy, three by hysterectomy plus radiation, one by radiation only, one by chemotherapy only. The survivors all had hysterectomies performed.

In Taylor and Norris's study[31] of 39 patients with leiomyosarcoma, 19 were found to have tumor confined to the uterus at the time of surgery. Local extension was present in 11 and five were inoperable. Thirty were treated with total abdominal hysterectomy and unilateral or bilateral salpingo-oophorectomy, and three had a supracervical hysterectomy. The patients were followed for 3 years and 10 months to 20 years. The results were as follows: three patients were living and well, two died without evidence of tumor, two were alive with tumor and 29 died of the disease.

The generally accepted therapy for leiomyosarcoma is simple total hysterectomy, usually with bilateral salpingo-oophorectomy. Following surgical treatment 20 to 25% of patients can be expected to survive 5 years. Pelvic recurrence is the most common initial indication of treatment failure. Intraperitoneal recurrence and distant metastases, particularly to lung, are next in frequency.

Autopsies on 15 patients who died of leiomyosarcoma[8] revealed 100% to have pelvic or intraabdominal visceral involvement, 80% to have lung or pleural metastases, 40% to have para-aortic nodal disease, 33% to have renal metastases, and 20% to have liver metastases.

A study by Laberge[16] suggests that, all other factors being equal, leiomyosarcomas which are primary in myometrium have a worse prognosis than those arising in leiomyomas.

# Endometrial Stromal Sarcoma

The stromal tumors are rare and they occur, as do smooth muscle tumors, in a wide and continuous spectrum of lesions from benign to malignant. The terms stromatosis, stromal nodule, and endolymphatic stromal myosis are used to designate the more benign variants and stromal sarcoma the more malignant. Endolymphatic stromal myosis has been discussed previously and will not be mentioned here except as it relates to stromal sarcoma. The cell of origin for these tumors is generally presumed to be the endometrial stromal cell.

## Clinical Findings

Norris and Taylor[23] reported on 53 cases of stromal tumors. The patients ranged from 17 to 61 years of age, averaging 45. Most were Caucasian. The commonest presenting symptom was vaginal bleeding, although several complained of pelvic or abdominal pain. On physical examination, 9 were found to have extrauterine extension of disease, and 3 patients had a "frozen pelvis," which means the pelvic organs were fixed in position due to extension of tumor to the pelvic side walls.

## Gross Appearance

Stromal sarcomas appear grossly as circumscribed or ill-defined uterine masses usually involving both endometrium and myometrium, although they may be confined to one or the other. They vary in size, usually from 2 to 20 cm, but tend to be smaller than leiomyosarcomas, averaging 5 to 6 cm in diameter. The cut surfaces reveal nodules which are homogeneous, grayish, tan, or yellow in color, and bulging. Often they project into the uterine cavity (Figure 17.7). Focal hemorrhage or degenerative changes may be present but are less common than in other uterine sarcomas.

## Microscopic Appearance and Prognosis

Histologically these tumors consist of uniform small cells with round or ovoid, closely packed nuclei, frequently monotonously similar in appearance. They have a small amount of pale, poorly defined cytoplasm (Figure 17.8). The cells closely resemble endometrial stromal cells. Occasionally, glands resembling endometrial glands are seen in stromal sarcomas (Figure 17.9). When the junction of the tumor with adjacent tissue is rounded or pushing, rather than irregular and infiltrating, the tumor usually shows no

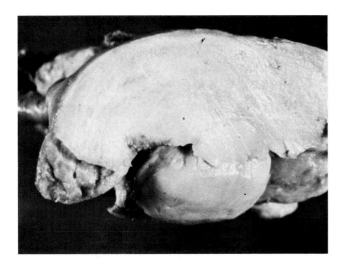

**17.7** Gross view of a submucosal stromal sarcoma, having no clear line of demarcation from subjacent myometrium. The uterus has been cut sagitally.

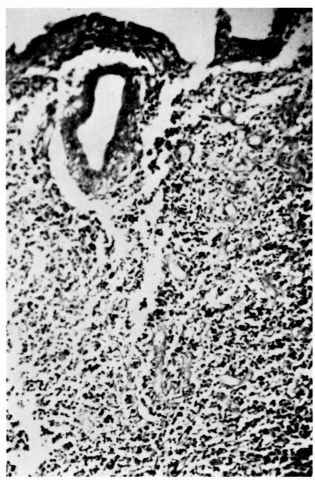

**17.9** Stromal sarcomas occasionally contain an endometrial type gland.

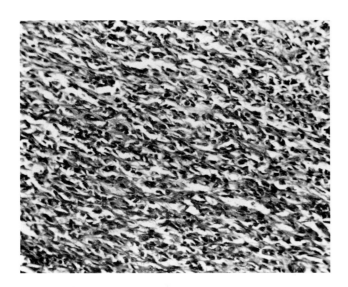

**17.8** Endometrial stromal sarcoma having small, closely packed ovoid nuclei and pale, poorly defined cytoplasm.

lymphatic or vascular invasion and has a low mitotic count. Such lesions have been found to behave benignly and have been termed stromal nodules.[23] Several sections are required to determine whether a mass has pushing or infiltrating margins, since one section may not show infiltration, whereas additional sections may reveal myometrial invasion. Although some stromal sarcomas may show considerable pleomorphism, this feature has not been found to correlate with behavior (Figure 17.10). Norris and Taylor[23] divided their cases showing infiltrating margins and lymphatic invasion into two groups. One group of 20 patients with tumors showing less than 10 mitoses per 10 HPF had an actuarial survival of 100% at 10 years. One patient in this group died of tumor after 12 years and 31% were alive with tumor. Those lesions showing lymphatic invasion but having low mitotic counts are examples of endolymphatic stromal myosis. The clinical progression of this disease is slow and indolent, characterized by very late recurrences and a relatively good progress. The second group of 15 patients had tumors with mitotic rates of 10 per 10 HPF or greater. The 5-year actuarial survival in this group was 55%.

Kempson[14] believes that stromal lesions having mitotic

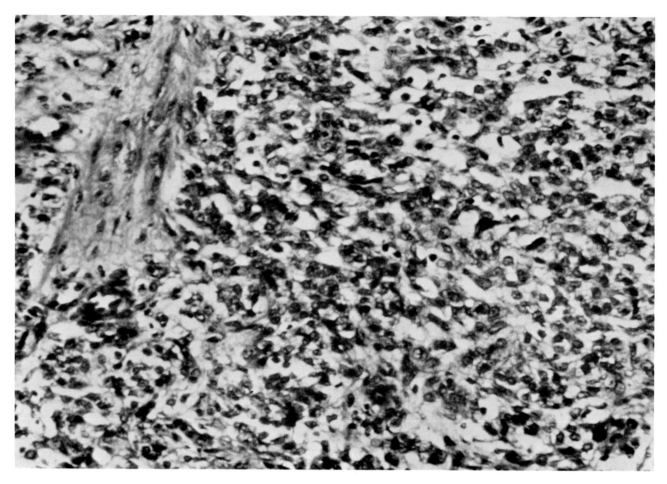

**17.10** Stromal sarcoma showing anaplasia. Pleomorphism is of less prognostic value than mitotic count.

counts of 20 or greater in 10 HPF should be designated as sarcomas, and those having less than 5 per 10 HPF should be designated endolymphatic stromal meiosis.

Based on these data, it is imperative to do routine mitotic counts on all stromal tumors to assist in the proper diagnosis and prognosis.

Occasionally, despite low mitotic counts, lesions will recur. A case in point is that of a 19-year-old woman, seen because of uterine bleeding. Curettage showed (Figure 17.11a) what was called an endometrial polyp with atypical stroma. A year later the patient again developed irregular vaginal bleeding and curettage showed a polypoid lesion with intact surface and atypical stroma (Figure 17.11b). Five years later, hysterectomy was performed because of persistent bleeding. The uterus revealed stromal sarcoma (Figure 17.11c). The lesion recurred 14 months later. This lesion was undoubtedly a low grade sarcoma from its

inception despite the fact that mitotic counts in the surgical material were found to be 1 per 10 HPF. Electron microscopic examination of the tumor (Figure 17.12) from the uterus revealed its fine structure to be characteristic of stromal sarcomas as described by Komorowski.[15] The cytoplasm of the stromal sarcoma cells are packed with microfilaments varying from 100 to 200 Å units in thickness. Lipid droplets and granular endoplasmic reticulum are present. Prominent cytoplasmic processes are also noted.

## Therapy

Patients with endolymphatic stromal myosis should be treated with simple total hysterectomy. Patients with stromal sarcoma do better if salpingo-oophorectomy is performed in addition to hysterectomy. If extrauterine disease is present, some patients may benefit from radiation therapy.[23] However, follow-ups on radiated patients were not sufficiently long for its effects to be properly evaluated.

# Malignant Mixed Müllerian Tumors

These sarcomas have challenged and fascinated pathologists since they were first described by Virchow in 1864. They have been referred to by a galaxy of terms including mesenchymal tumor, mesenchymal sarcoma, mixed mesodermal tumor, carcinosarcoma, dysontogenetic tumor, and many more, totalling 119.[17]

## Histogenesis

There are several theories regarding the histogenesis of these tumors. The first suggests that the tumor develops from embryonic rests deposited in the uterus during intrauterine development.[32] A second theory based on observations of the growth of endometrial cells in tissue culture[27] postulates an origin of mixed Müllerian tumors from endometrial and endocervical stroma. Another theory states this tumor is derived from a totipopential mesenchymal cell located just beneath the surface epithelium,[30] and this has become widely accepted. This theory has recently found support in an ultrastructural study of a mixed mesodermal tumor by Boram.[3] He demonstrated the stages in the development of differentiated myoblasts from primitive mesenchymal cells. The question of origin should probably remain an open one until more conclusive evidence is available.

## Incidence

Mixed Müllerian sarcomas account for 2 to 5% of all uterine malignancies.[10] In our laboratory the incidence has increased significantly in the past decade, and we currently see more mixed Müllerian tumors than leiomyosarcomas.

In an analysis of all admissions to the department of gynecology from 1957 to 1960, Chuang[6] found mixed mesodermal sarcomas to account for 2% of all uterine sarcomas. Of 118 cases of corpus sarcoma, 49 (41.5%) were mixed Müllerian (including carcinosarcoma), 48 were leiomyosarcomas, and 14 were stromal sarcomas.

## Clinical Features

The median age of patients with this tumor is about 68, with a range from 40 to 90. These tumors, therefore, usually occur in an older group than do leiomyosarcomas or stromal sarcomas. Almost all the patients are postmenopausal. The commonest presenting symptom, as with other sarcomas, is vaginal bleeding. Often too, however, the patients develop a brown discharge. Weight loss or abdominal pain is occasionally present. Some patients develop symptoms related to uterine enlargement such as urinary frequency. A few patients pass masses of necrotic tumor or, more often, a mass may protrude through the cervix into the vagina. Dilatation and curettage is a valuable diagnostic tool for mixed Müllerian tumors since they are always present within the endometrial cavity. Chuang[6] reports that 75% of curettages performed on patients with mixed Müllerian tumors accurately diagnosed mixed Müllerian tumors, and all but one diagnosed a malignant tumor.

Masterson[18] found that of 25 patients with mixed mesodermal tumors the mean parity was three. However, 40% were nulliparous and 24% had five or more children, so that the figures at both ends of the scale tend to be high. A history of prior radiation was found in five patients (20%). In 3 instances the radiation therapy was for benign bleeding, 16 to 23 years before. In two instances radiation therapy was administered for carcinoma (one cervical and one endometrial) 4 and 8 years earlier. Several other investigators have confirmed the use of prior radiation in significant numbers of these patients.[19]

## Gross Appearance

The typical gross appearance of mixed Müllerian tumors is quite diagnostic. The lesions are generally bulky, polypoid, and soft, often causing symmetrical enlargement of the uterus (Figure 17.13). They are usually attached at the fundus, by a broad or narrow base, filling and enlarging the uterine cavity. The outside of the tumor mass is variegated with some areas appearing gray or tan, soft and moist, other areas appearing red and hemorrhagic, and still others dark and necrotic or ulcerated (Figure 17.14). Upon opening the uterus, the tumors expand through the incision, as if having been compressed by the uterine wall (Figure 17.15). Although confined to the uterus in 10 out of 25 cases, and characterized by extra uterine extension in an equal number of cases,[19] most lesions confined to the uterus show significant myometrial penetration.

## Microscopic Appearance

By definition, carcinoma and sarcoma are present in all mixed Müllerian tumors. The sarcomatous element is

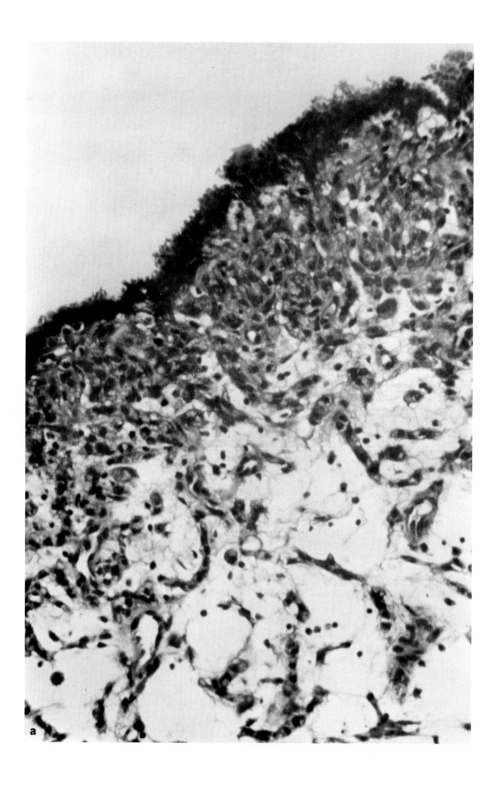

**17.11** Evolution of a case of low grade endometrial stromal sarcoma beginning in a patient at age 19.

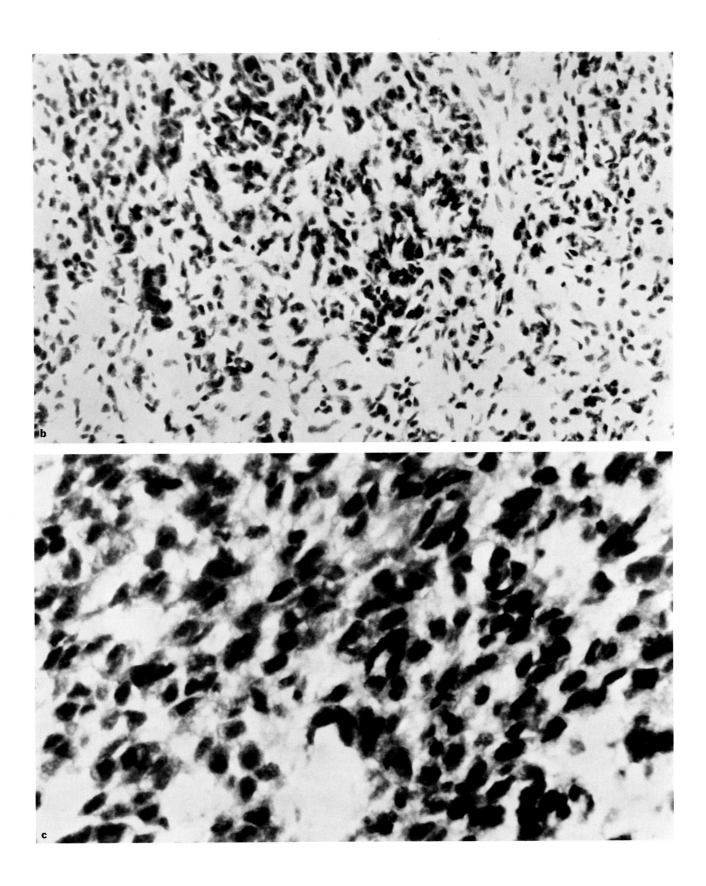

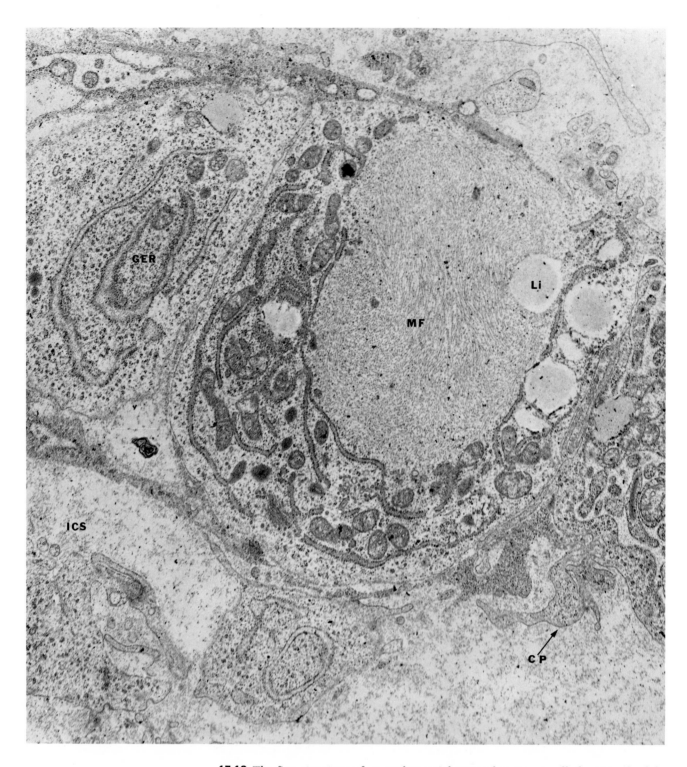

**17.12** The fine structure of an endometrial stromal sarcoma cell showing the following labeled organelles: GER represents granular endoplasmic reticulum, MF represents microfilaments, ICS represents the intercellular space, Li represents lipid droplets and CP represents cytoplasmic processes.

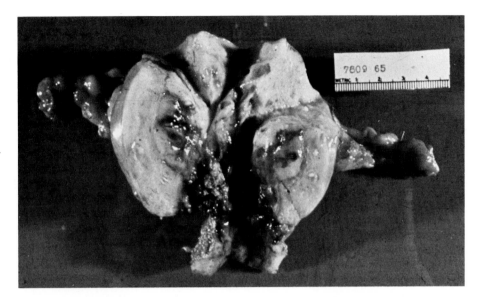

**17.13** A uterus containing a mixed Müllerian sarcoma showing globular enlargement.

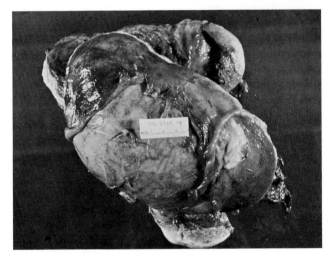

**17.14** The surface of mixed Müllerian tumors have a variegated appearance showing surface ulceration, hemorrhage, and necrosis.

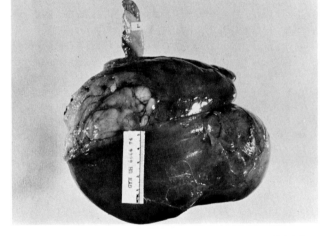

**17.15** Upon opening a uterus containing a mixed Müllerian tumor, the polypoid tumor mass literally burst free, as if compressed within the cavity.

usually predominant over the carcinomatous. The sarcoma often varies from areas which are bland and myxomatous in appearance to areas which are undifferentiated resembling fibroleiomyosarcoma. At times the sarcoma is very anaplastic with numerous tumor giant cells and mitoses. The carcinoma is usually gland forming. The glands are scattered and are often well differentiated, but they, too, may be bizarre and anaplastic. The glands often resemble endometrial glands. Occasionally areas of squamous differentiation, probably representing metaplasia of glandular

elements, are noted. Areas of undifferentiated carcinoma often blend and mix with anaplastic sarcoma so that it may be impossible to distinguish them (Figure 17.16).

A variety of differentiated sarcomas may be seen including leiomyosarcoma, rhabdomyosarcoma (Figure 17.17), chondrosarcoma (Figure 17.18), and osteogenic sarcoma (Figure 17.19), or, rarely, liposarcoma (Figure 17.20). These may be immature and poorly differentiated, or may be well differentiated and strongly resemble normal tissues. Occasionally rhabdomyoblasts, which are immature skele-

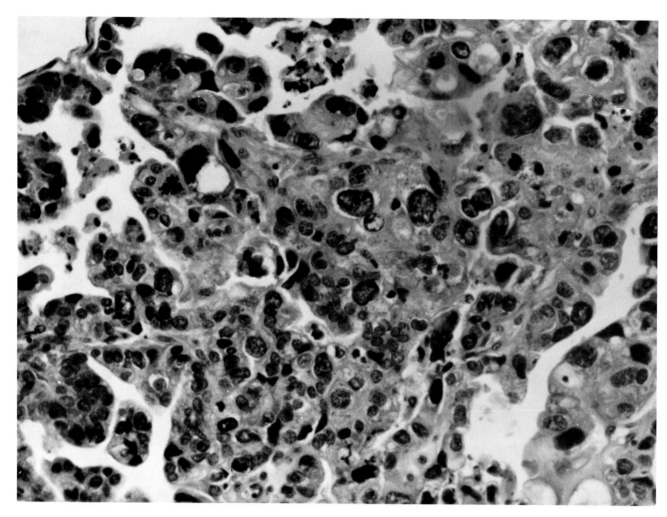

**17.16** The undifferentiated anaplastic sarcoma often blends intimately with anaplastic carcinoma making it difficult to separate the two.

tal muscle cells having a rectangular shape, abundant densely eosinophilic cytoplasm, and large hyperchromatic nuclei, will demonstrate cross striations (Figure 17.21).

An analysis of the various types of tissues present in 36 mixed Müllerian tumors was carried out by Kempson.[14] Twenty-one contained carcinoma and homologous sarcoma (carcinosarcomas) and 15 contained heterologous sarcoma. In the first group, 18 contained adenocarcinoma, five had squamous carcinoma, and two contained both adeno and squamous differentiation. Stromal sarcoma was present in 15 and leiomyosarcoma in nine, and three cases had both smooth muscle and stromal sarcoma. In the second group containing heterologous elements, chondrosarcoma was found in seven, rhabdomyosarcoma in six,

and bone in two. Eight contained stromal sarcoma and six leiomyosarcoma in addition to heterologous elements.

## Prognosis

It may be of more than academic interest to determine all the types of homologous and heterologous elements present in a mixed Müllerian tumor. Recent studies suggest that the types of tissues present may have some effect on 5-year survival. Therefore, numerous sections should be taken to ensure that all the tissue elements have been sampled. Norris and Taylor[24] and Norris and Roth[22] reported that patients with carcinosarcoma (carcinoma plus homologous sarcoma) have a somewhat better prog-

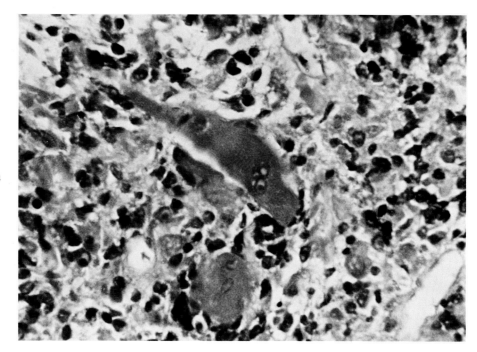

**17.17** A mixed Müllerian with scattered rhabdomyoblasts showing faint cross striations in the cytoplasm of the largest strap cell.

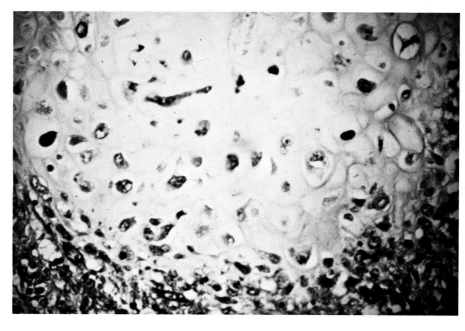

**17.18** An area of cartilagenous differentiation in a mixed Müllerian tumor.

nosis than patients having heterologous sarcoma. In addition all of the survivors with mixed mesodermal tumors contained cartilage and none contained striated muscle. On the other hand, Chuang[6] compared 5-year survivals in 29 patients with carcinosarcoma to 20 patients with mixed mesodermal tumors and found them to be 16 and 12%,

respectively. He concluded that there is no significant difference.

The single factor having the greatest effect on survival is the extent of the tumor at the time of diagnosis. All of the patients who survived 5 years in Chuang's study[6] had their tumors confined to the uterine corpus at the time of

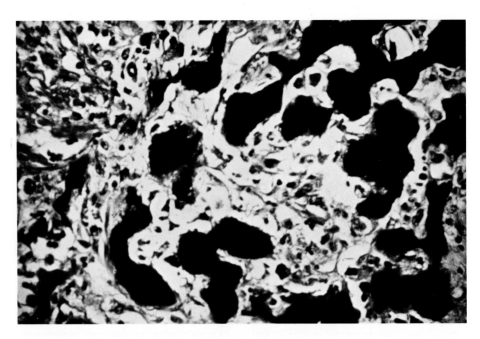

**17.19** An area of osteoid formation in a mixed Müllerian tumor.

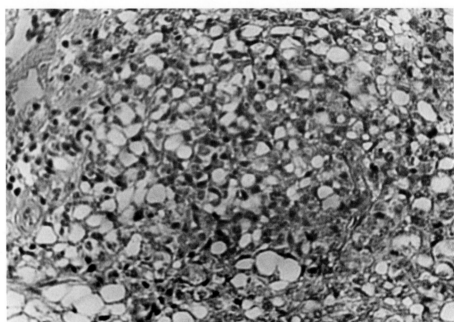

**17.20** Foci within this mixed Müllerian tumor showed well-differentiated liposarcoma.

diagnosis. This group had a 5-year survival of 30%. None of the patients with extrauterine extension survived 5 years. Kempson[14] found the 5-year survival for patients with carcinosarcoma to be 27% and for mixed Müllerian 15%, an insignificant difference. However, all the survivors in both groups had disease limited to the endometrium or inner half of the myometrium at the time of diagnosis.

Another feature of significance in determining prognosis is a history of prior radiation. Of eight patients with such a history in Chuang's series,[6] seven died within 8 months of diagnosis and the eighth developed inguinal node metastases.

In a review of the literature Alfonso[1] found that 57 out of 362 patients survived 5 years (15.7%). Survival rates

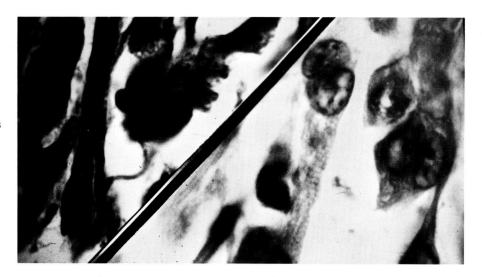

**17.21** Rhabdomyoblasts formed the predominant element in this mixed Müllerian tumor. Many of the strap cells showed cross striations.

were higher in younger women, and the best prognostic features were absent or minimal myometrial invasion and absence of extrauterine disease.

## Course and Treatment

Pelvic recurrence is common and usually occurs within 1 year following surgery. Pelvic lymph nodes are involved in most patients. Distant metastases are usually hematogenous and the sites most often involved are lungs and pleura, vagina, omentum, mesentery, ovaries, and extra pelvic lymph nodes.[1] The secondary tumor usually shows both carcinomatous and sarcomatous differentiation, although occasionally they are pure carcinoma or pure sarcoma. Vascular invasion is very often demonstrable on the slides of the original tumor.

Simple total hysterectomy and bilateral salpingo-oophrectomy is the preferred treatment for mixed Müllerian tumors. Since, depending on the series, 50 to 84%[6,14] of patients have extrauterine disease at the time of diagnosis, radiation therapy and chemotherapy should be considered as adjuvant therapy. Although these tumors have been considered to be radioresistant, some patients have shown a dramatic response.[12,20]

## Müllerian Adenosarcoma of the Uterus

A new and distinct type of tumor was described by Clement and Scully[7] characterized by benign epithelial elements and malignant stromal elements. They saw 10

such cases in a 12-year period at Massachusetts General Hospital. Nine had homologous sarcomas and one resembled an embryonal rhabdomyosarcoma. The patients were all Caucasian and had a median age of 71. Most presented with vaginal bleeding. There was no history of prior radiation. None of the patients had evidence of extrauterine spread. The lesions were all polypoid. Microscopic examination revealed vascular invasion in only one case. The microscopic appearance was reminiscent of cystosarcoma phylloides of the breast. The importance of this lesion is the fact that it has a much better prognosis than mixed Müllerian tumors in which the glandular element is malignant. Five of Clement's 10 patients had no recurrence 3 months to 7½ years after surgery. The other four patients developed vaginal recurrences at various intervals after surgery and the last patient developed intraabdominal recurrence and distant metastases.

## Primary Malignant Lymphoma of Uterus

Normal lymphoid follicles are commonly found in endometrium particularly during the childbearing years. Neumann[21] found follicles in curettings in 18 out of 300 cases, but when serial sectioning was done in 20 cases, 18 were found to contain lymphoid aggregates. The follicles tend to be small, located most often in the basal layer of the endometrium, and are usually seen during the late proliferative and early secretory phases. They tend to be larger at this time and to contain germinal centers.

The female reproductive tract may be involved by

lymphoma or leukemia as part of a generalized process. Rosenberg[28] found 40% of 1,269 autopsy cases of patients with lymphosarcoma had histologic involvement of the genital tract. However, primary involvement of the uterus is very rare. Chorlton[4] found 13 cases of patients at the AFIP (Armed Forces Institute of Pathology) whose initial presentation of lymphoma was in the female reproductive tract (excluding ovaries). Three out of the 13 involved the corpus. These patients ranged from 34 to 37 years of age. Two were staged as III and one was staged IV according to the FIGC clinical staging of lymphomas. All three received surgical therapy in which hysterectomy or uterine fundectomy was a part. Two were also given radiation therapy and one chemotherapy. All died from 4½ to 120 months after diagnosis.

# REFERENCES

1. Alfonso, J. F. Mixed mesodermal tumors of the uterus. West. J. Med. 120:17, 1974.

2. Bartsich, E. G., Bowe, E. T., and Moore, J. G. Leiomyosarcoma of the uterus. Obstet. Gynecol. 32:101, 1968.

3. Boram, L. H., Erlandson, R. A., and Hajdu, S. I. Mesodermal mixed tumor of the uterus. Cancer 30:1295, 1972.

4. Chorlton, I., Karnei, R. F. Jr., King, F. M., and Norris, H. J. Primary malignant reticuloendothelial disease involving the vagina, cervix, and corpus uteri. Obstet. Gynecol. 44:735, 1974.

5. Christopherson, W. M., Williamson, E. O., and Gray, L. A. Leiomyosarcoma of the uterus. Cancer 29:1512, 1972.

6. Chuang, J. T., Van Velden, D. J. J., and Graham, J. B. Carcinosarcoma and mixed mesodermal tumor of the uterine corpus. Obstet. Gynecol. 35:769, 1970.

7. Clement, P. B., and Scully, R. E. Mullerian adenosarcoma of the uterus. Cancer 34:1138, 1974.

8. Corscaden, J. A., and Singh, B. P. Leiomyosarcoma of the uterus. Am. J. Obstet. Gynecol. 75:149, 1958.

9. Crawford, E. J. Jr., and Tucker, R. Sarcoma of the uterus. Am. J. Obstet. Gynecol. 77:286, 1959.

10. Falkinburg, L. W., Hoey, W. O., Savran, J. and Stuart, J. R. Mesodermal mixed tumor of the corpus uteri. Am. J. Obstet. Gynecol. 90:450, 1964.

11. Fenton, A. N., and Burke, L. Sarcoma of the uterus. Am. J. Obstet. Gynecol. 63:158, 1952.

12. Henrichs, W. L., Climie, A. R. W., and Cook, J. C. Cure of primary mesodermal mixed tumor by radiotherapy. Obstet. Gynecol. 19:537, 1962.

13. Kempson, R. L., and Bari, W. Uterine sarcomas; classification, diagnosis and prognosis. Hum. Pathol. 1:331–349, 1970.

14. Kempson, R. L. The Uterus. Norris, H. J., Hertig, A. T., and Abell, M. R. Baltimore, Williams & Wilkins Company, 1973, Ch. 15, p. 303.

15. Komorowski, R. A., Garancis, J. C., and Clowry, L. J., Jr. Fine structure of endometrial stromal sarcoma. Cancer 26:1042, 1970.

16. Laberge, J. Prognosis of uterine leiomyosarcomas based on histopathologic criteria. Am. J. Obstet. Gynecol. 84:1833, 1962.

17. McFarland, J. Dysontogenic and mixed tumors of the urogenital region. Surg. Gynecol. Obstet. 61:42, 1935.

18. Masterson, J. G., and Kremper, J. Mixed mesodermal tumors. Am. J. Obstet. Gynecol. 104:693, 1969.

19. Mortel, R., Koss, L. G., Lewis, J. L. Jr., and D'Urso, J. R. Mesodermal mixed tumors of the uterine corpus. Obstet. Gynecol. 43:248, 1974.

20. Mortel, R., Nedwich, A., Lewis, G. C., Jr., et al. Malignant mixed Mullerian tumors of the uterine corpus. Obstet. Gynecol. 35:468, 1970.

21. Neumann, H. Zur Frage des Lymphatischen Apparatas in der Gebarmutterschleimhaut. Arch. Gynakol. 141:425, 1930.

22. Norris, H. J., Roth, E., and Taylor, H. B. Mesenchymal tumors of the uterus. II. A clinical and pathologic study of 31 mixed mesodermal tumors. Obstet. Gynecol. 28:57, 1966.

23. Norris, H. J., and Taylor, H. B. Mesenchymal tumors of the uterus. I. A clinical and pathological study of 53 endometrial stromal tumors. Cancer 19:755, 1966.

24. Norris, H. J., and Taylor, H. B. Mesenchymal tumors of the uterus. III. A clinical and pathologic study of 31 carcinosarcomas. Cancer 19:1459, 1966.

25. Novak, E., and Anderson, D. F. Sarcoma of the uterus. Am. J. Obstet. Gynecol. 34:740, 1937.

26. Ober, W. B. Uterine sarcomas. Histogenesis and taxonomy. Ann. N.Y. Acad. Sci. 75:568, 1959.

27. Papanicolaou, G. N., and Maddi, F. V. Observations on the behavior of human endometrial cells in tissue culture. Am. J. Obstet. Gynecol. 76:601, 1958.

28. Rosenberg, S. A., Diamond, H. D., and Carver, L. F. Lymphosarcoma: A review of 1269 cases. Medicine 40:31, 1961.

29. Spiro, R. H., and Koss, L. G. Myosarcoma of the uterus. Cancer 18:571, 1965.

30. Sternberg, W. H., Clark, W. H., and Smith, R. C. Malignant mixed Mullerian tumor. Cancer 7:704, 1954.

31. Taylor, H. B., and Norris, H. J. Mesenchymal tumors of the uterus. Arch. Pathol. 82:40, 1966.

32. von Conheim, J. Congenitales quergestreifter Muskel sarcoma der Nieren. Arch. Path. Anat. Physiol. 65:64, 1875.

James E. Wheeler, M.D., and
Luigi Mastroianni, Jr., M.D.

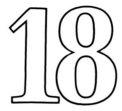

# Pathology of the Fallopian Tube

## Introduction

The biologic function of the fallopian tube, transport of sperm and ovum, may be seriously compromised or entirely destroyed by inflammatory processes or tubal pregnancy. Tumors may interfere with normal function or, if malignant, may lead to death. Although the etiology and pathophysiology of many tubal diseases are imperfectly understood at present, progress is certain to take place, if only against a background of thorough knowledge of normal anatomy, histology, and physiology.

## Anatomy

The normal fallopian tube extends from the area of its corresponding ovary anteriorly and medially to its terminus in the posterosuperior aspect of the uterine fundus. In an adult during the reproductive years its length is usually between 9 and 11 cm. The ovarian end as it opens to the pelvic portion of the peritoneal cavity is surrounded by about 25 irregular fingerlike extensions of the tube, the fimbriae. The fimbriated end, expanded like the bell of a trumpet initially, soon narrows to about 4 mm in outside diameter. The expanded end, or infundibulum is about 1 cm long and lies next to or within a few millimeters of the superolateral or tubal end of the ovary. It merges medially with the ampullary portion of the tube, which itself extends about 6 cm, passing anteriorly as it loops around the ovary. At a point characterized by relative thickening of the muscular wall, the isthmic portion begins and extends some 2 cm to the uterus. Within the myometrium, the tube extends as a 1-cm-long intramural segment until it joins the extension of the endometrial cavity at the uterotubal junction.

Throughout its extrauterine course the tube lies in a peritoneal fold along the superior margin of the broad ligament, the mesosalpinx. The arterial blood supply is ensured by a dual origin. A tubal branch of the uterine artery passes in the mesosalpinx laterally from the cornu of the uterus to anastomose with tubal branches of the ovarian artery. Venous drainage parallels the arterial supply via anastomosing tubal branches of uterine and ovarian veins, also located in the mesosalpinx. Tubal lymphatics pass laterally, accompanying the ovarian vessels. Hence, on the right side lymph drains into nodes in the area of the right renal vein and the inferior vena cava, whereas on the left lymph drains into nodes lying between the left ovarian vein and the left renal vein. Lymph also drains into presacral and common iliac nodes. It is apparent that lymphatic spread of tubal malignancy may reach extrapelvic sites early in its dissemination.

The nerve supply of the tube is both sympathetic and parasympathetic. Sympathetic fibers from $T_{10}$ through $L_2$ synapse in the celiac, aortic, renal, inferior mesenteric, cervicovaginal, and possibly presacral plexuses. Postsynaptic fibers pass into the myosalpinx, where they provide adrenergic innervation to the smooth muscle. The fact that isthmic and ampullary tubal muscle is innervated via presacral and ovarian plexuses, respectively, provides a possible neural explanation for differential myosalpingeal activity and formation of a physiologic sphincter. Sensory pain fibers pass along with the sympathetic nerves to the spinal cord at the level of $T_{10}$ to $T_{12}$. Parasympathetic fibers from the vagus nerve supply the extrauterine tube via postganglionic fibers from the ovarian plexus, whereas the intramural portion is innervated via $S_{2-4}$ parasympathetic fibers synapsing in the pelvic plexuses.

## Histology

A mucosal membrane, a wall of smooth muscle, and a serosal coat make up the three histologic layers of the tube.

The serosa is lined by flattened mesothelial cells. Beneath the mesothelium lies a small amount of connective tissue containing a few collagen fibers and blood vessels.

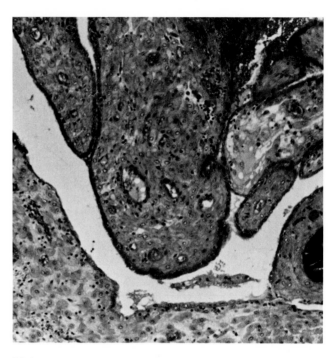

**18.1** Decidual reaction in tubal mucosa. The mucosal folds are swollen by a massive decidual reaction. Some degree of decidual change is found in the tips of the tubal folds in over 10% of normal pregnancies. Hematoxylin–eosin, ×100.

The tubal muscularis generally has but two layers, an outer longitudinal layer and an inner circular layer. However, at its uterine end, beginning in the intramural tube and extending about 1 cm, there is an inner longitudinal layer.

The outer longitudinal layer is easily overlooked, as it is composed of inconspicuous bundles of smooth muscle interspersed with loose connective tissue containing numerous small blood vessels. The circular layer forms the major muscle mass of the tube. Its thickness varies, being about 0.5 mm in the isthmus and only about 0.1 mm in the ampulla.

The mucosal layer lies directly on the muscularis. It consists of a luminal epithelial lining and a scanty underlying lamina propria containing vessels and spindly or angular cells. Although these stromal cells seem sparse, they are the cells that lead to focally recognizable decidua in 5 to 12% of pregnancies (Figure 18.1).[46,107] The mucosa increases significantly in its gross structural complexity as the lumen enlarges from uterine to ovarian end. The interstitial and intramural portion each contains about five or six blunt plicae, or folds. In the isthmus, the plicae

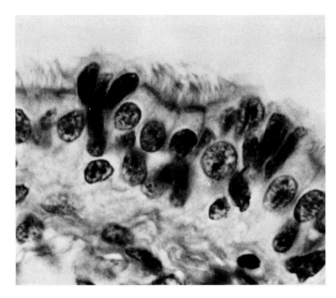

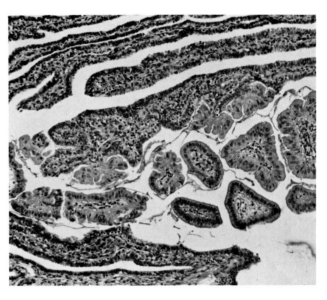

**18.2** Tubal epithelium. Ciliated cells are numerous. Secretory cells with columnar, somewhat compressed nuclei protrude above the level of the ciliated cells. Note the vacuolated apical cytoplasm of secretory cells. Hematoxylin–eosin, ×1,200.

**18.3** Benign oncocytic metaplasia. Cells with prominent eosinophilic cytoplasm form papillary projections or line modestly distorted plicae. Scattered lymphocytes are present in the plicae. Hematoxylin–eosin, ×380.

increase in height to more nearly occupy the larger lumen. A dozen or more plicae, some with secondary folds, are present. In the ampulla, the plicae are frondlike and delicate, and both secondary and tertiary branches may be appreciated. The infundibular plical pattern is similar.

The epithelial layer of the mucosa is composed of at least three histologic cell types: ciliated, secretory, and intercalary. About 20 to 30% of the cells contain prominent cilia[26] and about 55 to 65% are secretory. A pattern of increasing ciliated cells with increased proximity to the fimbriae is present in the rhesus monkey. Although some[33] have found the ciliated cells in humans to be apparently randomly and equally distributed throughout the isthmic, ampullary, and fimbriated portions, others[73] have found ciliated cells numerous and preferentially located at the apical portions of the plicae, especially in the fimbriae and ampulla. Ciliated cells in the isthmus are less frequent and occur in short strands. Ciliated cells are even scantier in the intramural tubal segment.

The ciliated cell itself is columnar, approximately 20 to 30 $\mu$ high and 9 to 12 $\mu$ wide (Figure 18.2). Each cell on its luminal surface contains about 50 cilia about 4-$\mu$ long.[33] Electron microscopic study reveals typical ciliary basal bodies and rootlets.[33] The nucleus is oval to round, is about 8 to 10 $\mu$ in greatest extent, and may lie parallel or perpendicular to the long axis of the cell. The chromatin

pattern is moderately granular. A distinct but small nucleolus is present.

The secretory cell is also columnar, approximately the same height as the ciliated cell but often narrower (Figure 18.2). Its nucleus is ovoid and perpendicular to the long axis of the cell. The chromatin pattern may be somewhat denser than that of the ciliated cell but its nucleolus is similar.

The intercalary or peg cell is a columnar cell that appears to be occupied mainly by a thin dark-staining nucleus. It is likely a morphologic variant of the secretory cell.[66]

In addition to the three epithelial types described above, a basally located cell with a rounded nucleus and dark-staining chromatin is present. Although this cell has been postulated to be a reserve cell and precursor of the other cell types,[75] recent electron microscopic evidence indicates that most, if not all, are actually lymphocytes.[67]

The tubal epithelium may undergo metaplastic changes without apparent reason. The metaplastic cells may be columnar and mucin secreting, resembling endocervical[113] or squamous epithelium.[75] Oncocytic metaplasia with marked cytoplasmic eosinophilia on routine hematoxylin and eosin staining may occur (Figure 18.3). Recent studies[65] have better delineated the amount of epithelial atypia that may be considered to be within normal

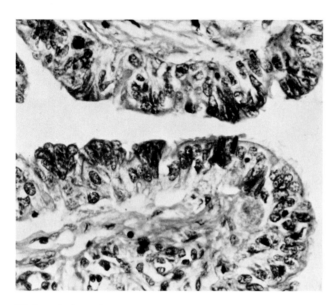

**18.4** Tubal epithelium. Crowding of nuclei and tufting of epithelial cells is a normal variant. Hematoxylin–eosin, ×380.

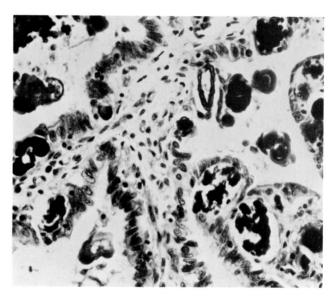

**18.5** Psammoma bodies in tubal epithelium. These calcific bodies may be found in chronic salpingitis or in relatively normal epithelium containing only rare lymphocytes. Hematoxylin–eosin, ×200.

limits. Focal nuclear crowding and tufting, for example, are frequent and normal (Figure 18.4) but mitoses are quite infrequent. Psammoma bodies are an occasional finding in chronic salpingitis but may be seen in otherwise normal appearing epithelium (Figure 18.5).

## Physiology

The characteristics of the tubal epithelium change during life. Ciliated cells appear during early fetal development[72] and persist until the postmenopausal years. At this time, as circulating estrogen levels drop, the cilia are gradually lost.[39] Estrogen therapy of postmenopausal women, however, restores both the cilia and the ability to transport particulate matter.[39,108] The demonstration of a specific estradiol receptor in the human tube[35] suggests that there is a direct action of estrogen on ciliogenesis.

The characteristics of the tubal epithelium change during the course of the menstrual cycle.[66] Early in the cycle the cells are low and the secretory cells appear relatively inactive. As the time of ovulation approaches, probably under the influence of increasing amounts of estrogen, the secretory cells become columnar and actually project beyond the ciliated cells (Figure 18.2). A discharge of PAS-positive material, probably glycogen, into the tubal lumen has been demonstrated.[36]

The cilia play a dominant role in tubal function at the time of ovulation. The cilia beat in synchronized waves in the direction of the uterus.[38] Once the ovum is released from its follicle, surrounded by an entourage of sticky cumulus cells, it is transported along the surface of the fimbriated end of the fallopian tube by the action of the cilia. Muscular contraction may also play a role in tubal transport. There is recent evidence that tubal contraction is affected by prostaglandins.[18] The newly released ovum is thus progressively moved along the fimbria to a point well within the ampullary portion of the fallopian tube in relatively short order. The cumulus cells with their characteristic tackiness are responsible for orderly progression of the ovum along the course of the tube.

During the course of ovum pickup there is likely a realignment of fimbriae in their relationship to the ovary itself. A distinct fimbria, the fimbria ovarica, runs from the tubal ostium to one pole of the ovary. At the time of ovulation it is thought that the muscle of the fimbria ovarica contracts, pulling the tube in the direction of the rupturing follicle. At the same time some muscular elements in the paraovarian tissue contract, pulling the ovary toward the tubal ostium. This realignment of fimbriae over the rupturing follicle has been observed in several laboratory species but, for technical reasons, it has not yet been satisfactorily evaluated in the human. Once safely within the tubal lumen the ovum is retained there for an interval of approximately 3 days,[20] after which it is delivered into the uterus.

Spermatozoa are transported upward through the uterus into the fallopian tube. The mechanisms by which they transverse the uterotubal junction and tubal isthmus in the face of a ciliary beat in a downward direction is still not understood. It is known, however, that spermatozoa can reach the tube within minutes after they are placed in the vagina in the human.[92] It is likely that the ferilizing spermatozoan is already present in the fallopian tube at the time the ovum arrives there.

The environment provided within the tubal lumen is of special importance in reproductive function. The fallopian tube does provide a temporary milieu for spermatozoa, the ovum, and finally the fertilized, cleaving ovum during its initial development. It therefore creates acceptable conditions for the fertilization process and for early development. The secretory cells certainly must play a role in the provision of suitable conditions for the processes that occur within the tubal lumen. Contents of the tubal fluid have been studied extensively in the rhesus monkey, but only limited observations have been carried out in the human.[22,55] The salient components of oviductal fluid include metabolic substrates, the most important of which are lactate and pyruvate; bicarbonate, which appears in tubal fluid as a result of carbonic anhydrase in the tubal epithelium; and electrolytes, including calcium.[63] Tubal fluid also contains trypsin inhibitors, which may influence the fertilization process.

The bicarbonate ion is in part responsible for dispersion of cells that surround the ovum. On reaching the level of the zona pellucida (a protein–mucopolysaccharide layer immediately surrounding the egg) the spermatozoan is able to penetrate by virtue of the presence of a trypsin-like enzyme in its head. Trypsin inhibitors appear in high concentration both before and after ovulation but for a matter of hours subsequent to ovulation they are at their lowest level of concentration.[94] Some investigators have speculated that trypsin inhibitors control the fertilization process so that ova which are aged and which are in the fallopian tube in the presence of a high concentration of inhibitors are protected from fertilization. Be that as it may, the 3-day residence in the fallopian tube apparently serves a useful function in several experimental mammals. When zygotes are removed prematurely from the tube and placed in the uterus, implantation is less likely.

Most of the work on tubal physiology has focused on its role in reproduction and only scanty information is available on the tubal immune system and its role in infection. The immunoglobulin IgG is present in tubal

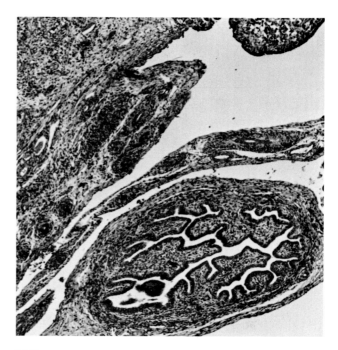

**18.6** Fetal tube, mesovarium, and portion of ovary. Tube is at lower right, ovary at upper right. Remnants of mesonephric tubules and duct may be identified as round or elongated oval cross sections surrounded by condensed, dark nuclei of their muscular coat. Hematoxylin–eosin, ×48.

fluid, but immunofluorescent studies show that the only significant tissue immunoglobulin is the secretory component of IgA. It is localized to the apical cytoplasm of the epithelial cells.[80]

## Benign Rests and Cysts

The Wolffian or mesonephric duct develops in close proximity to the fallopian tube (Figure 18.6) and remnants from it normally persist throughout adult life. These remnants consist of some 10 to 15 mesonephric tubules lying in the mesovarium. The tubules are lined by low columnar or cuboidal epithelium containing ciliated and nonciliated cells. There is only a thin, if any, muscular coat.[9] The tubules connect with the mesonephric duct, which runs parallel to the fallopian tube in the mesosalpinx. The duct is lined by nonciliated cuboidal or columnar cells surrounded by a relatively thick layer of first longitudinal and then circular smooth muscle. It is commonly seen on routine cross sections of tube lying outside the circular muscularis. Often a small group of

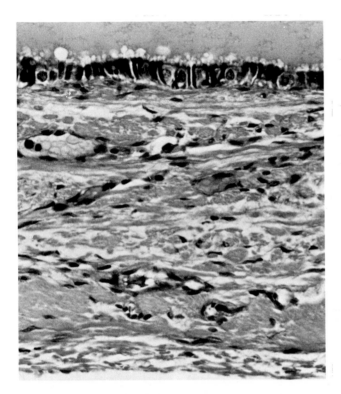

**18.7** Hydatid of Morgagni. Epithelial lining at the top contains epithelium similar to that of the tube. A few strands of smooth muscle in the wall are inapparent. Hematoxylin–eosin, ×327.

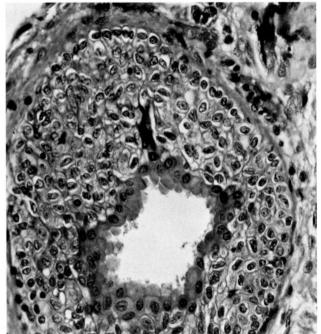

**18.8** Walthard rest. The most central epithelial cells have undergone columnar metaplasia. Nuclear grooves are visible in many of the other epithelial cells as dark lines in the long axis of the ovoid nuclei. Note the serosal surface at upper left. Hematoxylin–eosin, ×292.

ducts with thick muscle coats are seen together on section. This may be secondary to artifactual contraction and coiling of the duct on fixation.

Paratubal cysts may develop either of mesonephric (or Wolffian or Gartner's duct) origin, or of paramesonephric (or Müllerian or fallopian tube) origin.

The hydatid of Morgagni is by far the most common cyst. Grossly it is found dangling from one of the fimbriae. It is ovoid or round with a thin translucent wall and ranges from about 2 to 10 mm in diameter. It contains clear serous fluid. Histologically it has a thin fibrous wall lined by ciliated and nonciliated cells (Figure 18.7). Small epithelial-covered plicae may project into the cyst lumen. The nonciliated cells, unlike those of mesonephric origin, demonstrate distinct cyclic changes when examined by the electron microscope, indicating paramesonephric origin.[9] They are of little clinical significance.

Benign cysts originating in mesonephric ducts or tubules may form within the broad ligament or may extend from it to hang by a pedicle.[40] Grossly they may reach several centimeters in diameter and present clinically as an adnexal mass. Those of mesonephric tubular origin may be recognized by the presence of at least some ciliated cells in their single-layer epithelial lining. Their clinical importance, apart from symptoms of a pelvic mass, lies in the possibility of torsion and infarction. Because of its rarity, malignant degeneration is not a serious consideration.[41]

The tubal serosa, by invagination, may give rise to a number of benign inclusion cysts. The simplest is a 1- to 2-mm unilocular cyst lying directly beneath the serosal surface lined by mesothelial cells, a mesothelial inclusion cyst. By a process of metaplasia, these cysts may become filled with polygonal epithelial-like cells to form a Walthard rest. On gross examination a 1- to 2-mm yellowish-white nodule lies beneath the serosa. The cells of the rest often fully occupy it. Their nuclei are irregularly ovoid and a longitudinal nuclear groove gives them the "coffee-bean" appearance (Figure 18.8). Columnar metaplasia may occur in the rests and has no known significance. Both mesothelial inclusion cysts and Walthard rests are common incidental findings of no special clinical importance.

# Salpingitis

Salpingitis may be conveniently divided into three major types: acute, chronic, and granulomatous.

## Acute Salpingitis

Acute salpingitis is a purulent inflammatory process usually secondary to the introduction of bacteria from the uterine cavity into the tubal lumen. Although *Neisseria gonorrhoeae* has been considered the most common causative organism, recent meticulous bacteriologic studies indicate that anaerobic bacteria, especially *Bacteroides* sp. and peptostreptococci, are frequently present as well as such aerobes as *Escherichia coli*.[16,98,99,106] The presence in some of these women of serum antibodies against gonococcal pili, however, suggests that gonococci may initiate the process only to be supplanted by anaerobes.

Elegant *in vitro* studies by Ward and others[109] have clarified the likely initial steps in gonococcal infection. *Neisseria gonorrhoeae* perfused through the lumen of cultured whole tubes attach only to nonciliated cells. Within 3 hours microvilli from the cells appear to embrace the gonococci and adhere to them. The bacteria then penetrate both the cells and intercellular junctions with cell lysis and sloughing. Adjacent ciliated cells are also destroyed but are not invaded directly. Following cell lysis the bacteria penetrate the subepithelial connective tissue. During life this process is, naturally, considerably modified by the host response. A brisk diapedesis of granulocytes occurs from capillaries into the mucosa and lumen, and there is vascular engorgement and edema of all tubal layers (Figure 18.9). In severe cases transudation of plasma protein results in a fibrinous exudate on the serosal surface. As the lumen fills with granulocytes and cellular debris, and as the tube distends, pus may be seen dripping from the fimbriated end. The serosa reddens because of vascular dilatation and the tube attains the classic appearance of a "pus tube." The cell necrosis, distention of the tube, and focal peritonitis give rise to fever and abdominal pain. The gonococcus gains access to the tube most readily at the time of menstruation. Over the course of time, repeated invasions will result in recurrent symptoms as well as the anatomic changes of chronic salpingitis, discussed below.

Although *N. gonorrhoeae* spreads via the epithelial surface and thus causes mucosal changes, other bacteria present in the uterus, such as streptococci, tend to spread into the tube by vascular or lymphatic channels. This results in acute inflammation of the tubal wall with relative sparing of the mucosa.

Acute salpingitis appears to be increased about three-

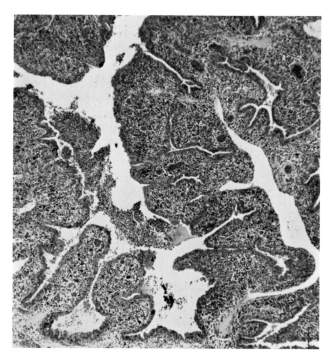

**18.9** Acute and chronic salpingitis. The plicae are broadened and blunted. Numerous granulocytes, lymphocytes, and plasma cells are present in the mucosa and many granulocytes are still present in the lumen. Hematoxylin–eosin, ×40.

fold in women using intrauterine contraceptive devices.[111] The reason for this is unknown, and nulliparous patients are disproportionately at risk.

Mycoplasma have been reported in both acute salpingitis and tuboovarian abscess.[10] Laparoscopically obtained pretreatment cultures from grossly infected tubes revealed *Mycoplasma hominis* in four of 50 patients. *Mycoplasma hominis* was present on the cervix of 54% of patients with lower genital tract infections or salpingitis but in only 4% of controls.[60,61] T-strain mycoplasma were isolated from the tubes of two additional patients, although the incidence of cervical T strain was about 45 to 55% in both infected patients and controls. The tubes examined have shown a moderate to marked infiltration with chronic inflammatory cells, some neutrophils, and focal epithelial ulceration.[10]

Almost no data on viral or chlamydial infection of the tube are available. Isolations of Coxsackie B5 and ECHO6 viruses have been reported from tubes with acute salpingitis, but no histologic data are available.[61]

An asymptomatic form of acute salpingitis is seen in tubes removed during postpartum ligation. Beginning about 5 hours after delivery and present up to 7 to 10 days

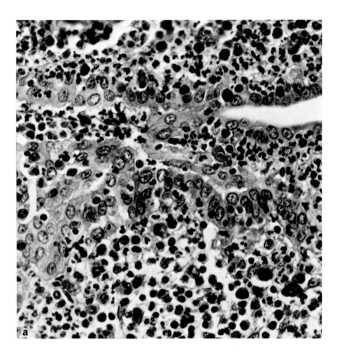

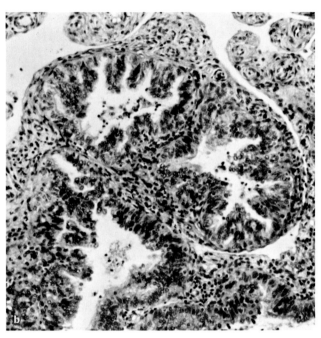

**18.10 a.** Acute and chronic salpingitis. Mucosal folds are distended with polymorphonuclear leukocytes, histiocytes, and a few lymphocytes and plasma cells. A few tiny fibrin strands lie in the lumen at left. Note the approximation of plicae and the suggestion of early adhesion at center. Hematoxylin-eosin, ×300.

**b.** Chronic salpingitis. Papillary ingrowth of reactive epithelial cells is prominent, but mitoses are absent. A few lymphocytes may be seen in the stroma. Hematoxylin–eosin, ×120.

later, a small or moderate number of acute or mixed acute and chronic inflammatory cells is found in the mucosa or lumen of 10% or more of specimens.[46,83] Attempts to culture aerobic or anaerobic bacteria[83,93] have been almost uniformly unsuccessful. The process may be regarded as secondary to the trauma of delivery and/or intrauterine tissue necrosis.

## Chronic Salpingitis

When acute salpingitis resolves through agent–host interaction, residual disease may be found in the fallopian tube. With acute inflammation, the mucosal plicae, possibly secondary to surface fibrin deposition, tend to adhere to one another (Figure 18.10a,b). Healing and organization then leads to permanent bridging between folds. In the classic case, this results in a "follicular salpingitis" (Figure 18.11). Plicae may retain much of their size and shape, but plasma cells and/or lymphocytes are still present in the mucosa. Often the height of the folds appears lowered or their intricate pattern, so prominent in the ampulla and infundibulum, is subtly altered. Fibrinous

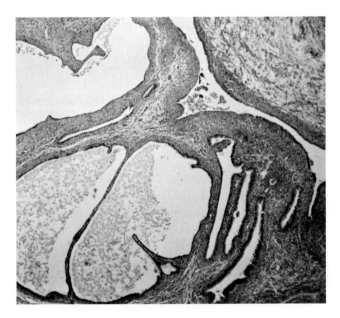

**18.11** Salpingitis follicularis. There is agglutination of plicae with the formation of dilated glandlike spaces between them. Hematoxylin-eosin, ×27.

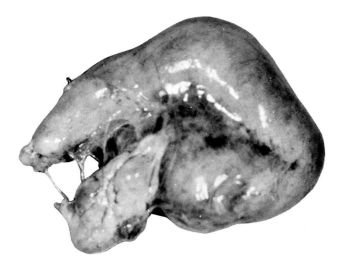

**18.12** Chronic salpingitis. Multiple, thin, fibrous adhesions are present between the tube and the ovary and between the ampulla and the infundibulum. The distal portion of the tube has a clubbed appearance because of obliteration of the tubal ostium. ×1.1.

adhesions between the serosa and surrounding peritoneal surfaces may organize into thin fibrous adhesions that, unless routinely looked for, are easily overlooked. Peritoneal inflammation may be widespread, and thin, "violin string" adhesions may form between liver and diaphragm. Agglutination of acutely inflamed fimbriae may be focal or massive. If severe enough, the bases of the fimbriae may coalesce in the center, with the fimbriae radiating outward like a daisy, or the tips of the fimbriae may adhere, blocking the lumen and causing a blunted end, the "clubbed" tube (Figure 18.12). The proximity of the ovary to the fimbriae allows multiple tuboovarian adhesions to form with occlusion of the tubal ostium. The ovary itself may then become more directly involved and a tuboovarian abscess may result (Figure 18.13).[104] If the fimbriae close before the ovary is seriously involved, the inflamed dilated tube forms a pyosalpinx full of acute and chronic inflammatory cells. As the inflammation subsides, the acute and most of the chronic inflammatory cells gradually disappear and the patient is left either with a severely scarred tube or with a hydrosalpinx.

## Hydrosalpinx

Hydrosalpinx is one of the complications of salpingitis. It is characterized by obliteration of the fimbriated end and dilation of the tube, usually the ampullary and infundibular portions. If the ovary is first involved by tuboovarian adhesions, the ovary may be compressed by the dilated tube. The dilated tube may resemble the chemist's retort and the wall is generally whitish, thin, and translucent, with occasional fibrous adhesions on its surface (Figure 18.14). The tube usually contains clear serous fluid with an

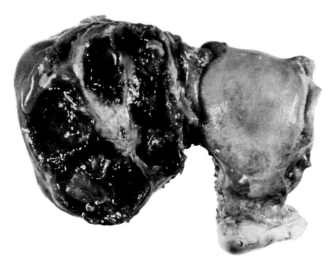

**18.13** Tuboovarian abscess. This posterior view shows a bisected tuboovarian abscess involving the entire left adnexa. The tube and ovary have been largely destroyed and replaced by a multiloculated mass containing foul-smelling pus lying in a shaggy-walled cyst. This lesion is associated with wearing of intrauterine contraceptive devices[103] as well as repeated bouts of tubal infection. Note smooth surface of uterus on right. ×0.6.

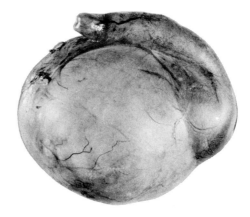

**18.14** Hydrosalpinx. The tube, especially in its ampullary portion, is dilated with total obliteration of the ostium. The wall is fibrous and translucent. ×0.6.

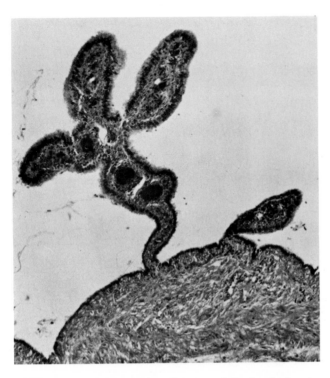

**18.15** Hydrosalpinx. Although most of the luminal epithelium is cuboidal or flattened, occasional plicae may remain with normal epithelial surface. Hematoxylin-eosin, ×95.

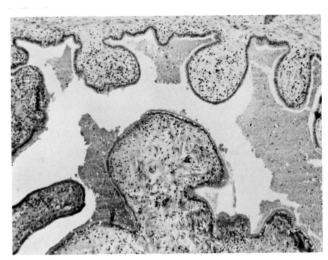

**18.16** Chronic salpingitis. Transitional stage between chronic salpingitis and hydrosalpinx. Marked blunting of plicae and only a scanty residual lymphocytic infiltrate. Hematoxylin–eosin, ×34.

electrolyte composition similar to serum but with a low protein content.[21] As a luminal communication can usually be demonstrated between dilated and nondilated portions of tube,[15,21] the etiology of the dilatation is obscure but may result in part from a sphincterlike action of the isthmus. The muscle wall is either thin and atrophic or replaced by collagenous connective tissue. The majority of the epithelial lining consists of low cuboidal cells but an occasional plica may persist with surprisingly intact columnar epithelium with histologically normal ciliated and secretory cells corresponding morphologically with the menstrual phase (Figure 18.15). The persistence of healthy appearing plicae suggests that pressure effects from the luminal fluid may not be responsible for the flattened and absent plicae. Instead, the preceding inflammatory process may have selectively damaged the tubal folds, resulting in uneven scarring and plical disappearance (Figure 18.16). A few lymphocytes may be found in the wall of the hydrosalpinx but are more commonly distinguished by their absence.

Complications of hydrosalpinx include a near impossibility of recovery of tubal function, even with expert surgery, and the possibility of tubal torsion with subsequent hemorrhagic infarction.[24]

# Granulomatous Salpingitis

Granulomatous inflammation of the fallopian tube may be provoked by a number of different organisms as well as by a variety of noninfectious processes. The histologic identification of one or more granulomas calls for immediate communication between pathologist and clinician and persistent attempts to determine the likely etiology.

## Tuberculous Salpingitis

*Mycobacterium tuberculosis,* historically, has been the predominant etiologic agent of granulomatous salpingitis. The incidence of tuberculous salpingitis in women studied for infertility ranges from about 1% in the United States to over 10% in India, whereas 10 to 20% of women who die from tuberculosis have tubal involvement.[87]

Primary infection of the genitalia, as by coitus with a partner with genitourinary tuberculosis, is extremely rare. Secondary spread, usually from a primary infection, is the normal route of infection. For reasons still unknown, the blood-borne organism preferentially lodges in the tubes rather than the other female genitalia. The primary pulmonary lesion may not be radiologically evident, but extrapulmonary involvement of the peritoneum, kidneys, or other site may be present. Lymphatic spread from primary intestinal tuberculosis[43] or direct spread from bladder or gastrointestinal tract may occur.

Although the earliest pathologic lesions are microscopic, with advancing disease the tube increases in diameter and may become nodular, mimicking salpingitis isthmica nodosa. In the more common adhesive type of the disease, multiple, dense adhesions may form between the tube and ovary and the fimbriae and ostium may be obliterated.[44] With the exudative type of disease, progressive distention mimics bacterial pyosalpinx. Hematosalpinx or hydrosalpinx may be found late in the disease process. In either form, serosal tubercles may be present.

The presence of an identifiable ostium and fimbriae in a grossly diseased tube has been regarded by some as characteristic of tuberculous salpingitis.[87]

The earliest microscopic lesions are mucosal with a typical granulomatous reaction of epithelioid cells and lymphocytes arranged in a nodular configuration. Giant cells are often seen, and central caseation, focal or massive, may be present. Immunosuppressive therapy may modify cellular immunity to a point where granulomas fail to form. With this clinical information, the mere finding of acute and chronic inflammatory cells should then lead to consideration of staining for acid-fast organisms.

From the mucosa, extension to the muscularis and serosa may occur.

Microscopically, as the tubercles enlarge, they may erode through the mucosa and discharge their contents into the tubal lumen (Figure 18.17). The mucosal inflammatory reaction leads to progressive scarring with plical distortion and conglutination. Large caseous nodules may form and coalesce, eventually filling the dilated tube. Ectopic calcification may occur in areas of fibrosis. As tubercles may not be present in a given section, the presence of caseation, fibrosis, or calcification in a tube may be the only histologic finding pointing to the necessity for more thorough study. The presence of severe mucosal atypicality in tuberculous salpingitis and confusion with adenocarcinoma has been stressed by numerous authors, but similar atypia may be found in chronic salpingitis (Figure 18.10b).[64] Complications of tuberculous salpingitis are several. Alteration in function is the rule. Sterility is almost universal because of the common bilaterality of the disease. Rarely, successful pregnancies occur but ectopic

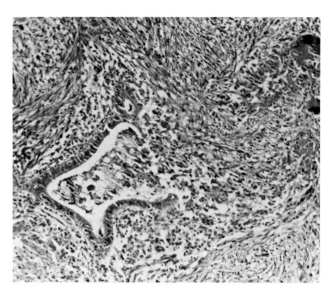

**18.17** Tuberculous salpingitis. Two giant cells are present in granulomas at upper right. There is necrosis and very early caseation in the center of the granulomas. One of the granulomas appears to be rupturing into a pocket of tubal epithelium, illustrating a mechanism whereby *M. tuberculosis* can reach the lumen and then seed the endometrial cavity. Hematoxylin–eosin, ×77.

tubal nidation is at least as common in the event fertilization is successful.[87]

Pelvic pain, sterility, or menstrual irregularities are the most common complaints. Because of repeated seeding of the endometrium from the infected tubes, mycobacterial culture and the histologic finding on currettage of endometrial tubercles are diagnostically useful. Laparoscopy and culdoscopy have been indicted as possibly causing bowel perforation in cases of extensive pelvic and peritoneal tuberculosis.

## Schistosomiasis

Although tubal bilharziasis must be one of the commonest causes of granulomatous salpingitis worldwide, it is rare in the United States. In Africa reported tubal infections may occur in as many as 20% of unselected women at autopsy.[37] The ova of *Schistosoma hematobium* are most common but *S. mansoni* eggs may be present in some women.[42] If granulomas are present and there is a suspicion of schistosomiasis, sodium hydroxide digestion of remaining tubal tissue may reveal ova.

Gross findings appear to be related to fibrosis surrounding the ova, producing a nodular or fibrotic tube. Ectopic pregnancy in an infected tube may precipitate its removal, but the granulomas themselves may not always cause sufficient damage to account for abnormal nidation.[7]

## Actinomycosis

Actinomycotic infections of the tube may occur, many of them associated with intrauterine contraceptive devices.[25,97]

Grossly, a large fibrous mass is present which often includes the ovary. The mass may appear simply to be a dilated tube or may be more obviously inflammatory by being bound down to pelvic structures with adhesions with or without fistula formation. Pus is present in the shaggy walled cavities within the tube. Anaerobic culture will permit growth of *Actinomyces israeli.* Microscopically, numerous histiocytes, plasma cells, and lymphocytes are present in the abscess walls, and gram-positive filamentous clumps, "sulfur granules," may be recognized in the pus. Complications in unrecognized cases may include dissemination to the liver and lung.

## Pinworm

The pinworm, *Enterobius vermicularis,* may migrate up the female genital tract, embed in the tube, and cause an imflammatory reaction. The tube may be involved with the ovary in what appears to be a tuboovarian abscess, or a fibrous nodular area may be present. Acute and chronic inflammatory cells may be found together with eosinophils, Charcot–Leyden crystals, and portions of gravid female worm. Ova may be released into the tissue, where they provoke a granulomatous reaction. The ova may be identified by their size (about 30 by 50 $\mu$) and ovoid asymmetrical shape[100] but may be obscured by calcification of granulomas. The ova may be widely disseminated in the peritoneum in the absence of histologic tubal involvement and the fibrous granulomas may simulate metastatic carcinoma.[34]

## Sarcoid

Sarcoidosis of the tube is rarely reported[44] and appears to accompany disseminated disease. One case[52] had gross tubal distention, tuboovarian adhesions, an ovarian abscess, and multiple serosal nodules, but bacterial salpingitis was not excluded as a cause. Histologically, noncaseating granulomas may be seen in the mucosa. Culture, special

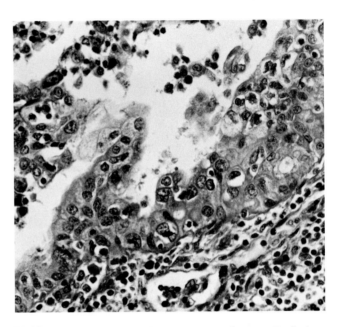

**18.18** Granulomatous salpingitis secondary to Crohn's disease. Underlying granulomas are not visible here, but severe chronic inflammation is present at the lower right. Epithelium is piled up and has marked nuclear atypia. This change should not be confused for carcinoma in situ. Hematoxylin–eosin, ×200.

stains, and clinical information is necessary to exclude other granulomatous diseases.

## Crohn's Disease

Crohn's disease of the ileum, colon, or appendix may secondarily involve the tube and ovary to produce a granulomatous salpingo-oophoritis.[11,114] Noncaseating granulomas may involve the entire thickness of the tubal muscularis as well as the mucosa. The epithelium may react with severe cellular atypia (Figure 18.18). Fistulas from bowel to tube may also occur.[19]

## Foreign Body

Foreign material may be introduced into the tube in the course of gynecologic investigation, especially hysterosalpingography. Lubricant jelly, mineral oil, and starch and talc powder may cause a lipoid or granulomatous salpingitis.[13,28] An intense phagocytic reaction to introduced lipid material causes accumulation of subepithelial foamy histiocytes (Figure 18.19). Talc may cause mucosal or serosal granulomas. A habit of examining all granulomas or

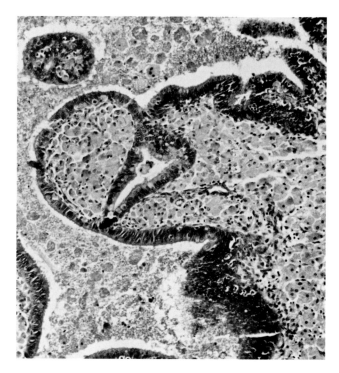

**18.19** Foreign body reaction in tubal mucosa. Hysterosalpingography or exposure to other foreign material may lead to an intense histiocytic reaction, as here, or to formation of foreign body granulomas. Hematoxylineosin, ×100.

foreign body reactions under polarized light is useful in the recognition of these processes.

Although other disease processes in the tube, such as leprosy,[113] may be mentioned on rare occasions as possible causes of granulomatous salpingitis, they are so infrequent as to be of little clinical or pathologic significance.

## Salpingitis Isthmica Nodosa

This peculiar condition consists of one or more outpouchings or diverticula of tubal epithelium in the isthmic region, often bilateral, and usually accompanied by nodular hyperplasia of the surrounding muscularis.

The etiology is presently unknown. The disease is found in women between the ages of 25 and 60 years, with the average age of discovery of about 30 years.[5] As the lesion is almost unknown prior to puberty and not found congenitally, attention has focused on other possible causes. These include postinflammatory distortion[89] and an adenomyosis-like process.[5,115] Against the proposed inflammatory etiology is the usual localization of nodu-

larity in the isthmic portion of the tube or immediately adjacent ampulla.[5] The majority of the ampulla is uninvolved, unlike the usual picture in inflammatory salpingitis. When salpingitis isthmica nodosa is associated with inflammatory salpingitis, such as pyosalpinx and hydrosalpinx, the inflammatory process is nearly as often contralateral as it is ipsilateral.[5] Although a few lymphocytes are found in the peridiverticular stroma, scarring is normally absent.

Evidence for a noninflammatory adenomyosis-like origin is more convincing. Moderate or large numbers of endometrial-like stroma cells accompany the diverticula in over half the cases.[5] As in uterine adenomyosis, the presence of glands appears to stimulate muscular growth with subsequent mural thickening. Unilateral tubal involvement is often accompanied by uterine adenomyosis on the same side.[115]

The external gross appearance consists of one or more nodular swellings in the isthmus up to 1 to 2 cm in diameter. The serosa is smooth. On section the tissue is firm and a sharp eye may pick out some of the dilated diverticula. Microscopically, the diverticula appear on the typical cross-section as dispersed glands of tubal epithelium surrounded by stout bands of muscularis (Figure 18.20). Diverticula may closely approach the serosal surface but do not normally connect with it. Endometrial-like stroma cells lying beneath the epithelial outpouchings may be abundant, sparse, or absent. If both glands and stroma are really apparent, a diagnosis of tubal endometriosis may well be considered. Because the underlying configuration is diverticular rather than glandular (Figure 18.21) and as the condition is not clearly related to pelvic endometriosis, it seems best to preserve the term "salpingitis isthmica nodosa" until the etiology is better understood.

The most serious clinical and pathologic complications of salpingitis isthmica nodosa are the high incidence of infertility and the strong association with ectopic pregnancy.[78] Inflammatory tubal disease may be associated with it ipsilaterally or contralaterally. A rare complication that we have seen recently is rupture of a deep diverticulum through the serosa with subsequent mild intraabdominal bleeding and pelvic pain.

## Torsion, Prolapse, and Intussusception

Among the various anatomical displacements of the tube, torsion is the commonest. The usual predisposing factors are cystic enlargement of the ipsilateral ovary, or

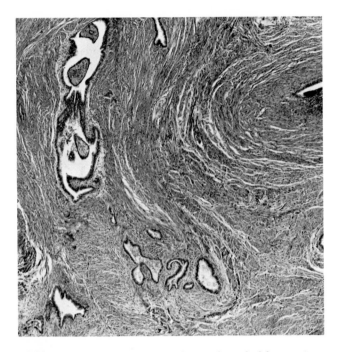

**18.20** Salpingitis isthmica nodosa. The tubal lumen is visible at the upper right. The cross-sectioned diverticula are widely separated by stout bands of smooth muscle. A few endometrial-like stromal cells are present at the lower right of the large central diverticulum. Hematoxylin–eosin, ×30.

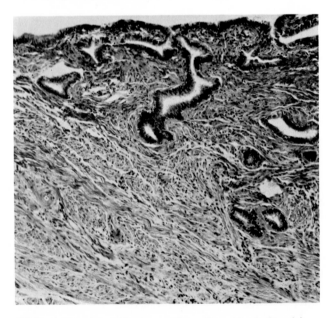

**18.21** Salpingitis isthmica nodosa. Diverticula lined by normal tubal epithelium extend into the muscularis. Note the lack of inflammation. Hematoxylin–eosin, ×75.

tubal enlargement secondary to hydro- or pyosalpinx,[53] but torsion may occur in the absence of apparent adnexal disease.

The typical patient is in the reproductive years and complains of the sudden onset of lower abdominal pain. At operation, the adnexa on one side are twisted in either direction, usually once or twice. Venous outflow is compromised early, and the resulting congestion may lead to arterial compression. The adnexa are often swollen and edematous with hemorrhagic infarction and gangrene, although prompt recognition and operation may lead to discovery of an earlier reversible state. A benign ovarian tumor is present in 40% of patients and malignant ovarian tumors in an additional 15%.[53] Paraovarian cysts are also associated with torsion. Undiagnosed torsion in the infant may result in resorption and total disappearance of the infarcted adnexa or in calcification of the necrotic tissue.[14]

Tubal prolapse into the vagina may rarely occur as a complication of hysterectomy, usually vaginal.[29,86]

Clinically this is characterized by vaginal discharge beginning a few days up to several years after hysterectomy. On examination, an excrescence is seen in the vaginal vault suggestive of granulation tissue or carcinoma. Fimbriae may be apparent grossly. Severe acute and chronic inflammation is present microscopically, and pseudogland formation by the tubal epithelium may mimic adenocarcinoma.[86]

Intussusception of the tube has been reported once.[2] A paraovarian cyst was engulfed by the end of the tube and pulled the fimbriated end into the ampulla. Simple eversion and cystectomy permitted tubal salvage.

## Endometriosis

Endometriosis may affect the tube in two anatomic locations with different consequences. First, the tubal lumen in the interstitial or isthmic segments may be totally filled by endometrial tissue (Figure 18.22) with resultant loss of function. This should be distinguished from focal extension of the endometrium into the interstitial portion of the tube, which displaces the lumen slightly without obliterating it. This finding is a normal anatomic variant.[56] Second, functional serosal implants may lead to repeated bouts of intralesional hemorrhage and fibrosis. This may result in periodic pelvic pain and sufficient scarring to account for infertility. During pregnancy a florid decidual reaction occurs in stromal cells of the serosal endometrial implants.

When glands and endometrial-like stroma cells are

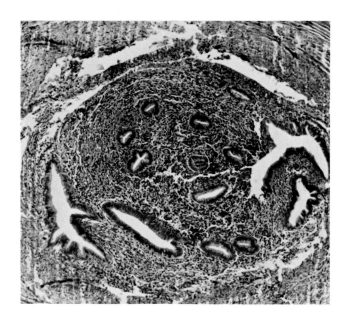

**18.22** Endometriosis. Endometrial glands and stroma completely fill the lumen of the isthmus. Hematoxylin–eosin, ×62.

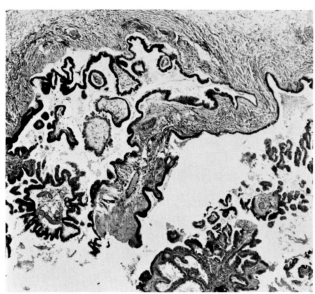

**18.23** Endosalpingiosis. Papillary projections from the surface of the ovary (top) are lined by benign tubal epithelium. A similar change on the omentum may be confused with metastatic disease. Hematoxylin–eosin, ×40.

found in the tubal muscularis, salpingitis isthmica nodosa should be strongly considered. However, if there is serosal disease, and if the glandular epithelium appears endometrial with near total absence of ciliated cells, then the diagnosis of tubal endometriosis seems preferable.

## Endosalpingiosis

Epithelium resembling that of the normal tube may be occasionally seen on ovarian or other peritoneal surfaces.[12,47] Such lesions are termed endosalpingiosis.[84] Grossly the affected areas may resemble implants of endometriosis. Microscopically there are delicate, occasionally branching fibrovascular fronds or papillae lined by secretory, ciliated, and intercalary cells similar to those of the normal tube. Two possible etiologies are metaplasia[12] and inflammation.[48] A metaplastic process of the coelomic lining partially reduplicating the embryologic development of the tubal epithelium could give rise to such a condition. Close association with endometriosis, another condition of possible metaplastic origin, does occur.[12]

Ruptured inflammatory adhesions between the tube and various pelvic sites could result in transfer of tubal epithelium to an extratubal site, and this would account for fimbrialike processes on the ovarian surface (Figure 18.23).[48]

Although the lesions appear histologically benign, if an ovarian tumor is present they may be mistaken for metastatic implants.[12]

## Infertility of Tubal Origin

Most of the diseases discussed in this chapter may result in sufficient anatomic distortion to cause infertility. Although purely physiologic causes of infertility, such as abnormal motility or abnormal tubal secretions may theoretically interfere with normal tubal function, such lesions have not yet been convincingly shown to occur in experimental animals or man in the absence of anatomically visible abnormality. Further investigation of these factors, however, might uncover new diseases of physiologic dysfunction. The same lines of investigation might also lead to new methods of prevention of pregnancy.

Contraception through interference with tubal function involves procedures designed to damage the tube either by surgical removal of a segment or the fimbriated end or by heat coagulation of a portion of the tube. Tubal resection is best confirmed by histologic demonstration of a complete cross section of tubal lumen. In spite of these procedures, spontaneous reanastomosis may occur in approxi-

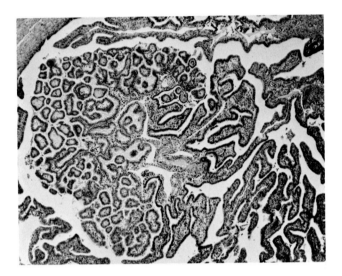

**18.24** Epithelial papilloma. A single layer of uniform cells lines a delicately branched papillary core. Hematoxylin–eosin, ×27.

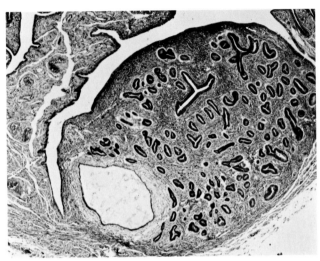

**18.25** Adenomyoma. A nodule of mixed simple glands and smooth muscle fibers protrudes into the tubal lumen. Hematoxylin–eosin, ×27.

mately 1% of all cases. The success of surgical reanastomosis in reestablishing a patent lumen varies with the extent of the initial procedure and the skill of the surgeon but is reported to be as high as 80%. Only 25 to 40% of the patients, however, will subsequently become pregnant. The incidence of ectopic pregnancy following reanastomosis is increased.

## Benign Tumors

Both benign and malignant tumors of the fallopian tube are uncommon. They are frequently mistaken for lesions of chronic salpingitis or pyosalpinx, both preoperatively and during the actual operative procedure itself. Benign tumors are most often of mesodermal origin and are usually small enough to be incidental findings at laparotomy.

### Benign Epithelial Tumors

Epithelial papillomas or polyps are rare. The only example acquired in our laboratory in the past 40 years was an incidental finding in a 42-year-old woman. It was composed of a delicate branching stromal stalk lined by a single layer of nonciliated columnar cells with regular nuclei (Figure 18.24). Whether or not these lesions have malignant potential is unknown. Because of the papillary proliferation that may accompany salpingitis (Figure 18.10b), one should be disinclined to diagnose a papilloma

in the presence of inflammatory cells or plical distortion secondary to previous inflammation.

### Benign Mesodermal Tumors

Tumors of smooth muscle origin, chiefly leiomyomas, may originate from the tubal muscularis, from smooth muscle of the broad ligament, or from walls of blood vessels in either location. Compared to the frequency of uterine leiomyomas, tubal leiomyomas are quite uncommon.[82] Microscopically they are similar to those found in the uterus and can undergo similar degenerative changes. Rarely, benign glands and smooth muscle may be so intimately involved in a tumor that a true adenomyoma is produced (Figure 18.25).

Other benign tumors of mesenchymal origin are rare. Hemangiomas,[27] lipomas,[23] and neural tumors[68,110] have been reported. Their microscopic appearance is identical to that of similar tumors appearing elsewhere in the body. Those whose pathology experience is limited to gynecologic tissue may wish to consult a general surgical pathologist for confirmation of some of these connective tissue tumors. Occasionally a benign fibroblastic or fatty tumor will contain a focus of cartilage.[3,69]

### Mesothelioma

Benign mesotheliomas (adenomatoid tumors) are the most frequent type of benign tubal tumor. Previously reported "lymphangiomas"[85] likely represent examples of this entity. They are usually only 1 cm in diameter, ap-

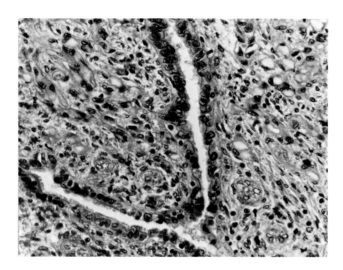

**18.26** Benign mesothelioma (adenomatoid tumor). The tumor infiltrates mucosal folds in a diffuse manner. Confusion with carcinoma is possible on frozen section. Note the intact epithelium of the tubal lumen. Hematoxylin–eosin, ×346.

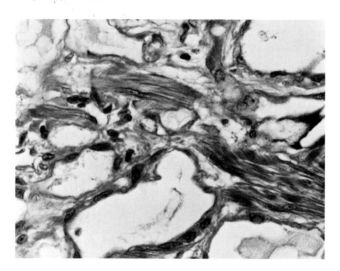

**18.27** Benign mesothelioma (adenomatoid tumor). Cuboidal or flattened mesothelial cells line dilated slitlike spaces. Penetration between small bundles of smooth muscle is seen here. Hematoxylin–eosin, ×346.

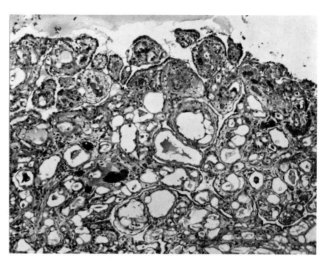

**18.28** Benign mesothelioma (adenomatoid tumor). Multiple connections with serosal surface are seen at the top. Cuboidal or flattened cells line round or slitlike spaces. Hematoxylin–eosin, ×54.

pearing as a nodular swelling beneath the tubal serosa, and are yellow or whitish gray on section. Similar lesions may be found on the uterine surface[105] and in the cul-de-sac.[113]

Their chief importance to the gynecologic pathologist is differentiation from carcinoma at the time of frozen section (Figure 18.26). Microscopically, multiple, small slitlike or ovoid spaces are seen lined by a single layer of low cuboidal or flattened endothelial-like cells (Figure 18.27). Connection with the serosa may be seen on a fortuitous section (Figure 18.28) but usually the serosa covers the lesion. The tumor may be large enough to displace the tubal lumen eccentrically and may grow into the supporting stroma of the luminal folds in an infiltrating manner (Figure 18.26). Histochemical studies[103] have shown hyaluronidase-digestable, alcian blue-positive material in the cells and spaces. No significant glycogen or intracellular mucin is present, as might be found in a tumor of Müllerian origin. Electron microscopy[32,103] supports a mesothelial origin for these lesions. Microvilli project from the cell surfaces. Bundles of tonofilaments are present and are occasionally attached to desmosomes. Desmosomes are numerous between cells but are absent along the basal lamina on which the cells lie. These features are not characteristic of endothelial or Müllerian epithelium but are seen in benign mesotheliomas[32] as well as in malignant mesotheliomas. Clinically they are asymptomatic and rarely, if ever, recur after adequate excision.

## Benign Teratoma

Benign tubal teratomas compose a distinct group of tumors. Grossly they are located most frequently in the lumen, often attached by a pedicle to the inner tubal wall. They may, however, be intramural or attached to the serosa. On section they are more often cystic than solid and tend to be either rather small (1 to 2 cm in diameter), or quite large (10 to 20 cm in diameter).[64] As in their ovarian counterparts, ecto-, meso-, and endodermal layers

357

are represented by well-differentiated mature elements. One lesion consisting entirely of mature thyroid tissue has been described in the tube of a woman without clinical hyperthyroidism.[49] An isolated nodule of pancreatic tissue has also been found beneath the tubal mucosa of one patient.[62] Immature or malignant tubal teratomas remain to be described.

Although recent evidence suggests that ovarian teratomas originate in abnormally developing ova,[95] no displaced primordial follicles or ova have been described in the tubal lumen, nor is there evidence of origin from implantation of a zygote. Over 10% are bilateral. Clinically the patient is frequently nulliparous and is most often in the fourth decade.

## Adrenal Rests

Adrenal cortical rests, if carefully looked for, may be found in the broad ligament in over 20% of women. They lie in the ligament "anywhere from its junction with the mesosalpinx to its lateral attachment to the pelvic wall"[30] adjacent to the ovarian vein and just beneath the peritoneum. Grossly they appear as yellow nodules or disks but may be obscured by fat. Medullary tissue is absent, but microscopically all three cortical layers are recognizable. This accessory tissue may hypertrophy secondary to adrenal destruction[50] or may, rarely, give rise to a functional cortical adenoma.[8]

## Hilus Cells

Nests of cells morphologically similar to ovarian hilus cells have been described in the midportion of the tube.[69] In the absence of Reinke crystalloids, close association with nonmyelinated nerve fibers, or histochemical studies, it is difficult to exclude the possibility of an adrenal rest. Hilus cell nests with Reinke crystalloids may be seen, however, in fimbrial stroma.[54]

## Wolffian Adenoma

A small group of distinctive tumors has been recently described located either within the leaves of the broad ligament or attached to the tube by a pedicle.[51] They may measure from 1.3 to 12 cm in greatest dimension and are lobulated with gross encapsulation. On section the consistency may be rubbery or friable, and cysts or calcification may be present. The microscopic picture varies widely. Solid masses of epithelial cells may be present or tubular

areas may be found similar to Pick's tubular adenoma. A sievelike pattern reminiscent of benign tubal mesotheliomas may also be seen. Microscopically the capsule is often breached by tongues of tumor and a solitary liver metastasis has been found in one case.[102] Hence the tumors are not as benign as originally proposed.[51] Patients have been from 29 to 58 years old and have presented either with abdominal pain and a palpable mass or else have had the tumor discovered as an incidental finding. Origin in other than Wolffian structures is thought to be unlikely.[51]

Besides tumors of smooth muscle origin, other tumors of the broad ligament, whether benign or malignant, are extremely uncommon.[41]

Two distinctly different multifocal lesions may involve the tubal serosa; mature glial implants, and leiomyomatosis peritonealis disseminata.

## Glial Implants

Occasionally, a mature solid ovarian[81] or nonovarian pelvic teratoma will be found accompanied by multiple implants of mature glial tissue. They are found on all peritoneal surfaces, including the tube and broad ligaments. The outcome following the removal of the teratoma is benign unless immature elements are present in the primary. One possible mechanism for the spread of this mature glial tissue is trauma to the capsule of the primary tumor.

## Leiomyomatosis Peritonealis Disseminata

A peculiar serosal change, often associated with pregnancy, has been described in a few women. This consists of nodules or plaquelike accumulations of spindle cells resembling fibroblasts or smooth muscle cells. These lesions may be found beneath the pelvic peritoneum, including that covering the tube and broad ligament. Their location and the occasional presence of decidualike cells has led to the proposal[71] that these lesions represent a fibroblastic metaplasia of extrauterine decidual tissue. As this change occurs on occasion in nonpregnant women,[101] this proposed origin is somewhat speculative, although decidual change may be seen in the absence of pregnancy. Mitoses tend to be quite frequent in these lesions, although nuclear atypia is not marked. Not every case has a perfectly benign course, as spread to the lung of nodules of mature smooth muscle fibers (benign metastasizing leiomyoma) may be seen, usually associated with pregnancy.[4]

# Malignant Tumors

Malignant tumors involving the tube are usually secondary to spread from carcinomas of the ovary or endometrium.[112] Peritoneal spread naturally involves the serosal surface, whereas lymphatic metastases from adjacent primary sites may involve the mucosa or muscularis as well.

Endolymphatic stromal myosis, originating in the uterus, may extend to involve the tubes and ovaries. Spread takes place by the extension of wormlike tongues of tumor along tubal lymphatics. Blood-borne metastases from breast carcinomas or other extrapelvic tumors may also occur.

On occasion, squamous carcinoma of the uterine cervix may spread in an *in situ* manner to involve the endometrial cavity, tubes, and even the ovarian surfaces.[79] Primary squamous carcinoma is a rarity.[58]

The presence of a large ovarian primary coupled with tumor in the lumen of the fallopian tube and tumor in the endometrial cavity suggests that the tubal lumen may serve as a conduit for tumor spread.

Primary malignancy of the fallopian tube, although less common than metastatic tumor, may present both clinical and pathologic diagnostic problems.

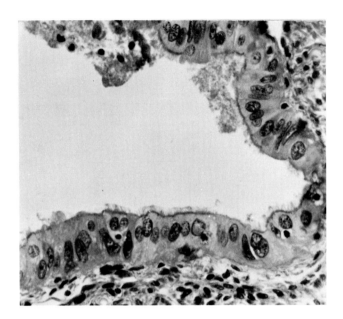

**18.29** Benign oncocytic metaplasia. Nuclear atypia and cell crowding in the absence of papillary formations and mitoses should not be confused with early carcinoma. Hematoxylin–eosin, ×385.

## Carcinoma in Situ

The great majority of primary malignant lesions of the fallopian tube are adenocarcinomas. Although the typical adenocarcinoma is rarely a diagnostic problem, a good deal of confusion has centered on what constitutes the earliest malignant change.[77] Previous authors[75,113] have illustrated cases in which tubal epithelium showed nuclear crowding and atypia and termed it carcinoma in situ. Moore and Enterline have recently reported similar epithelial changes in 18% of routinely accessioned salpingectomy specimens.[65] Frequently changes in their series were present in only one or two sections of the entirely blocked tube (Figures 18.3 and 18.4). Although the lesions were more common in tubes with salpingitis, 14% of otherwise normal tubes evinced changes consisting of nuclear crowding and stratification, loss of polarity, and nuclear atypia. Mitoses were quite sparse. Papillary formation with some bridging reminiscent of some forms of mammary papillomatosis occurred in a few cases. An oncocytic type of metaplasia with cytoplasmic acidophilia was occasionally present (Figures 18.3 and 18.29).

As noted previously, papillary formations with atypia are common in various forms of chronic salpingitis. Numerous mitoses or evidence of invasion would provide the surest proof of malignancy in these lesions.

Carcinoma in situ is apparently safely diagnosed only when exuberant papillary formations with mitoses and marked nuclear atypia are present, and one must question whether nonpapillary noninfiltrative lesions ever represent carcinoma in situ.

Startling epithelial changes that tend to mimic early papillary adenocarcinoma may be produced by accidental exposure of the specimen to heat.[17]

## Invasive Primary Tubal Adenocarcinoma

Unfortunately, primary tubal carcinoma is rarely found in the *in situ* stage. The typical patient is in her fifth or sixth decade and ordinarily presents with one or more of the classic signs or symptoms of invasive tubal carcinoma: clear or serosanguinous vaginal discharge, pelvic pain, or pelvic mass.[45,91] The diagnosis is rarely made prior to operation, but occasionally positive cytology associated with negative endometrial curettage will indicate the correct location of malignancy.[6]

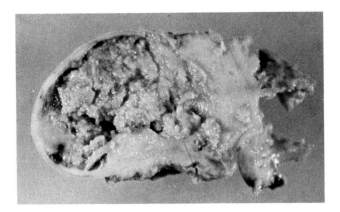

**18.30** Primary tubal adenocarcinoma. The tube is dilated and filled by papillary and solid tumor growth, which penetrates the muscularis along the lower margin of the specimen. ×1.6.

Pathologically, the tube is usually swollen secondary to advanced intraluminal growth. Hydrosalpinx or tubo-ovarian abscess are ruled out only after the specimen is opened. The lumen is usually filled and dilated by papillary or solid tumor (Figure 18.30). The fimbriated end is closed in about half the cases.[113]

Alveolar, papillary, and medullary patterns of tumor growth may be observed microscopically but mixtures are frequent. Disorganized piling up of cells with mitoses, nuclear pleomorphism, and hyperchromaticity is present in virtually all types (Figures 18.31 and 18.32). Abrupt transitions from normal to neoplastic epithelium may be found. Mucin production is usually inconspicuous but may rarely be prominent. Attempts to grade tumor anaplasia have not proved to be of prognostic value,[45] but staging (Table 18.1) clearly provides useful information.[90] Unfortunately, 5-year survival is not synonymous with cure. Nineteen percent of patients were alive but with tumor at 5 years.[90]

Bilateral tubal carcinoma is relatively common but the reason for this is unknown. A common carcinogenic stimulus could cause simultaneous development of tumor in both tubes, or a retrograde lymphatic spread following blockage by advanced tubal carcinoma of one side could lead to metastatic deposits contralaterally. Subsequent growth might then mimic a second primary. The fact that bilateral tubal carcinoma is present in only about 7% of stage 0–2 lesions but may be seen in as many as 30% of stage 3 and 4 lesions[90] suggests that metastatic spread in advanced lesions is an important cause of bilaterality.

Carcinomas other than adenocarcinomas are rare.

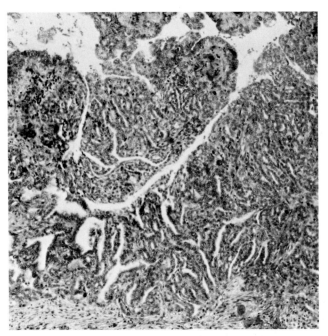

**18.31** Tubal adenocarcinoma. A papillary–alveolar pattern of intraluminal tumor growth is present. Note the invasion of the muscularis at lower right. Hematoxylin-eosin, ×75.

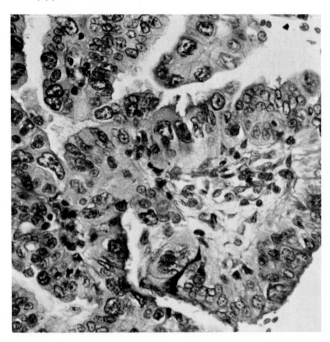

**18.32** Tubal adenocarcinoma. Papillary projections are lined by piled up epithelial cells, showing marked nuclear atypia. Mitoses are present in nearby areas. Hematoxylin-eosin, ×300.

**Table 18.1** Staging and survival in adenocarcinoma of the fallopian tube

| Stage | Definition | Number of patients | Percent 5-year survival without disease |
|-------|------------|--------------------|------------------------------------------|
| 0 | Carcinoma in situ | 11 | 82 |
| 1 | Tumor extends into submucosa or muscularis, not serosa | 13 | 53 |
| 2 | Tumor extends to serosa | 6 | 16 |
| 3 | Tumor extends to ovary and/or endometrium | 12 | 8 |
| 4 | Tumor extends beyond reproductive organs | 34 | 9 |

[a] After Schiller and Silverberg.[90]

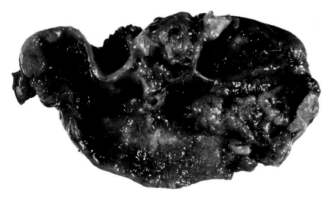

**18.33** Primary tubal carcinosarcoma. The dilated tube has been opened to illustrate the irregular intraluminal projections and a shaggy irregular mucosal surface (slightly reduced).

Adenoacanthomas or adenosquamous carcinomas are composed, respectively, of foci of benign or malignant appearing squamous epithelium within an adenocarcinoma.[45] Primary squamous and transitional cell carcinomas have been described.[31,58]

## Sarcomas

Sarcomas of the tube are exceedingly uncommon and may be pure or mixed with carcinomatous elements.

Pure sarcomas may be histologically classified if suffi-

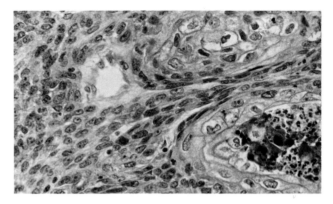

**18.34** Carcinosarcoma of the tube. Two ovoid islands of malignant squamous epithelium on the right lie in a stroma of leiomyosarcoma. Hematoxylin-eosin, ×219.

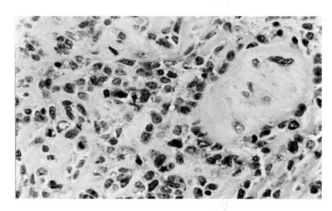

**18.35** Primary mixed mesodermal tumor of the tube. On the right, a relatively acellular nodule of osteoid may be seen lying in a sarcomatous background. Elsewhere, carcinomatous areas were present. Hematoxylin-eosin, ×277.

cient differentiation is present. Leiomyosarcomas[1] are perhaps the most common type and may arise from the tube or broad ligament. Chondrosarcomas have been described.[1,88] Carcinomas mixed with sarcomas containing only elements normally present in the fallopian tubes, such as smooth muscle, are termed carcinosarcomas (Figures 18.33 and 18.34). If heterologous elements not normally found in the tubes, such as cartilage or bone, are present the tumor is termed "mixed mesodermal tumor" (Figure 18.35).[116] The number of cases available is too few to prove any prognostic difference between these two groups.

As with tubal carcinomas, patients with sarcomas may have watery or bloody vaginal discharge and abdominal pain and may present with signs of intraperitoneal spread. Life span is usually measured in months.

## Lymphomas

Tubal involvement by lymphoma is rare and is almost invariably associated with simultaneous involvement of the ipsilateral ovary.[1] Undifferentiated carcinoma must be ruled out.

## Trophoblastic Tumors

Trophoblastic tubal tumors are exceedingly rare. Hydatiform moles usually occur as isolated growths but may be associated with intrauterine pregnancy.[96] Histologically their appearance is similar to intrauterine molar pregnancy. Clinically, perhaps one in 5,000 ectopic pregnancies will prove to be a mole.[49]

Choriocarcinoma of the tube occurs during the reproductive years and has often metastasized by the time of its discovery.[74] At least one case was associated with a simultaneous ectopic pregnancy.[57] Clinically the patient is believed to have an ectopic pregnancy. At operation a large and very hemorrhagic fleshy mass may have largely destroyed the tube. Histologically, the malignant trophoblastic proliferation is similar to that of uterine choriocarcinomas. Response to modern chemotherapy has been gratifying.[74]

# REFERENCES

1. Abrams, J., Kazal, H. L., and Hobbs, R. E. Primary sarcoma of the fallopian tube. *Am. J. Obstet. Gynecol.* 75:180, 1958.

2. Adams, B. E. Intussusception of a fallopian tube. *Am. J. Surg.* 118:591, 1969.

3. Bachmann, F. F. Ein chondrolipom des Eileiters. *Geburtshilfe Frauenheilkd* 21:975, 1961.

4. Barnes, H. M., and Richardson, P. J. Benign metastasizing fibroleiomyoma. *J. Obstet. Gynecol. Br. Commonw.* 80:569, 1973.

5. Benjamin, C. L., and Beaver, D. C. Pathogenesis of salpingitis isthmica nodosa. *Am. J. Clin. Pathol.* 21:212, 1951.

6. Benson, P. A. Cytologic diagnosis in primary carcinoma of fallopian tube. *Acta Cytol.* 18:429, 1974.

7. Bland, K. G., and Gelfand, M. The effects of schistosomiasis on the fallopian tubes in the african female. *J. Obstet. Gynaecol. Br. Commonw.* 77:1024, 1970.

8. Boularan, Cahuzac, Salvador, and Genesseau. Macrogénitosomie et gynandrie chez un sujet porteur de deux tumeurs cortico-surrénaliennes incluses dans les ligaments larges. *Annales d'Endocrinol.* 6:57, 1945.

9. Bransilver, B. R., Ferenczy, A., and Richart, R. M. Female genital tract remnants. An ultrastructural comparison of hydatid of Morgagni and mesonephric ducts and tubules. *Arch. Pathol.* 96:255, 1973.

10. Braun, P., and Besdine, R. Tuboovarian abscess with recovery of T. mycoplasma. *Am. J. Obstet. Gynecol.* 117:861, 1971.

11. Brooks, J. J., and Wheeler, J. E. Granulomatous salpingitis secondary to Crohn's disease. *Obstet. Gynecol.* (in press).

12. Burmeister, R. E., Fechner, R. E., and Franklin, R. R. Endosalpingiosis of the peritoneum. *Obstet. Gynecol.* 34:310, 1969.

13. Campbell, J. S., Nigam, S., Hurtig, A., Sahasrabudhe, M. R., and Marino, I. Mineral oil granulomas of the uterus and parametrium and granulomatous salpingitis with Schaumann bodies and oxalate deposits. *Fertil. Steril.* 15:278, 1964.

14. Case Records of the Massachusetts General Hospital (Case 9-1971). *N. Engl. J. Med.* 284:491, 1971.

15. Chevallier, G., and Parent, B. L'hydrosalpinx. Etude de 253 cas. *Presse Med.* 74:2035, 1966.

16. Chow, A. W., Malkasian, K. L., Marshall, J. R., and Guze, L. B. The bacteriology of acute pelvic inflammatory disease. *Am. J. Obstet. Gynecol.* 122:876, 1975.

17. Cornog, J. L., Curie, J. L., and Rubin, A. Heat artifact simulating adenocarcinoma of fallopian tube. *J.A.M.A.* 214:1118, 1970.

18. Coutinho, E. M., Maia, H. Jr., and Mattos, C. E. R. Contractility of the fallopian tube. *Gynecol. Invest.* 6:146, 1975.

19. Crohn, B. B., and Yarnis, H. *Regional Ileitis*, 2nd ed., New York, Grune and Stratton, 1958.

20. Croxatto, H. B., Diaz, S., Fuentealba, B., Croxatto, H. D., Carrillo, D., and Fabres, C. Studies on the duration of egg transport in the human oviduct. I. The time interval between ovulation and egg recovery from the uterus in normal women. *Fertil. Steril.* 23:447, 1972.

21. David, A., Garcia, C.-R., and Czernobilsky, B. Human hydrosalpinx. Histologic study and chemical composition of fluid. *Am. J. Obstet. Gynecol.* 105:400, 1969.

22. David, A., Serr, D. N., and Czernobilsky, B. Chemical composition of human oviduct fluid. *Fertil. Steril.* 24:435, 1973.

23. Dede, J. A., and Janovski, N. A. Lipoma of the uterine tube. *Obstet. Gynecol.* 22:461, 1963.

24. Diamant, Y. Z., Aboulafia, Y., and Raz, S. Torsion of hydrosalpinx. *Int. Surg.* 57:303, 1972.

25. Dische, F. E., Burt, J. M., Davidson, N. J. H., and Puntambekar, S. Tuboovarian actinomycosis associated with intrauterine contraceptive devices. *J. Obstet. Gynaecol. Br. Commonw.* 81:724, 1974.

26. Dudkiewicz, J. Quantitative and qualitative changes of epithelial cells of fallopian tubes in women according to the phase of menstrual cycle. A cytologic study. *Acta Cytol.* 14:531, 1970.

27. Ebrahimi, T., and Okagaki, T. Hemangioma of the fallopian tube. *Am. J. Obstet. Gynecol.* 115:864, 1973.

28. Elliott, G. B., Brody, H., and Elliott, K. A. Implications of "lipoid" salpingitis. *Fertil. Steril.* 16:541, 1965.

29. Ellsworth, H. S., Harris, J. W., McQuarrie, H. G., Stone, R. A., and Anderson, A. E. Prolapse of the fallopian tube following vaginal hysterectomy. *J.A.M.A.* 224:891, 1973.

30. Falls, J. L. Accessory adrenal cortex in the broad ligament. *Cancer* 8:143, 1955.

31. Federman, Q., and Toker, C. Primary transitional cell tumor of the uterine adnexa. *Am. J. Obstet. Gynecol.* 115:863, 1973.

32. Ferenczy, A., Fenoglio, J., and Richart, R. M. Observations on benign mesotheliomas of the genital tract (adenomatoid tumor). *Cancer* 30:244, 1972.

33. Ferenczy, A., and Richart, R. M. *Female Reproductive System: Dynamics of Scan and Transmission Electron Microscopy*, New York, J. Wiley, 1974, pp. 212–253.

34. Fitzgerald, T. B., Mainwaring, A. R., and Ahmed, A. Pelvic

peritoneal oxyuriasis simulating metastatic carcinoma. *J. Obstet. Gynaecol. Br. Commonw.* 81:248, 1974.

35. Flickinger, G. L., Muechler, E. K., and Mikhail, G. Estradiol receptor in the human fallopian tube. *Fertil. Steril.* 25:900, 1974.

36. Fredricsson, B. Histochemistry of the oviduct. *In* Hafez, E. S. E., and Blandau, R. J., eds. *The Mammalian Oviduct.* Chicago, University of Chicago Press, 1969.

37. Frost, O. Bilharzia of the fallopian tube. *S. Afr. Med. J.* 49:1201, 1975.

38. Gaddum-Rosse, P., and Blandau, R. J. *In vitro* studies on ciliary activity within the oviducts of the rabbit and pig. *Am. J. Anat.* 136:91, 1973.

39. Gaddum-Rosse, P., Rumery, R. E., Blandau, R. T., and Thiersch, J. B. Studies on the mucosa of postmenopausal oviducts: Surface appearance, ciliary activity, and the effect of estrogen treatment. *Fertil. Steril.* 26:951, 1975.

40. Gardner, G. H., Greene, R. R., and Peckham, B. M. Normal and cystic structures of broad ligament. *Am. J. Obstet. Gynecol.* 55:917, 1948.

41. Gardner, G. H., Greene, R. R., and Peckham, B. Tumors of the broad ligament. *Am. J. Obstet. Gynecol.* 73:536, 1957.

42. Gelfand, M., Ross, M. D., Blair, D. M., and Weber, M. C. Distribution and extent of schistosomiasis in female pelvic organs with special reference to the genital tract, as determined at autopsy. *Am. J. Trop. Med. Hyg.* 20:846, 1971.

43. Gravaller, J., Suranyi, S., and Berensci, G. Neue Gesichtpunkte in der Klinik der Genitaltuberkulose. *Zentralbl. Gynaekol.* 78:496, 1956.

44. Haines, M. Tuberculous salpingitis as seen by the pathologist and the surgeon. *Am. J. Obstet. Gynecol.* 75:472, 1958.

45. Hanton, E. M., Malkasian, G. D. Jr., Dahlin, D. C., and Pratt, J. H. Primary carcinoma of the fallopian tube. *Am. J. Obstet. Gynecol.* 94:832, 1966.

46. Hellman, L. M. Morphology of the human fallopian tube in the early puerperium. *Am. J. Obstet. Gynecol.* 57:154, 1949.

47. Henriksen, E. Struma salpingii. *Obstet. Gynecol.* 5:833, 1955.

48. Hertig, A. T., and Gore, H. Tumors of the female sex organs. Part 3. Tumors of the ovary and fallopian tube. in *Atlas of Tumor Pathology,* Series 1, Fasc. 33. Washington, D.C., Armed Forces Institute of Pathology, 1961, pp. 84–85.

49. Hertig, A. T., and Mansell, H. Tumors of the female sex organs. Part 1. Hydatiform mole and choriocarcinoma, in *Atlas of Tumor Pathology,* Series 1, Fasc. 33. Washington, D.C., Armed Forces Institute of Pathology 1956, pp. 62–63.

50. Karakascheff, K. I. Weitere Beiträge zur pathologischen Anatomie der Nebennieren. *Beitr Pathol.* 39:373, 1906.

51. Kariminejad, M. H., and Scully, R. E. Female adnexal tumor of probable Wolffian origin. *Cancer* 31:671, 1973.

52. Kay, S. Sarcoidosis of the fallopian tubes. *J. Obstet. Gynaecol. Br. Emp.* 63:871, 1956.

53. Lee, R. A., and Welch, J. S. Torsion of the uterine adnexa. *Am. J. Obstet. Gynecol.* 97:974, 1967.

54. Lewis, J. D. Hilus cell hyperplasia of ovaries and tubes. *Obstet. Gynecol.* 24:728, 1964.

55. Lippes, J., Ender, R. G., Pragay, O. A., and Bartholomew, W. R. The collection and analysis of human fallopian tube fluid. *Contraception* 5:85, 1972.

56. Lisa, J. R., Gioia, J. D., and Rubin, I. C. Observations on the interstitial portion of the fallopian tube. *Surg. Gynecol. Obstet.* 99:159, 1954.

57. Madden, S. Chorionepithelioma of the fallopian tube. *J. Obstet. Gynaecol. Br. Emp.* 57:68, 1950.

58. Malinak, L. J., Miller, G. V., and Armstrong, J. T. Primary squamous cell carcinoma of the fallopian tube. *Am. J. Obstet. Gynecol.* 95:1067, 1966.

59. Mallory, T. Case records of the Massachusetts General Hospital. *N. Engl. J. Med.* 213:1249, 1935.

60. Mårdh, P.-A., and Weström, L. Antibodies to *Mycoplasma hominis* in patients with genital infections and in healthy controls. *Br. J. Vener. Dis.* 46:390, 1970.

61. Mårdh, P.-A., and Weström, L. Tubal and cervical cultures in acute salpingitis with special reference to *Mycoplasma hominis* and T-strain mycoplasmas. *Brit. J. Vener. Dis.* 46:179, 1970.

62. Mason, T. E., and Quagliarello, J. R. Ectopic pregnancies in the fallopian tube. *Obstet. Gynecol.* 48:70s, 1976.

63. Mastroianni, L. Jr., and Komins, J. Capacitation, ovum maturation, fertilization and preimplantation development in the oviduct. *Gynecol. Invest.* 6:226, 1975.

64. Mazzarella, P., Okagaki, T., and Richart, R. M. Teratoma of the uterine tube. *Obstet. Gynecol.* 39:381, 1972.

65. Moore, S. W., and Enterline, H. T. Significance of proliferative epithelial lesions of the uterine tube. *Obstet. Gynecol.* 45:385, 1975.

66. Novak, E., and Everett, H. S. Cyclical and other variations in the tubal epithelium. *Am. J. Obstet. Gynecol.* 16:499, 1928.

67. Odor, D. L. The question of "basal" cells in oviductal and endocervical epithelium. *Fertil. steril.* 25:1047, 1974.

68. Okagaki, T., and Richart, R. M. Neurilemmoma of the fallopian tube. *Am. J. Obstet. Gynecol.* 106:929, 1970.

69. Outerbridge, G. W. Polypoid chondrofibroma of the fallopian tube associated with tubal pregnancy. *Am. J. Obstet. N.Y.* 70:173, 1914.

70. Palomaki, J. F., and Blair, O. M. Hilus cell rest of the fallopian tube. *Obstet. Gynecol.* 37:60, 1971.

71. Parmley, T. H., Woodruff, J. D., Winn, K., Johnson, J. W., and Douglas, P. H. Histogenesis of leiomyomatosis peritonealis disseminata (disseminated fibrosing deciduosis). *Obstet. Gynecol.* 46:511, 1975.

72. Patek, E., and Nilsson, L. Scanning electron microscopic observations on the ciliogenesis of the infundibulum of the human fetal and adult fallopian tube epithelium. *Fertil. Steril.* 24:819, 1973.

73. Patek, E., Nilsson, L., and Johannisson, E. Scanning electron microscopic study of the human fallopian tube. Report I. The proliferative and secretory stages. *Fertil. Steril.* 23:459, 1972.

74. Patton, G. W. Jr., and Goldstein, D. P. Gestational choriocarcinoma of the tube and ovary. *Surg. Gynecol. Obstet.* 137:608, 1973.

75. Pauerstein, C. J. *The Fallopian Tube: A Reappraisal.* Philadelphia, Lea & Febiger, 1974.

76. Pauerstein, C. J., and Woodruff, J. D. The role of the "indifferent" cell of the tubal epithelium. *Am. J. Obstet. Gynecol.* 98:121, 1967.

77. Pauerstein, C. J., and Woodruff, J. D. Cellular patterns in proliferative and anaplastic disease of the fallopian tube. *Am. J. Obstet. Gynecol.* 96:486, 1966.

78. Persaud, V. Etiology of tubal ectopic pregnancy. *Obstet. Gynecol.* 36:257, 1970.

79. Qizilbash, A. H., and DePetrillo, A. D. Endometrial and

tubal involvement by squamous carcinoma of the cervix. *Am. J. Clin. Pathol.* 64:668, 1975.

80. Rebello, R., Green, F. H. Y., and Fox, H. A study of the secretory immune system of the female genital tract. *Br. J. Obstet. Gynaecol.* 82:812, 1975.

81. Robboy, S. J., and Scully, R. E. Ovarian teratoma with glial implants on the peritoneum. *Hum. Pathol.* 1:643, 1970.

82. Roberts, C. L., and Marshall, H. K. Fibromyoma of the fallopian tube. *Am. J. Obstet. Gynecol.* 82:364, 1961.

83. Rubin, A., and Czernobilsky, B. Tubal ligation. A bacteriologic, histologic and clinical study. *Obstet. Gynecol.* 36:199, 1970.

84. Sampson, J. A. Postsalpingectomy endometriosis (endosalpingiosis). *Am. J. Obstet. Gynecol.* 10:649, 1930.

85. Sanes, S., and Warner, R. Primary lymphangioma of the fallopian tube. *Am. J. Obstet. Gynecol.* 37:316, 1939.

86. Sapan, I. P., and Solberg, N. S. Prolapse of the uterine tube after abdominal hysterectomy. *Obstet. Gynecol.* 42:26, 1973.

87. Schaefer, G. Tuberculosis of the female genital tract. *Clin. Obstet. Gynecol.* 13:965, 1970.

88. Scheffey, L. C., Lang, W. R., and Nugent, F. B. Clinical and pathologic aspects of primary sarcoma of the uterine tube. *Am. J. Obstet. Gynecol.* 52:904, 1941.

89. Schenken, J. R., and Burns, E. L. A study and classification of nodular lesions of the fallopian tube. *Am. J. Obstet. Gynecol.* 45:624, 1943.

90. Schiller, H. M., and Silverberg, S. G. Staging and prognosis in primary carcinoma of the fallopian tube. *Cancer* 28:389, 1971.

91. Sedlis, A. Primary carcinoma of the fallopian tube. *Obstet. Gynec. Surv.* 16:209, 1961.

92. Settlege, D. S. F., Motoshima, M., and Tredway, D. R. Sperm transport from the external cervical os to the fallopian tube in women. A time and quantitation study. *Fertil. Steril.* 24:655, 1973.

93. Spore, W. W., Moskal, P. A., Nakamura, R. M., and Mishell, O. R. Bacteriology of postpartum oviducts and endometrium. *Am. J. Obstet. Gynecol.* 107:572, 1970.

94. Stambaugh, R., Seitz, H. M., and Mastroianni, L. Jr. Acrosomal proteinase inhibitors in rhesus monkey (*Macaca mulatta*) oviduct fluid. *Fertil. Steril.* 25:352, 1974.

95. Stevens, L. C., and Varnum, D. S. The development of teratomas from pathogenetically activated ovarian mouse eggs. *Dev. Biol.* 37:369, 1974.

96. Sutherland, C. G. Tubal mole associated with intrauterine pregnancy. *Am. J. Obstet. Gynecol.* 65:1164, 1953.

97. Surur, F. Actinomycosis of the female genital tract. *N.Y. State J. Med.* 75:408, 1974.

98. Sweet, R. L. Anaerobic infections of the female genital tract. *Am. J. Obstet. Gynecol.* 122:891, 1975.

99. Swenson, R. M., Michaelson, T. C., Daly, M. J., and Spaulding, E. H. Anaerobic bacterial infections of the female genital tract. *Obstet. Gynecol.* 42:538, 1973.

100. Symmers, W. St. C. Pathology of oxyuriasis. *Arch. Pathol.* 50:475, 1950.

101. Taubert, H.-D., Wissner, S. E., and Haskins, A. L. Leiomyomatosis peritonealis disseminata. *Obstet. Gynecol.* 25:561, 1965.

102. Taxy, J. B., and Battifora, H. Female adnexal tumor of probable Wolffian origin. *Cancer* 37:2349, 1976.

103. Taxy, J. B., Battifora, H., and Oyasu, R. Adenomatoid tumors: A light microscopic, histochemical, and ultrastructural study. *Cancer* 34:306, 1974.

104. Taylor, E. S., McMillan, J. H., Greer, B. E., Droegemueller, W., and Thompson, H. E. The intrauterine device and tuboovarian abscess. *Am. J. Obstet. Gynecol.* 123:338, 1975.

105. Teilum, G. *Special Tumors of the Ovary and Testis.* Copenhagen, Munksgard, 1971, p. 298.

106. Thadepalli, H., Gorbach, S. L., and Keith L. Anaerobic infections of the female genital tract: Bacteriologic and therapeutic aspects. *Am. J. Obstet. Gynecol.* 117:1034, 1973.

107. Tilden, I. L., and Winstedt, R. Decidual reactions in fallopian tubes. *Am. J. Pathol.* 19:1043, 1943.

108. Verhege, H. G., and Brenner, R. M. Estradiol-induced differentiation of the oviductal epithelium in ovariectomized cats. *Biol. Reprod.* 13:104, 1975.

109. Ward, M. E., Watt, P. J., and Robertson, J. N. The human fallopian tube: A laboratory model for gonococcal infection. *J. Infect. Dis.* 129:650, 1974.

110. Weber, D. L., and Fazzini, E. Ganglioneuroma of the fallopian tube. *Acta Neuropathol.* 16:173, 1970.

111. Weström, L., Bengtsson, L. P., and Mårdh, P.-A. The risk of pelvic inflammatory disease in women using intrauterine contraceptive devices as compared to non-users. *Lancet* 2:221, 1976.

112. Woodruff, J. D., and Julian, C. G. Multiple malignancy in the upper genital canal. *Am. J. Obstet. Gynecol.* 103:810, 1969.

113. Woodruff, J. D., and Pauerstein, C. J. *The Fallopian Tube.* Baltimore, Williams and Wilkins, 1969.

114. Wlodarski, F. M., and Trainer, T. D. Granulomatous oophoritis and salpingitis associated with Crohn's disease of the appendix. *Am. J. Obstet. Gynecol.* 122:527, 1975.

115. Wrork, D. H., and Broders, A. C. Adenomyosis of the fallopian tube. *Am. J. Obstet. Gynecol.* 44:412, 1942.

116. Wu, J. P., Tanner, W. S., and Fardal, P. M. Malignant mixed mullerian tumor of the uterine tube. *Obstet. Gynecol.* 41:707, 1973.

Ancel Blaustein, M.D.

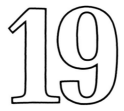

# Anatomy and Histology of the Human Ovary

## Gross Anatomy

### Orientation

The ovaries are two nodular bodies located one on either side of the uterus, attached to the broad ligament, and situated close to the lateral pelvic wall in a shallow depression called the ovarian fossa (Figure 19.1). The fossa is bounded by the external iliac vessels and the ureter. The anterior margin of the ovary is thin, straight, and attached to the posterior surface of the broad ligament by a fold of peritoneum referred to as the mesovarium. The posterior (free margin) is rounded, convex, and unattached. Besides the attachment to the broad ligament, the ovary is held in place by two ligaments, the uteroovarian ligament that is attached to the lateral angle of the uterus and a suspensory ligament that extends from the upper rounded pole of the ovary to the wall of the fallopian tube, immediately adjacent to the fimbriated end. The ovarian blood vessels are contained within the suspensory ligament.[21] The uteroovarian ligament contains some nonstriated muscle fibers.[28] Asymmetry is common, the right ovary usually being larger than the left.

### Ectopic Ovarian Tissue

Ectopic ovarian tissue[32] is uncommon but has been reported both in a retroperitoneal location and in the mesentery[1] of the sigmoid. It is divided into two categor-

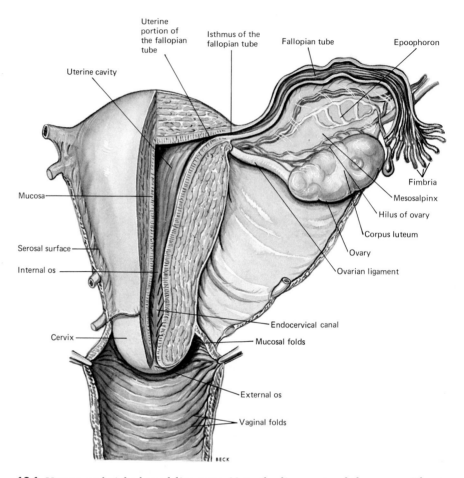

**19.1** Uterus and right broad ligament. Note the ligaments of the ovary. The ovarian vessels traverse the suspensory ligament.

[Adapted from *Gray's Anatomy of the Human Body,* 1973, courtesy of Lea & Febiger.]

ies: (1) supernumerary ovary and (2) accessory ovary. A supernumerary ovary[7,31,38] is by definition a third ovary that has no connection whatever with the normally located ovaries. This is in contrast to the accessory ovary, which is invariably situated near the normally placed ovary or is connected with it. The accessory ovary is a more frequent finding than the supernumerary ovary, according to Wharton.[44] He has also found additional congenital defects in three of four cases of supernumerary ovary and in an equal number with accessory ovary.[24]

## Blood Supply

### Arterial supply

The ovarian artery arises from the aorta[21] and, in the mesosalpinx, anastomoses with the uterine artery. Some branches supply the fallopian tube and others enter the mesovarium. They divide and become multiple in the hilum of the ovary. Within the hilus and in the medulla they are coiled (Figure 19.2). In the medulla each branch divides in two, and these traverse through to the cortex, giving off branches that divide into arterioles that freely anastomose and form arteriovenous anastomoses at the periphery of the cortex (Figure 19.3). Branches that supply the follicles give off end-arterial branches to the theca interna.

The coiled nature of the ovarian arteries is uniquely suited to increasing vascular surface when needed, such as with corpus luteum formation and in pregnancy.

### Venous drainage

The veins emerge from the hilus of the ovary as a pampiniform plexus.[21] The ovarian vein forms from the plexus, traverses the mesovarium, and enters the suspen-

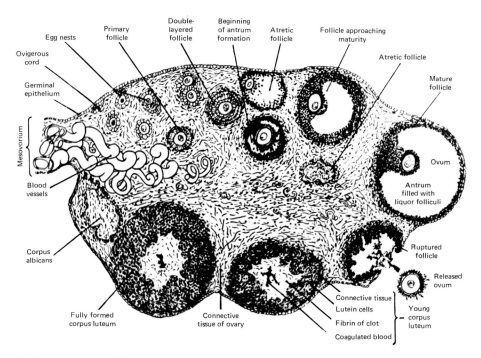

Primary follicle

Egg nests

Double-layered follicle

Beginning of antrum formation

Atretic follicle

Follicle approaching maturity

Ovigerous cord

Atretic follicle

Germinal epithelium

Mature follicle

Mesovorium

Ovum

Blood vessels

Antrum filled with liquor folliculi

Corpus albicans

Ruptured follicle

Released ovum

Connective tissue

Young corpus luteum

Lutein cells

Fully formed corpus luteum

Connective tissue of ovary

Fibrin of clot

Coagulated blood

**19.2** Note the coiled nature of the blood vessels in the hilus and medulla of the ovary.

[Reprinted by permission from B. M. Patten, in *Human Embryology*, Philadelphia, Blakiston. Courtesy of McGraw-Hill Book Company.]

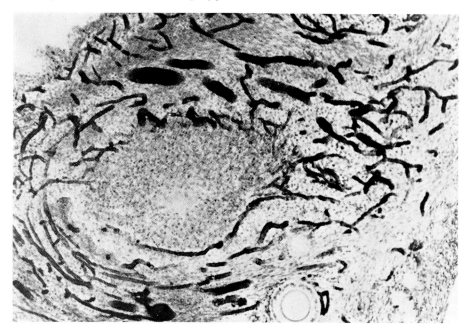

**19.3** Section of a portion of an ovary in which the blood vessels had been injected with colored gelatin prior to sectioning. Note the abundant capillary networks in relation to the growing follicles. ×26.

[Reprinted by permission from C. R. Leeson and T. S. Leeson, The female reproductive system, in *Histology*, Philadelphia, W. B. Saunders, 1970, pp. 416–425.]

sory ligament. The left ovarian vein empties into the left renal vein while the right ovarian vein drains into the inferior vena cava.

## Nerve Supply

The nerve supply arises from a sympathetic plexus[26] that is intimately enmeshed with the ovarian vessels in the infundibulopelvic ligament. They originate from the fibers of the renal and aortic plexuses as well as from the celiac and mesenteric ganglia. Nerve fibers (nonmedullated) follow the ovarian artery, dividing into delicate terminal plexuses that surround the arterioles and the outer surface of the follicles.

## Lymphatic Supply

COURSE OF LYMPHATICS WITHIN THE OVARY. Morris and Sass[33] found delicate nets of lymph vessels in the tunica albuginea and the theca interna and externa. The work of Anderson[2] has demonstrated anastomoses between the network serving the internal and the external theca. The follicle in its immature and mature states seems to lack lymphatic vessels, whereas the corpus luteum possesses numerous lymph vessels. The corpus albicans is surrounded by a lymph net immediately at its periphery.

EFFERENT LYMPH CHANNELS OF THE OVARY. There are four to six vessels leading from the hilus of the ovary and, with branches from the fallopian tube and the fundus of the uterus, these form the subovarian plexus of lymphatics that can be found under the hilus of the ovary (Figures 19.4 and 19.5). Channels from these run along the infundibulopelvic ligament to the upper aortic lymph nodes at the level of the lower renal pole. They have the appearance of "strings of beads."[14]

# Histology and Histochemistry

## Orientation

The ovary is covered by a layer of surface cells that are a modified form of peritoneal mesothelium. It covers the whole surface but is separated from the rest of the pelvic peritoneum by a distinct line of demarcation, known as the Farre–Waldeyer line, close to the hilus of the ovary. Surface cells are separated from the cortex by a tunica albuginea. The cortex houses the functional components, namely, the oocytes, follicles, and corpora lutea in varying

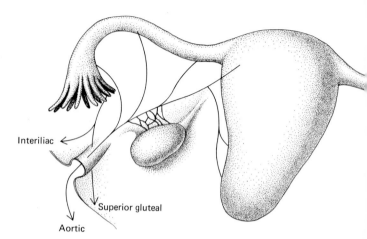

**19.4** A semischematic representation of the lymphatics of the ovary. Drainage trunks from the cornual region of the uterine fundus, the proximal portion of the fallopian tube, and the ovary combine in the mesovarium to form the subovarian plexus. Large trunks leave this plexus and are joined by additional lymphatic channels from the distal portion of the tube. They follow the ovarian vessels upward to terminate in the aortic nodes. Additionally, not shown here, a small collateral trunk from the ovary also bypasses the subovarian plexus and travels within the folds of the broad ligament to drain into the uppermost interiliac node.

[Reprinted by permission from A. A. Plentl and E. A. Friedman, eds., Lymphatic system of the female genitalia, in *Major Problems in Obstetrics and Gynecology*, Philadelphia, W. B. Saunders, 1971, Vol. 2.]

stages of development and regression. The stroma of the cortex is composed of a surface zone of compact fibrous connective tissue. Deep to this it is somewhat looser and more cellular. The medulla and hilus contain the arteries, veins, and nerve supply, as well as vestigial Wolffian duct remnants in the form of tubules lined by cuboidal cells and Leydig (hilar) cells.

### Surface epithelium

The surface of the ovary is covered by a single layer of cuboidal epithelium and occasional peglike cells (Figure 19.6). It is present on the fetal ovary and persists throughout life. It extends into deep clefts that form on the ovary (Figure 19.7). Nothing is known of the survival time of these cells or the site of their regeneration. Although they tend to be cuboidal, they are prone to undergo metaplasia to Müllerian epithelium. The commonest form of meta-

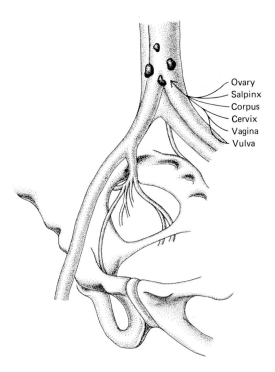

Ovary
Salpinx
Corpus
Cervix
Vagina
Vulva

**19.5** Schematic presentation of the aortic nodes shown here only in the lumbar region. This group, which drains lymph from the organs listed, includes all lymph nodes located superiorly, posteriorly, and laterally to the aorta over its entire abdominal course.

[Reprinted by permission from A. A. Plentl and E. A. Friedman, eds., Lymphatic system of the female genitalia, in *Major Problems in Obstetrics and Gynecology,* Philadelphia, W. B. Saunders, 1971, Vol. 2.]

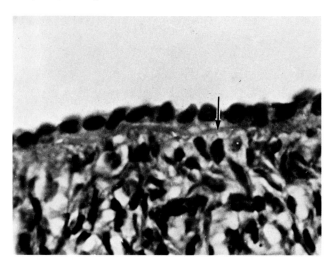

**19.6** Surface cells covering the ovary. At the tip of the arrow there is a thin tunica albuginea separating the surface cells from the cortex. ×200.

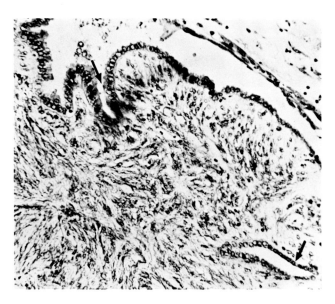

**19.7** Surface cells of the ovary growing into clefts in the ovarian surface (upper arrow). Lower arrow points to cysts in the cortex lined by surface cells. ×188.

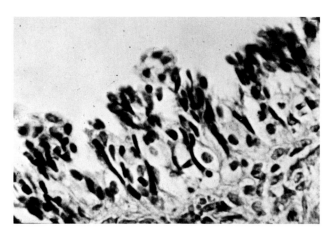

**19.8** Metaplasia of surface cells to those resembling endosalpinx. ×472.

plasia is to cells resembling endosalpinx (Figure 19.8), endometrium (Figure 19.9), and mucinous epithelium (Figure 19.10), in that order. Surface cells, by light microscopy, appear to be composed mostly of nucleus, and cell borders are not always clearly defined. Glycogen and ribonucleic acid is often present as fine cytoplasmic granules in the basal cytoplasm in adult ovaries at all ages. McKay *et al.*[30] found the cells to be enzymatically inert, but Blaustein[5] demonstrated the presence of 17$\beta$-steroid dehydrogenase in the cytoplasm in two instances; both in the ovaries of patients in their forties who had breast

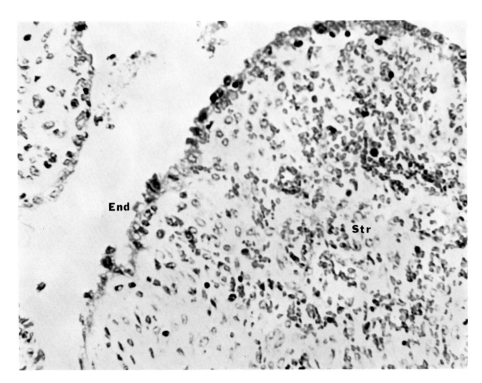

**19.9** Metaplasia of surface cells of the ovary to those resembling endometrium (End). ×100. Str, stroma.

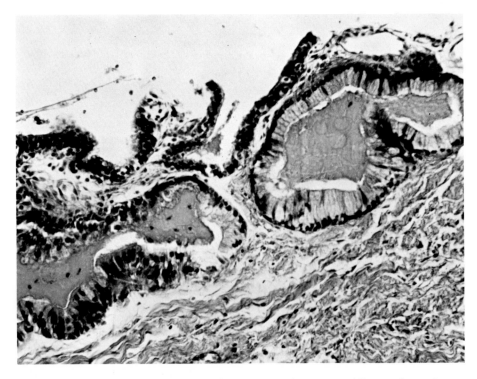

**19.10** Metaplasia of surface cells of the ovary to those resembling endocervix. ×170.

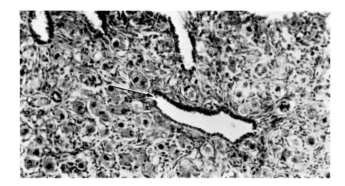

**19.11** Ovary of a newborn. Note early development of a cyst (arrow) lined by surface cells of the ovary.

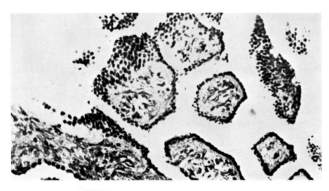

**19.12** Surface of the ovary. Note surface papillations composed largely of stroma and covered by surface cells.

cancer. Inclusion cysts composed of surface cells can be found at all ages, including the ovary of the newborn (Figure 19.11). Occasionally one finds wartlike excrescences composed of surface cells and stroma. These may be focal and of no significance and are most commonly found in the menopausal and postmenopausal ovary (Figure 19.12).

Transmission and scanning electron microscopy (TEM and SEM, respectively) suggest features that relate to active fluid and ion transport, which may occur through surface pinocytosis and intercellular spaces.[16,34,37] The characteristic features seen by SEM show dome-shaped apices covered by generally abundant surface microvilli (Figure 19.13). TEM shows cuboidal epithelium with numerous, often branching microvilli. The cytoplasm contains well-developed organelles that are perinuclear in position. Lateral plasma membranes are straight or convoluted, reinforced by luminal junctional complexes and scattered desmosomes. Occasionally they are widely separated, resulting in greatly dilated intercellular spaces. A well-defined basal lamina separates the cells from the underlying tunica albuginea (Figure 19.14).[16]

### Cortex, medulla, and hilus

The appearance of the cortex is dependent on the age of the ovary. In the newborn it is packed with oocytes and primitive follicles,[3] and during the reproductive period it contains follicles and corpora lutea in varying stages of

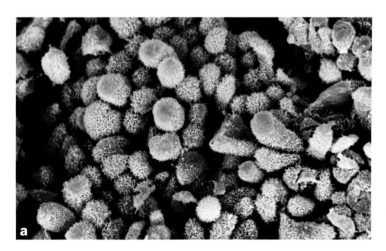
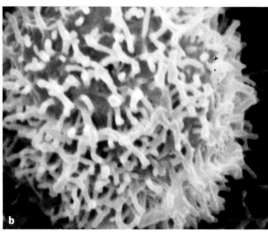

**19.13 a.** Scanning electron micrograph of the surface of the ovary. The characteristic features of the ovarian celomic epithelium include the presence of dome-shaped apices covered by generally abundant, surface microvilli. ×1,140. **b.** Detailed view of slender and often branching surface microvilli. ×12,000.

[Reprinted by permission from A. Ferenczy and R. M. Richart, *Female Reproductive System, Dynamics of Scan and Transmission Electron Microscopy*, New York, John Wiley & Sons, 1975.]

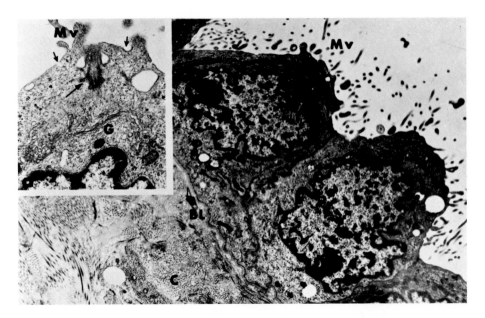

**19.14** Ovary from a 39-year-old woman. The low cuboidal surface epithelium has numerous, often branching, microvilli (Mv), and the cytoplasm contains well-developed organelles in a perinuclear location. G, Golgi. The nuclei have indented nuclear membranes and peripheral nucleoli. Lateral plasma membranes are straight or convoluted and reinforced by luminal junctional complexes and scattered desmosomes but are occasionally widely separated, resulting in greatly dilated intercellular spaces. A well-defined basal lamina (BL) separates the cells from the underlying collagenous corpus (C) albuginea. ×5,120.

[Reprinted by permission from A. Ferenczy and R. M. Richart, *Female Reproductive System, Dynamics of Scan and Transmission Electron Microscopy*, New York, John Wiley & Sons, 1975.]

maturation. It also contains scarred remnants of follicles that undergo atresia, corpora fibrosa, and scarred remnants of corpora lutea, called corpora albicantia. The postmenopausal cortex is composed mostly of scarred remnants.

The cells of the cortex are spindle-shaped and round fibroblast elements (Figures 19.15 and 19.16). They form the matrix in which the elements described above are found. Ultrastructural studies show cells with narrow cigar-shaped nuclei and a slender cytoplasm rich in ribosomes and microfilaments. There are rows of micropinocytic vesicles along the plasma membrane and clusters of mitochondria are often perinuclear in location[27] (Figure 19.17a,b).

Cortical stromal hyperplasia and conversion of islands of stromal cells to those resembling lutein epithelium (Figure 19.18) led to studies of ovarian enzyme activity.[39] Scully and Cohen[40] found disseminated nests of cells with oxidative-enzyme activity, equivalent quantitatively to that of the theca interna and hilus cells. Enzymatically active cells were always more numerous in the medulla than in

the cortex and, when they were scant, were almost always located in the medulla. The incidence of these cells, labeled EASC, was age related, being 18% in ages 15 to 40, 46% in women over the age of 50 years, and rose to 67% in the 61- to 86-year-old age group. EASC cells are not one and the same as luteinized stromal cells, although both often coexist. Normal ovaries show a higher incidence of EASC cells than luteinized cells. Mattingly and Huang[29] incubated tissue slices of menopausal and postmenopausal ovaries with pregnenolone-7H$^3$ and $\Delta^4$-androstene-3,17-dione-7H$^3$ precursors and the stromal cells had the capacity to produce dehydroepiandrosterone, androstenedione, and testosterone. Blaustein, Blaustein, and Gross[6] were able to grow cortical stromal cells in tissue culture and islands of cells were enzymatically active. All this suggests that whereas the follicle is the hormonally functional unit of the ovary, cortical medullary stroma is not inert and can, in certain endocrine states and advancing age, synthesize steroids.[15]

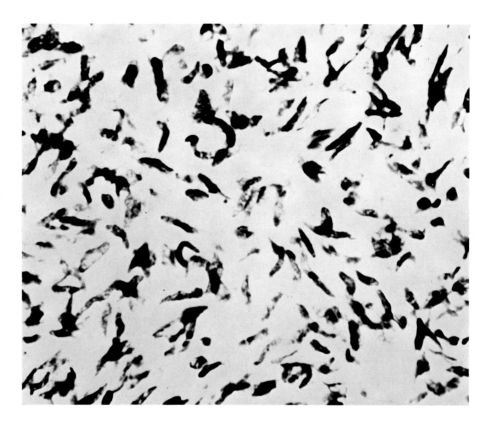

**19.15** Cortex of the ovary. The nuclei of the stromal cells are elongated and cigar shaped. ×200.

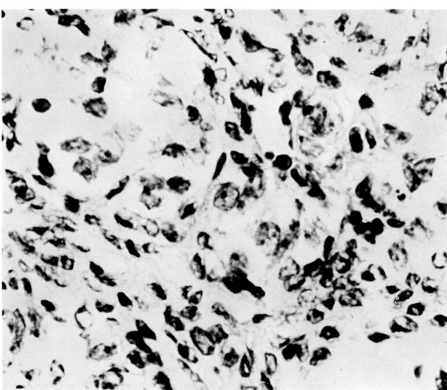

**19.16** Cortex of the ovary. In the deeper part of the cortex the nuclei of cells are oval and round. ×200.

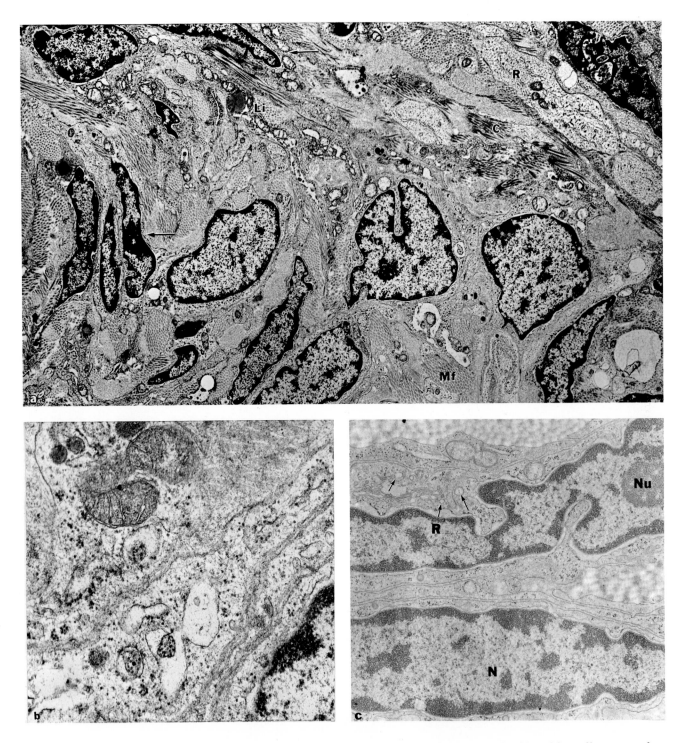

**19.17 a.** Ovarian stromal cells are spindle-shaped fibroblast-like cells arranged in a haphazard fashion. ×3,000. C, Collagen fibers; Mf, tropocollagen; R, free ribosomes; and Li, lipid inclusions. Perinuclear clustering of mitochondria (arrows). **b.** High-power view. ×25,000. **c.** Ovarian stroma. Arrows point to micropinocytic vesicles. ×12,000. N, nucleus; Nu, nucleolus; R, ribosomes.

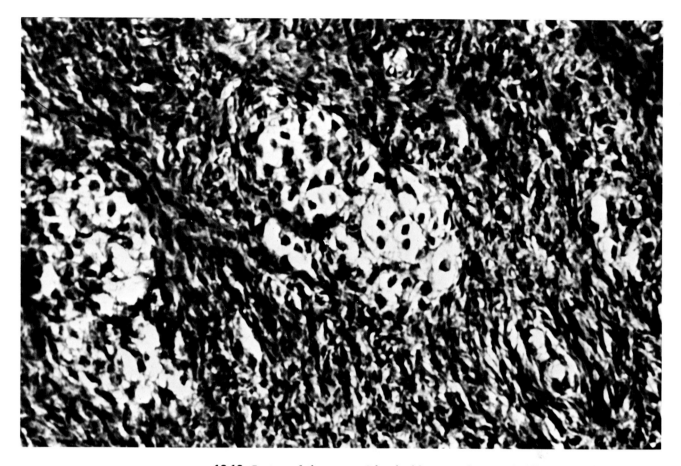

**19.18** Cortex of the ovary. Island of luteinized stromal cells in a zone of cortical stromal hyperplasia. The patient had a carcinoma of the breast. ×180.

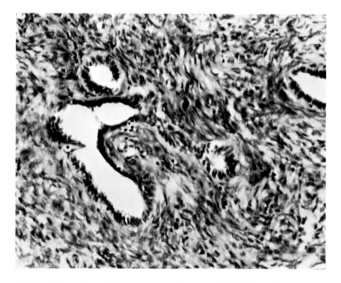

**19.19** Medulla of the ovary. Vestigial Wolffian duct remnants. ×100.

The medulla largely consists of blood vessels, lymphatic channels, and nerves, as well as occasional islands of the stromal cells just described. The hilus contains the above structures, stromal cells excepted. It also contains vestigial Wolffian ducts[17] lined by cuboidal epithelium (Figure 19.19) and hilar cells that are found in relation to the nerves and blood vessels (Figure 19.20a). These cells are round or oval, have well-defined nuclei and cytoplasm that is somewhat eosinophilic, and have a foamy appearance. Some, but not all, exhibit well-defined cell borders. The cells may contain crystalloids of Reinke and lipochrome pigment (Figure 19.20b).

## Structure of the Follicle

Primary or primitive follicles are numerous in the cortex of the ovary during the reproductive period. They consist of an oocyte surrounded by a single layer of flattened granulosa cells (Figure 19.21). Follicles that have

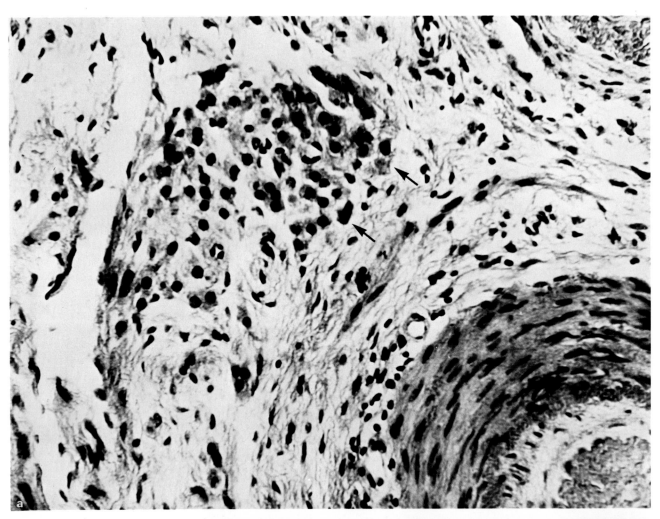

**19.20 a.** Perivascular cuffing of Leydig cells (arrows). ×146.
**b.** Hilus of the ovary. Leydig cells in clusters adjacent to blood vessels and nerves. Arrow points to Reinke crystals in a Leydig cell. ×200.

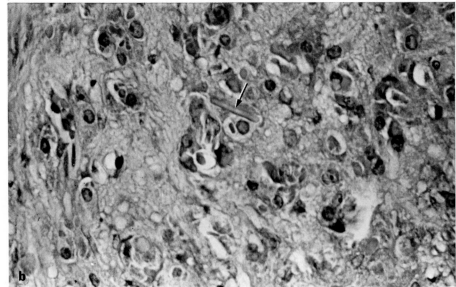

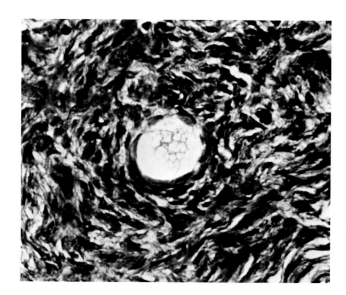

**19.21** Cortex of the ovary. Primitive follicle lined by pregranulosa cells. ×100.

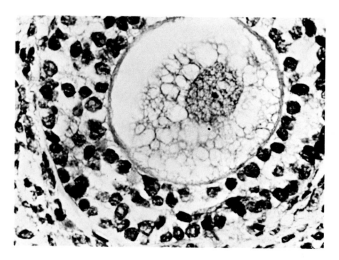

**19.22** Cortex of the ovary. Developing follicle. Germ cell contains a nucleus and nucleolus. The zona pellucida and corona radiata are distinct. ×400.

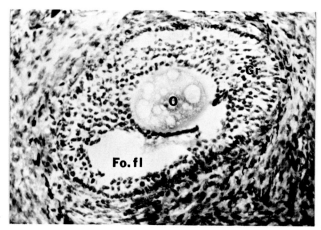

**19.23** Maturing follicle. Gr, granulosa cells; O, ovum; Fo.fl, follicular fluid.

been stimulated by pituitary follicle stimulating hormone (FSH) show hyperplasia of their cells to as many as four to six cells in depth. This is sometimes referred to as the germinal layer. These have divided by mitosis and form a stratified epithelium of low columnar cells around the sex cell, separated from it by an eosinophilic homogeneous band called the zona pellucida (Figure 19.22). The zona pellucida appears to derive from secretions from the endo-

plasmic reticulum of follicular cells. It is composed of mucopolysaccharide with a sialic acid component.[23] The first signs of its formation are isolated wedges of material between adjacent primary follicular cells, rather than a uniform deposit around the oocytes. When fully developed, it measures from 10 to 15 $\mu$ in thickness. The zona pellucida is surrounded by a pseudostratified layer of follicular cells called the corona radiata (Figure 19.22). Inside, the ovum can be found a well-defined nucleus, referred to as the germinal vesicle, and a nucleolus, called the germinal spot. Encircling the follicle is a cellular layer of stroma called theca interna. These cells, under the influence of FSH, synthesize estrogens.[11] It was initially believed that they independently elaborated estrogens, but experiments in which theca interna was implanted into the anterior chamber of the guinea pig eye, revealed that estrogens were only elaborated after the addition of granulosa cells. Therefore, it is believed that there is an interdependence of these two cell types and that their interaction is required to elaborate estrogens. There is a spherical distribution of theca interna about the follicle,[42,43] and at one point there is a cone-shaped clustering of these cells, with the apex directed toward the surface of the ovary. Strassman[42] suggested that this configuration of cells had as its purpose, the direction of the mature follicle to the surface. This is more supposition than fact.

### Mature Graafian follicle

The follicle that is under FSH stimulation increases in size; follicle cells secrete fluid,[36,38,45] which gradually forms a cavity (Figure 19.23). The ovum surrounded by

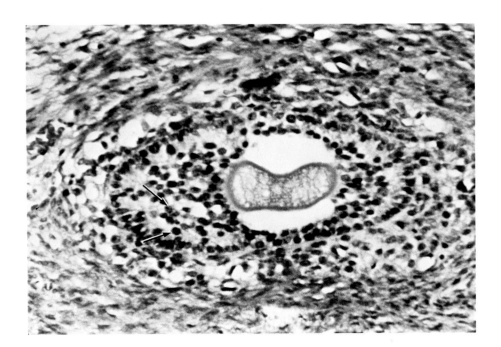

**19.24** Follicle showing Call–Exner bodies (arrows).

follicle cells projects into the lumen of the cavity and the hillock formed is referred to as the cumulus oophorus. Within the stratified layer of follicular cells there are isolated smaller accumulations of follicular fluid. Some are rounded and become surrounded by cells from pseudo-glandular structures called Call–Exner bodies[8] (Figures 19.24 and 19.25).

### Follicular atresia

Ova, oogonia, and primitive follicles undergo degeneration, but they are so small and scattered that they may not modify the microscopic appearance of the ovary as a whole. However, atresia of mature follicles is conspicuous and presents a variety of appearances depending on the stage of the follicle at the time degeneration begins and on the extent of the retrogressive change at the time (Figure 19.26). The determinant for atresia is not known. Furthermore, it is not known whether the ovum or the follicle cells are primarily affected. First evidences appear to be cessation of mitoses, pyknosis, and karyorrhexis in the follicular cells immediately adjacent to the lumen of vesicular follicles and external to the corona radiata. These nuclear fragments and pyknotic cells tend to float into the follicular liquor. The cells of the cumulus oophorus slough off, exposing the antral surface. The egg with the zona pellucida may float off into the follicular fluid and become infiltrated by leukocytes and fragment. The follicle

collapses, is invaded by fibroblastic connective tissue (Figure 19.27), and ends up as a small hyalinized structure akin to the corpus albicans, called a corpus fibrosum (Figure 19.28). However, they are usually considerably smaller than corpora albicantia.

## Structure of the Corpus Luteum

The life cycle of the corpus luteum commences immediately following ovulation and, in its early stage, none of the stigmata of corpus luteum is apparent.[4,8,12] Following extrusion of the ovum, the wall of the follicle collapses and the stigma, or site of ovulation, becomes plugged by fibrin and shortly by fibrous connective tissue. The microscopic appearance does not differ appreciably from the follicle before ovulation occurs (Figure 19.29). The granulosa cells now undergo proliferation and alteration to lutein cells that have as their role the production of progesterone. This is followed by vascularization, which is characterized by penetration of the granulosa by thin-walled blood channels arising from the vessels of the theca interna. These pass toward the lumen after filling it partially, or at times extensively, with blood. If the bleeding has been extensive, the corpus luteum can be dominated by the hematoma. The lutein cells become large and polyhedral. The cytoplasm is somewhat foamy and eosinophilic. Following bleeding into the lumen of the corpus luteum, the inner surface of the lutein cells becomes

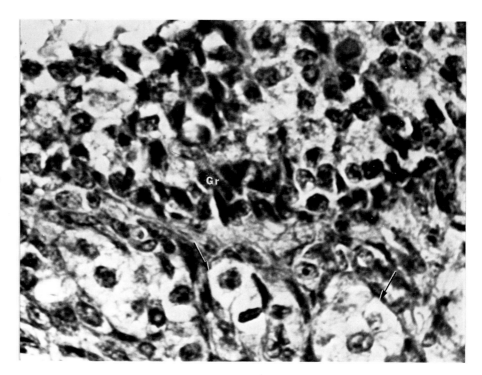

**19.25** Edge of maturing follicle. Granulosa cells (Gr) and luteinized theca interna (arrows).

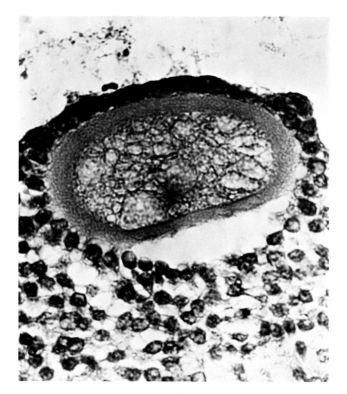

**19.26** Ovum in a follicle. Note degeneration of the zona pellucida in an egg undergoing degeneration. ×208.

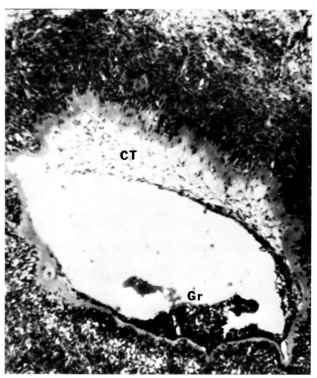

**19.27** Follicle undergoing atresia. Residual granulosa cells (Gr) and connective tissue proliferation (CT) are seen. ×190.

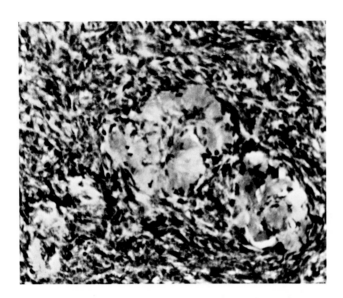

**19.28** Corpus fibrosum. Scarred remnant of an atretic follicle. ×80.

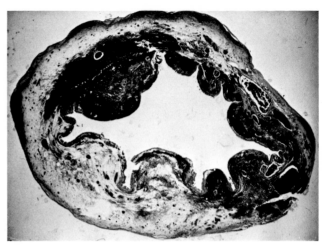

**19.29** Collapse of mature follicle from which a mature ovum has been discharged. The dark zone represents hemorrhage in the theca interna. This is the earliest stage in corpus luteum development. ×7.4.

covered by fibroblasts. The theca interna undergoes involution and now resembles fibrous connective tissue, except where it is incorporated into the septa that compartmentalize the corpus luteum. Here they retain their theca lutein configuration and are called paralutein cells (Figure 19.30). They function as endocrine cells that produce estrogens. The corpus luteum now is composed of a broad zone of cells traversed by the septa. This is now the period of maturation (Figure 19.31) and the paralutein cells increase in size and prominence. The layer of fibroblast cells covering the inner surface of the lutein cells is now mature fibrous connective tissue. Much, but not necessarily all, of the blood may be resorbed (Figure 19.32).

The corpus luteum at any of its stages can project on the surface of the ovary or be below the surface. At the height of its maturity, it may measure up to 2 cm in diameter. The broad festooned layer of lutein cells can vary in color from golden yellow to pale white, depending on how much carotin is present. There is every indication that beyond day 21 in the menstrual cycle, if fertilization and implantation has not taken place, the corpus luteum commences the stage of involution.[9,11] This phase is characterized by vacuoles of varying size forming in the luteal cells (Figure 19.33), with progressive hyalinization of the mass, and contraction, with the formation of a convoluted hyalinized lutein surrounding a central core of scar tissue, a corpus albicans (Figure 19.34). Carotin pigment is removed from the mass. Ultimately the corpus albicans undergoes resorption.

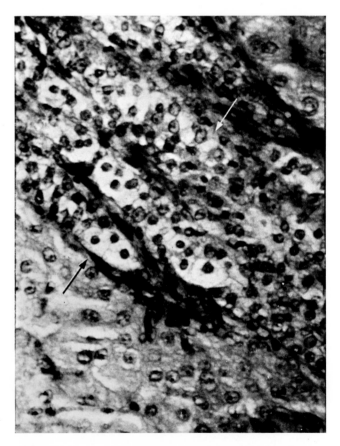

**19.30** Paralutein cells (arrows) in the trabeculae that separate lobules of the corpus luteum. ×240.

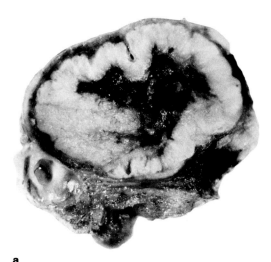

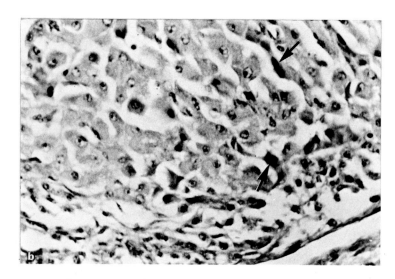

**19.31 a.** Mature corpus luteum cyst of ovary. ×4.3. **b.** Mature lutein cells and K cells (arrows) with dark nuclei and deeper eosinophilic cytoplasm.

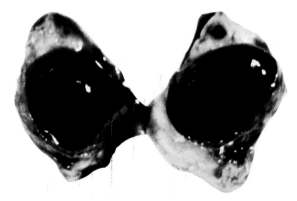

**19.32** Corpus hemorrhagicum. The cavity of the corpus luteum is filled with blood.

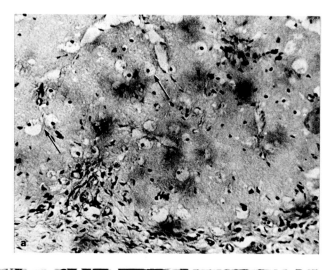

**19.33 a.** Corpus luteum cyst, regressing phase. Note the vacuoles (arrows) in corpus luteum cells. ×160. **b.** Corpus luteum cyst, regressing phase. Cells are now completely devoid of cytoplasm.

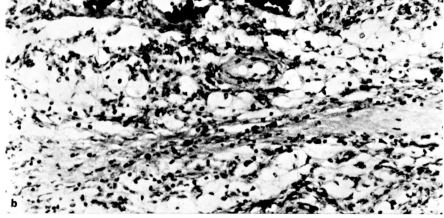

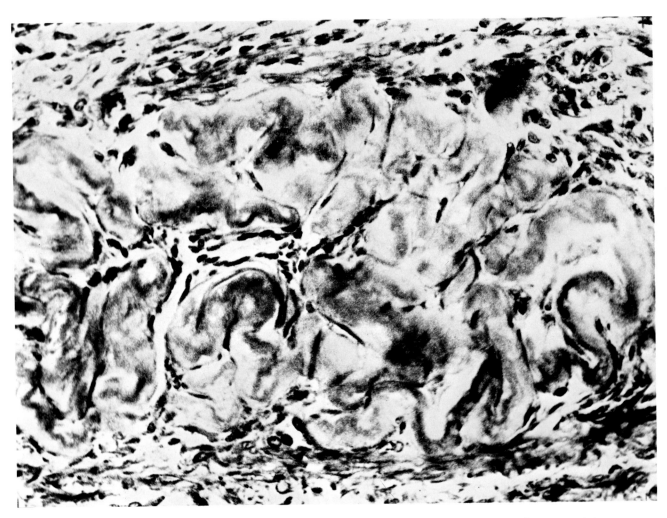

**19.34** Corpus albican body. Burnt out, fibrotic remnant of a corpus luteum. ×200.

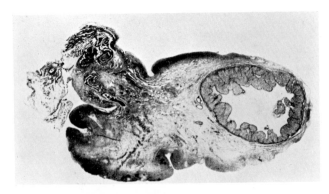

**19.35** Corpus luteum of pregnancy. Note that it occupies more than one-third of the ovary. ×8.

## The Ovary in Pregnancy

The corpus luteum of pregnancy is much larger than in the normal menstrual cycle.[13,19,35] It may constitute more than one-third of the ovary[18] (Figure 19.35). The festooned border can be very prominent or at times less marked if the central cavity is somewhat cystic. Paralutein tissue[20] is hyperplastic and the cells are larger in size than in the usual corpus luteum.[34] It persists, on the average, for 2½ months following pregnancy before it undergoes regression. Patches of decidual cells may be found on the surface or in the cortex (Figure 19.36). Grossly, they are white opalescent spots. Ectopic decidua[22,24,25] reflects the response of connective tissue to pregnancy hormones.

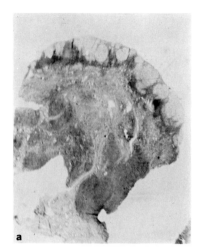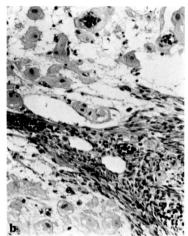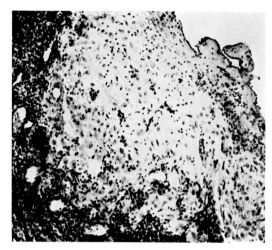

**19.36 a.** Surface of the ovary showing pale areas of deciduosis. **b.** High-power view of cells in (**a**). **c.** Deciduosis on the surface and in the cortex of the ovary in pregnancy. ×59.

[Reprinted by permission from H. Mosman and K. Duke, *Comparative Morphology of the Mammalian Ovary*, Madison, University of Wisconsin Press, 1973.]

**19.37** Ovary of a newborn female. Note its size in relation to the fallopian tube, the latter being almost equal in diameter. The cortex is filled with primitive ova. ×5.4.

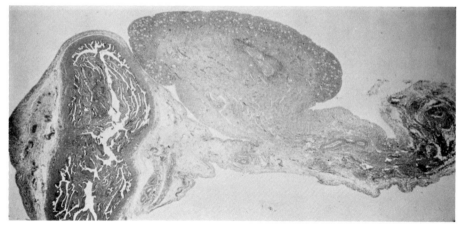

Similar nonspecific changes may be seen in the omentum, peritoneum, and mesoappendix.

Ovulation ceases during pregnancy and some follicles can be seen that have undergone atresia. It is in the pregnant ovary that one can appreciate the special character of the ovarian arterial supply, namely, its ability to uncoil and supply an increased surface with ease. The position of the ovary is altered by the enlarging uterus, which lifts it out of the true pelvis. During puerperium, the ovary reduces in size and returns to the true pelvis; after a time normal follicular activity returns.

# Alterations Induced by Age

*Newborn ovary*

The newborn ovary is an elongated structure 1.5 to 2 cm in length, 0.5 cm in width, and 1 to 3.5 mm in thickness, weighing between 0.3 and 0.4 g. Initially it lies in the false pelvis and only later in its growth phase does it move into the true pelvis. The surface is pinkish white and smooth, except for an occasional follicle that may be near the surface (Figure 19.37).

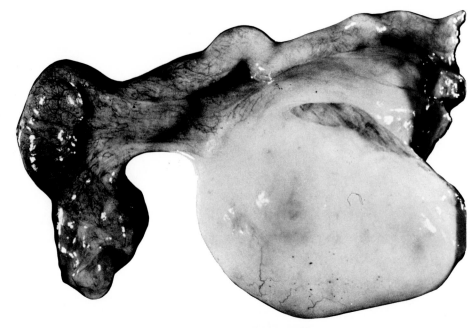

**19.38** Ovary of an adolescent aged 16. The surface is smooth and devoid of the scarring following multiple ovulations. ×8.3.

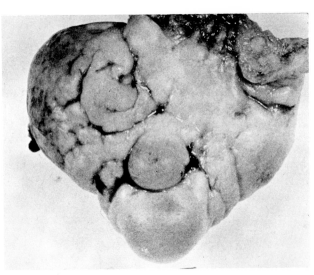

**19.39** Ovary of a female aged 38. The surface shows multiple scars and several follicle cysts. ×12.4.

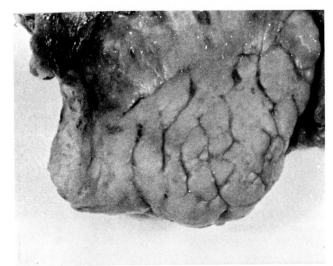

**19.40** Ovary of a female aged 62. The surface is cerebriform because of scarification. ×16.7.

### Adolescent ovary

There is a growth phase between birth and puberty, and at the commencement of menarche the ovary is large, largely because of cortical growth. It measures 3 to 3.5 cm in length and 1.5 to 2.0 cm in width and has increased considerably in thickness to 1.0 to 1.5 cm. Its weight now varies from 4 to 7 g. The surface is pearly gray (Figure 19.38); follicles are visible and there is a resemblance to

the polycystic ovary. In childhood the follicles tend to be atretic but in adolescence ovulation occurs, although the surface is still smooth.

### Ovary during reproductive period

The normal functioning ovary contains follicles and corpora lutea in varying stages of maturation and regression, as well as corpora albicantia and corpora fibrosa.

Scarred remnants of corpora lutea and follicles are also seen. During the reproduction period the surface becomes repeatedly scarred by ovulation, and by the fifth decade it has a cerebriform convoluted appearance (Figure 19.39).

### Postmenopausal ovary

The ovary is now nonfunctioning and again small. It may weigh from 1 to 2 g. The outer surface is cerebriform in appearance and the cut surface is essentially fibrotic (Figure 19.40).[41]

# REFERENCES

1. Abrego, D., and Ibrahim, A. Mesenteric supernumerary ovary. *Obstet. Gynecol.* 45(3):352, 1975.

2. Anderson, D. H. Lymphatics and blood vessels of the ovary of the sow. *Contr. Embryol. Carnegie Inst. (Washington, D.C.)* 18:135, 1927.

3. Baker, T. G. Quantitative and cytological study of germ cells in human ovaries. *Proc. R. Soc. Sec. B.* 158:417, 1963.

4. Blanchette, E. J. Ovarian steroid cells. II. The lutein cell. *J. Cell Biol.* 31:517, 1966.

5. Blaustein, A. Unpublished data, 1975.

6. Blaustein, R. L., Blaustein, A., and Gross, M. J. Oxidative enzyme activity of human ovarian stromal cells. *Obstet. Gynecol.* 36(2):269, 1970.

7. Burnett, J. E., Jr. Supernumerary ovary: A case report. *Am. J. Obstet. Gynecol.* 82:929, 1961.

8. Call, E., and Exner, S. Zur Kenttniss der Graafischen Follikels und des Corpus Luteum Biem Kaninchen, Sitzungsber. *Math. Naturwiss, KL Kaiser, Akad. Wiss. Wien* 11:321, 1875.

9. Chiquoine, A. D. The development of the zona pellucida of the mammalian ovary. *Am. J. Anat.* 105:149, 1960.

10. Corner, G. W. The sites of formation of estrogenic substances in the animal body. *Physiol. Rev.* 18:154, 1938.

11. Corner, G. W. Development, organization and breakdown of the corpus luteum in the rhesus monkey. *Contrib. Embryol. Carnegie Inst. (Washington, D.C.)* 31:112, 1945.

12. Corner, G. W., Jr. The histological dating of the human corpus luteum of menstruation. *Am. J. Anat.* 98:377, 1956.

13. Crisp, T. M., Dessouky, A. D., and Denys, F. R. Fine structure of the human corpus luteum of early pregnancy and during the progestational phase of the menstrual cycle. *Am. J. Anat.* 127:37, 1970.

14. Eichner, E., and Bove, E. R. In vivo studies on the lymphatic drainage of the human ovary. *Obstet. Gynecol.* 3:287, 1954.

15. Feinberg, R., and Cohen, R. B. A comparative histochemical study of the ovarian stromal lipid band, stromal thecal cell and normal ovarian follicular apparatus. *Am. J. Obstet. Gynecol.* 92:958, 1965.

16. Ferenczy, A., and Richart, R. M. *Female Reproductive System, Dynamics of Scan and Electron Microscopy.* New York, John Wiley & Sons, 1975.

17. Forbes, J. R. On the fate of the medullary cords of the human ovary. *Contrib. Embryol. Carnegie Inst. (Washington, D.C.)* 30:9, 1942.

18. Forleo, R. Anatomy of the human ovary during pregnancy. *B.I. Obstet. Gynecol.* 16:530, 1961.

19. Gillman, J., and Stein, H. B. Human corpus luteum of pregnancy. *Surg. Gynecol. Obstet.* 72:129, 1951.

20. Govan, A. D. T. Follicular activity in the human ovary in late pregnancy. *J. Endocrinol.* 48:235, 1970.

21. *Gray's Anatomy, Female Genital Organs.* 29th American Edition. Philadelphia, Lea & Febiger, Ch. 17, pp. 1317–1321.

22. Green, R. R., and Nelson, W. W. Decidual reaction in the ovary. *Quart. Bull. Northwest. Univ. Med. Sch.* 26:197, 1952.

23. Hertig, A. T., and Adams, E. C. Studies on the human oocyte and its follicle. I. Ultra-structural and histochemical observations on the primordial follicle stage. *J. Cell Biol.* 34:647, 1967.

24. Hogan, M. L., Barber, D. D., and Kaufman, R. H. Dermoid cyst in supernumerary ovary of the greater omentum: Report of a case. *Obstet. Gynecol.* 29:405, 1967.

25. Israel, S. L., Rubenstone, A., and Meranze, D. R. The ovary at term I. Decidua-like reaction and surface cell proliferation. *Obstet. Gynecol.* 3:399, 1965.

26. Jacobowitz, D., and Wallach, E. E. Histochemical and chemical studies of the autonomic innervation of the ovary. *Endocrinology* 81:1132, 1967.

27. Laffargue, P., Adichy-Benkoel, L., and Valette, C. Ultra structure of the ovarian stroma. *Am. Anat. Pathol. (Paris)* 13:381, 1968.

28. Leeson, C. R., and Leeson, T. S. The Female Reproductive System, in *Histology,* 2nd ed. Philadelphia, W. B. Saunders, 1970, pp. 416–425.

29. Mattingly, R. F., and Huang, W. Y. Steroidogenesis of menopausal and post-menopausal ovary. *Am. J. Obstet. Gynecol.* 103:679, 1969.

30. McKay, D. G., Pinkerton, J. H. M., Hertig, A. T., and Danziger, S. The adult human ovary—A histochemical study. *Obstet. Gynecol.* 18:13, 1961.

31. McNeill, J. Aberrant ovarian tissue in the round ligament of the uterus *J. Obstet. Gynaecol. Br. Commonw.* 38:608, 1931.

32. Mobius, W., Carol, W., and Schmid, H. H. Retroperitoneal Gelegenes Pseudomuzinkcystom, Von ektopischen Ovarial Gewebe Augehend. *Zentralblatt Gynakol.* 86:133, 1964.

33. Morris, B., and Sass, M. D. The formation of lymph in the ovary. *Proc. R. Soc. Sec. B* 164:577, 1966.

34. Motto, P., Cherney, D. D., and Didio, L. J. Scanning and transmission electron microscopy of the ovarian surface in mammals with special reference to ovulation. *J. Sub. Microse. Cytol.* 3:85, 1971.

35. Nelson, W. W., and Green, R. R. Histology of human ovary during pregnancy. *Am. J. Obstet. Gynecol.* 76:66, 1958.

36. Pankratz, D. S. Some observations on the Graafian follicles in an adult human ovary. *Anat. Rec.* 71:211, 1938.

37. Papadaki, L., and Beilby, J. O. W. The fine structure of the surface epithelium of the human ovary. *J. Cell Sci.* 8:445, 1971.

38. Printz, J. L., Choate, J. W., Townes, P. L., et al. The embryology of supernumerary ovaries. *Obstet. Gynecol.* 41:246, 1973.

39. Rice, B. F., and Savard, K. Steroid hormone formation in the human ovary. IV. Ovarian stromal compartment; formation of radio-active steroids from acetate-1-$^{14}$C and action of gonadotropins. *J. Clin. Endocrinol.* 26:593, 1966.

40. Scully, R. E., and Cohen, R. B. Oxidative-enzyme activity in normal and pathologic human ovaries. *Obstet. Gynecol.* 24:667, 1964.

41. Serment, H., Laffargue, P., and Vallette, C. The functional stroma of the menopausal ovary. *Press. Med.* 77:1653, 1969.

42. Strassman, E. L. The theca cone and its tropism toward the ovarian surface. A typical feature of growing human and mammalian follicles. *Trans. Am. Assoc. Obstet. Gynecol.* 53:11, 1940.

43. Strassman, I. O. The theca cone: The pathmaker of growing human and mammalian follicles. *Int. J. Fertil.* 6:135, 1961.

44. Wharton, L. R. Two cases of supernumerary ovary and one of accessory ovary with an analysis of previously reported cases. *Am. J. Obstet. Gynecol.* 78:1101, 1959.

45. Zacharias, F., and Jensen, C. E. Histochemical and physiochemical investigations on genuine follicular fluid. *Acta Endocrinol.* 27:343, 1958.

Ancel Blaustein, M.D.

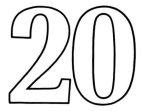

# Inflammatory Diseases of the Ovary

Inflammatory lesions of the ovary occur largely in relation to infection of the fallopian tube. The most common infecting agent is *Neisseria gonococcus* and the ovary is infected by contiguity. Oophoritis may follow endometrial curettage, cervical biopsy, or vaginal surgery, but this fortunately is a rare occurrence. The organisms in these cases are anaerobic and/or aerobic streptococci and enterococci and the pathway of infection is lymphatic or hematogenous. Occasionally oophoritis may be related to colonic diverticulitis or acute appendicitis, but in these conditions the ovary is usually focally involved by its proximity to the bowel and then only superficially. It is interesting to observe that despite extensive adhesions between the fallopian tube and ovary, follicles and corpora lutea can still be seen in varying stages of development and regression. There are, of course, instances in which abscesses develop and the whole ovary may be destroyed, but these appear to be infrequent.

## Acute Oophoritis

It is rare to receive specimens in this stage because surgery during this period is inadvertent. However, when acute oophoritis is found, the gross appearance of the ovary is far more striking than is the microscopic. It may be edematous, angry red in color, and have a thin layer of

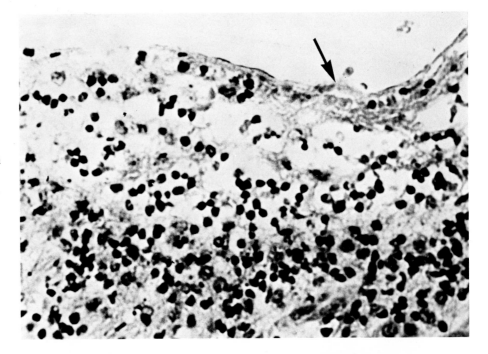

**20.1** Acute oophoritis. There is a thin layer of fibrin (arrow) on the surface. In the cortex there is edema, fibrin deposition, and a leukocytic infiltration.

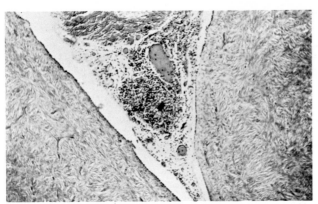

**20.2** Acute perioophoritis. There is fibrin and granulation tissue present in a surface cleft.

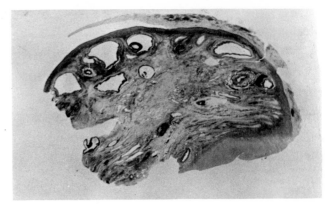

**20.3** Chronic perioophoritis. There is a layer of dense fibrous adhesions on the surface.

fibrin deposited on the surface. Microscopic examination (Figure 20.1) may only show mild subepithelial edema, superficial congestion, and a thin surface layer of fibrin. It is rare to see leukocytic infiltration. The residua of this degree of involvement are adhesive bands that in their early stage are quite vascular (Figure 20.2) and in the later stages are densely collagenous (Figure 20.3).

Transient oophoritis may occur in association with mumps and exanthemata. The mechanisms are not clearly understood but are never as destructive as in the male, where sterility may follow involvement of the testicle.

## Ovarian and Tubovarian Abscess

There are instances when bacteria enter a thin-walled or a ruptured follicle cyst or corpus luteum.[2] This is deeper penetration and can result in the whole ovary being edematous and congested and can result in abscess formation. The portal of entry is often confirmed by finding the abscess limited to a follicle or corpus luteum. The finding of an ovarian abscess in the absence of salpingitis can usually be related to recent pelvic surgery usually associated with manipulative procedures *per vaginum.*

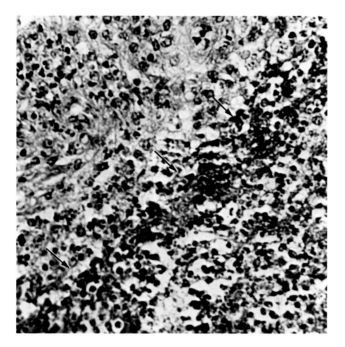

**20.4** Ovarian abscess. The border of the abscess cavity (tips of arrows) is clearly delineated. The cavity contains fibrin and leukocytes.

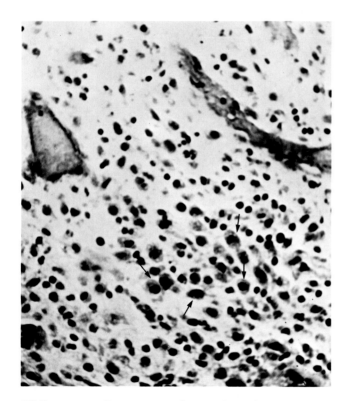

**20.5** Ovarian abscess. Granulation tissue is present. Numerous histiocytes (arrows) are seen.

The fallopian tube infected by *Neisseria gonococcus* tuberculosis results in destruction of the normal architecture with loss of function. In particular with gonococcal involvement, the tube, edematous and congested, adheres to the ovary and as the infection progresses can bind the two organs together into a distorted mass in which both can lose identifiable landmarks. The cut surface of a tubovarian mass usually reveals a fibrotic or sclerotic wall and a cavity that may contain purulent material. The appearance is dependent on the age of the lesion. Fresh tubovarian masses are deep red on their outer surfaces and are covered with fresh adhesions; the lumen of the mass is filled with purulent material.[4,5,6,11] Microscopic examination (Figure 20.4) reveals necrosis, leukocytic infiltration, granulation tissue (Figure 20.5), and foci of histiocytes (Figure 20.6). The histiocytes are lipid laden and have, on occasion, been mistaken for cells of a corpus luteum.

## Chronic Perioophoritis

Chronic inflammation of the ovary usually takes the form of extensive adhesions on the surface and adhesive bands may form pseudocystic spaces. Chronic inflammation may also induce some metaplastic changes in the surface epithelium adjacent to adhesions and the epithelium may look somewhat bizarre.

## Chronic Granulomatous Oophoritis

### Tuberculosis

Genital tuberculosis is still quite prevalent in India,[9,20] the Far East, the Middle East,[10] and the Carribean area. The incidence of involvement of the ovary is significantly lower than that of the fallopian tube. Ylinen,[20] in a review of 206 oophorectomies reported an incidence of 20.4%. In a comparable series of cases the fallopian tube was involved in 68.4%. The ovary is involved by contiguous spread from tuberculous salpingitis. A common hematogenous origin from a remote focus, generally situated in the lungs, is to be considered probable for genital tuberculosis in the majority of cases. The common clinical complaints are sterility, pelvic pain, poor general condition, fever, menstrual disturbances, and less often vaginal discharge. The fallopian tube may be functionally destroyed by tuberculosis and, when it is bound by adhesions to the ovary, the granulomata characteristic of tuberculosis can be found in the cortex of the ovary. Only rarely does the ovary reveal extensive caseation and abscess formation.

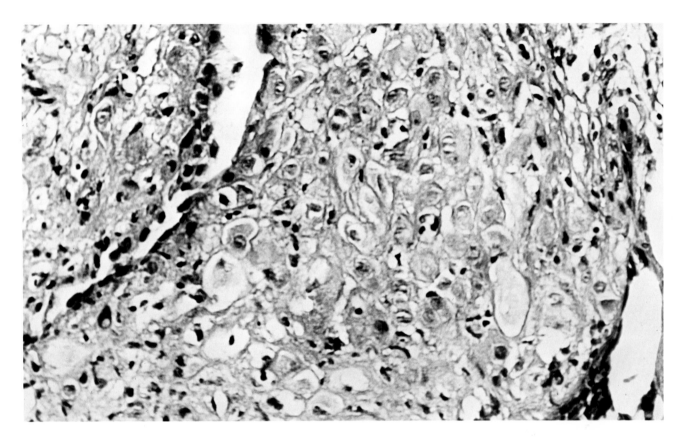

**20.6** Ovarian abscess. Healing stage. The cavity is filled with lipid-laden macrophages that have a pseudolutein appearance.

**20.7** Actinomycosis of ovary. There is a large abscess (arrow) present in the cortex. The cut surface is yellowish white and soft.

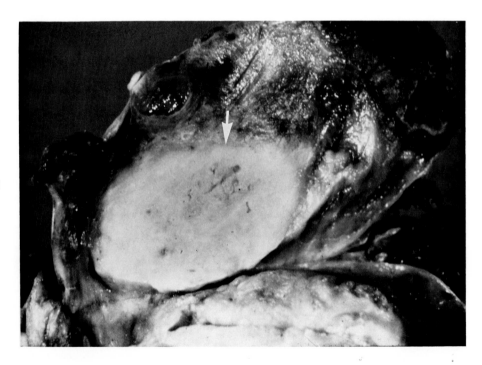

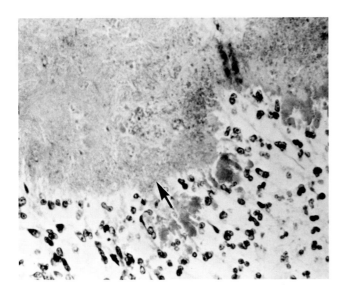

**20.8** Sulfurlike granule (tip of arrow) surrounded by leukocytes.

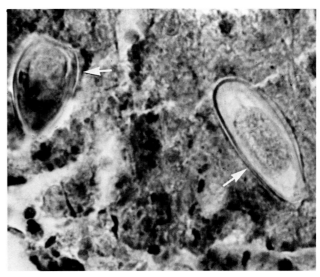

**20.9** Surface of ovary. Ova of *Enterobius vermiculosis* (arrows) seen within adhesions.

## Sarcoidosis

This is an uncommon disorder. It is a generalized disease of unknown etiology, frequently disseminated in various organs, most notably lungs and lymph nodes. Involvement of the female genital tract was first described by Longcope[13] in 1941. He found granulomas typical of sarcoidosis in curettings. Lesions have been described in the myometrium, cervix, fallopian tubes and, to a much lesser degree, in ovaries. Winslow and Funkhouser[19] described a case in which the ovary as well as the fallopian tube showed granulomatous lesions.

The diagnosis of sarcoidosis is usually made when acid-fast stains for tuberculosis are negative and the Kveim test is positive. In some areas, the diagnosis was made only after the patients failed to respond to antituberculous therapy. The disease is inconsequential in the female pelvis; it is not a cause of sterility and is usually self-limiting.

## Actinomycetes as a Cause of Oophoritis

*Actinomyces israeli* are saprophytic organisms in the anorectal area and have been reported to be responsible for ovarian abscess[3,7,14–17] (Figure 20.7). The appendix may be a nidus of infection and, in rare instances, a chronically infected appendix may be adherent to the ovary. The actinomycotic abscesses are usually not large. They are thin-walled and the lumen contains sulfurlike granules that contain the hyphae of *Actinomyces israeli* (Figure 20.8).

## Granulomatous Oophoritis due to *Enterobius vermicularis*

Granulomata in reaction to *Enterobius vermicularis* have been described beneath the fibrovascular adhesions associated with endometriosis[12] (Figure 20.9). They have not been found on normal ovaries, only in and around ovarian adhesions. The source of infection may be the anorectal area or an adherent retrocecal appendix laden with pin worms and showing acute or chronic inflammation.

## Genital Schistosomiasis and Oophoritis

Schistosomiosis involving the female genital tract has been reported in the Far East, Middle East, and South America.[1,8] There have been over 100 cases reported from Brazil. Infection has been described with *Schistosoma mansoni, S. japonicum,* and *S. haematobium.* Migration of the ova through the pelvic plexus of veins has been emphasized, localizing in the ovaries, fallopian tubes, cervix, vulva, vagina, and uterus. The rich network of venous anastomoses between the urinary bladder and the genital organs offer an explanation for the high incidence of genital manifestations in *S. haematobium. Schistosoma mansoni* are usually found in the portal venous system, but the imperfect quality of the valvular system and frequent anastomoses offer no obstacle for migration of ova from the portal veins to the venous canal system that normally drains the ovary. The involved ovary may be enlarged to as much as three times its normal size. The surface may show small, white nodules. Microscopic section reveals granulomata in which lie the ova, with abundant histiocytes, lymphocytes, and large numbers of eosinophils.

# REFERENCES

1. Bahary, C. M., Ovadia, Y., and Neri, A. *Schistosoma mansoni* of the ovary. *Am. J. Obstet. Gynecol. 98:*290, 1967.

2. Black, W. T. Abscess of ovary. *Am. J. Obstet. Gynecol. 31:*487, 1936.

3. Brenner, R. W., and Gehring, S. W. Pelvic actinomycosis in the presence of an endocervical contraceptive device. *Obstet. Gynecol. 29:*71, 1967.

4. Bruchner, W. M. Rupture of pyosalpinx as a cause of acute diffuse peritonitis. *Surg. Gynecol. Obstet. 14:*474, 1912.

5. Collins, C. G., Nix, F. G., and Cerha, H. T. Ruptured tubovarian abscess. *Am. J. Obstet. Gynecol. 72:*820, 1956.

6. Cummin, R. C. Abscess of ovary. *J. Obstet. Gynaecol. Br. Commonw. 58:*1025, 1951.

7. Duncan, J. A. Abdominal actinomycosis: Changing concepts. *Am. J. Surg. 110:*148, 1965.

8. Fernandes, M., and Lapa, R. Schistosomiosis of the ovary. *Ann. Brasil de Giec. 11:*427, 1941.

9. Gupta, S. Pelvic tuberculosis in women. *J. Obstet. Gynaecol., India 7:*181, 1957.

10. Halbrech, I. Sterility from healed genital tuberculosis. *Int. J. Fertil. Steril. 4:*50, 1959.

11. Koen, R. C. Ovarian abscess. *U.S.A.F.M.J. 8:*1664, 1957.

12. Lansman, H. H., Lapin, A., and Blaustein, A. Pelvic *enterobius vermicularis* granuloma associated with endometriosis. *Am. J. Obstet. Gynecol. 79:*1178, 1960.

13. Loncope, W. T. Sarcoidosis or besnier-Boeck Schaumann's disease: Frank Billings's lecture. *JAMA 117:*321, 1941.

14. Loth, M. F. Actinomycosis of the fallopian tube. *Am. J. Obstet. Gynecol. 72:*919, 1956.

15. McCarthy, J. Actinomycosis of the female pelvic organs with involvement of the endometrium. *J. Pathol. Bacteriol. 69:*173, 1955.

16. Perkin, G. W. Intra-uterine contraception. *Can. Med. Assoc. J. 94:*431, 1966.

17. Sweeney, D. F., and Blackwelden, T. F. Pelvic actinomycosis. Report of a case. *Obstet. Gynecol. 25:*690, 1965.

18. Wilson, J. R., and Black, J. R. Ovarian abscess. *Am. J. Obstet. Gynecol. 90:*34, 1964.

19. Winslow, R. D., and Funkhouser, J. W. Sarcoidosis of the female reproductive organs. *Obstet. Gynecol. 32:*285, 1968.

20. Ylinen, O. Genital tuberculosis in women. *Acta Obstet. Gynecol., Scand. 40,* 1961.

Ancel Blaustein

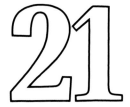

# Nonneoplastic Cysts of the Ovary

Nonneoplastic cysts are the commonest cause of ovarian enlargement. They are conveniently divided into inactive cysts and those that are capable of elaborating hormones having an end organ effect (see Table 21.1).

## Serous Inclusion Cyst

These are nonfunctional and commonly found after the menopause but may be seen as early as in the newborn (see p. 369). They may lie close to the surface or deep in the cortex and may vary in size from a few millimeters to several centimeters in diameter. They can be readily distinguished from parovarian cysts because the latter are located in the mesovarium.

Serous cysts may, at times, be large and unilocular and have a smooth, well-vascularized outer and inner surface (Figures 21.1 and 21.2). They contain thin watery fluid that may be clear, blood tinged, or grossly bloody, particularly if torsion of the cyst on its pedicle has occurred. Adhesions are absent. Smaller cysts may be multiple in the cortex. They are generally lined by cuboidal epithelium (Figure 21.3) but frequently parts of the cyst may be lined by metaplastic epithelium. The commonest form of metaplasia seen is that resembling endosalpinx. Other forms of metaplasia seen are endometrial and less often resemble endocervix. These cysts are devoid of hormonal activity and are not associated with abnormal uterine bleeding.

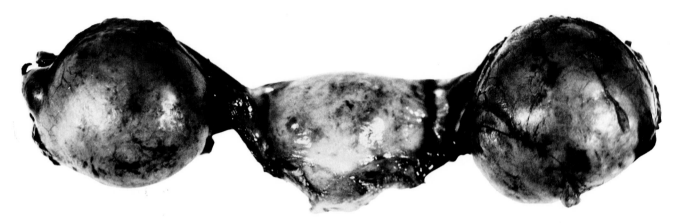

**21.1** Bilateral serous cysts of the ovary. The serosa is well vascularized.

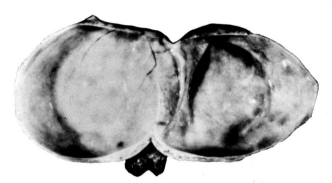

**21.2** Serous cyst of the ovary. Inner surface is smooth and well vascularized.

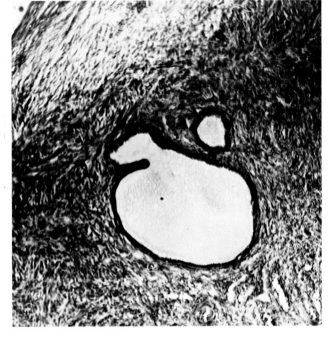

**21.3** Small serous inclusion cysts in the cortex of the ovary.

## Follicle Cyst

These are extremely common and are usually unilocular. They vary in size from 1 up to 5 cm in diameter and lie just beneath the surface of the ovary (Figure 21.4). The outer surface is smooth, the wall is thin, and the cyst usually contains clear watery fluid. Follicle cysts (Figure 21.5) are lined by a stratified layer of granulosa cells beneath which may be seen the cells of the theca interna. Granulosa cells are round and plump and have well-defined nuclei but poorly defined cytoplasmic borders. The surrounding theca interna cells are spindle shaped and they also have prominent nuclei and indistinct cytoplasmic borders.

If the cyst is large, the lining epithelium may be compressed by the fluid content and the granulosa layer may be obliterated (Figures 21.6 and 21.7), so that only theca interna or only hyalinized fibrous connective tissue may be seen. In the latter case, they are often called simple cysts,

**Table 21.1** Classification of nonneoplastic ovarian cysts

| Cyst | Hormone activity | Hormone |
|------|------------------|---------|
| Serous inclusion cyst | None | None |
| Follicle cyst | Possible | Estrogens |
| Corpus luteum cyst | Yes | Progesterone |
| Corpus albicans cyst | None | None |
| Theca lutein cyst | Yes | Estrogens |

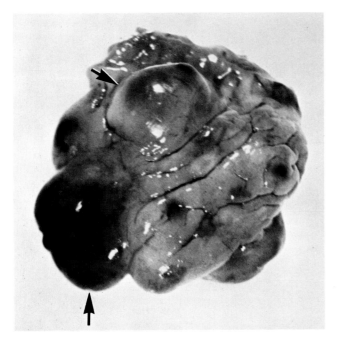

**21.4** Multiple small follicle cysts (arrows) bulging just beneath the cortex of the ovary.

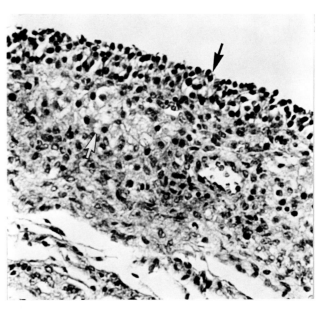

**21.5** Lining of a follicle cyst. Granulosa layer (dark arrow) is composed of a multicellular layer. Theca interna (light arrow) lies immediately beneath the granulosa cells.

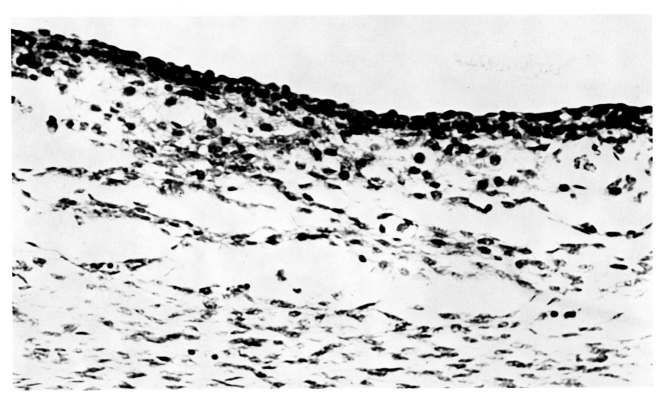

**21.6** Lining of a follicle cyst. Compression by the cyst content distorts the granulosa layer.

395

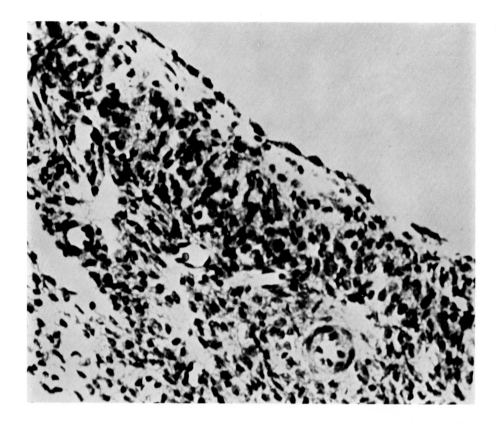

**21.7** Lining of a follicle cyst. Compression has resulted in a monolayer of flattened epithelium.

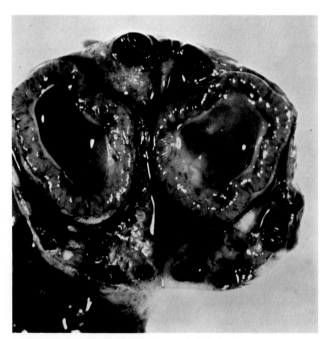

**21.8** Corpus luteum cyst. The border is composed of a corrugated layer of cells and a central cavity containing fibrin.

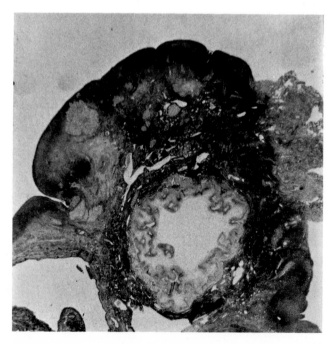

**21.9** Corpus albicans cyst. The lining of the cyst is composed of hyalinized connective tissue.

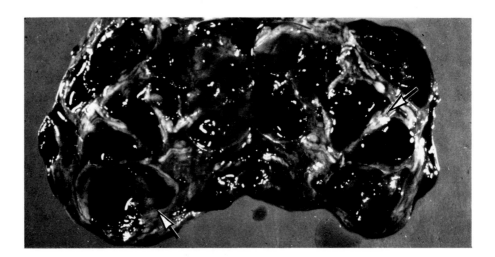

**21.10** Theca lutein cyst. Conglomerate of nodular masses (arrows). The cut surface is hemorrhagic.

because they cannot be distinguished from nonfollicular cysts. Follicle cysts usually undergo spontaneous involution, but they may persist and, uncommonly, may be lined by active, functional granulosa and/or thecal cells and contain estrogen-rich fluid.[1] Estrogens produced by an active follicle can result in endometrial hyperplasia and irregular uterine bleeding.

## Corpus Luteum Cyst

Corpora lutea normally develop, function, and regress in a cyclical pattern. Sometimes, however, organization of the central cavity is slow and a thin layer of fibroblastic connective tissue forms on the inner surface of the cyst (Figure 21.8). This results in delayed regression of luteal cells. Consequently, progesterone production persists, resulting in delayed menstruation followed by persistent uterine bleeding. Ultimately the luteal tissue is replaced by a hyalin-like tissue. If the cystic cavity persists, it is designated a corpus albicans cyst (Figure 21.9), which is nonfunctional. At times a corpus luteum cyst can rupture into the pelvic cavity. The amount of blood loss can be minimal but at times can be extensive enough to require the patient to be transfused.

## Theca Lutein Cyst

Theca lutein cysts, as the term implies, are dominated by theca interna. Granulosa cells are not increased in number and may even be atrophic. These cysts may be

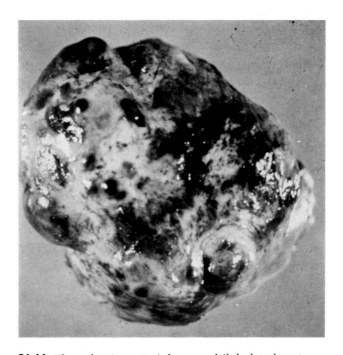

**21.11** Theca lutein cyst. A large multilobulated cyst.

quite small but in pregnancy, twinning, particularly in a hydatidiform mole, choriocarcinoma, and in patients receiving gonadotropin therapy they may form large nodular masses (Figures 21.10 through 21.12) that may, to the inexperienced observer, present a difficult diagnostic problem. The cut surface of the cyst is often partly yellow and partly hemorrhagic. Microscopic examination is characterized by hyperplasia of theca interna cells, often showing

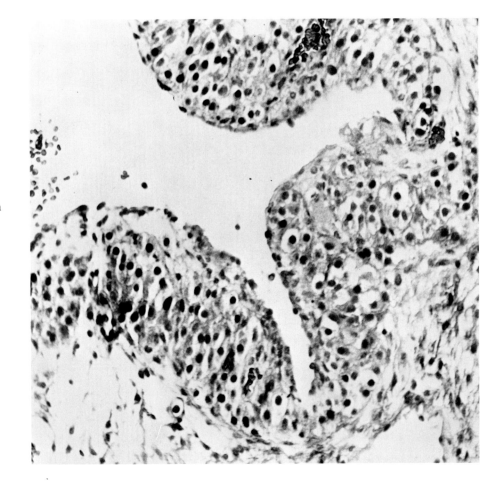

**21.12** Lining of a theca lutein cyst. Granulosa layer is atrophic and luteinized theca interna is the dominant cell type.

prominent luteinization. It is believed that these cysts result from excessive stimulation of the theca interna by unusually high levels of circulating gonadotropins, particularly in trophoblastic disease. Theca lutein cysts have been experimentally produced in animals by the injection of choriogonadotropins in large amounts.

## Polycystic (Sclerocystic) Ovaries and Hyperthecosis

Polycystic ovaries are less commonly found than single follicle cysts and they are certainly less well understood.[13,14,22] Both ovaries (Figure 21.13) tend to be almost uniformly involved and they resemble the pubescent ovary in the sense that they are two to five times the normal size.[24,35] The cysts may cause surface bulging but are often not fully appreciated prior to sectioning because of the thickening of the ovarian capsule (Figure 21.14).

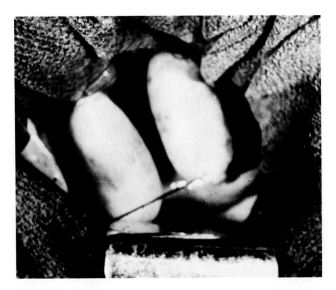

**21.13** Polycystic ovaries. They appear enlarged and have a pearly gray capsule.

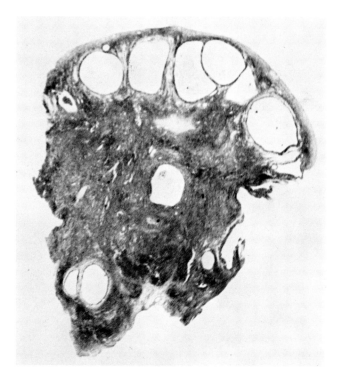

**21.14** Polycystic ovaries. Macrofollicle cysts lie beneath the thickened capsule.

Microscopic examination shows a dense eosinophilic tunica albuginea.[24] In the normal ovary, the tunica is thin and often indistinct. Here it is increased in thickness 10- to 15-fold (Figure 21.15). The cysts are lined by granulosa cells of varying thickness and beneath this there is usually a prominent layer of theca interna cells; the latter frequently show extensive luteinization. Corpora albicantia may be found. Atretic follicles are more abundant in the cortex (Figure 21.16). An important observation is the very striking hyperplasia and luteinization of theca interna surrounding the cysts and atretic follicles[11,33] (Figure 21.17). Cortical stroma itself may be hyperplastic[5,7,11] and also may show islands of luteinized cells.[30] This has been called by some hyperthecosis or thecomatosis[5,6,11,19,31,33,41] (Figure 21.18).

Ovaries containing multiple follicle cysts and other morphologc changes described above need not necessarily be associated with endocrine disorders. Endocrine abnormalities that do occur, however, fall into three broad categories.

1. Abnormal uterine bleeding associated with estrinism[22,30]
2. Stein–Leventhal syndrome—amenorrhea and sterility[18,23]
3. Virilism[5,8,9,12,16,17,21,25,38,39]

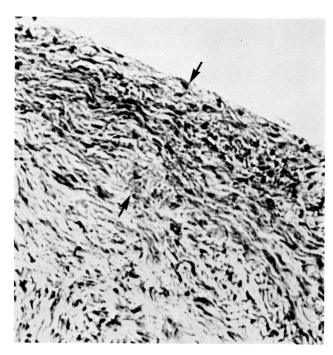

**21.15** Polycystic ovaries. The thickened capsule lies between the two arrows.

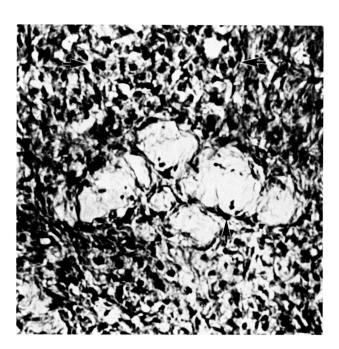

**21.16** Polycystic ovary. Cluster of atretic follicles (lower arrow). Luteinized stromal cells (upper two arrows) lie in close proximity.

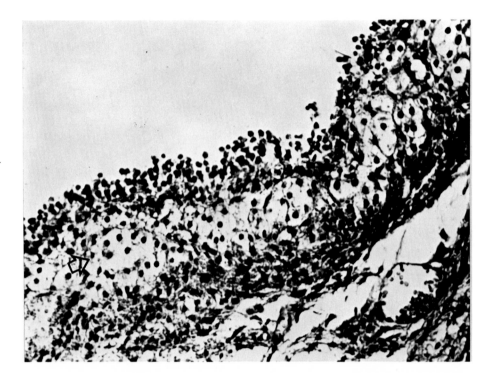

**21.17** Polycystic ovary. Luteinization of the theca interna is striking.

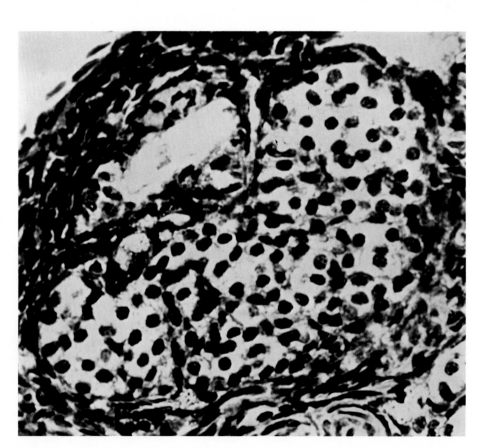

**21.18** Polycystic ovary. Stromal luteinization can be found in the cortex.

There is overlapping within these categories and a lack of uniformity in the menstrual history obtained and in the distribution and extent of the hirsutism. Endocrine abnormalities associated with polycystic ovaries are found only during the reproductive years.[22]

## Polycystic Ovaries in Association with Estrinism

The multiple follicle cysts in polycystic ovaries can result in endometrial hyperplasia and abnormal uterine bleeding similar to that found with single or multiple follicle cysts that may develop in normal ovaries. In cases of polycystic ovaries, endometrial hyperplasia can persist for long periods of time and atypical hyperplasia, as well as carcinoma, have been reported. There have also been reports of patients under 35 years of age with endometrial carcinoma. At laparotomy their ovaries frequently were polycystic.[22]

## Stein–Leventhal Syndrome

In 1934 Stein and Leventhal[36] described a syndrome characterized by secondary amenorrhea, sterility, and bilateral polycystic ovaries. Hirsutism in varying degrees may be present in fully 50% of cases. This syndrome occurs in young women in the second or third decade of life. Breast development may be normal or deficient. Obesity may or may not be present, the incidence being no greater than in the general population. The menstrual history is variable and is related to the duration of the abnormal physiologic state. Secondary amenorrhea[20] may follow normal menarche and normal early periods. In some cases there is a history of menstrual abnormalities since menarche, even though the patient may at times have normal periods. The usual history is one of development of oligomenorrhea that progresses to amenorrhea. There may be periods of frequent bleeding or even menorrhagia. After amenorrhea develops, scant bleeding may occur occasionally. Curettage performed at the time of bleeding, or at the time menstruation should occur, invariable shows proliferative endometrium or endometrial hyperplasia. This is the result of persistent anovulation. Basal body temperatures reveal a monophasic curve and the vaginal smears demonstrate estrogenic effects. In some patients ovulation may break through spontaneously and be followed by pregnancy. Stein and Leventhal have had cases where normal menstruation persisted once pregnancy had been achieved. It is a rare instance where a patient has had a pregnancy preceding the onset of the syndrome. Successful pregnancy, with a reversal to normal menses following wedge resection, has been reported in patients that had been amenorrheic for 10 years. The incidence of the classic syndrome is low and a review of 9,000 gynecologic laparotomies found six cases of the Stein–Leventhal syndrome. A study of 370 wives who complained of infertility found five with the syndrome, and culdoscopy performed on 316 patients complaining of infertility revealed polycystic ovaries in only nine. Culdoscopy and/or pneumoroentgenography are used to evaluate ovarian size. The gross and microscopic appearance of the ovaries conforms to that seen in all forms of polycystic ovarian syndrome.

## Association of Endometrial Carcinoma with Stein–Leventhal Syndrome

A number of authors[2,15,26,32,40] have described endometrial carcinoma in association with Stein–Leventhal syndrome. What percentage of cases of Stein–Leventhal syndrome shows endometrial carcinoma is not accurately known as yet. The significance of the association must await a significant statistical study.

## Virilism

This syndrome may be a part or extension of the Stein–Leventhal syndrome, but patients frequently present with complaints that primarily relate to virilism.[8,12] Hirsutism of a progressive nature, voice changes, and breast atrophy overshadow any concern for the associated oligo- and amenorrhea. The microscopic appearance of the ovary is dominated by hyperthecosis and stromal luteinization. There may or may not be follicular cysts.

## Endocrine Abnormalities in Polycystic Ovarian Syndrome

There are no consistent abnormalities found; no distinctive pre- or postoperative changes in urinary hormone excretion. Follicle-stimulating hormone (FSH) levels are in general in the normal range. In cases where luteinization of the theca interna and stroma is prominent, elevated pregnandiol excretion has, on occasion, been reported.[19,22] Urinary 17-ketosteroids may be normal or slightly elevated.[27] Elevations reported are rarely significant.[11,18] A significant number of investigations have now reported elevations of free or unbound testosterone levels as compared with protein-bound testosterone.[9,29,34] The unbound testosterone concentration appears to represent the physiologically effective circulating androgen and can explain the not uncommon patient with evidence of virilization and normal or only slightly elevated total serum testosterone concentration. Molar concentration of testosterone-binding protein in the serum of patients with polycystic ovarian syndrome is about half that of normal women in the reproductive age group. The etiology of the marked reduction in the levels of testosterone-binding protein in women with polycystic ovarian syndrome, as compared to the normal, is unclear. This may be a congenital defect that is possibly genetically transmitted or may be an alteration in androgen and/or estrogen production and metabolism.

## Etiology

The three clinical syndromes are associated with similar pathologic alterations in the ovaries; however, this need not suggest a common etiology. The factors that initiate the ovarian changes are unknown. Different investigators have suggested that there are hormonal abnormalities that commence at the level of the hypothalamus and pituitary gland.[10,21,22] A number have suggested that an imbalance of pituitary gonadotropins is an important factor.[29] One investigator was able to experimentally produce polycystic change by repeated injections of FSH into monkeys.[10] Other workers suggest that luteinizing hormone (LH) may be related to stromal luteinization.[10] Fairly consistent aberrations of testosterone metabolism probably account for any mascularizing changes that may be present.[9,17,21,37] There are cases of menstrual disorders with hirsutism or virilism in which 17-ketosteroids are elevated.[3] The adrenal gland in these cases is usually hyperplastic.[17] Scully[28] reported a case of progressive hirsutism in a young woman with elevated 17-ketosteroid excretion. Laparotomy revealed polycystic ovaries with striking theca and stroma–lutein cell formation. Adrenal exploration revealed hyperplasia of the cortex such as has been described in the adrenogenital syndrome. Some cases of Cushing's disease[17] have been described in which ovaries are polycystic and show hyperthecosis as well as stromal luteinization.

Bartuska *et al.*[4] have reported a few cases of polycystic ovaries that followed traumatic brain damage.

In summary, extraovarian factors, probably hormonal in nature, may initiate the syndrome; but the frequent return of the normal menstrual cycle and, indeed, the occurrence of pregnancy following wedge resection of the ovary underscore the importance of the role of the ovary itself.

# REFERENCES

1. Adair, F. L., and Watts, R. M. A study of the hormonal content of ovarian cyst fluids. *Am. J. Obstet. Gynecol.* 34:799, 1937.
2. Allan, M. S., and Hertig, A. M. Carcinoma of the ovary. *Am. J. Obstet. Gynecol.* 58:640, 1949.
3. Barlow, J. Adrenocortical influences on estrogen metabolism of normal females. *J. Clin. Endocrinol. Metab.* 24:586, 1964.
4. Bartuska, D. G., Eskin, B. A., Smith, E. M., et al. Brain damage, hypertrichosis, and polycystic ovaries. Clinical evaluation of seven cases. *Am. J. Obstet. Gynecol.* 99:387, 1967.
5. Beattie, M. K., Kay, W. W., Elton, A., and Hucker, A. C. Masculinization associated with luteinized microcysts of the ovary. *J. Obstet. Gynaecol. Br. Commonw.* 59:465, 1952.
6. Bigelow, B. Comparison of ovarian and endometrial morphology spanning the menopause. *Obstet. Gynecol.* 11:487, 1958.
7. Blaustein, R. L., Blaustein, A. U., and Gross, M. J. Oxidative enzyme activity in cells derived from the cortex of human ovary. *J. Obstet. Gynecol.* 36:269, 1970.
8. Culiner, A., and Shippel, S. Virilism and theca cell hyperplasia of the ovary. *J. Obstet. Gynaecol. Br. Commonw.* 46:439, 1949.
9. Easterling, W. E., Jr., Talbott, L. M., and Poher, H. D. Serum testosterone levels in the polycystic ovary syndrome. *Am. J. Obstet. Gynecol.* 120:385, 1974.
10. Evans, T. N., and Riley, G. M. Polycystic ovarian disease: A clinical experimental study. *Am. J. Obstet. Gynecol.* 80:873, 1960.
11. Feinberg, R. Thecosis: A study of diffuse stromal thecosis of the ovary and superficial collagenization with follicular cysts (Stein–Leventhal ovary). *Obstet. Gynecol.* 21:687, 1963.
12. Geist, S. H., and Gaines, J. A. Diffuse luteinization of the ovaries associated with the masculinization syndrome. *Am. J. Obstet. Gynecol.* 43:975, 1942.
13. Goldzieher, J. W., and Green, J. A. The polycystic ovary. I. Clinical and histologic features. *J. Clin. Endocrinol. Metab.* 22:325, 1962.
14. Ingersoll, F. N., and McDermott, W. V. Jr. Bilateral polycystic ovaries. Stein–Leventhal syndrome. *Am. J. Obstet. Gynecol.* 60:17, 1950.
15. Jackson, R.L., and Dockerty, M. B. Stein–Leventhal syndrome and endometrial cancer. *Am. J. Obstet. Gynecol.* 73:161, 1957.
16. Jeffcoute, T. A. The androgenic ovary with special reference to the Stein–Leventhal syndrome. *Am. J. Obstet. Gynecol.* 88:143, 1964.
17. Jones, H. W., Jr. The gynecologic aspects of adrenal hyperplasia and allied disorders. *Am. J. Obstet. Gynecol.* 68:1330, 1954.
18. Judd, H. L., Barnes, A. B., and Kliman, B. Long-term effect of wedge resection on androgen production in a case of polycystic ovarian disease. *Am. J. Obstet. Gynecol.* 110:1061, 1971.
19. Judd, H. L., Scully, R. E., Herbst, A. L., Yen, S. S. C., Ingersol, F. M., and Kliman, B. Familial hyperthecosis: Comparison of endocrinologic and histologic findings with polycystic ovarian disease. *Am. J. Obstet. Gynecol.* 117:976, 1973.
20. Kistner, R. W. in Disorders of menstruation, Danforth, D. N., ed. *Textbook of Obstetrics and Gynecology*, 2nd ed. New York, Harper and Row, 1971.

21. Klinefelter, H. F., Jr., and Jones, G. E. S. Amenorrhea due to polycystic ovaries (Stein–Leventhal syndrome). *J. Clin. Endocrinol. Metab.* 14:127, 1954.

22. Leventhal, M. L. The Stein–Leventhal syndrome. *Am. J. Obstet. Gynecol.* 76:825, 1958.

23. Leventhal, M. L. Functional and morphologic studies of the ovaries and supra-renal glands in the Stein–Leventhal syndrome. *Am. J. Obstet. Gynecol.* 84:154, 1962.

24. Leventhal, M. L., and Scommegna, A. Multiglandular aspect of Stein–Leventhal syndrome. *Am. J. Obstet. Gynecol.* 84:445, 1963.

25. Lynch, M. J., Kyle, P. R., Raphael, S. S., and Bruce-Lockhart, P. Unusual ovarian changes (hyperthecosis) in pregnancy. *Am. J. Obstet.* 77(2):335, 1959.

26. Roddick, J. W., and Green, R. R. Relation of ovarian stromal hyperplasia to endometrial carcinoma. *Am. J. Obstet. Gynecol.* 73:843, 1957.

27. Rosenfield, R. L. Plasma testosterone binding globular and indexes of the concentration of unbound plasma androgens in normal and hirsute subjects. *J. Clin. Endocrinol. Metab.* 32:717, 1971.

28. Scully, R. E., and Richardson, G. S. Luteinization of the stroma of metastatic cancer involving the ovary and its endocrine significance. *Cancer* 14:827, 1962.

29. Sherman, R. P., and Cox, R. I. Clinical and chemical correlations in the Stein–Leventhal syndrome. *Am. J. Obstet. Gynecol.* 92:747, 1965.

30. Sherman, R. P., and Cox, R. I. The enigmatic polycystic ovary. *Obstet. Gynecol. Surg.* 21:1, 1966.

31. Shippel, S. Ovarian theca cell. IV. Hyperthecosis syndrome. *J. Obstet. Gynaecol. Br. Commonw.* 62:321, 1955.

32. Sommers, S. C., Hertig, A. T., and Bengloff, H. Genesis of endometrial carcinoma. Cases 19 to 35 years old. *Cancer* 2:957, 1949.

33. Sommers, S. C., and Teloh, H. A. Ovarian stromal hyperplasia in breast cancer. *Arch. Pathol.* 53:106, 1952.

34. Southern, A. L., Gordon, G. G., Jochinoto, S., Olivo, J., Sherman, D. H., and Pinzon, G. Testosterone and adrostenedione metabolism in the polycystic ovary syndrome: Studies of the percentage binding of testosterone in plasma. *J. Clin. Endocrinol. Metab.* 29:1356, 1969.

35. Stein, I. F. Bilateral polycystic ovaries. Significance in sterility. *Am. J. Obstet. Gynecol.* 50:385, 1945.

36. Stein, I. F., and Leventhal, M. L. Amenorrhea associated with bilateral polycystic ovaries. *Am. J. Obstet. Gynecol.* 29:181, 1935.

37. Taymor, M., Clark, R., and Sturgis, S. H. The polycystic ovary. A clinical and laboratory study. *Am. J. Obstet. Gynecol.* 86:188, 1963.

38. Turner, S. J. Bilateral microcystic degeneration of the ovaries and the masculinizing syndrome. *Am. J. Obstet. Gynecol.* 46:295, 1943.

39. Vermeullen, A., Stoica, T., and Verdonck, L. The apparent free testosterone concentration an index of androgenecity. *J. Clin. Endocrinol. Metab.* 33:759, 1971.

40. Woll, E., Hertig, A. T., Smith, G. V., and Johnson, L. C. The ovary in endometrial carcinoma. *Am. J. Obstet. Gynecol.* 56:617, 1948.

41. Yin, P. H., and Sommer, S. C. Some pathologic correlations of ovarian stromal hyperplasia. *J. Clin. Endocrinol. Metab.* 21:472, 1961.

Ancel Blaustein, M.D.

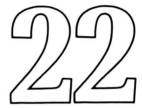

# Pelvic Endometriosis

## Ectopic Sites of Endometrium

Endometrium, the normal lining mucosa of the uterus, is found in a variety of ectopic sites (Figures 22.1 and 22.2).[9,20,21,42-45] Some of the extrauterine locations in which it has been found include (in order of frequency):

Ovaries (80% of all pelvic endometriosis)
Fallopian tubes, uterus, and cul de sac
Uterine ligaments[8]
Rectovaginal septum
Gastrointestinal tract
Cervix, vagina, and vulva
Skin, umbilicus, and incisional scars[12]
Inguinal region (including hernial sacs),[23] bladder wall,[16,24] kidney,[30] and pelvic lymph nodes
Extremities, lungs, pleura,[6,35] etc. (distant sites)

## Incidence

Kistner,[25,26] in a 10-year study of gynecologic laparotomies, reported that about 18% revealed microscopically proved endometriosis. The incidence rose to as high as 33⅓% when laparotomy for infertility was included.

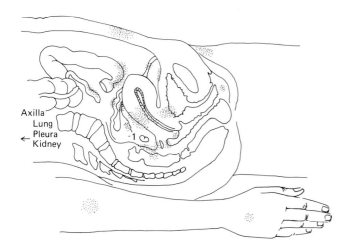

**22.1** Extrauterine locations in which endometriosis has been found. Lymph node (1).

[Reprinted by permission from C. Javert, Pathogenesis of endometriosis, *Cancer* 2:399, 1949.]

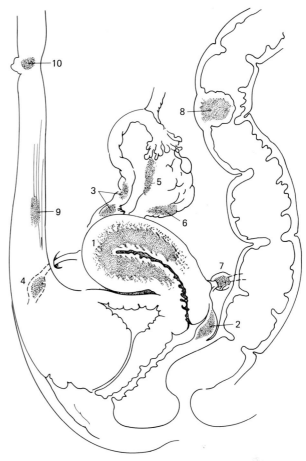

**22.2** Pelvic and abdominal sites of endometriosis.

[Reprinted by permission from C. Javert, Pathogenesis of endometriosis, *Cancer* 2:399, 1949.]

# Pathogenesis

The continuous cyclic homeoplastic activity of the benign endometrium makes it unlike most other tissues,[20,21] and it may be that this distinctive quality gives it the ability to disseminate in various channels and grow in heterotopic locations, producing lesions of endometriosis. Although it is usual for benign endometrium to remain localized in the uterus for long periods of time, direct myometrial extension (adenomyosis), exfoliation implantation, and lymphatic and hematogenous metastasis may occur (Figure 22.3).

The earliest theory to explain ectopic endometrium was that of Cullen[9] and separately von Recklinghausen.[49] Cullen[9] believed it originated in Müllerian rests and von Recklinghausen felt they were of Wolffian duct origin. These concepts today have few disciples. The theory of origin by celomic metaplasia first propounded by Ivanoff[19] is still regarded by many as one mechanism that results in endometriosis.[14,29] In 1922, Sampson[46] explained the histogenesis of endometriosis on the basis of regurgitation of endometrium through the fallopian tube and implantation of menstrual endometrium on pelvic organs. He[46] also suggested that lymphatic channels could be a route of dissemination. Numbers of authors have reported finding endometriosis in lymph nodes and Javert[20,21] reported a

case in which endometrium was found in a right ureteral lymph node (Figure 22.4) and another in a hypogastric lymph node (Figure 22.5). The extension of endometrial tissue to the broad ligament (Figure 22.6), such adjacent organs as the cervix (Figure 22.7), vagina (Figure 22.8), vulva, bladder, rectum, and pelvic lymph nodes may be via lymphatic channels (Figure 22.9). Sampson's concept of lymphatic dissemination of the endometrium is today accepted as the explanation for some of the ectopic sites of the endometrium. Dissemination by the hematogenous route is the only means of understanding endometriosis of the forearm,[3] thigh, and axilla[28] and multiple pulmonary lesions[6] and pleural involvement.[5]

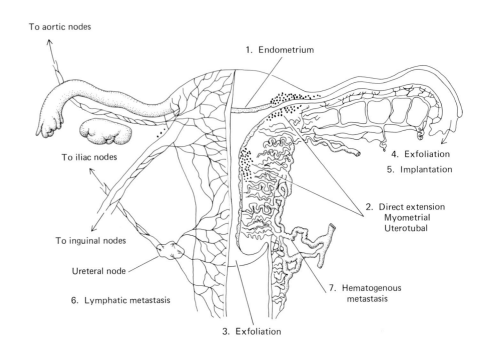

**22.3** Various channels of dissemination for benign endometrium.

[Reprinted by permission from C. Javert, Pathogenesis of endometriosis, *Cancer* 2:399, 1949.]

To aortic nodes

1. Endometrium

To iliac nodes

4. Exfoliation

5. Implantation

2. Direct extension
   Myometrial
   Uterotubal

To inguinal nodes

Ureteral node

7. Hematogenous metastasis

6. Lymphatic metastasis

3. Exfoliation

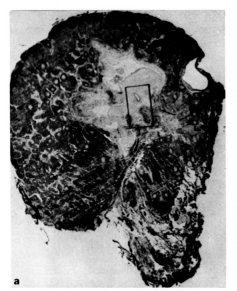
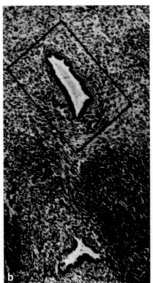
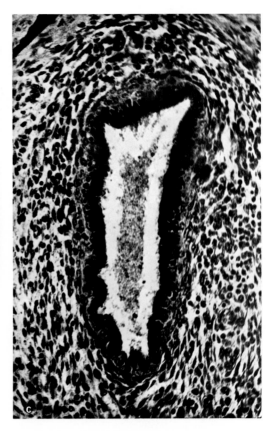

**22.4 a.** Low-power view of entire midportion of right ureteral lymph node showing islands of endometrial tissue within the hilum of the node. **b** and **c** are high-power views of the implant.

[Reprinted by permission from C. Javert, Pathogenesis of endometriosis, *Cancer* 2:399, 1949.]

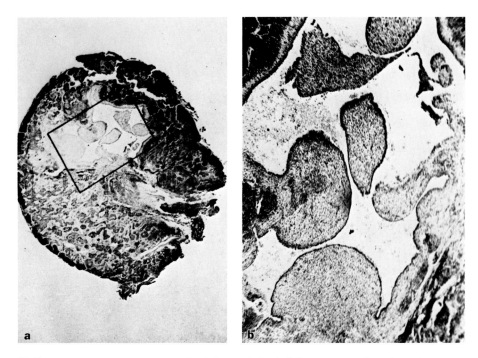

**22.5 a.** Endometrial tissue in the hilum of the left hypogastric lymph node. **b.** High-power view of area designated in (**a**).

[Reprinted by permission from C. Javert, Observations on the pathology and spread of endometriosis based on the theory of benign metastasis, *Am. J. Obstet. Gynecol.* 62:477, 1951.]

**22.6** Broad ligament. Macrophotograph showing lymphatic vessels containing endometrium in boxed area. Note implants (arrows).

[Reprinted by permission from C. Javert, Observations on the pathology and spread of endometriosis based on the theory of benign metastasis, *Am. J. Obstet. Gynecol.* 62:477, 1951.]

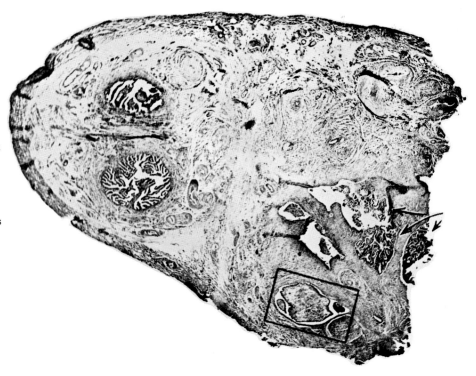

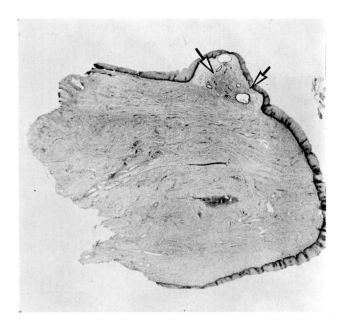

**22.7** Cervix showing endometriosis. Note implants (arrows).

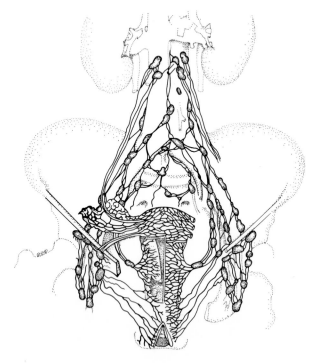

**22.9** Potential routes of benign lymphatic spread of endometrium.

[Reprinted by permission from C. Javert, Pathogenesis of endometriosis, *Cancer* 2:399, 1949.]

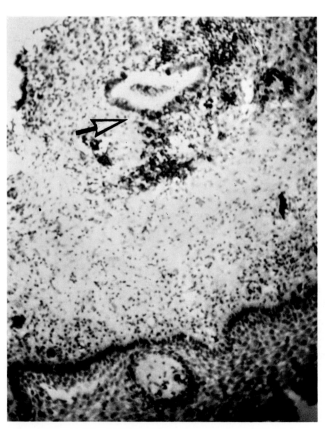

**22.8** Vagina. Note endometrial implants (arrow) beneath the vaginal mucosa.

# Symptomatology—Relationship to Pathologic Alterations

The symptoms include dysmenorrhea which appears to be related to implants on the uterosacral ligaments that swell just before and during menstruation.[18,38] It is perhaps the commonest complaint. Dyspareunia, rectal pain, tenesmus, and bloody stool (rare) may be present when there is extensive involvement of the rectovaginal septum.[1] Bowel involvement may be suspected if progressive intermittent cramping pain develops in the lower part of the abdomen.[4,7,10,13] This is usually associated with loss of appetite, nausea and vomiting, abdominal distension, and increasing constipation over a period of months.[7] The involvement of the urinary bladder[16] may occur and the patient may complain of frequency of urination, urgency, and rarely hematuria. Infertility[25,26] is the primary complaint in 30 to 40% of women with endometriosis. Fertility is felt to be reduced because of interference with tubal

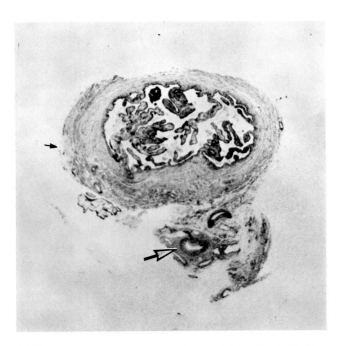

**22.10** Fallopian tube. Note endometrial implants (light arrow) and surface adhesions (dark arrow).

motility caused by adhesions and fibrotic changes resulting from implants involving these structures[25,26] (Figure 22.10). It is also thought that ovarian implants with concomitant exuberant adhesions interfere with maturation of ova. The cyclic activity of the ectopic endometrium with proliferation, engorgement, swelling, and menstruation results in extravasation of blood and release of iron, with subsequent formation of fibrosis and adhesions. Adhesions are mainly responsible for much of the symptomatology described. In the pelvis they result in tubovarian adhesions and adherence of ovaries to other adjacent structures. Adhesions on the bowel wall result in kinking, volvulus, intussusception, and partial and complete obstruction.

## Diagnosis

Extra pelvic lesions, such as those in the skin,[42] umbilicus, vulva, and incisional scars,[47] can be suspected because there may be a bluish discoloration of the skin over the lesion and prominence of pain that is cyclic with the menses. Lesions on the cervix are usually small and punctate and may have a red or blue appearance. Laparoscopy and culdoscopy are commonly used to visualize lesions on the fallopian tube, ovary, and uterine ligaments. Laparos-

copy may not be too useful in viewing the ovary if extensive adhesions are present. Most cases, although clinically suspected, are diagnosed at laparotomy.

## Pathologic Alterations in the Ovary

### Gross Findings

What one may observe depends on the site, extent, and age of the lesion. Fresh implants vary in color from raspberry red to blueberry blue, are small in size, and vary from 1 to 5 mm in diameter. They may be raised or dimpled lesions. As lesions increase in size and age, fibrous adhesions become more prominent. Endometrial cysts that in the early phase are small increase in size and are filled with old blood, which is brown in color and often inspissated (Figure 22.11).

Endometrial cysts may be single or frequently multiple.[39] They tend to increase in size with the bleeding that occurs during the menstrual cycle. The cyst wall, which may have initially been thin, becomes fibrotic and thick. The surface of older cystic lesions (Figure 22.12) show exuberant adhesions (arrows). Adhesions[33,36] are the hallmark of endometriosis. Adhesions are felt to be caused by the menstrual blood that escapes from the endometrial cyst, releasing its iron and perhaps other substances that are fibrogenic. Endometrial cysts in the ovary are usually small but can reach 15 to 20 cm in diameter. The cut surface usually shows a shaggy lining membrane that may have brown adherent deposits. The content is often dark brown and thick; the wall varies in thickness, depending on the age of the lesion, and there may be satellite cysts in the wall or on the surface.

### Microscopic Appearance

There is variation in the appearance of lesions. Endometrial glands and stroma may be seen on the surface of the ovary (Figure 22.13) or typical glands may be seen in the wall of an endometrial cyst (Figure 22.14). Other parts of the same cyst wall may only show a monolayer of endometrium and underlying stroma (Figure 22.15). Vessels in the stroma may contain coagulative thrombi (Figure 22.16) and infarction of the mucosa with sloughing occurring. The mucosa may also be obliterated by pressure atrophy of the blood in the cyst cavity, and the few remaining cells may have pyknotic nuclei and appear atypical (Figure 22.17). In some old cysts where the lining mucosa

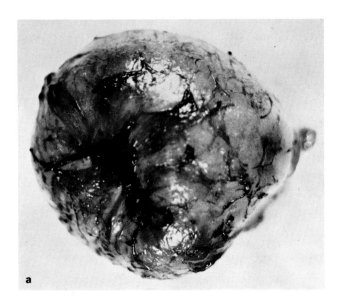

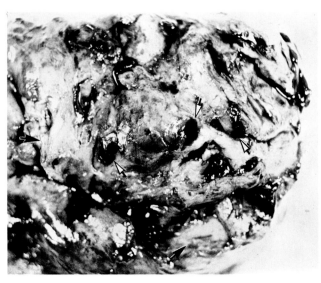

**22.12** Surface of the endometrioma of the ovary showing bluish-brown deposits (light arrows) surrounded by dense bands of connective tissue (dark arrows).

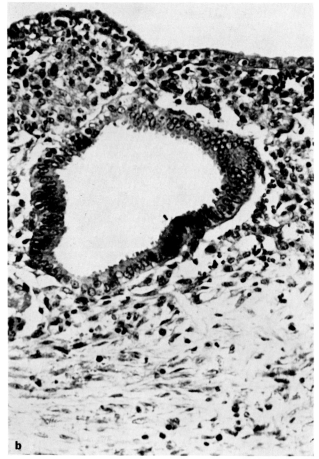

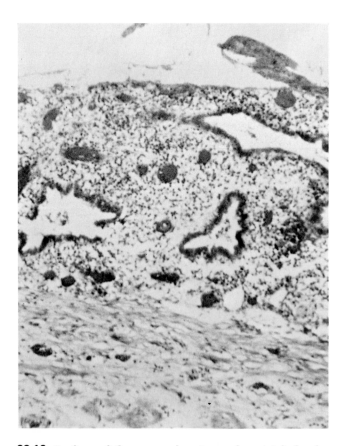

**22.11  a.** Endometrial cyst of the ovary. Note puckering and vascular-like surface implants. **b.** Endometrial gland surrounded by vascular stroma.

**22.13** Surface of the ovary showing endometrial glands and stroma.

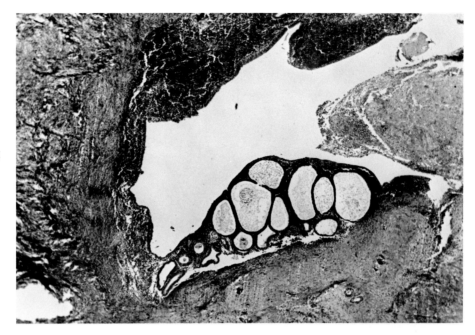

**22.14** Endometrial cyst showing lining epithelium composed of endometrial glands.

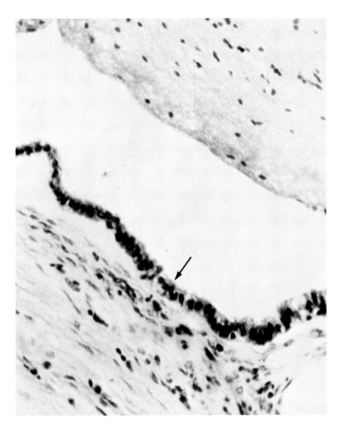

**22.15** Endometrial cyst of the ovary. Same cyst as in Figure 22.14 showing areas lined by a monolayer of endometrial cells (arrow).

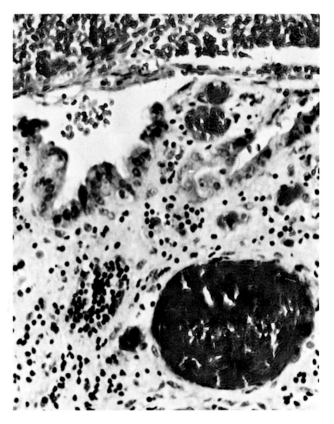

**22.16** Endometriosis of the ovary. Stromal vessels show coagulative thrombi with early sloughing of mucosa. Note extensive inflammatory cell infiltrate.

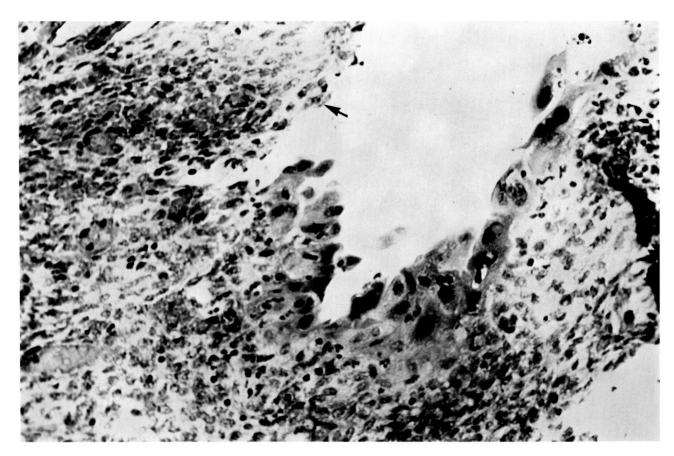

**22.17** Lining of endometrial cyst of ovary. Remaining epithelium have smaller, pyknotic nuclei. Mucosa is no longer present (arrow) in much of the cyst.

**22.18** Squamous metaplasia in an endometrioma of the ovary.

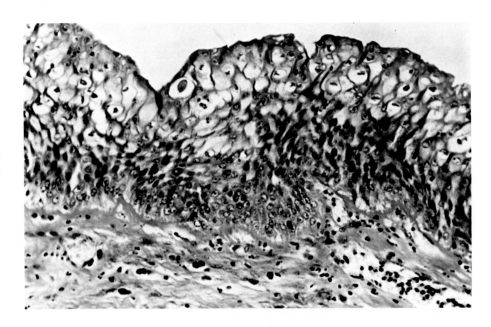

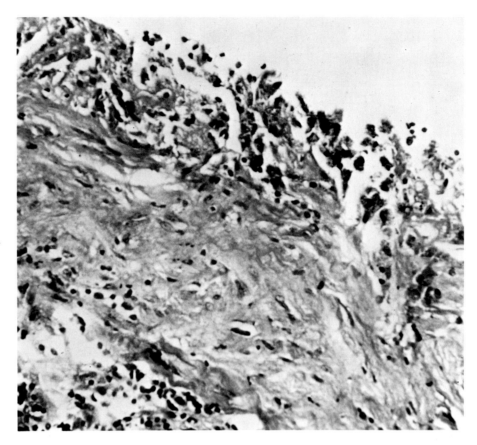

**22.19** Endometrioma of the ovary. Lining mucosa is denuded and replaced by macrophages laden with iron pigment interspersed in a fibrous stroma. Beneath this is dense collagenous connective tissue.

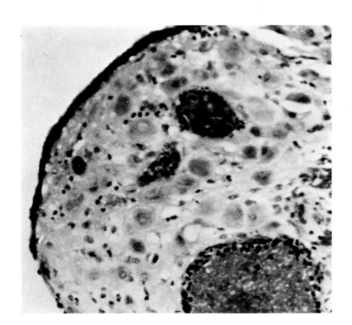

**22.20** Endometriosis of the ovary. Decidual alteration of stroma, produced by use of delalutin.

is smooth and pearly gray in appearance, microscopic study reveals metaplasia to squamous epithelium (Figure 22.18). At times sections of a cyst that have all the gross characteristics of endometriosis show only a thickened wall that may or may not have any surface mucosa but may be composed of macrophages laden with blood pigment interspersed in a fibroblastic stroma, and beneath this there is collagen (Figure 22.19). Even in the absence of endometrial epithelium, this lesion is now recognized as endometriosis. The term "presumptive endometriosis" has frequently been used as the diagnosis, but there is no reason not to simply refer to it as endometriosis. In the same cyst one can see this pattern, and in other parts of the cyst viable endometrium and/or glands as well as stroma may be found.

Pregnancy and progestational agents can induce a marked decidual response in the stroma (Figure 22.20). Some endometrial-like cysts are lined by epithelium resembling that of the fallopian tube and these lesions are referred to as "endosalpingiosis." The histogenesis of this type of lesion is undoubtedly by metaplasia.

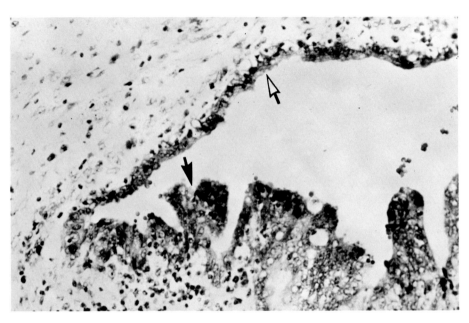

**22.21** Endometrioid carcinoma occuring in an endometrial cyst of the ovary. Normal appearing endometrium (light arrow) blends in with proliferative endometrium (dark arrow) and then merges imperceptibly with carcinoma.

## Endometrioid Carcinoma of the Ovary Arising from or Coexistent with Endometriosis

Sampson[41,42] was the first to recognize this association, and he believed that the carcinoma had its origin from abnormal endometrium in the ovary. It is most often difficult to say what percentage of endometrioid carcinomas of the ovary arise from ectopic endometrium, because in most instances there are no remaining traces of normal endometrium. There is, however, a small percentage of such tumors in which one can trace the transition of normal appearing ectopic endometrium (Figure 22.21) (light arrow) to proliferative hyperplastic endometrium (dark arrow), and the proliferative hyperplastic endometrium blends into adenocarcinoma (Figure 22.22). In the frankly malignant zone, there were several islands of clear cell carcinoma (Figure 22.23) (arrow), and the finding of islands of clear cell tumor in association with endometrioid carcinoma is not an unusual observation, although the relationship is not clear. In few cases, endometrioid carcinoma can be found in an ovarian cystic mass in which the cyst is largely lined by squamous epithelium (Figures 22.24 and 22.25). Well-differentiated endometriosis was found on the opposite ovary in this particular case. These rare combinations demonstrate the pluripotential nature of celomic epithelium.

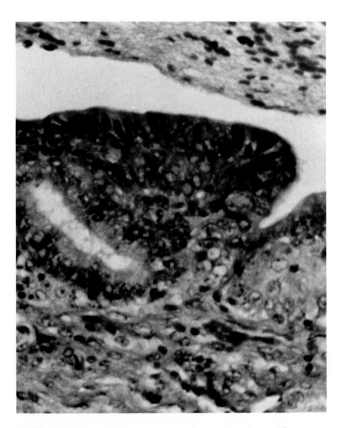

**22.22** Endometrioid carcinoma in continuity with proliferative endometriosis (ovary).

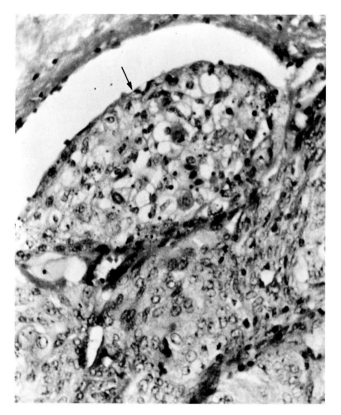

**22.23** Endometrioid carcinoma (same case as in Figure 22.22) with islands of clear cell carcinoma (arrow).

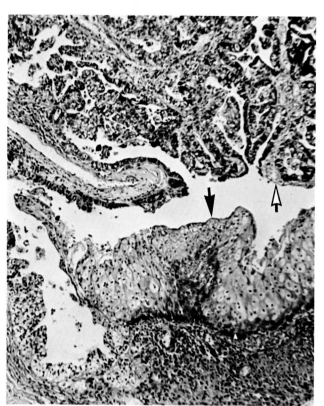

**22.24** Endometrioid carcinoma in ovary (light arrow) arising in a cyst largely lined by squamous epithelium (dark arrow).

**22.25** Endometrioid carcinoma (same case as in Figure 22.24) high-power view of the tumor.

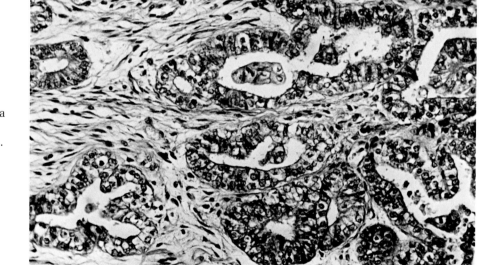

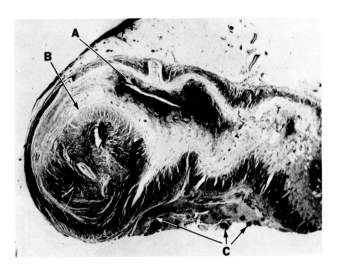

**22.26** Endometriosis of the appendix. **A**, **B**, and **C** are sites of endometrial implants in well of the appendix.

[Reprinted by permission from M. D. Senapti, Endometriosis of the appendix, *Br. J. Surg.* 41:330, 1953.]

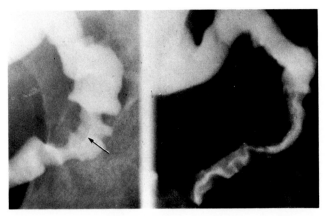

**22.27** Polypoid filling a defect in the terminal ileum. The mucosa overlying the lesion is intact.

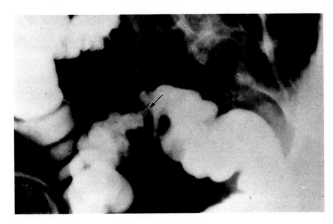

**22.28** Intramural lesion (arrow) producing appearance of carcinoma.

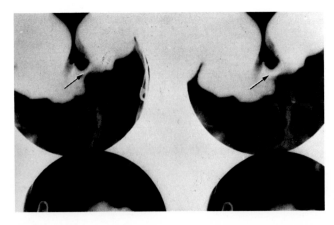

**22.29** Napkin-ringlike constriction (arrows) of the wall. Intramural endometriosis was present.

# Endometriosis Involving the Gastrointestinal System

Sampson[37] in 1922 described intestinal adenomas of endometrial origin. Macafee and Greer,[27] in a review of 7,177 cases of endometriosis, noted that 12% of patients had intestinal complaints and, of these, 72% of the lesions were in the rectosigmoid area and only 7% in the small bowel.[34] Appendiceal lesions (Figure 22.26) have been reported by Senapti.[48] The authors emphasize that most series of intestinal endometriosis include only those cases which have come to surgery. They speculate that the true incidence may, in fact, be much greater. It is also obvious that endometrial implants on the bowel wall may be asymptomatic and only be seen as incidental observations at surgery. Small bowel involvement is almost wholly limited to the ileum.[4,10] Only one case has been reported in the jejunum.[4]

## Clinical Manifestations and Diagnosis

The main symptoms and signs are those of intermittent obstruction of the small intestine.[4,32] The symptoms can be of acute or short duration or be chronic. The outstanding symptoms are usually accentuated with menstruation.

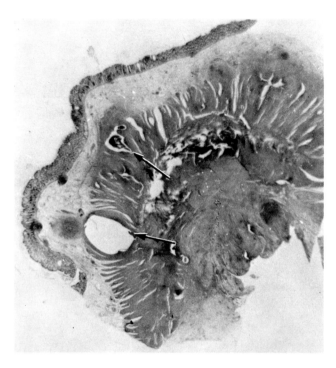

**22.30** Sigmoid colon. Endometrial implants (arrows) in the smooth muscle layer. There is a hypertrophy of muscle about the implants.

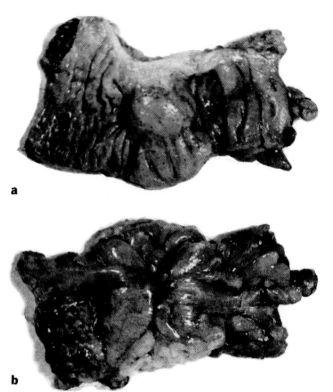

a

b

**22.31** Sigmoid colon. Lesions of endometriosis that on gross appearance have a high index of suspicion for carcinoma. In **a** there is a raised submucosal lesion and **b** puckering on the serosal surface.

[Reprinted by permission from C. R. W. Davis, W. Alexander, and R. E. Buenger, Surgery of endometriosis of the ileum and colon, Am. J. Surg. 105:263, 1963.]

Pelvic examination may reveal evidence of nodularity and thickening, suggestive of endometriosis. Radiographic studies may suggest the diagnosis preoperatively. In 10 cases studied by Davis, Alexander, and Buergen,[11] endometrioma was mentioned as a possible cause in four cases. Radiographic examination may reveal a polypoid filling defect (Figure 22.26) or luminal deformity (Figure 22.27). In both these cases the mucosa was seen to be intact. This is a useful clue because in carcinoma the mucosa is replaced by tumor. In the sigmoid colon, it can be difficult to exclude carcinoma by radiologic examination (Figure 22.28). Complete obstruction, volvulus, and intussusception have all been reported as a result of endometriosis.

## Gross and Microscopic Appearance

Surgical specimens show puckering of the serosa and extensive fibrosis in the serosa overlying a lesion. The cut surface usually reveals cysts that are intramural. The endometrial cysts appear to result in smooth muscle hyperplasia (Figure 22.29). At times the degree of fibrosis is so exten-

sive that the resected lesion may resemble carcinoma (Figure 22.31a,b).[2] However, the overlying mucosa is invariably intact. In some instances (Figure 22.30) the final diagnosis required microscopic examination.

Endometriosis in the rectovaginal septum[1,11,13,15,22] may result in fixation of pelvic organs, resembling the so-called frozen pelvis. Although ulceration of bowel mucosa is rare, rectal bleeding has been reported by Henrickson[16] in 19 of 21 cases. Microscopic examination of the lesions are essentially similar to those seen in other areas in the pelvis. Although the majority of patients with pelvic endometriosis are in the age range of 30 to 50 years, McKittrick[31] reported progressive lesions leading to bowel symptoms in a group of postmenopausal patients.

# REFERENCES

1. Ballon, H. C., Strean, G. J., and Simon, M. A. Obstructive ulcerated endometriosis of the rectum diagnosed by proctoscopic biopsy. *Can. Med. Assoc. J.* 74:817, 1956.

2. Benz, E. S., Dockerty, M. B., and Dixon, C. F. Polypoid endometrioma of colon; case in which unusual pathologic features were present. *Proc. Staff Meet., Mayo Clin.* 27:201, 1952.

3. Biebl, M. Bauchferne Endometriose am Unterarm und ihre Bedcutting fur eine neue Lehre von cincr einheitlich mesenchymalen Genese der Endometriosen allgemein. *Zentralbl. f. Chir.* 65:1026, 1938.

4. Bose, A., and Davson, J. Endometriosis of the small intestine. *Br. J. Surg.* 56:109, 1969.

5. Bungeler, W., and Fleury Silveira, D. Consideracos sobre a patogenia das endometrioses (a proposito de tres casos de endometriose externa). *Arq. de cir. clin. 3 exper.* 3:169, 1939; Abstr. in *Obstet. Gynecol. Surv.* 1:408, 1946.

6. Charles, D. Endometriosis and hemorrhagic pleural effusion. *Obstet. Gynecol.* 10:309, 1957.

7. Colcock, B. P., and Lamphier, T. A. Endometriosis. *Ann. Surg.* 131:507, 1950.

8. Cullen, T. S. Adeno-myoma of the round ligament. *Bull. Johns Hopkins Hosp.* 7:112, 1896.

9. Cullen, T. S. Discussion: Symposium on misplaced endometrial tissue. *Am. J. Obstet. Gynecol.* 10:732, 1925.

10. Cunningham, K., and Smith, K. V. A case of intussusception caused by endometriosis of ileum. *Br. J. Surg.* 36:50, 1948.

11. Davis, C., Alexander, R. W., and Buenger, R. E. Surgery of endometriosis of ileum and colon. *Am. J. Surg.* 105:250, 1963.

12. DeJong, J. Subserose adenomyomatose des dunndarms. *Virchows Arch. [Pathol. Anat. Physiol.]* 211:141, 1913.

13. Gray, L. A. Endometriosis of the bowel: Role of bowel resection, superficial excision and oophorectomy in treatment. *Am. Surg.* 177:380, 1973.

14. Gruenwald, P. Origin of endometriosis from mesenchyme of celomic walls. *Am. J. Obstet. Gynecol.* 44:470, 1942.

15. Hauck, A. E. Endometriosis of the colon. *Ann. Surg.* 151:896, 1960.

16. Henriksen, E. Primary Endometriosis of the urinary bladder: Report of one case. *JAMA* 104:1401, 1935.

17. Henricksen, E. Endometriosis. *Am. J. Surg.* 90:331, 1955.

18. Israel, S. L. *Menstrual Disorders and Sterility.* 5th ed. New York, Hoeber Medical Division, Harper & Row, 1967.

19. Ivanoff, N. S. K Voprosu ob adenomiomakh matki (Thesis). St. Petersburg K 897, 1907.

20. Javert, C. T. Pathogenesis of endometriosis based upon endometrial homeoplasia, direct extension, exfoliation, and implantation: Lymphocytic and hematogenous metastasis (including 5 case reports of endometrial tissue in pelvic lymph nodes). *Cancer* 2:399, 1949.

21. Javert, C. T. Observations on the pathology and spread of endometriosis based on the theory of benign metastasis. *Am. J. Obstet. Gynecol.* 62(3):477, 1951.

22. Jenkinson, E. L., and Brown, W. H. Endometriosis: A study of 117 cases with special reference to constricting lesions of the rectum and sigmoid colon. *JAMA* 122:349, 1943.

23. Jimenz, M., and Miles, R. M. Inguinal endometriosis. *Ann. Surg.* 151:193, 1960.

24. Keene, F. E. Perforating ovarian cysts (Sampson's) with invasion of the bladder wall, report of two cases. *Am. J. Obstet. Gynecol.* 10:619, 1925.

25. Kistner, R. W. Infertility with endometriosis: Plan of therapy. *Fertil. Steril.* 13:237, 1962.

26. Kistner, R. W. *Principles of Gynecology.* Chicago, Year Book, 1964.

27. Macafee, C. H. G., and Greer, H. L. H. Intestinal endometriosis. *J. Obstet. Gynaecol. Br. Commonw.* 67:538, 1960.

28. Mankin, Z. W. Beitrage zur Histogeneses der Endometriome mit Hinweis auf eine besonders selten vorkommende Lokalisation in mittleren Oberschenkeldrittel. *Arch. f. Gynak.* 159:671, 1935.

29. Mankin, Z. W. Beitrage zur histogeneses der Endometriome mit Hinweis auf eine besonders selten vorkommende Lokalisation in mittleren Oberschenkeldrittel. *Arch. f. Gynak.* 159:671, 1935.

30. Marshall, V. F. The occurrence of endometrial tissue in the kidney; case report and discussion. *J. Urol.* 50:652, 1943.

31. McKittrick, L. S. Discussion of Cattell's paper. *N. Engl. J. Med.* 217:16, 1937.

32. Melody, G. F. Endometriosis causing obstruction of the ileum. *Obstet. Gynecol.* 8:468, 1956.

33. Novak, E. Pelvic endometriosis. Spontaneous rupture of endometrial cysts, with a report of three cases. *Am. J. Obstet. Gynecol.* 22:826, 1931.

34. Rio, F. W., Edwards, D. L., Regan, J. F., and Schmutzer, K. J. Endometriosis of the small bowel. *Arch. Surg.* 101:403, 1970.

35. Ripstein, C. B., Rohman, M., and Wallach, J. B. Endometriosis involving the pleura. *J. Thoracic Surg.* 37:464, 1959.

36. Sampson, J. A. Perforating hemorrhagic (chocolate) cysts of the ovary; their importance and especially their relation to pelvic adenomas of endometrial type ("adenomyoma" of the uterus, rectovaginal septum, sigmoid, etc.). *Arch. Surg.* 3:245, 1921.

37. Sampson, J. A. Intestinal adenomas of endometrial type. *Arch. Surg.* 5:217, 1922.

38. Sampson, J. A. The life history of ovarian hematomas (hemorrhagic cysts) of endometrial (Mullerian) type. *Am. J. Obstet. Gynecol.* 4:451, 1922.

39. Sampson, J. A. Ovarian hematomas of endometrial type (perforating hemorrhagic cysts of the ovary) and implantation adenomas of endometrial type. *Boston M. & S. J.* 186:445, 1922.

40. Sampson, J. A. Benign and malignant endometrial implants in the peritoneal cavity and their relation to certain ovarian tumors. *Surg. Gynecol. Obstet.* 38:287, 1924.

41. Sampson, J. A. Endometrial carcinoma of the ovary, arising in endometrial tissue in that organ. *Arch. Surg.* 10:1, 1925.

42. Sampson, J. A. Heterotopic or misplaced endometrial tissue. *Am. J. Obstet. Gynecol.* 10:649, disc. 730–738, 1925.

43. Sampson, J. A. Inguinal endometriosis (often reported as endometrial tissue in groin, adenomyoma in groin and adenomyoma of round ligament). *Am. J. Obstet. Gynecol.* 10:462, 1925.

44. Sampson, J. A. Metastatic or embolic endometriosis, due to menstrual dissemination of endometrial tissue into the venous circulation. *Am. J. Pathol.* 3:93, 1927.

45. Sampson, J. A. Peritoneal endometriosis due to menstrual dissemination of endometrial tissue into the peritoneal cavity. *Am. J. Obstet. Gynecol.* 14:422, 1927.

46. Sampson, J. A. Development of the implantation theory for origin of peritoneal endometriosis. *Am. J. Obstet. Gynecol. 40*:549, 1940.

47. Sampson, J. A. Pathogenesis of postsalpingectomy endometriosis in laparotomy scars. *Am. J. Obstet. Gynecol. 50*:597, 1945.

48. Senapati, M. D. Endometriosis of the appendix. *Br. J. Surg. 4*:330, 1953.

49. von Recklinghausen, F. Ueber die venose Embolic und den regrograden Transport in den Venen und in den Lymphgefassen. *Virchows Arch. [Pathol. Anat.] 100*:503, 1885.

Lawrence R. Shapiro, M.D.

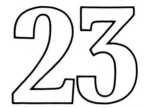

# Disorders of Female Sex Differentiation

This chapter deals with disturbances of female sex differentiation during embryogenesis and the resulting disorders of genetic, gonadal, and phenotypic sex. Because the embryologic details have been discussed in another chapter, they are only briefly reviewed. An understanding of the pathogenesis of abnormal sexual differentiation is essential as a basis of diagnosis and ultimate therapy.

## Normal Sexual Differentiation

The mechanisms of normal sexual differentiation in the mammalian embryo have been divided into three sequential processes, involving the establishment of genetic sex and the ultimate reflection of gonadal sex as phenotypic sex.[77-80]

Genetic sex is determined by the sex chromosome constitution established at the time of fertilization. In the mammal, the heterogametic sex is male (XY) and the homogametic sex is female (XX). The mechanism whereby genetic information determines that an indifferent gonad differentiates either into a testis in the male or an ovary in the female is not clearly understood; however, the translation of gonadal sex into phenotypic sex is a direct result of the type of gonad formed. During the course of sex differentiation, indifferent internal and external genital *anlage* are converted to a male or female form, and the ultimate functional characteristics are determined.[134]

In the absence of the testis, as in the normal female or

male embryos castrated prior to the onset of phenotypic sex differentiation, the development of phenotypic sex proceeds along female lines.[77-80] In order for a fetus to be masculinized, positive action by testicular hormones is required. Development of the female phenotype appears to be a passive process that does not require fetal gonadal hormone action; consequently, normal female phenotype appears to be neutral or "neuter."

Normally, phenotypic sex can be anticipated to conform ultimately to the chromosomal or genetic sex. A disturbance during embryogenesis of any step in the process of translation of genetic sex into gonadal sex and the ultimate determination of phenotypic sex results in a clinical disorder of sexual development.

Classification of disorders of sexual development based on the presumed site of action of abnormal genes during embryogenesis[58,134] has been modified to classify the disorders of female sex differentiation (Table 23.1). These disorders may be either genetic or sporadic in nature and are the result of disturbances in the processes of embryologic sexual differentiation.

The discussion of disorders of female sex differentiation will be divided into abnormal genetic sex differentiation, abnormal gonadal sex differentiation, and abnormal phenotypic sex differentiation (Table 23.1).

# Abnormal Genetic Sex Differentiation

## Monogenic Sex Disorders

At present no monogenic or single-gene disorders of genetic sex have been described or documented in man. The human syndromes that result from abnormalities in genetic sex appear to originate from sporadic chromosome aberrations resulting from either meiotic or mitotic aberrations involving the X and Y chromosomes or sex chromosome mosaicisms. Forms of gonadal dysgenesis in phenotypic females associated with an XX or XY sex chromosome constitution have been described and recessive inheritance has been suggested.[116,117] These forms of gonadal dysgenesis are discussed in greater detail in a following section.

## Cytogenetics and Sex Chromosome Disorders

The chromosomes contain the units of heredity, the genes, and they are responsible for transmitting genetic information from generation to generation. The chromo-

**Table 23.1** Classification of disorders of female sex differentiation

I. Abnormal genetic sex differentiation
   A. Monogenic—no disorders yet identified
   B. Sex chromosome abnormalities

II. Abnormal gonadal sex differentiation
   A. True hermaphroditism
   B. Gonadal dysgenesis

III. Abnormal phenotypic sex differentiation
   A. Male pseudohermaphroditism
   B. Female pseudohermaphroditism
   C. Defects of Wolffian–Müllerian duct development

somes are the organs of heredity or, more precisely, the organelles of heredity.[63]

As recently as 1956, our knowledge of human chromosomes and cytogenetics was minimal. As a result of technical advances at that time, the normal human chromosome number was reported and confirmed as being 46; prior to 1956, the normal human chromosome number was incorrectly thought to be 48.[48,128] As a result of these technical advances made in 1956, more information has been accumulated about human genetics and chromosome behavior than about the chromosomes of any organism, with the possible exception of *Drosophila* and some plant varieties.[63] In 1959, the first known human chromosome abnormality was described (trisomy 21),[87] and a case of a 45X female who had gonadal dysgenesis and Turner's stigmata was also reported.[49] These technical advances have enabled the study of human chromosomes during cell division and, more specifically, during the metaphase of mitosis. Photographs of human metaphase chromosomes (Figure 23.1) are utilized to construct karyotypes, and an assessment of an individual's cytogenetic constitution can be undertaken. The normal human karyotype has 46 chromosomes, with the 23 homologous pairs including 22 autosomes and a pair of sex chromosomes (Figure 23.2). With the advent of such differential staining techniques as fluorescence (Q bands) or the denaturation techniques (C bands and G bands), the study of human chromosomes has become more highly refined (Figure 23.3). Definite parameters for karyotypic analysis have been established,[11,12] and these include morphologic criteria as well as reproducible banding patterns for each chromosome. These banding characteristics enable exact identification of all chromosomes including the X and Y chromosomes. Prior to the advent of the banding techniques, it was not always possible to separate the X chromosome from the C group (6–12) and the Y chromosome was often difficult

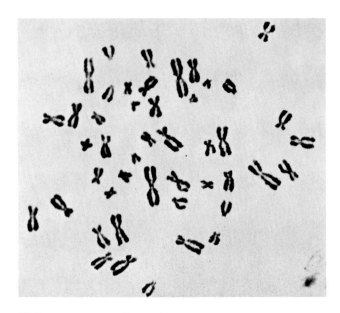

**23.1** Human metaphase chromosomes. ×1300.

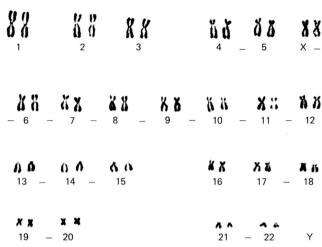

**23.2** Standard normal human female karyotype (46XX).

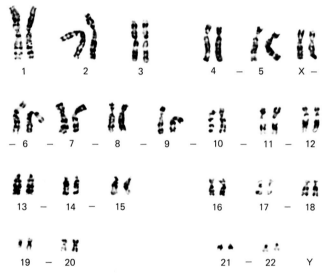

**23.3** Giemsa banded (G bands) normal human female karyotype (46XX). These chromosomes can be specifically identified and classified according to the Paris Conference.[12]

to distinguish from the number 21 and 22 chromosomes. In addition, it is now sometimes possible to detect small structural deletions or additions of chromosomal material with the use of the banding techniques.

In order to understand the underlying mechanisms of sex chromosome abnormalities, it is necessary to briefly review normal cellular mechanisms. The process of nuclear division in the somatic cells of the body is known as mitosis. The growth and repair of somatic tissues and somatic cells is accomplished by mitosis, and this involves equal division of the chromosomes in the nucleus followed by a division of the cell into two daughter cells (Figure 23.4). Mitosis is divided into a number of stages: interphase, prophase, metaphase, anaphase, and telophase. Although each of these stages can be clearly delineated, there is no specific dividing line between any of them. Mitosis is a continuous process and each step flows smoothly into the next. In the embryo, mitosis provides the normal means of growth and development. In an adult organism, when growth is complete, mitosis is most easily detected in those tissues with a high rate of cellular growth, such as bone marrow and peripheral blood. It is for this reason that peripheral blood is an excellent source for the study of human chromosomes. *In vitro,* human mitosis can be arrested during metaphase by a variety of mitotic arresting agents (colchicine, colcemid, and vinblastine), and it is during the metaphase state that cytogenetic studies are culminated (Figure 23.1).

Mitosis involves the replication of the genetic material, followed by the longitudinal division of the chromosome

into chromatids and the subsequent precise distribution of the chromatids to the two daughter cells, ensuring that each daughter cell has an identical genome. In this fashion, exact linear transmission of genetic material is accomplished from cell to cell and organism to organism.

Meiosis is that form of cellular division which occurs only in the germ cells and results in the formation of the gametes. Because it is the means by which the haploid gametes are formed, it is actually a reduction division (Figures 23.5 and 23.6). During the first meiotic division

**23.4** Schematic representation of normal mitosis. Stage I: A normal female zygote or cell containing 44 autosomes and an XX sex chromosome constitution (46XX). Stage II: Replication of each chromosome. Each chromosome is exactly duplicated and the two chromatids are connected by the centromere, which is represented by a solid dot. Stage III: Division of the centromere occurs, with disjunction (separation) of the chromatids resulting in equal diploid chromosome complements in each of two daughter cells identical to each other and to the cell of origin.

**23.5** Schematic representation of normal meiosis in the male (spermatogenesis). Stage I: One male germ cell containing 44 autosomes and an XY sex chromosome constitution (46XY). Stage II: Replication of each chromosome. Each chromosome is exactly duplicated and the two chromatids are connected by the centromere, which is represented by a solid dot. Stage III: First meiotic division. This is a reduction division in which the chromosome pairs separate but the centromeres do not divide. Stage IV: Second meiotic division. The centromeres divide, with disjunction (separation) of the chromatids resulting in four equal but not identical haploid gametes.

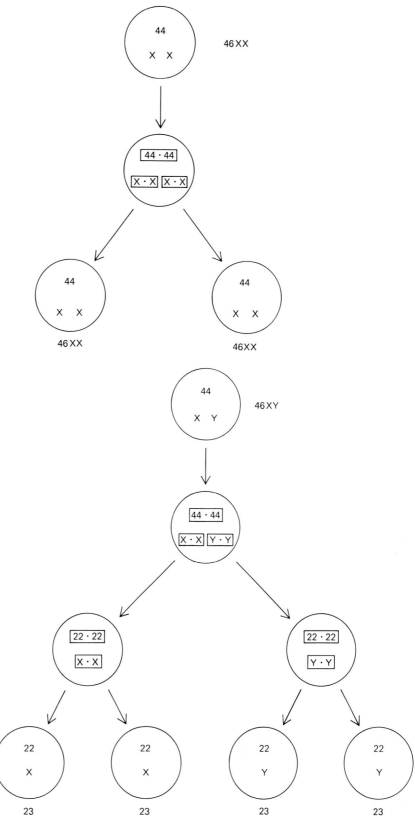

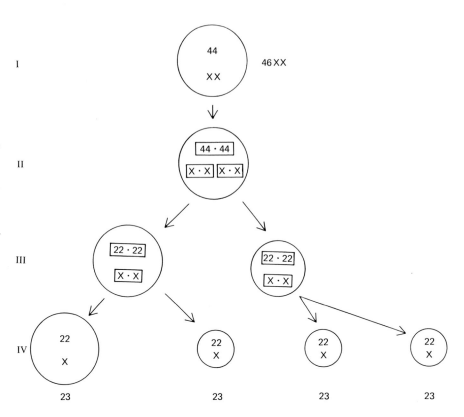

**23.6** Schematic representation of normal meiosis in the female (oogenesis). Stages I and II are identical to male meiosis (see Figure 23.5). Stage III: First meiotic division. This stage is similar to male meiosis except that a polar body is formed. A polar body has the same nuclear/chromosome complement but much less cytoplasm and is represented as being small in size. Stage IV: Second meiotic division. This is again similar to male meiosis except that three polar bodies result and they do not compete with the single gamete (egg) that is formed.

each chromosome reduplicates itself and the two chromatids remain attached at the centromere. In the first meiotic division the homologous chromosome pairs separate, but the chromatids remain intact. In the second meiotic division the centromeres divide, with separation of the chromatids giving rise to the formation of four equal but not identical gametes, each containing the haploid chromosome number (Figure 23.5). Meiosis in the female (oögenesis) gives rise to a polar body as a result of the first meiotic divison. The polar body has the same chromosome complement but much less cytoplasm than the actual gamete (ovum). Consequently, after the second meiotic division only one gamete (ovum) is formed, and three of the cells are polar bodies that do not compete with the resultant single ova (Figure 23.6).

Separation of the paired chromosome members during meiosis or of sister chromatids during mitosis or meiosis is known as disjunction. An error in the separation of the paired chromosome members or sister chromatid is known as nondisjunction. Meiotic nondisjunction can result in gametes lacking an autosome or sex chromosome (Figure 23.7), or in gametes with an extra autosome or sex chromosome (Figure 23.8). When gametes produced by meiotic nondisjunction are fertilized by normal gametes with

23 chromosomes, zygotes with either 45 or 47 chromosomes are formed.

Meiotic nondisjunction is a prefertilization event, but nondisjunction during mitosis (Figure 23.9) is a postfertilization event. Mitotic nondisjunction produces a variety of stem cells with different chromosome numbers. An organism with two or more types of stem cells or stem lines is termed a mosaic. A mosaic has cells with different karyotypes but of one genetic origin. If mitotic nondisjunction occurs during the first cell division of the zygote, two stem lines are simultaneously created (Figure 23.9); however, three stem lines can be produced by mitotic nondisjunction at a step beyond the first division of the zygote (Figure 23.10).

Another error of mitosis is the production of mosaicism by anaphase lag (Figure 23.11). Mitotic anaphase lag occurs after normal replication of the chromosomes, and one of the chromosomes fails to be incorporated into the one of the two daughter cells. This results in the creation of a hypodiploid stem and a normal stem line (Figure 23.11). Anaphase lag is a particularly significant mechanism with regard to the production of sex chromosome aberrations.

Sex chromosome mosaicism is important because the

**23.7** Meiotic nondisjunction in the female. A gamete with 22 instead of 23 chromosomes (missing an X) results when the X chromosomes fail to separate (nondisjoin) during the second meiotic division (IV) and both X chromosomes enter the polar body.

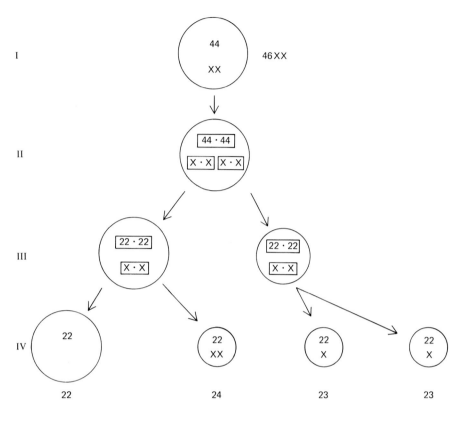

**23.8** Meiotic nondisjunction in the female. A gamete with 24 instead of 23 chromosomes (an extra X) results when the X chromosomes fail to separate (nondisjoin) during the second meiotic division (IV) and both X chromosomes enter the gamete.

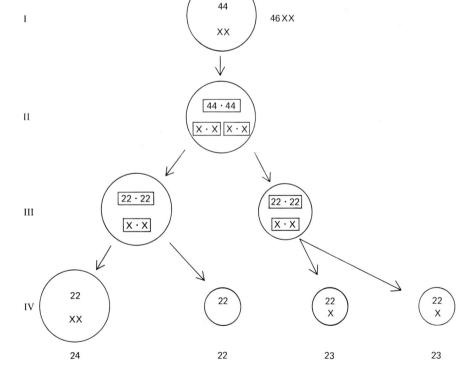

**23.9** Mitotic nondisjunction. Following normal replication of the chromosomes (II), the chromosomes do not divide normally and a two-cell-line mosaicism results (45X/47XXX).

**23.10** Mitotic nondisjunction. The type of mosaicism and the number of resultant cell lines depends on the timing of this mitotic error. If the nondisjunction occurs after at least one normal cell division, three cell lines are formed. The three cell lines include one normal line and two lines resulting from the same mechanism as represented in Figure 23.9.

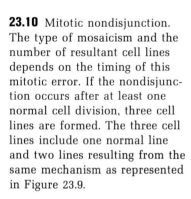

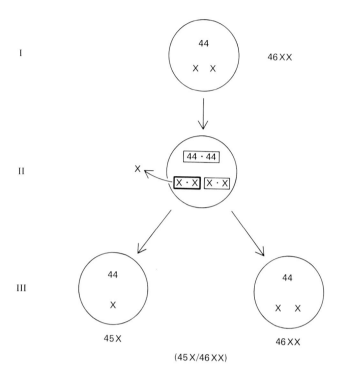

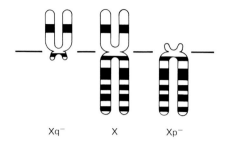

**23.12** X chromosome deletion. This loss of X chromosome material can involve either the short or the long arm. The X chromosomes are schematically represented with G bands according to the Paris Conference.[12] Xp − represents a short-arm deletion and Xq − a long-arm deletion (p = short arm; q = long arm).

**23.11** Mitotic anaphase lag. Following normal chromosomal replication in the zygote, one of the X chromosomes is lost when it is not incorporated into one of the two daughter cells. A two-cell-line mosaicism results and is represented as a 45X/46XX mosaicism.

potential variations of the mosaicism are unlimited. The mechanism producing the mosaicism may originate at a time that results in at least three stem lines. These lines may survive unequally in the organism as a whole or in different tissues. As a result, the expression of the various stem lines may be variable. In addition, because of the timing of the origin of the mosaicism, it is possible that sampling of any one tissue for chromosome analysis may not detect a significant mosaicism. The significance and examples of sex chromosome mosaicism are discussed at a later point in this chapter.

Structural anomalies of chromosomes, in particular the sex chromosomes, are also related to the pathogenesis of abnormal sexual differentiation. If one of the X chromosomes sustains a break with subsequent loss of chromosomal material, the loss of genetic material (deletion) may be detectable, especially with the use of banded chromosomes/karyotypes (Figure 23.12). The deletion of genetic material from an X chromosome may result in a clinical picture of abnormal sex differentiation. Another significant structural alteration of the X chromosome is the isochromosome. The isochromosome is considered to be the result of a misdivision of the centromere in meiosis or

mitosis. Transverse division, instead of the usual longitudinal division of the centromere, results in the formation of an unstable chromosome that may be subsequently converted to an isochromosome[63] (Figure 23.13). The transverse misdivision of the centromere of an X chromosome results in the formation of an X isochromosome composed of either two long or two short arms plus a chromosomal fragment that lacks a centromere and is known as an acentric fragment. The acentric fragment is unable to attach to the mitotic spindle and is lost. The result, in succeeding metaphases, is an X chromosome with two identical arms from the original X chromosome, and the acentric material is lost (Figure 23.13). Isochromosomes of both the long and short arms of the X chromosome are known (Figure 23.14) and are discussed in greater detail subsequently.

## Sex Chromatin

In 1949, Barr and Bertram reported a clump of chromatin visible in the nuclei of female cells but absent from those of males.[7] This mass of heteropyknotic or darkly staining material is known as the sex chromatin mass or the Barr body. The sex chromatin mass represents most or all of the second X chromosome of a female cell. If an individual has two X chromosomes, one of these is condensed into a form that is biochemically inert and this inactive chromosome forms the sex chromatin mass.[37,63] The buccal smear for sex chromatin determination is well established as a simple and inexpensive means for determining the number of X chromosomes present in a patient.[63,97] The number of X chromosomes minus one is the number of sex chromatin masses (Barr bodies) that is found.[95] Although the normal values for sex chromatin analysis of buccal mucosal cells may vary from laboratory

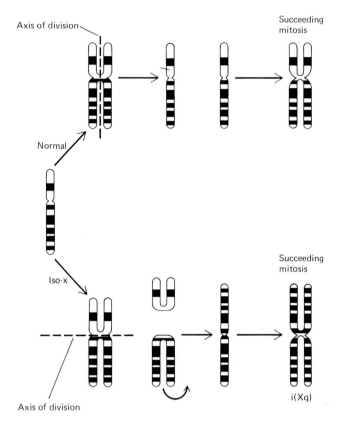

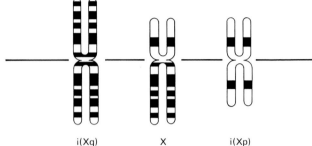

**23.14** Schematic representation of G banded X chromosomes according to the Paris Conference.[12] The normal X chromosome is between a long-arm X isochromosome [i(Xq)] and a short-arm X isochromosome [i(Xp)].

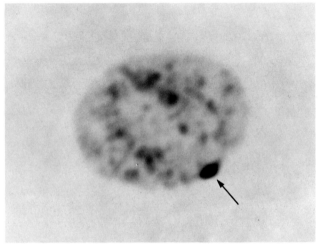

**23.15** A chromatin-positive nucleus from a buccal mucosal cell. The arrow indicates the sex chromatin mass (Barr body) at the nuclear membrane.

**23.13** Mechanism of isochromosome formation. The X chromosome is schematically represented with G bands according to the Paris Conference.[12] Normally the axis of division of the centromere is longitudinal, giving rise to two equal chromatids. In succeeding mitoses, the chromosome replicates and the process is repeated. In the formation of an isochromosome, the axis of division of the centromere is transverse. The short arms in a long-arm isochromosome [i(Xq)] do not contain the centromere (acentric) and are lost in the course of division. The long arms, containing the centromere, form a new chromosome with arms of equal lengths. In succeeding mitoses, the isochromosome replicates and is perpetuated.

to laboratory, a normal female (46XX) usually has one sex chromatin mass at the periphery of the nucleus in 20–35% of the buccal mucosal cells examined (Figure 23.15). A normal male (46XY) will be chromatin negative and have no sex chromatin mass. It is important that the sex chromatin analysis include the result as a percentage of positive and not just as positive or negative. A female who has significantly less than 20% chromatin-positive cells may be an example of mosaicism and have two cell lines, one of which contains only one X chromosome (45X/46XX).[95] The size of the sex chromatin body may also yield important information. Patients with long-arm X isochromosomes may have abnormally large sex chromatin bodies (Figure 23.16), and patients with partially deleted X chromosomes or short-arm X isochromosomes may have unusually small sex chromatin bodies.[41,63,74]

When a phenotypic female has two sex chromatin bodies, she must have three X chromosomes (47XXX), and when she has three sex chromatin masses she must have four X chromosomes (48XXXX) (Figure 23.17). Sex chromatin analysis may contribute significantly to the diagnosis and elucidation of any condition associated with

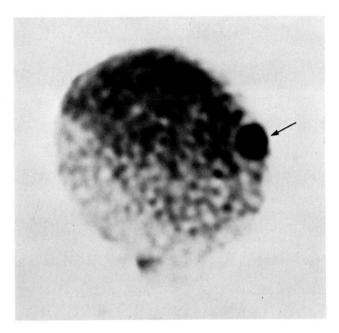

**23.16** A chromatin-positive nucleus from a buccal mucosal cell but the sex chromatin mass (indicated by the arrow) is markedly enlarged and represents a long-arm X isochromosome [i(Xq)].

[Courtesy of Patrick Wilmot, Ph.D.]

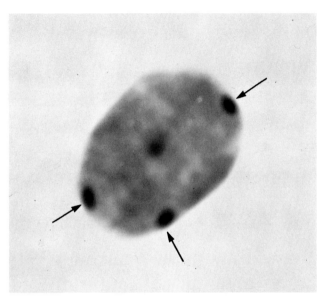

**23.17** A nucleus from a buccal mucosal cell with three sex chromatin masses (indicated by arrows) from a 48XXXX individual.

abnormal or ambiguous genitalia or abnormal sexual development.

The analysis of a buccal smear in the first 3 to 4 days of life can be quite difficult because a reduction in the percentage of sex chromatin bodies in the oral mucosal cells of newborn females has been observed.[52,71,122,127] It has been suggested that this decreased frequency of sex chromatin is an artifact and can be overcome by employing strict selection criteria for those nuclei which are examined and analyzed.[71]

## Sex Chromosome Abnormalities

Poly-X females (47XXX;48XXXX;49XXXXX) have been described but do not exhibit any gross deviation from the normal female phenotype.[100] Most affected individuals have regular menstrual cycles and normal physical development, although some cases have been reported with secondary amenorrhea and poorly developed secondary sexual characteristics.[100] Mental retardation is more frequent among poly-X females and it appears that the greater the number of excess X chromosomes the greater the degree of mental retardation, although exceptions have been noted.[13]

X chromosome monosomy (45X), mosaicism for X chromosome monosomy, and structural abnormalities of the X chromosome are discussed in detail under abnormal gonadal sex differentiation.

# Abnormal Gonadal Sex Differentiation

## True Hermaphroditism

True hermaphroditism refers to the presence of both ovarian and testicular tissue.[37,61,107] Internal and external differentiation may vary widely from almost normal female to male with some degree of hypospadias. Most true hermaphrodites are raised as males, but most have been found to be chromatin positive with a 46XX cytogenetic constitution.[37,107] In some cases of true hermaphroditism, testes may be found on one side and an ovary on the contralateral side, and in other cases the ovarian and testicular tissue are combined as an ovotestis (Figure 23.18). The gonads are usually found in the abdomen but can be anywhere along the tract of testicular descent, including a scrotum. A uterus is almost always present and the internal

**23.18** Ovotestis. Left arrow points to testicular tubular tissue. Right arrow points to an ovarian follicle.

[Courtesy of Dr. M. Melicow and reprinted by permission from A. Blaustein, R. Scully, B. Bigelow, R. Demopoulos, and F. Gorstein, *Audiovisual Seminars in Gynecologic Pathology. Pathology of the Ovary,* W. B. Saunders, 1974.]

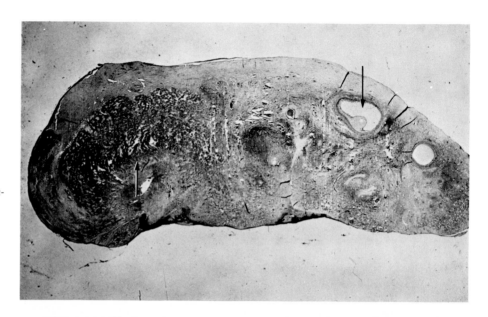

**23.19** True hermaphroditism. The following specimens were removed at surgery: uterus (U); testes (T); ovotestis (OT); and ovary (O).

[Courtesy of Dr. M. Melicow.]

ductal development usually corresponds with that of the adjacent gonad (Figure 23.19).[37,107]

At least 75% of true hermaphrodites are raised as males and hypospadias is almost always present in those patients raised as males.[107] The hypospadias found in true hermaphroditism is usually associated with complete or par-tial failure of fusion of the labioscrotal folds. Cryptorchidism and inguinal hernia are common findings in true hermaphrodites (Figure 23.20), and on close examination a great majority of true hermaphrodites have ambiguous genitalia.[37,61,107]

Although a few cases of true hermaphroditism have

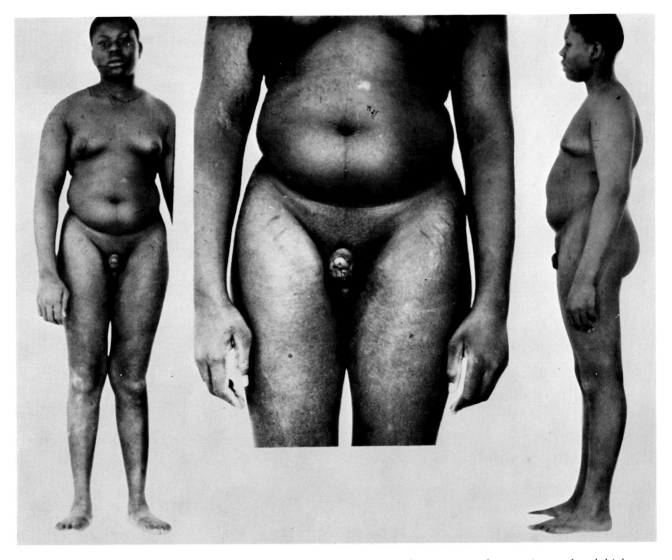

**23.20** True hermaphroditism. Note the prominent breasts, incomplete labial folds, and penis resembling an enlarged clitoris.

[Courtesy of Dr. M. Melicow and reprinted by permission from A. Blaustein, R. Scully, B. Bigelow, R. Demopoulos, and F. Gorstein, *Audiovisual Seminars in Gynecologic Pathology. Pathology of the Ovary,* W. B. Saunders, 1974.]

been reported with a 46XY karyotype, over 80% of true hermaphrodites are chromatin positive and about half have a nonmosaic 46XX karyotype. The remainder are chromosomal mosaics having an XX cell line.[107] The origin of testicular tissue in the absence of a Y chromosome is not clearly understood. It has been postulated that a Y-containing cell line may have been present but not detected, or that one of the X chromosomes of the 46XX true hermaphrodite may contain Y chromosomal testicular

differentiation genes that have been translocated by interchange between the X and Y chromosome.[39,107] Several 46XX/46XY patients have been shown to be chimeras who probably resulted from double fertilization.[107]

A familial form of true hermaphroditism has been reported in which the affected individuals characteristically have a 46XX karyotype but the gonads contain a mixture of testicular and ovarian tissue. A number of pedigrees

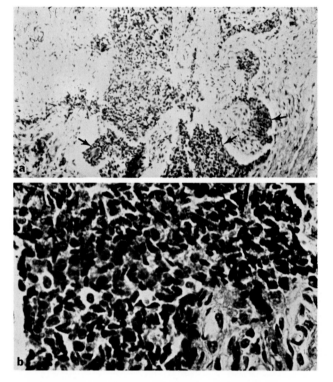

**23.21 a.** Streaks of theca interna tissue (arrows).
**b.** High-power view of **a**.

[Reprinted by permission from A. Blaustein, R. Scully,
B. Bigelow, R. Demopoulos, and F. Gorstein, *Audiovisual
Seminars in Gynecologic Pathology. Pathology of the Ovary,*
W. B. Saunders, 1974.]

have been reported in which multiple siblings have been affected, suggesting that this form of true hermaphrodism may be inherited in an autosomal recessive fashion.[10,23,94,108] In view of the diverse forms of true hermaphroditism, the etiology can be associated with both chromosomal aberrations and single-gene defects.[103]

A diagnosis of true hermaphroditism can be made only by the anatomic demonstration of both ovarian and testicular tissue. Sex assignment of these patients is best determined by their external genitalia.

## Gonadal Dysgenesis

Gonadal dysgenesis is characterized by replacement of the gonads by streaks of connective tissue containing no germ cells (Figure 23.21). Gonadal dysgenesis is usually associated with monosomy for the X chromosome (45X) or structural rearrangements of the X chromosome, but the abnormality may also be associated with normal male

(46XY) or female (46XX) sex chromosome constitutions.[107,116] When gonadal dysgenesis is also associated with short stature and other somatic abnormalities, Turner's syndrome is said to be present. In 1938, Turner described seven girls with sexual infantilism, short stature, and skeletal abnormalities.[129] In 1959, a case of a 45X female who had gonadal dysgenesis and Turner stigmata was reported.[49] Subsequently, other X chromosome complements associated with gonadal dysgenesis and Turner's stigmata were described and included structural rearrangements of the X chromosome, autosomal rearrangements, various types of mosaicism, and even normal male (46XY) or female (46XX) complements.

The terms "gonadal dysgenesis" and "Turner's syndrome" are often used interchangeably, but this may cause troublesome confusion. It has been suggested that the term "gonadal dysgenesis" be applied to any individual with streak gonads and the term "Turner's syndrome" be reserved only for those individuals with streak gonads, short stature, and other somatic anomalies.[116]

It has been shown that 22 pairs of normal autosomes and at least one normal X chromosome is essential for survival of the zygote. When the second sex chromosome is abnormal, gonadal dysgenesis or one of its variants results.[38] The abnormalities of the second sex chromosome can be characterized as being absent (monosomy) or structurally abnormal, or a combination of these factors may exist in some of the cells of the individual when that person is a mosaic.

## Gonadal Dysgenesis—45X (X-Chromosome Monosomy)

45X (X-chromosome monosomy) is the sex chromosome constitution most frequently associated with gonadal dysgenesis. The occurrence of the 45X complement is sporadic and, unlike other chromosome abnormalities, maternal age is not increased in the families of patients with 45X chromosome constitution.[37,107] The estimated incidence of 45X is wide ranging because both sex chromatin surveys and chromosome analyses of consecutive newborn populations have been employed. A reasonable estimate of the incidence of 45X seems to be 1/3,000 to 1/5,000 phenotypic female live births.[61,63,69,93]

Monosomy X can originate during oogenesis, during spermatogenesis, or as a postfertilization event. Studies in 45X individuals and their parents utilizing Xg blood groups have indicated that the loss of the paternal X chromosome is more common than the loss of the maternal X chromosome.[90,105,109] Although nonmosaic

X monosomy (45X) can be readily explained by either meiotic anaphase lag or meiotic nondisjunction, there are no direct data to substantiate that these are the causal mechanisms. If monosomy X arose as a result of a meiotic error during spermatogenesis, it would be necessary for a spermatoza nullisomic for a sex chromosome to fertilize a 23X gamete in order to have a resulting 45X zygote. This mechanism is theoretically possible but has not been proved. The high prevalence of mosaicism combined with the increased frequency of monozygotic twinning in siblings of 45X patients indicates that the abnormality giving rise to 45X is probably a postfertilization event related to cleavage and cell division of the zygote.[37,82,99] In most cases of mosaicism, the abnormal 45X cell line results from nondisjunction or anaphase lag in the zygote. Nonmosaic 45X individuals may also arise as a result of mitotic nondisjunction, and it has been postulated that a single event, such as chromosomal breakage, can produce both a structurally rearranged chromosome and an acentric fragment. If the acentric fragment is lost, a monosomic cell results.[57] If following the chromosome breakage only the 45X cell line survives, this may explain a nonmosaic 45X individual arising in the zygote as a result of a postfertilization event. The increased association of twinning with monosomy X[82,99] is an additional indication that 45X individuals may arise following fertilization.

A 45X karyotype has been found in approximately 5% of all spontaneous abortions and none of those has been found to be mosaic.[18,19] Based on this information, it has been estimated that nonmosaic 45X embryos come to term in only 2% of the cases and that 98% of 45X fetuses are spontaneously aborted during the first trimester.[69] Consequently, 45X is a potentially lethal chromosome constitution and an affected fetus is much more likely to survive if mosaicism is present.[69] The high frequency of mosaicism in patients found with 45X may readily explain the survival of these individuals.

Streak gonads appear identical histologically, regardless of the nature of the sex chromosome constitution of the affected individual.[42,75,116] In adults with gonadal dysgenesis, the gonads appear to be white fibrous streaks 2–3 cm long and about 0.5 cm wide.[116] The fibrous streaks are characterized by sheets and whorls of fibrous tissue and no germ cells are present. At the attachment of the streak gonad to the fallopian tubes, hilar cell and mesonephric remnants may persist.[107] Recent studies on the ovaries of 45X embryos have reported the presence of follicles that regress after several months of gestation.[119,120] By the time of birth the follicles are usually absent, but some 45X infants may have streak gonads containing degenerative germ cells. The germ cells completely disappear by the time of puberty. The 45X teenager has streak gonads that are not functional and are devoid of germ cells; however, her external genitalia, vagina, and uterus are normal, although infantile. Evidence of hypoestrinism is present in the 45X teenager, and there is no cornification of the vaginal epithelium and secondary sexual development usually does not occur. There is a sparsity of axillary and pubic hair and urinary estrogen excretion is reduced, whereas gonadotropin concentration is elevated.[107]

The Turner stigmata or Turner's syndrome is more frequently associated with 45X than with any other sex chromosome complement. The somatic anomalies that comprise Turner's syndrome form a characteristic clinical spectrum[35,37,62,64,88,100,116] (Table 23.2). None of these characteristics is pathognomonic or diagnostic nor do all of the characteristics occur in every patient. There is extensive phenotypic variability in 45X patients; however, the one finding that is not variable is significant shortness of stature.[40] Birth weight is frequently at or below the third percentile, whereas adult height usually ranges from 50 to 60 inches and is related somewhat to parental height.[21,88] It has been shown that the shortness of stature is not secondary to growth hormone deficiency,[31,50] although the growth retardation may be caused by a selective resistance of the skeleton to growth hormone.[28,132] An additional consideration as to the basis of the consistent growth retardation and shortness of stature may be that 45X cells tend to be less viable and do not survive in large numbers; consequently, there may be fewer cells in the 45X individual, resulting in shortness of stature. Although this is an intriguing consideration, there are no specific data to substantiate it.

In addition to the shortness of stature (Figure 23.22), individuals with Turner's syndrome have facies that are triangular in shape with a small chin (Figure 23.23), persistent epicanthal folds, and frequent ptosis. The ears tend to be prominent and occasionally abnormally shaped and the palate tends to be high arched and narrow. There is an increased incidence of otitis media and this may be related to the palatal anomalies.[107] The sclera generally have a bluish tint and strabismus is a frequent finding. The neck is short and broad (Figure 23.24) and as many as 46 to 50% of 45X patients have webbing of the neck (pterygium coli).[37,64,100,107,116] In infancy, the webbing may appear as loose redundant folds of skin around the neck,[115] but with growth the skin folds eventually become taut. The degree of webbing is variable. Individuals with Turner's syndrome have a low posterior hairline that ranges from heavy hair growth down to the first thoracic

433

**Table 23.2**  Partial list of somatic features of 45X (Turner's syndrome)[a]

*Growth*
  Decreased birth weight
  Decreased adult height (mean 141 ± 0.62 cm)

*Intellectual function*
  Verbal IQ greater than performance IQ
  Cognitive deficits (space–form–blindness)
  Immature personality (possibly secondary to short stature)

*Craniofacial*
  Premature fusion sphenoccipital and other sutures, producing brachycephaly
  Abnormal pinnae
  Retruded mandible
  Epicanthal folds (25%)
  High-arched palate (36%)
  Abnormal dentition
  Visual anomalies, usually strabismus (22%)
  Auditory deficits: sensorineutral or secondary to middle ear infections

*Neck*
  Pterygium coli (46%)
  Short, broad neck (74%)
  Low nuchal hair line (71%)

*Chest*
  Rectangular contour (shield chest) (53%)
  Apparent widely spaced nipples
  Tapered lateral ends of clavicle

*Cardiovascular*
  Aorta coarctation or ventricular septal defect (10–16%)

*Renal (38%)*
  Horseshoe kidneys
  Unilateral renal aplasia
  Duplication ureters

*Gastrointestinal*
  Telangiectasias

*Skin and Lymphatics*
  Pigmented nevi (63%)
  Lymphedema (38%) caused by hypoplasia in superficial vessels

*Nails*
  Hypoplasia or malformation (66%)

*Skeletal*
  Cubitus valgus (54%)
  Radial tilt of articular surface of trochlear
  Clinodactyly V
  Short metacarpals, usually IV (48%)
  Decreased carpal arch (mean angle 117%)
  Deformities of medial tibial condyle

[a] Modified from Simpson (Ref. 116).

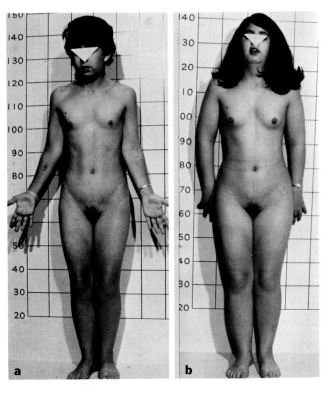

**23.22 a.** A 14-year-old girl with 45X Turner syndrome prior to therapy. Note lack of secondary sexual development and cubitus valgus. **b.** Same patient as in **a**, 1 year after cyclic estrogen–progesterone therapy. Note female fat distribution and breast development.

[Reprinted by permission from David L. Rimoin and R. Neil Schimke, *Genetic Disorders of the Endocrine Glands*, C. V. Mosby, 1971.]

vertebra (Figure 23.25) to a slightly lower hairline that ends in a trident (three points).[107] In 53 to 75% of 45X patients, the chest is broad and shieldlike, with widely spaced and often inverted nipples.[107,116] Multiple pigmented nevi are found in approximately 50 to 63% of the patients.[107,116] Lymphedema of the hands and feet at birth is an important presenting sign of Turner's syndrome and may be the only clue to its presence in the newborn period.[9,59,130] This lymphedema is apparently a result of hypoplasia of the superficial lymphatic channels.[9] The lymphedema usually regresses in infancy but may persist as fullness of the dorsum of the fingers and toes. Individuals with Turner's syndrome have fingernails that are hypoplastic, hyperconvex, and deep set at the base. The fifth finger is usually short and has clinodactyly.[107,116] The fourth and often the fifth metacarpals are short, producing a dimpled knuckle and a metacarpal sign. Other skeletal abnormalities have also been described.[3,45,83,84,85,116] Although

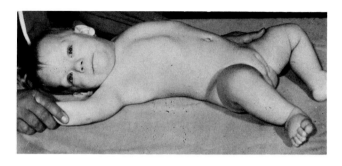

**23.23** Infant with 45X Turner syndrome. Note the peculiar facies and mild congenital lymphedema.

[Reprinted by permission from David L. Rimoin and R. Neil Schimke, *Genetic Disorders of the Endocrine Glands*, C. V. Mosby, 1971.]

cubitus valgus was described in all of Turner's original patients,[129] it has subsequently been found in approximately 54 to 60% of 45X patients.[107,116]

Kidney abnormalities, often asymptomatic and diagnosed only by x ray, occur in about 38 to 50% of patients with 45X.[27,33,106,116] The renal malformations range from unilateral renal agenesis to horseshoe kidneys, duplicated renal pelvis, bifid collecting system, or simple positional or rotational anomalies. The renal anomalies may be related to recurrent episodes of urinary tract infection, leading ultimately to chronic pyelonephritis and renal failure.[107] Approximately 10 to 16% of 45X patients have congenital heart disease, primarily coarctation of the aorta or ventricular septal defect. A group of less frequent abnormalities is associated with Turner's syndrome and

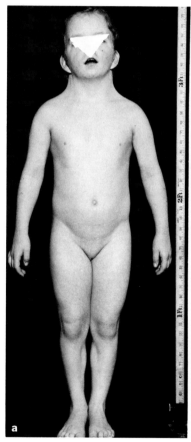
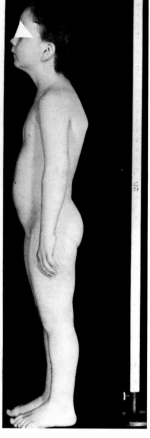
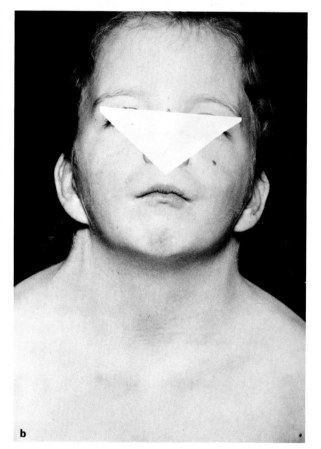

**23.24 a.** A 9-year-old girl with a 45X chromosome constitution and the classic features of the Turner syndrome. Note the short stature, shield chest with widely spaced nipples, webbed neck, and low-set ears. The profile view shows retrognathism. **b.** Close-up view of the 45X patient shown in **a**. Note the hairline extending down the ridge of the pterygium colli.

[Reprinted by permission from L. R. Neu and L. I. Gardner, Abnormalities of the sex chromosomes, in *Endocrine and Genetic Diseases of Childhood*, W. B. Saunders, p. 684, 1969.]

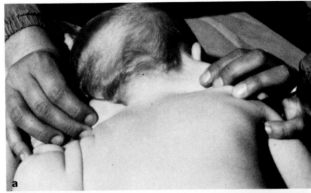

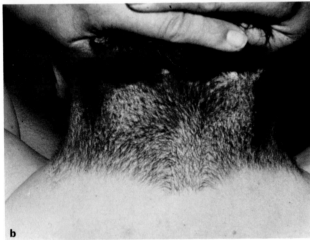

**23.25 a.** Infant with 45X Turner syndrome. Note loose folds of skin around the neck. **b.** 45X Turner syndrome with low, trident hairline.

[Reprinted by permission from David L. Rimoin and R. Neil Schimke, *Genetic Disorders of the Endocrine Glands*, C. V. Mosby, 1971.]

includes hemangiomas of the bowel resulting in upper gastrointestinal bleeding, keloid formation, and pyloric stenosis.[35,62,88]

Mental retardation is not a feature of Turner's syndrome, but cognitive defects may be present, and there is some discrepancy between the verbal and the performance IQ.[1,55,96,114]

Thyroiditis and thyroid autoantibodies have been described in patients with Turner's syndrome and in their mothers.[32,44,133] A prevalence of diabetes mellitus and abnormal glucose tolerance tests have also been described in these patients and their parents.[47]

The complete phenotype of Turner's syndrome is rarely present in any individual patient (Figure 23.26a,b). Undetected mosaicism is probably the cause of a significant part of this phenotypic variation. Clitoral hypertrophy associated with hilar cell hyperplasia has been found in some patients with a presumed 45X constitution. In most of these cases, one cannot discount the presence of a Y-containing cell line because it has not been systematically excluded. In addition, mosaicism (45X/46XX) may well explain those cases of apparent 45X patients who have had menstrual periods[38,40] and the presumed 45X patients who are fertile.[5,98]

## Gonadal Dysgenesis—Mosaicism for Monosomy X with Structurally Normal X Chromosomes

If such postfertilization mitotic errors as nondisjunction or anaphase lag occur, two or more cell lines may result and the affected individual is a mosaic. The exact chromosome constitution depends on the stage at which abnormal cell division occurs and on whether or not subsequent stem cells survive. The possibility that monosomic or normal cells may go undetected makes a phenotypic-karyotypic correlation extremely difficult.

The detection of mosaicism depends on the number of cells analyzed per tissue and the number of tissues analyzed. It has been calculated that the analysis of 50 cells without detection of at least one cell representing a minor cell line excludes any population of cells comprising at least 10% of all cells in the tissue studied.[116] If mitotic nondisjunction were to occur at an early stage in embryogenesis, analysis of a single tissue with random cell selection would probably be satisfactory; however, if a monosomy X cell line originated from nondisjunction or anaphase lag in an older embryo, it might pass undetected if only peripheral lymphocytes were studied. Another factor to be considered is that 45X/46XY mosaicism has been found to be present in lymphocytes but not in skin fibroblasts of some affected individuals.[43] In addition, although analysis of gonadal tissues should theoretically detect additional cases of mosaicisms this has not been borne out by actual experience.[116,117] It therefore appears that the most effective way to exclude or detect a mosaicism is to analyze at least 50 cells per tissue from each individual patient.

### 45X/46XX mosaic

These individuals have been found to have fewer anomalies than those with pure 45X. Patients with 45X/46XX have a higher percentage of menstruation and

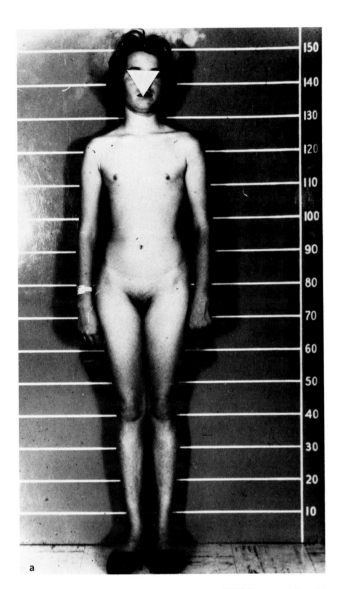
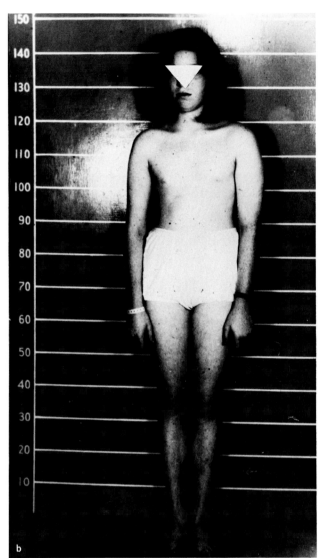

**23.26 a** and **b.** XX pure gonadal dysgenesis in two sisters. Both are infantile and amenorrheic; none has the somatic abnormalities of the Turner syndrome.

[Reprinted by permission from David L. Rimoin and R. Neil Schimke, *Genetic Disorders of the Endocrine Glands,* C. V. Mosby, 1971, and by courtesy of Dr. J. L. Simpson.]

a greater incidence of breast development; mean adult height is greater in mosaic than in nonmosaic patients. In addition, most of the somatic anomalies described in Turner's syndrome were less prevalent in 45X/46XX patients.[116]

### 45X/47XXX mosaic

This mosaic is less common than the 45X/46XX sex chromosome mosaicism.[26,64] Although it is reasonable to anticipate individuals with 45X/47XXX to also have fewer anomalies than those with 45X, it is difficult to make this determination because of the relatively few cases that have been reported.

### 45X/46XX/47XXX mosaic

In these individuals one would also anticipate the somatic abnormalities to occur with less frequency than in 45X; however, because this is a rare sex chromosome mosaicism, the actual phenotypic correlation of this mosaicism cannot be accurately determined. This three-cell-line mosaicism results from mitotic nondisjunction sometime after the first cleavage, with survival of original 46XX parental cells as well as the 45X and 47XXX daughter cells.

### 45X/46XY and 45X/47XYY mosaics

These individuals usually have genital ambiguity. The mixed gonadal dysgenesis phenotype with a unilateral streak gonad and contralateral testis is causally related to these mosaicisms.[29,37] Patients with 45X/46XY and 45X/47XYY mosaicism may also have bilateral streak gonads and associated Turner's stigmata. When this occurs, these patients are not clinically distinguishable from 45X individuals.

Dysgenetic tumors may arise in individuals who have streak gonads and a cell line containing a Y chromosome.[112] The prevalence of tumors in individuals with either 45X/46XY or 45X/47XYY mosaicism appears to be significant.[117] The tumors that arise from the gonads of such individuals are gonadoblastomas and dysgerminomas. Gonadoblastomas tend to be benign but are associated with malignant germ cell tumors,[112] whereas dysgerminomas are more often malignant.[54] Because such tumors may occur even during early childhood, removal of the gonad should be performed as soon after a Y chromosome-containing cell line is detected in an individual with gonadal dysgenesis.[113] In order to properly determine the risk of tumor formation in the gonad of a patient with gonadal dysgenesis, it is imperative that a complete chromosome analysis be undertaken. It is important that sex chromatin analysis not be exclusively utilized in individuals with Turner's stigmata. Sex chromatin analysis enables the detection of a single X chromosome but does not reliably determine the presence of a Y chromosome.

Other mosaic combinations with structurally intact X chromosomes have been reported, but these cases are too rare to adequately correlate their karyotypes and phenotypes.

## Gonadal Dysgenesis—X-Chromosome Structural Aberrations

A deletion of the short arm of the X chromosome [Xp−[11] or del(Xp)[12]] usually results in gonadal dysgenesis frequently associated with short stature and Turner's stigmata.[116] The morphology of reported Xp− chromosomes has been very similar, and often the proximal portion of the short arm of the X chromosome is all that is remaining (Figure 23.12).

The phenotype associated with Xp− is difficult to assess because of the frequency of associated mosaicism, usually 45X/46XXp−. All nonmosaic individuals are short and have some features of Turner's syndrome. Streak gonads are usually found in Xp− patients, but in some patients the presence of ovarian tissue has been postulated because those patients have menstruated.[116] This can be explained by the presence of a 46XX cell line (46XXp−/46XX) or by gonadal determinants present at several locations on the X short arm which are retained or lost according to the structural abnormality.

As discussed above, a misdivision through the centromere of a chromosome, in a tranverse rather than a longitudinal direction, results in an isochromosome (Figure 23.13). An isochromosome consists of two arms that are structurally identical and contain the same genes. A long-arm X isochromosome [Xqi[11] or i(Xq)[12]] consists of duplication of all the long arm of the X and deficiency of the entire short arm of the X (Figure 23.14). An isochromosome of the long arm of an X [i(Xq)] differs from a deletion of the short arm of an X (Xp−) in that the entire short arm of the X is deleted in an isochromosome and there is a duplication of the long arm (Figures 23.14, 23.27, and 23.28). The i(Xq) chromosome is most often paternal in origin.[109] Because mosaicism is frequently observed with the i(Xq) chromosome, it is probable that the paternal X chromosome undergoes rearrangement during early embryogenesis.[57] An alternative possibility is that the long-arm X isochromosome may arise as a meiotic error with a subsequent 45X line resulting during embryogenesis (mitosis) giving rise to a 45X/46X,i(Xq) mosaicism. All patients with long-arm isochromosome [46X,i(Xq)] have streak gonads, short stature, and Turner's stigmata. Primary amenorrhea and hypoestrinism are also prominent findings.[116]

The complete lack of gonadal development in individuals with i(Xq) contrasts with the findings in those patients with Xp−. It has been suggested that gonadal determinants are present at several different locations on the short arm of the X, including a locus on the portion of the short arm normally retained in Xp− but lost in an i(Xq).[116] An additional factor to be considered is that mosaicism (46XXp−/46XX) may occur more frequently than realized and be related to the less complete involvement in gonadal development with Xp−. It should be observed that duplication of the gonadal determinants on the long arm of the X in i(Xq) does not compensate for

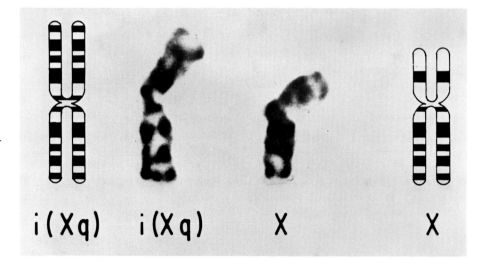

**23.27** A G banded karyotype of an individual with a long-arm X isochromosome (indicated by arrow) but otherwise normal karyotype [46X,i(Xq)].

[Courtesy of Patrick Wilmot, Ph.D.]

**23.28** Partial karyotype from Figure 23.27, comparing the actual G banded chromosomes with schematic counterparts according to the Paris Conference.[12]

the deficiency of the gonadal determinants on the lost X short arm. From the foregoing, it seems reasonable to state that the gonadal determinants on the long and short arms of the X chromosome have different functions and/ or operate by different mechanisms. The range of clinical findings associated with 45X and 46X,i(Xq) are extremely similar; however, the prevalence of thyroid autoantibodies and Hashimoto's thyroiditis is higher in patients with i(Xq) than in other X-chromosome abnormalities.[32]

Deletion of the X long arm [46XXq−[11] or 46Xdel(Xq)[12]] is found either as a single-cell line or as a mosaicism with monosomic cells (45X/46XXq−). Because of the frequent incidence of mosaicism, phenotypic–karyotypic correlations are not easily determined. It has been postulated that loss of some material of the X long arm (Xq−) produces gonadal dysgenesis but not short stature or other somatic features of Turner's syndrome.[38,42]

Most patients with X long-arm deletions (46XXq−) (Figure 23.12) and short-arm isochromosome X [(46X,i(Xp)[12]], in whom the long arm of the X has been lost (Figure 23.14), have primary amenorrhea and hypoestrinism with presumably streak gonads.[116] Because breast development caused by the stimulation of ovarian steroids seems to occur more often in individuals with 46XXq− than 45X individuals, it is possible that more than one gonadal determinant exists on the long arm of an X as has been discussed for the short arm of the X. Long-arm deletions of the X are not strictly associated with short stature and those patients with Xq− who have short stature may have an undetected monosomic line (45X/46XXq−). Undetected monosomy seems likely in those patients with long-arm deletions who are short and have one or more anomalies of Turner's syndrome. Short-arm isochromosome X [46X,i(Xp)] occurs with less frequency than long-arm isochromosome X, and it may be difficult to cytogenetically distinguish between a short-arm isochromosome X and certain long-arm deletions.[116] Five patients with short-arm isochromosome X [46X,i(Xp)] have been reported and reviewed, and all the individuals had primary amenorrhea, hypoestrinism with no breast development, normal stature, and several somatic abnormalities found in Turner's syndrome. Normal stature in these individuals supports the postulate that the long arm of the X contains gonadal but no statural determinants.[38,42] Because of the very rare nature of the short-arm isochromosome X, it is difficult to compare these patients to those with other structural aberrations.

Deletions of the short arm of the X chromosome and long-arm X isochromosomes both involve loss of short-arm material and both result in short stature, Turner's stigmata, and gonadal dysgenesis. Patients with deletion of the long arm or with short-arm X isochromosome both have loss of long-arm X chromosome material and may only have simple gonadal dysgenesis with normal stature and no somatic abnormalities associated with Turner's syndrome. Consequently, it has been postulated that the genes responsible for the short stature and congenital anomalies of Turner's syndrome are located on the short arm of the X chromosome.[38] It has recently been pointed out, however, that patients with long-arm deletions of the X chromosome may also have short stature and Turner's

stigmata but not as frequently as 45X patients.[68] It has been suggested that the reduced frequency of somatic anomalies and short stature may be secondary to bias of ascertainment because it is easier to detect a short-arm deletion than a long-arm deletion.[68] As stated above, gonadal determinants appear to be present on both the long and short arms of the X although more than a single determinant may exist on each arm. Each of these gonadal determinants on the long and short arms of the X chromosome may have different functions, each essential for normal ovarian development.[116] It is apparent that the X short arm contains determinants which, when lost, result in short stature and somatic anomalies comprising Turner's syndrome. Whether or not the X long arm contains stature and somatic determinants remains to be seen and is somewhat controversial at this time.

Other X-chromosome structural abnormalities, such as centric fragments and ring X chromosomes, have been described.[24] These types of abnormalities are frequently associated with monosomic cells in affected individuals and this makes meaningful phenotypic–karyotypic correlation extremely difficult.

X-autosome translocation has been associated with a wide range of phenotypes, including gonadal dysgenesis.[110] The phenotypic–karyotypic correlation of translocations involving an autosome and an X chromosome is dependent on the amount of X chromosome material lost and on which arm of the X chromosome is involved.

## Gonadal Dysgenesis—Autosomal Chromosomal Abnormalities

Autosomal chromosomal aberrations have been associated with gonadal dysgenesis; however, the relationship is not clear. Prior to the advent of banding techniques, errors in identification of translocations involving the X chromosome and autosomes could easily occur (Figure 23.29). With the use of the banding techniques, more exact identification of structural aberrations and translocations has become possible (Figure 23.30). The significance of autosomal abnormalities in individuals with gonadal dysgenesis remains to be determined. One of the possible explanations is coincidence. An autosomal aberration associated with an XX sex chromosome constitution might be detected only because of the individual's presenting complaints related to the gonadal dysgenesis. Hemizygosity for a mutant gene producing gonadal dysgenesis in the presence of two X chromosomes is another possibility. If it were shown that the same autosome was consistently

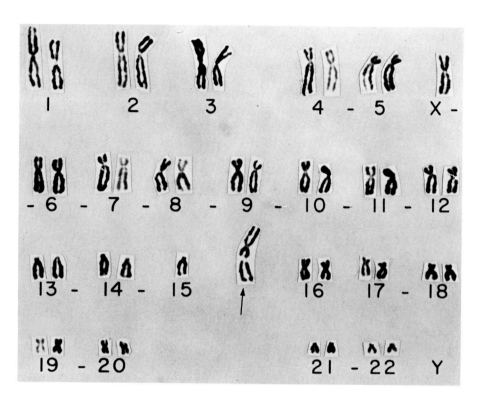

**23.29** Standard karyotype of a 17-year-old female with normal stature, primary amenorrhea, and poorly developed secondary sex characteristics. The karyotype was interpreted, prior to banding, as a translocation between a number 15 and an X chromosome. The arrow indicates the translocation chromosome. The gaps on the long arms are achromatic gaps and the long arms are continuous. The involvement of the X chromosome was thought to be responsible for the clinical picture.

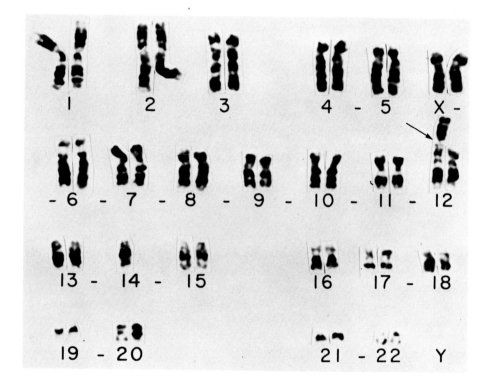

**23.30** G banded karyotype of same patient as in Figure 23.29. Correction of the karyotype revealed two normal X chromosomes with a 12/14 translocation. The arrow indicates the translocation chromosome.

involved, the possibility of hemizygosity would deserve strong consideration. If the mutant gene for gonadal dysgenesis, in the presence of two X chromosomes, were shown to be recessive and to occur on a specific autosome, this gene might be expressed if the portion of the homologous chromosome containing the allele was in some way deleted. Deletion of the homologous chromosome would allow the recessive mutant gene to be expressed in the hemizygous state. Because the few cases of autosomal abnormalities that have been associated with gonadal dysgenesis have shown no convincing pattern and/or have not been studied with the banding techniques, no specific conclusions can be drawn at this time.

## Pure Gonadal Dysgenesis—46XX or 46XY

Pure gonadal dysgenesis refers to those phenotypic females with gonadal dysgenesis, primary amenorrhea, hypoestrinism, and associated poorly developed secondary sexual development who do not have somatic abnormalities of Turner's syndrome and who have normal stature.[65,70,123] The designation "pure gonadal dysgenesis" should be reserved for those patients with 46XX or 46XY gonadal dysgenesis who have normal stature and no somatic anomalies of Turner's syndrome.[117] Individuals who contain XX or XY cell lines as part of a mosaicism related to gonadal dysgenesis generally are not classified as "pure gonadal dysgenesis" because of the variability of the association of Turner's stigmata associated with the mosaicism.

### 46XX pure gonadal dysgenesis

These patients are phenotypic females with streak gonads, primary amenorrhea, lack of secondary sexual characteristics, normal stature, and evidence of hypoestrinism. The Turner's stigmata are not found, but the gonadal lesion is identical to that seen in the 45X Turner's syndrome. A uterus and tubes are always present but are usually juvenile and the genitalia are of normal female configuration. Hirsuitism and virilization do not generally occur with 46XX gonadal dysgenesis.[37,61,107]

This syndrome is generally not recognized prepubertally because genital and somatic development is usually normal until the time of puberty. The usual presenting complaint is that of primary amenorrhea and lack of secondary sexual development. The 46XX gonadal dysgenesis can be distinguished from other forms of pure gonadal dysgenesis and testicular feminization by the finding of a pure 46XX chromosome constitution. It can be distinguished from

isolated gonadotropin deficiency by the elevated gonadotropin levels associated with streak gonads.[61,107]

Because of the finding of 46XX gonadal dysgenesis in multiple siblings and because of an increased frequency of parental consanguinity, an autosomal recessive mode of inheritance has been postulated.[16,22,34,117] Although the presence of an undetected mosaicism (45X/46XX) may explain some of the cases of apparent 46XX gonadal dysgenesis, the presence of multiple affected siblings, an increased incidence of consanguinity, and the finding of only 46XX cells in over 50 cells in more than one tissue clearly establishes this syndrome as a distinct entity inherited in an autosomal recessive fashion.[111] The association of 46XX gonadal dysgenesis and deaf-mutism in two families suggests that there may be at least two distinct autosomal recessive varieties of 46XX gonadal dysgenesis.[22,102]

### 46XY pure gonadal dysgenesis

These patients are also phenotypic females with bilateral streak gonads, primary amenorrhea, evidence of hypoestrinism with deficient secondary sexual development.[15] This syndrome differs from 46XX gonadal dysgenesis because there is frequent clitoral enlargement and virilization at the time of puberty; moreover, there is an increased frequency of gonadal neoplasia. Because these features are variable, many of the patients who have been reported as 46XY gonadal dysgenesis may represent undetected 45X/46XY mosaicism. Plasma and urinary gonadotropin levels are elevated at or after puberty and increased levels of plasma testosterone have been found in those patients who were virilized at the time of puberty.[107]

As discussed above, neoplasia of the streak gonads frequently occurs in patients with an XY cell line and 46XY gonadal dysgenesis follows this rule.[15,17,20,25,30,46,51,53,61,107,126] Based on reports of multiple affected siblings, concordant monozygotic twins, and affected individuals in several different sibships of a kindred with transmission through unaffected females, it has been suggested that 46XY gonadal dysgenesis is inherited either as an X-linked recessive or as a sex-limited autosomal dominant trait. There is no increased incidence of parental consanguinity with 46XY gonadal dysgenesis.[4,8,15,17,20,25,36,51,61,124,126] There has been no report of both 46XX and 46XY gonadal dysgenesis occurring in the same family and 46XY gonadal dysgenesis differs from 46XX gonadal dysgenesis in that deaf-mutism has not been found in patients with the XY gonadal dysgenesis. The 46XY gonadal dysgenesis can be differentiated from the testicular feminization syndrome because of the finding of streak gonads instead of testes, the presence of uterus and tubes, and virilization at or after puberty with 46XY gonadal dysgenesis.

## Mixed Gonadal Dysgenesis

Mixed gonadal dysgenesis is a group of disorders associated with asymmetrical gonadal development. A testis is found on one side and a streaklike gonad on the other. Mixed gonadal dysgenesis has been described above in relation to sex chromosome mosaicism, particularly of the 45X/46XY type. Because 45X/46XY mosaicism can also occur in males with bilateral testes as well as in females with bilateral streak gonads and associated Turner's stigmata, the chromosomal findings do not allow for a specific diagnosis of this syndrome. In order for mixed gonadal dysgenesis to be diagnosed, anatomic and histologic examination of the asymmetrical gonads is required.

## Gonadal Dysgenesis—An Overview

The major underlying cause of gonadal dysgenesis is an abnormality of the second sex chromosome in some or all of the cells of the affected individual. In at least half of the patients, the gonadal dysgenesis is caused by an absence of the second sex chromosome.[37] In a small percentage of patients, a structural aberration of the second X chromosome with loss of genetic material is responsible for the gonadal dysgenesis. In at least one-third of the cases, sex chromosome abnormalities appear as components of mosaicism. It is clear that a number of phenotypic–karyotypic correlations can readily be ascertained:

1. Short stature and somatic abnormalities, currently referred to as Turner's syndrome, are more frequent and more pronounced in patients with a 45X chromosome constitution.
2. Patients with short-arm X-chromosome deletions (Xp−) are less severely involved than those with monosomy for the X chromosome. In each of these, the findings probably result from a loss of genetic material on the short arm of the X with subsequent monosomy for some genes on the short arm.
3. The long arm of the X chromosome appears to be necessary for normal ovarian development but less critical for normal stature and causal relationship to Turner's stigmata. This is controversial and not yet fully resolved.
4. Mosaicism results in an unpredictable combination of the features of the different stem cells present. There is

no direct correlation between the relative number of the various stem cells or the tissues involved and the ultimate phenotypic expression.

It may be difficult to understand why monosomy X or structural aberrations of the X chromosome result in gonadal dysgenesis and Turner's syndrome when one considers that one X chromosome in the normal female is inactivated. This inactivated X chromosome is represented by the tightly clumped DNA of the sex chromatin mass which is heteropyknotic. This denser and darker staining DNA is also known as heterochromatin, which is considered to be inactive.[63] According to the theory proposed by Lyon,[91] "Lyonization" of the X chromosome occurs during fetal life and results in inactivation of either the maternally derived or the paternally derived X chromosome.

In order to understand why patients with monosomy X or structurally abnormal X chromosomes have gonadal dysgenesis, consideration of several facts is necessary. Lyonization does not occur immediately at conception. The sex chromatin mass or Barr body in human nuclei appears sometime between the twelfth and sixteenth days of embryogenesis; consequently, there is a significant period of time during which both X's are active.[37,63] It is also possible that not all loci on the heterochromatic, or inactivated, X chromosome in adult human females are inactivated.[104] It also appears that the mechanism of X inactivation does not occur equally in all tissues of the organism. For example, no Barr body is seen in certain critical cells, such as oocytes.[56] It is probably for these reasons that individuals with monosomy X or structural aberrations of the X chromosome develop gonadal dysgenesis despite the fact that a second X chromosome is inactivated in a normal 46XX female.

It is reasonable to anticipate, with the refinement of the newer cytogenetic techniques, additional information regarding the pathogenesis of gonadal dysgenesis to become available and an even better understanding of the various structural aberrations and their relationship to gonadal dysgenesis to be achieved.

# Abnormalities of Phenotypic Sex Differentiation

The disorders of genital development that reflect disturbances in the internal or external endocrinologic environment of the fetus are expressed as phenotypic abnormalities of sex differentiation. In all of these conditions, the chromosomes appear normal and correspond to the gonadal sex. Those syndromes that fall into this category are all forms of pseudohermaphroditism. A true hermaphrodite has gonadal tissue of both sexes, whereas the pseudohermaphrodite has gonadal differentiation compatible with the sex chromosome constitution but some of the genital appearance of the opposite sex. A male pseudohermaphrodite is a patient who has testes but in whom the genital development is not compatible with the gonadal sex. Accordingly, the female pseudohermaphrodite has ovaries but is virilized to certain degree. From a phenotypic standpoint, the male pseudohermaphrodite has incomplete virilization, whereas the female pseudohermaphrodite has varying degrees of virilization.[37]

## Male Pseudohermaphroditism

Male pseudohermaphroditism is a condition in which the gonads are exclusively testes but the genital ducts or external genitalia are not fully masculinized and appear to some degree to possess the phenotypic appearance of a female. A male pseudohermaphrodite may range from an individual who appears to be female to a male with only mild hypospadius or cryptorchidism. This discussion is limited to those cases in which the phenotype simulates a female.

### Testicular feminization

This condition (feminizing testes), in its complete form, represents an end organ insensitivity to androgenic hormones, and it is one of the better known and distinctive disorders of sex differentiation. Patients with testicular feminization are phenotypic females who appear normal at birth and have a 46XY chromosome constitution. As many as 1 to 2% of female children with inguinal hernias have the syndrome of testicular feminization.[81] As a result, some of the patients are seen by physicians in childhood because of an inguinal hernia, but most patients are not seen until puberty.[37] The growth and development of patients with testicular feminization are usually normal,[37] although there is an indication that patients with testicular feminization may be taller than the average for women.[37]

By the time of puberty most patients become quite feminine and the breasts develop at the expected time and usually attain normal size; however, even when the breasts are large there is usually a decrease of glandular tissue and the nipples are usually small with pale areolae.[37,61,107]

A striking feature of this disorder is a marked lack of body hair, including a total absence of axillary and pubic

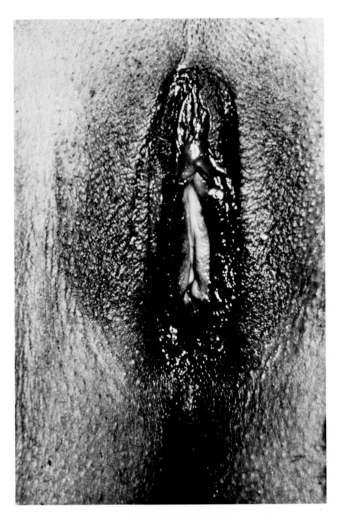

**23.31** Testicular feminization. Note absence of pubic hair.

[Reprinted by permission from A. Blaustein, R. Scully, B. Bigelow, R. Demopoulos, and F. Gorstein, *Audiovisual Seminars in Gynecologic Pathology. Pathology of the Ovary,* W. B. Saunders, 1974.]

hair (Figure 23.31). The external genitalia appear quite normal, although the labia minora are usually underdeveloped and the vagina ends as a blind pouch, which is shallow. The clitoris is normal or small and the uterus is absent, although there may be some vestigial Müllerian remnants.[37,61,107] In patients with testicular feminization, the testes may be intraabdominal (Figure 23.32) but are often located in a hernia sac. Histologic sections of the testes reveal seminiferous tubules (Figure 23.33) but no spermatogenesis. In older patients with testicular feminization there is a significant incidence of neoplasia in the testes.[37,61,107]

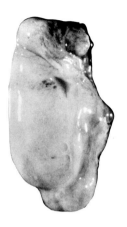
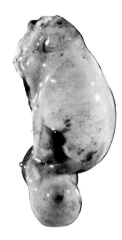

**23.32** Right and left testicles in a case of testicular feminization.

[Reprinted by permission from A. Blaustein, R. Scully, B. Bigelow, R. Demopoulos, and F. Gorstein, *Audiovisual Seminars in Gynecologic Pathology. Pathology of the Ovary,* W. B. Saunders, 1974.]

The phenotype of testicular feminization is the result of androgen insensitivity (testosterone). The pathophysiology of this resistance is unknown. The only feature of male development that is found in affected persons is suppression of Müllerian duct development with subsequent absence of the uterus and fallopian tubes.[37,61,107] The complete absence of external genital development is entirely explained by the absence of end organ androgen effect and is also associated with the absence of body and sexual hair. The apparent breast development in these patients has been attributed to the action of estrogen unopposed by androgen. An additional possibility for the spontaneous breast development is that the abnormal testes may fail to control or suppress whatever causes gynecomastia in the normal pubertal male.[37]

Patients with testicular feminization are chromatin negative and have a normal 46XY karyotype. Incidence figures for testicular feminization and analysis of pedigrees of involved families suggests an X-linked recessive inheritance or a sex-limited autosomal dominant trait. An X-linked recessive trait manifested in the male is easily understood, for the abnormal gene is present in the hemizygous state because there is only one X chromosome. A sex-limited disorder is carried on an autosome and becomes apparent in only one sex because of factors relating to its expression.[37] Studies of animal models of testicular feminization have revealed marked similarities to the human syndrome. It is considered likely that testicular

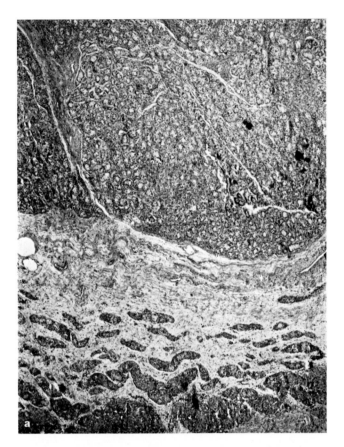

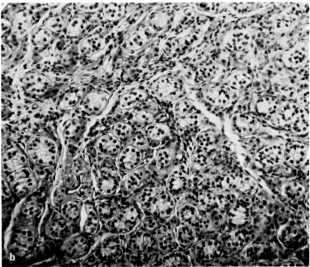

**23.33 a.** Tubular adenoma in testicular feminization. **b.** High-power view of **a**.

[Reprinted by permission from A. Blaustein, R. Scully, B. Bigelow, R. Demopoulos, and F. Gorstein, *Audiovisual Seminars in Gynecologic Pathology. Pathology of the Ovary,* W. B. Saunders, 1974.]

feminization in man is caused by absent or defective cytoplasmic androgen receptors.[6,61,92]

### The incomplete syndrome of testicular feminization

This is a variant of the syndrome of complete testicular feminization. Affected individuals have some phallic enlargement associated with labioscrotal fusion. If the labioscrotal fusion is severe enough, the vaginal orifice is obscured, with preservation of the urogenital sinus. Although breast development usually occurs in these patients at adolescence, feminization is less complete than in the complete testicular feminization syndrome. Hirsuitism or true virilization may occur in addition to the development of female sexual characteristics.[61] Because the incomplete syndrome of testicular feminization is a variant of the syndrome of feminizing testes, it can probably be explained on the basis of varying degrees of androgen insensitivity.[61]

### Male pseudohermaphroditism with normal virilization at puberty

This configuration has been described in familial forms of male pseudohermaphroditism without defective androgen syntehsis or defective end organ response. In these patients, both secretion of testosterone and the response of androgen-responsive target organs appear to be entirely normal and adequate virilization occurs at puberty. These individuals are uniformly 46XY and only male internal genital ducts are present. These patients encompass the full range of external sexual ambiguity, ranging from mild hypospadius and a normal sized phallus to individuals who resemble females with slight clitoral enlargement and incomplete masculinization of the urogenital sinus.[37,61,107] The more severe familial forms constitute a clinically distinctive entity and should be distinguished from the milder forms. One such familial entity was recently reported in which males were born with ambiguous external genitalia but with subsequent virilization at puberty. Biochemical evaluation revealed a marked decrease in plasma dihydrotestosterone secondary to a decrease in steroid 5-α-reductase activity. *In utero*, the decrease in dihydrotestosterone results in incomplete masculinization of the external genitalia. This condition is apparently inherited in an autosomal recessive fashion.[72]

### Pseudovaginal perineoscrotal hypospadius

This condition is characterized by ambiguous female-like genitalia in otherwise normal males (Figure

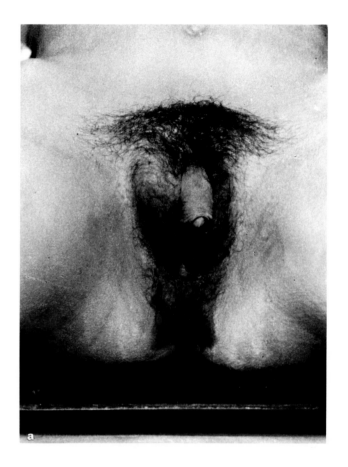

23.34a,b,c).[61,73,101,107,118] The genitalia have a blind perineal opening, cleft scrotum, and severe hypospadius with a perineal urethral opening. The phallus is usually mistaken for an enlarged clitoris; consequently, these patients are usually raised as females although complete masculinization takes place at the time of puberty. No breast enlargement or other evidence of female secondary sexual development occurs at the time of virilization. Individuals with this syndrome are sex chromatin negative and have a 46XY chromosome constitution. Their testes are normal and are found in the labioscrotal folds. Normal epididymis, vas deferens, and seminal vesicles have been found in most cases. Testicular endocrine function has been found to be completely normal.[61,107]

The pseudovaginal perineoscrotal hypospadius syndrome represents a localized congenital abnormality of the urogenital sinus and external genitalia in otherwise normal males. Differentiation between this syndrome and the incomplete form of testicular feminization can be very difficult before puberty. Because the pseudovaginal perineoscrotal hypospadius syndrome has been described in multiple siblings and in association with consanguinity, it

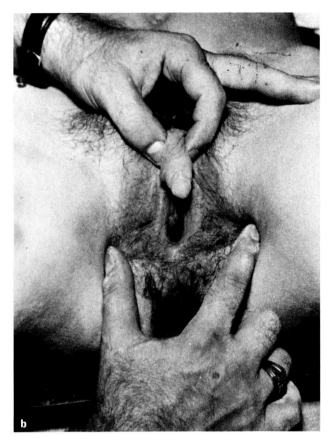
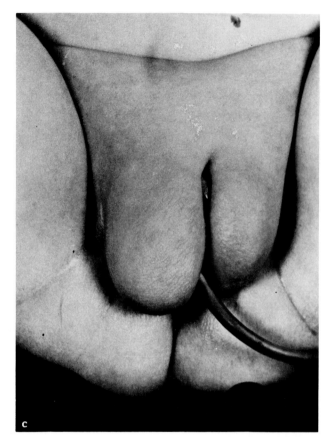

**23.34** Pseudovaginal perineoscrotal hypospadias. **a** and **b.** Pubertal individual with genital ambiguity and virilization. Note the small hypospadic penis resembling an enlarged clitoris, and the pseudovaginal opening. **c.** Infant sibling of patient in **a** and **b**. Note the ambiguous genitalia and testes within the labioscrotal folds. The catheter is in the pseudovaginal opening.

[Reprinted by permission from David L. Rimoin and R. Neil Schimke, *Genetic Disorders of the Endocrine Glands,* C. V. Mosby, 1971, and by courtesy of Dr. J. L. Simpson.]

is felt that it is inherited as an autosomal recessive trait.[60,118] Because individuals with this syndrome have genitalia that resemble those of a normal female and reconstructive surgery to create a functioning penis is difficult or impossible, most of these individuals are raised as females.

Male pseudohermaphroditism can also be associated with several types of adrenal hyperplasia: 3-$\beta$-hydroxysteroid deficiency (type IV), 17-hydroxylase deficiency (type V), and lipoid hyperplasia of the adrenal (type VI).[61,107] These rare and relatively complex endocrinologic syndromes are not within the scope of this discussion, and the interested reader should refer to a complete discussion of the adrenal gland for additional details.[61,89,107,125,135]

## Female Pseudohermaphroditism

Female pseudohermaphrodites are genetic and gonadal females with varying degrees of external genital masculinization. Female pseudohermaphroditism is most frequently caused by congenital adrenal hyperplasia.[37,61,107]

### Congenital adrenal hyperplasia

Congenital adrenal hyperplasia is a hereditary adrenal disorder in which defective hydrocortisone biosynthesis leads to overproduction of androgen. This excess of androgen results in virilization of the female fetus and is the most frequent cause of ambiguous genitalia in the newborn period. It is noteworthy that it is the only condition involving ambiguous genitalia in which an entirely normal sex role and fertility can be achieved with appropriate therapy. It is also the only condition involving ambiguous genitalia in which the life of the patient is at risk.[37,61,107] The newborn female infant with congenital adrenal hyperplasia always has some perceptible abnormality of the external genitalia. The degree of masculinization is variable; however, the internal development of the female with congenital adrenal hyperplasia is entirely normal regardless of the degree of external virilization.[37] The uterus, fallopian tubes, and upper vagina develop normally and the Wolffian primordia regress completely. The ovaries are morphologically normal. When the abnormal adrenal function is controlled by proper therapy, many of these patients may have normal reproductive function. Patients who are untreated and who are raised as females show the effects of excess androgen in their growth, general appearance, and genitalia. They grow faster and develop a muscularity and hirsuitism suggestive of early male adolescence in their first years of life. Their voices deepen and they may develop acne and ultimately facial hair. Premature closure of the epiphyses secondary to the growth effect of the androgen occurs, and the child who seems to be tall during her early years later becomes shorter than her peers.[37] The clitoris continues to enlarge during childhood but no further anatomic change occurs in the external genitalia. The onset of puberty is delayed or does not occur, and the patient may go through life with short stature, primary amenorrhea, and varying degrees of virilization with no specific medical problems unless acute adrenal insufficiency is precipitated.[37]

Six major types of congenital adrenal hyperplasia have been described and each has a distinctive clinical picture and specific biochemical abnormality.[61] Each of the six types of congenital adrenal hyperplasia is transmitted in an autosomal recessive fashion and all six types have impaired cortisone formation in common. Consequently, hyperplasia of the adrenal cortex results from hypersecretion of ACTH through the negative-feedback mechanism.[61] Types I, II, and III are predominantly virilizing disorders resulting in female pseudohermaphroditism, and types IV, V, and VI have been briefly mentioned in relation to male pseudohermaphroditism.

### Type I: Partial $C_{21}$ hydroxylase defect

This condition involves a partial defect in $C_{21}$ hydroxylation, and this leads to simple virilism. Aldosterone secretion in these patients is normal or increased and there is no salt-losing tendency.[61]

### Type II: Complete $C_{21}$ defect

The salt-losing variant of congenital adrenal hypoplasia is caused by a more complete block in $C_{21}$ hydroxylation. In these patients aldosterone secretion is impaired but not lacking. Patients with type II congenital adrenal hyperplasia are likely to have severe salt-losing crises and often die in the early weeks of life unless they are properly diagnosed and adequately treated. Types I and II account for over 90% of the patients with congenital adrenal hyperplasia.[61]

### Type III: $C_{11}$ hydroxylase defect

A defect in hydroxylase at $C_{11}$ leads to the hypersecretion of 11-deoxycorticosterone (DOC) and 11-deoxycortisol (compound S) in addition to adrenal androgens. Patients with this condition have hypertension and virilization.[61] A detailed discussion of the biochemistry, pathophysiology, and pathogenesis of congenital adrenal hyperplasia is beyond the scope of this discussion, and the interested reader is referred to sources that deal with the adrenal gland in detail.[61,89,107,125,135]

# Nonadrenal Female Pseudohermaphroditism— Maternal Androgens and Progestogens

Nonadrenal female pseudohermaphroditism is rare but deserves brief mention. Virilization of babies born to mothers treated with either progesterone or estrogen or both during pregnancy has been noted. Because all normal babies develop in mothers who are secreting large quantities of both of these hormones, the mechanism of virilization in these cases is obscure.[37,61] In rare cases, masculinization of the female fetus can occur if the mother is suffering from a virilizing ovarian or adrenal tumor or if she develops virilism from any other cause during the course of pregnancy.

Female pseudohermaphroditism arising from accidental early exposure to androgens is the most easily treated of all types of ambiguous genital development. No hormonal therapy is necessary and masculinization during the postnatal period does not occur. The female secondary sex characteristics develop at the usual time of puberty, and surgical correction of the external genitalia restores feminine appearance and permits normal sexual function.[37,61,107]

## Defects of Wolffian–Müllerian Duct Development

Errors in phenotypic sex can also result from developmental defects in the differentiation of the Wolffian–Müllerian duct system.

The Rokitansky–Küster–Hauser syndrome is an example of abnormal Müllerian duct development. It is characterized by congenital absence of the uterus and vagina in otherwise normal females with functional ovaries and 46XX chromosome constitution.[2,14,66,67,76,86,131,134] The disorder is surprisingly common and, after Turner's syndrome, has been estimated to be the second most frequent cause of primary amenorrhea in young women.[134] Some females with this syndrome have been noted to manifest a variety of skeletal abnormalities as well as a conductive hearing loss.[134] The cause of the Rokitansky–Küster–Hauser syndrome has been considered to be a single early primary defect in the migration of the caudal mesoderm.[121] Most cases of this syndrome are sporadic, although several well-documented familial cases have been recorded and the pedigree patterns suggest an autosomal recessive trait.[2,76,134] It has been suggested that the importance of the familial form of this disorder is the demonstration of an abnormal gene that prevents uterine and vaginal development. Consequently, there must be at least one normal gene the product of which is critical to development of the Müllerian duct and early migration of the caudal mesoderm.[134]

## REFERENCES

1. Alexander, D., and Money, J. Reading ability, object constancy, and Turner's syndrome. *Percept. Mot. Skills* 20:981, 1965.

2. Anger, D., Hemet, J., and Ensel, J. Forme familiale du syndrome de Rokitansky–Küster–Hauser. *Bull. Fed. Soc. Gynecol. Obstet. Lang. Fr.* 18:229, 1966.

3. Archibald, R. M., Finby, N., and deVito, F. Endocrine significance of short metacarpals. *J. Clin. Endocrinol.* 19:1313, 1959.

4. Back, F., Karl, H. L., and Macias-Alvarez, I. Familial XY gonadal dysgenesis. *Lancet.* 2:635, 1968.

5. Bahner, F., Schwarz, G., Harnden, D. G., Jacobs, P. A., Heinz, H. A., and Walter, K. A fertile female with XO sex chromosome constitution. *Lancet* 2:100, 1960.

6. Bardin, C. W., Bullock, L., Blackburn, W. R., Sherins, R. J., and Vanha-Perttula, T. Testosterone metabolism in the androgen-insensitive rat: A model for testicular feminization, in Bergsma, D., ed.: *Part X. The Endocrine System, Birth Defects: Original Article Series.* Baltimore, Williams and Wilkins Co., for the National Foundation-March of Dimes, 1971, Vol. VII, No. 6, pp. 185–192.

7. Barr, M. L., and Bertram, E. G. A morphological distinction between neurones of the male and female, and the behavior of the nucleolar satellite during accelerated nucleoprotein synthesis. *Nature* (London) 163:676, 1949.

8. Barr, M. L., Carr, D. H., Plunkett, E. R., Soltan, H. C., and Weins, R. G. Male pseudo hermaphroditism and pure gonadal dysgenesis in sisters. *Am. J. Obstet. Gynecol.* 99:1047, 1967.

9. Benson, P. F., Gough, M. H., and Polani, P. E. Lymphangiography and chromosome studies in females with lymphoedema and possible ovarian dysgenesis. *Arch. Dis. Child.* 40:27, 1965.

10. Berger, R., Abonyi, D., Nodot, A., Vialatte, S., and LeJeune, J. Hermaphrodisme vrai et "Garcon XX" dans une Fratrie. *Res. Eur. Etudes. Clin. Biol.* 15:330, 1970.

11. Bergsma, D., ed. *Chicago Conference: Standardization in Human Cytogenetics, Birth Defects: Original Article Series.* White Plains, The National Foundation-March of Dimes, 1966, Vol. II, No. 2.

12. Bergsma, D., ed. *Paris conference (1971): Standardization in Human Cytogenetics, Birth Defects: Original Article Series.* White Plains, The National Foundation-March of Dimes, 1972, Vol. VIII, No. 7.

13. Blackston, R. D., and Chen, A. T. L. A case of 48, XXXX female with normal intelligence. *J. Med. Genet.* 9:230, 1972.

14. Bloch, P., Curchod, A., and Cordey, R. Confection d'un neo-vagin par dedoublement du ligament large dans un cas de Rokitansky–Küster–Hauser. *Gynaecologia* 151:113, 1961.

15. Boczkowski, K. Further observations on the syndrome of pure gonadal dysgenesis. *Am. J. Obstet. Gynecol.* 106:1177, 1970.

16. Boczkowski, K. Pure gonadal dysgenesis and ovarian dysplasia in sisters. *Am. J. Obstet. Gynecol.* 106:626, 1970.

17. Brogger, A., and Strand, A. Contribution to the study of the so called pure gonadal dysgenesis. *Acta Endocrinol.* 48:490, 1965.

18. Carr, D. H. Chromosome studies in spontaneous abortions. *Obstet. Gynecol.* 26:308, 1965.

19. Carr, D. H. Cytogenetic aspects of induced and spontaneous abortions. *Clin. Obstet. Gynecol.* 15:203, 1972.

20. Chemke, J., Carmichael, R., Stewart, J. M., Greer, R. H., and Robinson, A. Familial XY gonadal dysgenesis. *J. Med. Genet.* 7:105, 1970.

21. Chen, A. T., Chan, Y. K., and Falek, A. The effects of chromosome abnormalities on birth weight in man. I. Sex chromosome disorders. *Hum. Hered.* 21:543, 1971.

22. Christakos, A. C., Simpson, J. L., Younger, J. B., and Christian, C. D. Gonadal dysgenesis as an autosomal recessive condition. *Am. J. Obstet. Gynecol.* 104:1027, 1969.

23. Clayton, G. W., Smith, J. F., and Rosenberg, H. S. Familial true hermaphroditism in pre- and post-pubertal genetic females. Hormonal and morphologic studies. *J. Clin. Endocrinol.* 18:1349, 1958.

24. Cohen, M. M., Sandberg, A. A., Takagi, N., et al. Autoradiographic investigations of centric fragments and rings in patients with stigmata of gonadal dysgenesis. *Cytogenetics* (Basel) 6:254, 1967.

25. Cohen, M. M., and Shaw, M. W. Two XY siblings with gonadal dysgenesis and a female phenotype. *N. Engl. J. Med.* 272:1083, 1965.

26. Court Brown, W. M., Harnden, D. G., Jacobs, P. A., Maclean, N., and Mantle, D. J. *Abnormalities of the Sex Chromosome Complement in Man.* Med. Res. Council, Spec. Rept. Ser. No. 305. London, Her Majesty's Stationery Office, 1964.

27. Dalla Palma, L., Cavina, C., and Borghi, A. Radiological

aspects of the urinary tract in Turner's syndrome. *Radiol. Clin. Biol.* 36:328, 1967.

28. Daughaday, W. H., Laron, Z., Pertzelan, A., and Heins, J. N. Defective sulfation factor generation: A possible etiological link in dwarfism. *Trans. Assoc. Am. Physicians* 82:129, 1969.

29. Davidoff, F., and Federman, D. D. Mixed gonadal dysgenesis. *Pediatrics* 52:725, 1973.

30. Dewhurst, C. J., Paine, C. G., and Blank, C. E. An XY female with absent gonads and vestigial pelvic organs. *J. Obstet. Gynaecol. Br. Commonw.* 70:675, 1963.

31. Donaldson, C. L., Wegienka, L. C., Miller, D., and Forsham, P. H. Growth hormone studies in Turner's syndrome. *J. Clin. Endocrinol.* 28:383, 1968.

32. Doniach, D., Roitt, I. M., and Polani, P. E. Thyroid antibodies and sex chromosome anomalies. *Proc. R. Soc. Med.* 61:278, 1968.

33. Egli, F., and Stalder, G. Malformations of kidney and urinary tract in common chromosomal aberrations. I. Clinical studies. *Humangenetik* 18:1, 1973.

34. Elliot, G. A., Sandler, A., and Rabinowitz, D. Gonadal dysgenesis in three sisters. *J. Clin. Endocrinol.* 19:995, 1959.

35. Engel, E., and Forbes, A. P. Cytogenetic and clinical findings in 48 patients with congenitally defective or absent ovaries. *Medicine* 44:135, 1965.

36. Espiner, E. A., Veale, A. M. O., Sands, V. E., and Fitzgerald, P. H. Familial syndrome of streak gonads and normal male karyotype in five phenotypic females. *N. Engl. J. Med.* 283:6, 1970.

37. Federman, D. D. *Abnormal Sexual Development.* Philadelphia, W. B. Saunders Co., 1968.

38. Ferguson-Smith, M. A. Karyotype-phenotype correlations in gonadal dysgenesis and their bearing on the pathogenesis of malformations. *J. Med. Genet.* 2:142, 1965.

39. Ferguson-Smith, M. A. X-Y chromosomal interchange in the aetiology of true hermaphroditism and of XX Klinefelter's syndrome. *Lancet* 2:475, 1966.

40. Ferguson-Smith, M. A. Phenotypic aspects of sex chromosome aberrations. *Birth Defects: Original Article Series* 5:3, 1969.

41. Ferguson-Smith, M. A. Chromosomal abnormalities. II. Sex chromosome defects. *Hosp. Pract.* 5:88, 1970.

42. Ferguson-Smith, M. A., Alexander, D. S., Bowen, P., et al. Clinical and cytogenetical studies in female gonadal dysgenesis and their bearing on the cause of Turner's syndrome. *Cytogenetics* 3:355, 1964.

43. Ferrier, P. E., Ferrier, S. A., and Kelley, V. C. Sex chromosome mosaicism in disorders of sexual differentiation: incidence in various tissues. *J. Pediat.* 76:739, 1970.

44. Fialkow, P. J. Genetic aspects of autoimmunity. *Prog. Med. Genet.* 7:117, 1969.

45. Finby, N., and Archibald, R. M. Skeletal abnormalities associated with gonadal dysgenesis. *Am. J. Roentgenol.* 89:1222, 1963.

46. Fischer, P., Golab, E., and Holzner, H. XY gonadal dysgenesis and malignancy. *Lancet* 2:110, 1969.

47. Forbes, A. P., and Engle, E. The high incidence of diabetes mellitus in 41 patients with gonadal dysgenesis and their close relatives. *Metabolism* 12:428, 1963.

48. Ford, C. E., and Hamerton, J. L. The chromosomes of man. *Nature* (London) 178:1010, 1956.

49. Ford, C. E., Jones, K. W., Polani, P. E., et al. A sex-chromosome anomaly in a case of gonadal dysgenesis (Turner's syndrome). *Lancet* 1:711, 1959.

50. Fraccaro, M., Gemzell, C. A., and Lindsten, J. Plasma level of growth hormone and chromosome complement in four patients with gonadal dysgenesis (Turner's syndrome). *Acta Endocrinol.* 34:496, 1960.

51. Frasier, S. D., Bashore, R. A., and Mosier, H. D. Gonadoblastoma associated with pure gonadal dysgenesis in monozygous twins. *J. Pediatr.* 64:740, 1964.

52. Frasier, S. D., Crudd, F. S. Jr., and Farrell, F. J. Buccal smears in the newborn female. *J. Pediatr.* 65:222, 1964.

53. Freeman, M. V. R., and Miller, O. J. XY gonadal dysgenesis and gonadoblastoma: Report of a case. *Obstet. Gynecol.* 34:478, 1969.

54. Gallagher, H. S., and Lewis, R. P. Sequential gonadoblastoma and choriocarcinoma. *Obstet. Gynecol.* 41:123, 1973.

55. Garron, D. C., and Vander Stoep, L. R. Personality and intelligence in Turner's syndrome. A critical review. *Arch. Gen. Psychiat.* (Chicago) 21:339, 1969.

56. Gartler, S. M., Liskay, R. M., Campbell, B. K., et al. Evidence for two functional X chromosomes in human oocytes. *Cell Differ.* 1:215, 1972.

57. German, J. Abnormalities of human sex chromosomes. V. A unifying concept in relation to the gonadal dysgeneses. *Clin. Genet.* 1:15, 1970.

58. Goldstein, J. L., and Wilson, J. D. Hereditary disorders of sexual development in man. *In* Motulsky, A. G., and Lenz, W., eds.: *Birth Defects.* Amsterdam, Excerpta Medica, 1974, pp. 165–173.

59. Gordon, R. R., and O'Neill, E. M. Turner's infantile phenotype. *Br. Med. J.* 1:483, 1969.

60. Green, O. C., Miller, R. R., Garcia, O., and Hamwi, C. J. Virilizing male pseudohermaphroditism associated with abnormal testicular function. *J. Clin. Endocrinol.* 29:728, 1969.

61. Grumbach, M. M., and Van Wyk, J. J. Disorders of sex differentiation. *In* Williams, R. H., ed.: *Textbook of Endocrinology,* 5th ed. Philadelphia, W. B. Saunders Co., 1974, pp. 423–501.

62. Haddad, H. M., and Wilkins, L. Congenital anomalies associated with gonadal aplasia. Review of fifty-five cases. *Pediatrics* 23:885, 1959.

63. Hamerton, J. L. *Human Cytogenetics.* New York, Academic Press, 1971, Vol. 1.

64. Hamerton, J. L. *Human Cytogenetics.* New York, Academic Press, 1971, Vol. 2.

65. Harnden, D. G., and Stewart, J. S. S. The chromosomes in a case of pure gonadal dysgenesis. *Br. Med. J.* 2:1285, 1959.

66. Hauser, G. A., Keller, M., Keller, T., and Wenner, R. Das Rokitansky-Küster Syndrom. *Gynaecologia* 151:111, 1961.

67. Hauser, G. A., and Schreiner, W. E. Das Mayer-Rokitansky-Küster-Syndrom. Uterus bipartitus solidus rudimentarius cum vagina solida. *Schweiz. Med. Wochenschr.* 91:381, 1961.

68. Hecht, F., Jones, D. L., Delay, M., et al. Xq− Turner's syndrome: Reconsideration of hypothesis that Xp− causes somatic features in Turner's syndrome. *J. Med. Genet.* 7:1, 1970.

69. Hecht, F., and MacFarlane, J. P. Mosaicism in Turner's syndrome reflects the lethality of XO. *Lancet* 2:1197, 1969.

70. Hoffenberg, R., and Jackson, W. P. U. Gonadal dysgenesis in normal looking females. *Br. Med. J.* 1:1281, 1957.

71. Hsu, L. Y. F., Klinger, H. P., and Weiss, J. Influence of nuclear selection criteria on sex chromatin frequency in oral mucosal cells of newborn females. *Cytogenetics* 6:371, 1967.

72. Imperato-McGinley, J., Guerrero, L., Gautier, T., and Peter-

son, R. E. Steriod 5-α-reductase deficiency in man: An inherited form of male pseudohermaphroditism. *Science* 186:1213, 1974.

73. Inhorn, S. L., and Opitz, J. M. Abnormalities of sex development. *In* Bloodworth, J. M. B., ed.: *Endocrine Pathology.* Baltimore, Williams and Wilkins, 1968, p. 529.

74. Jacobs, P. A., Harnden, D. G., Court Brown, W. M., Goldstein, J., Close, H. G., MacGregor, T. N., MacLean, N., and Strong, J. A. Abnormalities involving the X chromosome in women. *Lancet* 1:1213, 1960.

75. Jones, H. W. Jr., Ferguson-Smith, M. A., and Heller, R. H. The pathology and cytogenetics of gonadal agenesis. *Am. J. Obstet. Gynecol.* 87:578, 1963.

76. Jones, H. W. Jr., and Mermut, S. Familial occurrence of congenital absence of the vagina. *Am. J. Obstet. Gynecol.* 114:1100, 1972.

77. Jost, A. Problems of fetal endocrinology: The gonadal and hypophyseal hormones. *Recent Prog. Res.* 8:379, 1953.

78. Jost, A. Recherches sur la differenciation sexuelle de l'embryon de lapin. *Arch. Anat. Microsc. Morphol. Exp.* 36:271, 1946–1947.

79. Jost, A. The role of fetal hormones in prenatal development. *In Harvey Lectures,* Series 55. New York, Academic Press, 1959–1960, pp. 201–225.

80. Jost, A. A new look at the mechanisms controlling sex differentiation in mammals. *Johns Hopkins Med. J.* 130:38, 1972.

81. Kaplan, S. A., Snyder, W. H. Jr., and Little, S. Inguinal hernias in females and the testicular feminization syndrome. *Am. J. Dis. Child.* 117:243, 1969.

82. Karp, L., Bryant, J. I., Tagatz, G., et al. The occurrence of gonadal dysgenesis in association with monozygotic twinning. *J. Med. Genet.* 12(1):70, 1975.

83. Kosowicz, J. Changes in medial tibial condyle—a common finding in Turner's syndrome. *Acta Endocrinol. (kbh.)* 31:321, 1959.

84. Kosowicz, J. The deformity of the medial tibial condyle in nineteen cases of gonadal dysgenesis. *J. Bone Joint Surg. [Am.]* 42-A:600, 1960.

85. Kosowicz, J. The carpal sign in gonadal dysgenesis. *J. Clin. Endocrinol.* 22:949, 1962.

86. Leduc, B., Van Campenhout, J., and Simard, R. Congenital absence of the vagina. Observations on 25 cases. *Am. J. Obstet. Gynecol.* 100:512, 1968.

87. Lejeune, J., Gautier, M., and Turpin, R. Etude des chromosomes somatique de neuf enfants mongoliens. *C. R. Acad. Sci. [D] (Paris)* 248:1721, 1959.

88. Lemli, L., and Smith, D. W. The XO syndrome; a study of the differential phenotype in 25 patients. *J. Pediatr.* 63:577, 1963.

89. Liddle, G. W., and Melmon, K. L. The adrenals. *In* Williams, R. H., ed.: *Textbook of Endocrinology,* 5th ed. Philadelphia, W. B. Saunders Co., 1974, pp. 233–322.

90. Lindsten, J., Bowen, P., Lee, C. S. N., McKusick, V. A., Polani, P. E., Wingate, M., Edwards, J. H., Hamper, J., Tippett, P., Sanger, R., and Race, R. R. Source of the X in XO females: The evidence of Xg. *Lancet* 1:558, 1963.

91. Lyon, M. F. Sex chromatin and gene action in the mammalian X-chromosome. *Am. J. Hum. Genet.* 14:135, 1962.

92. Lyon, M. F., and Hawkes, S. G. X-linked gene for testicular feminization in the mouse. *Nature* (London) 227:1217, 1970.

93. Mikamo, K., and de Watteville, H. Incidence of sex chromosomal anomalies in newborn infants. *Int. J. Fertil.* 14:95, 1969.

94. Milner, W. A., Garlick, W. B., Fink, A. J., and Stein, A. A. True hermaphrodite siblings. *J. Urol.* 79:1003, 1968.

95. Mittwoch, U. Sex chromatin. *J. Med. Genet.* 1:50, 1964.

96. Money, J., and Granoff, D. IQ and the somatic stigmata of Turner's syndrome. *Am. J. Ment. Defic.* 70:69, 1965.

97. Moore, K. L., and Barr, M. L. Smears from the oral mucosa in the detection of chromosomal sex. *Lancet* 2:57, 1955.

98. Nakashima, I., and Robinson, A. Fertility in a 45,X female. *Pediatrics* 47:770, 1971.

99. Nance, W. E., and Uchida, I. Turner's syndrome, twinning, and an unusual variant of glucose-6-phosphate dehydrogenase. *Am. J. Hum. Genet.* 16:380, 1964.

100. Neu, R. L., and Gardner, L. I. Abnormalities of the sex chromosomes. *In* Gardner, L. I., ed.: *Endocrine and Genetic Diseases of Childhood.* Philadelphia, W. B. Saunders Co., 1969, pp. 682–703.

101. Nowakowski, H., and Lenz, W. Genetic aspects in male hypogonadism. *Rec. Progr. Horm. Res.* 17:53, 1961.

102. Perez-Ballester, B., Greenblatt, R. B., and Byrd, J. R. Familial gonadal dysgenesis. *Am. J. Obstet. Gynecol.* 107:1262, 1970.

103. Polani, P. E. Hormonal and clinical aspects of hermaphroditism and the testicular feminizing syndrome in man. *Philos. Trans. R. Soc. Lond.* (B) 259:187, 1970.

104. Polani, P. E., Angell, R., Giannelli, F., et al. Evidence that the Xg locus is inactivated in structurally abnormal X chromosomes. *Nature* (London) 227:613, 1970.

105. Race, R. R., and Sanger, R. Xg and sex-chromosome abnormalities. *Br. Med. Bull.* 25:99, 1969.

106. Reveno, J. S., and Palubinskas, A. J. Congenital renal abnormalities in gonadal dysgenesis. *Radiology* 86:49, 1966.

107. Rimoin, D. L., and Schimke, R. N. *Genetic Disorders of the Endocrine Glands.* Saint Louis, The C. V. Mosby Co., 1971.

108. Rosenberg, H. S., Clayton, G. W., and Hsu, T. C. Familial true hermaphroditism. *J. Clin. Endocrinol.* 23:203, 1963.

109. Sanger, R., Tippet, P., and Gavin, J. Xg groups and sex abnormalities in people of northern European ancestry. *J. Med. Genet.* 8:417, 1971.

110. Sarto, G. E., Therman, E., and Patau, K. X inactivation in man: A woman with t(Xr−;12q+). *Am. J. Hum. Genet.* 25:262, 1973.

111. Schlegel, R. J., Neu, R. L., Leao, J. C., and Gardner, L. I. XX sex chromosomes in cells cultured from "streak gonads" and in peripheral leukocytes. *J. Clin. Endocrinol.* 27:1588, 1967.

112. Scully, R. E. Gonadoblastoma. *Cancer* 25:1340, 1970.

113. Segall, M., Shapiro, L. R., Freedman, W., and Boone, J. A. XO/XY gonadal dysgenesis and gonadoblastoma in childhood. *Obstet. Gynecol.* 41:536, 1973.

114. Shaffer, J. W. A specific cognitive deficit observed in gonadal aplasia (Turner's syndrome). *J. Clin. Psychol.* 18:403, 1962.

115. Shapiro, L. R., Hsu, L. Y. F., and Hirschhorn, K. Extra posterior cervical skin. A possible sign of chromosomal aberration in infancy. *J. Pediatr.* 77:690, 1970.

116. Simpson, J. L. Gonadal dysgenesis and abnormalities of the human sex chromosomes: Current status of phenotypic-karyotypic correlations. *In* Bergsma, D., ed.: *Genetic Forms of Hypogonadism.* Miami, Symposia Specialists, 1975, pp. 23–59.

117. Simpson, J. L., Christakos, A. C., Horwith, M., and Silverman, F. S. Gonadal dysgenesis in individuals with apparently normal chromosomal complements: Tabulation of cases and compilation of genetic data. *In* Bergsma, D., ed.: *Part X. The Endocrine System, Birth Defects: Original Article Series.* Baltimore, Williams and Wilkins Co., for The National Foundation–March of Dimes, 1971, Vol. VII, No. 6, pp. 215–228.

118. Simpson, J. L., New, M., Peterson, R. E., and German, J. Pseudovaginal perineo-scrotal hypospadius (PPSH) in sibs. *In* Bergsma, D., ed.: *Part X. The Endocrine System, Birth Defects: Original Article Series.* Baltimore, Williams and Wilkins Co., for The National Foundation–March of Dimes, 1971, Vol. VII, No. 6, pp. 140–144.

119. Singh, R. P., and Carr, D. H. The anatomy and histology of XO human embryos and fetuses. *Anat. Rec. 155:*369, 1966.

120. Singh, R. P., and Carr, D. H. Anatomic findings in human abortions of known chromosomal constitution. *Obstet. Gynecol. 29:*806, 1967.

121. Smith, D. W., Bartlett, C., and Harrah, L. M. Duhamel anomalad and monozygotic twinning: An association between two malformations. *Birth Defects Conference.* Kansas City, 1975, p. 92 (abstact).

122. Smith, D. W., Marden, P. M., McDonald, M. J., and Speckhard, M. Lower incidence of sex chromatin in buccal smears of newborn females. *Pediatrics 30:*707, 1962.

123. Sohval, A. R. The syndrome of pure gonadal dysgenesis. *Am. J. Med. 38:*615, 1965.

124. Stanesco, V., Maxmilian, C., Florea, I., and Ciovirnache, M. Trois soeurs avec dysgenesie gonadale pure et caryotype XY. *Ann. Endocrinol. 29:*449, 1968.

125. Stempfel, R. S., Jr. Disorders of sexual development. *In* Gardner, L. I., ed.: *Endocrine and Genetic Disease of Childhood.* Philadelphia, W. B. Saunders Co., 1969, pp. 500–521.

126. Sternberg, W. H., Barclay, D. L., and Kloepfer, H. W. Familial XY gonadal dysgenesis. *N. Engl. J. Med. 278:*695, 1968.

127. Taylor, A. I. Sex chromatin in the newborn. *Lancet 1:*912, 1963.

128. Tjio, J. H., and Levan, A. The chromosome number of man. *Hereditas 42:*1, 1956.

129. Turner, H. H. Syndrome of infantilism, congenital webbed neck, and cubitus valgus. *Endocrinology 23:*566, 1938.

130. Ullrich, O. Turner's syndrome and status Bonnevie-Ullrich: A synthesis of animal phenogenetics and clinical observations on a typical complex of developmental anomalies. *Am. J. Hum. Genet. 1:*179, 1949.

131. Van Campenhout, J., and Leduc, B. Unusual features in the Rokitansky–Küster–Hauser syndrome. *Lancet 2:*928, 1971.

132. Willemse, C. H. A patient suffering from Turner's syndrome and acromegaly. *Acta Endocrinol. 39:*204, 1962.

133. Williams, E. D., Engel, E., and Forbes, A. P. Thyroiditis and gonadal dysgenesis. *N. Engl. J. Med. 270:*805, 1964.

134. Wilson, J. D., and Goldstein, J. L. Classification of heriditary disorders of sexual development. *In* Bergsma, D., ed.: *Genetic Forms of Hypogonadism.* Miami, Symposia Specialists, 1975, pp. 1–16.

135. Zurbrügg, R. P. Congenital adrenal hyperplasia. *In* Gardner, L. I., ed.: *Endocrine and Genetic Diseases of Childhood.* Philadelphia, W. B. Saunders Co., 1969, pp. 407–428.

Bernard Czernobilsky, M.D.

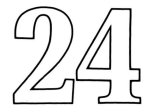

# Primary Epithelial Tumors of the Ovary

## Introduction

In the histogenetic classification of ovarian neoplasms the epithelial tumors belong to the group of "tumors of surface-epithelial and ovarian-stromal origin,[95] also known as tumors of "paramesonephric celomic (germinal, Müllerian)" derivation.[51] These constitute the majority of ovarian neoplasms.

Although the origin of the majority of these tumors from the capsular or so-called germinal epithelium and the underlying stroma has been accepted by most authorities, the evidence supporting this histogenesis varies in the individual tumors from fairly conclusive to merely circumstantial. In this discussion this aspect is considered separately with each of the neoplasms. It should be emphasized that the histologic pleomorphism and heterogeneity encountered in this group of tumors by no means contradict their common origin. Although the ovary is not of Müllerian origin, the source of these neoplasms, namely, the germinal epithelium is derived from the celomic epithelium, which in the embryo gives rise to the Müllerian duct; this latter as is well known, forms the fallopian tubes, uterine body, cervix, and part of the vagina with their large variety of epithelia. The presence of different epithelial elements in these tumors therefore can be satisfactorily explained; however, the cause for the great neoplastic potential of the ovarian germinal epithelium has not yet been elucidated.

**Table 24.1   Primary epithelial tumors of the ovary**

I. Serous tumors
   A. Serous cystadenoma
   B. Borderline serous cystadenoma
   C. Serous cystadenocarcinoma
   D. Cystadenofibroma
   E. Adenofibroma
   F. Malignant adenofibroma

II. Mucinous tumors
   A. Mucinous cystadenoma
   B. Borderline mucinous cystadenoma
   C. Mucinous cystadenocarcinoma

III. Endometrioid tumors
   A. Endometrioma
   B. Endometrioid carcinoma

IV. Clear cell carcinoma

V. Brenner tumors
   A. Benign Brenner tumor
   B. Proliferating Brenner tumor
   C. Malignant Brenner tumor

VI. Mixed epithelial and mesenchymal tumors
   A. Carcinosarcoma
   B. Mixed mesodermal tumor

VII. Adenomatoid tumor

VIII. Adenocarcinoma not otherwise classifiable

Table 24.1 lists the order in which the various epithelial tumors are discussed in this chapter. This is a simplified version of the listing of "Common Epithelial Tumours" in the "Histologic Classification of Ovarian Tumours" issued by the World Health Organization (Table 24.2). This listing although complete in its enumeration of all possible variations and combinations of epithelial neoplasms would unnecessarily complicate the presentation of our material and be too cumbersome for the purpose of this chapter. As is evident from Table 24.1 most of the tumors can be divided into benign and malignant forms. In addition, there are "borderline" situations, which according to Scully[95] exist in almost all of the listed neoplasms. However, because borderline and proliferating forms of epithelial ovarian neoplasia have been adequately studied in the serous, mucinous, and Brenner tumors only, detailed discussion of this feature will be limited to these three neoplasms.

Admixtures of histologic elements from various epithelial ovarian tumors within a given tumor are very common and constitute further proof of their common derivation.

Hence, separate listings of all possible histologic combinations for each of the tumors are not feasible. Instead, neoplasms are classified according to their predominant component, with mention of mixed forms whenever relevant.

A clear-cut distinction between functioning and nonfunctioning ovarian tumors is no longer possible since it is now well known that almost all ovarian neoplasms including primary epithelial tumors are capable of endocrine activity. The morphologic expression of this activity is the presence of luteinized and or enzymatically active stromal cells (EACS) within the ovaries harboring the epithelial neoplasms. In order to avoid repetitions, therefore, these particular histologic features of all these neoplasms are dealt with in one separate section at the end of the chapter.

**Table 24.2   Histologic classification of ovarian tumors: Common "epithelial" tumors[a]**

I. Serous tumors
   A. Benign
      1. Cystadenoma and papillary cystadenoma
      2. Surface papilloma
      3. Adenofibroma and cystadenofibroma
   B. Of borderline malignancy (carcinomas of low malignant potential)
      1. Cystadenoma and papillary cystadenoma
      2. Surface papilloma
      3. Adenofibroma and cystadenofibroma
   C. Malignant
      1. Adenocarcinoma, papillary adenocarcinoma, and papillary cystadenocarcinoma
      2. Surface papillary carcinoma
      3. Malignant adenofibroma and cystadenofibroma

II. Mucinous tumors
   A. Benign
      1. Cystadenoma
      2. Adenofibroma and cystadenofibroma
   B. Of borderline malignancy (carcinomas of low malignant potential)
      1. Cystadenoma
      2. Adenofibroma and cystadenofibroma
   C. Malignant
      1. Adenocarcinoma and cystadenocarcinoma
      2. Malignant adenofibroma and cystadenofibroma

III. Endometrioid tumors
   A. Benign
      1. Adenoma and cystadenoma
      2. Adenofibroma and cystadenofibroma

B. Of borderline malignancy (carcinomas of low malignant potential)
    1. Adenoma and cystadenoma
    2. Adenofibroma and cystadenofibroma
C. Malignant
    1. Carcinoma
       a. Adenocarcinoma
       b. Adenoacanthoma
       c. Malignant adenofibroma and cystadenofibroma
    2. Endometrioid stromal sarcomas
    3. Mesodermal (Müllerian) mixed tumors, homologous and heterologous

IV. Clear cell (mesonephroid) tumors
    A. Benign: adenofibroma
    B. Of borderline malignancy (carcinomas of low malignant potential)

V. Brenner tumors
    A. Benign
    B. Of borderline malignancy (proliferating)
    C. Malignant

VI. Mixed epithelial tumors
    A. Benign
    B. Of borderline malignancy
    C. Malignant

VII. Undifferentiated carcinoma

VIII. Unclassified epithelial tumors

---

[a] From *International Histological Classification of Tumours, No. 9: Histological Classification of Ovarian Tumours, 1973.* [Reproduced by permission of the copyright holder, World Health Organization.]

# Serous Tumors

## Serous Cystadenoma

It is quite obvious that the benign serous cystadenoma originates in the germinal epithelium of the ovary. These tumors possess the same histologic structures as the common germinal epithelium inclusion cysts, which arise through invaginations of the surface epithelium.[80] For example, serous cystadenomas may develop either in pre-existing germinal epithelium inclusion cysts or in the germinal surface epithelium itself.

These are common tumors, forming about 23% of all benign ovarian neoplasms.[4] The majority of these neoplasms are encountered between the ages of 30 and 40 years,[51] although they can even occur in infancy.[72] In about 20% of the cases the tumors are bilateral.[46]

Grossly, these are cystic, often large neoplasms filled with clear serous liquid, although occasionally one may also encounter a more stringy mucous material.[95] Therefore, the diagnosis cannot be established from the nature of the fluid but should be based on the histologic features of the epithelial lining cells. The external surface of the cyst is smooth and glistening, often with a marked vascular pattern (Figure 24.1). The majority of these neoplasms are unilocular but multilocular forms do exist. The inner lining either is entirely flat or may present areas with grossly visible papillary projections (Figure 24.2). In the benign serous cystadenomas the papillary projections practically never cover the entire inner surface of the tumor. Whenever this occurs the tumor is either frankly malignant or of the borderline variety.

On microscopic examination, the predominant lining

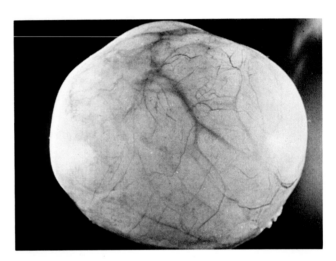

**24.1** External surface of a serous cystadenoma demonstrating a smooth capsule with prominent vasculature.

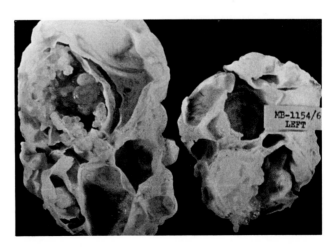

**24.2** Cut surface of a serous cystadenoma showing a multilocular structure with papillary areas.

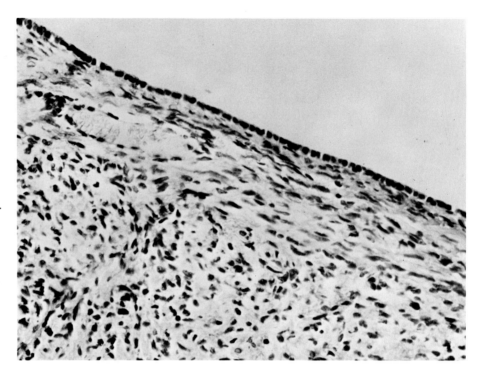

**24.3** Low cuboidal epithelial lining cells of serous cystadenoma. Hematoxylin–eosin, ×250.

cell of both the smooth and papillary areas consists of a single layer of regular cuboidal epithelium, with basally arranged uniform nuclei. However, as in other Müllerian neoplasms, a variety of epithelial cells, such as columnar, cuboidal, mucous-secreting, ciliated, clear, and hobnail, are frequently encountered (Figures 24.3 through 24.5). In large cysts under pressure, the epithelium is usually cuboidal, probably as a result of compression by the fluid. The luminal border of these cells contains diastase-resistant periodic acid Schiff (PAS), mucicarmine- and alcian blue-positive material. Mitoses are not encountered. Psammoma bodies, which are rounded microscopic calcifications formed most likely as a result of degenerative changes, are frequently present within the papillary projections (Figure 24.6). The stroma of the cyst wall as well as that of the papillary projections consists of connective tissue with scattered blood vessels. It is occasionally edematous and hyalinized.

Ultrastructural studies of the epithelial lining cells of serous cystadenomas[37] reveal generally uniform oval nuclei, with only mild irregularities of nuclear borders and relatively homogenous central chromatin, which is condensed along the periphery. Microvilli and cilia are present along the luminal border. Interdigitations are prominent and numerous (Figure 24.7). Of all the above, the absence of prominent nuclear irregularity and the presence of

marked complex cell interdigitations seem to characterize the benign serous cystadenomas as compared to borderline and malignant lesions.[37]

Because the serous cystadenomas are perfectly benign neoplasms, surgical ablation constitutes adequate therapy.

## Borderline Serous Cystadenoma

Although borderline serous cystadenomas, also known as facultative or potentially malignant, were reported in the early 1950s,[55,117] these tumors were only incorporated in the classification of the International Federation of Gynecology and Obstetrics (FIGO) in 1964.[89]

The two main parameters that characterize these lesions and made them occupy an intermediate position between the benign serous cystadenomas and the frankly malignant serous cystadenocarcinomas are their histologic features and prognostic aspects.

Grossly, the borderline tumors are similar to the previously described benign serous cystadenomas with papillary projections, but the borderline tumors possibly show an increased incidence of bilaterality. In addition, the papillary component in the borderline lesions is usually more abundant than in the perfectly benign serous cystadenomas[58] (Figure 24.8).

The histologic criteria characterizing the borderline

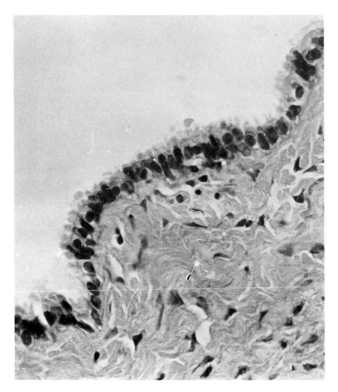

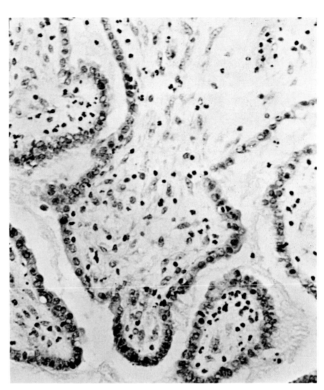

**24.4** Columnar and ciliated epithelial cells lining a serous cystadenoma. Hematoxylin–eosin, ×400.

**24.5** Papillary serous cystadenoma lined by a variety of epithelial cells. Hematoxylin–eosin, ×250.

**24.6** Psammoma bodies in the wall of a serous cystadenoma demonstrating the typical concentric arrangement. Hematoxylin–eosin, ×400.

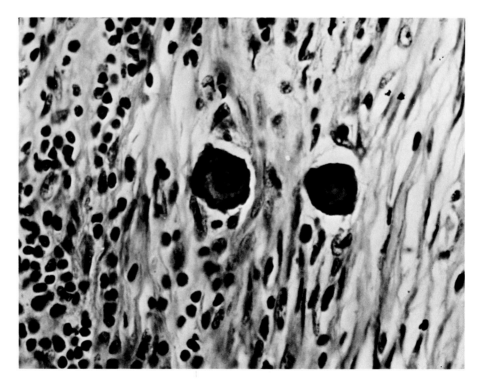

**24.7** Electron micrograph of serous cystadenoma with slightly irregular nuclear borders, numerous cell membrane interdigitations (Id), desmosomes (D), and terminal bars (Tb). Cytoplasm includes supranuclear Golgi complex (G), round to oval mitochondria (Mi), and dense bodies (DB). ×16,720.

[Reprinted by permission from B. Gondos, Electron microscopic study of papillary serous tumors of the ovary, *Cancer* 27:1455, 1971, J. B. Lippincott.]

tumors can be summarized as follows: stratification of the epithelial lining of the papillae; formation of microscopic papillary projections or tufts arising from the epithelial lining of the papillae; epithelial pleomorphism; atypicality; and mitotic activity (Figures 24.9 and 24.10). According to Janovski and Paramanandhan[51] at least two of the above features must be present in order for the tumor to quality as borderline. Fisher et al.[33] specify that the number of mitoses in this lesion should be less than one per high-power field. From the above, it becomes evident that except for the absence of stromal invasion in

the borderline serous cystadenoma, there are no clear-cut histologic differences between this tumor and a well-differentiated serous cystadenocarcinoma. It should be emphasized, however, that because of the pronounced papillary structure of these tumors, the aspect of invasion is often difficult to evaluate. According to Fisher et al.,[33] a desmoplastic reaction of the stroma of the papillary projections is more frequent in the borderline and frankly malignant tumors than in the benign serous cystadenoma.

In an electron microscopic investigation of papillary serous tumors of the ovary,[37] two borderline lesions stud-

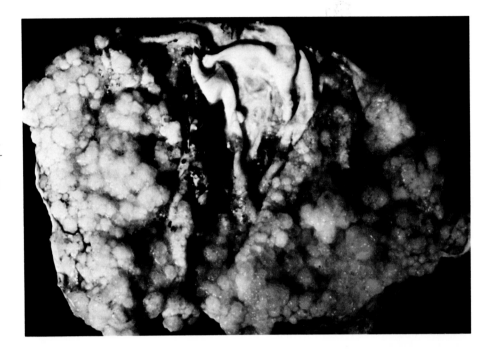

**24.8** Borderline serous cystadenoma showing an exuberant growth of papillary projections arising in large areas of inner lining.

ied showed a marked degree of nuclear infolding, which also characterized the nuclei of serous cystadenocarcinomas (Figure 24.11). In contrast, the epithelial cells of borderline tumors did show cilia, which were absent in the frankly malignant neoplasms. Interdigitations were less prominent than in the benign serous cystadenomas.

As has been mentioned before, the prognostic aspect of the borderline lesion, as compared to that of frank carcinoma, has been used as one of the distinguishing features between the two. In the Fisher et al.[33] series none of the patients with borderline tumors died of their disease within 5 years, whereas during the same period of time the mortality rate of serous cystadenocarcinoma was 50%. Santesson and Kottmeier[89] reported a 10-year survival for borderline serous cystadenoma of 76%, with the corresponding figure of 13% for serous cystadenocarcinoma.

We believe that although the borderline serous cystadenoma appears to be a well-established entity, it remains a controversial one. This is because the criteria of borderline malignancy vary, ranging from individual cellular changes[33,51] to cases with peritoneal implants that apparently regress after removal of the primary tumors.[108] Although there is no doubt that there exists a group of low-grade malignant tumors among the serous cystadenocarcinomas of the ovary, it is doubtful whether qualifying terms of "borderline," "facultative," or "potentially malignant" are the appropriate ones. This is more than a seman-

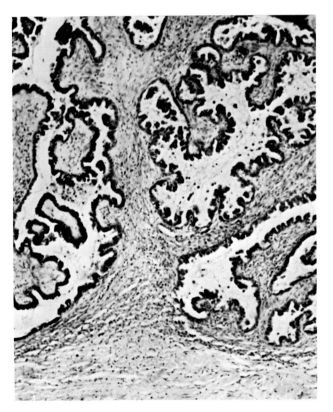

**24.9** Irregular papillary growth in a borderline serous cystadenoma. Hematoxylin–eosin, ×42.

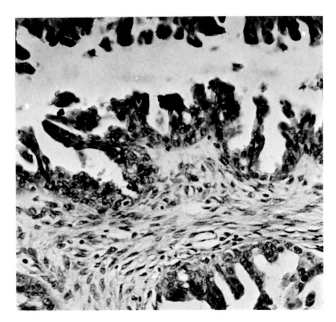

**24.10** Detail of the epithelial lining in a borderline serous cystadenoma showing stratification, pleomorphism, and tuft formations. Hematoxylin–eosin, ×250.

tic problem because therapy and prognostication is often determined by the pathologist's terminology. Therefore, a tumor classified as essentially benign, regardless of a variety of qualifying terms, is sometimes being dealt with conservatively, even in those cases in which circumstances justify a more radical approach. Because many of the histologic features and prognostic aspects of the borderline serous cystadenomas are closer to malignant than benign tumors, it may perhaps be preferable to classify them as well-differentiated, low-grade, noninvasive serous cystadenocarcinomas.

Treatment should strive to completely extirpate the tumor, if unilateral, provided a thorough examination, including biopsy of the contralateral ovary, reveals no neoplasm there. In cases of bilateral involvement, papillary projections on the external surface of the tumor, or peritoneal spread, a more radical surgical approach, such as total hysterectomy with bilateral tuboophorectomy, is advocated. This therapy will be curative in most patients with localized borderline serous cystadenomas. Recurrences, peritoneal seeding, and death occur mostly in those patients who because of the assumption that this tumor is essentially benign have been inadequately treated.

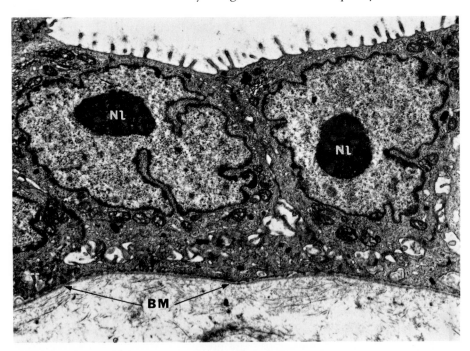

**24.11** Electron micrograph of a borderline serous cystadenoma showing deep nuclear indentations, prominent regular nucleoli (Nl), and smooth basal lamina (BM). ×6,045.

[Reprinted by permission from B. Gondos, Electron microscopic study of papillary serous tumors of the ovary, *Cancer* 27:1455, 1971, J. B. Lippincott.]

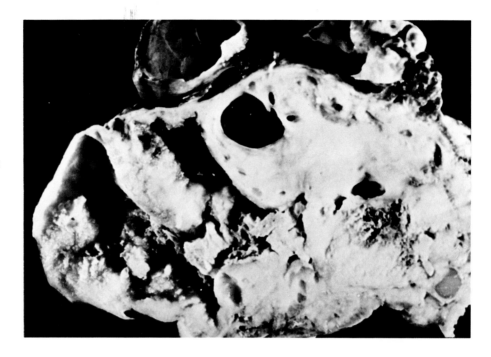

**24.12** Cut surface of a serous cystadenocarcinoma showing a partly cystic neoplasm with large areas of solid and friable tumor masses.

## Serous Cystadenocarcinoma

These are the most common malignant ovarian tumors, comprising approximately 40% of the total.[88] They are bilateral in about 50% of the cases[51] and occur most frequently between the ages of 40 and 60 years.[51]

According to Allen and Hertig,[1] 56.2% of these tumors measure over 15 cm in diameter, 39.9% from 5 to 15 cm, and 3.9% less than 5 cm in diameter. These are primarily cystic, multiloculated tumors, although the soft, friable, proliferating papillae may fill the entire cavity (Figure 24.12). In contrast to the benign serous cystadenomas, the malignant tumors are always extensively papillary. Fluid if present is usually turbid or bloody. The external surface is smooth or may present papillary projections, which are the result of penetration of the tumor through the cyst wall.

Histologically the serous cystadenocarcinomas can be divided into well-differentiated, moderately well-differentiated, and poorly differentiated varieties. These correspond to grades I, II, and III reported by Allan and Hertig.[1]

In the well-differentiated serous cystadenocarcinomas, the papillary structures are well formed, with prominent fibrous stalks. This pattern is less regular in the moderately well-differentiated tumors, where the papillae are more crowded together and individual stalks cannot always be made out. In the poorly differentiated tumors the papillary pattern is usually obliterated to a great extent and the tumor appears to be made up of solid sheaths of cells

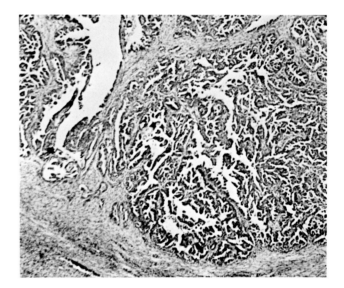

**24.13** Well-differentiated serous cystadenocarcinoma with crowded, irregular papillary structures pushing and invading into the surrounding stroma. Hematoxylin–eosin, ×40.

(Figures 24.13 through 24.15). Histologic grading is therefore primarily based on the papillary pattern and not on the epithelial lining cells, which may show various degrees of atypism, pleomorphism, mitotic activity, and admixtures with epithelia of other Müllerian neoplasms in

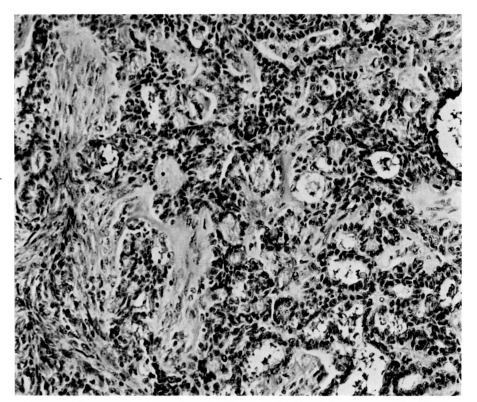

**24.14** Moderately well-differentiated serous cystadenocarcinoma with a prominent cellular stroma. Hematoxylin–eosin, ×250.

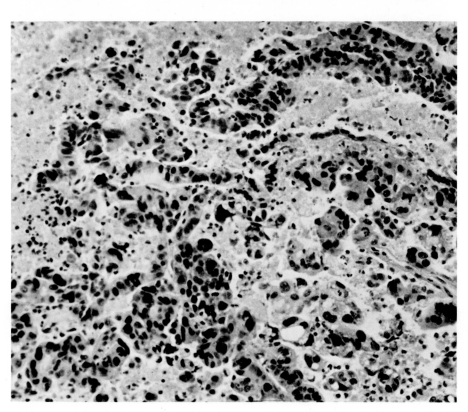

**24.15** Poorly differentiated serous cystadenocarcinoma showing highly anaplastic tumor cells with only a suggestion of papillary arrangement. Hematoxylin–eosin, ×250.

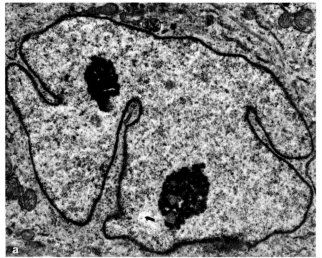

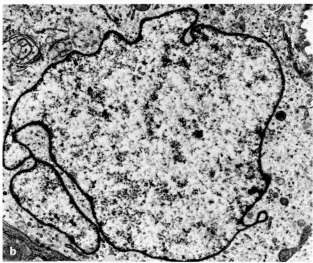

**24.16** Electron microphotograph of the nuclei of serous cystadenocarcinoma, showing multiple deep indentations and prominent nucleoli (**a**), ×9,490, and irregular lobulation (**b**), ×9,855.

[Reprinted by permission from B. Gondos, Electron microscopic study of papillary serous tumors of the ovary, *Cancer* 27:1455, 1971, J. B. Lippincott.]

all of the three grades. Furthermore, capsular invasion also, occurs, regardless of histologic grading. According to Aure et al.,[7] psammoma bodies were found in 32.5% of serous cystadenocarcinomas. In addition, a significantly higher survival rate was found in cases with such calcifications than in those without. The authors propose that the development of psammoma bodies reflects a specific tumor–host reaction. Here too as in the benign and borderline lesions, the luminal border of the epithelial cells stain positively with diastase-resistant PAS, mucicarmine, and alcian blue stains.

The ultrastructural characteristics of the epithelium of these tumors[37] include marked nuclear irregularity, a decreased amount of cell membrane interdigitation, and reduced cilia (Figure 24.16). As mentioned before, these features differ significantly from those of the benign serous cystadenoma but present many similarities to the borderline lesions. Ferenczy et al.[31] described both endometrial- and endocervical-type cells in the well-differentiated tumors. These authors postulate that the latter is the source of the occasional mucin production seen in these neoplasms.

Clinical staging of the lesion, usually done at time of initial surgery, appears to be of primary prognostic significance.[9] Histologic differentiation and grading is of much less value in predicting the outcome of the disease. Because early detection methods, which are of crucial importance, have not improved significantly, the prognosis of serous cystadenocarcinomas remains poor with an overall 5-year survival rate of less than 20%.[89] The scope of this chapter does not allow for any detailed discussion of modalities of therapy. Radical surgery with radiotherapy remains the main method of treatment in most of the cases, supplemented lately by chemotherapeutic agents, especially in more advanced clinical stages.[9]

## Cystadenofibroma

This is the one neoplasm in the entire group of epithelial tumors in which the origin from the ovarian surface epithelium and underlying stroma can be most easily traced. Nevertheless, cystadenofibromas occupy an equivocal position among ovarian tumors. Although some look on them as mere variants of serous cystadenomas,[58] others consider them as fairly common tumors.[65] In the Czernobilsky et al.[20] series, cystadenofibromas constituted 46.5% of all benign ovarian cystic serous tumors. According to Scott,[94] over 90% of the patients were 40 years old and older. This was not borne out in the more recent series,[20] where the patients ages ranged from 15 to 65 with a mean of 30.7 years.

Because small papillary projections arising from the ovarian surface are fairly common, it is advisable not to make a diagnosis of cystadenofibroma if the lesion is less than 1 cm in diameter. In the Czernobilsky et al.[20] series, the tumors varied in size from 1 to 20 cm, with a mean of 9 cm. These neoplasms are cystic, with small, tight clusters

**24.17** Cystadenofibroma showing tight clusters of firm, short, rounded papillary structures arising from the cyst wall.

[Reprinted by permission from B. Czernobilsky, R. Borenstein, and M. Lancet, Cystoadenofibroma of the ovary. A clinicopathologic study of 34 cases and comparison with serous cystadenoma, *Cancer* 34:1971, 1974, J. B. Lippincott.]

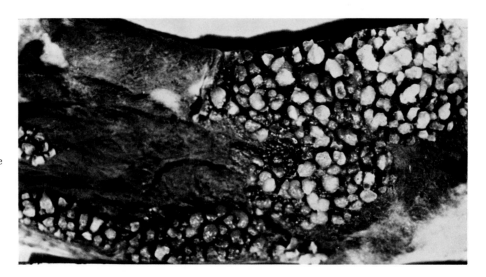

**24.18** Papillary projections of cystadenofibroma consisting of broad, fibrous structures lined by epithelial cells. Hematoxylin-eosin, ×40.

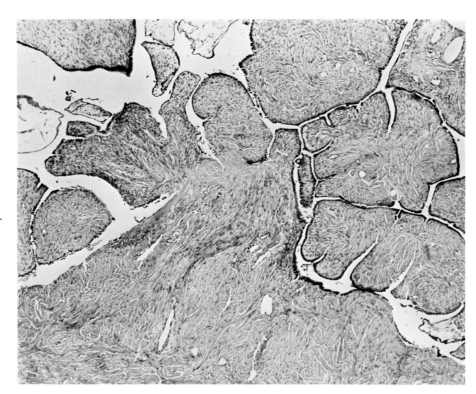

of short, rounded papillary structures (Figure 24.17). In contrast, the papillary projections of the serous cystadenomas are softer and more elongated and usually occupy larger areas of the inner cyst lining. Some of the cystadenofibromas are multiloculated. The intracystic fluid is of the serous, clear type. Bilaterality varies in different reports from 5.8%[20] to 15%.[47]

The epithelium lining the cyst wall and its papillary projections is similar to that of the serous cystadenomas and includes cuboidal, columnar, ciliated, hobnail, and clear cells (Figures 24.18 through 24.20). No atypism or mitotic figures are present. As in the other papillary tumors, psammoma bodies are occasionally found. We found no borderline tumors among our cases studied.[20] The

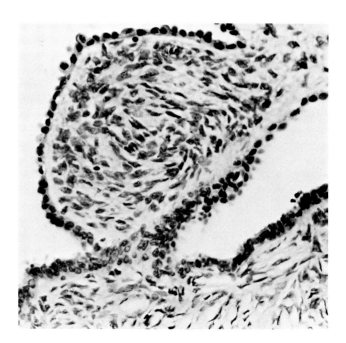

**24.19** Cuboidal, columnar, and hobnail-type epithelial lining of a cystadenofibroma. Hematoxylin–eosin, ×250.

[Reprinted by permission from B. Czernobilsky, R. Borenstein, and M. Lancet, Cystoadenofibroma of the ovary. A clinicopathologic study of 34 cases and comparison with serous cystadenoma, *Cancer 34:*1971, 1974, J. B. Lippincott.]

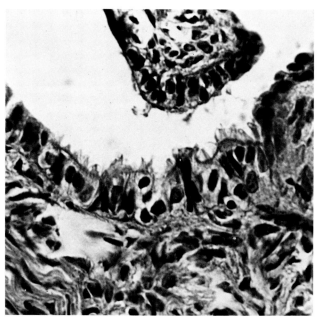

**24.20** Ciliated cells with interspersed clear cells lining a cystadenofibroma. Hematoxylin–eosin, ×400.

[Reprinted by permission from B. Czernobilsky, R. Borenstein, and M. Lancet, Cystoadenofibroma of the ovary. A clinicopathologic study of 34 cases and comparison with serous cystadenoma, *Cancer 34:*1971, 1974, J. B. Lippincott.]

epithelium presents the same staining reactions with PAS, mucicarmine, and alcian blue stains as it does in the serous tumors.

The stroma of the papillary structures ranges from highly cellular fibrous to almost acellular hyalinized tissue. Severe stromal edema is a common finding (Figure 24.21). A highly characteristic feature is a narrow, acellular zone of connective tissue situated between the epithelial lining cells and the fibrous stroma of the papillae (Figure 24.22). This was present in about one-third of the cases in the Czernobilsky et al.[20] series. This same acellular zone is also present in the cortex of the normal ovary (Figure 24.23). Occasionally, the cyst wall presents thickened areas, which are composed of fibrous stroma and glandular spaces lined by the same type of epithelium as the papillary projections. These are still classified as cystadenofibroma, because the diagnosis of adenofibroma is reserved to grossly solid or predominantly solid tumors only (Table 24.3).

Transmission electron micrography of this tumor[31] demonstrates mature ciliated cells with numerous supranuclear mitochondria and cross-striated ciliary rootlets (Figure 24.24).

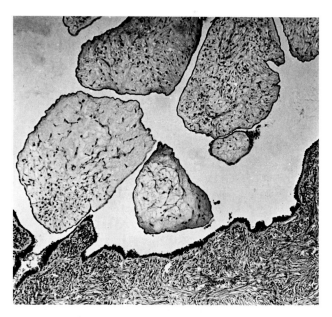

**24.21** Markedly edematous papillary formations arising in the wall of a cystadenofibroma. Hematoxylin–eosin, ×31.

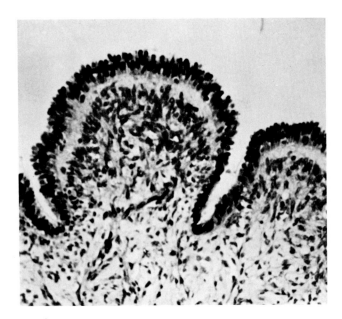

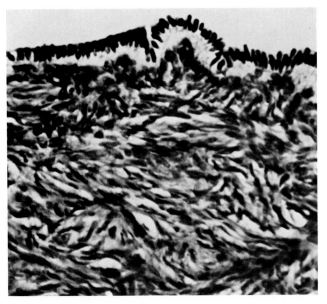

**24.22** Narrow, acellular zone of connective tissue situated between the epithelial lining and the fibrous stroma of the papillae in a cystadenofibroma. Hematoxylin–eosin, ×100.

[Reprinted by permission from B. Czernobilsky, R. Borenstein, and M. Lancet, Cystoadenofibroma of the ovary. A clinicopathologic study of 34 cases and comparison with serous cystadenoma, *Cancer 34*:1971, 1974, J. B. Lippincott.]

**24.23** Acellular zone of connective tissue underneath the surface epithelium of a normal ovary. Hematoxylin–eosin, ×100.

[Reprinted by permission from B. Czernobilsky, R. Borenstein, and M. Lancet, Cystoadenofibroma of the ovary. A clinicopathologic study of 34 cases and comparison with serous cystadenoma, *Cancer 34*:1971, 1974, J. B. Lippincott.]

**24.24** Electron micrograph of mature ciliated cells with supranuclear mitochondria and lipid droplets (Li), similar to those of normal oviductal mucosa, which are characteristic of the lining cells of cystadenofibroma. ×4,437.

[Courtesy of Dr. A. Ferenczy.]

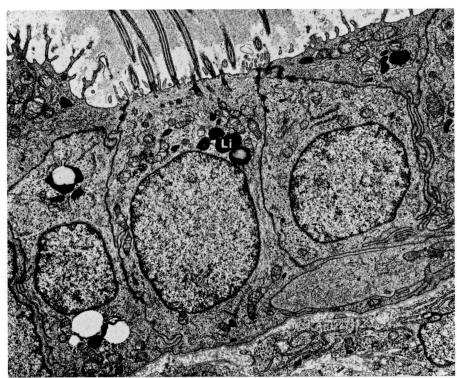

**Table 24.3** Microscopic features of 34 cystadenofibromas and 39 cystadenomas[a]

| Features | Cystadeno-fibroma (no. of cases) | Cystadenoma (no. of cases) |
|---|---|---|
| Papillary projections | 34 | 14 |
| Epithelial lining | | |
|   Cuboidal | 34 | 39 |
|   Columnar | 22 | 20 |
|   Cilia | 11 | 10 |
|   Hobnail | 7 | 8 |
|   Clear | 4 | 1 |
|   Pseudostratification | 6 | 8 |
|   Psammoma bodies | 10 | 5 |
|   Tufting | 0 | 6 |
|   Atypism | 0 | 5 |
|   Mitoses | 0 | 5 |
|   Borderline malignancy | 0 | 3 |
| Stroma | | |
|   Spindle cells | 34 | 32 |
|   Collagen | 27 | 28 |
|   Hyaline | 15 | 3 |
|   Edema | 18 | 10 |
|   Subepithelial acellular layer | 11 | 1 |

[a] Each tumor presenting more than one cell type. [Reprinted by permission from B. Czernobilsky et al., *Cancer* 34:1970, 1974, J. B. Lippincott.]

Because cystadenofibromas are perfectly benign tumors, surgical removal of the lesion constitutes adequate therapy. Furthermore, because of characteristic macro- and microscopic appearance of these tumors, the pathologist should be able to arrive at a correct diagnosis when a frozen section is requested in the operating room, thus saving the patient unnecessary extensive surgery.

In conclusion, we believe that in spite of the many similarities between cystadenofibromas and serous cystadenomas, the former represents a distinct entity and so should be separately classified. The typical macro- and microscopic appearance of its papillary projections separates the cystadenofibroma from the serous cystadenomas. Furthermore, the cystadenofibroma, with its easily traceable origin from the ovarian surface, can be considered the prototype of ovarian neoplasms of germinal epithelium and underlying stroma origin and as such alone deserves a place in the histogenetic classification of ovarian tumors.

## Adenofibroma

The adenofibroma is a benign, solid, ovarian neoplasm composed of dense, fibrous connective tissue with interspersed glandular spaces of various sizes. Occasionally the latter may grow to become macroscopically visible. The lesion is often described together with the cystadenofibroma and considered as a solid variant of the latter.[47,80] Others treat these solid or predominantly solid neoplasms as a separate entity,[18,112] a course that we prefer to follow in our department. Nevertheless, there seems to be no doubt concerning the germinal epithelium–cortical stromal origin of this tumor, although this is more easily demonstrable in the previously described cystadenofibroma.

Because these tumors are usually discussed together with cystadenofibromas, reliable incidence figures are not available. It is quite apparent, however, that the solid adenofibroma is a rare neoplasm. In the Timonen and Purola[112] series patients' ages ranged from 23 to 70 years, with 50% of the tumors occuring over the age of 50.

As in the cases of cystadenofibromas, we do not consider the microscopic or tiny cortical adenofibromas as neoplasms. This was also the approach used by Timonen and Purola,[112] who separated these lesions into "small adenofibroma-like formations in the ovarian cortex" and "benign tumors."

Grossly these are solid or predominantly solid tumors ranging in size from 1 to about 15 cm. Except for the presence of tiny scattered cystic dots, the solid adenofibromas are similar to ovarian fibromas. About 20% of the tumors are bilateral, whereas 25% showed microscopic cortical adenofibromas in the contralateral ovary.[112]

Microscopically, the cystic spaces are lined by a variety of epithelia, similar to that described in the cystadenofibromas, with a predominance of the cuboidal type. Atypism and mitotic figures are not present. The cellularity of the stroma varies too, from highly cellular fibrous to almost acellular hyalinized areas (Figures 24.25 and 24.26). The luminal border of the epithelial cells, as well as the intraluminal fluid, stain positively with PAS, diastase-resistant, mucicarmine, and alcian blue stains.

Treatment should be conservative and removal of the tumor is curative.

## Malignant Adenofibroma

This appears to be an extremely rare tumor. Up to 1970 only 30 such cases were reported.[18,71,86,112] Because in the malignant adenofibromas it is the epithelial and not the

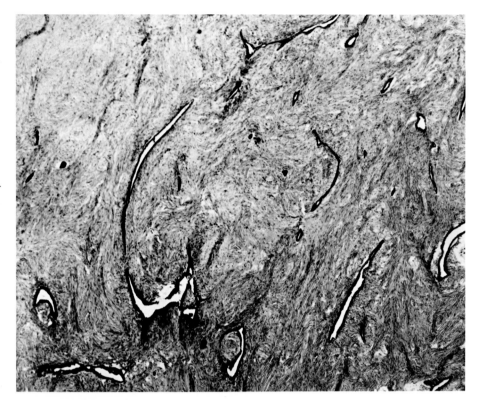

**24.25** Fibrous stroma with compressed slitlike glandular spaces in an adenofibroma. Hematoxylin–eosin, ×40.

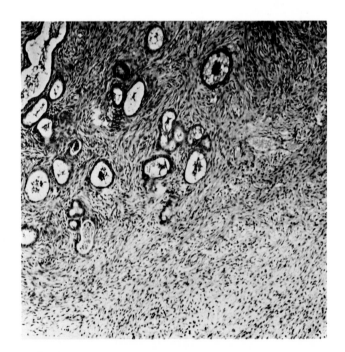

**24.26** Cellular stroma with rounded glands in an adenofibroma. Hematoxylin–eosin, ×100.

fibrous element that is malignant, a more accurate term would have been "adenocarcinofibroma." In contrast to the benign cystadeno- and adenofibromas the patients with the malignant neoplasms are all over the age of 40 years.[18,86,112]

On gross examination these tumors do not differ in any significant way from the benign adenofibromas. These, too, are solid lesions in which tiny cystic structures can be discerned. Five of the 10 reported cases by Timonen and Purola[112] and one of the three cases reported by Compton and Fink[18] were bilateral. The contralateral ovary occasionally contains benign adenofibromas.[18,112]

Microscopically, the glandular component of the tumor shows malignant characteristics, such as epithelial atypism, mitotic activity, piling up of epithelial layers, irregular glandular outlines, and invasive features (Figure 24.27). As in the other epithelial tumors of the ovary, because the epithelial element may vary considerably and include cuboidal, columnar, mucinous, clear, and hobnial cells, it may be difficult to reach the correct diagnosis. Differential diagnosis between this tumor and the parvilocular cystoma variant of the clear cell carcinoma may become particularly problematic, especially as the epithelial elements in the

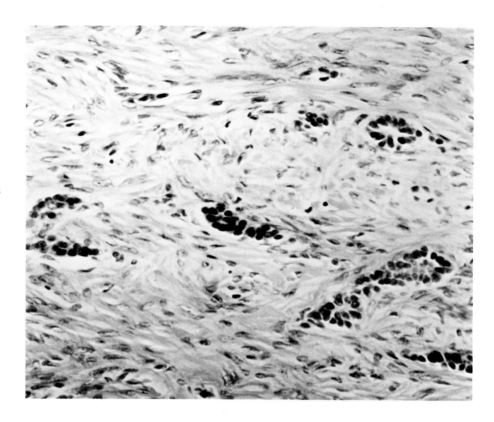

**24.27** Malignant adenofibroma showing malignant epithelial nests in the dense fibrous stroma. Hematoxylin–eosin, ×100.

latter can also be of a mixed variety. The diagnosis of malignant adenofibroma can be reached with more certainty, therefore, if in addition to the malignant features the tumor has preserved some of the benign components of an adenofibroma.

Because this tumor is a frank ovarian carcinoma, total hysterectomy with bilateral salpingo-oophorectomy is the treatment of choice. Postoperative radiation and chemotherapy has sometimes been added to the surgical treatment.[18,112] Five patients with malignant adenofibromas died within 1 year following surgical extirpation.[86,112] As in the ovarian malignancies, the extent of the tumor at time of operation to a large extent determines the prognosis.

# Mucinous Tumors

## Mucinous Cystadenoma

Whereas the origin of the serous tumors from the germinal epithelium is generally accepted, the histogenesis of mucinous tumors is more problematic.[83] The finding of goblet cells, argentaffin cells,[34] and Paneth cells[96] in some mucinous tumors, as well as the presence of cystic teratomas in about 5% of mucinous tumors,[17] has raised the possibility that mucinous neoplasms represent a teratoma in which the endodermal element alone has persisted.[17] However, the not infrequent admixture of elements from Müllerian-type neoplasms, such as serous, endometrial, and Brenner tumors, within mucinous cystadenomas[17,95] and the observation that germinal epithelium may undergo mucinous metaplasia[61,113] do support a Müllerian origin of mucinous tumors. In spite of conflicting reports as to the chemical similarities or differences between intestinal mucin and that contained with mucinous ovarian tumors,[17,35] the prefix "pseudo-" for the latter has by now been abandoned.

Mucinous cystadenomas comprise about 20% of all benign ovarian neoplasms.[54] The tumor is most frequent during the third to fifth decade,[47] although it does occur as well in young women. In the Jensen and Norris[52] series, mucinous cystadenomas constituted about 47% of benign epithelial tumors in patients less than 20 years of age.

Grossly these are cystic, frequently multiloculated tumors (Figure 24.28) ranging in diameter from 1 to 50 cm,

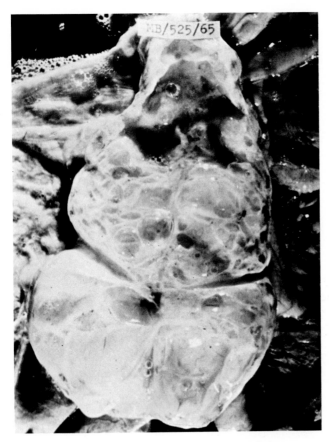

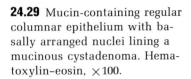

**24.28** Cystic multiloculated mucinous cystadenoma.

with the majority measuring 15 to 30 cm in diameter.[17] The external surface is that of an opaque or translucent cyst under pressure. On cut section the lining is usually smooth, although occasionally raised papillary areas can be identified. The cysts contain a thick, stringy material but here too, as in the serous cystadenomas, the diagnosis should only be established after microscopic examination of the neoplasms instead of from the gross appearance of the intracystic fluid, which can be misleading.[95] About 5% of the tumors are bilateral.[36]

On microscopic examination the characteristic lining of the mucinous cystadenoma is that of a single layer of tall, columnar epithelium with clear, homogenous cytoplasm and basally regularly arranged uniform nuclei with interspersed goblet cells (Figure 24.29). The entire cytoplasm, as well as the luminal content, stains positively with mucicarmine, PAS, and alcian blue stains. The stromal component is made up of fibrous tissue of varying cellularity.

Electron microscopic studies[29,60] have revealed that there exist two types of mucinous cells in these tumors. In 13 out of 17 mucinous cystadenomas studied by Langley et al.,[60] the epithelium resembled that of the endocervix, whereas in the remaining four cases it was of gastrointestinal type (Figure 24.30). Fenoglio et al.[29] reported pure endocervical and a mixed intestinal–endocervical type of mucinous cystadenomas. The latter authors do not consider the mixture of these cellular elements as contrary to

**24.29** Mucin-containing regular columnar epithelium with basally arranged nuclei lining a mucinous cystadenoma. Hematoxylin–eosin, ×100.

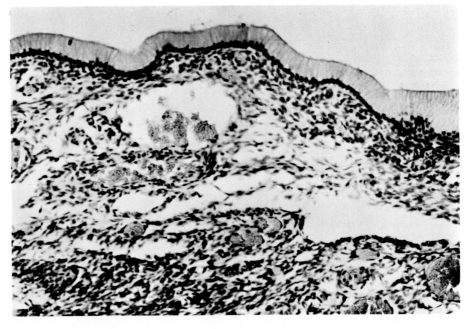

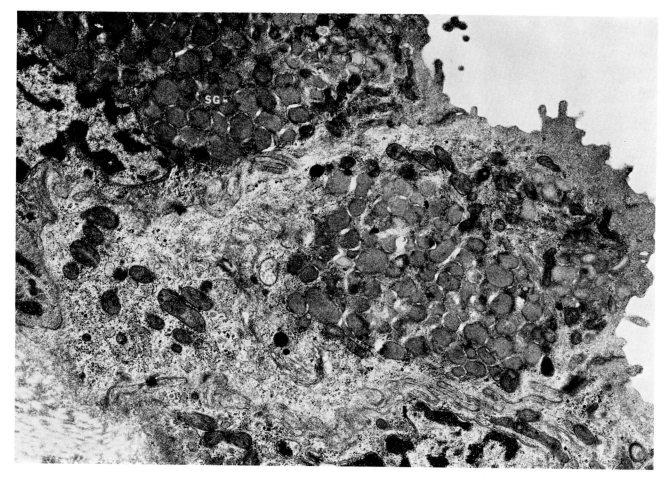

**24.30** Electron micrograph of the cells of a mucinous cystadenoma packed with mucin-containing secretory granules (SG) compressing the nucleus in the left upper corner of the photograph. These cells are similar to those found in normal endocervix. ×8,858.

[Courtesy of Dr. A. Ferenczy.]

the germinal epithelial origin of these neoplasms, for the metaplastic potential of this epithelium is well documented.

In these benign tumors removal of the involved ovary constitutes adequate therapy, provided the opposite ovary is carefully examined in order to rule out the presence of bilateral neoplasms. This should be done despite the fact that bilaterality in mucinous tumors is much less common than in the serous neoplasms.

One of the serious complications of ovarian mucinous cystadenomas is the appearance of pseudomyxoma peritonei in about 2 to 5% of the cases.[100,116] This consists of massive gelatinous accumulations, often arranged in a locular fashion in the peritoneal cavity, similar to that occasionally observed with mucoceles of the appendix. As

a matter of fact, appendiceal mucoceles, ovarian mucinous tumors, and pseudomyxomas peritonei do occasionally occur together in the same patient,[100] making it sometimes difficult if not impossible to determine the primary lesion. It is believed that the mucous-producing cells that implant on the peritoneal surfaces and secrete the vast amount of mucus reach the abdominal cavity through rupture of the ovarian cyst wall, although such a perforation is not always demonstrable. Microscopic dissection of the mucinous material through the cyst wall may constitute another such pathway.

Histologically, the extraovarian peritoneal epithelial implants are similar to the epithelium found within the ovarian mucinous cystadenomas, namely, strips of a single layer of mature, uniform, columnar or goblet-type epithe-

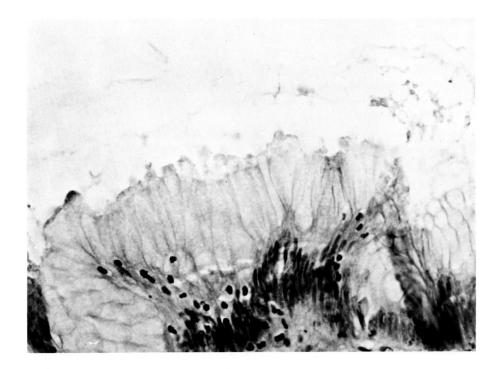

**24.31** Layer of mucinous cells attached to the peritoneal surface in a case of pseudomyxoma peritonei. Hematoxylin-eosin, ×100.

lium filled with mucus and basally arranged regular nuclei (Figure 24.31). As in the benign mucinous cystadenomas, no atypism or mitotic activity is encountered, and this in spite of the aggressive behavior and often dismal clinical outcome of these lesions. Individual epithelial cells are also found to be floating free within the gelatinous masses. In many instances the enormous masses of mucus present make it difficult to identify cellular elements.

Treatment is primarily surgical and, because of the recurrent nature of the lesion, often necessarily repetitive. Intraperitoneal alkylating agents have been used with some success, whereas the use of x-ray therapy, radioactive materials, and mucolytic agents has been disappointing.[62] Nevertheless, a 45% 5-year and 40% 10-year survival has been reported.[64]

## Borderline Mucinous Cystadenoma

Most of the reports of borderline malignancy in ovarian neoplasms have dealt with serous cystadenomas.[89,117] In studies dealing with borderline mucinous cystadenomas,[8,33,44,89] criteria have been similar to those used in borderline serous tumors, namely, histologic features and a prognosis superior to that of frank mucinous cystadenocarcinomas.

As histologic criteria of borderline mucinous tumors vary considerably, so do incidence figures of this neoplasm, which range from 17 to 52% of all mucinous carcinomas.[8,33,75,89] In the most recent series by Hart and Norris[44] 14% of all benign and malignant mucinous tumors belonged to the borderline group. According to Aure et al.[8] the mean age of patients with borderline tumors was lower than that of patients with frank carcinoma. Hart and Norris[44] found an age distribution of 9 to 70 years with a median of 35 years, which did not differ from the mean age of their patients with frank mucinous cystadenocarcinoma.

Grossly these neoplasms do not differ significantly from their benign counterpart. These are multilocular, cystic, frequently voluminous masses, with a smooth outer surface. The inner lining is also similar to that of the benign mucinous cystadenomas and is generally smooth, although papillary structures and solid thickening of the capsule have been observed in about 13 and 50%, respectively.[44] In the same series bilateral ovarian tumors were present in 8% of cases with borderline mucinous cystadenomas, although in 57% of these the tumor in the contralateral ovary was a perfectly benign mucinous cystadenoma.

Microscopically, in contrast to the benign mucinous cystadenomas the epithelial lining of the borderline tumors is characterized by stratification of two to three layers. Whereas in the benign tumors the cells show no atypism or pleomorphism, the epithelium of the borderline lesions does demonstrate atypism, with irregular, hyperchromatic nuclei and enlarged nucleoli. Mitotic figures are also encountered. Gland formations and a micro-

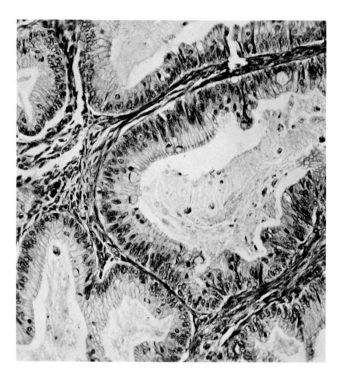

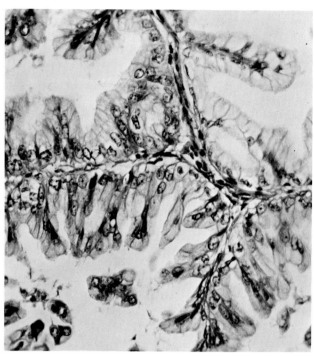

**24.32** Borderline mucinous cystadenoma showing strati-fied mucinous epithelium with atypical nuclei. Hema-toxylin–eosin, ×265.

[Reprinted by permission from W. R. Hart and H. J. Norris, Borderline and malignant mucinous tumors of the ovary. Histo-logic criteria and clinical behavior, *Cancer 31*:1031, 1973, J. B. Lippincott.]

**24.33** Tufting of mucinous cells in a borderline muci-nous cystadenoma. Hematoxylin–eosin, ×395.

[Reprinted by permission from W. R. Hart and H. J. Norris, Borderline and malignant mucinous tumors of the ovary. Histo-logic criteria and clinical behavior, *Cancer 31*:1031, 1973, J. B. Lippincott.]

scopic filigree pattern similar to the tufting described in the borderline cystadenomas is a characteristic feature of these tumors (Figures 24.32 and 24.33). Capsular invasion is absent. The stroma of this tumor does not differ from that of the benign variety.

In cases in which the tumor is present in one ovary only, unilateral salpingo-oophorectomy appears to be ade-quate therapy. Santesson and Kottmeier reported 68% 10-year survival in borderline tumors, in contrast to 34% in true carcinomas.[89] In the Hart and Norris[44] series 94% of the patients were alive and well during a followup period ranging from 1.7 to 28.4 years with a mean of 8.6 years. However, one should emphasize that in the latter series three patients with borderline mucinous cystadenomas died of metastatic tumor 1, 1.2, and 7.3 years, respectively, after treatment.

In conclusion it should be stated that although the diagnosis of borderline serous cystadenomas is often diffi-cult, it is even more controversial with regard to mucinous tumors. In the latter neoplasms the problem of stromal

invasion is particularly difficult to evaluate.[95] Hence, Hart and Norris[44] do not place absolute reliance on the pres-ence of stromal invasion for a diagnosis of mucinous cystadenocarcinoma. This, together with the fact that in most series of borderline mucinous cystadenomas some of the patients do die of metastatic tumor, raises the question of whether these tumors should not have been classified as well-differentiated, low-grade, noninvasive mucinous car-cinomas, rather than as borderline mucinous cystadenoma, which may imply benignity. This problem of classification has also been discussed in the section on serous tumors but appears to be even more pertinent in the mucinous group.

## Mucinous Cystadenocarcinoma

Mucinous cystadenocarcinoma constitute 3%[4] to 10%[51] of all malignant primary ovarian neoplasms. Most of the patients with this tumor are in their fourth to sixth decades, although the median age in the Hart and Norris[44] series was 35 years.

473

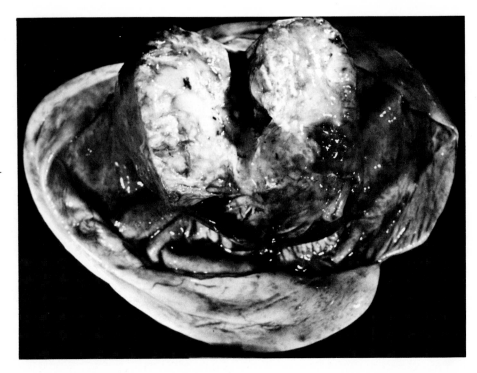

**24.34** Mucinous cystadenocarcinoma with a large solid tumor arising from the cyst lining.

As in the case with benign and borderline cystadenomas, the frank mucinous cystadenocarcinomas are grossly cystic, multiloculated neoplasms that may reach 50 cm in diameter. Solid areas and papillary projections are more frequent than in the benign and borderline lesions (Figure 24.34). Bilaterality figures of mucinous cystadenocarcinomas vary considerably in different series. According to Hart and Norris[44] only about 5% of the tumors are bilateral, whereas Cariker and Dockerty[17] have reported a 23.4% and Woodruff et al.[116] a 50% incidence of bilaterality. The medium figure is the generally accepted one.

Histologically the mucinous cystadenocarcinomas can be divided into well-, moderately well-, and poorly differentiated patterns. In some of the older series[1,17] well-differentiated or grade I carcinomas include lesions that are now generally classified as borderline tumors. The above-mentioned histologic differentiation relates primarily to the glandlike structures of the tumor, which are well formed; lined by tall columnar, mucin-producing cells with few mitoses in the well-differentiated group; more irregular and lined by atypical epithelium with more numerous mitoses in the moderately well-differentiated tumors; and difficult to identify, with highly atypical cells, in the poorly differentiated neoplasms. Definite stromal invasion is characterized by irregular cords and glands scattered throughout the stroma, sometimes arranged in back-to-back fashion (Figure 24.35). These features however may be lacking in some of the malignant mucinous tumors and hence a diagnosis of malignancy is now being based on stratification of epithelial lining cells exceeding three layers, in addition to invasion.[44] These epithelial cells demonstrate large nuclei with prominent nucleoli and diminished or occasionally absent intracytoplasmic mucin. Mitoses can be numerous. The stroma of the tumor is usually composed of dense, cellular fibrous tissue.

Ultrastructural studies of this tumor[31] revealed cells similar to those found in mucin-producing colonic adenocarcinoma.

The treatment of choice of mucinous cystadenocarcinoma is hysterectomy with bilateral salpingo-oophorectomy, which can be followed by radiation or chemotherapy. According to Cariker and Dockerty[17] the overall 5-year survival of patients with this tumor is 63.9%, whereas Santesson and Kottmeier[89] reported a 40% survival. This discrepancy may result from the fact that borderline tumors are included among carcinomas in the former series but are separately dealt with in the latter publication.

The various clinical and pathologic parameters of pseudomyxoma peritonei, which have been dealt with in the section on mucinous cystadenoma, are essentially the same, regardless of whether the primary tumor is a be-

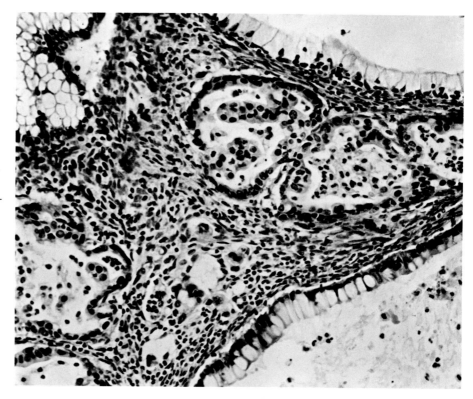

**24.35** Mucinous cystadenocarcinoma showing benign histologic areas with obvious stromal invasion by malignant elements. Hematoxylin–eosin, ×250.

nign mucinous cystadenoma or a mucinous cystadenocarcinoma. The only significant difference resides in the histologic appearance of the mucous-producing cells of the extraovarian lesions, which tend to show benign features in the former and malignant characteristics in the latter tumors.[100]

## Endometrioid Tumors

### Endometrioma

In the ovary endometriosis can present as microscopic foci of endometrial tissue or in the form of macroscopically visible cystic structures. The term "endometrioma," which implies a benign neoplasm, has been applied only to the grossly visible lesions, although both forms are obviously of the same origin. As is well known, the problem of the histogenesis of endometriosis is a complex and still unsettled one. Here we shall restrict ourselves to a brief discussion of the origin of ovarian endometriosis. Hertig and Gore[49] enumerate four main concepts concerning the origin of endometriosis: (1) embryonic rests; (2) transtubal transport of endometrial fragments in menstrual blood, with subsequent implantation; (3) celomic metaplasia; and (4) lymphatic or vascular dissemination. These authors dismiss all but one, namely, the celomic metaplasia theory. They base their conclusions mainly on the known Müllerian potential of the celomic epithelium. Gricouroff,[40] in contrast, supports Halban's theory of lymphatic metastasis[41] because in his opinion it has the advantage of supplying a sole satisfactory explanation for the presence of endometriosis at any site. At present, however, it is generally accepted that ovarian endometriosis originates in the germinal epithelium. Observations of transformation of this epithelium into endometrial-type cells, as well as of direct transition of the germinal epithelium into inclusion cysts lined by endometrial cells, are commonplace and supply tangible evidence in favor of the germinal epithelial theory of ovarian endometriosis.

Because most reports of ovarian endometriosis deal with both the micro- and macroscopic types of endometriosis, incidence figures relating solely to the so-called endometrioma are difficult to obtain. In general it is stated that endometriosis occurs most frequently between 30 and 40 years of age and that in the United States it seems to be more prevalent among White patients.[80]

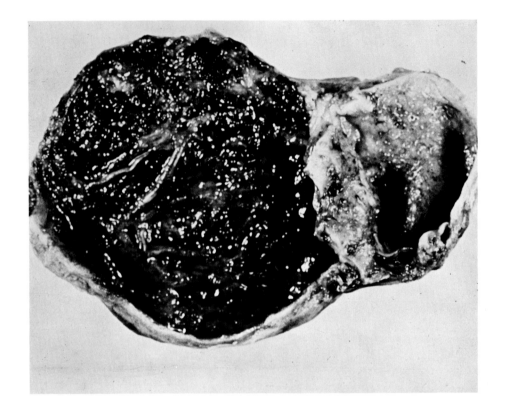

**24.36** Opened endometrioma showing a large cyst lined by hemorrhagic tissue.

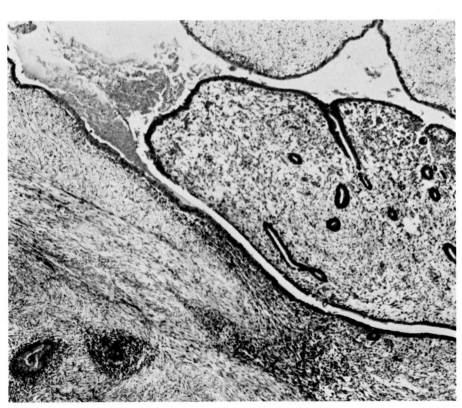

**24.37** Wall of endometrioma lined by endometrial-type epithelium with underlying endometrial stroma. Note the polypoid projections of endometrial tissue projecting into the cyst lumen. Hematoxylin–eosin, ×40.

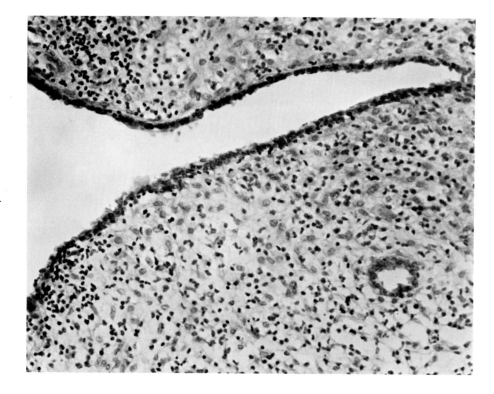

**24.38** Patient on progesterone medication showing decidual reaction of the stroma in ovarian endometrioma. Hematoxylin–eosin, ×250.

Grossly these are cysts varying in size from a few millimeters to 10 cm in diameter. They are often adherent to surrounding structures. The lumen usually contains blood of varying color depending on the amount and age of the hemorrhage. In most instances it is dark brown—hence the term "chocolate cyst." The inner lining also varies in color from pink to brown. It can be smooth or thick and velvety depending on the amount of endometrial and or granulation tissue present. Rarely papillary projections can be made out in these benign cysts (Figure 24.36). In at least 50% of cases both ovaries are involved.[47]

On microscopic examination it is unusual to find the three cardinal features of endometriosis in each case. These consist of endometrial epithelium, endometrial-type stroma, and evidence of repeated hemorrhage in the form of hemosiderin laden macrophages within the cyst wall (Figure 24.37). According to Hertig and Gore[47] it is actually the endometrial stroma that is pathognomonic of endometriosis, providing, of course, that its typical features can be demonstrated, which is the exception rather than the rule. It is not usual for the endometrioma to participate in the normal cyclic changes of the uterus, and in patients of progesterone medication predecidual transformation of the stroma of the lesion may occur (Figure 24.38). In the more advanced endometriomas some or even all of the typical histologic features are obliterated by repeated hemorrhages, leaving a cyst lining consisting of inflammatory cells and macrophages only. Obviously, many intermediary cases do exist in which one or the other histologic feature is still recognizable.

Although a "borderline" type of endometrioma, which showed proliferating, papillary, but not invasive histologic features, was described in 1961,[88] this appears to be of such rarity that no additional clinicopathologic data are available. For the moment at least, therefore, no meaningful discussion of such an entity is feasible.

Treatment is either hormonal or surgical with good results with both modalities. Prognosis is good but because ovarian endometrioma should be regarded as a benign neoplasm possessing a malignant counterpart a more careful followup of these patients is indicated.

## Endometrioid Carcinoma

Endometrioid carcinoma of the ovary is defined as a primary ovarian carcinoma that is histologically identical to endometrial adenocarcinoma or adenoacanthoma. This entity was well described in 1925 by Sampson,[87] who insisted on the origin of this tumor from preexisting ovarian endometriosis. Since then, endometriosis has repeatedly been stressed as the source of this neoplasm, although this cannot be proved in each case.[25-27,38] In the Czernobilsky et al. series of 75 cases of endometrioid carcinoma[23] about 17% presented with endometriosis in the ovary harboring the neoplasm. However in only three of these 13 cases was there continuity between the endometriosis and the endometrioid carcinoma. It is of course possible that the tumor destroys the preexisting endometriosis or the link of the neoplasm to it. Furthermore, because the germinal epithelium is now being considered the source of ovarian endometriosis,[47] it can directly give rise to endometrioid carcinoma without first passing through the stage of a benign endometrioma.

The reported incidence of endometrioid carcinoma of the ovary ranges from 10 to 24.4%[99] of all primary ovarian adenocarcinomas.[63] It is now considered to constitute the second in frequency among primary ovarian adenocarcinomas with an incidence of about 20%,[23] the first being the serous cystadenocarcinoma. The mean age of the patients with this neoplasm is about 53 years.[23,63]

Grossly, the majority of the endometrioid carcinomas are primarily cystic, ranging in size from 2 to 35 cm. Frequently, friable soft or papillary structures partly fill the lumen. In some instances the neoplasm is completely solid with necrotic or hemorrhagic areas (Figure 24.39). At time of surgery about 30 to 50% of the tumors are bilateral, with about half of the patients belonging to clinical stages I and II.[23,95]

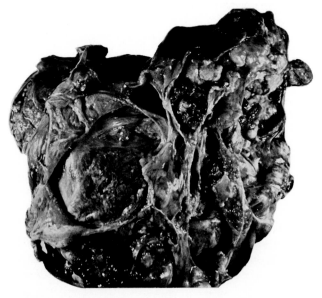

**24.39** Endometrioid carcinoma with multilocular cystic structures partly filled with soft and papillary tumor tissue.

[Courtesy of Dr. H. T. Enterline.]

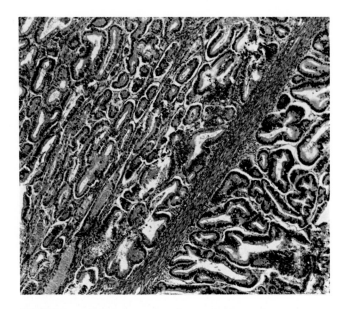

**24.40** Well-differentiated endometrioid carcinoma. Hematoxylin–eosin, ×50.

[Reprinted by permission from B. Czernobilsky, B. B. Silverman, and H. T. Enterline, Clear-cell carcinoma of the ovary. A clinicopathologic analysis of pure and mixed forms and comparison with endometrioid carcinoma, *Cancer* 25:762, 1970, J. B. Lippincott.]

When the same histologic grading that is used for endometrial adenocarcinoma,[80] is applied, endometrioid carcinoma ranges from grade 1 to grade 4 according to the degree of differentiation of the glandular components (Figures 24.40 and 24.41). Over 50% of these neoplasms belong to the better differentiated grades 1 and 2.[23,63] The stromal element is not different from that encountered in endometrial adenocarcinoma. Although the endometrial-like character is most readily recognizable in the well-differentiated tumors, it may prove to be difficult if not impossible to identify in the poorly differentiated grades 3 and 4 of the neoplasm. In these cases one should be able to demonstrate foci of better differentiated endometrioid carcinoma before reaching the latter diagnosis. In the absence of such areas of definite endometrioid carcinoma within poorly differentiated adenocarcinomas, a diagnosis of "adenocarcinoma not otherwise classifiable" is required.

Because papillary formations do occur in endometrial adenocarcinomas they can also be observed in endometrioid carcinoma. Occasionally psammoma bodies can also appear.[23] In these cases the differential diagnosis between endometrional and serous cystadenocarcinoma may prove to be a difficult one. Special stains are not contribu-

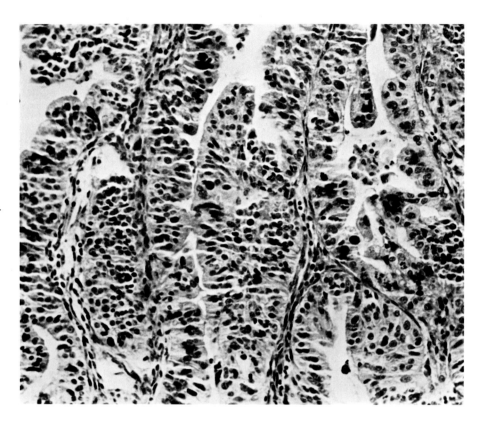

**24.41** Moderately well- to poorly differentiated endometrioid carcinoma. Hematoxylin-eosin, ×250.

tary because the luminal border of the epithelium in both endometrioid carcinoma and serous cystadenocarcinoma stain positively with diastase-resistant PAS, mucicarmine, and alcian blue stains. Here too the presence of typical areas of endometrioid carcinoma adjacent to the papillary components facilitates reaching the correct diagnosis. Furthermore, the epithelial cells lining the papillary structures of endometrioid carcinomas, in contrast to those of serous cystadenocarcinomas, are predominantly columnar and pseudostratified, with prominent elongated hyperchromatic nuclei. In this respect ultrastructural studies can be of help, because in endometrioid carcinoma these show features indistinguishable from those of endometrial adenocarcinoma but different from those seen in serous cystadenocarcinoma[19] (Figure 24.42).

Apart from the above-described papillary structures, which may be present in endometrioid carcinoma of the ovary but which constitute an integral part of the neoplasm, there are many instances in which endometrioid carcinomas contain additional histologic elements clearly belonging to other types of Müllerian neoplasms. For example, among the 75 cases of endometrioid carcinoma described by Czernobilsky et al.,[23] 18 showed elements of clear cell carcinoma, seven of serous cystadenocarcinomas, and one an anaplastic carcinoma (Figure 24.43).

As in endometrial adenocarcinoma, the presence of squamous elements in endometrioid carcinomas warranting a diagnosis of adenoacanthoma is very common. In our series,[23] this feature was present in almost 50% of the cases (Figure 24.44). Because histologic criteria of adenoacanthoma vary, the incidence of this type of endometrioid carcinoma also varies in different series.[27,38] In contrast to those who restrict this term to histologically perfectly benign squamous areas within an adenocarcinoma,[74] we, as Tweeddale et al.,[114] use it in a broader way, including tumors that show squamous, squamoid, and atypical, possibly malignant squamous nests.

One of the most interesting features of this neoplasm is the frequent finding of a concomitant endometrial carcinoma. This was observed in 14.6% of the patients in the Czernobilsky et al.[23] series and in more than 50% by Dockerty.[26] Although it is often difficult to establish whether these ovarian and endometrial cancers are independent primaries or metastatic from each other, we have concluded, as have Campbell et al.,[16] that these are independent primary tumors. This is borne out by the good survival data of these patients, which is not consistent with metastatic disease,[57] as well as by the usual focal noninvasive nature of the endometrial carcinoma (Figure 24.45).

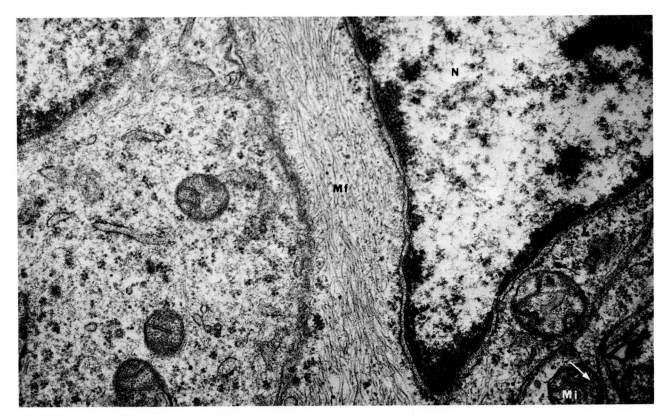

**24.42** Electron micrograph of a well-differentiated endometrioid carcinoma showing the characteristic perinuclear (N) microfilament (Mf). Note the mitochondria (Mi) in close apposition (arrow) with parallel membranes of granular endoplasmic reticulum. ×25,750.

[Courtesy of Dr. A. Ferenczy.]

**24.43** Endometrioid carcinoma (upper aspect of photograph) mixed with clear cell carcinoma elements (lower aspect). Hematoxylin–eosin, ×121.

[Reprinted by permission from B. Czernobilsky, B. B. Silverman, and J. J. Mikuta, Endometrioid carcinoma of the ovary. A clinicopathologic study of 75 cases, *Cancer* 26:1141, 1970, J. B. Lippincott.]

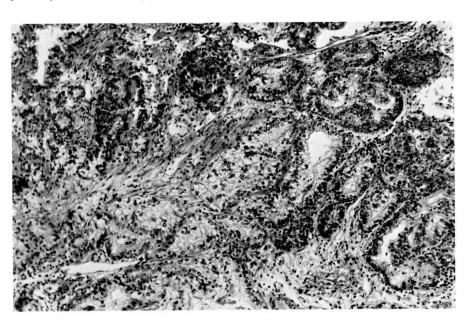

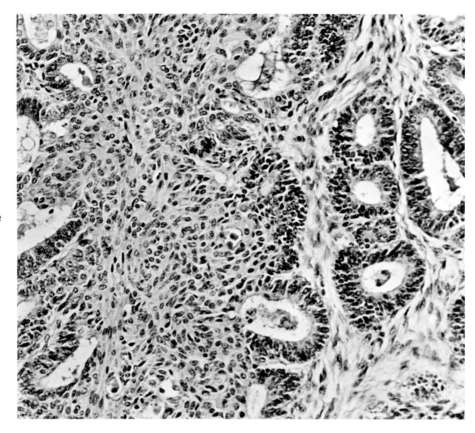

**24.44** Adenoacanthoma demonstrating typical endometrioid carcinomatous glands with large area of squamoid epithelium. Hematoxylin–eosin, ×278.

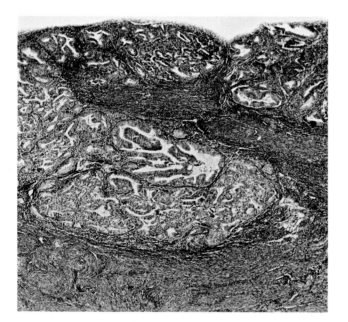

**24.45** Superficial small fundal endometrial adenocarcinoma in a patient with endometrioid carcinoma of the ovary. Hematoxylin–eosin, ×52.

Total hysterectomy with bilateral salpingo-oophorectomy constitutes the major modality of treatment of endometrial carcinoma. Survival does not seem to be affected by supplementary radiation or chemotherapy.[23]

Most authors have stressed the better prognosis of endometrioid carcinoma as compared to that of other ovarian cancers.[63,93] According to Santesson and Kottmeier, about 55% and close to 40% of the patients survive 5 and 10 years, respectively, after institution of treatment, whereas the 5-year survival of patients with serous cystadenocarcinoma is less than 20%.[89] The 5- and 10-year cumulative survival rates of endometrioid carcinoma listed by Czernobilsky et al.[23] were 40 and 32.7%, respectively. A more detailed analysis of survival rates as related to clinical staging and histologic grading[23] revealed a 5-year survival figure of 92.5% in stage I, which dropped to 27.8% in stage II, and was even lower in more advanced clinical stages. There was no good correlation between survival rates and histologic gradings. Prognosis was not influenced by admixture with other tumors of Müllerian origin or by the presence of a synchronous endometrial carcinoma (Tables 24.4 and 24.5). These data

**Table 24.4** Five-year cumulative survival figures of all the patients with endometrioid carcinoma of the ovary as compared to their various subdivisions[a]

| Clinical stage | Entire series (%) | "Mixed" endometrioid (%) | "Pure" endometrioid (%) | Adenoacanthoma (%) | Endometrioid without squamous (%) | Endometrioid with endometrial carcinoma (%) | Endometrioid without endometrial carcinoma (%) |
|---|---|---|---|---|---|---|---|
| I | 92.5 (31) | 88.9 (10) | 93.8 (21) | 93.3 (19) | 90.9 (12) | 80 (5) | 94.9 (26) |
| II | 27.8 (5) | 25 (4) | 100 (1) | 50 (2) | 0 (3) | — | 27.8 (5) |
| III | 3.7 (33) | 11 (9) | 0 (24) | 0 (11) | 5.5 (22) | 25 (4) | 3.5 (29) |
| IV | 0 (6) | 0 (3) | 0 (3) | 0 (4) | 0 (2) | 0 (2) | 0 (4) |
| Total | 40.5 (75) | 40.8 (26) | 39.9 (49) | 51.5 (36) | 29.8 (39) | 45.5 (11) | 39.7 (64) |

[a] Numbers in parentheses indicate number of patients in each clinical stage. [Reprinted by permission from B. Czernobilsky et al., *Cancer* 26:1141, 1970, J. B. Lippincott.]

**Table 24.5** Comparison of cumulative 5-year survival of patients with endometrioid carcinoma of the ovary by histologic grading and clinical staging[a]

| Clinical stage | Histologic grading | | | | All histologic grades combined (%) |
|---|---|---|---|---|---|
| | 1 (%) | 2 (%) | 3 (%) | 4 (%) | |
| I | 100 (11) | 83.6 (15) | 100 (3) | 100 (2) | 92.5 (31) |
| II | — | 100 (1) | 0 (4) | — | 27.8 (5) |
| III | 0 (5) | 0 (12) | 0 (9) | 21.4 (7) | 3.7 (33) |
| IV | — | 0 (1) | 0 (4) | 0 (1) | 0 (6) |
| Total | 67.3 (16) | 44.5 (29) | 13.2 (20) | 37.5 (10) | 40.5 (75) |

[a] Numbers in parentheses indicate number of patients. [Reprinted by permission from B. Czernobilsky et al., *Cancer* 26:1141, 1970, J. B. Lippincott.]

again emphasize that in ovarian carcinomas the one parameter which above all others determines the ultimate outcome is the extent of the tumor as evidenced at the time treatment is initiated.

## Clear Cell Carcinoma

The histogenesis of this tumor has been the subject of much controversy. For many years it was considered to be of mesonephric origin and hence also acquired the name of "mesonephroma".[78,79,92] The conclusion that this neoplasm is of mesonephric derivation is based on histologic grounds only, because the clear cells that make up the majority of these tumors resemble those that line the renal tubules. The occasional presence of structures resembling primitive glomeruli, or so-called "glomerular bodies," in these tumors gave further support to the mesonephric theory. Teilum eventually reclassified some of these neoplasms as "endodermal sinus tumors," which belong to the germ cell category of ovarian neoplasms.[109] The mesonephric histogenetic theory of what is now being called clear cell carcinoma continued to be questioned over the years by many authors who favored a Müllerian rather than a mesonephric origin.[25,63,105,107] Scully and Barlow,[97] in 1967, published a report establishing the relationship of clear cell carcinoma to Müllerian-type neoplasms on the following bases: (1) the high incidence of pelvic endometriosis in cases of ovarian clear cell carcinoma, (2) the coexistence of endometrioid and clear cell carcinomas, (3) the observation that clear cell carcinoma occasionally arises from the epithelium of the endometrioma, and

(4) the fact that a clear cell-type carcinoma of the uterine corpus originates in the endometrium, where mesonephric remnants are not located. Other authors have consequently confirmed these observations.[22] Furthermore, recent ultrastructural studies[31,104] have supplied additional data in support of the germinal epithelium origin of clear cell carcinoma. This, of course, does not exclude the existence of true mesonephric tumors within the immediate vicinity of the ovary—but these must be very rare lesions and, as has been shown in other than ovarian locations, do not necessarily present the characteristic clear cells that are the hallmark of the so-called ovarian mesonephroma.[67]

Although according to Scully[95] clear cell tumors may exist in benign, borderline, and frankly malignant forms, there is only a rare mention in the literature of the former two. For example, Anderson and Langley[3] and Hayes[45] describe benign mesonephromas that are characterized by little epithelial proliferation, prominent stroma, and apparent cure of the patient. Borderline cases are only alluded to and not reported as such.

Clear cell carcinomas of the ovary constitute about 5%[59] to 11%[22] of all primary ovarian carcinomas. The mean age of patients with this tumor is 54 years, with a range from about 40 to 78 years.[22,59]

Grossly, these tumors vary in size from 2 to 30 cm in diameter.[22,32] Most are partially cystic, with yellow, white, gray, and hemorrhagic areas. Forty percent are bilateral[22,32] (Figure 24.46).

The predominant histologic pattern is that of tubules, grandular areas, and cysts scattered within varying amounts of stroma. The characteristic epithelial cells lining these structures consist of (1) so-called hobnail or peg cells, which possess large prominent nuclei projecting toward the lumen; (2) cuboidal, columnar, or pavement-shaped cells with completely clear cytoplasm; and (3) cells similar to these latter ones but with single, sharply defined intracytoplasmic vacuoles (Figures 24.47 and 24.48). Occasional clear cells demonstrate intracytoplasmic PAS-positive diastase-resistant material but in most instances there is some intraluminal and luminal border positive staining with mucicarmine, diastase-resistant PAS, and alcian blue. Glandular cystic structures with intraluminal papillary projections showing resemblance to glomerular structures and Arias–Stella-type endometrial glands are occasionally observed (Figure 24.49). Another pattern is that of dense fibrous stroma, with scattered cystic cavities lined by hobnail and other clear cells, called "parvilocular cystoma" (Figure 24.50).

One of the interesting features of clear cell carcinoma is the frequent admixture with elements from other Müllerian-type neoplasms, which seems to be even more prominent in this neoplasm than in the other tumors of germinal epithelial origin. For example, in the Scully and Barlow series,[97] 12% of the tumors were mixed with endometrioid carcinoma and Kurman and Craig[59] found clear cell carcinoma in association with various types of primary epithelial carcinomas, although the most common admixture was the endometrioid and serous carcinomas. Of the 39 clear cell carcinomas described by Czernobilsky et al.[22] only 12 were of the "pure" type and the rest were

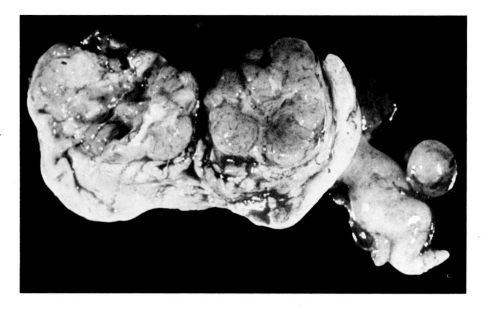

**24.46** Cut surface of a predominantly solid clear cell carcinoma.

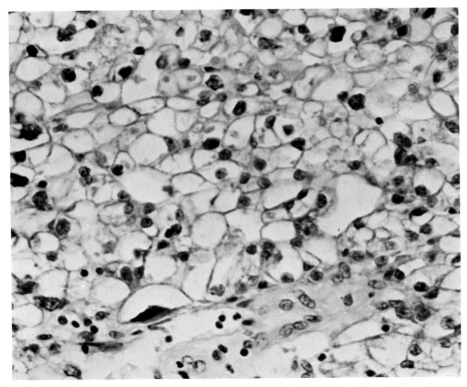

**24.47** Typical cells of a clear cell carcinoma with pleomorphic nuclei. Hematoxylin–eosin, ×263.

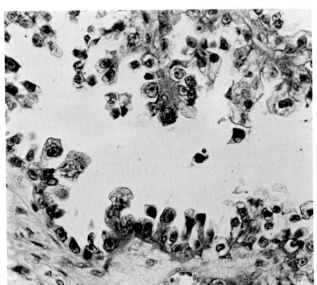

**24.48** Hobnail-shaped clear cells in a clear cell carcinoma. Hematoxylin-eosin, ×300.

[Reprinted by permission from B. Czernobilsky, B. B. Silverman, and H. T. Enterline, Clear-cell carcinoma of the ovary. A clinicopathologic analysis of pure and mixed forms and comparison with endometrioid carcinoma, *Cancer* 25:762, 1970, J. B. Lippincott.]

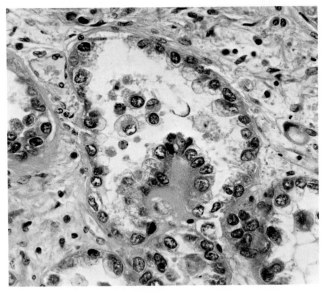

**24.49** Glandular structure with intraluminal projection referred to as glomerular body in clear cell carcinoma. Hematoxylin-eosin, ×300.

[Reprinted by permission from B. Czernobilsky, B. B. Silverman, and H. T. Enterline, Clear-cell carcinoma of the ovary. A clinicopathologic analysis of pure and mixed forms and comparison with endometrioid carcinoma, *Cancer* 25:762, 1970, J. B. Lippincott.]

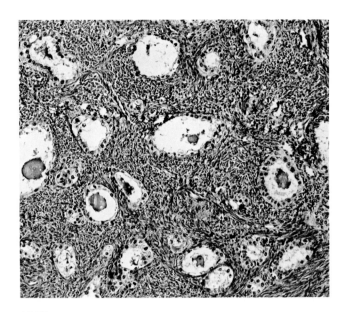

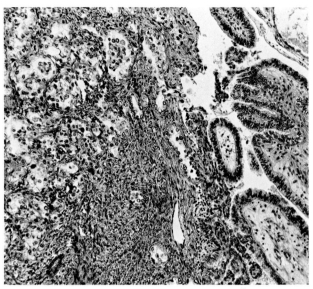

**24.50** Clear cell carcinoma with a dense fibrous stroma containing cystic cavities lined by clear cells. This is referred to as parvilocular cystoma. Hematoxylin–eosin, ×100.

[Reprinted by permission from B. Czernobilsky, B. B. Silverman, and H. T. Enterline, Clear-cell carcinoma of the ovary. A clinicopathologic analysis of pure and mixed forms and comparison with endometrioid carcinoma, *Cancer* 25:762, 1970, J. B. Lippincott.]

**24.51** Clear cell carcinoma (left side of photomicrograph) with associated papillary serous cystadenocarcinoma. Hematoxylin–eosin, ×85.

[Reprinted by permission from B. Czernobilsky, B. B. Silverman, and H. T. Enterline, Clear-cell carcinoma of the ovary. A clinicopathologic analysis of pure and mixed forms and comparison with endometrioid carcinoma, *Cancer* 25:762, 1970, J. B. Lippincott.]

mixed with other Müllerian neoplasms, especially with endometrioid and serous cystadenocarcinomas (Figure 24.51). From the above it follows that clear cell carcinomas are indeed of germinal epithelium origin and seem to be most closely related to endometrioid carcinoma.

Electron microscopic studies of the clear cells from this tumor[31,104] revealed prominent aggregates of glycogen particles in close relationship with stacked granular endoplasmic reticulum, and other features that are common to clear cell carcinomas of endometrial, cervical, and vaginal origin (Figures 24.52 and 24.53).

The treatment of choice is total hysterectomy with bilateral tubo-oophorectomy. Postoperative irradiation, chemotherapy, intraperitoneal radioactive gold, phosphorus, or nitrogen do not appear to significantly affect the course of the disease.[32]

The 5-year survival of patients with pure and mixed clear cell carcinoma in the Czernobilsky et al.[22] series was 41 and 34%, respectively, with 10-year survival figures of 32 and 28%. These figures did not differ significantly from those of a group of patients with endometrioid carcinomas

that was compared to the former patients (Figure 24.54). The clinical stage of the lesion, however, played a most significant role in the prognosis. Those with tumors limited to one ovary had a 5-year survival of 80.5%, as compared to a 11.2% survival with more extensive neoplasms. Similar observations were made by Kottmeier[56] and by Kurman and Craig,[59] with overall 5-year survival figures ranging from 39 to 27%, respectively. It is therefore obvious that the prognosis of clear cell carcinoma is much superior to that of serous cystadenocarcinomas, although approaching that of endometrioid carcinoma.

# Brenner Tumor

## Benign Brenner Tumor

In 1907, Dr. Fritz Brenner described an ovarian tumor that he named "oophoroma folliculare,"[14] postulating a granulosa cell origin. Since then, numerous histogenetic theories have been advanced, probably more so than for any other single ovarian neoplasm.

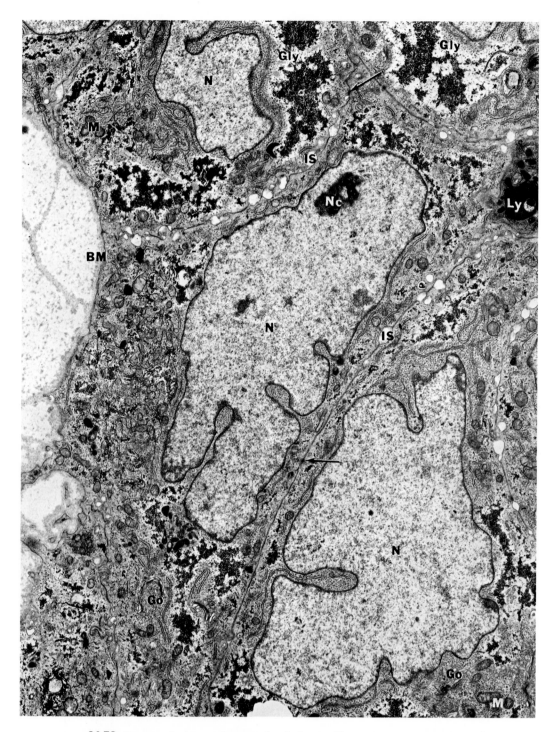

**24.52** Survey electron micrograph of clear cell carcinoma. Basement membrane (BM) separates the neoplastic cells from the stroma. Desmosomes are frequent (arrows). Clusters of glycogen (Gly), lysosomes (Ly), Golgi complexes (Go), mitochondria (M), and numerous intercellular spaces (IS) are noted. Nuclei (N) are rather large and lobular and sometimes contain a coiled nucleolus (Nc), ×5,580.

[Reprinted by permission from H. Salazar et al., Human ovarian neoplasms: Light and electron microscopic correlations, *Obstet. Gynecol.* 44:551, 1974, Harper and Row.]

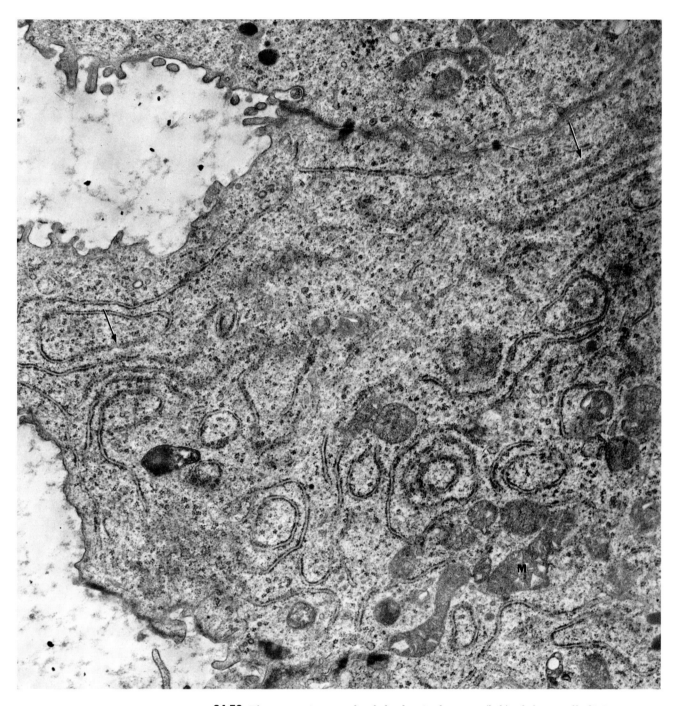

**24.53** Electron micrograph of the luminal aspect (left) of three cells lining a tubule of clear cell carcinoma. Note the "hobnail" arrangement of cells and the
short, thick microvilli. Terminal tight junctions and desmosomes are seen between the cells. Mitochondria (M) and lamellae of granular endoplasmic reticulum, some of which are stacked in parallel rows (arrows), are prominent as are
ribosomes and glycogen granules, ×20,000.

[Reprinted by permission from S. G. Silverberg, Ultrastructure and histogenesis of clear cell
carcinoma of the ovary, *Am. J. Obstet. Gynecol. 115*:394, 1973, C. V. Mosby.]

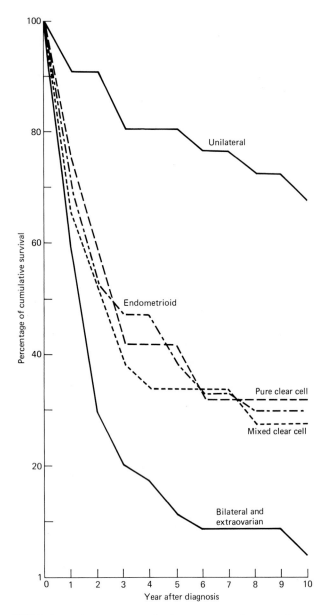

**24.54** Cumulative survival of patients with pure clear cell carcinoma, mixed clear cell carcinoma (a combination of focal and predominant clear cell groups), and endometrioid carcinoma of the ovary. The "unilateral" line refers to a combination of all types of neoplasms confined to one ovary. The "bilateral and extraovarian" group includes tumors of all types either unilateral with spread beyond the ovary, or bilateral with or without spread beyond the ovary.

[Reprinted by permission from B. Czernobilsky, B. B. Silverman, and H. T. Enterline, Clear-cell carcinoma of the ovary. A clinicopathologic analysis of pure and mixed forms and comparison with endometrioid carcinoma, *Cancer* 25:762, 1970, J. B. Lippincott.]

The granulosa cell theory, which was first mentioned by Brenner himself and which was based on a superficial resemblance of the epithelial elements of the neoplasm to granulosa cells, can now be definitely refuted in the light of ultrastructural studies.[12] Greene[39] suggested a possible origin from ovarian stroma, a theory that is not tenable because of the lack of similarity between the epithelial and stromal elements of the tumor in spite of the continuity between the reticulum fibers of the stroma and those present within the epithelial nests. Schiller's mesonephric theory[10,91] was supported by the frequent occurrence of this tumor near the rete ovarii and its histologic similarity to urinary tract epithelium. Here too, however, ultrastructural studies revealed no similarities between the epithelium of Brenner tumors and that of mesonephric remnants.[13] The latter study also refuted a possible origin of the Brenner tumor from paramesonephric remnants.[36] Another theory, that of metaplasia of mucinous epithelium,[91] was based on the not infrequent association of mucinous cystadenomas and Brenner tumors. However, careful observations suggest that mucinous cells present within epithelial nests of Brenner tumors are the result of mucinous metaplasia rather than the source of the Brenner epithelium. Because of the occasional presence of heterologous epithelia in Brenner tumors, a teratomatous origin has also been suggested,[53] but here too the metaplastic theory seems to be more tenable. The Walthard cell nest theory was advanced as early as 1932 by Meyer.[68] These nests are most commonly found on the surface of the fallopian tubes, mesosalpinx, mesovarium, and occasionally in the ovarian hilus, all being sites in which Brenner tumors are not usually located. Nevertheless, there exists a striking histologic similarity among the Walthard cell nests, urothelium, and the epithelium of the Brenner tumor, on both light and electron microscopic examination.[12] These observations in no way contradict the now generally accepted theory that Brenner tumors arise from the germinal epithelium of the ovary, a theory based on observations of continuity between the germinal epithelium and that of the Brenner tumor.[5] It is therefore believed that Brenner tumors are derived from the germinal epithelium of the ovary, which through a metaplastic process forms the typical urothelial-like epithelial elements of the neoplasm as well as Walthard cell nests, providing a common denominator for the morphologic similarities among these seemingly unrelated epithelial elements.[13,105]

According to Jondahl et al.,[53] the rate of incidence among all ovarian tumors is 1.7%, although some consider it to be even less frequent. These authors also reported a bilaterality of 6.5% and an age range from 6 to 81 years, with 50.5% of the patients over 50 years. In Silverberg's

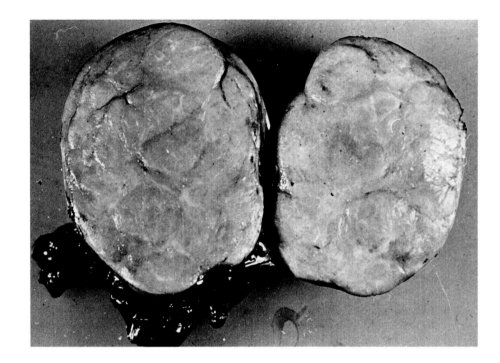

**24.55** Cut section of a solid, nodular Brenner tumor.

[Courtesy of Dr. H. T. Enterline.]

series[103] the tumors had a left-sided predominance, bilaterality was 3.7%, and only 31.5% of the patients were postmenopausal.

The majority of Brenner tumors are solid and firm, with a gray-white and whorled cut surface (Figure 24.55). They vary in size from microscopic tumors to huge masses, most of the larger ones measuring 2 to 8 cm in diameter. The frequency of microscopic lesions explains the common incidental discovery of this tumor. Frequently, small cystic structures can be made out in these solid tumors but occasionally the entire neoplasm is grossly cystic. Brenner tumors are not encapsulated but do produce compression of the surrounding ovarian tissue.

On microscopic examination, Brenner tumors are comprised of solid to partly cystic epithelial nests surrounded by a stroma composed of bundles of tightly packed spindle-shaped cells. The epithelial cells are polygonal and of squamoid type, with pale, eosinophilic cytoplasm and oval nuclei that have distinct nucleoli and longitudinal grooving, the so-called "coffee-bean" appearance (Figures 24.56 and 24.57). Mitotic figures and epithelial atypism are not identified. The nuclear grooving is also present in Waldhard cell nests, being caused by a peculiar infolding of the nuclei,[6] and can be observed in other epithelial or mesothelial cells as well. Some of the epithelial cells may undergo mucinous metaplasia and also contain small amounts of glycogen.

The association of Brenner tumors with other cystic neoplasms, especially mucinous cystadenomas and cystic teratomas, is well known. In Silverberg's[103] study such an association was observed in the ipsilateral ovary in 19 out of 60 cases. Six of these were mucinous cystadenomas and three were cystic teratomas.

Fine structural studies of Brenner tumors[12,84] showed similarities between their epithelial elements and those of urothelium and Waldhard cell nests (Figures 24.58 and 24.59), an observation that as stated before is consistent with the histogenetic theory of metaplasia of the germinal epithelium.

Treatment of the benign form of Brenner tumor consists of simple excision, which is curative.

## Proliferating Brenner Tumors

In 1971, Roth and Sternberg[85] described three unusual Brenner tumors that on the basis of histologic characteristics were named "proliferating" and placed as an intermediate neoplasm between the benign and malignant forms.

The patients reported by Roth and Sternberg[85] were 78, 66, and 59 years old. The ovarian tumors were all unilateral and cystic and measured from about 12 to 25 cm in diameter. Papillary projections into the cyst's lumen could be grossly recognized in two of the cases.

On microscopic examination the papillary portions of the tumors, as well as parts of the cystic areas, were lined by eight to 20 layers of well-differentiated transitional-type

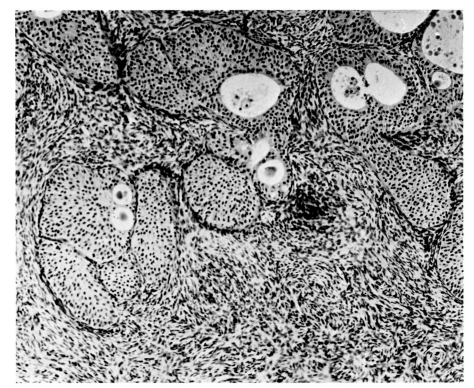

**24.56** Brenner tumor showing a solid and partly cystic epithelial nest in the dense fibrous stroma. Hematoxylin–eosin, ×113.

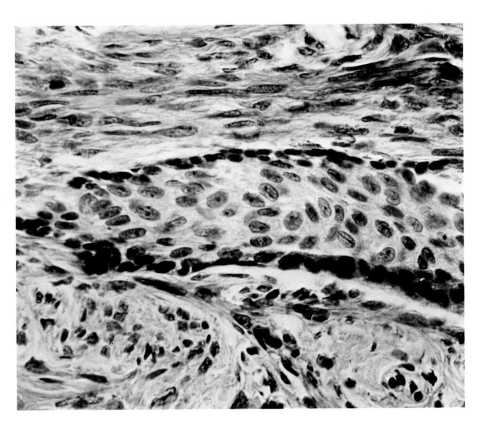

**24.57** Detail of an epithelial nest of a Brenner tumor demonstrating typical longitudinal grooving or coffee-bean appearance of the nuclei. Hematoxylin–eosin, ×400.

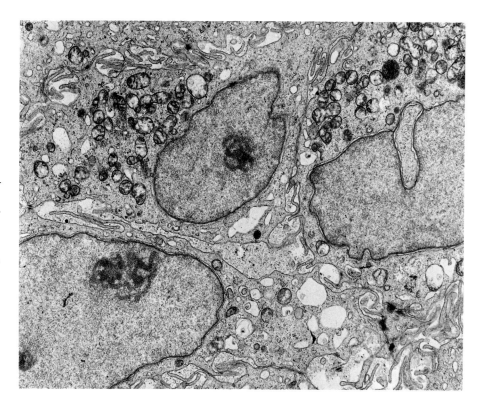

**24.58** Electron micrograph of the epithelial cells of a Brenner tumor. The nuclei are irregular and have evenly distributed chromatin and a prominent nucleolus. A cytoplasmic invagination into the nucleus is present in the cell on the right. Intercellular spaces are abundant. ×10,800.

[Reprinted by permission from L. M. Roth, Fine structure of the Brenner tumor, *Cancer* 27:1482, 1971, J. B. Lippincott.]

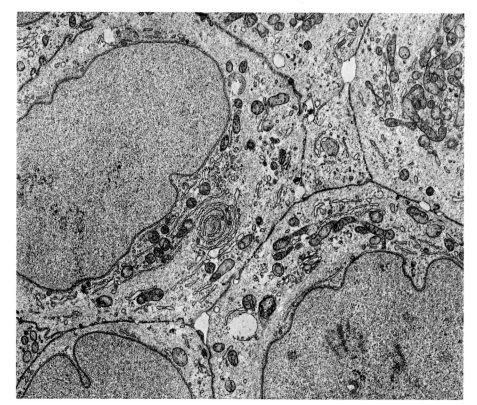

**24.59** Electron micrograph of the urothelial cells of the human urinary bladder. Note the general similarity to the epithelium of the Brenner tumor. The cells show a greater uniformity. Intercellular spaces, less abundant than in the Brenner tumor, are present at the angles between adjacent cells. A cytoplasmic invagination into the nucleus is present in the lower left hand corner. ×9,200.

[Reprinted by permission from L. M. Roth, Fine structure of the Brenner tumor, *Cancer* 27:1482, 1971, J. B. Lippincott.]

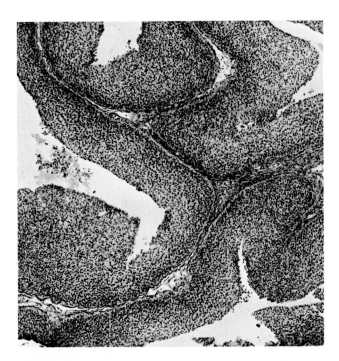

**24.60** Multilayered epithelium lining the cystic areas of a proliferating Brenner tumor. Hematoxylin–eosin, ×56.
[Courtesy of Dr. H. J. Norris.]

epithelium with only mild focal atypia (Figures 24.60 and 24.61). A few normal mitotic figures occurred. There was no stromal invasion. Adjacent to these areas, typical Brenner tumors were observed in all the three cases. Because of the close association with Brenner tumors and the urothelial characteristics of the proliferating elements, Roth and Sternberg considered these lesions to represent a proliferating variant of Brenner tumors and found a few additional cases among previously reported malignant Brenner tumors. None of their patients developed recurrences.

Miles and Norris[69] and Hallgrimson and Scully[42] reported 14 additional cases of proliferating Brenner tumors. Here too, as in the Roth and Sternberg[85] series, most of these tumors were large and cystic, with polypoid masses projecting into the lumen.

Treatment consisted of total abdominal hysterectomy with bilateral salpingo-oophorectomy and unilateral salpingo-oophorectomy. Followup, which ranged from 1 month to 18 years, revealed no recurrences in any of the patients.

In conclusion, proliferating Brenner tumors are histologically as well as clinically benign neoplasms and the decision by Hallgrimson and Scully[42] to classify them as

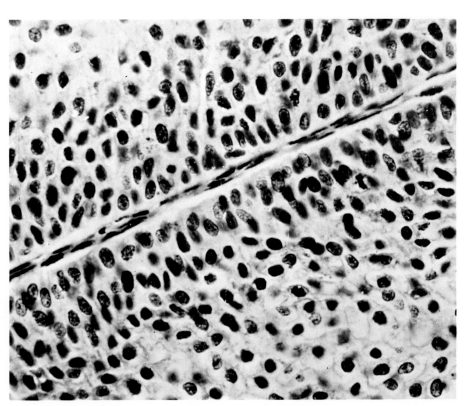

**24.61** Atypism of the epithelial elements of a proliferating Brenner tumor. Hematoxylin–eosin, ×400.

"borderline" was admittedly prompted by a desire to comply with the nomenclature originally proposed by the International Federation of Gynecology and Obstetrics. In reality, they differ from the borderline serous and mucinous cystadenomas, because the latter demonstrate a number of malignant histologic and clinical features, whereas so far, at least, this has not been observed in the proliferating Brenner tumors.

## Malignant Brenner Tumor

This is a rare neoplasm, with only about 41 cases reported up to 1973.[69] The true incidence of this tumor is difficult to establish but histologic changes suggestive of malignancy have been found by Woodruff and Acosta[115] in eight out of 90 Brenner tumors. Some of these lesions may possibly be reclassified now as benign proliferating Brenner tumors, whereas others may actually have been carcinomas arising in associated cystadenomas and not in the Brenner tumor itself. The same can also be said for Idelson's series of 25 cases.[50] Malignant Brenner tumors make up 5% of all Brenner tumors in the Miles and Norris[69] series, but here too this may not constitute the true incidence because of the consultative nature of their material.

Because of the many controversial aspects of this tumor, it is important to adopt strict histologic criteria before reaching such a diagnosis. These criteria based on the work by Hull and Campbell[49] are as follows: (1) Frankly malignant histologic features must be present; (2) there must be intimate association between the malignant element and a benign Brenner tumor; (3) mucinous cystadenomas should preferably be absent or must be well separated from both the benign and the malignant Brenner tumor; and (4) stromal invasion by epithelial elements of the malignant Brenner tumor must be demonstrated.

The average age of patients with malignant Brenner tumor is 60.3 years.[50] These are usually large, partly cystic tumors. The cystic portions are frequently lined by friable, polypoid masses. The majority of these tumors seem to arise on the left side.

Microscopically, malignant Brenner tumors demonstrate transitional cell-type adenocarcinoma, moderate to severe atypism, and mitotic activity (Figure 24.62 and 24.63). There can also be squamous metaplasia and frank squamous carcinoma within the epithelial nests. Capsular and sometimes vascular invasion is common. Stromal invasion is difficult to evaluate because of the basic architecture of Brenner tumors, in which epithelial nests are scattered throughout the stroma.

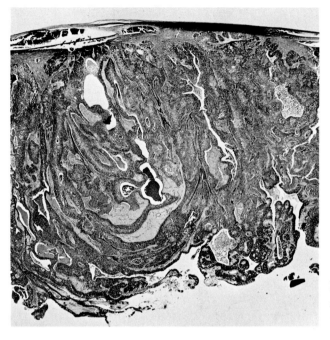

**24.62** Low-power view of a malignant Brenner tumor showing marked proliferation of the epithelium. Hematoxylin-eosin, ×12.

[Reprinted by permission from P. A. Miles and H. J. Norris, Proliferative and malignant tumors of the ovary, *Cancer* 30:174, 1972, J. B. Lippincott.]

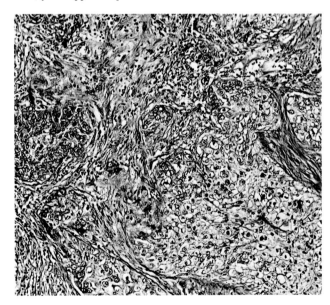

**24.63** Malignant Brenner tumor showing the marked atypism of the epithelial nests with a resemblance to transitional cell carcinoma. Hematoxylin-eosin, ×100.

[Courtesy of H. J. Norris.]

Treatment consists in most instances of total hysterectomy with bilateral tubo-oophorectomy. Of 16 patients with followup in Idelson's[50] series four were alive and well from 1 to 3 years after the diagnosis was established. Of the eight patients with malignant Brenner tumors in the Hallgrimson and Scully publication,[42] two died and one was alive with residual cancer. Three of Miles' and Norris' seven patients died of their disease from 3 months to 2 years after its removal.[69]

# Mixed Epithelial and Mesenchymal Tumors

In this group of neoplasms are included carcinosarcomas and mixed mesodermal tumors. Because of their common origin and certain histologic similarities, these two tumors have in the past been described together. However, because of differences of survival in these two types of tumors and distinctive histologic features, a separate discussion of carcinosarcomas and mixed mesodermal tumors seems now justified.

Because both types of mixed epithelial and mesenchymal tumors occur in the uterus, where they arise from the endometrium,[76,77] it can be assumed that in the ovary as well they are Müllerian-type neoplasms, originating either in preexisting endometriosis[90] or in the multipotential germinal epithelium. As endometriosis is rarely identified in ovaries harboring this neoplasm and because of the advanced age of these patients, in whom endometriosis is usually no longer active, the germinal epithelial histogenetic theory is by far the most attractive. It is for this reason that in the new classification of ovarian tumors these mixed neoplasms are now being listed with tumors of surface epithelial origin.[95]

## Carcinosarcoma

Because of the great rarity of this neoplasm, its incidence cannot be established. This is a tumor of the elderly, the ages ranging from 43 to 78 years and with a median age of 57 years.[6] Most of the tumors are unilateral, large, partly cystic neoplasms, with a median diameter of 15 cm. The solid portions often demonstrate necrotic areas and hemorrhages[90] (Figure 24.64).

The typical microscopic appearance is that of an admixture of malignant epithelial and stromal elements. The epithelial component is most frequently an adenocarcinoma of varying differentiation, occasionally with intracellular mucinous material. The adenocarcinomatous portion

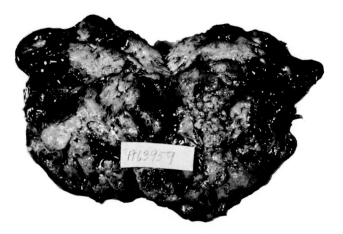

**24.64** Cross section of a carcinosarcoma showing solid, cystic, and hemorrhagic areas.

[Reprinted by permission from B. Czernobilsky and G. C. La-Barre, Carcinoma and mixed mesodermal tumor of the ovary. A clinicopathologic analysis of 9 cases, *Obstet. Gynecol.* 31:21, 1968, Harper and Row.]

can also demonstrate papillary and squamous features (Figure 24.65). This component is usually sharply demarcated from the surrounding stroma, although transitions between the two components of the tumor can occasionally be observed. The stroma in carcinosarcomas is predominantly made up of tightly packed hyperchromatic spindle cells with numerous mitoses (Figure 24.66).

Carcinosarcomas must be differentiated from ovarian adenocarcinomas with prominent stroma. In the latter lesions the stroma may be extremely cellular but does not show the marked pleomorphism and mitotic activity that characterize the stromal sarcomatous elements of the carcinosarcomas.

The treatment consists of total hysterectomy with bilateral tubo-oophorectomy, sometimes complemented by adjunctive postoperative irradiation and chemotherapy.

As stated before, one of the reasons justifying a separate discussion of carcinosarcomas and mixed mesodermal tumors has been the better prognosis in the former. This difference in prognosis was first observed by Norris et al.[76,77] who studied similar tumors arising in the endometrium. In the Czernobilsky and Labarre[21] series, behavioral differences between these two types of neoplasms in the ovary could not be established, possibly because of the small number of patients. However, in the larger series by Dehner et al.,[24] the authors could confirm that patients with ovarian carcinosarcomas did indeed have a better prognosis than those with mixed mesodermal tumors. Both are highly malignant tumors but the median survival

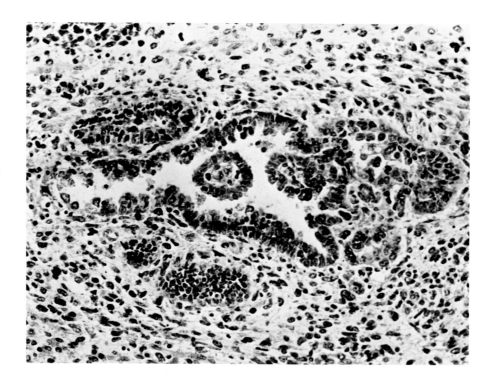

**24.65** Adenocarcinoma with a surrounding sarcomatous stroma in a carcinosarcoma. Hematoxylin–eosin, ×250.

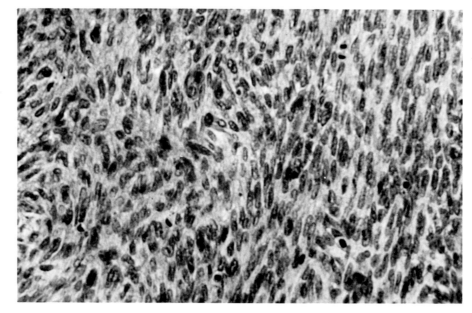

**24.66** Area of pure stromal sarcoma in a carcinosarcoma. Hematoxylin–eosin, ×190.

[Reprinted by permission from B. Czernobilsky and G. C. LaBarre, Carcinosarcoma and mixed mesodermal tumor of the ovary. A clinicopathologic analysis of 9 cases, *Obstet. Gynecol. 31:21,* 1968, Harper and Row.]

for patients with ovarian carcinosarcoma was 12 months, as compared to a 6-month survival for those with mixed mesodermal tumors. The tumors disseminate widely but the most common site is that of peritoneal seeding.[24] At autopsy the sarcomatous element is the predominating one in the various sites in which the tumor is found.[21,24]

## Mixed Mesodermal Tumors

Here too, because of the rarity of the tumor, no incidence figures are available. In the Dehner et al.[24] series the mean age was 53 years. Only one of their 14 patients and one of the 21 patients reported by Fenn and Abell[28] were

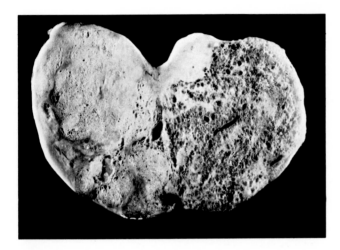

**24.67** Mixed mesodermal tumor showing a mixture of solid and cystic areas.

[Courtesy of Dr. H. J. Norris.]

below the age of 40. Nulliparity seems to be an important clinical feature in patients with this neoplasm.[2,21,24]

The gross appearance of the mixed mesodermal tumors is similar to that of the carcinosarcoma, all being unilateral, large, partly cystic neoplasms with a median diameter of 13.6 cm[24] (Figure 24.67).

The microscopic feature that distinguishes them from carcinosarcomas is the stromal component. In mixed mesodermal tumors the stroma presents malignant, heterogenous elements in addition to the spindle cell areas. These

consist most commonly of cartilage, striated muscle, and osteoid.[24] The epithelial elements are similar to those of the carcinosarcoma (Figures 24.68 and 24.69).

Because of the mixture of epithelial and heterogenous elements, mixed mesodermal tumors must be distinguished from malignant teratomas. In mixed mesodermal tumors there is complete absence of any orderly or organized arrangement of the heterologous stromal elements, all features that are usually present in malignant ovarian teratomas. In addition, mixed mesodermal tumors with neuroepithelial elements, which are commonplace in malignant teratomas, have never been described. Whereas the epithelial structures in mixed mesodermal tumors are frank adeno- or squamous carcinomas, these are usually representative of the respiratory or gastrointestinal tracts in malignant teratomas. Finally, malignant teratomas are tumors of young women, in contrast to mixed mesodermal tumors, which with very few exceptions appear in older women only.

Treatment of these lesions is similar to that of carcinosarcomas, namely, predominantly surgical. In the Dehner et al.[24] series prognosis of patients with this neoplasm was worse than for patients with carcinosarcoma. The median survival was 6 months, in contrast to the 12-month survival with carcinosarcoma. These authors also reported that at the end of a 15-month actuarial survival period 50% of patients with carcinosarcomas were alive, compared to only 14% with mixed mesodermal tumors. The observation by Norris et al.[76,77] that in uterine mixed mesoder-

**24.68** Mixed mesodermal tumor with a malignant glandular structure surrounded by highly atypical cartilage and smooth muscle (right side of photomicrograph). Hematoxylin–eosin, ×131.

[Reprinted by permission from B. Czernobilsky and G. C. LaBarre, Carcinosarcoma and mixed mesodermal tumor of the ovary. A clinicopathologic analysis of 9 cases, *Obstet. Gynecol.* 31:21, 1968, Harper and Row.]

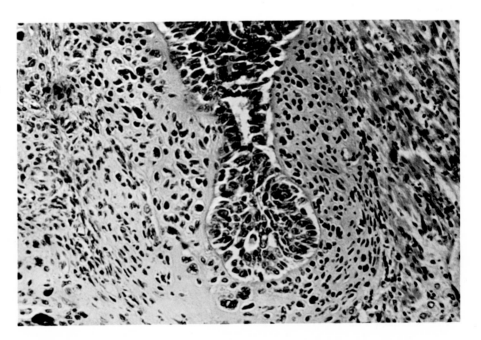

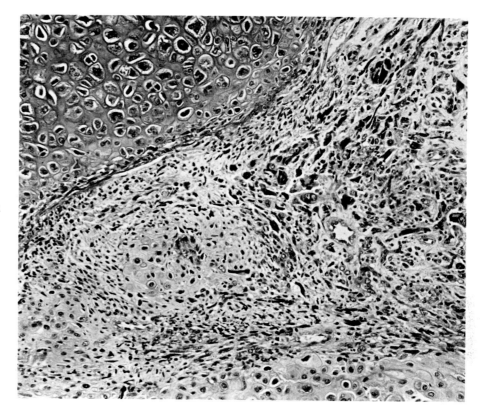

**24.69** Detail of sarcomatous elements in mixed mesodermal tumor showing chondrosarcoma and anaplastic sarcoma. Hematoxylin–eosin, ×100.

mal tumor the presence of cartilage and absence of striated muscle were favorable findings could not be confirmed in the ovarian tumors of this type.

## Adenomatoid Tumor

The adenomatoid tumor, which is infrequently found in the epididymis, fallopian tubes, and serosal aspect of the uterus, is one of the rarest of ovarian neoplasms. It has only been recently included in the new classification among the tumors of germinal epithelium origin.[51] Nevertheless, the histogenesis of this neoplasm in both males and females is still highly controversial. Lymphangiomatous,[102] mesonephric,[110] Müllerian,[112] and mesothelial[30,66] theories have been proposed. Of these, the latter is now being favored on the basis of morphologic,[43] histochemical,[15] and ultrastructural observations.[30] The ovarian adenomatoid tumor can therefore be considered a mesothelioma, being composed of ovarian surface lining cells without stromal participation. At this juncture it is of interest to note that according to Parmley and Woodruff[81] all primary epithelial ovarian neoplasms are actually meso-

theliomas because of their derivation from the germinal epithelium, which represents the mesothelium of the ovary. About six cases have to date been briefly mentioned or described in the literature.[30,102] The patients were in their third and fourth decade and the tumors were for the most part incidental discoveries. The lesions were well-circumscribed, solid, grayish-yellowish nodules, ranging from 0.5 to 1.5 cm in diameter and often situated in the hilar region of the ovary.

Microscopically these tumors are composed of cuboidal or low columnar vacuolated cell-lined spaces or solid cords of cells in collagenous or hyalinized connective tissue stroma (Figure 24.70). The cells lining the channels possess brush borders and stain weakly with PAS and mucicarmine stains. Hyaluronic acid is present in the intercellular spaces.[15] Ultrastructural studies[30] have revealed abundant microvilli, bundles of cytoplasmic filaments, dilated intercellular spaces, and scanty micropinocytic vesicles (Figure 24.71), which are all features of normal mesothelial cells.

These are benign neoplasms and their simple removal, which is usually carried out because of unrelated genital lesions, is curative.

497

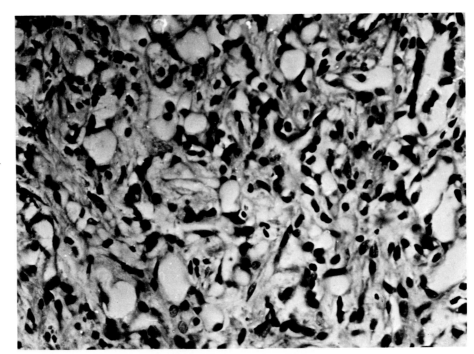

**24.70** Adenomatoid tumor demonstrating spaces lined by columnar and cuboidal cells. Hematoxylin–eosin, ×250.

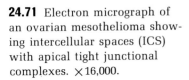

**24.71** Electron micrograph of an ovarian mesothelioma showing intercellular spaces (ICS) with apical tight junctional complexes. ×16,000.

[Reprinted by permission from A. Ferenczy and M. Richart, Observations on benign mesothelioma of the genital tract (adenomatoid tumor). A comparative ultrastructural study, *Cancer* 30:244, 1972, J. B. Lippincott.]

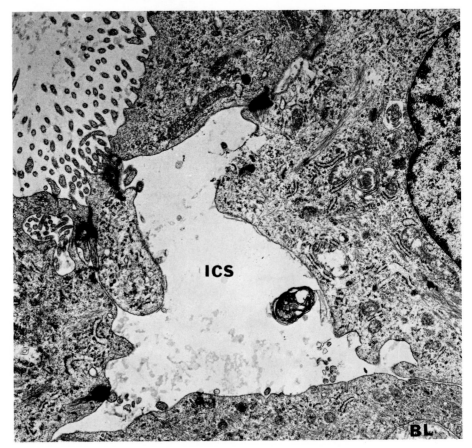

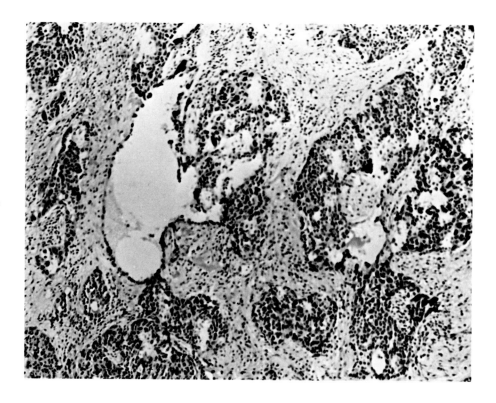

**24.72** Solid and cystic nest of unclassifiable adenocarcinoma. Hematoxylin–eosin, ×100.

## Adenocarcinoma Not Otherwise Classifiable

In contrast to the preceding categories of primary epithelial tumors of the ovary, each of which represents a distinct type of neoplasm, this last grouping is of malignant tumors that because of a lack of any specific microscopic features and/or presence of histologic anaplasia cannot be classified under any of the previously discussed headings. Because the basic histologic structure of these neoplasms is carcinomatous, they are classified with the epithelial tumors, although the severe anaplasia that characterizes many of these tumors may make the differential diagnosis between unclassifiable adenocarcinomas and tumors of other origins, especially poorly differentiated granulosa cell tumors, a difficult task.[95] The above not withstanding, it becomes quite obvious from a thorough study of the unclassifiable adenocarcinomas that most of them represent poorly differentiated serous cystadenocarcinomas and endometrioid carcinomas. This is also borne out by the fact that these two latter neoplasms constitute about 60% of all the malignant primary epithelial tumors of the ovary. Therefore, either a papillary or a solid glandular pattern predominates in the unclassifiable tumors (Figure 24.72). In the Santesson and Kottmeier[89] series, they constituted 5.2% of all the primary malignant epithelial ovarian neoplasms.

As are most highly malignant ovarian neoplasms, the unclassifiable tumors are usually large, partly cystic masses with areas of necrosis and hemorrhage. According to Kottmeier,[57] 54% of these tumors are bilateral. At the time of discovery many of these carcinomas have spread beyond the ovaries and their prognosis is even poorer than that of serous cystadenocarcinomas.[95]

## Luteinized and Enzymatically Active Stromal Cells in Primary Ovarian Epithelial Tumors

A careful histologic examination of the stroma adjacent to or forming part of the various primary ovarian epithelial tumors reveals in many instances single or groups of lipid-containing luteinized cells (Figures 24.73 and 24.74). It was speculated that the ovarian neoplasia stimulated the stromal cells to differentiate into such thecal or luteinized elements.[73] In 1958, Hughesdon[48] described serous, mucinous, clear cell, and endometrioid tumors, all of

20. Czernobilsky, B., Borenstein, R., and Lancet, M. Cystadenofibroma of the ovary. A clinicopathologic study of 34 cases and comparison with serous cystadenoma. *Cancer* 34:1971, 1974.

21. Czernobilsky, B., and LaBarre, G. C. Carcinosarcoma and mixed mesodermal tumor of the ovary. A clinicopathologic analysis of 9 cases. *Obstet. Gynecol.* 31:21, 1968.

22. Czernobilsky, B., Silverman, B. B., and Enterline, H. T. Clear-cell carcinoma of the ovary. A clinicopathologic analysis of pure and mixed forms and comparison with endometrioid carcinoma. *Cancer* 25:762, 1970.

23. Czernobilsky, B., Silverman, B. B., and Mikuta, J. J. Endometrioid carcinoma of the ovary. A clinicopathologic study of 75 cases. *Cancer* 26:1141, 1970.

24. Dehner, L. P., Norris, H. J., and Taylor, H. B. Carcinosarcomas and mixed mesodermal tumors of the ovary. *Cancer* 27:207, 1971.

25. DeSanto, D. A., Bullock, W. K., and Moore, F. J. Ovarian cystomas. *Arch. Surg.* 78:98, 1959.

26. Dockerty, M. B. Primary and secondary ovarian adenoacanthoma. *Surg. Gynecol. Obstet.* 99:392, 1954.

27. Fathalla, M. F. Malignant transformation in ovarian endometriosis. *J. Obstet. Gynaecol. Br. Commonw.* 74:85, 1967.

28. Fenn, M. E., and Abell, M. R. Carcinosarcoma of the ovary. *Am. J. Obstet. Gynecol.* 110:1066, 1971.

29. Fenoglio, C. M., Ferenczy, A., and Richart, R. M. Mucinous tumors of the ovary. Ultrastructural studies of mucinous cystadenomas with histogenetic considerations. *Cancer* 36:1709, 1975.

30. Ferenczy, A., Fenaglio, J., and Richart, R. M. Observations on benign mesothelioma of the genital tract (adenomatoid tumor). A comparative ultrastructural study. *Cancer* 30:244, 1972.

31. Ferenczy, A., and Richart, R. M. *The Female Reproductive System. Dynamics of Scan and Transmission Electron Microscopy.* New York, John Wiley and Sons, 1974, pp. 287–309.

32. Fine, G., Clarke, H. D., and Horn, R. C. Mesonephroma of the ovary. A clinical, morphological, and histogenetic appraisal. *Cancer* 31:398, 1973.

33. Fisher, E. R., Krieger, J. S., and Skirpan, P. J. Ovarian cystoma. Clinicopathologic observations. *Cancer* 8:437, 1955.

34. Fox, H., Kazzaz, B., and Langley, F. A. Argyrophil and argentaffin cells in the female genital tract and ovarian mucinous cysts. *J. Pathol. Bacteriol.* 88:479, 1964.

35. Garcia-Bunnel, R., and Morris, B. Histochemical observation on mucin in human ovarian neoplasms. *Cancer* 17:1108, 1964.

36. Goldman, R. L. A Brenner tumor of the testis. *Cancer* 26:853, 1970.

37. Gondos, B. Electron microscopic study of papillary serous tumors of the ovary. *Cancer* 27:1455, 1971.

38. Gray, L. A. and Barnes, M. L. Endometrioid carcinoma of the ovary. *Obstet. Gynecol.* 29:694, 1967.

39. Greene, R. R. The diverse origins of Brenner tumors. *Am. J. Obstet. Gynecol.* 64:878, 1952.

40. Gricouroff, G. Endometrioid tumor of the ovary, in Gentil, F., and Junqueira, A. C., eds.: *Ovarian Cancer,* UICC Monograph Series, Vol. 11. New York, Springer Verlag, 1968, pp. 22–39.

41. Halba, J. Hysteroadenosis metastatica. *Arch. Gynäk.* 124:457, 1925.

42. Hallgrimson, J., and Scully, R. E. Borderline and malignant Brenner tumors of the ovary. A report of 15 cases. *Acta Pathol. Microb. Scand. A (Suppl. 80),* 233:56, 1972.

43. Hanrahan, J. B. A combined papillary mesothelioma and adenomatoid tumor of the omentum; report of a case. *Cancer* 16:1497, 1963.

44. Hart, W. R., and Norris, H. J. Borderline and malignant mucinous tumors of the ovary. Histologic criteria and clinical behaviour. *Cancer* 31:1031, 1973.

45. Hayes, D. Mesonephroid tumors of the ovary. *J. Obstet. Gynaecol. Br. Commonw.* 79:728, 1972.

46. Herbert, P. A. *Gynecological and Obstetrical Pathology.* Philadelphia, C. V. Mosby, 1953, p. 458.

47. Hertig, A. T., and Gore, H. *Atlas of Tumor Pathology.* Section IX, Fascicle 33. Tumors of the Female Sex Organs. Part 3: Tumors of the Ovary and Fallopian Tube. Washington, D.C., Armed Forces Institute of Pathology, 1961, p. 77.

48. Hughesdon, P. E. Thecal and allied reactions in epithelial ovarian tumors. *J. Obstet. Gynaecol. Br. Commonw.* 65:702, 1958.

49. Hull, M. G. R., and Campbell, G. R. The malignant Brenner tumor. *Obstet. Gynecol.* 42:527, 1973.

50. Idelson, M. G. Malignancy in Brenner tumors of the ovary, with comments on histogenesis and possible estrogen production. *Obstet. Gynecol. Surv.* 18:246, 1963.

51. Janovski, N. A., and Paramanandhan, T. L. *Ovarian Tumors. Tumors and Tumor-like Conditions of the Ovaries, Fallopian Tubes and Ligaments of the Uterus.* Stuttgart, Georg Thieme, 1973, p. 9.

52. Jensen, R. D., and Norris, H. J. Epithelial tumors of the ovary. Occurrence in children and adolescents less than 20 years of age. *Arch. Pathol.* 94:29, 1972.

53. Jondahl, W. H., Dockerty, M. D., and Randall, C. M. Brenner tumors of the ovary: A clinicopathologic study of 31 cases. *Am. J. Obstet. Gynecol.* 60:160, 1950.

54. Kent, S. W., and McKay, D. G. Primary cancer of the ovary. *Am. J. Obstet. Gynecol.* 80:430, 1960.

55. Kottmeier, H. L. The classification and treatment of ovarian tumors. *Acta Obstet. Gynecol. Scand.* 31:313, 1952.

56. Kottmeier, H. L. The diagnosis and treatment of ovarian malignancies. *Arch. Pathol.* 37:51, 1965.

57. Kottmeier, H. L. Surgical management—conservative surgery. Indications according to the type of the tumor, in Gentil F., and Junqueira, A. C., eds.: *Ovarian Cancer.* UICC Monograph Series, Vol. 11, New York, Springer-Verlag, 1968, pp. 157–164.

58. Kraus, F. T. *Gynecologic Pathology.* St. Louis, C. V. Mosby, 1967, p. 333.

59. Kurman, R. J., and Craig, J. M. Endometrioid and clear cell carcinoma of the ovary. *Cancer* 29:1653, 1972.

60. Langley, F. A., Cummins, P. A., and Fox, H. An ultrastructural study of mucin secreting epithelia in ovarian neoplasms. *Acta Pathol. Microbiol. Scand.* (Suppl. 80,) 233:76, 1972.

61. Lauchlan, S. L. Histogenesis and histogenetic relationship of Brenner tumors. *Cancer* 19:1628, 1966.

62. Limber, G. K., King, R. E., and Silverberg, S. G. Pseudomyxoma peritonaei. A report of ten cases. *Ann. Surg.* 178:587, 1973.

63. Long, M. E., and Taylor, H. C. Endometrioid carcinoma of the ovary. *Am. J. Obstet. Gynecol.* 90:936, 1964.

64. Long, R. T., Spratt, J. S., and Dowling, E. Pseudomyxoma peritonaei: New concepts in management with a report of 17 patients. *Am. J. Surg.* 117:162, 1969.

65. Malloy, J. J., Dockerty, M. B., Welch, J. S., and Hunt, A. B. Papillary ovarian tumors. I. Benign tumors and serous and mucinous cystadenocarcinomas. *Am. J. Obstet. Gynecol.* 93:867, 1965.

66. Masson, P., Riopelle, J. L., and Simard, L. G. Le mesotheliome benin de la sphere genitale. *Rev. Can. Biol. 1:720, 1942.*

67. McGee, C. T., Cromer, D. W., and Greene, R. R. Mesonephric carcinoma of the cervix—differentiation from endocervical adenocarcinoma. *Am. J. Obstet. Gynecol. 84:358, 1962.*

68. Meyer, R. Über verschiedene Erscheinungsformen der als typus Brenner bekannten Eierstockgeschwulst, ihr absonderung von den Granulosa-Zell tumoren und zuordnung unter andere Ovarialgeschwülste. *Arch. Gynaek. 148:541, 1932.*

69. Miles, P. A., and Norris, H. J. Proliferative and malignant Brenner tumors of the ovary. *Cancer 30:174, 1972.*

70. Ming, S. C., and Goldman, H. Hormonal activity of Brenner tumors in postmenopausal women. *Am. J. Obstet. Gynecol. 83:666, 1962.*

71. Minkowitz, S., and Cohen, H. M. Adenocarcinoma within serous cystadenofibroma of the ovary. *N.Y. State J. Med. 66:529, 1966.*

72. Moore, J. G., Schifrin, B. S., and Erez, S. Ovarian tumors in infancy, childhood and adolescence. *Am. J. Obstet. Gynecol. 93:850, 1965.*

73. Morris, J. M., and Scully, R. E. *Endocrine Pathology of the Ovary.* St. Louis, C. V. Mosby, 1958, pp. 131–139.

74. Ng, A. B. P. Mixed carcinoma of the endometrium. *Am. J. Obstet. Gynecol. 102:506, 1968.*

75. Nieminen, U., and Purola, E. Stage and prognosis of ovarian cystadenocarcinomas. *Acta Obstet. Gynecol. Scand. 49:49, 1970.*

76. Norris, H. J., Roth, E., and Taylor, H. B. Mesenchymal tumors of the uterus. II. A clinical and pathologic study of 31 mixed mesodermal tumors. *Obstet. Gynecol. 28:57, 1966.*

77. Norris, H. J., and Taylor, H. B. Mesenchymal tumors of the uterus. III. A clinical and pathologic study of 31 carcinosarcomas. *Cancer 19:1459, 1966.*

78. Novak, E., Woodruff, J. D., and Novak, E. R. Probable mesonephric origin of certain female genital tumors. *Am. J. Obstet. Gynecol. 68:1222, 1954.*

79. Novak, E. R., and Woodruff, J. D. Mesonephroma of the ovary—thirty-five cases from the ovarian tumor registry of the American Gynecological Society. *Am. J. Obstet. Gynecol. 77:632, 1959.*

80. Novak, E. R., and Woodruff, J. D. *Novak's Gynecologic and Obstetric Pathology with Clinical and Endocrine Relations,* 7th ed. Philadelphia, W. B. Saunders, 1974, pp. 365–366.

81. Parmley, T. H., and Woodruff, J. D. The ovarian mesothelioma. *Am. J. Obstet. Gynecol. 120:234, 1974.*

82. Pfleiderer, A., and Teufel, G. Incidence and histochemical investigation of enzymatically active cells in stroma of ovarian tumors. *Am. J. Obstet. Gynecol. 102:997, 1968.*

83. Reagan, J. W. Histopathology of ovarian pseudomucinous cystadenoma. *Am. J. Pathol. 25:689, 1949.*

84. Roth, L. M. Fine structure of the Brenner tumor. *Cancer 27:1482, 1971.*

85. Roth, L. M., and Sternberg, W. H. Proliferating Brenner tumors. *Cancer 27:687, 1971.*

86. Rothman, D., and Blumenthal, H. T. Serous adenofibroma and cystadenofibroma of the ovary. Report of five cases with malignant change in one. *Obstet. Gynecol. 14:389, 1959.*

87. Sampson, J. A. Endometrial carcinoma of the ovary arising in endometrial tissue in that organ. *Arch. Surg. 10:1, 1925.*

88. Santesson, L. Suggested classification of ovarian tumors.

Paper presented at the meeting of the Cancer Committee of the International Federation of Gynecologists and Obstetricians. Stockholm, Sweden, August 24–26, 1961.

89. Santesson, L., and Kottmeier, H. L. General classification of ovarian tumors, in Gentils F., and Junqueira, A. C. eds.: *Ovarian Cancer,* UICC Monograph Series. Vol. 11. New York, Springer-Verlag, 1968, pp. 1–8.

90. Saunders, P., and Price, A. B. Mixed mesodermal tumor of the ovary arising in pelvic endometriosis. *Proc. R. Soc. Med. 63:1050, 1970.*

91. Schiller, W. Zur histogenese der Brennerschen ovarial tumoren. *Arch. Gynaekol. 157:65, 1934.*

92. Schiller, W. Mesonephroma ovarii. *Am. J. Cancer 35:1, 1939.*

93. Schüller, E. F., and Kirol, P. M. Prognosis in endometrioid carcinoma of the ovary. *Obstet. Gynecol. 27:850, 1966.*

94. Scott, R. B. Serous adenofibromas and cystadenofibromas of the ovary. *Am. J. Obstet. Gynecol. 43:733, 1942.*

95. Scully, R. E. Recent progress in ovarian cancer. *Hum. Pathol. 1:73, 1970.*

96. Scully, R. E. Germ cell tumors of the ovary, in Sturgis, S. H., and Taymor, M. L., eds.: *Progress in Gynecology.* New York, Grune and Stratton, 1970, Vol. V, p. 343.

97. Scully, R. E., and Barlow, J. F. "Mesonephroma" of ovary. Tumor of müllerian nature related to the endometrioid carcinoma. *Cancer 20:1405, 1967.*

98. Scully, R. E., and Cohen, R. B. Oxidative-enzyme activities in normal and pathologic human ovaries. *Obstet. Gynecol. 24:667, 1964.*

99. Scully, R. E., Richardson, G. S., and Barlow, J. F. The development of malignancy in endometriosis. *Clin. Obstet. Gynecol. 9:384, 1966.*

100. Shanks, H. G. I. Pseudomyxoma peritonei. *J. Obstet. Gynaecol. Br. Commonw. 68:212, 1961.*

101. Sharman, A., and Sutherland, A. M. A case of serous adenofibroma of the ovary. *J. Obstet. Gynaecol. Br. Emp. 54:382, 1947.*

102. Siddall, R. S., and Clinton, W. R. Lymphangioma of the ovary. *Am. J. Obstet. Gynecol. 34:306, 1937.*

103. Silverberg, S. G. Brenner tumor of the ovary. A clinicopathologic study of 60 tumors in 54 women. *Cancer 28:588, 1971.*

104. Silverberg, S. G. Ultrastructural and histogenesis of clear cell carcinoma of the ovary. *Am. J. Obstet. Gynecol. 115:394, 1973.*

105. Sternberg, W. Nonfunctioning ovarian neoplasms, in Grady, H. G., and Smith, D. E., eds.: *International Academy of Pathology Monograph, The Ovary.* Baltimore, Williams & Wilkins, 1963, pp. 209–254.

106. Sundarasivarao, D. Müllerian vestiges and benign epithelial tumors of epididymis. *J. Pathol. Bacteriol. 66:417, 1953.*

107. Tarridge, J., and Kingsley, W. B. "Mesonephroma" of the ovary. A report of five cases. *Cancer 22:1208, 1968.*

108. Taylor, C. H. Studies in the clinical and biological evolution of adenocarcinoma of the ovary. *J. Obstet. Gynaecol. Br. Commonw. 66:827, 1959.*

109. Teilum, G. Endodermal sinus tumors of the ovary and testis. Comparative morphogenesis of the so-called mesonephroma ovarii (Schiller) and extra embryonic (yolk-sac-allantoic) structures of the rat's placenta. *Cancer 12:1092, 1959.*

110. Teilum, G. Histogenesis and classification of mesonephric tumors of the female and male genital system and relationship to

benign so-called adenomatoid tumors (mesotheliomas). *Acta Pathol. Microbiol. Scand. 34*:431, 1954.

111. Thompson, J. D. Primary ovarian adenoacanthoma. Its relationship to endometriosis. *Obstet. Gynecol. 9*:403, 1957.

112. Timonen, S., and Purola, E. Adenofibroma and cystadenofibroma of the ovary. *Ann. Chir. Gynaecol. Fenn. (Suppl. 56) 154*:5, 1967.

113. Towers, R. P. A note on the origin of the pseudomucinous cystadenoma of the ovary. *J. Obstet. Cynaecol. Br. Emp. 63*:253, 1956.

114. Tweeddale, D. N., Early, L. S., and Goodsitt, E. S. Endometrial adenoacanthoma. A clinical and pathologic analysis of 82 cases with observations on histogenesis. *Obstet. Gynecol. 23*:611, 1964.

115. Woodruff, J. D., and Acosta, A. A. Variations in the Brenner tumors. *Am. J. Obstet. Gynecol. 83*:657, 1962.

116. Woodruff, J. D., Bie, L. S., and Sherman, R. J. Mucinous tumors of the ovary. *Obstet. Gynecol. 16*:699, 1960.

117. Woodruff, J. D., and Novak, E. R. Papillary serous tumors of the ovary. *Am. J. Obstet. Gynecol. 67*:1112, 1954.

118. Woodruff, J. D., Williams, T. J., and Goldberg, B. Hormone activity of the common ovarian neoplasm. *Am. J. Obstet. Gynecol. 87*:679, 1963.

Robert E. Scully, M.D.

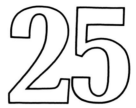

# Sex Cord–Stromal Tumors

## Classification and Nomenclature

This category of ovarian tumors includes all those that contain granulosa cells, theca cells and their luteinized derivatives, Sertoli cells, Leydig cells, and fibroblasts of gonadal stromal origin, singly or in several combinations and in varying degrees of differentiation. The generic terms that have been most widely applied to these tumors reflect differing views of gonadal embryology. Those investigators who are convinced that all the cell types listed above, including granulosa and Sertoli cells, are derived from the mesenchyme or "specialized stroma" of the genital ridge have proposed the terms mesenchymomas[3] and gonadal stromal tumors for these neoplasms.[24,27] In contrast, others, recognizing that embryologists disagree on the role of the coelomic epithelium in the formation of the sex cords which are the proximal precursors of the granulosa and Sertoli cells, prefer to leave open the possibility that these cell types are ultimately derived from the coelomic epithelium and have favored the term sex cord–mesenchyme tumors[20,36] or sex cord–stromal tumors.[40] In the developing testis the sex cords are clearly distinguishable by the fifth week of embryonic life as slender columns of primitive Sertoli cells, but similar cords, at least in the sense of thin columns, are not encountered in the developing ovary; instead, packets or lobules of small pregranulosa cells enveloping germ cells become evident later in embryonic life. For that reason, the term sex cords has been

**Table 25.1** Sex cord-stromal tumors

A. GRANULOSA-STROMAL CELL TUMORS
1. Granulosa cell tumor
2. Tumors in the thecoma-fibroma group
   (a) thecoma
   (b) fibroma
   (c) unclassified
B. ANDROBLASTOMAS; SERTOLI-LEYDIG CELL TUMORS
1. Well differentiated
   (a) tubular androblastoma; Sertoli cell tumor [tubular adenoma of Pick]
   (b) tubular androblastoma with lipid storage; Sertoli cell tumor with lipid storage [folliculome lipidique of Lecène]
   (c) Sertoli–Leydig cell tumor [tubular adenoma with Leydig cells]
   (d) Leydig cell tumor; hilus cell tumor
2. Of intermediate differentiation
3. Poorly differentiated [sarcomatoid]
4. With heterologous elements
C. GYNANDROBLASTOMA
D. UNCLASSIFIED

criticized as inaccurate to describe the progenitors of the granulosa cells. Nevertheless, the traditional usage of this designation by embryologists and the lack of a better one justify its retention. The adoption of the term sex cord–stromal tumors, which has been recommended by the World Health Organization (WHO),[40] has the advantage of acknowledging the presence in all tumors in this general category of derivatives of one or two of the three major components of the developing gonads, namely, the sex cords and the stroma. The offspring of the former, the granulosa and Sertoli cells, are typically arranged in epithelial configurations, whereas those of the stroma, which lies between the sex cords in the developing gonad, have the appearance of cellular gonadal stroma or its specialized derivatives, the theca and Leydig cells.

Most sex cord–stromal tumors are composed of ovarian cell types, but some contain only elements of testicular type; rarely cells and patterns of growth characteristic of both gonads are present in a single tumor. On occasion, when the cells are immature, when their appearance is intermediate between those of male and female cell types, or when the characteristic architectural patterns of the testis or ovary are not reproduced by the tumor, it may be impossible to determine whether it belongs in the granulosa-stromal cell or Sertoli–Leydig cell category; in such cases the term sex cord-stromal tumor, unclassified, is used. The classification of sex cord–stromal tumors adopted by WHO is presented in Table 25.1.

Sex cord–stromal tumors as a group account for approximately 5% of all ovarian tumors, but functioning forms comprise only 1 to 2%. Five to 10% of ovarian cancers belong in the sex cord–stromal category and most of these are granulosa cell tumors, which are of a low grade of malignancy.

# Granulosa–Stromal Cell Tumors

This category includes all ovarian tumors composed of granulosa cells and cells of ovarian stromal derivation, theca cells, and fibroblasts, singly or in any combination and in varying degrees of differentiation.

## Granulosa Cell Tumor

This may be composed almost entirely of granulosa cells or contain a large component of theca cells and/or fibroblasts as well. The granulosa cell tumor is the most common form of estrogenic ovarian tumor, accounting for 1 to 2% of all ovarian tumors and 5 to 10% of all ovarian cancers.

Five percent of granulosa cell tumors are diagnosed before the age of normal puberty, and most of these are associated with isosexual precocity, accounting for 10% of the cases of that syndrome in the female.[12,14,23,39] (The more common form of isosexual precocity is of central origin with premature release of gonadotropins from the anterior pituitary gland; this type is usually constitutional, or idiopathic.) The precocity caused by a granulosa cell tumor is more specifically designated pseudoprecocity because there is no associated ovulation or progesterone production, precluding the possibility of pregnancy, which exists, in contrast, in cases of true sexual precocity. Typically, pseudoprecocity is heralded by development of the breasts; this is followed by the appearance of pubic and axillary hair, stimulation and enlargement of the external and internal secondary sex organs, irregular uterine bleeding, and a whitish vaginal discharge, which is believed to originate in the endocervical glands. Skeletal development is typically accelerated. In most of the cases the precocity has its onset before the age of 5 years.

Ninety-five percent of granulosa cell tumors are distributed more or less evenly among premenopausal and postmenopausal women. Estrogenic changes of clinical significance are usually present, but the precise proportion of tumors that secrete hormones is difficult to establish because often a specimen of endometrium is not available for an evaluation of estrogenic stimulation. The typical appearance of an endometrium associated with a granulosa cell tumor is that of cystic hyperplasia with or without varying degrees of precancerous atypicality (adenomatous hyperplasia; atypical hyperplasia; carcinoma *in situ*).[11] Invasive carcinoma of the endometrium, which is usually well differentiated, has been reported in from slightly less than 5 to slightly more than 25% of the cases; these widely varying frequencies can be partly attributed to differing views of the dividing line between markedly atypical hyperplasia and carcinoma *in situ,* on the one hand, and grade I adenocarcinoma, on the other.

The endometrial changes are manifested clinically in younger women by metropathia hemorrhagica, characterized by irregular, excessive uterine bleeding, but amenorrhea, lasting from months to years, may be the only estrogenic manifestation or may precede the abnormal bleeding. Postmenopausal bleeding is the most common endocrine symptom in older women, in whom carcinoma of the endometrium is encountered more often than in the younger age group.[11] Occasionally, swelling and tenderness of the breasts are prominent symptoms. Elevated levels of estrogens have been reported in the blood and urine,[46] and vaginal cytologic smears typically show an increased maturation of the squamous epithelial cells.[13] Alterations resembling those seen in a secretory endometrium have been observed rarely in association with granulosa cell tumors, suggesting the possibility of a significant production of progesterone by the neoplasm, and on exceptional occasions virilization has been the sole endocrine manifestation.[26]

Granulosa cell tumors vary in size from those that are too small to be felt on pelvic examination (10 to 15%)[8] to very large masses that distend the abdomen; one of the largest recorded weighed 34 pounds.[7] At surgery they may appear predominantly solid or cystic and are unilateral in over 95% of the cases.[20] Sectioning a solid granulosa cell tumor shows a gray or yellow color, depending on cellularity and lipid content, and a soft or firm consistence depending on relative proportions of cells and fibromatous stroma (Figure 25.10a, Plate VIII). Areas of necrosis and hemorrhage are not uncommon. More frequently the tumor forms a predominantly cystic mass in which numerous compartments, typically filled with fluid or clotted blood, are separated by bridges of solid tissue (Figure 25.1). An interesting clinical corollary of this gross appearance is the presentation of 10 to 15% of granulosa cell tumors not in the form of an overt endocrine disturbance

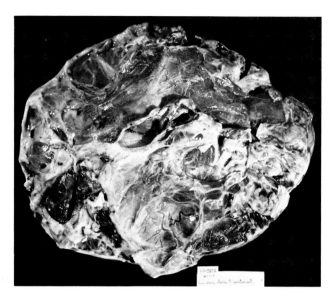

**25.1** Sectioned surface of a granulosa cell tumor. Numerous cysts, some of which are filled with clotted blood, are evident.

[Reprinted by permission from Case Records of the Massachusetts General Hospital, Case 89-1961, N. Engl. J. Med. 265:1213, 1961.]

but as a result of rupture of a cystic compartment with hemoperitoneum. A rare granulosa cell tumor simulates a serous cystadenoma on gross examination, forming a large mass composed of one or more thin-walled cysts separated by little or no solid tissue (Figure 25.10b, Plate VIII).

On microscopic examination the granulosa cells grow in a wide variety of patterns, which are commonly admixed (Figure 25.2). Microfollicular, macrofollicular, trabecular, insular, and/or solid tubular arrangements are characteristic of the more highly differentiated tumors. The microfollicular pattern, which is the single most distinctive, features multiple small cavities containing eosinophilic fluid and often one or a few degenerating nuclei (Figure 25.3); these spaces, designated Call–Exner bodies, are separated by well-differentiated granulosa cells, the pale, angular, and often grooved nuclei of which are arranged haphazardly in relation to one another and to the cavities. It is most important to distinguish Call–Exner bodies from the glands of adenocarcinomas and carcinoids and the hyaline bodies of similar size that are seen in gonadoblastomas[38] and sex cord tumors with annular tubules,[37] because all these tumors have clinical implications that differ considerably from those of the granulosa cell tumor. The glands of adenocarcinomas and primary or metastatic carcinoids are generally lined by cells that have a

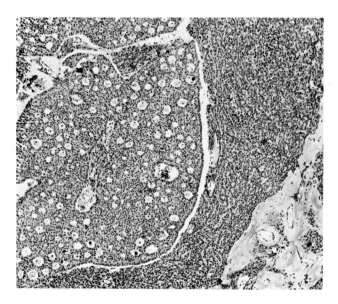

**25.2** Granulosa cell tumor. ×55. A microfollicular pattern is present on the left, and a watered silk pattern on the right.

[Reprinted by permission from J. McL. Morris and R. E. Scully, *Endocrinology of the Ovary*, St. Louis, C. V. Mosby, 1958.]

more orderly arrangement than that of granulosa cells. The lumens in adenocarcinomas are often filled with thick mucus, whereas those of carcinoids typically contain an eosinophilic secretion, which is sometimes calcified; the nuclei of adenocarcinomas are usually more highly malignant in appearance than those of the granulosa cell tumor, whereas those of the carcinoid have a characteristic round contour and coarse chromatin. The hyaline bodies of the gonadoblastoma and sex cord tumor with annular tubules are denser than Call–Exner bodies and can sometimes be observed to be continuous with hyaline thickenings of the basement membrane along the periphery of the tumor cell nests. These bodies also often undergo calcification; other characteristic features of these tumors are even more helpful in the differential diagnosis.

The macrofollicular pattern is characterized by cysts lined by well-differentiated granulosa cells, beneath which theca cells are usually present (Figure 25.4). One or both of these cell layers may be luteinized (i.e., accumulate abundant cytoplasm so that they resemble cells of the corpus luteum). The degree of differentiation in the walls of the cysts may be so marked that a high-power distinction from a nonneoplastic follicle cyst may be difficult, but

**25.3** Granulosa cell tumor, microfollicular pattern. ×460. Call–Exner bodies are surrounded by granulosa cells with disoriented angular nuclei.

[Reprinted by permission from R. E. Scully and J. McL. Morris, Functioning ovarian tumors, *in* J. V. Meigs and S. H. Sturgis, eds., *Progress in Gynecology*. Vol. 3. New York, Grune and Stratton, 1957, pp. 20–34.]

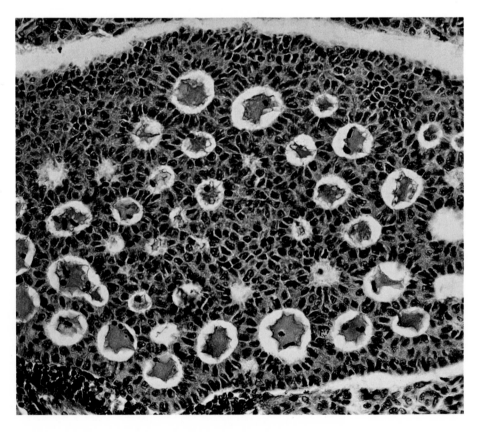

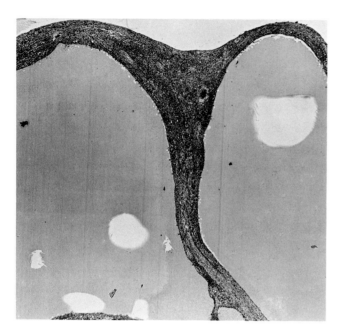

**25.4** Granulosa cell tumor, macrofollicular pattern. ×29.

[Reprinted by permission from Case Records of the Massachusetts General Hospital, Case 89-1961, N. Engl. J. Med. 265:1213, 1961.]

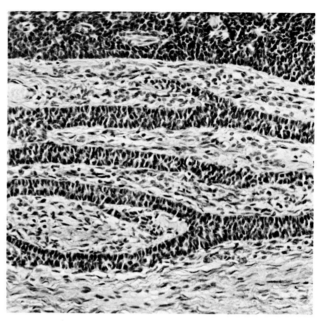

**25.5** Granulosa cell tumor, trabecular pattern. ×200.

[Reprinted by permission from S. F. Serov, R. E. Scully, and L. H. Sobin, *International Histological Classification of Tumours. No. 9. Histological Typing of Ovarian Tumours*, Geneva, WHO, 1973.]

practically this problem rarely exists when the cysts are viewed in the context of the clinical, gross, and other microscopic findings. The trabecular and insular forms are characterized by cords and islands of granulosa cells separated by a fibromatous or thecomatous stroma (Figures 25.5 and 25.6), whereas the solid tubular pattern features elongated tubules with peripherally arranged nuclei and central masses of cytoplasm; rarely a few hollow tubules or glandlike structures are encountered.

The less well-differentiated forms of granulosa cell tumor typically have watered silk (moire silk), gyriform, and/or diffuse (sarcomatoid) patterns (Figures 25.2 and 25.7). The first two patterns are manifested by undulating or zigzag rows of granulosa cells, generally in single file, whereas the diffuse form appears as a monotonous cellular growth resembling a low-grade round cell sarcoma; mitoses may be numerous. The unfortunate misinterpretation of an undifferentiated carcinoma as a diffuse granulosa cell tumor is one of the most frequent in ovarian tumor pathology. If the clinical course of the patient is atypically malignant for a granulosa cell tumor, the possibility of such a misdiagnosis must be considered. The single best criterion for distinguishing these two tumors is the appearance of the nuclei, which are typically uniform, pale,

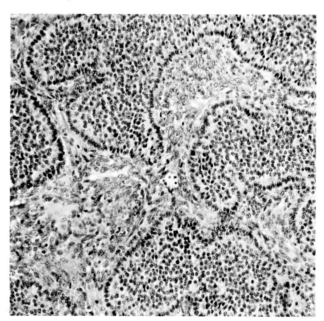

**25.6** Granulosa cell tumor, trabecular and insular patterns. ×160.

[Reprinted by permission from Case Records of the Massachusetts General Hospital, Case 89-1961, N. Engl. J. Med. 265:1213, 1961.]

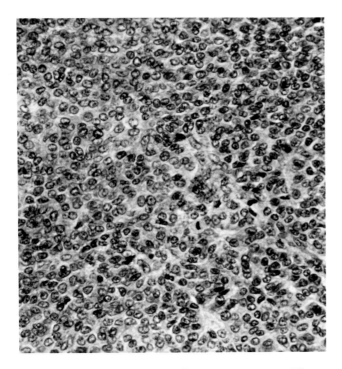

**25.7** Granulosa cell tumor, diffuse pattern. ×300. The nuclei are pale and oval.

[Reprinted by permission from Case Records of the Massachusetts General Hospital, Case 45292, *N. Engl. J. Med.* 261:149, 1959.]

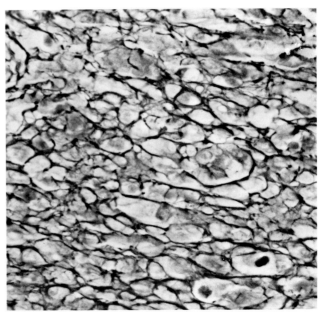

**25.8** Pattern of reticulin in thecoma. ×600.

[Reprinted by permission from S. F. Serov, R. E. Scully, and L. H. Sobin, *International Histological Classification of Tumours. No. 9. Histological Typing of Ovarian Tumours,* Geneva, WHO, 1973.]

and often grooved in granulosa cell tumors and are of unequal size and shape, hyperchromatic, and rarely grooved in undifferentiated carcinomas; atypical mitoses are often found in the latter as well.

Most granulosa cell tumors contain theca cells in varying quantities (Figure 25.6), and this has led to frequent usage of the term granulosa–theca cell tumors. Although this designation accurately describes the cellular content of many of these neoplasms, the simple term granulosa cell tumor is more widely accepted. Also, it is possible that the theca cell element, at least in some cases, represents a response of the ovarian stroma to the growth of granulosa cells within it rather than a truly neoplastic proliferation. Evidence favoring such an interpretation includes the nonspecific presence of thecalike cells in a variety of ovarian tumors, both benign and malignant, primary and metastatic, and the observation that theca cells may disappear from a granulosa cell tumor once it has extended beyond the ovary. It seems likely, however, that those tumors in which the theca cell element is prominent or even preponderant are truly mixed neoplasms. The theca

cells in granulosa cell tumors may resemble theca externa or theca interna cells and may be luteinized. In some tumors, particularly those with a diffuse pattern, differentiation of the granulosa and theca cell elements may be difficult or impossible. In such cases a reticulum stain can be helpful; just as in a developing graafian follicle, so in a granulosa cell tumor, the fibrils invest theca cells individually (Figure 25.8); in contrast, the granulosa cell layer of a follicle, which is not vascularized, contains no fibrils, and in the granulosa cell component of a tumor the reticulum is sparse, being typically confined to perivascular zones (Figure 25.9). Several histochemical reactions for steroid hormone-producing cells, particularly those that demonstrate various types of lipid content and enzyme activity, are characteristically positive in the theca cell element and negative in the granulosa cell component of a mixed tumor. This has led some observers to conclude that the theca cells probably produce the estrogens in granulosa cell tumors. Additional evidence in favor of this conclusion is the observation that granulosa cell tumors that recur outside ovarian tissue are typically not estrogenic.[9] In some instances, however, histochemical and other evidence has suggested a role for the granulosa cells in estrogen secretion.

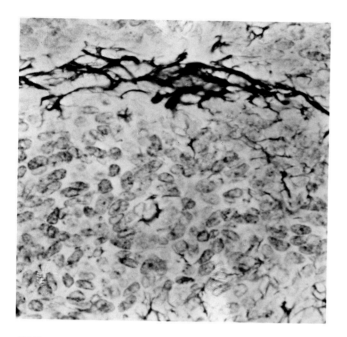

**25.9** Pattern of reticulin in granulosa cell tumor. ×560.
[Reprinted by permission from S. F. Serov, R. E. Scully, and L. H. Sobin, *International Histological Classification of Tumours. No. 9. Histological Typing of Ovarian Tumours*, Geneva, WHO, 1973.]

One variety of granulosa cell tumor that merits special attention is the type that is observed almost always in children and only rarely in older patients; its distinctive appearance and age distribution have led us to propose for it the designation juvenile granulosa cell tumor.[6] Two patterns are most commonly encountered: one of large follicles with thick walls and cavities, smaller than those seen in the adult macrofollicular form, and the other a disorderly pattern in which granulosa and theca cells are inextricably mixed. Other features of this type of tumor are a marked luteinization and lipid content of one or both elements, nuclei that are more hyperchromatic and immature than in the adult forms of granulosa cell tumor, and a generally more malignant appearance than the latter.

After the removal of a granulosa cell tumor, the manifestations of hyperestrinism typically regress. If the uterus has been conserved in a young woman, estrogen withdrawal bleeding typically occurs in 1 or 2 days and regular menses ensue shortly thereafter. No matter what its microscopic pattern, the granulosa cell tumor has to be considered one of a low grade of malignancy because it may extend beyond the ovary or recur after apparently successful operative removal. Its spread is largely within the pelvis and lower abdomen; distant metastases are rare, although

they have been reported in many sites. Although recurrences may appear within 5 years, often they are not evident until a much longer postoperative interval has elapsed, and numerous cases have been reported in which the tumor has reappeared two or even three or more decades after the initial therapy. The optimal treatment of the granulosa cell tumor in the menopausal or postmenopausal woman is total hysterectomy and bilateral salpingo-oophorectomy. In younger women and children in whom the preservation of fertility is an important consideration, removal of only the tumor and the adjacent fallopian tube is justifiable if no spread beyond the ovary is demonstrable and the opposite ovary is shown by biopsy to be uninvolved. Recurrences have often been treated successfully by reoperation, radiation therapy, or a combination thereof. Too little information is available on the chemotherapy of granulosa cell tumors to evaluate the comparative merits of various agents, but several of these have been used with varying success.[18,42] The 10-year salvage figures that have been recorded in the literature have varied widely from under 60 to over 90%[2,10,25,41] and progressive declines in survival have been documented after longer followup periods. Only one center has been able to correlate the microscopic pattern of the tumor and its prognosis, demonstrating a significantly greater frequency of late recurrences in cases with a diffuse pattern[17]; other investigators have commented on the frequency of a mixture of patterns in the same tumor, making a subdivision according to pattern impractical.

## Tumors in the Thecoma–Fibroma Group

These tumors are composed exclusively or almost exclusively of theca cells and/or fibroblasts of ovarian stromal origin; the presence of a few small nests of granulosa cells does not exclude a neoplasm from this category.

### Thecoma

This is composed of stromal cells that have become laden with lipid so that they bear a resemblance to theca cells; varying numbers of fibroblasts are also present in the tumor. The thecoma is only one-third as common as the granulosa cell tumor, is characteristically accompanied by estrogenic manifestations, and occurs at an older average age than the granulosa cell tumor, being very rare prior to puberty.

Thecomas range in size from small, impalpable tumors to large, solid masses; their consistence is firm and fibrous and their color, typically yellow or orange (Figure 25.10c,

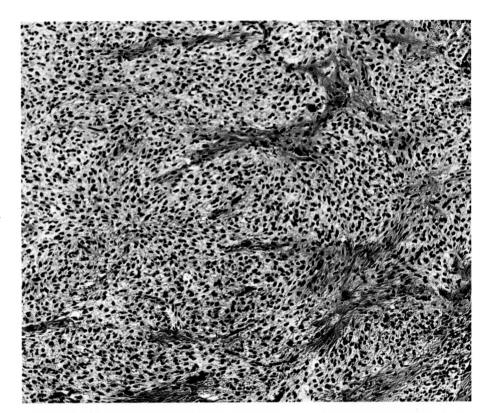

**25.11** Thecoma. ×133.

[Reprinted by permission from J. McL. Morris and R. E. Scully, *Endocrine Pathology of the Ovary,* St. Louis, C. V. Mosby, 1958.]

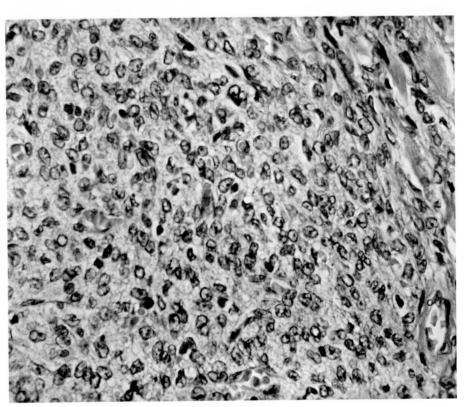

**25.12** Thecoma. ×425.

PLATE IX

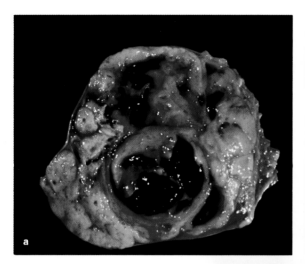

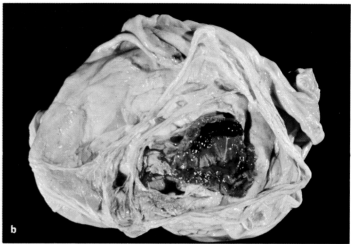

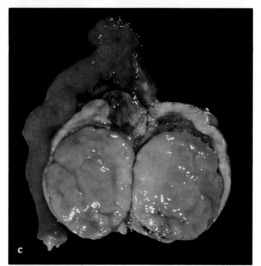

**25.10 a.** Sectioned surface of a solid granulosa cell tumor with focal hemorrhage. **b.** Opened unilocular-cystic granulosa cell tumor resembling serous cystadenoma. **c.** Sectioned surfaces of a thecoma. **d.** Sectioned surfaces of a fibroma.

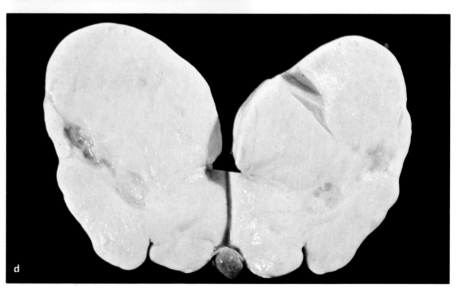

PLATE X

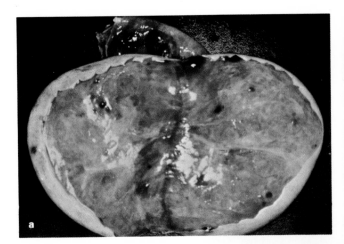

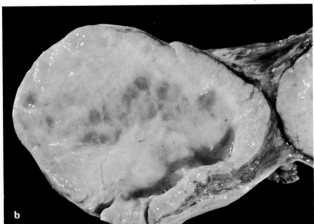

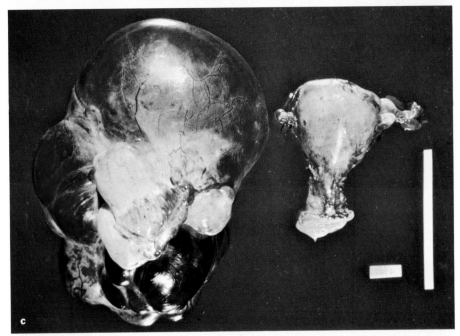

**25.16 a.** Sectioned surfaces of an ovary involved by massive endema. **b.** Sectioned surface of a sclerosing stromal tumor with areas of edema and cyst formation. **c.** Multicystic Sertoli–Leydig cell tumor with uterus. Cysts were filled with blood.
**d.** Sectioned surface of a hilus cell tumor.

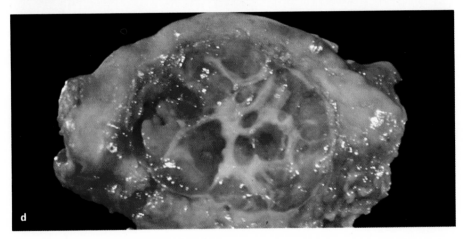

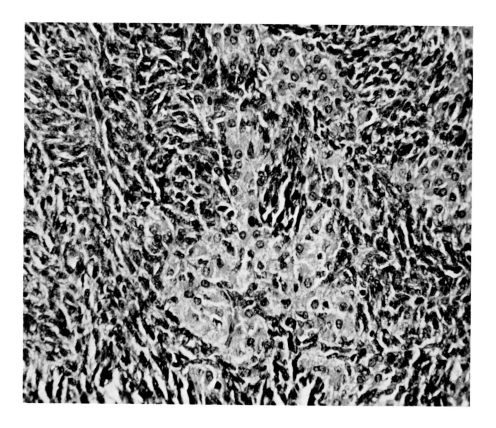

**25.13** Luteinized thecoma. ×291.

Plate IX), although in some cases it is whitish with only a tinge of yellow. Microscopic examination reveals two forms. The more common is characterized by ill-defined masses of rounded, lipid-rich, vacuolated cells separated by a fibromatous component (Figures 25.11 and 25.12). The second form, called a luteinized thecoma, has the basic appearance of a fibroma or a typical thecoma, but lutein cells are scattered singly or in nests throughout the tumor (Figure 25.13). This tumor has to be distinguished from the stromal–Leydig cell tumor,[45] which can be diagnosed only if crystalloids of Reinke are identified in the cytoplasm of the lutein-like cells. It is, indeed, possible that a number of "luteinized thecomas" are stromal–Leydig cell tumors that do not happen to contain crystalloids. A third type of neoplasm that belongs conceptually in the thecoma category but is included among the lipid cell tumors for purposes of differential diagnosis is the fully luteinized form, which has been called a stromal luteoma.[35] Possibly, many tumors in the lipid cell category, which are composed exclusively of cells resembling lutein cells, are stromal luteomas, but it is only when the tumor develops within the ovarian stroma, away from the hilus, and small islands of lutein cells are found elsewhere in the stroma of both ovaries that a definitive diagnosis of this subtype of lipid cell tumor can be made.

The thecoma is almost always unilateral and almost never malignant. Several tumors have been reported as malignant thecomas in the literature, but at least some of these are better interpreted as endocrinologically inactive fibrosarcomas or diffuse forms of granulosa cell tumor. In cases in which the preservation of fertility is important, a thecoma can be treated adequately by oophorectomy. However, total hysterectomy with bilateral salpingo-oophorectomy is indicated in most menopausal or postmenopausal women.

*Fibromas*

These tumors, which are composed of spindle cells forming collagen, account for 4% of all ovarian tumors. They occur in both young and old females but are most frequent during middle age, with an average age of 48 years; less than 10% of the cases are encountered under the age of 30 years.[21] The fibroma is not associated with steroid hormone production but it may be a component of two unusual clinical syndromes, the Meigs' syndrome[19]

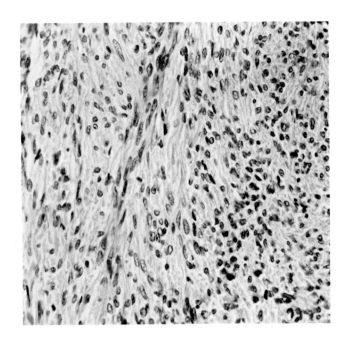

**25.14** Fibroma. ×325.

[Reprinted by permission from S. F. Serov, R. E. Scully, and L. H. Sobin, *International Histological Classification of Tumours. No. 9. Histological Typing of Ovarian Tumours,* Geneva, WHO, 1973.]

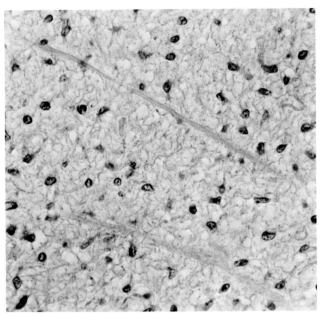

**25.15** Edematous fibroma. ×350.

[Reprinted by permission from S. F. Serov, R. E. Scully, and L. H. Sobin, *International Histological Classification of Tumours. No. 9. Histological Typing of Ovarian Tumors,* Geneva, WHO, 1973.]

and the basal cell nevus syndrome.[1] The former, which is characterized by the presence of ascites and pleural effusion in association with a fibromatous tumor of the ovary and a disappearance of the fluid after the removal of the ovarian tumor, has been reported in association with a very small percent of ovarian fibromas[21]; ascites alone has been seen in approximately 10 to 15% of the cases.[33] The most widely accepted explanation of the Meigs' syndrome is the seepage of fluid from the tumor through its capsule into the peritoneal cavity and its transfer therefrom into one or both pleural cavities either via lymphatics or a communication between the abdominal and pleural cavities, such as the foramen of Bochdalek.[19] The hereditary basal cell nevus syndrome is characterized by the presence of keratocysts of the jaw, basal cell carcinomas appearing early in life, a variety of other abnormalities, and often ovarian fibromas.[1]

The fibroma ranges in size from microscopic to very large; the smaller tumors are not uncommon, and for statistical purposes no tumor should be categorized as a fibroma unless it is 3 cm or more in diameter. Sectioning a fibroma reveals hard, flat, chalky-white surfaces that have a whorled appearance (Figure 25.10d). Areas of edema, occasionally with cyst formation, are commonly encountered. Focal or diffuse calcification and bilaterality are

observed in less than 10% of all the cases,[43] but these are characteristic features of the fibromas associated with the basal cell nevus syndrome. Microscopic examination reveals intersecting bundles of spindle cells producing collagen (Figure 25.14). Occasionally, a storiform pattern similar to that of the dermatofibrosarcoma protuberans is encountered. Many tumors show varying degrees of intercellular edema fluid, which may have a myxoid appearance (Figure 25.15).[33] The presence of bands of hyalinized fibrous tissue is not uncommon; and the cytoplasm of the neoplastic cells may contain small quantities of lipid.

The fibroma must be distinguished from massive edema (Figure 25.16a, Plate X) and stromal hyperplasia of the ovaries. The former is a uni- or bilateral disorder characterized by a nonneoplastic proliferation of ovarian stromal cells with marked intercellular edema.[4,16] Unlike the edematous fibroma, which displaces such ovarian structures as follicles, corpora lutea, and corpora albicantia, these structures are incorporated within the edematous tissue in cases of massive edema (Figure 25.17). Stromal hyperplasia, in contrast to the ovarian fibroma, is typically bilateral and is characterized by a multinodular or diffuse proliferation of closely packed, small stromal cells with minimal collagen formation.

Ovarian fibromas are benign, but the precise dividing

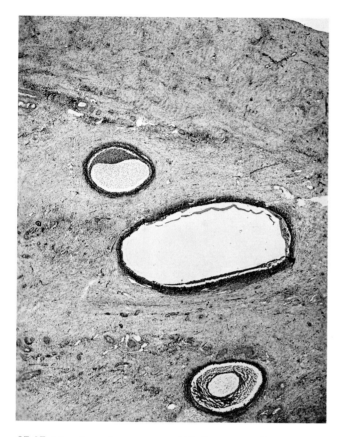

**25.17** Massive edema. ×16. Follicles are within edematous stroma.

[Reprinted by permission from S. F. Serov, R. E. Scully, and L. H. Sobin, *International Histological Classification of Tumours. No. 9. Histological Typing of Ovarian Tumours*, Geneva, WHO, 1973.]

line between them and the very rare fibrosarcoma of stromal cell origin has not been clearly established because of the infrequency of the latter. Occasional mitoses may be found in fibromatous tumors that are clinically benign, but a rare tumor with relatively few mitoses may recur after operative removal, particularly if it is adherent to surrounding structures. Exceptional tumors of apparent stromal cell origin are obviously malignant on microscopic examination as well as in their clinical behavior.

*Unclassified Tumors*

Tumors in the intermediate zone between fibromas and thecomas account for approximately 10% of all the cases in the general category and most of them are impossible to classify further. Such tumors are made up of cells having some but not all the features of theca cells, containing small to moderate amounts of lipid and presenting no more than equivocal evidence of estrogen secretion. One interesting subtype in the unclassified category, which is not specified in the WHO classification, is the sclerosing stromal tumor.[5] This neoplasm has been encountered in patients in the second and third decades in over 80% of 30 personally observed cases and has been associated with equivocal evidence of estrogen secretion in only a few instances. On gross examination it is almost always predominantly solid, characteristically forming a discrete mass, sharply demarcated from the adjacent ovarian tissue. Its sectioned surface is basically solid and whitish but typically shows foci of yellow discoloration and areas of edema and cyst formation (Figure 25.16b, Plate X). Microscopic examination shows a number of distinctive features: a pseudolobular pattern in which cellular nodules are separated from one another by less cellular areas of densely collagenous or edematous connective tissue (Figure 25.18); sclerosis within the nodules; prominent thin-walled vessels in some of the nodules (Figure 25.19); and a jumbled pattern of fibroblasts and rounded, lipid-laden, vacuolated cells within the nodules (Figure 25.20); occasionally, the vacuolated cells may have a signet cell appearance, creating some confusion with a Krukenberg tumor.

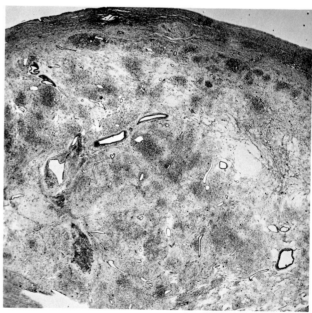

**25.18** Sclerosing stromal tumor. ×11. Cellular pseudolobules are separated by edematous hypocellular tumor.

[Reprinted by permission from A. Chalvardjian, and R. E. Scully, Sclerosing stromal tumors of the ovary, *Cancer* 31:664, 1973.]

**25.19** Sclerosing stromal tumor.
×173. The pseudolobule is
richly vascularized.

[Reprinted by permission from
A. Chalvardjian and R. E. Scully,
Sclerosing stromal tumors of the
ovary, *Cancer 31*:664, 1973.]

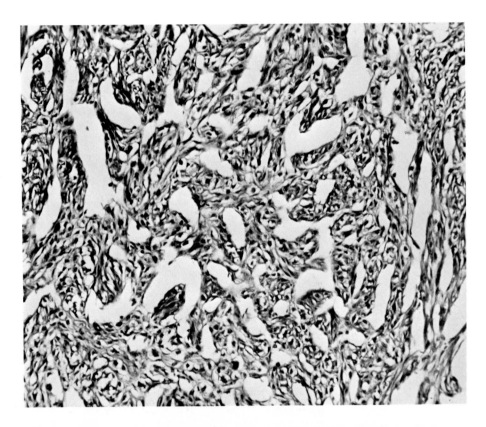

**25.20** Sclerosing stromal tumor.
×440. Spindle cells are mixed
with large, rounded vacuolated
cells.

[Reprinted by permission from
A. Chalvardjian and R. E. Scully,
Sclerosing stromal tumors of the
ovary, *Cancer 31*:664, 1973.]

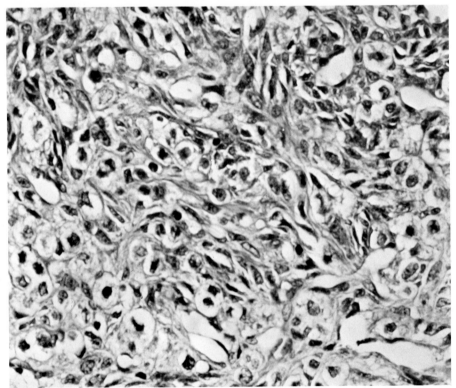

516

# Sertoli–Leydig Cell Tumors (Androblastomas)

These tumors contain Sertoli cells and/or Leydig cells in varying proportions and varying degrees of differentiation. Because the less well-differentiated neoplasms within this category may recapitulate the development of the testis, the terms androblastomas and arrhenoblastomas have been used as synonyms for Sertoli–Leydig cell tumors. However, their connotation of associated masculinization is misleading because some of these tumors have no endocrine manifestations and others may even be accompanied by an estrogenic syndrome. Nevertheless, WHO has selected androblastomas as an alternate term for Sertoli–Leydig cell tumors.[40] These neoplasms account for less than 1/2% of all ovarian tumors but are among the most fascinating from both pathologic and clinical viewpoints.[24,28,29,31,34,48,49] They occur in all age groups but are most often encountered in young women, who usually become virilized. Typically a patient who has been having normal periods begins to have oligomenorrhea followed within a few months by amenorrhea. There is a concomitant loss of female secondary sex characteristics with atrophy of the breasts and disappearance of normal bodily contours. Progressive masculinization is heralded by hirsutism, with temporal balding, deepening of the voice, and enlargement of the clitoris in its wake. The androgen secretion by the tumor may also result in erythrocytosis. Plasma testosterone and/or androstenedione levels are typically elevated[30,31] but the urinary 17-ketosteroid values are usually normal or only slightly raised; occasionally a very high level of 17-ketosteroids has been recorded. Tests involving attempted stimulation by tropic hormones and suppression by gonadal and adrenal cortical steroids have not yet proved reliable diagnostically in differentiating these tumors from those of the adrenal cortex.[15] Many Sertoli–Leydig cell tumors have no endocrine manifestations, and still others have been associated with various estrogenic syndromes, including isosexual precocity and abnormal postpubertal uterine bleeding.[48,49] The degree of correlation between the cellular composition of these tumors and the type of associated endocrine effect is discussed below in the context of the various subtypes.

Sertoli–Leydig cell tumors may vary as greatly in gross appearance as granulosa cell tumors and thecomas; indeed, these neoplasms cannot be distinguished on gross examination alone (Figure 25.16c, Plate VIII). Sertoli–Leydig cell tumors have been classified by WHO both on the basis of their degree of differentiation and the presence or absence of heterologous elements (Table 25.1).[40] The pure or almost pure well-differentiated Sertoli cell tumors have been divided into two categories based on their lipid content. The Sertoli cell tumor (tubular androblastoma) is characterized by solid or hollow tubules, composed of or lined by cells that resemble to varying degrees well-differentiated Sertoli cells, with few or no Leydig cells between the tubules (Figure 25.21). The Sertoli cells may contain some but not large amounts of lipid; this tumor may be inactive or may produce estrogens. The Sertoli cell tumor with lipid storage, or tubular androblastoma with lipid storage, is characterized by solid tubules and more diffuse, discrete masses of well-differentiated Sertoli cells, the cytoplasm of which is highly vacuolated and contains very large quantities of lipid (Figures 25.22 and 25.23). This tumor, which was initially described by Lecène and considered to be a lipid-rich granulosa cell tumor (*folliculome lipidique*), has been associated with estrogenic manifestations.[48,49] The well-differentiated Sertoli–Leydig cell tumor is simply a Sertoli cell tumor that contains more than a minimal component of Leydig cells, which resemble those of the testis and have occasionally been shown to contain crystalloids of Reinke (Figures 25.24 and 25.25). Tumors of this type are often nonfunctioning but may be virilizing or occasionally estrogenic.

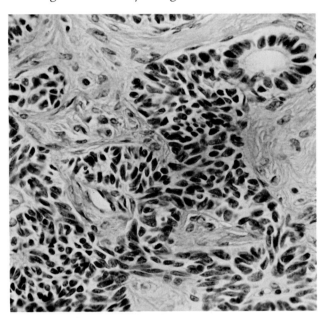

**25.21** Sertoli cell tumor. ×350.

[Reprinted by permission from S. F. Serov, R. E. Scully, and L. H. Sobin, *International Histological Classification of Tumours. No. 9. Histological Typing of Ovarian Tumours*, Geneva, WHO, 1973.]

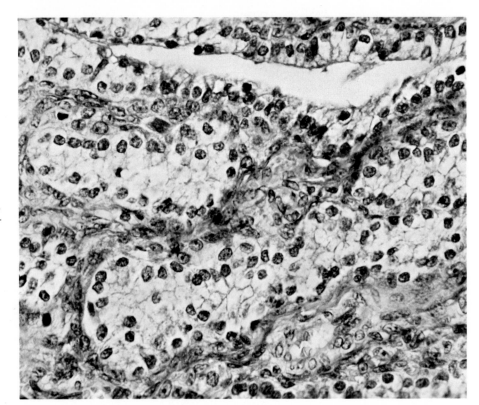

**25.22** Sertoli cell tumor with lipid storage. ×95.

[Reprinted by permission from S. F. Serov, R. E. Scully, and L. H. Sobin, *International Histological Classification of Tumours. No. 9. Histological Typing of Ovarian Tumours*, Geneva, WHO, 1973.]

**25.23** Sertoli cell tumor with lipid storage. ×445.

[Reprinted by permission from S. F. Serov, R. E. Scully, and L. H. Sobin, *International Histological Classification of Tumours. No. 9. Histological Typing of Ovarian Tumours*, Geneva, WHO, 1973.]

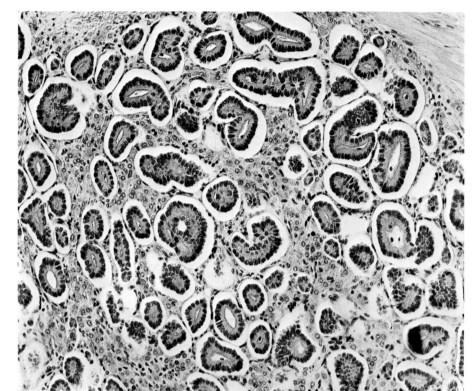

**25.24** Sertoli–Leydig cell tumor, well differentiated. ×160.

[Reprinted by permission from J. McL. Morris and R. E. Scully, *Endocrine Pathology of the Ovary*, St. Louis, C. V. Mosby, 1958.]

**25.25** Sertoli–Leydig cell tumor. ×690. Arrows point to crystalloids of Reinke.

[Reprinted by permission from R. E. Scully, Androgenic lesions of the ovary, *in* H. Grady and D. E. Smith, eds., *The Ovary*. International Academy of Pathology Monograph No. 3. Baltimore, Williams and Wilkins, 1962, Chapter 9.]

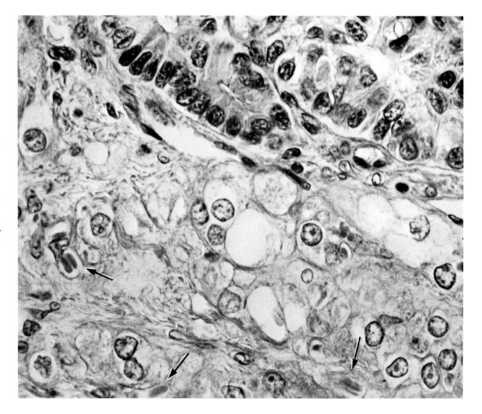

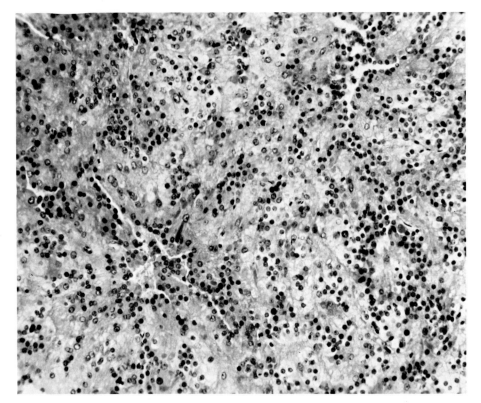

**25.26** Hilus cell tumor. ×184.

[Reprinted by permission from R. E. Scully, Androgenic lesions of the ovary, *in* H. Grady and D. E. Smith, eds., *The Ovary*. International Academy of Pathology Monograph No. 3. Baltimore, Williams and Wilkins, 1962, Chapter 9.]

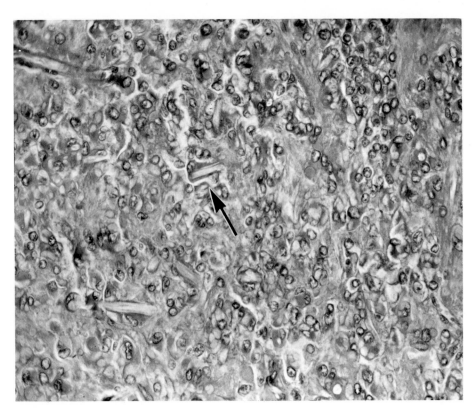

**25.27** Hilus cell tumor. ×320. Arrow points to crystalloids of Reinke.

[Reprinted by permission from J. McL. Morris and R. E. Scully, *Endocrine Pathology of the Ovary*, St. Louis, C. V. Mosby, 1958.]

The pure, well-differentiated Leydig cell tumor may result in some instances from a one-sided development of a Sertoli–Leydig cell tumor; in other cases it may arise directly from ovarian stromal cells.[32] However, most such tumors appear to originate in the ovarian hilus from hilus cells (hilar Leydig cells), which have been demonstrated as an embryologic remnant in 80 to 85% of adult ovaries, usually in relation to nonmedullated nerve fibers.[44] Leydig cell or hilus cell tumors, which typically form small red to brown nodules centered in the hilar region (Figure 25.16d, Plate VIII), also have to be considered in the context of lipid cell tumors (tumors of uncertain origin composed only of cells resembling adrenal cortical, lutein, and Leydig cells[47]) and can be isolated with certainty from this more general category only if specific crystalloids of Reinke are demonstrable in the cytoplasm of some of the neoplastic cells. Fewer than 25 such cases have been reported. It is possible, however, that a number of lipid cell tumors are hilus cell tumors but cannot be recognized as such in the absence of crystalloids; this possibility is suggested by the fact that crystalloids of Reinke have been found in no more than 40% of Leydig cell tumors of the testis.[22] On microscopic examination the cells of hilus cell tumors typically have a diffuse pattern; often distinctive cellular zones with nuclear crowding alternate with zones poor in nuclei (Figures 25.26 and 25.27); occasionally, the tumor cells contain large amounts of lipochrome pigment. These neoplasms, which are encountered in a slightly older age group than Sertoli–Leydig cell tumors in general, are typically virilizing but may have estrogenic manifestations as well.

Sertoli–Leydig cell tumors of intermediate and poor differentiation form a continuum characterized by a variety of patterns and combinations of cell types and can be regarded as grade II and grade III tumors in the more general category rather than subtypes of distinctive appearance. Often a tumor exhibits intermediate differentiation in one area and poor differentiation in another, and both Sertoli cells and Leydig cells, singly or in combination, may be characterized by varying degrees of immaturity. Only the more common of the many patterns are discussed here. In the tumors of intermediate differentiation immature Sertoli cells with small, round, oval, or angular nuclei are arranged typically in ill-defined masses, solid tubules, nests, and thin cords resembling the sex cords of the embryonic testis (Figure 25.28). These structures are separated by a fibromatous stroma that contains clusters of well-differentiated Leydig cells (Figure 25.29). Occasionally thin-walled cysts lined by flattened Sertoli cells create a thyroidlike appearance. The Sertoli and Leydig cell ele-

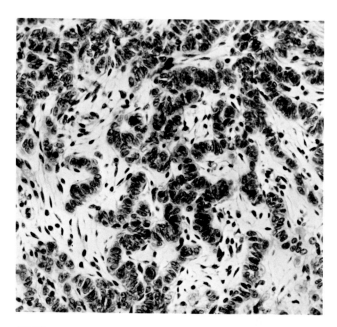

**25.28** Sertoli cell element of Sertoli–Leydig cell tumor of intermediate differentiation. ×250. The arrangement suggests that of testicular sex cords.

[Reprinted by permission from S. F. Serov, R. E. Scully, and L. H. Sobin, *International Histological Classification of Tumours. No. 9. Histological Typing of Ovarian Tumours*, Geneva, WHO, 1973.]

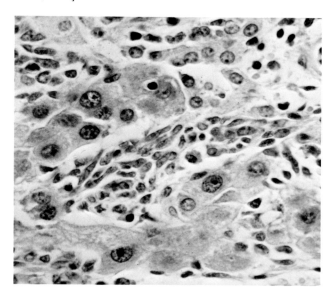

**25.29** Sertoli–Leydig cell tumor of intermediate differentiation. ×500.

[Reprinted by permission from S. F. Serov, R. E. Scully, and L. H. Sobin, *International Histological Classification of Tumours. No. 9. Histological Typing of Ovarian Tumours*, Geneva, WHO, 1973.]

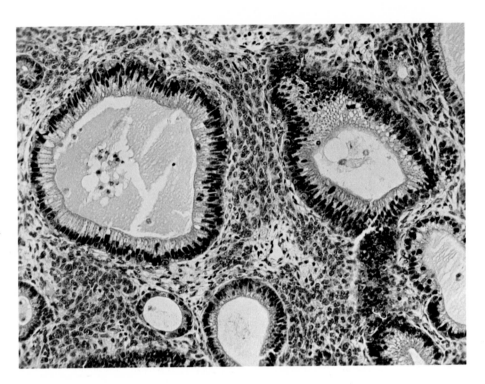

**25.30** Sertoli–Leydig cell tumor with heterologous elements. ×167. Mucinous glands lie in background of a more typical intermediate pattern.

[Reprinted by permission from S. F. Serov, R. E. Scully, and L. H. Sobin, *International Histological Classification of Tumours. No. 9. Histological Typing of Ovarian Tumours,* Geneva, WHO, 1973.]

ments, singly or together, may contain varying and sometimes large amounts of lipid in the form of small or large droplets. In certain cases the Leydig cell component may exist in the form of a densely cellular stroma, or well-formed Leydig cells may exhibit marked nuclear atypicality. Certain pure or relatively pure Sertoli cell tumors and perhaps a rare, relatively pure Leydig cell tumor may appropriately be placed in the poorly differentiated category. Poorly differentiated Sertoli–Leydig cell tumors were originally classified as sarcomatoid because, aside from the presence of specifically diagnostic elements, they resemble fibrosarcomas; however, rare Sertoli cell carcinomas also belong in the poorly differentiated category. Sertoli–Leydig cell tumors of intermediate and poor differentiation are usually virilizing but, like the better differentiated forms, can be nonfunctioning or estrogenic.

Sertoli–Leydig cell tumors with heterologous elements may contain a variety of unusual cell types, but the degree of differentiation of the tumor is probably of greater importance than its content of unexpected tissues in determining its prognosis. The most commonly encountered foreign elements are glands and cysts lined by moderately to well-differentiated mucinous epithelial cells (Figure 25.30); occasionally argentaffin cells can be demonstrated among the mucinous elements, and on rare occasions a Sertoli–Leydig cell tumor has included a carcinoid. The stromal compartment of these tumors may contain islands of cartilage and skeletal muscle elements. Occasionally the sarcomatoid variety has large areas of embryonal rhabdomyosarcoma. We have also seen a rare combination of Sertoli–Leydig cell tumor and neuroblastoma. Despite the wide variety of unexpected tissues in occasional examples of Sertoli–Leydig cell tumor, in no case have areas of the latter been encountered in an otherwise typical ovarian teratoma.

Generally the distinctive patterns and cell types of Sertoli–Leydig cell tumors enable one to make a diagnosis with ease, but difficulties exist in certain cases. As discussed below, an intermediate morphologic zone exists between tumors composed of male cell types and those containing granulosa and theca cells. Another occasional source of confusion is the endometrioid carcinoma, which may have small tubular structures resembling those of a Sertoli cell tumor; moreover, the tubular glands of the Sertoli cell tumor may be larger than usual, simulating those of the well-differentiated endometrioid carcinoma. The appearance of squamous differentiation or mucous secretion is helpful in diagnosing an endometrioid carcinoma, but in their absence it may be impossible to decide whether a tumor with a pattern intermediate between that of the typical Sertoli cell tumor and that of the well-differentiated endometrioid carcinoma belongs definitively in either category. Finally, because a variety of tumors that stimulate proliferation of the ovarian stroma are accompanied by virilization, the presence of the latter alone does not establish a diagnosis of Sertoli–Leydig cell tumor.

After the removal of a virilizing Sertoli–Leydig cell tumor, the menses characteristically resume in about 4 weeks. In most cases the excess hair diminishes, but often incompletely. Clitoromegaly and particularly deepening of the voice are less apt to regress. Sertoli–Leydig cell tumors vary widely in their degree of differentiation. Well-differentiated forms rarely exhibit a malignant behavior, whereas the poorly differentiated tumors, which resemble sarcomas or carcinomas, may have a rapidly malignant course. Pelvic and intraabdominal spread is much more common than distant metastasis.

The overall 5-year survival rate of patients with Sertoli–Leydig cell tumors has been reported to be in the range of slightly under 70 to slightly over 90%.[28,29] Because these tumors occur predominantly in young women and are bilateral in fewer than 5% of the cases, conservative removal of the tumor and adjacent fallopian tube is justifiable if the preservation of fertility is an important consideration and there is no evidence of extension beyond the involved ovary.

# Gynandroblastoma

This extremely rare tumor has been greatly overdiagnosed. According to WHO, the term should be used only if clearly recognizable, well-differentiated female and male cellular elements each form significant components of a neoplasm (Figure 25.31). Occasional foci of female-type cells in an otherwise typical Sertoli–Leydig cell tumor, or of male cell types in a granulosa–stromal cell tumor, do not constitute sufficient evidence for this diagnosis. It goes without saying that in view of the proved capacity of tumors of male cell types to produce estrogens and of tumors of female cell types to produce androgens, the nature of the hormones secreted by a tumor should not determine its diagnosis.

# Unclassified Sex Cord–Stromal Tumors

This ill-defined group of tumors, which comprises less than 10% of those in the sex cord–stromal category, can be defined as neoplasms in which no clearly predominant pattern of male or female differentiation or clear predominance of male or female cell types is recognizable. This

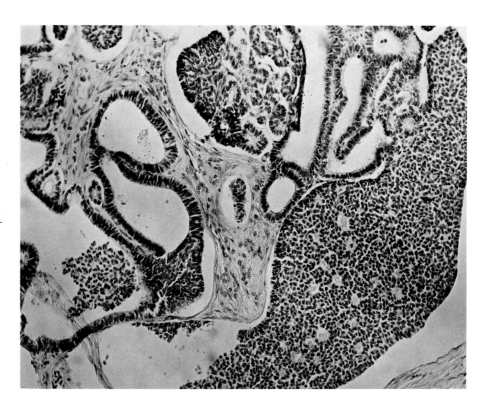

**25.31** Gynandroblastoma. ×160.

[Reprinted by permission from R. E. Scully, Androgenic lesions of the ovary, *in* H. Grady and D. E. Smith, eds., *The Ovary.* International Academy of Pathology Monograph No. 3. Baltimore, Williams and Wilkins, 1962, Chapter 9.]

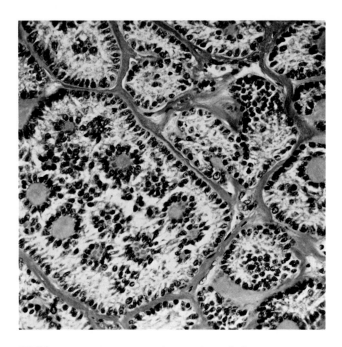

**25.32** Sex cord tumor with annular tubules. ×239.

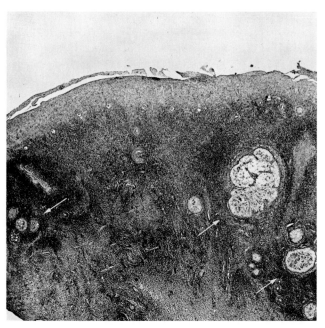

**25.33** Sex cord tumor with annular tubules. ×23. Multicentric foci (arrows) are evident in this case, which was associated with the Peutz–Jeghers syndrome.

[Reprinted by permission from R. E. Scully, Sex cord tumor with annular tubules. A distinctive ovarian tumor of the Peutz–Jeghers syndrome, *Cancer* 25:1107, 1970.]

grouping gives the pathologist an opportunity to segregate neoplasms of uncertain type that might elicit a diagnosis of granulosa cell tumor from one pathologist and Sertoli cell tumor from another if a more specific diagnosis were required. The boundary lines between these tumors and granulosa–stromal cell tumors, on the one hand, and Sertoli–Leydig cell tumors, on the other, are of necessity vague because interpretations of overlapping patterns and closely similar cell types are by their very nature subjective.

One recurring pattern within the category that is unclassified according to the WHO schema is distinctive enough to have given a subgroup of these tumors the more specific designation sex cord tumor with annular tubules.[37] This neoplasm is characterized by simple and complex annular tubules. The simple tubules have the shape of a ring or wheel, with nuclei oriented around the periphery and a central round body of hyalinized material of basement membrane origin; an intervening anuclear cytoplasmic zone forms the major component of the ring or wheel. The complex annular tubules are made up of intercommunicating rings revolving around multiple hyaline bodies (Figure 25.32). Tumors containing these structures have been called Sertoli cell tumors by some observers and granulosa cell tumors by others, but the pattern is intermediate and the cell type indifferent. A study of tumorlets of this type suggests an origin in the ovarian cortex from granulosa cells, but the differentiation of the

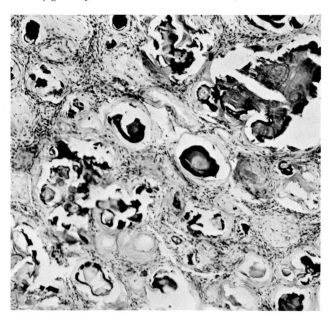

**25.34** Sex cord tumor with annular tubules. ×76. Extensive calcification of epithelial nests has occurred in this tumor, which was associated with the Peutz–Jeghers syndrome.

neoplastic cells is more in the direction of Sertoli cells. These rare tumors may be estrogenic or nonfunctioning. They may form large masses and have on occasion exhibited a malignant behavior with extraovarian extension and metastasis. When they have been multiple, usually in the form of tumorlets (Figure 25.33), they have almost always been complicated by calcification (Figure 25.34) and have been documented to be associated with the Peutz–Jeghers syndrome (mucocutaneous melanin pigmentation and intestinal hamartomatous polyposis); indeed, on occasion their detection provides the first evidence of the disease.

# Conclusion

Sex cord-stromal tumors are difficult to classify precisely and are characterized by a spectrum of morphologic and physiologic patterns; their behavior varies from benign to highly malignant. Their complexity is an invitation to sophisticated morphologic and physiologic approaches to improve our understanding of them.

# REFERENCES

1. Berlin, N. I., Van Scott, E. J., Clendenning, W. E., Archard, H. O., Block, J. B., Witkop, C. J., and Haynes, H. A. Basal cell nevus syndrome. *Ann. Intern. Med.* 64:403, 1966.

2. Burslem, R. W., Langley, F. A., and Woodcock, A. S. A clinicopathological study of oestrogenic ovarian tumours. *Cancer* 7:552, 1954.

3. Busby, T., and Anderson, G. W. Feminizing mesenchymomas of the ovary. *Am. J. Obstet. Gynecol.* 68:1391, 1954.

4. Case Records of the Massachusetts General Hospital. Case 24, 1971. *N. Engl. J. Med.* 284:1369, 1971.

5. Chalvardjian, A., and Scully, R. E. Sclerosing stromal tumors of the ovary. *Cancer* 31:664, 1973.

6. Dickersin, G. R., and Scully, R. E. The juvenile granulosa cell tumor. Report of 20 cases and review of the literature. In preparation, 1976.

7. Dockerty, M. B., and MacCarty, W. C. Granulosa cell tumors; with the report of a 34-lb. specimen and a review. *Am. J. Obstet. Gynecol.* 37:425, 1939.

8. Fathalla, M. F. The occurrence of granulosa and theca tumors in clinically normal ovaries. A study of 25 cases. *J. Obstet. Gynaecol. Br. Commonw.* 74:279, 1967.

9. Fathalla, M. F. The role of the ovarian stroma in hormone production by ovarian tumors. *J. Obstet. Gynaecol. Br. Commonw.* 75:78, 1968.

10. Fox, H., Agrawal, K., and Langley, F. A. A clinicopathologic study of 92 cases of granulosa cell tumor of the ovary with special reference to the factors influencing prognosis. *Cancer* 35:231, 1975.

11. Gusberg, S. B., and Kardon, P. Proliferative endometrial response to theca–granulosa cell tumors. *Am. J. Obstet. Gynecol.* 111:633, 1971.

12. Iturzaeta, N., Kenny, F. M., and Sieber, W. Precocious pseudopuberty due to granulosa cell tumor in three girls. *Am. J. Dis. Child.* 114:39, 1967.

13. Johnston, W. W., Goldston, W. R., and Montgomery, M. S. Clinicopathologic studies in feminizing tumors of the ovary. III. The role of genital cytology. *Acta Cytol.* 15:334, 1971.

14. Jolly, H. *Sexual Precocity. A Personal Study of 69 Patients.* American Lecture Series, Springfield, Ill., Charles C Thomas, 1955.

15. Judd, H. L., Spore, W. W., Talner, L. B., Rigg, L. A., Yen, S. S. C., and Benirschke, K. Preoperative localization of a testosterone-secreting ovarian tumor by retrograde venous catherization and selective sampling. *Am. J. Obstet. Gynecol.* 120:91, 1974.

16. Kalstone, C. E., Jaffe, R. B., and Abell, M. R. Massive edema of the ovary simulating fibroma. *Obstet. Gynecol.* 34:564, 1969.

17. Kottmeier, H. L. *Carcinoma of the Female Genitalia.* The Abraham Flexner Lectures, Series No. 11, Baltimore, Williams and Wilkins, 1953.

18. Malkasian, G. D. Jr., Webb, M. J., and Jorgensen, E. O. Observations on chemotherapy of granulosa cell carcinomas and malignant ovarian teratomas. *Obstet. Gynecol.* 44:885, 1974.

19. Meigs, J. V. Fibroma of the ovary with ascites and hydrothorax. Meigs' syndrome. *Am. J. Obstet. Gynecol.* 67:962, 1954.

20. Morris, J. McL., and Scully, R. E. *Endocrine Pathology of the Ovary.* St. Louis, C. V. Mosby Co., 1958, 151 p.

21. Morrison, C. W., and Woodruff, J. D. Fibrothecoma and associated ovarian stromal neoplasia. *Obstet. Gynecol.* 23:344, 1964.

22. Mostofi, F. K., and Price, E. B. Jr. Tumors of the male genital system. *Atlas of Tumor Pathology*, Second Series, Fascicle 8. Washington, D.C., Armed Forces Institute of Pathology, 1973.

23. Niswander, K. R., Courey, N. G., and Woodward, T. Precocious pseudopuberty caused by ovarian tumors. *Obstet. Gynecol.* 26:381, 1965.

24. Norris, H. J., and Chorlton, I. Functioning tumors of the ovary. *Clin. Obstet. Gynecol.* 17:189, 1974.

25. Norris, H. J., and Taylor, H. B. Prognosis of granulosatheca tumors of the ovary. *Cancer* 21:255, 1968.

26. Norris, H. J., and Taylor, H. B. Virilization associated with cystic granulosa tumors. *Obstet. Gynecol.* 34:629, 1969.

27. Novak, E. R., Kutchmeshgi, J., Mupas, R. S., and Woodruff, J. D., et al. Feminizing gonadal stromal tumors. *Obstet. Gynecol.* 38:701, 1971.

28. Novak, E. R., and Long, J. H. Arrhenoblastoma of the ovary. *Am. J. Obstet. Gynecol.* 92:1082, 1965.

29. O'Hern, T. M., and Neubecker, R. D. Arrhenoblastoma. *Obstet. Gynecol.* 19:758, 1962.

30. Osborn, R. H., and Yannone, M. E. Plasma androgens in the normal and androgenic female: A review. *Obstet. Gynecol. Surv.* 26:195, 1971.

31. Prunty, F. T. G. Hirsutism, virilism and apparent virilism and their gonadal relationship. Part 1. *J. Endocrinol.* 38:85, 1967.

32. Roth, L. M., and Sternberg, W. H. Ovarian stromal tumors containing Leydig cells. II. Pure Leydig cell tumor, non-hilar type. *Cancer* 32:952, 1973.

33. Samanth, K. K., and Black, W. C. Benign ovarian stromal tumors associated with free peritoneal fluid. *Am. J. Obstet. Gynecol.* 107:538, 1970.

34. Scully, R. E. Androgenic lesions of the ovary. In Grady, H. G., and Smith, D. E., eds. *The Ovary.* International Academy of

Pathology Monograph No. 3, Baltimore, Williams and Wilkins, 1962, pp. 143–174.

35. Scully, R. E. Stromal luteoma of the ovary. A distinctive type of lipoid-cell tumor. *Cancer 17*:769, 1964.

36. Scully, R. E. Sex cord–mesenchyme tumours. Pathologic classification and its relation to prognosis and treatment. *In* Junqueira, A. C., and Gentil, F., eds. *Ovarian Cancer.* IUCC Monograph Series, Vol. II. Heidelberg, Springer-Verlag, 1968, pp. 40–56.

37. Scully, R. E. Sex cord tumor with annular tubules. A distinctive ovarian tumor of the Peutz–Jeghers syndrome. *Cancer 25*:1107, 1970.

38. Scully, R. E. Gonadoblastoma. A review of 74 cases. *Cancer 25*:1340, 1970.

39. Serment, H. L., Laffargue, P., Piana, L., and Blanc, B. Ovarian hormone tumors of female children. *Int. J. Gynaecol. Obstet. 8*:409, 1970.

40. Serov, S. F., Scully, R. E., and Sobin, L. H. *International Histological Classification of Tumours*, No. 9. *Histological Typing of Ovarian Tumours.* Geneva, World Health Organization, 1973.

41. Sjostedt, S., and Wahlen, T. Prognosis of granulosa cell tumors. *Acta Obstet. Gynecol. Scand. 40*:1, 1961.

42. Smith, J. P., and Rutledge, F. Chemotherapy in the treatment of cancer of the ovary. *Am. J. Obstet. Gynecol. 107*:691, 1970.

43. Sotto, L. S. J., Postoloff, A. V., and Carr, F. A case of calcified ovarian fibroma with ossification. *Am. J. Obstet. Gynecol. 71*:1355, 1956.

44. Sternberg, W. H. The morphology, endocrine function, hyperplasia and tumors of the human ovarian hilus cells. *Am. J. Pathol. 25*:493, 1949.

45. Sternberg, W. H., and Roth, L. M. Ovarian stromal tumors containing Leydig cells. 1. Stromal–Leydig cell tumor and nonneoplastic transformation of ovarian stroma to Leydig cells. *Cancer 32*:940, 1973.

46. Targett, C. S. Estrogen excretion in a case of theca–granulosa cell tumor. *Am. J. Obstet. Gynecol. 119*:859, 1974.

47. Taylor, H. B., and Norris, H. J. Lipid cell tumors of the ovary. *Cancer 20*:1953, 1967.

48. Teilum, G. Classification of testicular and ovarian androblastoma and Sertoli cell tumors. *Cancer 11*:769, 1958.

49. Teilum, G. *Special Tumors of Ovary and Testis. Comparative Pathology and Histological Identification.* Philadelphia, Lippincott, 1971.

A. Talerman, M.D.,
M.R.C. Path.

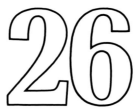

# Germ Cell Tumors of the Ovary

## Classification

This group of ovarian neoplasms is composed of a number of histologically different tumor types and embraces all the neoplasms considered to be ultimately derived from the primitive germ cells of the embryonic gonad. The concept of germ cell tumors as a specific group of gonadal neoplasms has evolved in the last three decades and has become generally accepted. This concept is based primarily on the common histogenesis of these neoplasms, on the relatively frequent presence of histologically different tumor elements within the same tumor mass, on the presence of histologically similar neoplasms in extragonadal locations along the line of migration of the primitive germ cells from the wall of the yolk sac to the gonadal ridge,[244] and on the remarkable homology between the various tumor types in the male and the female. In no other group of gonadal neoplasms is this homology better illustrated. Although the strong morphologic resemblance between the testicular seminoma and its ovarian counterpart the dysgerminoma was noted soon after these neoplasms were first described, for a long time there was no agreement as to their histogenesis. Nevertheless, these were the first neoplasms to become accepted as originating from germ cells. However, it was not until the studies by Teilum[212,213] on the homology of ovarian and testicular neoplasms, the studies by Friedman and Moore[66] and Dixon and Moore,[52] on testicular tumors, and those by

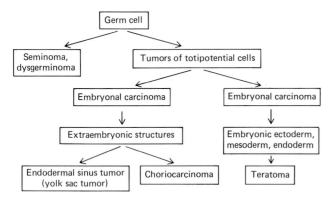

**26.1** The histogenesis and interrelationship of tumors of germ cell origin.

[Modified from G. Teilum, Classification of endodermal sinus tumour (mesoblastoma vitellinum) and so-called "embryonal carcinoma" of the ovary, *Acta Pathol. Microbiol. Scand.* 64:407, 1965.]

Friedman[65] on related extragonadal neoplasms that the germ cell origin of other neoplasms belonging to this group was suggested. These views were supported by the embryologic studies by Witschi[244] and Gillman,[70] and later by the experimental work of Stevens[198-200] and Pierce and his collaborators[156-158,161,162] on germ cell tumors in rodents. The histogenesis and the interrelationship of the various types of germ cell neoplasms as has been suggested by Teilum[217] is shown in Figure 26.1.

A number of classifications of germ cell neoplasms of the ovary have been proposed over the years,[84,96,184-186,190,215,218] each one becoming more detailed and encompassing newly established entities. Some years ago a panel of pathologists was established under the auspices of the World Health Organization in order to formulate an acceptable histologic classification of ovarian neoplasms to be used throughout the world. The classification proposed[190] divides the germ cell tumors into a number of groups and also includes neoplasms composed of germ cells and sex cord stroma derivatives. The classification used in this text is a slight modification of this classification[190] and is as follows:

I. *Germ cell tumors*
   A. Dysgerminoma
   B. Endodermal sinus tumor
   C. Embryonal carcinoma
   D. Polyembryoma
   E. Choriocarcinoma
   F. Teratomas
      1. Immature (solid, cystic, or both)

   2. Mature
      a. Solid
      b. Cystic
         i. Mature cystic teratoma (dermoid cyst)
         ii. Mature cystic teratoma (dermoid cyst) with malignant transformation
   3. Monodermal or highly specialized
      a. Struma ovarii
      b. Carcinoid
      c. Struma ovarii and carcinoid
      d. Others
   G. Mixed forms (tumors composed of types A through F in any possible combination)
II. *Tumors composed of germ cells and sex cord stroma derivatives*
   A. Gonadoblastoma
   B. Mixed germ cell–sex cord stroma tumor

# Germ Cell Tumors

## Dysgerminoma

*Synonyms*

Germinoma, disgerminoma,[131] ovarian seminoma,[126] gonocytoma,[213] embryonal carcinoma with lymphoid stroma.[60]

Although the term dysgerminoma was first introduced by Meyer[131] in 1931, ovarian neoplasms showing this histologic pattern had been recognized earlier. Chenot[35] in 1911 was the first to note their occurrence and their similarity to the testicular seminoma described some years earlier.[36] In view of the strong resemblance to their testicular counterpart the tumor was named ovarian seminoma by Masson[126] and this became the most popular term until its replacement by dysgerminoma. It is still widely used in the French literature. The term disgerminoma, as was originally suggested by Meyer,[131] and which later became dysgerminoma, has over the years gained almost universal acceptance.

*Histogenesis*

Dysgerminoma is composed entirely of germ cells, which show morphologic, including ultrastructural,[88,101,113,145] and histochemical[117,118] similarity to primordial germ cells. The cells of dysgerminoma are considered to be in an early and sexually indifferent stage of differentiation. They are arrested at a developmental stage at which they have not yet gained the ability for further differentiation. They are therefore sexually and hormonally inert. An origin from the primordial germ cells that migrate to the ovary during early embryogenesis from their site of origin in the wall of the yolk sac[244] is the most widely accepted view of the histogenesis of dysgerminoma. It is supported by the occurrence of homologous neoplasms in the testis (seminoma) and along the migration route of the primordial germ cells from the wall of the yolk sac to the primitive gonad, in the mediastinum, retroperitoneum, posterior abdominal wall, and sacrococcygeal region.[65,70]

The presence of sex chromatin bodies (Barr bodies) in the cells of dysgerminoma is a matter of controversy. Sex chromatin bodies were said to be present in the cells of a number of dysgerminomas by some investigators,[226] whereas others[8] could not identify them. The latter view is more in accordance with an origin from the primordial germ cells. The finding of twice the amount of DNA in the nuclei of dysgerminoma cells as compared with the nuclei of lymphocytes in all the cases studied[8] further supports the origin from primordial germ cells, which have the same amount of DNA in their nuclei (twice the amount present in normal diploid cells).

### Incidence

Dysgerminoma is an uncommon tumor accounting for 1 to 2% of primary ovarian neoplasms, and for 3 to 5% of ovarian malignancies.[133,142,174] Although until 1950 only 427 cases have been recorded in the literature,[133] at least as many cases have been reported since. Dysgerminoma may occur at any age from infancy to old age and the reported cases ranged between the age of 7 months[30] and 70 years,[133] but the majority of cases occur in adolescence and early adult life.[8,49,84,104,133,139,150,171,185,186,189,209] In view of this the tumor has been called carcinoma puellarum.[138] Dysgerminoma occurs not infrequently before puberty[1,30] but is rare after menopause.[49,185] Most cases occur in the second and third decades; nearly half the patients are under 20 years of age and 80% are under 30 years.[8,31,85,133,174,209,227] Therefore dysgerminoma is one of the most common malignant ovarian neoplasms of childhood, adolescence, and early adult life.[1,8,30,49,133,137,174] Dysgerminoma has been reported in siblings,[209] as well as in mother and daughter.[95]

The incidence of dysgerminoma in different parts of the world is not known, as most cancer registry reports do not differentiate between the various types of ovarian neoplasms.[111] In some countries there are considerable regional variations.[19] Although the majority of reports emanate from Europe and North America, dysgerminoma has been encountered in all parts of the world and in all races. A high incidence has been reported from Japan[85] and in a study from Bombay, India.[97]

### Clinical aspects

Although Meyer,[131] when describing dysgerminoma, emphasized the frequent occurrence of this neoplasm in pseudohermaphrodites, and patients with other forms of sexual maldevelopment, the great majority of patients with dysgerminoma are normally developed and sexually normal adolescent or young adult females.

The symptomatology of dysgerminoma is not distinctive and is similar to that observed in patients with other solid ovarian neoplasms.[8,49,133,174] The duration of symptoms is usually short and despite this the tumor is often large, indicating a rapid growth of the tumor.[174,209] The most common presenting symptoms are abdominal enlargement and presence of a mass in the lower abdomen, which is sometimes associated with abdominal pain that may be caused by torsion. Loss of weight may also be an accompanying symptom. In a number of cases the tumor has been found incidentally. In these cases the tumor is usually small. Sometimes the tumor may be detected during pregnancy.[8,49,150,174,209,227] In such cases it may be discovered as an incidental finding or may be obstructing labor.[174] Dysgerminoma is one of the two most common ovarian neoplasms observed in pregnancy, the other being serous cystadenoma.[84] The relatively common finding of dysgerminoma in pregnant patients is nonspecific and relates to the age of the patients.

Dysgerminoma may also be discovered incidentally in patients investigated for primary amenorrhea, and in these cases it is not infrequently associated with gonadoblastoma.[177,178,187] Occasionally menstrual and endocrine abnormalities may be the presenting symptom,[49] but this tends to be more common in patients with dysgerminoma combined with other neoplastic germ cell elements, especially choriocarcinoma. In children, precocious sexual development may occur.[1,27,30,84]

### Macroscopic appearances

Dysgerminoma is usually unilateral and tends to occur more often in the right ovary,[133,174,189,209] which is affected in approximately 50% of cases, whereas the left is affected in 30 to 35% and bilateral involvement occurs in 15 to 17%.[133,174] An incidence of bilateral involvement has been reported higher in some series[143,150,209] and

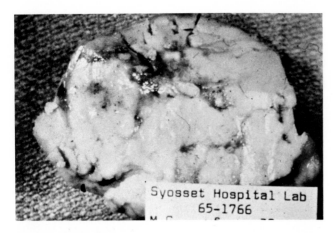

**26.2** Dysgerminoma. The cut surface is solid in consistency. There is some hemorrhage present.

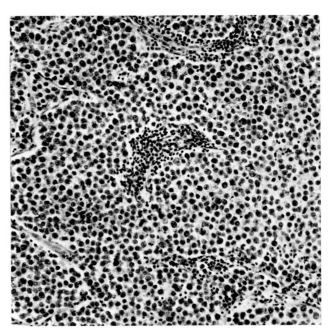

**26.3** Dysgerminoma composed of large aggregates of uniform cells surrounded by delicate strands of connective tissue containing lymphocytes. Hematoxylin–eosin, ×140.

lower in others.[8,49,128] The predilection of dysgerminoma for the right ovary has been considered to have some bearing on the histogenesis of the tumor[174] in view of the anatomic observations indicating slower differentiation and maturation of the right gonad as compared to the left. Others are doubtful whether such a histogenetic relationship exists.[59] Higher incidence of bilateral tumors is observed in patients with dysgerminoma associated with gonadoblastoma, the dysgerminoma arising from and overgrowing the gonadoblastoma.[177,178,187,202]

Pure dysgerminomas are solid tumors, which are round, oval, or lobulated, with a smooth, gray-white, slightly glistening fibrous capsule. They vary in size from small lesions a few centimeters in diameter to large masses measuring 50 cm across[8,30] and filling the pelvic and abdominal cavities. Tumors weighing in excess of 5 kg have been described.[133] Compressed ovarian tissue may be seen surrounding small tumors, but in large tumors it is not discernible. The capsule is usually intact but may be ruptured, especially in large tumors. This may lead to the formation of adhesions between the tumor and the surrounding structures. The consistency of dysgerminoma varies from firm and rubbery, in the small- and medium-sized tumors, to soft in the large ones. On cut surface (Figure 26.2) the tumor is solid and varies in color from gray-pink to pink and from yellow to light tan. Red, brown, or yellow discoloration caused by hemorrhage or necrosis is also seen, especially in large tumors. This may sometimes lead to the formation of small cysts, but cystic areas are only occasionally seen in pure dysgerminoma. Presence of cystic areas should alert the observer to the possibility that other neoplastic elements may be present in

association with the dysgerminoma. In view of the important prognostic implications concerning the presence of other neoplastic elements, judicious sampling of the different parts of the tumor and especially of the less typical areas is recommended.

*Microscopic appearances*

Dysgerminoma exhibits very distinctive histologic appearances. It is homologous and histologically identical with the classic seminoma of the testis. It is composed of aggregates, islands or strands, of large uniform cells surrounded by varying amounts of connective tissue stroma containing lymphocytes (Figures 26.3 and 26.4). The cells are large and measure from 15 to 25 $\mu$ across. They are oval or round and have usually distinguishable cytoplasmic borders (Figure 26.5). In very well-fixed material the cell boundaries are well defined. The cells contain an ample amount of pale, slightly granular eosinophilic or clear cytoplasm. The centrally located vesicular nucleus is large, occupying nearly half the cell. The nucleus is oval or round; has a sharp nuclear membrane and an ample amount of somewhat unevenly dispersed finely granular chromatin; and contains usually one, but sometimes two,

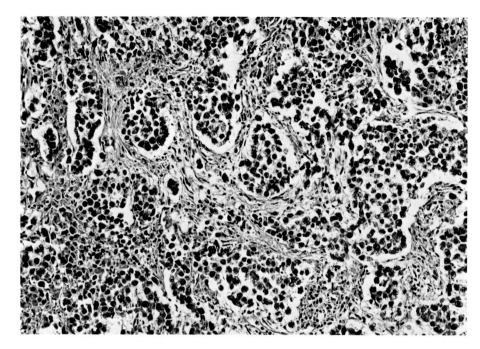

**26.4** Dysgerminoma composed of islands of tumor cells surrounded by connective tissue stroma containing lymphocytes. Hematoxylin–eosin, ×189.

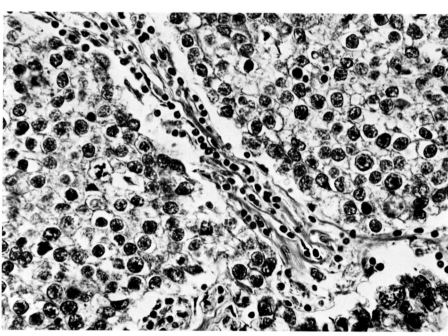

**26.5** Dysgerminoma showing the cellular composition and a connective tissue septum infiltrated by lymphocytes. An abnormal mitosis is seen to the left of center. Hematoxylin–eosin, ×388.

prominent eosinophilic nucleoli. Some variation in the size of the cells and nuclei and in the amount of nuclear chromatin is usually seen. Large or giant uninucleate tumor cells, which in all other respects resemble typical dysgerminoma cells, may be seen (Figure 26.6). Mitotic activity is almost always detectable (Figures 26.5 and 26.6)

and may vary from slight to brisk. This difference in mitotic activity may be observed not only in different tumors but also in different parts of the same tumor.

The cytoplasm of the tumor cells contains glycogen, which can be demonstrated with the periodic acid-Schiff (PAS) reaction, and this can be used as an aid in diagnosis.

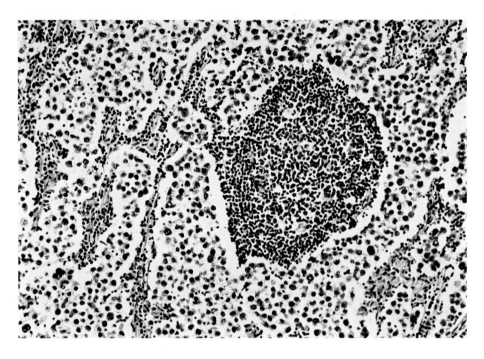

**26.6** Dysgerminoma showing a slight variation in size of the cells, a large uninucleate cell, and a mitosis in the center. Hematoxylin–eosin, ×388.

**26.7** Dysgerminoma showing a large collection of lymphocytes and the fine connective tissue septa surrounding the tumor cells. Hematoxylin–eosin, ×143.

The amount of glycogen in tumor cells is variable and in view of this the PAS reaction may vary from strong to very weak. Lipid is also present in the cytoplasm of the tumor cells and can be demonstrated in frozen tissue with the aid of lipid stains. The cells of dysgerminoma, as do the primordial germ cells, show a positive alkaline phosphatase reaction beneath the cytoplasmic rim[117] and in general show similar histochemical reactions to those of primordial germ cells. An increased amount of DNA, double the amount present in normal somatic cells, has been observed in the nuclei of dysgerminoma using densitometry.[8]

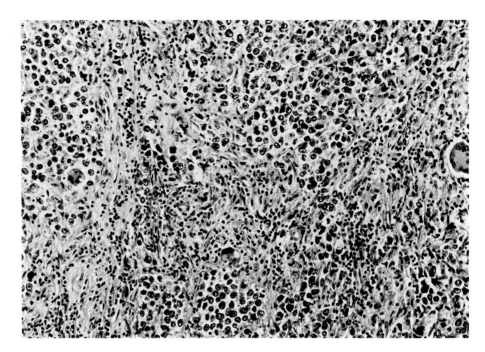

**26.8** Dysgerminoma showing a granulomatous reaction with foreign body and Langhans giant cells. Hematoxylin–eosin, ×143.

The stroma that surrounds the tumor cells is composed of connective tissue, which may be hyalinized. It is almost always infiltrated by lymphocytes. The lymphocytic infiltration may vary from slight to marked and large collections of lymphocytes may be present (Figure 26.7). Occasionally lymphoid follicles containing germinal centers may be seen. Plasma cells and eosinophils are not infrequently seen within the connective tissue stroma. Granulomatous reaction is also not infrequently seen and this manifests itself as collections of histiocytes surrounded by lymphocytes, plasma cells, and occasional giant cells both of the Langhans and foreign body types (Figure 26.8). The connective tissue stroma shows considerable variation in its appearance and amount. The latter tends to determine the pattern of the tumor, and thus, depending on the amount of stroma, the tumor cells, form large aggregates, smaller nests, islands, cords, or strands. The stroma varies from a fine, delicate fibrovascular network to large, fibrous strands or broad, fibrous, often hyalinized septa. It can be loose and edematous or dense and hyalinized. Occasionally the amount of stroma may be very large and this leads to wide separation of the nests of tumor cells (Figure 26.4). At the opposite end of the spectrum there are tumors that are very cellular and contain only an imperceptible amount of stroma. There may be a considerable variation in the amount of stroma in various parts of the same tumor.

Foci of necrosis and hemorrhage are frequently found and may be of considerable size in large tumors or in tumors affected by torsion. Small foci of hyalinization may also be present, but large hyalinized areas, such as observed sometimes in testicular seminoma, are uncommon. Calcification is only occasionally seen in dysgerminoma. It presents as small untidy spots or flecks of calcified material, which are found in association with necrosis, hemorrhage, fibrosis, or hyalinization. Occasionally relatively large, round, or ovoid calcified bodies are found, which may indicate the presence of a "burnt out" gonadoblastoma[187] (Figure 26.9). In a few cases of pure dysgerminoma, there may be in places, small collections of giant cells, some of which may be forming large syncytial masses, resembling syncytiotrophoblast of a choriocarcinoma but differing from the latter in the complete absence of cytotrophoblast (Figure 26.10). Some of these tumors have been found to be associated with elevation of urinary and serum chorionic gonadotropins, and presence of chorionic gonadotropin in the giant cells has been demonstrated by immunofluorescence.

Dysgerminoma may be associated with other neoplastic germ cell elements. Recent studies indicate a greater frequency of these mixed tumors[8,30,95,150,174,175,209,227,246] as compared to earlier reports.[133] This change is considered to result from a more detailed examination of the tumors and from a better recognition of the fact that germ cell tumors may be composed of histologically different neoplastic elements occurring in combination. For example, dysgerminoma may be combined with teratoma (Fig-

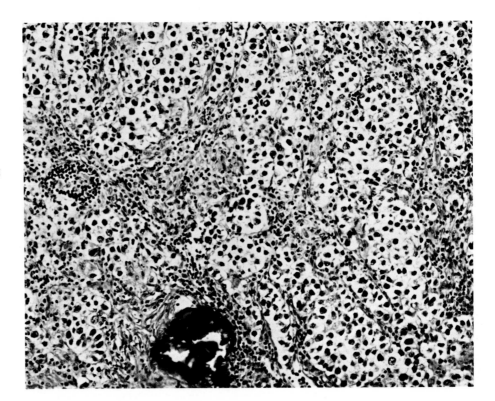

**26.9** Dysgerminoma containing a large calcified concretion. Nests of gonadoblastoma were found in other parts of the tumor. Hematoxylin–eosin, ×165.

ure 26.11), endodermal sinus tumor (Figure 26.12), embryonal carcinoma, and choriocarcinoma. Some tumors may contain all these neoplastic germ cell elements. The association of dysgerminoma with gonadoblastoma is frequent, occurring in 50% of cases of gonadoblastoma.[187] Histologically the other neoplastic germ cell elements may be intimately admixed with the dysgerminoma (Figure 26.11), or may be found adjacent to the dysgerminoma and separated from it by a fibrous septum (Figure 26.12). Endodermal sinus tumor elements and choriocarcinoma may be affected by hemorrhage and necrosis and a thorough search by extensive sampling, may be necessary to confirm their presence.

The cells of dysgerminoma, when studied with the electron microscope,[44,88,101,113,145] have been found to resemble closely the cells of classic testicular seminoma,[155] and when studied with the light microscope, resemble germ cell neoplasms in other locations showing similar histologic pattern,[106,165] as well as normal maturing germ cells in the ovary.[75,83] Slight ultrastructural differences have been noted between individual germ cells present within a tumor, as well as between those present in the different tumors studied. It is likely that some of these differences are related to the degree of differentiation and maturity of the tumor cells.

### Behavior

Dysgerminoma is a malignant neoplasm capable of metastatic and local spread. In spite of its less aggressive behavior as compared with other malignant germ cell neoplasms and its marked radiosensitivity, which are important factors concerning therapy and prognosis, the malignant potential of dysgerminoma should not be minimized. Dysgerminoma is a rapidly growing neoplasm, but metastatic spread does not occur very early in the course of the disease, although it is not possible to predict this in individual cases. When the tumor is freely mobile, its capsule is only rarely broken through, but large tumors may be adherent to the surrounding structures or may rupture.[49,174] Rupture may occur either spontaneously, or at operation. This leads to spillage of the tumor contents and peritoneal implantation and has serious prognostic consequences.[49,174] Penetration of the ovarian capsule by the tumor and formation of adhesions to the surrounding structures and organs may lead to their becoming infiltrated by the tumor.

Metastatic spread occurs via the lymphatic system, and the lymph nodes in the vicinity of the common iliac arteries and the terminal part of the abdominal aorta are first affected. Occasionally, there may be marked enlarge-

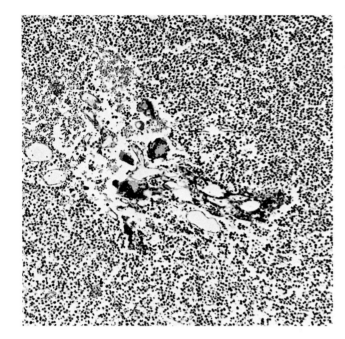

**26.10** Dysgerminoma containing collections of giant cells forming large syncytial masses resembling syncytiotrophoblast. Hematoxylin–eosin, ×62.

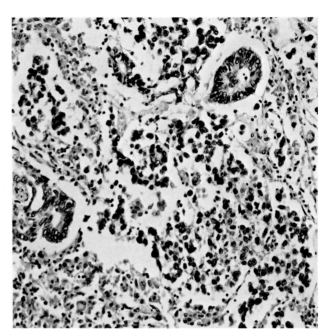

**26.11** Dysgerminoma intimately admixed with immature teratoma composed of primitive glandular epithelium. Hematoxylin–eosin, ×144.

[Reprinted by permission from A. Talerman, W, T. Huyzinga, and T. Kuipers. Dysgerminoma. Clinicopathologic study of 22 cases, *Obstet. Gynecol.* 41:137, 1973.]

**26.12** Dysgerminoma admixed with endodermal sinus tumor. Note the fibrous septum separating the two elements. Hematoxylin–eosin, ×71.

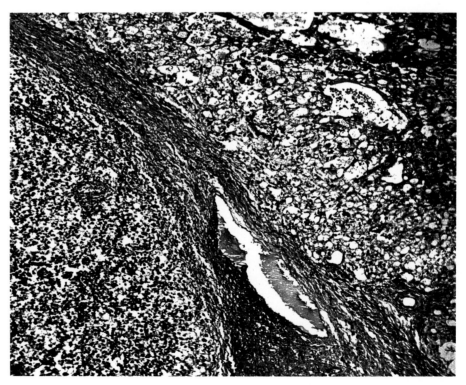

ment of these lymph nodes, with formation of large masses. Usually the enlargement is slight to moderate and can be detected by lymphangiography. From the abdominal lymph nodes, the tumor spreads to the mediastinal and supraclavicular lymph nodes. Hematogenous spread to distant organs occurs later and any organ may be affected, although involvement of the liver, lungs, and bones tends to be most common.[8,49,84,133,174] In cases of pure dysgerminoma, the metastases usually present a similar histologic appearance to the primary tumor, but occasionally, tumors composed of pure dysgerminoma may be associated with metastases composed of other neoplastic germ cell elements. This metastatic pattern is much more commonly observed in combined tumors. It has been suggested that cellular tumors with small amounts of stroma, slight lymphocytic infiltration, and associated with cellular atypia and high mitotic activity tend to be more aggressive,[8,49] but in view of the inconstancy of these findings, marked histologic variations within the same tumor, and its radiosensitivity, there is at present no good evidence that the behavior of an individual tumor can be assessed from its histologic appearance.[59,174,209] This does not apply to dysgerminomas admixed with other more malignant neoplastic germ cell elements; in these cases the outcome is unfavorable.[8,30,49,104,150,175,209,227]

## Prognosis

The prognosis of patients with pure dysgerminoma is now considered to be favorable. Although earlier reports indicated that the prognosis was poor and that the 5-year survival was only 27%,[133] more recent studies have reported a very much better prognosis for pure dysgerminoma with a 5-year survival of 75 to 90%.[8,30,31,49,120,227] At the same time the 5-year survival of patients with unilateral encapsulated dysgerminoma has been reported to be in excess of 90%,[8,31,49,120] although the patients were treated conservatively and had 18 to 52% recurrence rate. The recurrences were treated successfully with radiation therapy. The unfavorable prognostic parameters include presence of metastases at the time of diagnosis, presence of adhesions and spread into adjacent structures and organs, bilaterality, and large size of the tumor.[30,31,49,150,209] It should be noted that none of these parameters is by itself considered to indicate a hopeless outcome and many patients with these findings have been cured of their disease with radiotherapy. Some investigators consider that patients aged less than 20 years[31,49,128,150] as well as patients older than 40 years[31,128,150] have a worse prognosis. Others[8,30] do not regard age as important in this connection.

There is general agreement that presence of other neoplastic germ cell elements has a very adverse effect on prognosis.[8,30,150,174,175,209,227] Unlike patients with pure dysgerminoma, patients with tumors containing other malignant neoplastic germ cell elements have very poor prognosis and only a few survive 2 years from diagnosis.[8,30,150,175,227,246] As far as recurrences of dysgerminoma are concerned, 80% occur in the first 2 years after diagnosis[150] and it has been reported that more than 75% occur in the first year.[31,49]

## Therapy

Dysgerminoma, like its testicular counterpart the classic seminoma, is a very radiosensitive tumor. Although there is at present full agreement concerning the treatment of patients with bilateral or disseminated dysgerminoma, as well as patients with unilateral encapsulated tumors no longer desirous of having children, full agreement as to the treatment of a young patient with unilateral encapsulated pure dysgerminoma is still lacking. Patients belonging to the former groups are treated by radical operative procedure, namely, hysterectomy and bilateral salpingo-oophorectomy followed by radiation therapy to the abdominal and in some centers to the mediastinal lymph nodes. As far as the latter group is concerned, three different therapeutic approaches have been advocated. One advocates radical surgery and radiotherapy similar to that described above for patients with more extensive involvement.[61,236] The arguments in favor of the radical treatment are based on the fact that in spite of the radiosensitivity of dysgerminoma the survival of patients with this neoplasm has been poor, only 27 to 40% of patients surviving 5 years.[133,150,189] It should be noted that these results are based on earlier reported series, which include cases of dysgerminoma associated with other malignant germ cell tumors and cases of disseminated disease. The opposite view advising conservative therapy in such cases is held by those advocating unilateral oophorectomy, or salpingo-oophorectomy, wedge biopsy of the remaining ovary, careful followup of the patient, and treatment by radiotherapy of any metastases or recurrences if these occur.[8,30,185,186] The arguments in favor of this mode of therapy are based on very much better 5-year survival figures exceeding 90% described in recent series dealing solely with similar cases.[8,49,120] The advantages of this mode of treatment are that fertility is preserved and that there are no genetic hazards associated with administration of radiotherapy, a factor which at present is impossible to assess accurately. If metastases or recurrences develop they can be controlled successfully by radiotherapy. The third approach also advocates conservative therapy similar to that mentioned above but, in order to decrease and prevent the formation of metastases and recurrences, radiotherapy is administered to the abdominal lymph nodes on the ipsilateral side while the remaining ovary is shielded. There is evidence that this approach tends to decrease the risk of metastases and recurrences.[31,209] It is suggested by the advocates of conservative surgery without radiotherapy that this risk is not very serious, especially as the metastases or recurrences can be treated by radiotherapy when they develop.[8,30,49,185,227] The conservative approach to the therapy of unilateral encapsulated dysgerminoma has been gaining ground over the years and this approach is strongly recommended, but each individual case should be considered on its merits. It should be noted that before this mode of treatment can be considered the opposite ovary must be normal, there should be no evidence of spread of the tumor in the abdominal cavity, and the abdominal and pelvic lymph nodes must be free from metastases on inspection and lymphangiography. In addition to this the patient must be chromatin positive and have a normal female 46XX karyotype. The treatment of patients with dysgerminoma occurring in dysgenetic gonads must be radical in view of the high risk of the development of bilateral neoplasms in these patients and in view of the fact that the gonads are hormonally and functionally inactive. In view of the marked radiosensitivity of dysgerminoma, chemotherapy is only occasionally employed in the treatment of this tumor. Chemotherapy provides effective treatment and can be used either in conjunction with radiotherapy or in cases that for some reason cannot be controlled with radiotherapy, as well as in cases of disseminated disease. The chemotherapeutic agents that can be employed include chlorambucil, cyclophosphamide, methotrexate, actinomycin D, and combinations of these agents.

### Endocrine aspects

In the great majority of cases dysgerminoma is not associated with endocrine manifestations. Occasional cases have been described where the tumor was associated with elevated urinary chorionic gonadotropins, positive pregnancy tests, or signs of precocious puberty, and these manifestations have disappeared following excision of the tumor. Although in these cases the tumor has been said to be a pure dysgerminoma,[81,134] the possibility of admixture with choriocarcinomatous elements that have not been detected, perhaps because of inadequate sampling, is

the most likely explanation.[59,84,150,174] However, there remains a very small group of cases where in spite of a careful search, trophoblastic elements have not been found. In one case the tumor has been assayed for gonadotropin, with negative results.[98]

The presence of choriocarcinoma in association with dysgerminoma is not frequent but most of the reported series contain cases of this type.[95,150,175,209,227,246] Recently, occasional cases of pure dysgerminoma, containing multinucleate syncytiotrophoblastic giant cells but lacking cytotrophoblastic elements, have been noted to be associated with gonadotropin production. Although some cases of dysgerminoma showing these histologic appearances were recognized previously, evidence of gonadotropin production by the syncytiotrophoblastic giant cells was obtained only recently. This provides another possible explanation, apart from the presence of true choriocarcinomatous elements for the occasional presence of endocrine activity in cases of dysgerminoma. Dysgerminoma associated with evidence of virilization is mostly found in association with gonadoblastoma in patients with pure or mixed gonadal dysgenesis.

### Genetic aspects

When Meyer[131] described dysgerminoma, he observed that the tumor frequently occurred in hermaphrodites, pseudohermaphrodites, and patients with underdeveloped or malformed genitalia. In fact, 27 out of 48 cases collected by Meyer[131] occurred in sexually abnormal patients and this relationship was strongly emphasized. Although subsequent authors supported Meyer's contention about the very close association between dysgerminoma and developmental and sexual abnormalities, later reports, although accepting the existence of this relationship, suggested that it is not as close as had been postulated and stated that the majority of patients with dysgerminoma were normally developed females without any sexual abnormalities.[133,139,150,171,174,189,191] Most patients with dysgerminoma do not exhibit any menstrual abnormalities and are either capable of bearing or have actually borne children.[8,31,49] In a number of cases the diagnosis has been made during pregnancy.[8,31,49,104,174,209,227] A number of patients have become pregnant and have had normal offspring following therapy.[8,31,69,209,234] The majority of recent reports emphasize the occurrence of dysgerminoma in normal female patients[8,31,49,95,104,209,227] and some have even cast doubt on the relationship with developmental and sexual abnormalities.[8]

The common association of dysgerminoma with gonadoblastoma, a tumor that nearly always occurs in patients with dysgenetic gonads,[177,178,187] indicates that there is a relationship between dysgerminoma and genetic and somatosexual abnormalities. As the treatment of normal patients with dysgerminoma should be conservative, if possible, and as the treatment of patients with dysgerminoma associated with gonadoblastoma is radical because of the frequent occurrence of bilateral tumors and the absence of normal gonadal function, investigation of the genotype and karyotype of all patients with dysgerminoma, especially those with evidence of virilization or developmental and menstrual abnormalities, is strongly recommended. This is also very important in prepubertal patients, as in these patients other signs of abnormal function, such as primary amenorrhea, virilization, and absence of normal sexual development, are lacking. It must be emphasized that in patients who are sexually and genetically abnormal, the excision of the tumor is not associated with reversion to a normal state and substitution hormonal therapy must be administered. Adequate radical treatment in these cases prevents development of a tumor in the opposite gonad or leads to the removal of a clinically inapparent lesion that may subsequently prove lethal.[67]

## Endodermal Sinus Tumor

*Synonyms*

Yolk sac tumor, mesonephroma,[180] embryonal carcinoma, mesoblastoma vitellinum, mesoblastoma, Teilum tumor.

### Nomenclature and histogenesis

Endodermal sinus tumor is a malignant germ cell neoplasm that is considered to arise from the undifferentiated and multipotential embryonal carcinoma by selective differentiation toward yolk sac or vitelline structures, in the same way as nongestational choriocarcinoma differentiates toward trophoblastic structures. The concept of endodermal sinus tumor, its morphologic identity, and its establishment as a specific entity in the classification of germ cell neoplasms have resulted from the studies by Teilum, stretching over nearly three decades.[213,214,216,217,219] This concept has received strong support from the experimental studies of the neoplastic rodent yolk sac by Pierce and his collaborators.[156-158,161,162]

An ovarian neoplasm that showed the histologic appearances of endodermal sinus tumor and another, quite different, ovarian neoplasm composed of clear and hobnailed cells and that showed papillary pattern in places were grouped together by Schiller[180] and designated as a mesonephroma of the ovary, because of the presence of structures resembling immature glomeruli. Other investigators,[102] in spite of careful studies, have been unable to demonstrate the mesonephric origin of this tumor and have considered it as an endothelioma of the ovary, as suggested earlier.[182] In 1946, Teilum[213] indicated that the tumor described as mesonephroma[180,181] included two different and distinct entities with different histogenesis, histologic pattern, age incidence, and clinical behavior. One of these entities was found to be highly malignant, occurred in young patients, was found to be homologous with certain testicular neoplasms, and was considered to be of germ cell origin.[213] In addition to the terms mesonephroma[180,181] and endothelioma,[102,182] these tumors have been designated as embryonal carcinoma[1,135] because of certain similarities to the embryonal carcinoma of the testis.[52] Although embryonal carcinoma showing the histologic patterns resembling the typical embryonal carcinoma of the testis[52] is occasionally seen in ovarian tumors, the majority of ovarian tumors of this type show a distinctive pattern with differentiation toward yolk sac or vitelline structures.[91,93,216,217,219] They differ from the undifferentiated embryonal carcinoma,[52] although they resemble closely the endodermal sinus tumor or yolk sac tumor of both infantile[30,156,219] and adult testis.[156,206,216,217,219,248] It is now generally accepted that the term endodermal sinus tumor is much more correct and specific than the term embryonal carcinoma, on both morphologic and histogenetic grounds, and that the latter term should be used only to designate ovarian neoplasms showing the typical histologic patterns of the embryonal carcinoma as described in testicular tumors.[52]

The not infrequent combination of endodermal sinus tumor elements in ovarian tumors with other neoplastic germ cell elements[24,30,91,135,175,209,246] is one of the arguments in favor of the germ cell origin of this neoplasm. Endodermal sinus tumor, either pure or combined with other neoplastic germ cell elements, has been encountered in extragonadal locations where germ cell tumors are known to occur, such as the mediastinum,[92,211] the sacrococcygeal region,[37,92,94,166] the pineal gland,[3,23] and the vagina.[94,232]

### Incidence

Endodermal sinus tumor is an uncommon ovarian neoplasm, although more than 100 cases have been reported.[62] Its exact incidence is difficult to assess because it is a relatively recently established entity, and over the years it has been diagnosed under a variety of names and has been occasionally misinterpreted as a benign neoplasm. Because of its specific age incidence, however, it may be considered as one of the more common highly malignant ovarian neoplasms of childhood, adolescence, and early adult life and it is being diagnosed with greater frequency nowadays. Although most reports are concerned with Caucasians, endodermal sinus tumor has been encountered in other races.[91,135,246] The reported age distribution of patients with endodermal sinus tumor ranges from 16 months[91] to 46 years,[94] but most patients have been under 26 years of age.[91,135,175,217,219,246]

### Clinical aspects

The symptomatology is nonspecific and is usually that associated with the presence of a lower abdominal or pelvic mass.[30,91,135,175,246] The majority of patients present with symptoms of abdominal enlargement, usually of short duration, frequently associated with abdominal pain that occasionally may be acute and may lead to the diagnosis of acute abdominal emergency.[18,135,175] This is usually caused by torsion of the tumor.[91,135,175] Occasional cases have been encountered during pregnancy.[30,91,135,246] The presence of endodermal sinus tumor is not associated with endocrine symptoms,[30,91,135,175] although endocrine symptoms may be present if the tumor is combined with choriocarcinoma.[175] On clinical examination a tumor mass is usually palpable and is frequently of considerable size.[18,30,91,135,175] In recent years increased levels of $\alpha$-fetoprotein (AFP) have been found in sera of patients with endodermal sinus tumor[12,13,94,208,221,238] and this is now considered a useful diagnostic test for the presence of endodermal sinus tumor elements in a primary tumor, its metastases, and recurrences.

### Macroscopic appearances

Endodermal sinus tumors are usually unilateral.[30,91,135,175,246] They are bilateral in less than 10% of cases.[135,175] Bilaterality must be differentiated from metastatic spread to the contralateral ovary, which is not infrequent. Endodermal sinus tumor shows a certain predilection for the right ovary.[30,91,135,175] The tumor is usually large, varying in size from 3 to 30 cm in diameter and in the majority of cases being in excess of 10 cm.[18,30,91,135,175] It is usually encapsulated round, oval, or globular; firm, smooth, or somewhat lobulated; and gray-yellow, with areas of hemorrhage and cystic or

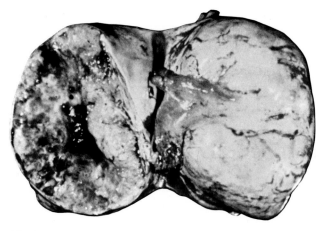

**26.13** Endodermal sinus tumor. It is oval-shaped, encapsulated, with a central area of cystic degeneration.

[Courtesy of R. Scully, M.D.]

gelatinous necrosis (Figure 26.13). It may form adhesions to the surrounding organs and structures and invade them. On sectioning it is mainly solid, but cystic spaces are frequently present. The fluid present in the cysts may also be gelatinous. Necrosis and hemorrhage may be marked, especially in large tumors, and may alter the appearances. Presence of other neoplastic germ cell elements, especially teratoma, may alter the appearance accordingly.

### Microscopic appearances

Endodermal sinus tumor exhibits a range of histologic patterns that differ considerably from each other and, although all the different patterns are frequently observed in the same tumor, one or two may predominate. Five principal microscopic patterns have been described by Teilum:[217-219]

1. *Microcystic* (Figure 26.14) *and myxomatous* (Figure 26.15) *pattern* composed of a loose vacuolated network, with small cystic spaces or microcysts forming a honeycomb pattern. The microcysts are lined by flat, pleomorphic, mesothelial-like cells, with large hyperchromatic or vesicular nuclei that show brisk mitotic activity. There is usually some variation in the size of the cysts (Figure 26.14). In the underlying capillary spaces hematopoiesis may be seen. The vacuolated network may contain pale, PAS-positive, mucinous material, forming small lakes or precipitates, as well as small, round, brightly eosinophilic PAS-positive and diastase-resistant globules or droplets. These globules are also found within the cytoplasm of the tumor cells

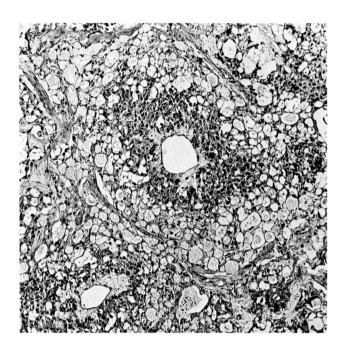

**26.14** Endodermal sinus tumor showing microcystic pattern. A labyrinthine structure composed of tumor cells radiating around a blood vessel resembling a perivascular formation is seen to the right of center. Hematoxylin–eosin, ×75.

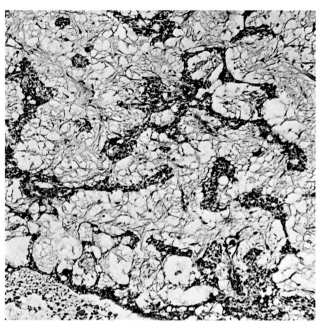

**26.15** Endodermal sinus tumor showing myxomatous pattern. Small collections of epithelial-like cells forming strands or glandlike structures are seen within the myxomatous tissue. Hematoxylin–eosin, ×60.

(Figure 26.16). Hyaline eosinophilic PAS-positive basement membrane material may also be seen in places and may be conspicuous in some tumors, the bands of hyaline material being surrounded by tumor cells (Figure 26.17). Areas composed of fine, loose myxomatous tissue containing alveolar spaces (Figure 26.18); occasional glandlike structures lined by cuboidal epithelium (Figure 26.19); and small cellular aggregates, often merging with the microcystic or other patterns, are also present (Figure 26.20). The loose myxomatous pattern was considered to be analogous to the magma reticulare or the extraembryonic mesoderm of the exocoelom[219] and the presence of this pattern led to the recognition of the mesoblastic nature of this tumor.[214]

2. *Endodermal sinus pattern* composed of perivascular formations (Figure 26.21), consisting of a narrow band of connective tissue with a capillary blood vessel in the center; lined by a layer of cuboidal or low columnar embryonal epithelial-like cells; with large, slightly vesicular nuclei, prominent nucleoli, and showing mitotic activity. The surrounding capsular sinusoid space is lined by a single layer of flat cells with prominent hyperchromatic nuclei. These characteristic perivascular

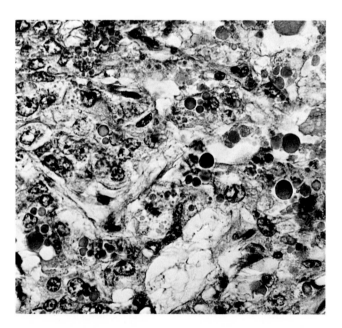

**26.16** Endodermal sinus tumor showing numerous round hyaline globules present both inside and outside the cells. Larger precipitates of this material are seen at the upper right. Hematoxylin–eosin, ×460.

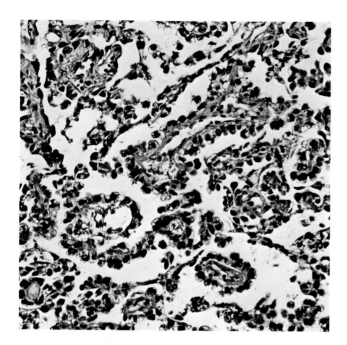

**26.17** Endodermal sinus tumor showing papillary pattern. The papillae are composed of hyaline material lined by tumor cells. Hematoxylin–eosin, ×235.

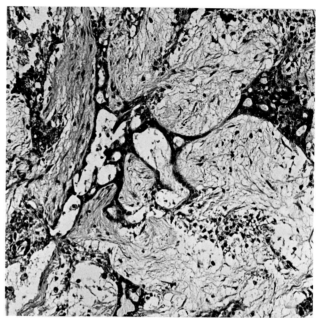

**26.18** Endodermal sinus tumor showing loose myxomatous pattern containing numerous cavities and channels. Note hyaline material at the top left. Hematoxylin–eosin, ×150.

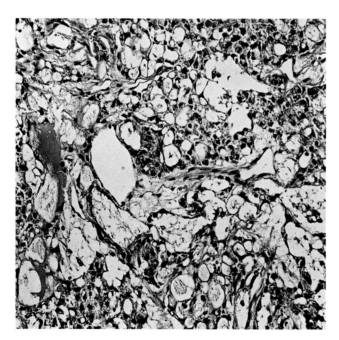

**26.19** Endodermal sinus tumor showing small cellular aggregates, microcysts, and myxomatous tissue. Mucinous material is also seen. Hematoxylin–eosin, ×150.

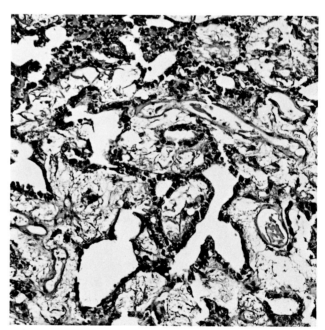

**26.20** Endodermal sinus tumor composed of myxomatous tissue containing glandular and alveolar spaces and channels. Hematoxylin–eosin, ×60.

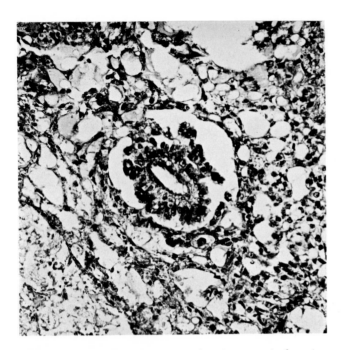

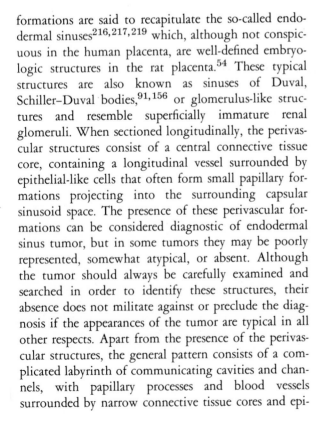

**26.21** Endodermal sinus tumor showing a typical perivascular formation (Schiller–Duval body). Hematoxylin–eosin, ×150.

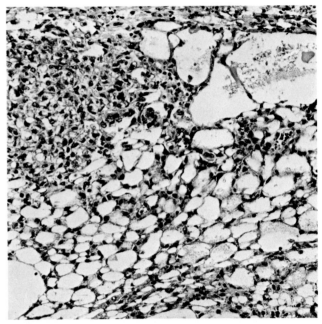

**26.22** Endodermal sinus tumor showing solid and microcystic pattern. Hematoxylin–eosin, ×150.

formations are said to recapitulate the so-called endodermal sinuses[216,217,219] which, although not conspicuous in the human placenta, are well-defined embryologic structures in the rat placenta.[54] These typical structures are also known as sinuses of Duval, Schiller–Duval bodies,[91,156] or glomerulus-like structures and resemble superficially immature renal glomeruli. When sectioned longitudinally, the perivascular structures consist of a central connective tissue core, containing a longitudinal vessel surrounded by epithelial-like cells that often form small papillary formations projecting into the surrounding capsular sinusoid space. The presence of these perivascular formations can be considered diagnostic of endodermal sinus tumor, but in some tumors they may be poorly represented, somewhat atypical, or absent. Although the tumor should always be carefully examined and searched in order to identify these structures, their absence does not militate against or preclude the diagnosis if the appearances of the tumor are typical in all other respects. Apart from the presence of the perivascular structures, the general pattern consists of a complicated labyrinth of communicating cavities and channels, with papillary processes and blood vessels surrounded by narrow connective tissue cores and epi-

thelial-like cells radiating into the surrounding stroma, resembling the typical perivascular formations but differing from them by the absence of the sinusoid space[219] (Figure 26.14).

3. *Solid cellular pattern* (Figure 26.22) composed of aggregates of small epithelial-like polygonal cells with clear cytoplasm, large vesicular or pyknotic nuclei, and prominent nucleoli, and exhibiting brisk mitotic activity.

4. *Alveolar–glandular or cystic pattern* (Figure 26.23) composed of alveolar, glandlike, or larger cystic spaces and cavities lined by flat or cuboidal epithelial-like cells with large, prominent nuclei and surrounded by myxomatous stroma or cellular aggregates. Some of these spaces may be lined by more than one layer of cells and sometimes the lining cells form small papillary projections protruding into the lumen. The layer of cells lining these spaces may be continuous with the lining of the perivascular sinusoid spaces.[216] Glandlike formations lined by columnar or cuboidal epithelial-like cells may be seen and in some tumors may be prominent and may form bizarre patterns (Figure 26.19).

5. *The polyvesicular vitelline tumor pattern*[217-219] composed of numerous cysts or vesicles surrounded by compact

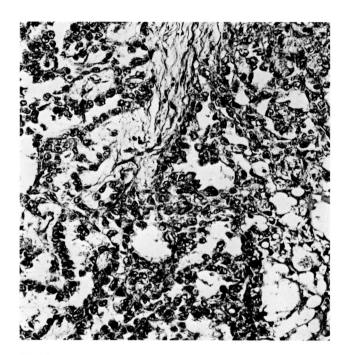

**26.23** Endodermal sinus tumor showing glandular alveolar pattern. Hematoxylin–eosin, ×235.

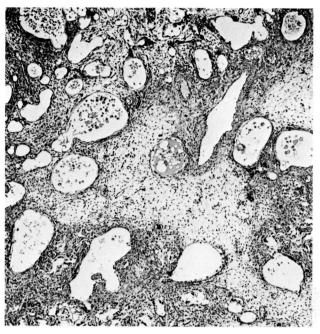

**26.24** Endodermal sinus tumor showing polyvesicular vitelline pattern. Hematoxylin–eosin, ×60.

connective tissue stroma (Figures 26.24 and 26.25). The vesicles are lined partly by columnar or cuboidal epithelial cells, frequently showing basal or paraluminal vacuolation, and partly by flat mesothelial-like cells (Figure 22.25). The individual vesicles or cysts vary in size and shape and contain invaginated protrusions into the lumen. The wall of the cyst may show a constriction dividing the part lined by the mesothelial cells from that lined by the columnar or cuboidal epithelium (Figure 26.25). This is considered to reflect the embryologic conversion of the primary yolk sac into the secondary yolk sac.[217-219] Occasionally the whole tumor may exhibit the polyvesicular vitelline pattern and such tumors have been designated as polyvesicular vitelline tumors.[217,219]

Small eosinophilic, PAS-positive, diastase-resistant droplets or globules may be present either within the tumor cells or outside them and in some tumors may be numerous and prominent (Figure 26.16). They may be observed in tumors exhibiting all the histologic patterns described above and their identification is a helpful diagnostic feature. They are considered to be secreted by the tumor cells and accumulate within the cytoplasm. As the amount of secretion increases, the cell becomes distended and ruptures,

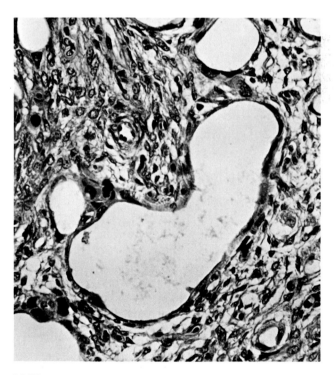

**26.25** Endodermal sinus tumor with polyvesicular vitelline pattern showing a typical vesicle. Hematoxylin–eosin, ×185.

discharging its contents into the surrounding tissue. This explains the presence of these globules outside the cells and the presence of pale eosinophilic, slightly PAS-positive material. Recently the significance of these globules in endodermal sinus tumor has been further enhanced by demonstrating with immunofluorescent techniques that they contain α-fetoprotein.[94,220] The presence of hyaline PAS-positive material forming bands or of connective tissue cores surrounded by tumor cells is not an infrequent finding in endodermal sinus tumor; in some tumors it may be a prominent feature, the tumor cells resting on and surrounding the bands of hyaline material (Figures 26.17 and 26.18). There may be an increased amount of the eosinophilic, PAS-positive globules described above in the vicinity of the hyaline bands and this suggests a relationship between these two features and a possibility of a common origin.[217,219] The hyaline PAS-positive material in endodermal sinus tumor has been found to be similar to the hyaline material produced by mouse teratocarcinoma during its conversion to ascitic form and this is considered to be a strong argument in favor of the yolk sac origin of the tumor.[156-158,161] The cells of endodermal sinus tumor, when examined with the electron microscope, resemble the ultrastructural appearance of the normal human yolk sac.[94,219]

### Differential diagnosis

Before it was recognized as a specific entity, endodermal sinus tumor was included with neoplasms composed of clear or parvilocular cells in the group of neoplasms of the ovary designated as mesonephroma[180,181] or was grouped together with embryonal carcinoma of the ovary.[1,30,135] It is with these two histogenetically different neoplasms that the endodermal sinus tumor may be confused. The clear cell or mesonephroid tumors of the ovary show much more regular tubular pattern; lack the honeycomb network composed of microcysts; and, although papillary projections are present, they are often lined by clear cells and are more frondlike. The typical perivascular formations, endodermal sinuses, or Schiller–Duval bodies present in endodermal sinus tumor are absent. The epithelial cells lining the tubules are cuboidal with clear cytoplasm or are hobnailed with nuclei bulging into the lumen. Areas composed of large polygonal cells with clear cytoplasm and small, dark, uniform, centrally situated nuclei resembling those of renal carcinoma are present. As these cells line cystic spaces they frequently proliferate in a papillary fashion or form solid aggregates. When the mesonephric tumor is composed entirely of tubules or spaces, confusion may arise with polyvesicular vitelline pattern, but the epithelial lining is different and is usually composed of the projecting hobnail cells and not of the two types of epithelia seen in the different parts of a vesicle forming part of the polyvesicular vitelline pattern. The cystic spaces are more tubular and less vesicle-like. The clear cell or mesonephroid tumors occur also in other parts of the female genital tract, they usually occur in older patients, and they are associated with much more favorable prognosis.[135,140,219]

The embryonal carcinoma,[52] which is uncommon in the ovary,[91,135,185,216-219] lacks the specific patterns observed in the endodermal sinus tumor and in its undifferentiated form is composed of aggregates of primitive embryonal cells forming a syncytial arrangement. The tumor cells are frequently larger than those seen in the solid cellular aggregates in endodermal sinus tumor. The cytoplasm is more granular, there is more marked cellular and nuclear pleomorphism, and the nucleoli are more prominent. Even when the tumor is somewhat more differentiated, with the embryonal cells forming cords, tubules, or papillae and lining clefts or spaces, it still lacks the typical patterns associated with endodermal sinus tumor. Endodermal sinus tumor, because of its cystic pattern and presence of numerous small blood vessels, has been confused with vascular tumors, but careful examination reveals that the pattern is more cystic and the absence of a true vascular pattern is confirmed by reticulin stains.

### Behavior

Endodermal sinus tumor of the ovary is a highly malignant neoplasm, metastasizing early and invading the surrounding structures and organs. Local invasion and intracoelomic spread, frequently lead to extensive involvement of the abdominal cavity by tumor deposits. Endodermal sinus tumor metastasizes first via the lymphatic system to the paraaortic and common iliac lymph nodes and then to the mediastinal and supraclavicular lymph nodes. Hematogenous spread occurs later and metastases are found in the lungs, liver, and other organs. The tumor is very aggressive locally, and spread beyond the ovary is observed in a considerable number of cases at the time of operation.[30,135,175,246] Recurrences in the pelvis are very frequent, even when the tumor and the affected adnexa have been excised completely.[91,135,246] They usually appear within a few weeks or months following excision of the primary tumor.

## Prognosis

The prognosis of patients with endodermal sinus tumor of the ovary irrespective of treatment is distinctly unfavorable,[1,30,91,135,175,219,246] most patients dying of the disease within 12 to 18 months of diagnosis. There are only a few known 5-year survivors.[91,185,209,246] The majority of these patients had tumors confined to the ovary, and in a number of these cases the tumor was composed of endodermal sinus tumor admixed with other neoplastic germ cell elements; frequently with dysgerminoma.[91,185,209,246] However, it should be noted that the clinical course in most patients with tumors composed of endodermal sinus tumor associated with dysgerminoma or other neoplastic germ cell elements does not differ materially from that in patients with pure endodermal sinus tumor.[30,91,135,175]

## Therapy

The treatment of patients with endodermal sinus tumor of the ovary has so far been disappointing. It is primarily surgical as the tumor is not sensitive to radiation therapy,[30,91,135,175,185,219,246] although there may be an initial response.[18,175] Although extensive surgery has been advocated, there is now evidence that radical surgery is of little avail and may not be justified since it does not improve the prognosis.[91] The small number of long-term survivors are mainly patients with tumors confined to the ovary, most of whom have been treated by unilateral adnexectomy.[30,91,135,185,246] Although single-agent chemotherapy or combinations of two or sometimes three agents has been tried without much success, in recent years there have been optimistic reports of sustained remissions, in some patients treated by surgery and chemotherapy using a combination of actinomycin D, 5-fluorouracil, and cyclophosphamide.[62,195] Although it is still too early to assess the value of this mode of therapy, its success at least in some cases may lead to the reassessment of the value of radical surgery and of radiotherapy, which may be useful in reducing the amount of tumor tissue as an adjunct to chemotherapy.

## α-Fetoprotein

α-Fetoprotein (AFP), an α-globulin, was first identified as a specific constituent of normal human fetal serum by Bergstrand and Czar[21] in 1956. In the human embryo, serum AFP reaches its maximum concentration of about 3,000 mg/liter at about 12 to 13 weeks of gestation. Its level then decreases slowly until birth, when the concentration is in the region of 55 mg/liter. After birth, AFP disappears from the serum and 3 weeks following full-term delivery it can only be detected in very small amounts (0 to 15 ng/ml) by radioimmunoassay. The sites of AFP synthesis in the fetus in the human and other mammalian species have been studied by Gitlin and his collaborators,[71-73] who have demonstrated conclusively that during fetal life AFP is produced by the yolk sac, liver, and gastrointestinal tract. They also have shown that AFP synthesis starts in the yolk sac.

In recent years there has been a considerable interest in the histologic aspects of germ cell neoplasms associated with raised serum AFP, and the histologic appearances of the germ cell tumors in patients with elevated serum AFP either are composed entirely of or contain endodermal sinus tumor elements.[12,13,94,208,221,238] Elevation of serum AFP level has not been observed in patients with pure dysgerminoma or seminoma,[194,208] mature cystic teratoma of the ovary,[12] or embryonal carcinoma and teratoma of the testis,[208] nor in patients with ovarian tumors not of germ cell origin, including sex cord stroma tumors.[208] Using immunofluorescent techniques, AFP has been identified in the cells of endodermal sinus tumor and in the eosinophilic, PAS-positive, diastase-resistant globules present both inside and outside the tumor cells.[94,220] Large amounts of AFP have been extracted from tumor tissue in endodermal sinus tumors of the ovary and testis.[220,238] The results of these studies indicate that endodermal sinus tumor elements are associated with AFP synthesis. In view of the fact that normal yolk sac in the human and other mammalian species has been conclusively shown to be associated with AFP synthesis,[73] it is reasonable to assume that tumors differentiating toward yolk sac or vitelline structures, such as endodermal sinus tumor, may also be capable of AFP synthesis in the same way as choriocarcinoma is capable of producing chorionic gonadotropin. This recent hypothesis[94,208,221] may not only explain the selective synthesis of AFP by some germ cell tumors but also give further support to the view that endodermal sinus tumor is a germ cell neoplasm resulting from differentiation of primitive embryonal elements in the direction of yolk sac or vitelline structures.

From the practical point of view serum AFP determination is considered to be a useful diagnostic test in patients with endodermal sinus tumor. It is also of value in monitoring the results of therapy and in detecting metastases and recurrences, although it should be noted that in the latter a normal result may not always imply the

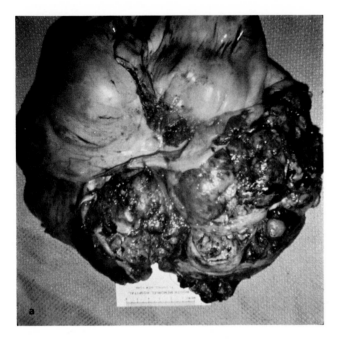 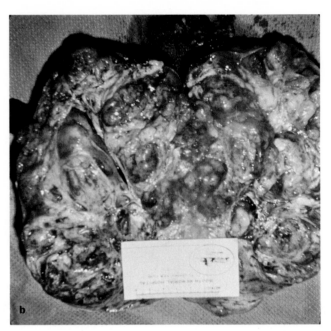

**26.26 a.** Embryonal carcinoma. A large lobular mass that is partially encapsulated. **b.** The cut surface is red-gray to gray-white in color. There are areas of hemorrhage and necrosis.

absence of active disease but only the absence of the tumor element associated with AFP synthesis. Preoperatively, if the tumor contains endodermal sinus tumor elements, the AFP can be detected in the serum and estimated by simple methods as the quantities of AFP present are relatively large. The AFP level falls postoperatively and, if there are no metastases, it reaches normal levels within 4 or 5 weeks. In these cases its monitoring requires more sophisticated methods of estimation capable of detecting very small amounts of AFP (most accurate of which is the radioimmunoassay). This is also necessary in the followup of patients in order to detect the presence of metastases or recurrences as early as possible. It is therefore considered that serum AFP estimation is a very useful diagnostic and prognostic test in patients with tumors containing endodermal sinus tumor elements.

## Embryonal Carcinoma

The term embryonal carcinoma in this chapter includes only ovarian neoplasms showing histologic appearances resembling those observed in the majority of embryonal carcinomas occurring in the testis of adults.[52] Dixon and Moore[52] consider embryonal carcinoma as both a morphologic and a conceptual entity, and this interpretation is

being followed. Embryonal carcinoma is considered to be the least differentiated form of germ cell tumor capable of differentiation. It may differentiate either toward somatic structures (teratomatous tumors of various degrees of differentiation), or toward extraembryonal structures, forming yolk sac or vitelline structures (endodermal sinus tumor) or trophoblastic structures (choriocarcinoma) (Figure 26.1). Although embryonal carcinoma shows similar appearances and is considered to be homologous with its testicular counterpart, it is very rare in the ovary both as a component of mixed germ cell tumors and even more so as a pure entity, whereas tumors showing this histologic pattern are relatively frequent in the testis. The reason for this major difference is unknown. Only one case of embryonal carcinoma of the ovary has been found in the archives of the Armed Forces Institute of Pathology, as compared to 27 cases of endodermal sinus tumor, and it was combined with other neoplastic germ cell elements.[135] Embryonal carcinoma has also been observed in association with gonadoblastoma.[187,205] The age incidence, clinical presentation, and findings are similar to those observed in patients with other malignant germ cell neoplasms, such as endodermal sinus tumor, immature teratoma, and dysgerminoma, the tumor occurring in children and young adults. Embryonal carcinoma is hormonally inert.

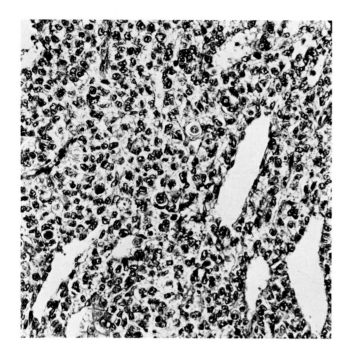

**26.27** Embryonal carcinoma showing mainly solid pattern. The tumor was admixed with teratoma and endodermal sinus tumor. Hematoxylin–eosin, ×150.

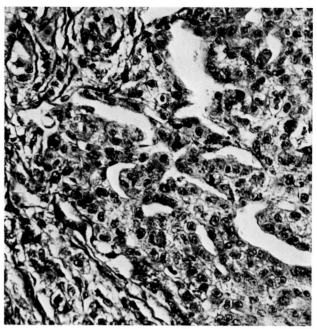

**26.28** Embryonal carcinoma forming clefts and spaces. Hematoxylin–eosin, ×235.

[Reprinted by permission from A. Talerman. Gonadoblastoma associated with embryonal carcinoma, *Obstet. Gynecol.* 43:138, 1974.]

### Macroscopic appearances

As embryonal carcinoma is usually a component of mixed germ cell tumors, the appearances of the tumor vary according to the type and amount of the different components present. On sectioning, the embryonal carcinomatous component is solid, gray-white, and slightly granular, with foci of necrosis and hemorrhage in the larger tumors (Figure 26.26a,b).

### Microscopic appearances

In its most primitive and undifferentiated form, embryonal carcinoma is composed of solid aggregates of epithelial-like, medium to large, polygonal or ovoid cells, containing an ample amount of somewhat pale eosinophilic granular cytoplasm and poorly distinguishable cytoplasmic borders and frequently forming a syncytial arrangement (Figure 26.27). The cells have a large, prominent, centrally situated, and somewhat irregular vesicular or hyperchromatic nucleus with a fine nuclear membrane and containing frequently more than one nucleolus. Mitotic activity is usually brisk, and abnormal mitoses are frequently seen. Cellular and nuclear pleo-

morphism is usually marked. Giant cells and multinucleated cells may be seen. In the slightly better differentiated tumors the cells, apart from forming solid areas, also tend to line clefts and spaces and form papillae (Figure 26.28). The cells appear more epithelial than those of the most undifferentiated type, being more cuboidal or columnar in shape and showing more regular arrangement, mutual orientation, and a suggestion of a formation of a cellular layer (Figure 26.28). Although there is a suggestion of glandular differentiation, true glandular formations are absent. The papillae are composed of solid collections of cells or may contain a cystic space or a small vessel surrounded by tumor cells. They must be differentiated from perivascular formations observed in endodermal sinus tumor. Foci of necrosis and hemorrhage are frequently seen.

Embryonal carcinoma may be present in the form of small solid aggregates or of pseudoglandular or cleftlike formations surrounded by better differentiated malignant teratomatous elements showing somatic differentiation. It may coexist with other neoplastic germ cell elements, such as endodermal sinus tumor, immature or mature teratoma, choriocarcinoma, polyembryoma, or dysgerminoma. It may be occasionally confused with the latter and differentiation from it is very important because of a totally different prognosis and response to treatment. It is usually the solid primitive type of embryonal carcinoma that is more likely to be confused with dysgerminoma, as the presence of clefts, alveoli, or cell-lined spaces militates against the diagnosis of dysgerminoma. The cells of embryonal carcinoma are usually larger and show much more marked cellular and nuclear pleomorphism. Mitotic activity is usually more prominent and bizarre mitoses are more frequent. The nuclear membrane is less sharp and the nuclei are more irregular, are larger, and contain usually more than one dark hyperchromatic nucleolus, in contrast to the rounded, prominent, usually single, and frequently eosinophilic nucleolus of dysgerminoma. The presence of connective tissue stroma infiltrated by lymphocytes and granulomatous reaction are prominent features of dysgerminoma. Their usual, although not invariable, absence in embryonal carcinoma is an important differentiating feature.

### Behavior and prognosis

Embryonal carcinoma of the ovary, as its testicular counterparts, is a highly malignant neoplasm. It is aggressive locally, spreads extensively in the abdominal cavity, and metastasizes early. The metastatic spread is similar to that observed with other germ cell neoplasms, taking place first via the lymphatic system and later by hematogenous spread. The prognosis is distinctly unfavorable.

### Therapy

The primary treatment of embryonal carcinoma is surgical. As the tumors are usually unilateral, conservative treatment is advocated if the tumor is localized to the ovary. Embryonal carcinoma is not radiosensitive but may respond to high doses of radiation. Chemotherapy in the form of a combination of three therapeutic agents, such as that used in the treatment of embryonal carcinoma of the testis,[6,196] may be of value, although this is difficult to assess in view of the rarity of the tumor.

## Polyembryoma

### Synonyms

Polyembryonic embryoma,[192] malignant teratoma with embryoid bodies.[17]

Polyembryoma is a very rare ovarian germ cell neoplasm composed of numerous embryoid bodies resembling morphologically normal presomite embryos. Similar homologous neoplasms occur more frequently in the human testis,[17,58,59,219] although pure polyembryoma is altogether rare. A more common finding is the presence of occasional or a number of embryoid bodies in a germ cell tumor composed of various other elements. All but one of the reported ovarian polyembryomas were combined with other neoplastic germ cell elements.[17]

### Histogenesis

There are conflicting views as to the origin of embryoid bodies. It has been suggested that they arise by parthenogenetic development from primitive germ cells present in malignant teratoma, indicating the mode of origin of teratomatous tumors, and so this may be considered as a model of their histogenesis.[124,154,192] Other investigators question this view and the whole idea that embryoid bodies bear a close similarity to early human embryos on the basis that embryoid bodies never appear to develop beyond the 18-day stage.[17,241,242] They consider that embryoid bodies probably develop transiently by bizarre differentiation, possibly in response to local release of organizers in malignant teratomas of the gonads. Another view that has been advanced accepts the morphologic similarities between the early embryo and the embryoid bodies, although disputing their parthenogenetic origin.[58,157,158,198,199] It considers that embryoid bodies are formed after initiation of teratogenesis, most likely from multipotential malignant embryonal cells present in a tumor, and not directly from germ cells.[200] This is supported by the observations of the development of embryoid bodies from undifferentiated embryonal cells in strain 129 mice. The tumor, a teratoma that had been serially transplanted for many years, was considered to be devoid of germ cells.[157,158,198,199] These findings are in accordance with the view that embryoid bodies probably persist only transiently within the tumor and while new embryoid bodies are being formed others lose their identity and their multipotential cells undergo further differentiation.[59] Although the origin and development of embryoid bodies are still a matter of dispute, the view that they originate from multipotential malignant embryonal cells, which is supported by experimental observations,[157,158,198,199] appears to be the most favored at present.

### Incidence

Only seven cases of ovarian polyembryoma have been recorded.[17] In six of these cases the polyembryoma was associated with other neoplastic germ cell elements, mainly immature, or with mature teratoma and in the remaining case the tumor was a pure polyembryoma.[17] All these tumors occurred in young patients or in patients in the reproductive age group.[17,153,192] The oldest patient was 38 years old.[192]

The clinical findings are similar to those observed in patients with other malignant germ cell neoplasms of the ovary.

### Macroscopic appearances

Polyembryoma is usually unilateral. Macroscopically the tumor resembles other malignant germ cell tumors, varying in size from relatively small, 9.5 cm in longest diameter,[17] to tumors filling almost the whole abdominal cavity and invading the surrounding structures.[192] The tumor is usually solid and contains hemorrhagic and necrotic areas.

### Microscopic appearances

Polyembryoma is composed of numerous embryoid bodies and the better differentiated ones are composed of an embryonic disc, amniotic cavity, and yolk sac, surrounded by primitive extraembryonic mesenchyme (Figure 26.29). Sometimes trophoblastic differentiation may be seen in the vicinity of the embryoid body. When the embryoid bodies are less well formed they are composed of a medullary plate and amnion associated with blastocystic space or with extraembryonic mesenchyme. They may have two or more amniotic cavities and share a single yolk sac cavity or vice versa. There may be a considerable disproportion between the two cavities and the cavities may be malformed. There may be a considerable variation in size between the different embryoid bodies; some may be more primitive and others appear to be better developed. Some embryoid bodies may be severely malformed and show bizarre appearances (Figure 26.30). None of the embryoid bodies appear to have developed beyond the 18-day stage. The embryonic disc of a classic embryoid body is lined on one side by cuboidal epithelial cells of uniform size, resembling endoderm, and on the other by tall columnar epithelium, resembling ectoderm; the latter merges with low cuboidal epithelium lining the rest of the cavity, which resembles the amnion. The cavity resembling the yolk sac is on the opposite side of the embryonic disc from the amnion (Figure 26.29). The embryoid bodies are surrounded by extraembryonic mesenchyme, which is composed of either closely or more loosely packed spindle-shaped cells of regular appearance (Figure 26.29) and showing occasional mitotic figures. Loose myxomatous areas may be present (Figure 26.30). Teratomatous struc-

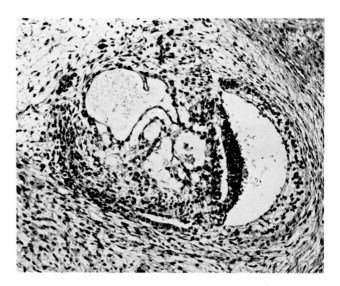

**26.29** Polyembryoma. Embryoid body showing amniotic cavity (right), embryonic disc (center), and atypical yolk sac (left). Hematoxylin–eosin, ×148.

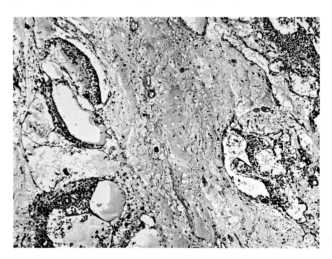

**26.30** Polyembryoma. Embryoid bodies showing bizarre appearances. Hematoxylin–eosin, ×54.

tures in various stages of differentiation are frequently seen interspersed among the embryoid bodies. In one reported case[17] chorionic gonadotropin and human placental lactogen were demonstrated within syncytiotrophoblastic cells, which were present in the vicinity of the embryoid bodies. Cytotrophoblastic cells were not identified in this tumor.

### Behavior and prognosis

Polyembryoma is a highly malignant germ cell neoplasm and in the majority of cases it has been associated with invasion of adjacent structures and organs and extensive metastases, which were mainly confined to the abdominal cavity.[192] One patient with a relatively small mobile tumor, absence of capsular penetration, and no evidence of metastases has survived more than 5 years,[17] but the other patients with polyembryoma have died of their disease.

### Therapy

The primary treatment of polyembryoma is surgical and, as the tumor is usually unilateral unless there is spread beyond the ovary, excision of the tumor and the adjoining adnexa is the treatment of choice. The tumor is not sensitive to radiotherapy and its response to chemotherapy is not known.

## Choriocarcinoma

### Synonyms

Chorioncarcinoma, chorionepithelioma, teratomatous choriocarcinoma.

Choriocarcinoma of the ovary may originate in three different ways:

1. As a primary gestational choriocarcinoma associated with ovarian pregnancy
2. As metastatic choriocarcinoma from a primary gestational choriocarcinoma arising in other parts of the genital tract, mainly the uterus
3. As a germ cell tumor differentiating in the direction of trophoblastic structures, usually admixed with other neoplastic germ cell elements

In each case it is very important to ascertain the mode of origin of the tumor, as apart from the histogenetic aspects there are important practical therapeutic and prognostic considerations. Choriocarcinoma of the ovary may also be divided into two broad groups of gestational choriocarcinoma, encompassing the first two groups mentioned above and the nongestational choriocarcinoma, a germ cell tumor differentiating toward trophoblastic structures. As this chapter deals solely with germ cell tumors, only the nongestational choriocarcinoma is discussed here.

### Incidence

Pure ovarian choriocarcinoma of germ cell origin is a very rare neoplasm and even the presence of choriocarcinomatous elements admixed with other neoplastic germ cell elements is considered to be rare in ovarian tumors.[59] In the majority of cases the tumor is admixed with other neoplastic germ cell elements, and their presence is diagnostic of nongestational choriocarcinoma, except for the remote possibility of the tumor being a gestational choriocarcinoma metastatic to an ovarian germ cell tumor. The presence of other neoplastic germ cell elements is a particularly helpful diagnostic feature in postmenarchal patients, in whom exclusion of gestational origin of the tumor may be difficult. In view of this it is considered that nongestational choriocarcinoma may be diagnosed with confidence in postmenarchal patients and not only in young children as has been considered earlier.[144] At least 50 cases of ovarian germ cell tumors containing choriocarcinoma have been reported.[27,48,105,107,125,144,175,230,246] The tumor, in common with other malignant germ cell neoplasms, occurs in children and young adults. Its occurrence in children has been emphasized and in some series 50% of cases occurred in children who had not reached puberty.[125] This high incidence in children may result from the previous reluctance of making the diagnosis in adults.

### Clinical aspects

The clinical findings in patients with ovarian nongestational choriocarcinoma are similar to those observed in patients with other malignant ovarian germ cell neoplasms, except that they may be modified by the endocrine activity of the tumor, which secretes chorionic gonadotropins. This is particularly noticeable in prepubertal children, who show evidence of isosexual precocious puberty with mammary development, growth of pubic and axillary hair, and uterine bleeding. Adult patients may present with signs of ectopic pregnancy. Because the nongestational choriocarcinoma, like its gestational counterpart, is associated with increased production of chorionic gonadotropins, estimation of urinary or plasma chorionic gonadotropins is a very useful diagnostic test in these cases as the circulating amounts of these hormones are greatly increased. These tests are very useful in the diagnosis of choriocarcinoma and its differentiation from other ovarian tumors. They are useful in monitoring the progress of the disease and its response to therapy, as well as in detecting metastases and recurrences containing choriocarcinomatous tissue. It should be noted that normal levels of chorionic gonadotropins do not exclude the presence of metastases or recurrences composed of other neoplastic germ cell elements. Chorionic gonadotropins can be extracted from tumor tissue and their presence within tumor tissue can be demonstrated by immunofluorescence.

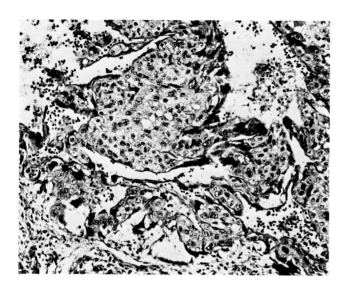

**26.31** Choriocarcinoma showing a cytotrophoblast composed of medium-sized cells, situated centrally, and a syncytiotrophoblast composed of very large multinucleated cells, situated peripherally. Hematoxylin–eosin, ×188.

## Macroscopic appearances

The tumor is usually unilateral, solid, gray-white, and hemorrhagic. Necrosis may also be in evidence. The tumors are usually of considerable size. As most of these tumors are composed of a combination of neoplastic germ cell elements, the appearances tend to vary according to the elements present in the tumor.

## Microscopic appearances

Choriocarcinoma is composed of two types of cells, the cytotrophoblast and the syncytiotrophoblast, and both should be present if a definite diagnosis is to be made (Figure 26.31). The cytotrophoblast is composed of medium-sized polygonal, round, or oval cells with clear cytoplasm, sharp nuclear borders, and centrally situated, small, round, and hyperchromatic nuclei or larger vesicular nuclei containing nucleoli and showing brisk mitotic activity. The syncytiotrophoblast is composed of large or very large basophilic, vacuolated cells with irregular outlines and, although frequently elongated, they may vary in shape. These cells contain multiple hyperchromatic nuclei, varying in shape and size, or large masses of chromatin. The cytotrophoblastic cells are usually disposed centrally within a tumor mass and are partly or completely surrounded by irregular collections or layers of the syncytiotrophoblastic

cells (Figure 26.31). There is a considerable variation in the pattern and in the ratio of the two components in different parts of the same tumor and in different tumors. The tumor cells form solid aggregates, nearly always associated with hemorrhage and necrosis, which may be so extensive that the tumor tissue is hardly recognizable. The tumor tissue may be seen on the outside of a hemorrhagic area and may form a projection into the hemorrhagic mass. When the tumor is combined with other neoplastic germ cell elements, the choriocarcinoma may form small nodules associated with hemorrhage and surrounded by other neoplastic germ cell elements. The presence of other neoplastic germ cell elements within the tumor is a frequent finding.

It appears that the cytotrophoblast is the more primitive element and the syncytiotrophoblast is formed from it either directly or indirectly. The syncytiotrophoblast is the differentiated, nondividing, hormone-secreting component. These findings are supported by electron microscopic and histochemical studies.[159,160]

## Behavior and prognosis

Nongestational choriocarcinoma of the ovary is a highly malignant germ cell neoplasm. It invades the adjacent structures and organs, spreads widely throughout the abdominal cavity, and metastasizes via both the lymphatics and the blood vessels. Although gestational choriocarcinoma tends to spread primarily via the blood stream, nongestational choriocarcinoma shows lymphatic and intraabdominal spread and hematogenous spread may not be so marked. The prognosis of patients with choriocarcinoma is unfavorable but may be somewhat better than of patients with endodermal sinus tumor. In one large series there were four survivors out of 12 patients with tumors containing choriocarcinoma, as compared with five out of 35 patients with tumors containing endodermal sinus tumor.[246]

## Therapy

Unlike gestational choriocarcinoma, the treatment of which has been revolutionized by the discovery that it responds to methotrexate, nongestational choriocarcinoma does not respond to this drug.[107,185,219,246] As these tumors are also not radiosensitive the treatment is primarily surgical. Although occasional therapeutic successes have been achieved[48,230,246] these usually have been in patients with small tumors and the successful treatment has consisted of unilateral ovariectomy or adnexectomy.

More recently, in spite of the lack of success with single-agent chemotherapy using methotrexate, a combination therapy using a few chemotherapeutic agents has been tried with some success in a number of cases.[27,74,235] In view of this it is hoped that this mode of therapy, together with surgery and in conjunction with radiotherapy, which may be used to reduce the tumor bulk in inoperable cases, can alter the poor prognosis of patients with nongestational choriocarcinoma.

## Teratoma

### Classification

Ovarian teratomas have usually been divided into two main groups. One includes the great majority of cases (99%) composed of the cystic and mature forms, also known as dermoid cysts; the remaining very small group is composed of the solid and immature forms.[59,84,138,142,218] Tumors composed entirely, or to a large extent of thyroid tissue, known as struma ovarii, were included in the larger group of dermoid cysts or were sometimes classified separately. In recent years more detailed classifications of ovarian teratoma have been proposed, taking into account new information that has come to light concerning the morphology and behavior of this group of neoplasms.[96,184–186,190]

The classification adopted in this chapter is the one recently proposed by the WHO Ovarian Tumor Panel[190] and the ovarian teratomas have been divided into the following subgroups:

1. Immature
2. Mature
   a. Solid
   b. Cystic
      i. Mature cystic teratoma (dermoid cyst)
      ii. Mature cystic teratoma (dermoid cyst) with malignant transformation
3. Monodermal and highly specialized
   a. Struma ovarii
   b. Carcinoid
   c. Struma ovarii and carcinoid
   d. Others

### Histogenesis

The origin of teratomas has been a matter of interest, speculation, and dispute for centuries. In the past many theories have been advanced to explain their origin, including witchcraft, nightmares, and many other bizarre causes.[25] In more recent times three main theories have been put forward. Of these the most recently propounded theory is the parthenogenic theory, which suggests an origin from the primordial germ cell. It has been steadily gaining support and is now generally accepted. The other two theories, one suggesting an origin from blastomeres segregated at an early stage of embryonic development and the second suggesting an origin from embryonal rests, have few adherents nowadays.[59,142] Support for the germ cell theory has come from the anatomic distribution of the tumors, which occur along the line of migration of the primordial germ cells from the yolk sac to the primitive gonad, and from the fact that the tumors occur most commonly during the years of reproductive activity. Support also comes from animal experiments in which cystic teratomas can be produced only during the period of reproductive activity of the gonad, as in roosters injected with zinc and copper salts,[11,33] and from the nuclear sexing and karyotyping of teratomas. It has been shown that cells of ovarian teratomas are always chromatin positive, unlike the cells of testicular teratomas, which may be chromatin negative, chromatin positive, or mixed in this order.[226] The karyotypes of all benign ovarian teratomas studied have been found to be 46XX.[41,68,110,167] Further support for the germ cell theory of origin has come from the recent work of Linder and his collaborators.[108–110] They have studied the histogenesis of mature cystic teratoma of the ovary using both cytogenetic techniques and the electrophoretic variants of four enzymes in normal as well as in tumor cells. They have demonstrated that these tumors are of germ cell origin and arise from a single germ cell after the first meiotic division.[110]

### Immature teratoma

Immature teratomas are composed of tissues derived from the three germ layers—ectoderm, mesoderm, and endoderm—and, in contrast to the very much more common mature teratoma, they contain immature or embryonal structures. Mature tissues are frequently present and sometimes may predominate. In these cases the tumor should be differentiated from a mature teratoma with malignant transformation. The presence of immature or embryonal elements as opposed to the neoplastic transformation of mature tissues differentiates between these two types of neoplasm.

INCIDENCE. The immature teratoma of the ovary is an uncommon tumor, comprising less than 1% of teratomas of the ovary.[29,34,121,141,246] In contrast to the mature cystic teratoma, which is encountered most frequently during the reproductive years but occurs at all ages, the immature teratoma has a very specific age incidence, occurring most commonly in the first two decades of life and being almost unknown after the menopause.[29,30,121,246] In view of this, teratomas occurring in childhood, adolescence, and early adult life should always be very carefully examined and thoroughly sampled.

CLINICAL ASPECTS. The tumor is usually asymptomatic until it reaches a considerable size. It tends to grow rapidly and may manifest itself as a pelvic or lower abdominal mass. It may cause pressure symptoms, abdominal heaviness, or pain or it may undergo torsion, causing acute abdominal pain.

MACROSCOPIC APPEARANCES. The tumor is usually unilateral[29,30,34,141,243,246] but occasionally may be bilateral or may coexist with benign cystic teratoma in the opposite ovary.[243] The tumors are usually large, varying in size from 9 to 28 cm in the longest diameter.[30] They may form a round, oval, or lobulated soft or firm mass (Figure 26.32). The tumor is often prone to perforate its capsule, which is not always well defined.[29,30,243] It tends to form adhesions to the surrounding structures and to invade locally.[29,30] The tumor is predominantly solid but frequently contains cystic structures.[29,30,34,121,243] Occasionally it may be predominantly cystic with solid areas present in the cyst wall.[30,115,228] The cut surface is usually variegated, trabeculated, and lobulated, varying in color from gray to dark brown. Occasionally foci of cartilage or bone may be recognizable and hair may be present. The cystic areas are usually filled with serous or mucinous fluid, colloid, or fatty material.

MICROSCOPIC ASPECTS. The tumor is composed of a variety of immature and mature tissues derived from the three germ layers. Occasionally the tumor may be composed of a small number of tissues, although usually derivatives of all the three germ layers are present. Ectoderm is usually represented by nervous tissue and brain tissue. Glia, ganglion cells, neuroblastic tissue (Figure 26.33), neuroepithelium, nerve trunks, and ocular structures are often represented. Skin elements (Figure 26.33), including pilosebaceous units, sweat glands, and hair, are not infrequently present. Mesodermal elements include fibrous connective tissue; cartilage (Figure 26.33); bone; muscle, usually smooth but occasionally striated; lymphoid tissue; and undifferentiated embryonic mesenchyme. Endodermal elements are usually represented by tubules

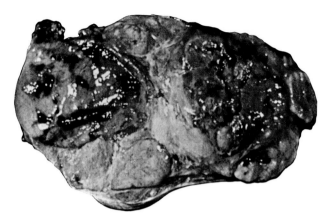

26.32 Immature teratoma. A large lobulated, firm to soft tumor mass. There are areas of hemorrhage and necrosis.

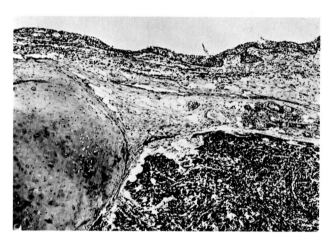

26.33 Immature teratoma showing both solid and cystic areas. The tumor was mainly composed of neuroblastic tissue (right). Note the squamous epithelium, adnexal glands, and cartilage. Hematoxylin–eosin, ×48.

lined by columnar, sometimes ciliated, epithelium. Occasionally gastrointestinal or bronchial epithelium may be present. All these tissues, which may be in stages of maturity varying from embryonic to mature, are scattered haphazardly throughout the tumor and so differ from the orderly organoid arrangement seen in a mature teratoma. In cases where the tumor is composed mainly of mature tissues, differentiation from mature teratoma may be difficult and patients have been diagnosed as having a benign lesion, only to return within a short time with recurrence. In a number of such cases review of the material taken from the original tumor has revealed immature elements. Therefore, careful examination and thorough sampling of the tumor are strongly recommended. Immature teratoma may be combined with other neoplastic germ cell elements, such as endodermal sinus tumor, dysgerminoma, embryonal carcinoma, choriocarcinoma, and polyembryoma. It can therefore form a part of a malignant germ cell tumor composed of two or more neoplastic germ cell elements (mixed germ cell tumor). Immature teratoma has been reported to develop from the germ cell element of gonadoblastoma.[187]

Immature solid teratoma must be differentiated from the mixed mesodermal tumor, which although occurring most frequently in the uterus also occurs in the ovary. Mixed mesodermal tumor is composed of derivatives of Müllerian mesoderm, a primitive structure that gives rise both to the stroma and epithelium of the endometrium. The monodermal origin of mixed mesodermal tumor distinguishes it from teratoma.[210] Mixed mesodermal tumor occurs most frequently in postmenopausal women between the ages of 50 and 70 years and, unlike solid immature teratoma, only occasionally occurs in younger patients. The tumor is composed of sarcomatous and carcinomatous tissue. The carcinoma is invariably an adenocarcinoma, squamous cell carcinoma, or adenosquamous carcinoma and the sarcomatous elements may be composed of a wide variety of tissues, including leiomyosarcoma, chondrosarcoma, rhabdomyosarcoma, fibrosarcoma, undifferentiated sarcomatous tissue, and myxomatous tissue. Derivatives of the three germ layers are absent in mixed mesodermal tumor and neuroectodermal derivatives, prominent in solid immature teratoma, are never seen. Mixed mesodermal tumor does not exhibit the great variety of tissues present in a teratoma, and the tissues present in a mixed mesodermal tumor generally form more typical sarcomatous or carcinomatous pattern.

BEHAVIOR. Immature teratoma is a malignant neoplasm that usually grows rapidly, penetrates its capsule, and forms adhesions to the surrounding structures. It spreads throughout the peritoneal cavity by implantation. It metastasizes first to the retroperitoneal, paraaortic, and more distant lymph nodes and later to the lungs, liver, and other organs. Peritoneal implants and metastases are not infrequently present at operation for the removal of the primary tumor.[29,30,243] Excision of the tumor is usually followed by a local recurrence, which occurs within a few weeks or months. Recurrences usually occur within the first year following the primary treatment and patients free from recurrence for 12 to 18 months survive.[29,30] Rupture of the tumor with spillage of the contents during opera-

tion is not infrequent and tends to be associated with poor outcome. The metastases and peritoneal implants may be composed of different tissues, and thus their teratomatous nature is readily apparent, but they may also be composed of a single tissue. The histologic appearances of the metastases and of the peritoneal implants may or may not reflect the appearances of the primary tumor.

PROGNOSIS. On the whole treatment is unsatisfactory and prognosis is poor, and less than 20% of patients survive 5 years after operation.[29,34,121] Better results have been claimed in cases where the only immature element was neurogenic.[121,246] It has been suggested that there is a relationship between the histologic appearances of the tumor and prognosis.[228] For example, poorly differentiated tumors have been found to have worse prognosis, whereas a more favorable outcome has been observed in the better differentiated ones.[228,243] A histologic grading has been proposed that may be of value for prognostic purposes.[228] Although the presence of this relationship is not accepted by some investigators[29,30] there is evidence that in uncomplicated cases such a relationship exists.[243]

THERAPY. The recommended treatment of immature teratoma has been bilateral adnexectomy and hysterectomy,[29,84] but it has become apparent that as the tumors are only occasionally bilateral there is no advantage in performing a radical operation unless the opposite ovary and uterus are involved.[30,185,243,246] Although radiation therapy is frequently used to treat immature teratoma, the tumor does not respond to radiotherapy.[29,30,122] The response to chemotherapy, using a combination of agents, is at present being evaluated and occasional therapeutic successes have been reported.[122,246]

### Solid mature teratoma

#### Synonyms

Solid adult teratoma, benign solid teratoma.

Solid mature teratoma is a very rare ovarian neoplasm and a very uncommon type of ovarian teratoma. The age incidence is similar to the age incidence of solid immature teratoma, the tumor occurring mainly in children and young adults.[151,228,243] The majority of solid ovarian teratomas are composed at least partly of immature tissues and are therefore considered to be malignant. The occasional cases of solid ovarian teratoma composed entirely of mature tissues have been usually included in this group and thus misinterpreted as malignant. At the same time this practice has improved the survival statistics, which are generally very poor in patients with immature ovarian teratoma. Solid mature teratoma is composed entirely of mature tissues derived from the three germ layers. Very rigid diagnostic criteria must be strictly adhered to and the examination and sampling of the tumor must be very thorough, as inclusion of cases with immature elements completely changes the prognosis of this neoplasm, which otherwise is excellent.[141,151,228,243,246] Neurogenic elements, which are one of the most common tissues present in this tumor, may often be the cause of difficulties in this context.[185] The presence of immature neural elements immediately excludes the tumor from this group, as by definition only tumors composed entirely of mature tissues may be included.

MACROSCOPIC APPEARANCES. The tumors are usually large, do not show any specific features, and show similar appearance to the majority of solid teratomas, which are composed of immature tissues. They grow slowly in comparison with immature solid teratoma, but as they are usually discovered after they have reached a considerable size this feature is of little help in diagnosis. In all reported cases of solid mature teratoma the tumor has been unilateral.[141,151,228,243,246]

MICROSCOPIC APPEARANCE. The tumor is composed of a variety of tissues derived from the three germ layers and arranged in an orderly manner resembling the much more common mature cystic teratoma, except that they form a solid pattern, or at least a predominantly solid pattern. The tumor is composed entirely of mature tissues (Figures 26.34 and 26.35). Sometimes neurogenic elements may predominate (Figure 26.35).

THERAPY AND PROGNOSIS. As the tumor is unilateral, oophorectomy or unilateral adnexectomy is the treatment of choice, resulting in a complete cure.[151,228,243,246]

Occasionally solid mature teratoma may be associated with peritoneal implants composed entirely of mature glial tissue (Figure 26.36) and in spite of extensive involvement, which may be present, and irrespective of the mode of therapy employed the prognosis is excellent.[168] Presence of peritoneal implants composed entirely of mature glial tissue may occasionally be observed in patients with immature solid teratoma and with mature cystic teratoma. The prognosis is likewise excellent.[168]

### Mature cystic teratoma

*Synonyms*

Dermoid cyst, dermoid, adult cystic teratoma, benign cystic teratoma.

Mature cystic teratoma of the ovary, or dermoid cyst, has been known since the times of antiquity. The tumor is composed of well-differentiated derivatives of the three germ layers—ectoderm, mesoderm, and endoderm—with ectodermal elements predominating. In its pure form ma-

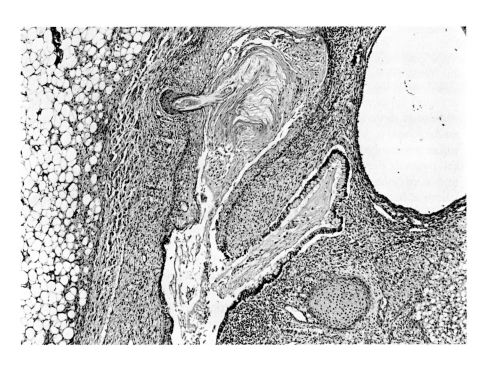

**26.34** Mature solid teratoma composed of squamous and glandular epithelium, adipose and fibrous tissue, and cartilage. Hematoxylin-eosin, ×61.

ously termed dermoid mamilla, dermoid protuberance, Rokitansky's protuberance, embryonic node, dermoid nipple, and so on. The hair present in the tumor arises from this protuberance and when bone or teeth are present they tend to be located within this area, which is composed of a variety of different tissues and is one of the sites that should always be carefully sampled when the tumor is being examined. Mature cystic teratomas contain macroscopically recognizable and well-formed teeth in 31% of cases.[25] Phalanges, long, and other bones; parts of the rib cage; loops of intestine; and even fetuslike structures are occasionally encountered.[9]

MICROSCOPIC APPEARANCES. The outer side of the cyst wall is composed of ovarian stroma, which may often be fibrosed and hyalinized, making its recognition difficult. The cavity of the cyst is lined mainly by skin and in small tumors cutaneous structures may form the entire lining. The skin is lined by keratinized squamous epithelium (Figures 26.38 and 26.39) and contains usually abundant sebaceous and sweat glands (Figure 26.38). Hair and other dermal appendages are usually present. Occasionally the cyst wall may be lined by bronchial or gastrointestinal epithelium or epithelium of columnar or cuboidal type, and the squamous epithelium may be present only in the region of the dermoid protuberance. Sometimes there may be loss of the lining epithelium caused by desquamation and this may be associated with foreign body giant cell reaction. The latter may be seen in other parts of the tumor as a reaction to the contents of the tumor. Foreign body giant cell reaction may also be seen when the contents of the tumor are spilled, leading to the formation of adhesions. The area around the dermoid protuberance may contain a large variety of tissues derived from the three germ layers. Ectodermal tissue is usually most abundant and is usually represented by squamous epithelium and other skin derivatives, brain tissue, glia, neural tissue, retina, choroid plexus, and ganglia. Mesodermal tissue is represented by bone, cartilage (Figure 26.39), smooth muscle, and fibrous and fatty tissue and endodermal tissue is represented by gastrointestinal and bronchial epithelium and glands, thyroid, and salivary gland tissue. In a careful study of 100 cases, ectodermal structures were found in 100%, mesodermal in 93%, and endodermal in 71% of cases, and it was considered that the presence of mesodermal and endodermal derivatives would have been higher had more sections been examined.[25] The various tissues present in mature cystic teratoma show an orderly organoid arrangement forming cutaneous, bronchial, and gastrointestinal tissues, as well as bone and other structures.

Although these tissues may be scattered diffusely, they do not exhibit the disorderly haphazard arrangement that is observed in immature teratoma.

Mature cystic teratoma must be differentiated from the rare cases of fetus *in fetu,* considered most likely to be caused by an inclusion of a monozygotic diamniotic twin. Fetus *in fetu* can be distinguished from a teratoma by its location in the retroperitoneal space, presence of vertebral organization with formation of limb buds, and a well-developed organ system. Fetus *in fetu* shows better organization than the most differentiated teratomas.[79,112] Like mature cystic teratoma, fetus *in fetu* is a benign lesion.

THERAPY. The treatment of choice for an uncomplicated mature cystic teratoma is the excision of the affected ovary. In young patients, if the tumor is small and conservation of a part of the ovary is possible, excision of the tumor may be the treatment of choice, usually resulting in a complete cure. Local recurrences following conservative treatment for mature cystic teratoma are very uncommon and occur in less than 1% of cases.[56]

COMPLICATIONS. Mature cystic teratoma of the ovary may be associated with complications in a number of cases. In view of the fact that in many of these cases the condition is amenable to cure, their recognition is of considerable importance. These complications can be classified as follows:

a. Torsion
b. Rupture
c. Infection
d. Hemolytic anemia
e. Development of malignancy

Torsion is the most frequent complication.[34,146,153] It has been observed in 16.1% of cases in one large series.[153] This complication tends to be more common during pregnancy and puerperium.[119,153] Mature cystic teratoma is said to comprise from 22 to 40% of ovarian tumors in pregnancy, and from 0.8 to 12.8% of reported cases of mature cystic teratoma have occurred in pregnancy.[34,153] The fact that these tumors when they occur during pregnancy are more liable to be associated with this complication is of considerable importance. Torsion is also more common in children and younger patients.[146,153] The patients usually present with severe acute abdominal pain and the condition is considered as an acute abdominal emergency. Excision of the affected ovary or salpingo-oophorectomy is the treatment of choice.

Torsion tends to predispose to rupture of the tumor.

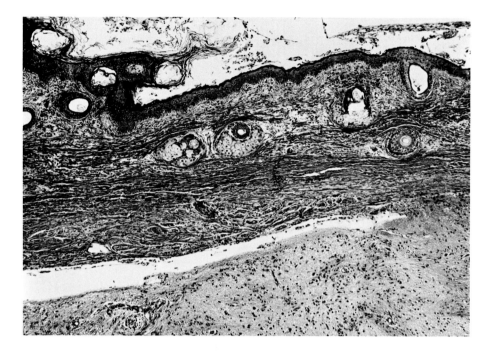

**26.38** Mature cystic teratoma. The lining of the cyst is composed of skin with its appendages. Mature neural tissue is seen beneath the cutaneous structures. Hematoxylin–eosin, ×61.

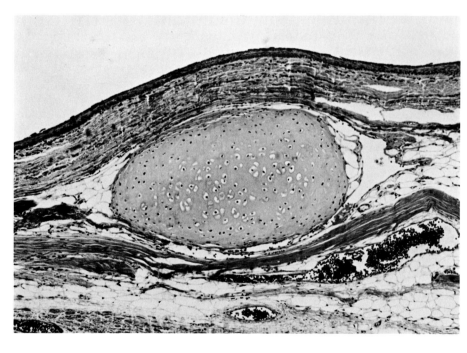

**26.39** Mature cystic teratoma lined by squamous epithelium and containing cartilage, muscle, and fatty tissue. Hematoxylin–eosin, ×95.

Rupture of mature cystic teratoma is an uncommon complication,[2] occurring in approximately 1% of cases.[119,153] It is much more common during pregnancy and may manifest itself during labor.[119,146] The immediate result of the rupture may be shock or hemorrhage, especially during pregnancy or labor, but the prognosis even in these cases is usually favorable. Rupture of the tumor into the peritoneal cavity may be followed by chemical peritonitis, caused by the spillage of the contents of the tumor. It produces a marked granulomatous reaction and leads to the formation of dense adhesions throughout the peritoneal cavity. Rupture of the tumor may occasionally be followed by formation of glial implants on the peritoneum. This occurs when the tumor contains mature neuroglial elements and spillage leads to deposition of numerous small nodules composed of mature glia in the peritoneal cavity. In spite of the wide dissemination of these deposits throughout the peritoneal cavity, the prognosis is favorable and simple surgical excision of the primary tumor is considered to be an adequate form of therapy.[168] Mature cystic teratoma may rupture not only into the peritoneal cavity but also into the adjacent organs, usually into the bladder or the rectum. More than 30 such cases have been reported.[45]

Infection is an uncommon complication of mature cystic teratoma and occurs in approximately 1% of cases.[119] The infecting organism is usually a coliform, but *Salmonella* infection causing typhoid fever has also been reported.[86]

Autoimmune hemolytic anemia has been noted occasionally in patients with teratoma of the ovary, mainly in mature cystic teratoma. Excision of the tumor in these cases resulted in the disappearance of the anemia and a complete cure.[15,22,46,47] Eighteen cases of benign cystic teratoma and seven other cystic ovarian tumors associated with this complication have been reported.[22] The patients present with symptoms and signs of progressive anemia, which may be moderate or severe. It is accompanied by reticulocytosis, spherocytosis, and increased osmotic fragility. Normoblasts may be present in the peripheral blood. The indirect serum bilirubin is elevated and the direct antiglobulin test (Coombs' test) is positive, indicating the presence of autoantibodies which react with the patient's red blood cells. The platelets are normal in number. The spleen may be palpable but is only slightly enlarged. Steroids are only transiently effective in treating the disease and splenectomy has no effect on the progress of the disease.[22] Excision of the ovarian tumor leads to the permanent disappearance of the anemia.[22,46,47] The following possible pathogenetic mechanisms have been suggested:[22]

1. Presence in the tumor of substances that are antigenically different from the host and that stimulate the production by the host of antibodies, which cross-react with her own red blood cells
2. Antibody production by the tumor directed specifically against the host's red blood cells and resembling the graft versus host reaction
3. Coating of red blood cells with products secreted by the tumor and resulting in changed red blood cell antigenicity

In view of this, pelvic and radiologic examination is indicated in a young woman with autoimmune hemolytic anemia, which does not respond to steroid treatment, as it may help to detect an ovarian teratoma and prevent an unnecessary splenectomy.[46,185]

### Mature cystic teratoma (dermoid cyst) with malignant transformation

INCIDENCE. Malignant transformation is an uncommon complication of mature cystic teratoma. It occurs in approximately 2% of cases,[38,119,152,153] although in a recent report the incidence was almost 4%.[147] The age of patients with this complication as reported in the literature ranges from 19 to 88 years.[153] Malignant transformation in mature cystic teratoma is usually observed in postmenopausal patients.[38,103,119,147,152,153]

CLINICAL ASPECTS. Clinically this tumor cannot be readily differentiated from an uncomplicated mature cystic teratoma or other ovarian tumor, although evidence of its rapid growth, pain, loss of weight, and other systemic symptoms are in favor of the presence of a malignant tumor. Sometimes the tumor may be found as an incidental observation. We have encountered, at autopsy, a large mature cystic teratoma containing a squamous cell carcinoma (Figure 26.40) in the left ovary of a 56-year-old woman.

MACROSCOPIC APPEARANCES. The tumor is frequently larger than an average mature cystic teratoma.[34] It may exhibit a more solid appearance but differentiation cannot be made on macroscopic grounds. Malignant transformation in mature cystic teratoma tends to occur in patients with unilateral tumors.[152,153]

MICROSCOPIC APPEARANCES. The tumor exhibits malignant transformation in one of its constituent tissues, most frequently the squamous epithelium (Figure 26.40) with formation of a typical squamous cell carcinoma.[34,38,147,152] Any of the tissues present in a mature cystic teratoma may undergo malignant transformation and a variety of malignant tumors have been reported, including carcinoid tumor, thyroid carcinoma, basal cell carcinoma (Figure 26.41), adenocarcinoma of the intestinal epithelium, malignant melanoma, leiomyosarcoma, and chondrosarcoma.[38,59,84,103,119,123,152,153,242] The malignant element invades other parts of the tumor and its wall (Figure 26.40), which it tends to perforate. Invariably only one tissue element becomes malignant and the pres-

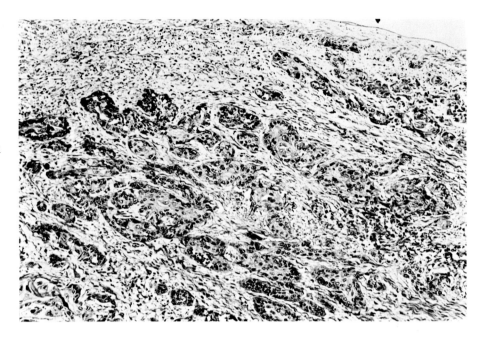

**26.40** Squamous cell carcinoma arising in and invading a mature cystic teratoma. Surface of the ovary is seen at top right. Hematoxylin–eosin, ×76.

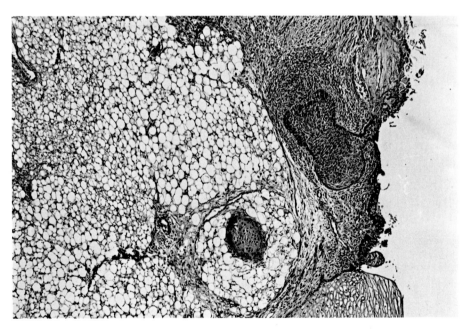

**26.41** Basal cell carcinoma arising in a mature cystic teratoma. Hematoxylin–eosin, ×77.

ence of many different malignant elements indicates that the tumor is an immature teratoma and not a mature cystic teratoma that has undergone malignant transformation.

BEHAVIOR. The mode of spread of the malignant tumor differs from that observed in other tumors of germ cell origin. The tumor spreads by direct invasion and perito-

neal implantation and generally does not metastasize to the lymph nodes.[152] Extensive local invasion and absence of lymph node involvement is usually observed at laparotomy.[147] Hematogenous dissemination is uncommon.

PROGNOSIS. The prognosis of patients with mature cystic teratoma with malignant transformation is unfavorable.[38,147,152,153] There are only 15 to 30.8% 5-year survivors.[152,153] Better prognosis has been reported when the malignant element is a squamous cell carcinoma confined to the ovary and is excised without spillage of the contents. In such cases the 5-year survival is 63%.[152] There have been no 5-year survivors when the malignant element was an adenocarcinoma or a sarcoma.[152]

THERAPY. The advocated treatment is hysterectomy and bilateral adnexectomy.[84] As the tumors are usually unilateral, however, in cases where there is no penetration of the capsule and no involvement of the adjacent structures a more conservative surgical procedure may be just as effective. If the tumor has spread beyond the confines of the ovary and there is involvement of the adjacent structures, however, a more radical procedure with resection of the tumor and the involved structures or viscera is advocated.[147] Response to radiation and chemotherapy is unsatisfactory.[147]

### Struma ovarii

Thyroid tissue is a relatively frequent constituent of mature cystic teratoma and has been demonstrated in 5 to 20% of cases.[185,186] Struma ovarii is considered as a one-sided development of a teratoma, as a tumor in which the thyroid tissue has overgrown all other tissues, or one in which only the thyroid tissue has developed. The term struma ovarii should be reserved only for tumors composed either entirely or predominantly of thyroid tissue or for those in which thyroid tissue can be recognized macroscopically.

INCIDENCE. Struma ovarii is uncommon and comprises 2.7% of ovarian teratomas.[80] The age incidence of patients with struma ovarii is generally the same as that of patients with benign cystic teratoma. The age of patients as reported in the literature ranges from 6 to 74 years and the majority of patients have been encountered during the reproductive years.[43,136,193,245,247]

CLINICAL ASPECTS. There are usually no specific symptoms and on the whole the clinical findings are similar to those observed in patients with benign cystic teratoma. The only differences are that in some cases struma ovarii has been associated with enlargement of the thyroid gland and in other cases there has been clinical evidence that the struma ovarii has been responsible for the development of thyrotoxicosis, this has not been confirmed by laboratory tests, as these were not performed preoperatively.[136,185,193,247] Some cases of thyrotoxicosis have been associated with struma ovarii which has also showed changes of thyroid hyperactivity.[80,172] The ectopic thyroid

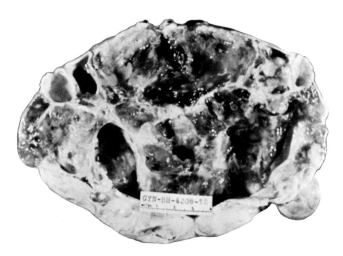

**26.42** Struma ovarii. The cut surface shows compartments of amber-colored thyroid tissue separated by thick fibrous septae.

[Courtesy of B. Bigelow, M.D.]

tissue present within struma ovarii may therefore be the subject of the same physiologic and pathologic changes as thyroid gland. Although the true thyroid nature of the tissue present in struma ovarii was not accepted initially, its true thyroid composition has been demonstrated conclusively.[55,163,193]

MACROSCOPIC APPEARANCES. Struma ovarii is usually unilateral[43,136,247] but, in one report, in 15% of cases the contralateral ovary also contained a teratoma and this tumor contained thyroid tissue in some of the cases.[193] Earlier reports have stated that in 50% of cases struma ovarii has been associated with a mature cystic teratoma, in 31% with a cystadenoma, and only in 17% was thyroid tissue the sole constituent.[193] More recent reports indicate a predominance of pure struma ovarii over those associated with mature cystic teratoma and a paucity of cases associated with cystadenoma.[136,247]

Struma ovarii may vary in size but usually measure less than 10 cm in diameter. It tends to be larger if it is associated with other elements. The surface is usually smooth, and prior to sectioning the tumor shows similar appearances to mature cystic teratoma. Occasionally adhesions may be present. The cut surface of the tumor may be composed entirely of light tan glistening thyroid (Figure 26.42) tissue or may consist of thyroid tissue associated with other tissues. Hemorrhage, necrosis, and foci of fibrosis may be present. Solid tumors with small amounts of colloid appear less glistening and more fleshy.

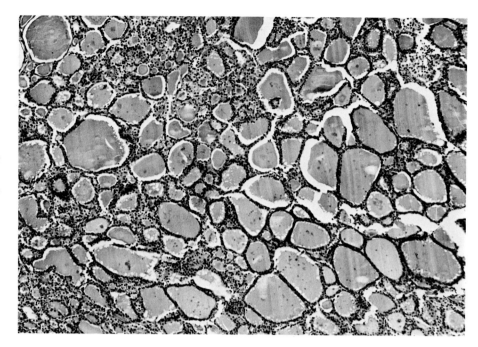

**26.43** Struma ovarii. The tumor is composed of normal thyroid tissue. Hematoxylin–eosin, ×76.

MICROSCOPIC APPEARANCES. The tumor shows similar appearances to those observed in mature thyroid tissue. The tumor is composed of acini of various sizes, lined by a single layer of columnar or flattened epithelium (Figure 26.43). The acini contain eosinophilic, PAS-positive colloid. The intensity of the staining may vary. There may be a considerable variation in the size of the acini, which may be very large, containing a large amount of colloid, or may be very small. Occasionally the lining of the acini may be columnar, containing small papillary projections not unlike those seen in hyperactive thyroid gland. Sometimes the appearances may resemble those of nodular adenomatous goiter. Adenoma-like lesions may be observed. Struma ovarii showing appearances suggestive of Hashimoto's thyroiditis has also been reported.[57]

BEHAVIOR. Most cases of struma ovarii are benign and can be treated by excision of the ovary or by unilateral salpingo-oophorectomy. In a small number of cases there are complications, the most important being the development of malignancy and the presence of ascites or ascites associated with pleural effusion. Ascites may be found in 17% of cases of struma ovarii and its presence does not indicate that the tumor is malignant.[193] Struma ovarii may be associated with ascites and pleural effusion, producing a "pseudo-Meigs syndrome."[100,185] The tumor in these cases is benign. The cause of the ascites and pleural effusion has not been fully elucidated. In the majority of re-ported cases tumor excision led to complete remission.[185]

Malignant change in struma ovarii is uncommon. In a number of reported cases, the diagnosis was based on the histology of the tumor and there were no metastases or other features of malignancy. A number of other reported cases were examples of struma ovarii and carcinoid.[185,186] Only 17 of 45 reported cases of malignant struma ovarii were associated with metastases.[76,136,185,186,247] The presence of metastases is an unequivocal proof of the malignant nature of the tumor. The malignant struma ovarii usually shows follicular pattern, but papillary carcinoma is also observed. We have encountered a 26-year-old patient with a mature cystic teratoma containing thyroid tissue and a typical well-differentiated papillary adenocarcinoma of the thyroid (Figure 26.44), which was associated with metastases in the paraaortic lymph nodes. The patient was well and symptom free 3½ years after excision of the tumor followed by laparotomy and dissection of the paraaortic lymph nodes, as well as a course of radiation therapy. There was no evidence of metastases elsewhere.

The metastatic spread of malignant struma ovarii frequently affects the peritoneum, where sometimes the deposits may show a histologically benign appearance (benign strumosis).[185,186] Prognosis in these cases is generally favorable and is compatible with long survival. Other routes of spread are via the lymphatics to the paraaortic and other lymph nodes and via the bloodstream to the lungs and bones. In these cases the prognosis is less

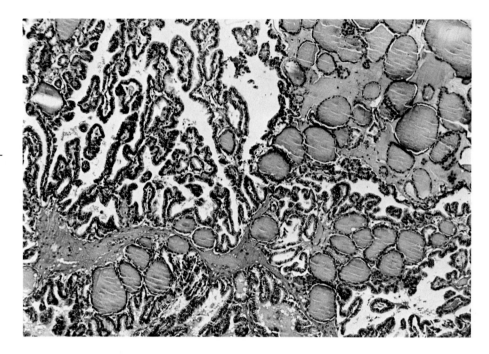

**26.44** Papillary carcinoma arising in thyroid tissue present in a mature cystic teratoma. Hematoxylin–eosin, ×76.

favorable. Treatment consists of surgery and administration of radioactive iodine ($^{131}$I) and other agents used in the treatment of thyroid malignancy, including radiation therapy.

### Carcinoid

Primary ovarian carcinoid tumors usually arise in association with gastrointestinal or respiratory epithelium present in a mature cystic teratoma. They may also be observed within a solid teratoma or a mucinous tumor or they may occur in an apparently pure form.[185,186,229] The latter are considered to arise either as a one-sided development of a teratoma or from argentaffin cells present within the ovary.

INCIDENCE. Primary ovarian carcinoid tumors are uncommon. Nearly 50 cases have been reported,[164] but the number of unreported cases reaches more than half this number.[169] The age distribution of patients with ovarian carcinoid is similar to that of patients with mature cystic teratoma, although the average age is higher. Many patients are postmenopausal.

CLINICAL ASPECTS. One-third of the reported cases have been associated with the typical carcinoid syndrome, in spite of the absence of metastases.[164] This is in contrast to intestinal carcinoids, which are associated with the syndrome only when there is metastatic spread to the liver. One reason for this difference is that the blood flow from the ovary goes directly into the systemic circulation and does not pass through the liver. The liver inactivates the substances produced by the tumor, and the blood coming from the ovary is not subjected to this action. The presence or absence of symptoms of carcinoid syndrome is also dependent on the number of secreting tumor cells. The fact that functioning ovarian carcinoid tumors have all measured approximately 10 cm in diameter, with only one exception,[176] indicates the presence of a large tumor mass capable of producing a large amount of secretion, whereas intestinal carcinoids are usually smaller. The excision of the tumor has been associated with rapid remission of the symptoms in all the described cases and the disappearance of 5-hydroxyindolylacetic acid (5-HIAA) from the urine. This provides further proof of the activity of the ovarian tumor. If the tumor is nonfunctioning, there are no specific features and the presentation is the same as in cases of mature cystic teratoma.

MACROSCOPIC APPEARANCES. The tumor shows similar appearances to those of mature cystic teratoma within which it is usually found. The same applies if the tumor is associated with a solid teratoma, or a mucinous tumor. If the carcinoid is not associated with other tissue elements the tumor is solid. The carcinoid may vary in size from microscopic to large and is solid and homogeneous (Fig-

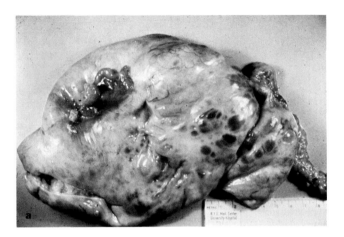
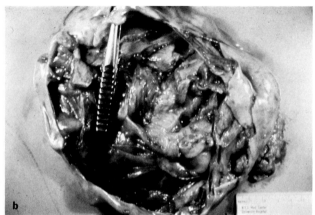

**26.45 a.** Carcinoid of the ovary. It is oval-shaped and encapsulated. **b.** The cut surface is yellow to brown in color. It is largely cystic.

[Courtesy of B. Bigelow, M.D.]

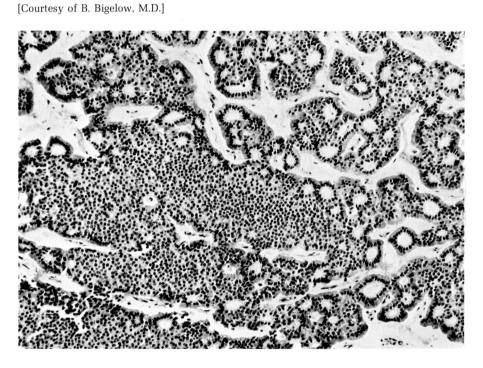

**26.46** Primary ovarian carcinoid showing the typical solid and acinar patterns of midgut carcinoids. Hematoxylin–eosin, ×153.

ure 26.45a,b). Its color may vary from light brown to yellow or pale gray. Primary ovarian carcinoids are practically always unilateral, although they may be associated with a benign cystic teratoma in the contralateral ovary.

MICROSCOPIC APPEARANCES. The primary ovarian carcinoid usually shows typical appearances associated with midgut carcinoids.[240] The tumor is composed of collections of small acini and solid nests of polygonal cells with ample amount of cytoplasm and round or oval centrally located hyperchromatic nuclei (Figure 26.46). The cyto-

plasm is basophilic or amphophilic and may contain red, brown, or orange argentaffin granules (Figure 26.47), which are demonstrated in the great majority of cases of primary ovarian carcinoids.[169] Ultrastructurally the cells of the ovarian carcinoid show similar appearances to those of carcinoid tumors from other locations.[229] Primary carcinoid of the ovary must be differentiated from metastatic carcinoid of the ovary, which is usually of gastrointestinal origin and practically always affects both ovaries unlike the primary ovarian carcinoid which is unilateral.[169] Macroscopically the metastatic carcinoid is composed of tumor

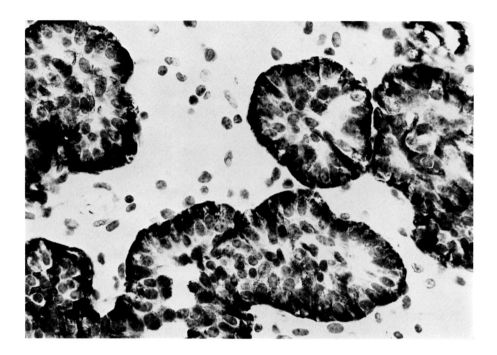

**26.47** Ovarian carcinoid. The tumor cells contain numerous argentaffin granules stained black. Masson–Fontana, ×388.

nodules, whereas primary ovarian carcinoid forms a single homogeneous mass. When other teratomatous elements are associated with primary ovarian carcinoid they are a very helpful distinguishing feature.[169] Primary ovarian carcinoid may sometimes be confused with Brenner tumor, but the appearances of the cell nests and the grooved "coffee-bean" nuclei of the cells of Brenner tumor are against the diagnosis of a carcinoid, whereas the typical small acinar pattern and the presence of argentaffin reaction are in favor of a carcinoid. Confusion with granulosa cell tumor may also arise and Call–Exner bodies may be confused with carcinoid acini, but the cells of the carcinoid tumor usually show acinar pattern and contain more cytoplasm and argentaffin granules.[169,229] Cystic areas that may be present in a granulosa cell tumor are nearly always absent in a carcinoid. Occasionally ovarian carcinoid may be confused with a Krukenberg tumor, but the latter is usually bilateral and may be larger and the cellular appearances are different. The cells of Krukenberg tumor tend to merge with the stroma, are larger, and show greater pleomorphism, a signet-ring appearance, and more brisk mitotic activity. Acinar pattern is less evident. Demonstration of argentaffin granules, which can be detected in the majority of ovarian carcinoids, confirms the diagnosis. These granules can be identified even more easily with the aid of the electron microscope and the tumor cells present characteristic ultrastructural appearances.[229]

BEHAVIOR AND PROGNOSIS. The primary ovarian carcinoids are only occasionally associated with metastases. This has been observed in three out of 47 reported cases.[164] In the cases where the tumor has metastasized, widespread metastases have developed after a number of years, the patients dying with extensive metastatic disease.[169] The prognosis after excision of the primary tumor is very favorable and in the great majority of cases is complete cure.

## Struma ovarii and carcinoid

*Synonym*

Strumal carcinoid.

Struma ovarii and carcinoid is an uncommon variant of struma ovarii. It is composed of thyroid tissue intimately admixed with carcinoid tumor showing ribbon or cordlike pattern. It has become recognized as a separate entity only in recent years.[185,186,190] The histologic pattern of struma ovarii, merging imperceptibly with carcinoid tumor that exhibited the ribbonlike pattern observed in hindgut carcinoids,[240] had been recognized previously.[76,89,103,163,245,247] However, it was usually interpreted as a carcinoma developing in a struma ovarii, although the resemblance to a carcinoid tumor was noted in some cases.[76,103]

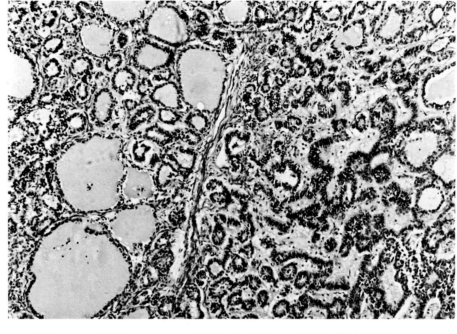

**26.48** Struma ovarii and carcinoid. The carcinoid forms long narrow cords and ribbons (right) merging with thyroid follicles (left). Hematoxylin–eosin, ×102.

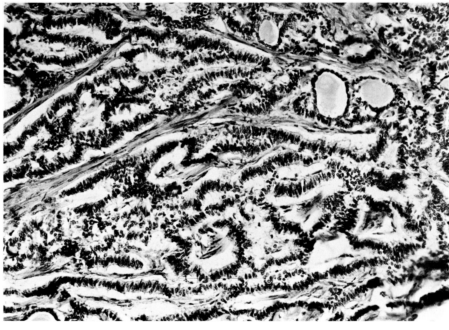

**26.49** Struma ovarii and carcinoid. The carcinoid is composed of columnar or cuboidal epithelial cells forming narrow winding cords and ribbons. Thyroid follicles are also seen. Hematoxylin–eosin, ×240.

Struma ovarii and carcinoid is rare and only a few cases have been reported. This tumor has the same age incidence as struma ovarii and is usually not associated with any specific clinical findings. In one reported case it was associated with virilization.[50] Like hindgut carcinoids, and unlike the primary ovarian carcinoid, struma ovarii and carcinoid is not associated with the carcinoid syndrome.

Macroscopically this tumor is similar to struma ovarii. Microscopically the tumor is composed of thyroid follicles containing colloid that merge with ribbons of neoplastic cells usually set in dense fibrous tissue stroma (Figures 26.48 and 26.49). The thyroid follicles are often small in size at the junction between the two types of tissue. The carcinoid is usually composed of long, winding or straight ribbons of columnar cells with elongated hyperchromatic nuclei (Figure 26.49). It may also be composed of small islands of tumor cells separated by dense fibrous tissue stroma from each other, from the long ribbons of carcinoid cells, and from the thyroid follicles (Figure 26.48). Slight mitotic activity is present in the carcinoid part of the lesion. In some cases argentaffin granules have been identified in the carcinoid cells.[7,185,186] The latter have been found to exhibit similar ultrastructural appearances to those seen in medullary carcinoma of the thyroid, including the presence of neurosecretory granules.[7] In one tumor, amyloid deposits were identified and were verified both histochemically and ultrastructurally.[7] This ultrastructural similarity between the cells of medullary carcinoma of the thyroid and carcinoid tumors has been noted previously.[28,77] Although carcinoid tumors have not been observed in the thyroid gland, one case of medullary carcinoma of the thyroid has been associated with the carcinoid syndrome.[132] It has been suggested that struma ovarii and carcinoid may originate from the parafollicular cells and may therefore be analogous in this respect to the medullary carcinoma of the thyroid.[7]

Struma ovarii and carcinoid should be distinguished from carcinoma of the thyroid arising in struma ovarii with which it has often been confused. The latter has the typical appearances observed in carcinoma of the thyroid and exhibits usually the follicular or papillary pattern.

Struma ovarii and carcinoid has been only once associated with metastases and even in this case the patient was apparently cured by a combination of surgery and radiation therapy.[247] All other cases have followed a benign course.[185,186] It is of interest that carcinoid tumors of hindgut origin are not associated with metastases and follow a benign course.[239]

### Other types of monodermal teratoma

The mucinous tumors of the ovary are usually described with the epithelial neoplasms and are considered to be derived from the germinal epithelium of the ovary. They are usually grouped together with the epithelial and not with the germ cell neoplasms of the ovary, but there are undoubtedly some cases where the tumor is of germ cell origin, forming a monodermal teratomatous neoplasm in which the mucinous element has outgrown all the other tissues in the same manner that in a pure struma ovarii the thyroid tissue has outgrown all the other tissues. The presence of occasional teratomatous tumors composed mainly of mucinous (intestinal type) epithelium of endodermal derivation and only a small amount of other tumor elements, as well as a 5% association of mature cystic teratoma with mucinous cystadenoma, tends to support this mode of origin for at least some mucinous tumors. Mucinous epithelium resembling intestinal epithelium has been observed in association with struma ovarii and with struma ovarii and carcinoid. In these cases it was the only other tissue element present. The mucinous epithelium frequently contains goblet cells and so shows greater resemblance to the intestinal than to the endocervical epithelium. In 21% of cases the epithelium lining mucinous tumors of the ovary contains argentaffin granules.[63] In occasional cases Paneth cells are also present.[185] These findings are considered to be a strong argument in favor of the derivation of at least some mucinous ovarian tumors from the intestinal type of epithelium and their teratomatous and therefore germ cell origin.

Mucinous tumors of the ovary are discussed fully with tumors of epithelial derivation, but a probable teratomatous or germ cell origin of some of these neoplasms should be recognized and noted, especially as they may probably represent the largest group of monodermal teratomatous neoplasms. It is possible that studies of the type undertaken by Linder, using both chromosomal and isoenzyme techniques,[110] may help to clarify the origin of mucinous tumors of the ovary and confirm that some of these tumors are of germ cell origin.

Other rare examples of monodermal teratomatous neoplasms observed in the ovary include the epidermoid cyst, which is lined by epidermis without appendages; the sebaceous gland tumor[201]; the melanotic tumor, resembling the "retinal anlage" tumor[82]; and the possible benign cystic counterpart of the latter.[5] Monodermal teratomatous origin of some malignant connective tissue tumors is very difficult to prove because of the occurrence of connective tissue neoplasms derived from normal ovarian tissue. Monodermal teratomatous origin of tumors derived from ectodermal or endodermal tissues is more easily acceptable, and there may be as yet undescribed tumors of this type.

## Mixed Germ Cell Tumors

Mixed germ cell tumors are tumors composed of more than one neoplastic germ cell element, such as dysgerminoma combined with teratoma, endodermal sinus tumor, choriocarcinoma, embryonal carcinoma, or polyembryoma, as well as any other possible combination of these tumor types. This group includes only neoplasms composed entirely of neoplastic germ cell elements and does not include the gonadoblastoma and mixed germ cell–sex cord stroma tumor, which in addition to germ cells contains sex cord stroma derivatives as an integral component. The relatively frequent finding of different neoplastic germ cell elements in gonadal tumors of germ cell origin is considered to be a strong argument in favor of the common histogenesis of this group of neoplasms. The various tumor elements present in these tumors may be intimately admixed (Figure 26.11) or may form separate areas adjacent to each other and separated by fibrous septa (Figure 26.12). Although many ovarian tumors belonging to this group are classified according to the predominant element present, it is emphasized that when these tumors are examined all areas of varying appearance should be carefully sampled and thoroughly analyzed. All the neoplastic germ cell elements observed within the tumor, however small, should be mentioned and described and, if possible, their relative size estimated. The importance of this practice is by no means only academic, as the behavior and treatment of neoplasms belonging to this group vary considerably, and the presence of a small area composed of a more malignant element may alter the therapeutic approach and the prognosis. The presence of more malignant elements within a tumor is usually associated with more aggressive behavior of the tumor, unsatisfactory response to therapy, and poor prognosis.[8,150,175,209,227] The different response to treatment and the different behavior of some cases of dysgerminoma described in the past may have been at least in some cases a result of the presence within the tumor of other neoplastic germ cell elements that have not been identified. Although in the past mixed germ cell tumors were considered to be uncommon[133] they tend to figure much more frequently in recent reports.[8,29,30,85,91,135,175,209,227,246] This is probably because of a more careful and extensive examination of the tumor.

# Tumors Composed of Germ Cells and Sex Cord Stroma Derivatives

## Gonadoblastoma

*Synonyms*

Dysgenetic gonadoma,[130] gonocytoma,[222] tumor of dysgenetic gonad.[39]

*Terminology*

In 1953, Scully[183] described two patients with a distinct steroid-secreting gonadal tumor, which he named gonadoblastoma. The tumor was composed of germ cells and sex cord stroma derivatives, resembling immature granulosa, and Sertoli cells. One of the tumors also contained stromal elements indistinguishable from lutein or Leydig cells. Both tumors occurred in phenotypic females who were chromatin negative and had abnormal sexual development. The exact nature of the gonads in which the tumors had originated could not be determined. In both patients the tumors were bilateral and contained deposits of or were partly overgrown by dysgerminoma. Both patients showed evidence of virilization and the tumor was considered to be capable of steroid hormone secretion. The tumor was named gonadoblastoma because it appeared to recapitulate the development of the gonads and because it occurred in individuals with abnormal sexual development and in gonads the nature of which could not be determined.[187]

In 1960, Teter[222] proposed a new classification of neoplasms containing germ cells and their endocrine relationships, based on the term gonocytoma, which had been introduced previously.[213] Teter assigned neoplasms containing germ cells to one of four groups, depending on the number of cell types present and on the endocrine properties of these cell types:

*Gonocytoma 1.* A tumor composed entirely of germ cells and corresponding to dysgerminoma or seminoma and not capable of endocrine activity.

*Gonocytoma 2.* A tumor composed of germ cells and sex cord stroma derivatives and of immature Sertoli or granulosa cells. This tumor, when hormonally active, is feminizing; otherwise it is inert.

*Gonocytoma 3.* A tumor composed of germ cells, immature granulosa or Sertoli cells, and lutein or Leydig cells and hormonally either virilizing or inert. This tumor was considered to correspond to the classic gonadoblastoma.[183]

*Gonocytoma 4.* A pure germ cell tumor (dysgerminoma) with clinical symptoms of virilism caused by overgrowth of androgenic interstitial (Leydig) cells adjacent to the germ cell tumor or present in the contralateral gonad.

This classification was an attempt to correlate the histologic, endocrine, clinical, and genetic aspects of this group of neoplasms. Unfortunately the differences between some of the groups are not very clear and have not always been clearly illustrated in the reported cases. The histologic findings did not always correlate well with the endocrine, genetic, and clinical aspects of the cases; in view of this, although the attempt to classify these neoplasms in this way was commendable, the results were far from satisfactory, Although in subsequent years the term gonadoblastoma became the most widely accepted term denoting this tumor, Teter's classification[222] received considerable attention. In 1970, Scully[187] in an extensive study of the subject presented convincing arguments against Teter's classification and considered it unjustifiable on both pathologic and clinical grounds. Further support for Scully's view came from other investigators,[90,203,204] who, although agreeing that there are other types of tumors composed of germ cells and sex cord stroma derivatives apart from the classic gonadoblastoma, considered that the division of this group of neoplasms into four subgroups[222] was not justifiable. These views are also supported by the present basic concept that the classification of gonadal tumors should be based as far as possible on the morphologic features and histogenesis and not on endocrine, clinical, and genetic considerations.

In view of its distinctive histologic appearance, which distinguishes it from any other gonadal neoplasm, gonadoblastoma is considered to be a separate and specific entity. The neoplastic nature of gonadoblastoma has been questioned because some lesions are very small and may undergo complete regression from hyalinization and calcification and because when malignancy supervenes it usually manifests itself as germ cell neoplasia in spite of the fact that gonadoblastoma is composed of two or three cell types. When the tumor metastasizes, gonadoblastoma as such has never been observed in the metastases. Nevertheless, gonadoblastoma shows exactly the same pattern in the very small lesions, "bisexual formations,"[225] as in the large ones, including mitotic activity in the germ cell element, as well as early overgrowth by dysgerminoma. The association with dysgerminoma is seen in 50% of cases[187] and the presence of other more malignant germ cell tumors is seen in a further 10%.[187,205] In view of this, the concept that gonadoblastoma represents an *in situ* germ cell malignancy[187] is considered to be justified.

### Incidence

The exact incidence of gonadoblastoma is not known. Although more than 100 cases have been reported it is considered to be uncommon. Gonadoblastoma is usually seen in young patients, occurring most frequently in the second and somewhat less frequently in the third and first decades in this order. All the reported cases occurred in patients under 30 years of age. Gonadoblastoma is much more common in phenotypic females than in phenotypic males, the ratio being 4:1.[187]

### Clinical aspects

Patients with gonadoblastoma usually present with primary amenorrhea, virilization, or developmental abnormalities of the genitalia and the discovery of gonadoblastoma is made in the course of investigations of these conditions. Another not infrequent mode of presentation is the presence of a gonadal tumor. The gonadoblastoma, which forms part of the tumor in these cases, is discovered on histologic examination. The majority of patients with gonadoblastoma (80%) are phenotypic females and the remainder are phenotypic males with cryptorchidism, hypospadias, and female internal secondary sex organs. Among the phenotypic females, 60% are virilized and the remainder are normal in appearance.[187] The majority of the phenotypic female patients exhibit poor genital development, and breast development is often poor even among the nonvirilized females. Although primary amenorrhea is a very common presenting symptom among phenotypic females with gonadoblastoma, some patients have episodes of spontaneous cyclical bleeding, but in the majority of these patients the episodes are usually sporadic and the bleeding scanty. A few patients menstruate normally.[187] The virilization present in phenotypic female patients with gonadoblastoma does not usually regress after excision of the tumor, although this has been seen in occasional cases and in a few additional cases there was partial regression. Although most patients have gonadal dysgenesis, gonadoblastoma has been described in one patient, who has had two normal pregnancies following the excision of a dysgerminoma containing a small focus of gonadoblastoma. This patient was chromatin positive and had a 46XX karyotype.[20] Gonadoblastoma has also been reported in a true hermaphrodite[148] and in two patients with normally descended testes.[90,207]

### Macroscopic appearances

Gonadoblastoma has been found more often in the right gonad than in the left and has been bilateral in 38% of cases.[187] Recent reports suggest a higher incidence of bilateral involvement. Although many tumors are recognized on gross examination, in a number of cases the lesion is detected only on histologic examination. This may be the case with bilateral tumors, only one of which may be recognized macroscopically. In the majority of cases the gonad of origin is indeterminate because it is overgrown by the tumor. When the nature of the gonad can be identified, it is usually a streak or a testis. The contralateral gonad in these cases may be a streak or a testis, and the former is more likely to harbor a gonadoblastoma.[187]

Pure gonadoblastoma varies in size from a microscopic lesion to 8 cm in diameter, most tumors measuring a few centimeters. When gonadoblastoma becomes overgrown by dysgerminoma (Figure 26.50) or other malignant germ cell tumor elements, much larger tumors may be observed.[187,205] The macroscopic appearance of the tumor varies to some extent according to the presence of hyalinization and calcification, as well as overgrowth by dysgerminoma. Gonadoblastoma is a solid tumor and presents a smooth or slightly lobulated surface. It varies from soft and fleshy to firm and cartilaginous. It is speckled with calcific granules and may be almost completely calcified. Calcification has been recognized on gross examination in 45% of cases and in more than 20% it has been detectable radiologically.[187] The tumor varies in color from gray or yellow to brown and on cross section it appears to be somewhat granular.

Although the external sex organs in patients with gonadoblastoma present a wide variety of appearances from normal to completely ambiguous, the secondary internal sex organs consist almost always of a uterus, which is hypoplastic in the majority of cases, and of two or occasionally one normal fallopian tube. This is also seen in the phenotypic males. Male secondary internal sex organs, such as the epididymis, vas deferens, and prostate, are found occasionally in the virilized phenotypic females and are always found in the phenotypic male pseudohermaphrodites.[187]

*Microscopic appearances*

Gonadoblastoma is composed of collections of cellular nests surrounded by connective tissue stroma (Figure 26.51). The nests are solid, usually small, and oval or round but occasionally may be larger and elongated. The cellular nests contain a mixture of germ cells and sex cord stroma derivatives resembling immature Sertoli and granulosa cells (Figure 26.52). The germ cells are large and round, with pale or slightly granular cytoplasm and large round vesicular nuclei, often with prominent nucleoli

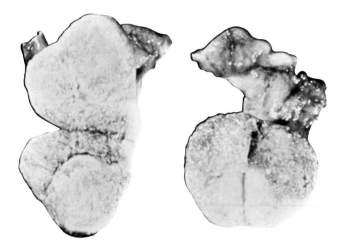

**26.50** Gonadoblastoma with dysgerminoma. The outer surface is smooth; the cut surface solid, granular, and yellow-brown in color.

[Courtesy of R. Scully, M.D.]

showing appearances and histochemical reactions similar to the germ cells of dysgerminoma or seminoma. The germ cells show mitotic activity in most cases, which may be marked in some. They are intimately admixed with immature Sertoli and granulosa cells, which are smaller and epithelial-like. The latter are round or oval and have dark, oval or slightly elongated carrot-shaped nuclei. Mitotic activity is not seen in these cells. The immature Sertoli and granulosa cells are arranged within the cell nests in three typical patterns (Figure 26.52):

1. They line in a coronal pattern the periphery of the nests.
2. They surround individual or collections of germ cells in the same way as the follicular epithelium surrounds the ovum of the primary follicle.
3. They surround small round spaces, containing amorphous hyaline, eosinophilic, and PAS-positive material, that resemble Call–Exner bodies.

The connective tissue stroma surrounding the cellular nests frequently contains collections of cells indistinguishable from Leydig cells or luteinized cells of ovarian stromal origin (Figure 26.53). There is considerable variation in the number of these cells from case to case and whereas in some cases they are numerous, in others they are identified with difficulty. Although in many cases the cells are indis-

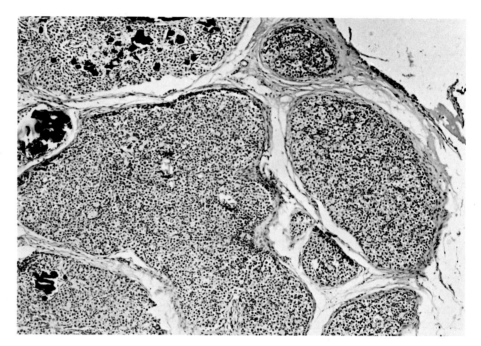

**26.51** Gonadoblastoma showing the cellular nests surrounded by connective tissue stroma. Note foci of calcification (heavy black areas). Hematoxylin–eosin, ×61.

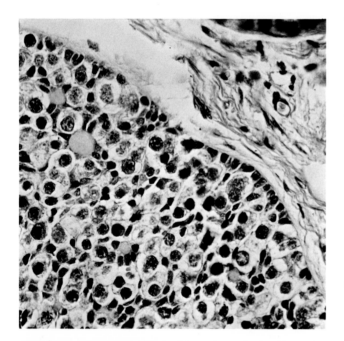

**26.52** Gonadoblastoma nest composed of large germ cells intimately admixed with smaller sex cord stroma derivatives. Hyaline Call–Exner-like bodies are also seen. Hematoxylin–eosin, ×460.

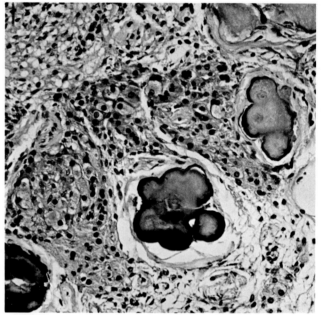

**26.53** Gonadoblastoma. Calcified nest surrounded by connective tissue containing numerous Leydig or lutein-like cells. Same case as Figure 26.52. Hematoxylin–eosin, ×235.

tinguishable from Leydig cells and may contain lipochrome granules, Reinke crystalloids, which are specifically diagnostic of Leydig cells, have never been identified in their cytoplasm. The Leydig or lutein-like cells are identi-

fied in 66% of cases and they are present nearly twice as frequently in older patients than in those 15 years or younger.[187] The presence of Leydig or lutein-like cells it not necessary for the diagnosis of gonadoblastoma. The connective tissue stroma surrounding the cellular nests may be scanty or abundant and may vary from dense and hyalinized to cellular, resembling ovarian stroma. These latter appearances are more common in tumors that either have arisen in or are suspected to originate in a gonadal streak.[187] Occasionally the stroma may be loose and edematous. The basic composition of gonadoblastoma, consisting of the two cell types with the Leydig or lutein-like cells present in the stroma, has been confirmed by electron microscopy.[44,88,114] Although there is agreement concerning the nature of the germ cells, the nature of the stromal cells is in dispute. They are considered by some to be Sertoli cells or their precursors,[114] whereas others consider them as primitive sex cord stroma cells and are unable to differentiate them further.[44,88] The nature of the amorphous, hyaline, eosinophilic material forming Call–Exner-like bodies is also a matter of dispute. It is considered to be either of basement membrane origin[44,114] or composed of fibrillar material formed by the stromal cells before they undergo fragmentation and cell death.[88]

The basic histologic appearances of gonadoblastoma may be altered and distorted by three processes, namely, hyalinization, calcification, and overgrowth by dysgerminoma.[187] Hyalinization takes place by coalescence and extension of the hyaline Call–Exner-like bodies within the nests and of the basement membranelike band of similar material present around the nest. The hyaline material replaces tumor cells and the whole nest may be affected and replaced. Calcification is a common feature (Figures 26.51 and 26.53) and is seen in 81% of cases[187]; it usually begins in the Call–Exner-like bodies with formation of small calcific spherules that are frequently laminated, resembling psammoma bodies (Figure 26.53). The process continues with enlargement and fusion of the calcified bodies and calcification of the hyalinized material, resulting in formation of a calcified mass embracing the whole nest. The process may extend to the stroma, which may also undergo hyalinization and calcification. In such cases, tumor cells become very scarce or absent and the presence of smooth, rounded, calcified masses may be the only evidence that gonadoblastoma has been present (Figure 26.9). Although this finding is not considered to be diagnostic of gonadoblastoma, it has been called a "burnt out" gonadoblastoma,[187] is a strong argument in favor of the diagnosis, and indicates that a careful search for more viable areas of the tumor should be made.

Gonadoblastoma is frequently overgrown by dysgerminoma (Figure 26.54). This is seen in 50% of cases.[187] The overgrowth by dysgerminoma may vary from the presence of a small collection of germ cells in the stroma outside the gonadoblastoma nests to massive overgrowth of the

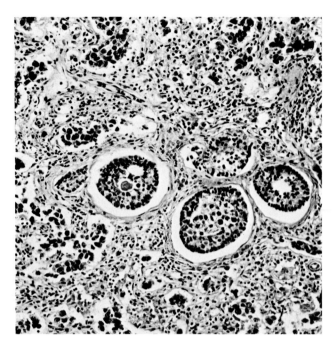

**26.54** Gonadoblastoma nests surrounded by dysgerminoma. Hematoxylin–eosin, ×140.

[Reprinted by permission from A. Talerman. Gonadoblastoma and dysgerminoma in two siblings with dysgenetic gonads. *Obstet. Gynecol.* 38:416, 1971.]

whole tumor, in which occasional nests of gonadoblastoma may be seen. The dysgerminoma in these cases shows the typical appearances of and cannot be distinguished from pure dysgerminoma or seminoma, either microscopically or ultrastructurally.[44,88] Gonadoblastoma may be associated with and overgrown by other more malignant germ cell neoplasms, such as immature teratoma, endodermal sinus tumor, embryonal carcinoma, and choriocarcinoma. This occurs in 10% of cases.[205]

Gonadoblastoma, because of its distinctive histologic pattern and its cellular composition, cannot be easily confused with any of the well-recognized gonadal neoplasms. The gonadal tumors with which confusion may arise are all newly recognized entities and may be related to it. For example, confusion may arise with the mixed germ cell–sex cord stroma tumor,[203,204] which shares with gonadoblastoma the unique distinction of being composed of germ cells and sex cord stroma derivatives but shows more varied appearance, completely different histologic pattern, absence of calcification and hyalinization, a more pronounced proliferative activity involving also the sex cord stroma derivatives, the tendency to occur in normal gonads, and other genetic, endocrine, and somatic differences. The other lesion resembling gonadoblastoma is the ovarian sex cord tumor with annular tubules,[188] which occurs in patients with Peutz–Jeghers syndrome. This lesion is composed of tubules lined by Sertoli and granulosa-like cells; contains similar round, eosinophilic, and hyaline Call–Exner-like bodies; and tends to calcify in the same manner as gonadoblastoma. The basic difference from gonadoblastoma is the absence of germ cells.

### Prognosis

The prognosis of patients with pure gonadoblastoma is excellent, provided the tumor and the contralateral gonad, which may be harboring a macroscopically undetectable gonadoblastoma, are excised. When gonadoblastoma is associated with or overgrown by dysgerminoma, the prognosis is still excellent. Metastases tend to occur later and more infrequently than in dysgerminoma arising *de novo*. All patients with gonadoblastoma and dysgerminoma with known followup, including the occasional cases with metastases,[1,179] are alive and well following treatment, except for one patient who died with disseminated dysgerminoma.[224] The picture is totally different when gonadoblastoma is associated with more malignant germ cell neoplasms, such as embryonal carcinoma, endodermal sinus tumor, choriocarcinoma, and immature teratoma, and none of these patients survived longer than 18 months.[205]

### Therapy

As gonadoblastoma occurs almost entirely in patients with dysgenetic gonads, which are not capable of normal function and therefore are expendable, and as gonadoblastoma may act as a source from which malignant germ cell neoplasms may originate, there is general agreement that excision of the gonads is the treatment of choice.[178,187,205,224] This applies not only to the gonad that appears to be abnormal but also to the contralateral gonad, however normal or small it may be. If one of the gonads is not excised the risk of a malignant neoplasm developing is considerable, although the time interval may vary.[177] There is no complete agreement whether the uterus should be excised together with the gonads. It has been considered that for psychologic reasons it should be left *in situ* if possible so that periodic bleeding simulating menstruation can take place on estrogen–progesterone substitution therapy. However, as estrogen administration is associated with a risk of development of endometrial carcinoma,[42] excision of the uterus together with the gonads has been advocated.[178]

### Endocrine aspects

The association of gonadoblastoma with endocrine abnormalities has been noted when the original two cases were described.[183] In view of the fact that gonadoblastoma occurs almost entirely in patients with gonadal dysgenesis, the defective gonadal development present in these patients should not be confused with the presence of endocrine effects, which are associated with the tumor and are not a result of the abnormal gonadal development. Although the virilization produced by the tumor may regress following the excision of the tumor, there is no further gonadal development and the gonadal abnormalities remain.

Although originally the exact source of the steroid hormone production was not known, the interstitial cells resembling Leydig or lutein cells were considered to be the most likely source of the androgens.[183] Further observations have shown that the presence of Leydig or lutein-like cells is not always associated with the presence of virilization, although they are more frequently encountered in tumors from virilized phenotypic female patients than in those from nonvirilized females. The possibility that the tumor may secrete estrogens, as evidenced by complaints of hot flashes and other menopausal symptoms following the excision of the tumor, has also been noted.[187] Originally the evidence of hormone secretion was mainly clinical, usually evidenced by virilization occurring after puberty and manifesting itself as masculine body contour, hirsutism, and clitoromegaly. The biochemical tests were not performed initially in many cases. In the cases where they were performed, the urinary 17-ketosteroids and the 17-ketogenic steroids were usually normal. Slight elevation of the urinary 17-ketosteroid excretion was noted in some cases.[40,116] The gonadotropins when estimated, were usually elevated and this was considered an important diagnostic criterion,[222] but as this finding, although frequent, is not invariable, it is not necessary for the diagnosis. In recent years it has been shown that gonadoblastoma is capable of producing testosterone from progesterone *in vitro*.[14,16,78,114,170] Production of estrogens from progesterone by gonadoblastoma has also been observed.[78,114] Evidence of testosterone secretion *in vivo* in patients with gonadal dysgenesis has been presented.[99,237] Androgen and estrogen formation from progesterone *in vitro* has been demonstrated in a streak gonad that did not contain any Leydig and lutein cells microscopically but from the description may have contained a small "burnt out" gonadoblastoma.[114] Although *in vitro* testosterone formation has been ascribed to the Leydig or lutein-like cells present in the gonadoblastoma,[14,170] the demonstration of steroid production by a streak gonad that did not contain Leydig or lutein cells indicates that the stromal tissue also has the capability of steroid synthesis.[114]

In spite of all these advances in the study and understanding of the hormonal aspects of gonadoblastoma and dysgenetic gonads, considerable problems remain, the most important being why some patients become virilized and others do not. Although there is a relationship between the virilization of patients with gonadoblastoma and the presence of Leydig or lutein-like cells, this relationship is not constant. It may be that the reason is quantitative and that the amount of the steroid secretion may be inadequate to produce virilization because of a small cell mass. Another possible reason is that the steroid metabolic pathways may be different and that gonadoblastoma may produce different steroid hormones or different quantities of various steroid hormones. Some of these hormones may be metabolically nonfunctioning and therefore unassociated with endocrine side effects, whereas the metabolically active steroids may be associated with evidence and visible signs of endocrine activity.[114]

### Genetic aspects

Gonadoblastoma occurs almost entirely in patients with pure or mixed gonadal dysgenesis or in male pseudohermaphrodites. Occasional patients are of short stature and may have other stigmata of Turner's syndrome.[177] The majority of patients are chromatin negative. This has been observed in 89% of cases.[187] Nearly all the patients with gonadoblastoma whose karyotype was recorded (96%) were found to have a Y chromosome. Of the 68 recorded karyotypes only three did not contain a Y chromosome.[177] Two patients had 46XX karyotype[20,173] and one of these was fertile[20]; one patient had a 45X/46XX mosaicism.[149] The most frequently encountered karyotype was 46XY, which was seen in half the cases, and this was followed by 45X/46XY mosaicism, which was seen in a quarter of the cases. The remainder showed many different forms of mosaicism.[177] Six patients had morphologic abnormalities of the Y chromosome. In 25 patients with gonadal dysgenesis and dysgerminoma, 96% had a Y chromosome. The karyotype was 46XY in 60% followed by 45X/46XY in 24%. The remainder showed various forms of mosaicism.[177] One patient had 45X monosomy and Turner's syndrome. All other patients with features of Turner's syndrome had various forms of mosaicism containing a Y chromosome. The similarity between the distribution of the karyotypes in the gonadoblastoma group and patients

with dysgerminoma and gonadal dysgenesis is striking, and 62% of the former group and 45% of the latter had clitoral hypertrophy.[177]

### Familial aspects

Family history of gonadal dysgenesis has been noted in at least nine reports of patients with gonadoblastoma.[202] Evidence of gonadal dysgenesis affecting three generations of a family of a patient with gonadoblastoma was obtained in two instances.[4,16] Gonadoblastoma has been reported in one pair of twins[64] and in three pairs of siblings.[4,26,202] All these patients had 46XY karyotype. These findings indicate that there is a strong family incidence of gonadal dysgenesis and gonadoblastoma. It has been postulated that the mode of inheritance is either an X-linked recessive gene or an autosomal sex-linked mutant gene.[16,177,178,197]

## Mixed Germ Cell–Sex Cord Stroma Tumor

### Synonyms

Epithelioma Pflügerien,[127] Pflügerome,[32] mixed germ cell tumor,[90] gonocytoma II.[222,223]

### Terminology

The descriptive term "mixed germ cell–sex cord stroma tumor" was originally intended to embrace all the tumors composed of these cell types, including the gonadoblastoma. In view of the fact that the latter term is now so well established, it is considered that "mixed germ cell–sex cord stroma tumor" should be reserved for tumors composed of these cell types, which exhibit distinctive histologic appearances differing from those of a gonadoblastoma. Although "mixed germ cell–sex cord stroma tumor" may be somewhat cumbersome, it has been chosen because it is purely descriptive, differentiating this entity from other gonadal neoplasms.[203,204] This term is considered to be preferable to the term Pflügerome[32] or epithelioma Pflügerien[127] because they imply a possible origin from Pflüger's tubes (germ cell clusters in a granulosal envelope that are formed during gonadal embryogenesis and may persist into infancy). As there is no good evidence for this mode of origin and as there is some doubt as to the formation of Pflüger's tubes during human embryogenesis the term Pflügerome is not considered to be very satisfactory. The term "mixed germ cell tumor"[90] is considered to be unsatisfactory because it implies a tumor composed of a mixture of different types of neoplastic germ cell elements and this term is used in this context in the classification of ovarian tumors proposed by the WHO ovarian tumor panel.[190]

### Incidence

These neoplasms are rare and only a few adequately documented cases have been recorded, although it is likely that some cases may not have been recognized and have been classified with tumors of germ cell origin or with sex cord stroma tumors. This is supported by the fact that since this neoplasm has been recognized as a specific entity, a few well-documented and so far unreported cases have been encountered. Tumors of this type have been observed more frequently in normal phenotypic female patients but have also been encountered in normal adult males. All the known cases in females, except one, were encountered in children in the first decade. Two cases occurred in infants under 1 year old.[51,204] In one less typical case, the tumor occurred in a girl of 16 years who was postpubertal.[90] Therefore the age incidence of patients with this neoplasm differs from that of patients with gonadoblastoma.

### Clinical aspects

In contrast to patients with gonadoblastoma, the patients with this neoplasm are normal phenotypic female children, and the main presenting symptom has been the presence of an abdominal tumor, sometimes complicated by torsion and presenting with symptoms of acute abdominal emergency. Only one patient was postmenarchal and the mestrual periods, which had started at the age of 13 years, were associated with menorrhagia.[90] One 8-year-old patient exhibited signs of precocious puberty for 3 years prior to the discovery of a large ovarian tumor. The other patients did not have endocrine abnormalities. The somatosexual development of all the patients has been normal, and there was no evidence of any abnormalities affecting the gonads and the external genitalia.

### Macroscopic appearances

The tumors encountered have been relatively large, varying in size from 7.5 to 18 cm in diameter and weighing from 100 to 1,050 g. In the only known case where the tumor was associated with other neoplastic germ cell elements it measured 30 cm in diameter.[90] The tumor was found to be unilateral in all cases except one,[90] and the contralateral gonad has always been described as a normal ovary. In some cases where biopsy was performed this was

confirmed on microscopic examination. In the only case where the contralateral ovary was affected[90] the tumor was associated with dysgerminoma, embryonal carcinoma, and endodermal sinus tumor. It was stated that the tumor may have been either primary or metastatic.[90] As mixed germ cell–sex cord stroma tumor has never been observed in extragonadal locations and in metastases, it is considered that in this case[90] the ovarian involvement was probably primary and not metastatic.

The tumor is usually round or oval, firm in consistency, and surrounded by a smooth, slightly glistening gray or gray-yellow capsule. In all cases except one, the tumor was solid. In one case it was partly solid and partly cystic, containing a number of cystic spaces that varied in size. The cut surface of the tumor is uniformly gray to gray-pink or yellow to pale brown. Calcified areas and foci of necrosis have not been observed on gross examination. The fallopian tubes and the uterus have always been found to be normal. There have been no abnormalities affecting the external genitalia.

### Microscopic appearances

The tumor is composed of germ cells and sex cord stroma derivatives, intimately admixed with each other. The tumor cells form two different histologic patterns, which in places may be seen to intermingle with each other. One is composed of long, narrow, ramifying cords or trabeculae (Figure 26.55), which in places tend to expand forming wider columns and larger round or oval cellular aggregates surrounded by connective tissue stroma (Figure 26.56). The other consists of tubular structures devoid of a lumen and surrounded by a fine connective tissue network (Figures 26.57 and 26.58). In some places the tubular pattern is less obvious and the tumor forms small clusters or larger round or oval cellular masses surrounded by connective tissue stroma. The latter varies in amount and appearance and tends to be more abundant in tumors showing mainly the cordlike or trabecular pattern (Figure 26.55), whereas the tubular variety tends to be more cellular and contains less connective tissue (Figures 26.57 and 26.58). The stroma may vary from loose and edematous (Figure 26.55) to dense fibrous and hyalinized (Figure 26.56). The former is seen more often where the cordlike pattern is most prominent, whereas the latter surrounds the larger cellular aggregates. In one case only a few very small collections of Leydig or lutein-like cells were observed,[203] but in all the remaining cases these cells were not identified.

The two cellular elements present in the tumor, the

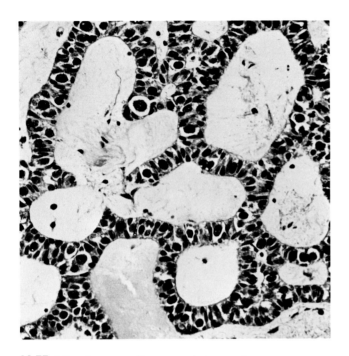

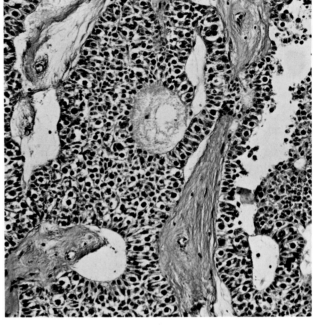

**26.55** Mixed germ cell–sex cord stroma tumor composed of long ramifying cords. Note the large germ cells and smaller sex cord stroma derivatives, and the loose connective tissue stroma. Hematoxylin–eosin, ×300.

**26.56** Mixed germ cell–sex cord stroma tumor composed of large cellular aggregates and more slender cords. Note the hyaline connective tissue stroma. Hematoxylin–eosin, ×150.

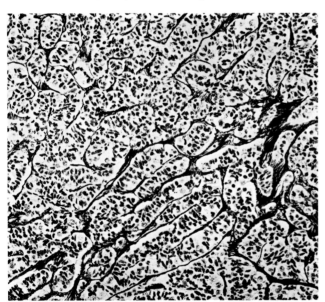

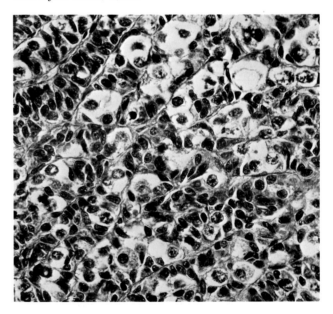

**26.57** Mixed germ cell–sex cord stroma tumor composed of solid tubules surrounded by fine connective tissue septa. Gomori's reticulin, ×140.

[Reprinted by permission from A. Talerman. A mixed germ cell–sex cord stroma tumor in a normal female infant. *Obstet. Gynecol.* 40:473, 1972.]

**26.58** Mixed germ cell–sex cord stroma tumor showing the tubular pattern and cellular composition. Hematoxylin–eosin, ×385.

[Reprinted by permission from A. Talerman. A mixed germ cell–sex cord stroma tumor in a normal female infant. *Obstet. Gynecol.* 40:473, 1972.]

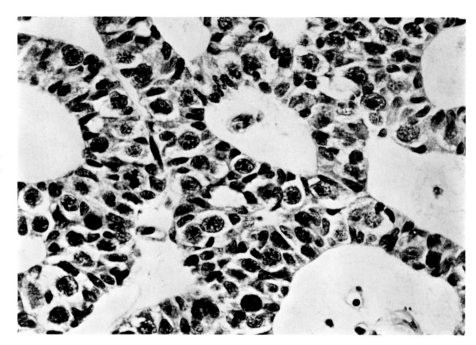

**26.59** Mixed germ cell–sex cord stroma tumor showing the cord-like pattern and cellular composition. Tripolar mitosis is seen to the left of center. Hematoxylin–eosin, ×490.

germ cells and the sex cord stroma derivatives, are intimately admixed together. The sex cord stroma derivatives are arranged peripherally in a single file, forming long rows at the periphery of the cords (Figures 26.55 and 26.59) or lining peripherally the tubular structures (Figure 26.58), as well as surrounding individual or groups of germ cells within the small clusters or larger aggregates. The germ cells resemble those observed in dysgerminoma and gonadoblastoma in all respects, including histochemical reactions. They show brisk mitotic activity (Figure 26.59). The sex cord–stroma derivatives tend to resemble Sertoli cells more than granulosa cells. They show slight mitotic activity. The tumor does not show hyalinization, calcification, or the regressive changes observed in some gonadoblastomas and appears to be actively proliferative. There is some variation in the cellular content in some parts of the tumor; in some areas there is a preponderance of germ cells, whereas in others the sex cord stroma derivatives predominate. However, the intimate admixture of these two cell types is seen everywhere. All the tumors except one showed solid pattern, although occasional small clefts were present. In the remaining tumor there were many cystic spaces of varying size, which were lined by flattened epithelium, devoid of epithelial lining, or lined by the sex cord stroma derivatives and resembled the cystic spaces observed in some cystic sex cord stroma tumors. The hyaline Call-Exner-like bodies observed in

gonadoblastoma and calcific concretions were observed in only one case.[90] This differed from all the remaining cases in other respects, namely, in the presence of bilateral involvement and the presence of other neoplastic germ cell elements. This tumor[90] showed closer histologic resemblance to gonadoblastoma than all the other tumors. Normal ovarian tissue as evidenced by the presence of normal ovarian stroma and at least some primordial follicles has been identified in all cases, including a case where it could not be identified in the original sections available.[203] In some cases Graafian follicles were also present.[204] In other cases tumor deposits were found very close to the surface of the ovary and there was capsular invasion. Apart from the case where the tumor was admixed with other neoplastic germ cell elements and there were metastases and recurrences,[90] mixed germ cell–sex cord stroma tumor has never been associated with metastases, and this tumor pattern has never been observed in metastases or extragonadal sites. The histologic appearances of this tumor have been described in detail some years ago.[203,204] Originally it was considered that the tumor might consist of two specific varieties, each with a different histologic pattern. Subsequently it has become apparent that these two histologic patterns may be present in the same tumor and can be seen to intermingle and merge with each other.

Histologically this tumor is most likely to be confused with gonadoblastoma. It can be differentiated from it by the presence of a different histologic pattern; greater proliferative activity, including that of the sex cord stroma derivatives; absence of calcification and hyalinization within the tumor; and in the majority of cases by the absence of Leydig or lutein-like cells. Macroscopically the tumors are generally larger. The gonad of origin is a normal ovary, and there is no evidence of gonadal dysgenesis or any somatosexual abnormalities. The patients are chromatin positive and have normal female 46XX karyotype. There is no evidence of virilization and if there are signs of abnormal endocrine activity they manifest themselves as feminization. Occasionally, if the germ cells are relatively scanty, the tumor may be included with the sex cord stroma tumors of the ovary, but the presence of germ cells should alert the observer to the true identity of the tumor. If the sex cord stroma derivatives are either few in number, are missed, or are disregarded, the tumor may be included with the germ cell tumors, but the presence of sex cord stroma elements intimately admixed with the germ cells should indicate its true identity.

### Prognosis and therapy

Although the biologic behavior of this neoplasm is not known with certainty, the prognosis of patients with mixed germ cell–sex cord stroma tumor of the ovary seems to be favorable. In all cases except one,[90] which differed from all the others in many respects, there has been no recurrence or metastases following excision of the affected adnexa, and the patients are well and free of disease for periods varying from 1 to 8 years. In all these cases the tumor was confined to the ovary, was fully mobile, and was excised completely. In one case the patient probably had the tumor for 3 years prior to its excision, and there was no evidence of metastases in the abdominal cavity and the biopsy of the contralateral ovary revealed normal appearances. In one case[90] the tumor was very large; was associated with highly malignant neoplastic germ cell elements, involvement of the other ovary, metastases, and recurrences; and the patient died with widespread intraabdominal disease.

As the patients with this tumor are young, normally developed female children and as the prognosis is generally favorable, the treatment of choice is conservative. If there is no involvement of adjacent organs and structures, oophorectomy or excision of the affected adnexa is considered to be adequate. Careful examination of the abdomen and a biopsy of the contralateral ovary are recommended. Following this procedure the patient should be fully investigated and this should include chromosome studies. If the karyotype is 46XX and if no other abnormalities are detected further therapy is not necessary, although a careful long-term followup is essential.

### Endocrine aspects

The majority of patients with mixed germ cell–sex cord stroma tumor did not exhibit any endocrine abnormalities, as observed clinically. In the majority of cases tests of hormonal function were not performed preoperatively. In cases where they were performed postoperatively they were found to be normal. In a recently encountered case, the patient, an 8-year-old girl, exhibited signs of precocious puberty manifesting as mammary development and menstrual bleeding for 3 years prior to the diagnosis of a large ovarian tumor. There was an increased urinary estrogen excretion. Following the excision of the ovarian tumor there was a cessation of the uterine bleeding and the urinary estrogens became normal. There was no evidence of virilization in any of the cases. These findings indicate that female patients with this neoplasm either do not have any associated endocrine abnormalities or if these are present they manifest themselves as feminization.

### Genetic aspects

Five female patients with this neoplasm who have had genotype and karyotype determinations have been found chromatin positive and have the normal female chromosome complement of 46XX; some other patients who did not have chromosome studies were chromatin positive.[90] Therefore, there is no evidence that patients with this tumor have chromosomal abnormalities or gonadal dysgenesis.

# REFERENCES

1. Abell, M. R., Johnson, V. J., and Holtz, F. Ovarian neoplasms in childhood and adolescence. Part 1. Tumors of germ cell origin. Am. J. Obstet. Gynecol. 92:1059, 1965.

2. Abitol, M. M., Pomerance, W., and Mackles, A. Spontaneous intraperitoneal rupture of benign cystic teratomas. Review of literature and report of two cases. Obstet. Gynecol. 13:198, 1959.

3. Albrechtsen, R., Klee, J. G., and Moller, J. E. Primary intracranial germ cell tumours, including five cases of endodermal sinus tumour. Acta Pathol. Microbiol. Scand. 80A Suppl., 233:32, 1972.

4. Allard, S., Cadotte, M., and Boivin, Y. Dysgenesie gonadique pure familiale et gonadoblastome. L'Union Medicale du Canada 101:448, 1972.

5. Andersen, M. C., and Mc.Dicken, I. W. Melanotic cyst of the ovary. *J. Obstet. Gynaecol. Br. Commw.* 78:1047, 1971.

6. Ansfield, F. J., Korbitz, B. C., Davis, H. L., and Ramirez, G. Triple drug therapy in testicular tumors. *Cancer* 24:442, 1969.

7. Arhelger, R. B., and Kelly, B. Strumal carcinoid. Report of a case with electron microscopical observations. *Arch. Pathol.* 97:323, 1974.

8. Asadourian, L. A., and Taylor, H. B. Dysgerminoma. An analysis of 105 cases. *Obstet. Gynecol.* 33:370, 1969.

9. Azoury, R. S., Jubayli, N. W., and Barakat, B. Y. Dermoid cyst of the ovary containing fetus-like structure. *Obstet. Gynecol.* 42:887, 1973.

10. Azzopardi, J. G., and Hou, L. T. Intestinal metaplasia with argentaffin cells in cervical adenocarcinoma. *J. Pathol. Bacteriol.* 90:686, 1965.

11. Bagg, H. J. Experimental production of teratoma testis in a fowl. *Am. J. Cancer* 26:69, 1936.

12. Ballas, M. Yolk sac carcinoma of the ovary with alpha-fetoprotein in serum and ascitic fluid demonstrated by immuno-osmophoresis. *Am. J. Clin. Pathol.* 57:511, 1972.

13. Ballas, M. The significance of alpha-fetoprotein in the serum of patients with malignant teratomas and related gonadal neoplasms. *Am. J. Clin. Lab. Sci.* 4:267, 1974.

14. Bardin, C. W., Rosen, S., Le Maire, W. J., Tjio, J. H., Gallup, J., Marshall, J., and Savard, K. *In vivo* and *in vitro* studies of androgen metabolism in a patient with pure gonadal dysgenesis and Leydig cell hyperplasia. *J. Clin. Endocrinol. Metab.* 29:1429, 1968.

15. Barry, K. G., and Crosby, W. H. Autoimmune hemolytic anemia arrested by removal of ovarian teratoma: Review of the literature and report of a case. *Ann. Int. Med.* 47:1002, 1957.

16. Bartlett, D. J., Grant, J. K., Pugh, M. A., and Aherne, W. A familial feminizing syndrome. A family showing intersex characteristics with XY chromosomes in three female members. *J. Obstet. Gynaecol. Brit. Commw.* 75:199, 1968.

17. Beck, J. S., Fulmer, H. F., and Lee, S. T. Solid malignant ovarian teratoma with "embryoid bodies" and trophoblastic differentiation. *J. Pathol.* 99:67, 1969.

18. Beilby, J. O. W., and Todd, P. J. Yolk sac tumour of the ovary. *J. Obstet. Gynaecol. Brit. Commw.* 81:90, 1974.

19. Berg, J. W., and Baylor, S. M. The epidemiologic pathology of ovarian cancer. *Hum. Pathol.* 4:537, 1973.

20. Bergher de Bacalao, E., and Dominguez, I. Unilateral gonadoblastoma in a pregnant woman. *Am. J. Obstet. Gynecol.* 105:1279, 1969.

21. Bergstrand, C. G., and Czar, B. Demonstration of a new protein fraction in serum from human fetus. *Scand. J. Lab. Invest.* 8:174, 1956.

22. Bernstein, D., Naor, S., Rikover, M., and Manahem, H. Hemolytic anemia related to ovarian tumor. *Obstet. Gynecol.* 43:276, 1974.

23. Bestle, J. Extragonadal endodermal sinus tumours originating in the region of the pineal gland. *Acta Pathol. Microbiol. Scand.* 74:214, 1968.

24. Bettinger, H. F., and Jacobs, H. Mesonephroma ovarii. *Med. J. Aust.* 1:100, 1948.

25. Blackwell, W. J., Dockerty, M. B., Masson, J. C., and Mussey, R. D. Dermoid cysts of the ovary; clinical and pathological significance. *Am. J. Obstet. Gynecol.* 51:151, 1946.

26. Boczkowski, K., Teter, J., and Sternadel, Z. Sibship occurrence of XY gonadal dysgenesis with dysgerminoma. *Am. J. Obstet. Gynecol.* 113:952, 1972.

27. Borushek, S., Berger, I., Echt, C., and Gold, J. J. Functioning malignant germ cell tumor of the ovary in a 4½ year old girl. *Cancer* 18:1485, 1965.

28. Braunstein, H., Stephens, C. L., and Gibson, R. L. Secretory granules in medullary carcinoma of the thyroid. Electronmicroscopic demonstration. *Arch. Pathol.* 85:306, 1968.

29. Breen, J. L., and Neubecker, R. D. Malignant teratoma of the ovary. An analysis of 17 cases. *Obstet. Gynecol.* 21:669, 1963.

30. Breen, J. L., and Neubecker, R. D. Ovarian malignancy in children with special reference to the germ cell tumors, *in* Weyer, E. H., ed.: *Pediatric and Adolescent Gynecology.* Ann. N.Y. Acad. Sci. 142:658, 1967.

31. Brody, S. Clinical aspects of dysgerminoma of the ovary. *Acta Radiol. (Stockholm)* 56:209, 1961.

32. Cabanne, F. Gonadoblastomes et tumeurs de l'ebauche gonadique. *Ann. Anat. Pathol. (Paris)* 16:387, 1971.

33. Carleton, R. L., Friedman, N. B., and Bomze, E. J. Experimental teratomas of testis. *Cancer* 6:464, 1953.

34. Caruso, P. A., Marsh, M. R., Minkowitz, S., and Karten, G. An intense clinicopathologic study of 305 teratomas of the ovary. *Cancer* 27:343, 1971.

35. Chenot, M. Contribution à l'étude des épithéliomas primitifs de l'ovaire. Thesis, Paris, 1911.

36. Chevassu, M. Tumeurs du Testicule. Thesis, Steinhall, Paris, 1906.

37. Chretien, P. B., Milam, J. D., Foote, F. W., and Miller, T. R. Embryonal adenocarcinomas (a type of malignant teratoma) of the sacrococcygeal region. Clinical and pathologic aspects of 21 cases. *Cancer* 26:522, 1970.

38. Climie, A. R., and Heath, L. P. Malignant degeneration of benign cystic teratoma of the ovary. Review of the literature and report of a chondrosarcoma and a carcinoid tumor. *Cancer* 22:824, 1968.

39. Collins, D. H., and Symington, T. Sertoli cell tumour, *in* Collins, D. H., and Pugh, R. C. B., eds.: *The Pathology of Testicular Tumours.* Edinburgh and London, Livingstone Ltd., 1965, pp. 52–61.

40. Cooperman, L. R., Hamlin, J., and Elmer, N. Gonadoblastoma: A rare ovarian tumor with characteristic roentgen appearance. *Radiology* 90:322, 1968.

41. Corfman, P. A., and Richart, R. M. Chromosome number and morphology of benign cystic teratomas. *New Engl. J. Med.* 271:1241, 1964.

42. Cutler, B. S., Forbes, A. P., Ingersoll, F. M., and Scully, R. E. Endometrial carcinoma after stilbestrol therapy in gonadal dysgenesis. *New Engl. J. Med.* 287:628, 1972.

43. Dalgaard, J. B., and Wetteland, P. Struma ovarii. A follow-up study of 20 cases. *Acta Chir. Scand.* 112:1, 1956.

44. Damjanov, I., Drobnjak, P., and Grizelj, V. Ultrastructure of gonadoblastoma. *Arch. Pathol.* 99:25, 1975.

45. Dandia, S. D. Rectovesical fistula following an ovarian dermoid with recurrent vesical calculus. A case report. *J. Urol.* 97:85, 1967.

46. Davidsohn, I., Kovarik, S., and Stejskal, R. Immunological aspects. Influence of prognosis and treatment, *in* Gentil, F., and Junqueira, A. C., eds.: *Ovarian Cancer.* U.I.C.C. Monograph Se-

ries, Vol. 11. Berlin, Heidelberg, New York, Springer-Verlag, 1968, pp. 105–121.

47. Dawson, M. A., Wilimer, T., and Yarbro, J. W. Hemolytic anemia associated with an ovarian tumor. *Am. J. Med. 50:552,* 1971.

48. De Haan, Q. C. Non-gestational choriocarcinoma of the ovary. *Obstet. Gynecol. 26:708,* 1965.

49. De Lima, F. A. O. Disgerminoma do Ovario, contribucao para o seo estudo anatomo-clinico. Thesis, Sao Paulo, Brazil, 1966.

50. Dikman, S. H., and Toker, C. Strumal carcinoid of the ovary with musculinization. *Cancer 27:925,* 1971.

51. Diligent, E. Gonadoblastomes et dysgenesies pseudo-gonadoblastiques. Thesis, Nancy, 1971.

52. Dixon, F. J., and Moore, R. A. Tumors of the Male Sex Organs. *Atlas of Tumor Pathology,* Sect. VIII, Fasc. 31b and 32. Washington, D.C., Armed Forces Institute of Pathology, 1952.

53. Duhig, J. T. An unusual adenocarcinoma of the ovary. *Am. J. Obstet. Gynecol. 77:201,* 1959.

54. Duval, M. Le placenta de rongeurs. *J. Anat. Physiol. (Paris)* 27:515, 1891.

55. Emge, L. A. Functional and growth characteristics of struma ovarii. *Am. J. Obstet. Gynecol. 40:738,* 1940.

56. Engel, T., Greeyley, A. V., and Sweeney, W. J. III. Recurrent dermoid cysts of the ovary. Report of 2 cases. *Obstet. Gynecol.* 26:757, 1965.

57. Erez, S. E., Richart, R. M., and Shettles, L. B. Hashimoto's disease in a benign cystic teratoma of the ovary. *Am. J. Obstet. Gynecol.* 92:273, 1965.

58. Evans, R. W. Developmental stages of embryo-like bodies in teratoma testis. *J. Clin. Pathol. 10:31,* 1957.

59. Evans, R. W. *Histological Appearances of Tumours,* 2nd ed. Edinburgh and London, Livingstone, 1966.

60. Ewing, J. *Neoplastic Diseases,* 4th ed. Philadelphia, W. B. Saunders, 1940, pp. 641, 672.

61. Felmus, L. B., and Pedowitz, P. Clinical malignancy of endocrine tumors of the ovary and dysgerminoma. *Obstet. Gynecol. 29:344,* 1968.

62. Forney, J. P., Di Saia, P. J., and Morrow, C. P. Endodermal sinus tumor. A report of two sustained remissions treated postoperatively with a combination of actinomycin D, 5-fluorouracil and cyclophosphamide. *Obstet. Gynecol. 45:186,* 1975.

63. Fox, H., Kazzaz, B., and Langley, F. A. Argyrophil and argentaffin cells in the female genital tract and in ovarian mucinous cysts. *J. Pathol. Bacteriol. 88:479,* 1964.

64. Frazier, S. D., Bashore, R. A., and Mosier, H. D. Gonadoblastoma associated with pure gonadal dysgenesis in monozygous twins. *J. Pediatr. 64:740,* 1964.

65. Friedman, N. B. The comparative morphogenesis of extragenital and gonadal teratoid tumors. *Cancer 4:265,* 1951.

66. Friedman, N. B., and Moore, R. A. Tumors of the testis. A report of 922 cases. *Mil. Surgeon 99:573,* 1946.

67. Galager, H. S., and Lewis, R. P. Sequential gonadoblastoma and choriocarcinoma. *Obstet. Gynecol. 41:123,* 1973.

68. Galton, M., and Benirschke, K. 46 chromosomes in an ovarian teratoma. *Lancet 2:761,* 1959.

69. Gans, B., Bahary, C., and Levie, B. Ovarian regeneration and pregnancy following massive radiotherapy for dysgerminoma. Report of a case. *Obstet. Gynecol. 22:596,* 1963.

70. Gillman, J. The development of the gonads in man with

consideration of the role of fetal endocrines and the histogenesis of ovarian tumors. *Contrib. Embryol. 32:83,* 1948.

71. Gitlin, D., and Boesman, M. Sites of serum alpha-fetoprotein synthesis in the human and in the rat. *J. Clin. Invest.* 46:1010, 1967.

72. Gitlin, D., and Pericelli, A. Synthesis of serum albumin, pre-albumin, alpha-fetoprotein, alpha-1-antitrypsin, and transferrin by the human yolk sac. *Nature 228:995,* 1970.

73. Gitlin, D., Pericelli, A., and Gitlin, G. Synthesis of alpha-fetoprotein by liver, yolk sac and gastro-intestinal tract of the human conceptus. *Cancer Res. 32:979,* 1972.

74. Goldstein, D. P., and Piro, J. A. Combination chemotherapy in the treatment of germ cell tumors containing choriocarcinoma. *Surg. Gynecol. Obstet. 134:61,* 1972.

75. Gondos, B., Bhiraleus, P., and Hobel, C. J. Ultrastructural observations on germ cells in human fetal ovaries. *Am. J. Obstet. Gynecol. 110:644,* 1971.

76. Gonzalez-Angulo, A., Kaufman, R., Braungardt, C. D., Chapman, F. C., and Hinshaw, A. J. Adenocarcinoma of thyroid arising in struma ovarii (malignant struma ovarii). Report of two cases and review of the literature. *Obstet. Gynecol. 21:567,* 1963.

77. Gonzalez-Licea, A., Hartman, W. H., and Yardley, J. H. Medullary carcinoma of the thyroid. Ultrastructural evidence of its origin from the parafollicular cell and its possible relation to carcinoid tumors. *Am. J. Clin. Pathol. 49:512,* 1968.

78. Griffiths, K., Grant, J. K., Browning, N. C. K., Whyte, W. G., and Sharp, J. L. Steroid synthesis *in vitro* by tumor tissue from dysgenetic gonad. *J. Endocrinol. 34:155,* 1966.

79. Grosfeld, J. L., Stepita, D. S., Nance, W. E., and Palmer, C. G. Fetus-in-Fetu. An unusual cause for an abdominal mass in infancy. *Ann. Surg. 180:80,* 1974.

80. Gusberg, S. B., and Danforth, D. N. Clinical significance of struma ovarii. *Am. J. Obstet. Gynecol. 48:537,* 1944.

81. Hain, A. M. An unusual case of precocious puberty associated with ovarian dysgerminoma. *J. Clin. Endocrinol. 9:1349,* 1949.

82. Hameed, K., and Burslem, M. R. G. A melanotic ovarian neoplasm resembling the "retinal anlage" tumor. *Cancer 25:564,* 1970.

83. Hertig, A. T., and Adams, C. E. Studies on the human oocyte and its follicle. 1. Ultrastructural and histochemical observations on primordial follicle stage. *J. Cell. Biol. 34:647,* 1967.

84. Hertig, A. T., and Gore, H. Tumors of the female sex organs. Part 3. Tumors of the ovary and Fallopian tube. *Atlas of Tumor Pathology,* Section 9, Fasc. 33. Washington D.C., Armed Forces Institute of Pathology, 1961.

85. Higuchi, K., and Kato, T. Dysgerminoma of the ovary. *J. Jap. Obstet. Gynecol. Soc. 5:206,* 1958.

86. Hingorani, V., Narula, R. K., and Bhalla, S. *Salmonella typhi* infection in an ovarian dermoid. Report of a case. *Obstet. Gynecol. 22:118,* 1963.

87. Hou, L. T., and Azzopardi, J. G. Muco-epidermoid metaplasia and argentaffin cells in nephroblastoma. *J. Pathol. Bacteriol. 93:477,* 1967.

88. Hou-Jensen, K., and Kempson, R. L. The ultrastructure of gonadoblastoma and dysgerminoma. *Hum. Pathol. 5:79,* 1974.

89. Hughesdon, P. E. Two cases of struma ovarii showing the histogenesis of thyroid and thymus in ovarian teratoma. *J. Pathol. Bacteriol. 70:35,* 1955.

90. Hughesdon, P. E., and Kumarasamy, T. Mixed germ cell

tumors (gonadoblastomas) in normal and dysgenetic gonads. *Virchow's Arch. Pathol. Anat.* 349:258, 1970.

91. Huntington, R. W. Jr., and Bullock, W. K. Yolk sac tumors of the ovary. *Cancer* 25:1357, 1970.

92. Huntington, R. W. Jr., and Bullock, W. K. Yolk sac tumors of extragonadal origin. *Cancer* 25:1368, 1970.

93. Huntington, R. W. Jr., Morgenstern, N. L., Sargent, J. A., Giem, R. N., Richards, A., and Hanford, K. C. Germinal tumors exhibiting the endodermal sinus pattern of Teilum in young children. *Cancer* 16:34, 1963.

94. Itoh, T., Shirai, T., Naka, A., and Matsumoto, S. Yolk sac tumor and alpha-fetoprotein: Clinicopathological study of four cases. *Gann* 65:215, 1974.

95. Jackson, S. M. Ovarian dysgerminoma. *Brit. J. Radiol.* 40:459, 1967.

96. Janovski, N. A., and Paramanandhan, T. L. *Ovarian tumors. Tumors and tumor-like conditions of the ovaries, Fallopian tubes and ligaments of the uterus.* Stuttgart, Georg Thieme, 1973.

97. Jatoi, A. F. Dysgerminoma of the ovary (A study of 23 cases). *J. Postgrad. Med.* 5:22, 1959.

98. Jedberg, H. Some clinical aspects of dysgerminoma ovarii. *Acta Obstet. Gynecol. Scand.* 28:194, 1949.

99. Judd, H. L., Scully, R. E., Atkins, L., Neer, R. M., and Kliman, B. Pure gonadal dysgenesis with progressive hirsutism. *New Engl. J. Med.* 282:881, 1970.

100. Kawahara, H.: Struma ovarii with ascites and hydrothorax. *Am. J. Obstet. Gynecol.* 85:85, 1963.

101. Kay, S., Silverberg, S. G., and Schatzki, P. F. Ultrastructure of an ovarian dysgerminoma. Report of a case featuring neurosecretory-type granules in stromal cells. *Am. J. Clin. Pathol.* 58:458, 1972.

102. Kazancigil, T. R., Laquer, W., and Ladewig, P. Papillo-endothelioma of the ovary; report of three cases and discussion of Schiller's "mesonephroma ovarii". *Am. J. Cancer* 40:199, 1940.

103. Kelley, R. R., and Scully, R. E. Cancer developing in dermoid cysts of the ovary. A report of 8 cases including a carcinoid and a leiomyosarcoma. *Cancer* 14:989, 1961.

104. Koller, O., and Gjonnes, H. Dysgerminoma of the ovary. *Acta Obstet. Gynecol. Scand.* 43:268, 1964.

105. Larson, N. E., Dockerty, M. B., and Pratt, J. H. Primary mixed choriocarcinoma and dysgerminoma of the ovary. Report of a case. *Proc. Mayo Clinic* 33:341, 1958.

106. Levine, G. D. Primary thymic seminoma—a neoplasm ultrastructurally similar to testicular seminoma and distinct from epithelial thymoma. *Cancer* 31:729, 1973.

107. Liebert, K. I., and Stent, L. Dysgerminoma of the ovary with chorionepithelioma. *J. Obstet. Gynaecol. Brit. Emp.* 77:627, 1960.

108. Linder, D. Gene loss in human teratomas. *Proc. Natl. Acad. Sci. U.S.* 63:699, 1969.

109. Linder, D., and Power, J. Further evidence for postmeiotic origin of teratomas in the human female. *Ann. Hum. Genet.* 34:21, 1970.

110. Linder, D., McCaw, B. K., and Hecht, F. Parthenogenic origin of benign ovarian teratoma. *New Engl. J. Med.* 292:63, 1975.

111. Lingeman, C. H. Etiology of cancer of the human ovary. A review. *J. Natl. Cancer Inst.* 53:1603, 1974.

112. Lord, J. M. Intra-abdominal foetus in fetu. *J. Pathol. Bacteriol.* 72:627, 1956.

113. Lynn, J. A., Varon, H. H., Kingsley, W. B., and Martin, J. H. Ultrastructure and biochemical studies of estrogen-secreting capacity of a "non-functional" ovarian neoplasm (dysgerminoma). *Am. J. Pathol.* 51:639, 1967.

114. Mackay, A. M., Pattigrew, N., Symington, T., and Neville, A. M. Tumors of dysgenetic gonads (gonadoblastoma). Ultrastructural and steroidogenic aspects. *Cancer* 34:1108, 1974.

115. McCullough, C. D., and Hardart, F. Neuroblastomatous transformation in a benign cystic teratoma. *Obstet. Gynecol.* 21:259, 1963.

116. McDonough, P. G., Greenblatt, R. B., Byrd, J. R., and Hastings, E. V. Gonadoblastoma (Gonocytoma III). Report of a case. *Obstet. Gynecol.* 29:54, 1967.

117. McKay, D. G., Hertig, A. T., Adams, E. C., and Danziger, S. Histochemical observations on the germ cells of human embryos. *Anat. Rec.* 117:201, 1953.

118. McKay, D. G., Pinkerton, J. H. M., Hertig, A. T., and Danziger, S. The adult human ovary: A histochemical study. *Obstet. Gynecol.* 18:13, 1961.

119. Malkasian, G. D. Jr., Dockerty, M. B., and Symmonds, R. E. Benign cystic teratomas. *Obstet. Gynecol.* 29:719, 1967.

120. Malkasian, G. D. Jr., and Symmonds, R. E. Treatment of the unilateral encapsulated germinoma. *Am. J. Obstet. Gynecol.* 90:379, 1964.

121. Malkasian, G. D. Jr., Symmonds, R. E., and Dockerty, M. B. Malignant ovarian eratomas. Report of 31 cases. *Obstet. Gynecol.* 25:810, 1965.

122. Malkasian, G. D. Jr., Webb, M. J., and Jorgensen, E. O. Observations on chemotherapy of granulosa cell carcinoma and malignant ovarian teratoma. *Obstet. Gynecol.* 44:885, 1974.

123. Marcial-Rojas, R. A., and de Arellano, R. G. A. Malignant melanoma arising in a dermoid cyst of the ovary. *Cancer* 9:523, 1956.

124. Marin-Padilla, M. Origin, nature and significance of the "embryoids" of human teratomas. *Virchow's Arch. Pathol. Anat.* 340:105, 1965.

125. Marrubini, G. Primary chorionepithelioma of the ovary. Report of two cases. *Acta Obstet. Gynecol. Scand.* 28:251, 1949.

126. Masson, P.: Seminomes ovariennes. *Bull. Soc. Anat. (Paris)* 87:402, 1912.

127. Masson, P. Epitheliomas pflügeriens, *in Diagnostics de laboratoire. Les tumeurs.* Paris, Maloine, 1923.

128. Mathieu, J., and Planchu, M. Le prognostic et le traitement du seminome de l'ovaire. Les oestrogenes out-ils place dans le traitement du seminome en general? *Lyon Chir.* 45:76, 1950.

129. Matz, M. H. Benign cystic teratomas of the ovary. *Obstet. Gynecol. Surv.* 16:591, 1961.

130. Melicow, M. M., and Uson, A. C. Dysgenetic gonadomas and other gonadal neoplasms in intersex. *Cancer* 12:552, 1959.

131. Meyer, R. The pathology of some special ovarian tumors and their relation to sex characteristics. *Am. J. Obstet. Gynecol.* 22:697, 1931.

132. Moertel, C. G., Beahrs, O. H., Woolner, L. B., and Tyce, G. M. "Malignant carcinoid syndrome" associated with non-carcinoid tumors. *New Engl. J. Med.* 273:244, 1965.

133. Mueller, C. W., Topkins, P., and Lapp, W. A. Dysgerminoma of the ovary. An analysis of 427 cases. *Am. J. Obstet. Gynecol.* 60:153, 1950.

134. Neigus, I. Ovarian dysgerminoma with chorio-

nepithelioma. *Am. J. Obstet. Gynecol.* 64:422, 1952.

135. Neubecker, R. D., and Breen, J. L. Embryonal carcinoma of the ovary. *Cancer* 15:546, 1962.

136. Nieminen, I., Von Numers, C., and Widholm, O. Struma ovarii. *Acta Obstet. Gynecol. Scand.* 42:399, 1964.

137. Norris, H. J., and Jensen, R. D. Relative frequency of ovarian neoplasms in children and adolescents. *Cancer* 30:713, 1972.

138. Novak, E. *Gynecologic and Obstetric Pathology,* 3rd ed. Philadelphia, W. B. Saunders, 1952.

139. Novak, E., and Gray, L. A. Dysgerminoma of the ovary. *Am. J. Obstet. Gynecol.* 35:925, 1938.

140. Novak, E., Woodruff, J. D., and Novak, E. R. Probable mesonephric origin of certain female genital tumors. *Am. J. Obstet. Gynecol.* 68:1224, 1954.

141. Novak, E. R. Solid teratoma of the ovary, with report of five cases. *Am. J. Obstet. Gynecol.* 56:300, 1948.

142. Novak, E. R., and Woodruff, J. D. *In* Novak, E. R., ed. *Gynecologic and Obstetric Pathology,* 6th ed. Philadelphia, W. B. Saunders, 1967, p. 367.

143. Nystrom, C. Dysgerminoma of the ovary. *Acta Obstet. Gynecol. Scand.* 35:385, 1956.

144. Oliver, H. M., and Horne, E. O. Primary teratomatous chorionepithelioma of the ovary. Report of a case. *New Engl. J. Med.* 239:14, 1948.

145. Overbeck, L., and Philipp, E. Die Ultrastruktur des Disgerminoms im Ovar. Zugleich ein Beitrag zur Histogenese des Tumors. *Z. Geburtschilfe Gynaekol.* 170:125, 1969.

146. Pantoja, E., Noy, M. A., Axtmayer, R. W., Colon, F. E., and Pelegrina, I. Ovarian dermoids and their complications. Comprehensive historical review. *Obstet. Gynecol. Surv.* 30:1, 1975.

147. Pantoja, E., Rodriguez-Ibanez, I., Axtmayer, R. W., Noy, M. A., and Pelegrina, I. Complications of dermoid tumors of the ovary. *Obstet. Gynecol.* 45:89, 1975.

148. Park, I. J., Pyeatte, J. C., Jones, H. W., and Woodruff, J. D. Gonadoblastoma in a true hermaphrodite with 46XY genotype. *Obstet. Gynecol.* 40:466, 1972.

149. Patel, S. K., and Prentice, S. A. Gonadoblastoma—distinctive ovarian tumor. *Arch. Pathol.* 94:165, 1972.

150. Pedowitz, P., Felmus, L. B., and Grayzel, D. M. Dysgerminoma of the ovary. Prognosis and treatment. *Am. J. Obstet. Gynecol.* 70:1284, 1955.

151. Peterson, W. F. Solid histologically benign teratomas of the ovary. A report of four cases and review of the literature. *Am. J. Obstet. Gynecol.* 72:1094, 1956.

152. Peterson, W. F. Malignant degeneration of benign cystic teratomas of the ovary; a collective review of the literature. *Obstet. Gynecol. Surv.* 12:793, 1957.

153. Peterson, W. F., Prevost, E. C., Edmunds, F. T., Huntley, J. M. Jr., and Morris, F. K. Benign cystic teratomas of the ovary. A clinico-statistical study of 1007 cases with review of the literature. *Am. J. Obstet. Gynecol.* 70:368, 1955.

154. Peyron, A. Faits nouveaux relatifs à l'origine et à l'histogenese des embryomes. *Bull. Ass. Franc. Cancer* 28:658, 1939.

155. Pierce, G. B. Jr. Ultrastructure of human testicular tumors. *Cancer* 19:1963, 1966.

156. Pierce, G. B. Jr., Bullock, W. K., and Huntington, R. W. Jr. Yolk sac tumors of the testis. *Cancer* 25:644, 1970.

157. Pierce, G. B. Jr., and Dixon, F. J. Testicular teratomas.

1. Demonstration of teratogenesis by metamorphosis of multipotential cells. *Cancer* 12:573, 1959.

158. Pierce, G. B. Jr., and Dixon, F. J. Testicular teratomas. 2. Teratocarcinoma as ascitic tumor. *Cancer* 12:584, 1959.

159. Pierce, G. B. Jr., and Midgley, A. R. The origin and function of human syncytiotrophoblastic giant cells. *Am. J. Pathol.* 43:153, 1963.

160. Pierce, G. B. Jr., Midgley, A. R., and Beals, T. F. An ultrastructural study of differentiation and maturation of trophoblast of the monkey. *Lab. Invest.* 13:451, 1962.

161. Pierce, G. B. Jr., Midgley, A. R., Sri Ram, J., and Feldman, J. D. Parietal yolk sac carcinoma. Clue to the histogenesis of Reichert's membrane of the mouse embryo. *Am. J. Pathol.* 41:549, 1964.

162. Pierce, G. B. Jr., and Verney, E. L. An in vitro and in vivo study of differentiation in teratocarcinomas. *Cancer* 14:1017, 1961.

163. Plaut, A. Ovarian struma: A morphologic, pharmacologic, and biologic examination. *Am. J. Obstet. Gynecol.* 25:351, 1933.

164. Qizilbash, A. H., Trebilcock, R. G., Patterson, M. C., and Lamont, K. G. Functioning primary carcinoid tumor of the ovary. A light and electronmicroscopic study with review of the literature. *Am. J. Clin. Pathol.* 62:629, 1974.

165. Ramsey, H. J. Ultrastructure of a pineal tumor. *Cancer* 18:1014, 1965.

166. Rao, N. R., Veliath, G. D., and Srinivasan, M. An unusual case of sacrococcygeal mesonephroma (Schiller). *Cancer* 17:1604, 1964.

167. Rashad, M. H., Fathalla, M. F., and Kerr, M. C. Sex chromatin and chromosome analysis in ovarian teratomas. *Am. J. Obstet. Gynecol.* 96:461, 1966.

168. Robboy, S. J., and Scully, R. E. Ovarian teratoma with glial implants on the peritoneum. An analysis of 12 cases. *Hum. Pathol.* 1:643, 1970.

169. Robboy, S. J., Scully, R. E., and Norris, H. J. Carcinoid metastatic to the ovary. A clinicopathologic analysis of 35 cases. *Cancer* 33:798, 1974.

170. Rose, L. I., Underwood, R. H., Williams, G. H., and Pincus, G. S. Pure gonadal dysgenesis. Studies of *in vitro* androgen metabolism. *Am. J. Med.* 57:957, 1974.

171. Sailer, S.: Ovarian dysgerminoma. *Am. J. Cancer* 38:473, 1940.

172. Sailer, S. Struma ovarii. *Am. J. Clin. Pathol.* 13:271, 1943.

173. Salet, J., de Gennes, L. J., de Grouchy, J., Musset, R., Pelissier, C., Yaneva, H., Sebaoun, M., and Netter, A. A propos d'un cas de gonadoblastome 46XX. *Ann. Endocrinol.* (Paris) 31:927, 1970.

174. Santesson, L. Clinical and pathological survey of ovarian tumours treated at the Radiumhemmet. 1. Dysgerminoma. *Acta Radiol.* (Stockholm) 28:643, 1947.

175. Santesson, L., and Marrubini, G. Clinical and pathological survey of ovarian embryonal carcinomas, including so-called "mesonephromas" (Schiller) or "mesoblastomas" (Teilum) treated at the Radiumhemmet. *Acta Obstet. Gynecol. Scand.* 36:399, 1957.

176. Saunders, A. M., and Hertzman, V. O. Malignant carcinoid teratoma of the ovary. *Can. Med. Ass. J.* 83:602, 1960.

177. Schellhas, H. F. Malignant potential of the dysgenetic gonad. Part 1. *Obstet. Gynecol.* 44:298, 1974.

178. Schellhas, H. F. Malignant potential of the dysgenetic gonad. Part 2. *Obstet. Gynecol.* 44:455, 1974.

179. Schellhas, H. F., Trujillo, J. M., Rutledge, F. N., and Cork, A. Germ cell tumors associated with XY gonadal dysgenesis. *Am. J. Obstet. Gynecol. 109*:1197, 1971.

180. Schiller, W. Mesonephroma ovarii. *Am. J. Cancer 35*:1, 1939.

181. Schiller, W. Histogenesis of ovarian mesonephroma. *Arch. Pathol. 33*:443, 1942.

182. Schmitz, E. F. Malignant endothelioma of perithelioma type in the ovary. *Am. J. Obstet. Gynecol. 9*:247, 1925.

183. Scully, R. E. Gonadoblastoma. A gonadal tumor related to dysgerminoma (seminoma) and capable of sex hormone production. *Cancer 6*:455, 1953.

184. Scully, R. E. Germ cell tumors of the ovary and Fallopian tube. *In* Meigs, J. V., and Sturgis, S. H., eds. *Progress in Gynecology.* New York, Grune and Stratton, 1963, Vol. 4, pp. 335–347.

185. Scully, R. E. Germ cell tumors of the ovary. *In* Sturgis, S. H., and Taymor, M. L., eds. *Progress in Gynecology.* New York, Grune and Stratton, 1970, Vol. 5, pp. 329–348.

186. Scully, R. E. Recent progress in ovarian cancer. *Hum. Pathol. 1*:73, 1970.

187. Scully, R. E. Gonadoblastoma. *Cancer 25*:1340, 1970.

188. Scully, R. E. Sex cord tumor with annular tubules. A distinctive ovarian tumor of the Peutz-Jeghers syndrome. *Cancer 25*:1107, 1970.

189. Seegar, G. E. Ovarian dysgerminomas. *Arch. Surg. 37*:697, 1938.

190. Serov, S. F., Scully, R. E., and Sobin, L. H. *Histological typing of ovarian tumors. International histological classification of tumors,* No. 9. Geneva, World Health Organization, 1973.

191. Sjovall, A. Disgerminome des Ovariums. *Acta Obstet. Gynecol. Scand. 23*:585, 1943.

192. Simard, L. C. Polyembryonic embryoma of the ovary of parthenogenetic origin. *Cancer 10*:215, 1957.

193. Smith, F. G. Pathology and physiology of struma ovarii. *Arch. Surg. 53*:603, 1946.

194. Smith, J. B., and O'Neill, R. T. Alpha-fetoprotein. Occurrence in germinal cell and liver malignancies. *Am. J. Med. 51*:767, 1971.

195. Smith, J. P., Rutledge, F. N., and Sutow, W. W. Malignant gynecologic tumors in children. Current approaches to treatment. *Am. J. Obstet. Gynecol. 116*:261, 1963.

196. Solomon, J., Steinfeld, J. L., and Bateman, J. R. Chemotherapy of germinal tumors. *Cancer 26*:747, 1967.

197. Sternberg, W. H., Barclay, D. L., and Kloepfer, H. W. Familial XY gonadal dysgenesis. *New Engl. J. Med. 278*:695, 1968.

198. Stevens, L. C. Embryology of testicular teratomas in strain 129 mice. *J. Natl. Cancer Inst. 23*:1249, 1959.

199. Stevens, L. C. Embryonic potency of embryoid bodies derived from a transplantable testicular teratoma of the mouse. *Develop. Biol. 2*:285, 1960.

200. Stevens, L. C. The biology of teratomas including evidence indicating their origin from primordial germ cells. *Ann. Biol. 1*:585, 1962.

201. Strauss, A. F., and Gates, H. S. Giant sebaceous gland tumor of the ovary. *Am. J. Clin. Pathol. 41*:78, 1964.

202. Talerman, A. Gonadoblastoma and dysgerminoma in two siblings with dysgenetic gonads. *Obstet. Gynecol. 38*:416, 1971.

203. Talerman, A. A distinctive gonadal neoplasm related to gonadoblastoma. *Cancer 30*:1219, 1972.

204. Talerman, A. A mixed germ cell–sex cord stroma tumor in a normal female infant. *Obstet. Gynecol. 40*:473, 1972.

205. Talerman, A. Gonadoblastoma associated with embryonal carcinoma. *Obstet. Gynecol. 43*:138, 1974.

206. Talerman, A. The incidence of yolk sac tumor (endodermal sinus tumor) elements in germ cell tumors of the testis in adults. *Cancer 36*:211, 1975.

207. Talerman, A., and Delemarre, J. F. M. Gonadoblastoma associated with embryonal carcinoma in an anatomically normal male. *J. Urol. 113*:355, 1975.

208. Talerman, A., and Haije, W. G. Alpha-fetoprotein and germ cell tumors: A possible role of yolk sac tumor in production of alpha-fetoprotein. *Cancer 34*:1722, 1974.

209. Talerman, A., Huyzinga, W. T., and Kuipers, T. Dysgerminoma. Clinicopathologic study of 22 cases. *Obstet. Gynecol. 41*:137, 1973.

210. Taylor, C. W. Mullerian mixed tumor. *Acta Pathol. Microbiol. Scand., 80A Suppl.,* 233:48, 1972.

211. Teilmann, I., Kassis, H., and Pietra, G. Primary germ cell tumour of the anterior mediastinum with features of endodermal sinus tumour (mesoblastoma vitellinum). *Acta Pathol. Microbiol. Scand. 70*:267, 1967.

212. Teilum, G.: Homologous tumours in ovary and testis; contribution to classification of gonadal tumours. *Acta Obstet. Gynecol. Scand. 24*:480, 1944.

213. Teilum, G. Gonocytoma; homologous ovarian and testicular tumours; 1; with discussion of "mesonephroma ovarii" (Schiller: Amer. J. Cancer 1939). *Acta Pathol. Microbiol. Scand. 23*:242, 1946.

214. Teilum, G. "Mesonephroma ovarii" (Schiller) extraembryonic mesoblastoma of germ cell origin in ovary and testis. *Acta Pathol. Microbiol. Scand. 27*:249, 1950.

215. Teilum, G. Classification of ovarian tumours. *Acta Obstet. Gynecol. Scand. 31*:292, 1952.

216. Teilum, G. Endodermal sinus tumors of the ovary and testis. Comparative morphogenesis of the so-called mesonephroma ovarii (Schiller) and extraembryonic (Yolk sac-allantoic) structures of the rat's placenta. *Cancer 12*:1092, 1959.

217. Teilum, G. Classification of endodermal sinus tumour (mesoblastoma vitellinum) and so-called "embryonal carcinoma" of the ovary. *Acta Pathol. Microbiol. Scand. 64*:407, 1965.

218. Teilum, G. Tumours of germinal origin, *in* Gentil, F., and Junqueira, A. C., eds.: *Ovarian Cancer,* U.I.C.C. Monograph Series. Berlin, Heidelberg, New York, Springer-Verlag, 1968, Vol. 11, pp. 58–73.

219. Teilum, G. *Special Tumors of the Ovary and Testis. Comparative histology and identification.* Copenhagen, Munksgaard Co., 1971.

220. Teilum, G., Albrechtsen, R., and Norgaard-Pedersen, B. Immunofluorescent localization of alpha-fetoprotein synthesis in endodermal sinus tumor (yolk sac tumor). *Acta Pathol. Microbiol. Scand. 82A*:586, 1974.

221. Teilum, G., Albrechtsen, R., and Norgaard-Pedersen, B. The histogenetic-embryologic basis for reappearance of alpha-fetoprotein in endodermal sinus tumors and teratomas. *Acta Pathol. Microbiol. Scand. 83A*:80, 1975.

222. Teter, J. A new concept of classification of gonadal tumors arising from germ cell (gonocytoma) and their histogenesis. *Gynaecologia (Basel) 150*:84, 1960.

223. Teter, J. A mixed form of feminizing germ cell tumor (gonocytoma II). *Am. J. Obstet. Gynecol. 84:*722, 1962.

224. Teter, J. Prognosis, malignancy and curability of the germ cell tumor occurring in dysgenetic gonads. *Am. J. Obstet. Gynecol. 108:*894, 1970.

225. Teter, J. and Boczkowski, K. Occurrence of tumors in dysgenetic gonads. *Cancer 20:*1301, 1967.

226. Theiss, E. A., Ashley, D. J. B., and Mostofi, F. K. Nuclear sex of testicular tumors and some related ovarian and extragonadal neoplasms. *Cancer 13:*323, 1959.

227. Thoeny, R. H., Dockerty, M. B., Hunt, A. B., and Childs, D. S. Jr. Study of ovarian dysgerminoma with emphasis on the role of radiation therapy. *Surg. Gynecol. Obstet. 113:*692, 1961.

228. Thurlbeck, W. M., and Scully, R. E. Solid teratoma of the ovary. *Cancer 13:*804, 1960.

229. Toker, C. Ovarian carcinoid. A light and electron microscopic study. *Am. J. Obstet. Gynecol. 103:*1019, 1969.

230. Turner, H. B., Douglas, W. M., and Gladding, T. C. Choriocarcinoma of the ovary. *Obstet. Gynecol. 24:*918, 1964.

231. Uzisima, H. Ovarian dysgerminoma associated with virilization. Report of a case. *Cancer 9:*736, 1956.

232. Vawter, G. F. Carcinoma of the vagina in infancy. *Cancer 18:*1479, 1965.

233. Wheatley, V. R. Further observations on the nature of the dermoid cyst fat. *J. Invest. Dermatol. 29:*445, 1957.

234. Whelton, J. A., and Fallon, R. J. Successful pregnancy after surgery and supervoltage therapy for metastatic dysgerminoma. *New Eng. J. Med. 271:*145, 1964.

235. Wider, J. A., Marshall, J. R., Bardin, C. W., Lipsett, M. B., and Rose, G. T. Sustained remissions after chemotherapy for primary ovarian cancers containing choriocarcinoma. *New Engl. J. Med. 280:*1439, 1969.

236. Wider, J. A., and O'Leary, J. A. Dysgerminoma: a clinical review. *Obstet. Gynecol. 31:*560, 1968.

237. Wieland, R. G., Ekstrom, B., and Vorijs, N. $C_{19}O_2$ Steroid secretion by dysgenetic gonads. *Obstet. Gynecol. 32:*643, 1968.

238. Wilkinson, E. J., Friedrich, E. G., and Hosty, T. A. Alphafetoprotein and endodermal sinus tumor of the ovary. *Am. J. Obstet. Gynecol. 116:*711, 1973.

239. Williams, E. D. Histogenesis of medullary carcinoma of the thyroid. *J. Clin. Pathol. 19:*114, 1966.

240. Williams, E. D., and Sandler, M. Classification of carcinoid by embryologic grouping. *Lancet 1:*238, 1963.

241. Willis, R. A. *The Borderland of Embryology and Pathology.* London, Butterworth, 1958.

242. Willis, R. A. *Pathology of Tumours,* 4th ed. London, Butterworth, 1967.

243. Wisniewski, M., and Deppisch, L. M. Solid teratomas of the ovary. *Cancer 32:*440, 1973.

244. Witschi, E. Migration of the germ cells of human embryos from the yolk sac to the primitive gonadal folds. *Contrib. Embryol. 32:*69, 1948.

245. Woodruff, J. D., and Markley, R. L. Struma ovarii. Demonstration of both pathologic change and physiologic activity; report of four cases. *Obstet. Gynecol. 9:*707, 1957.

246. Woodruff, J. D., Protos, P., and Peterson, W. F. Ovarian teratomas. Relationship of histologic and ontogenic factors to prognosis. *Am. J. Obstet. Gynecol. 102:*702, 1968.

247. Woodruff, J. D., Rauh, J. T., and Markley, R. L. Ovarian struma. *Obstet. Gynecol. 27:*194, 1966.

248. Wurster, K., Hedinger, C., and Meienberg, O. Orchioblastomatous foci in testicular teratoma of adults. *Virchow's Arch. Pathol. Anat. 357:*231, 1972.

M. R. Abell, M.D., Ph.D.

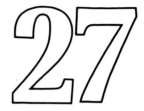

# Ovarian Neoplasms of Childhood and Adolescence

Before I build a wall I'd ask to know
what I was walling in or walling out.

"Mending Walls" by Robert Frost

## Introduction

Ovarian neoplasms occurring in children and adolescents during the first two decades of life comprise a very special group of lesions. They are special not because of any major histologic differences in types of neoplasms as compared with those of adults, but because of the clinical and therapeutic implications. In the treatment of these young patients it is essential that whenever possible ovarian tissue be preserved in order to insure future normal physical development and child-bearing potential. However, it is equally essential that the malignant neoplasms be appropriately eradicated. Too often, in the past, children and young women have been unnecessarily castrated on the basis that an ovarian tumor in this age group, particularly when solid, is malignant and requires radical surgery. It is mandatory that ovarian neoplasms in children and adolescents be accurately classified and their natural history clearly understood.

Although ovarian neoplasms are uncommon during the first two decades of life, they are the most frequently encountered genital neoplasms for that age period.[12] It is difficult to determine from the literature how frequently they do occur as some reports include nonneoplastic cysts in their compilations and the age ranges of the patients often differ. Lindfors,[92] in a study of girls 0 to 14 years of age, found the annual incidence of ovarian tumors in Helsinki to be 2.6 per 100,000. It is estimated that one ovarian neoplasm is encountered for every 3,000 to 5,000 hospital admissions of patients under 20 years of age. Ein et al.[46] reported 75 ovarian tumors in patients up to 15 years of age, including 26 nonneoplastic cysts, during a 44-year period at The Hospital for Sick Children, Toronto. The malignant ovarian lesions comprised between 0.5 and 1% of all malignant neoplasms in children in the hospital during this period. In two large series of ovarian neoplasms in patients less than 20 years of age, 55%[112] and 29%[4] were malignant or potentially malignant.

The proportion of ovarian tumors that occurs during the first two decades of life varies with the type of institution reporting, but it is usually 5 to 10%.[4,112] Approximately one-fifth of these occur before menarche. A small group of tumors, especially malignant germ cell neoplasms, appears during the first year of life but thereafter is very infrequent, until near menarche when a progressive increase in occurrence begins (Figure 27.1). The occurrence in the first year of life suggests a maternal hormonal influence. The increased occurrence, which begins just before menarche and continues thereafter, suggests that hormonal factors activated at that time are important in the pathogenesis of all types of ovarian neoplasms. A study by Li et al.[88] of United States mortality rates for ovarian cancers among girls 0 to 19 years of age from 1950 to 1968 showed no increase in ovarian cancer in contrast to a two- to three-fold increase in adults observed since 1930.[62] Malignant neoplasms had a low frequency during the first decade of life but progressively increased thereafter.

## Clinical Manifestations

The commonest presenting complaint is lower abdominal or pelvic pain, with abdominal enlargement being next in frequency.[45,46,64,66,76,92,145] Acute severe or intermittent pain, especially if associated with nausea and vomiting, suggests torsion of the ovarian pedicle. Acute appendicitis is a common clinical diagnosis and in adolescents with abdominal enlargement, pregnancy is often suspected. Menstrual irregularities after menarche include hypermenorrhea, oligomenorrhea, and dysmenorrhea. Isosexual precosity may be a presenting complaint in the prepubertal child but rarely occurs before 4 years of age.[159] The rare functioning tumor may cause masculinization in the adolescent. General ill feeling, malaise, abdominal pain, nausea, and vomiting are more likely to occur with malignant neoplasms.[45]

The ovarian mass can often be detected by abdominal or rectal examination. It is usually relatively nontender unless there is torsion of the ovarian pedicle or the neoplasm is malignant. Large tumors may cause pressure

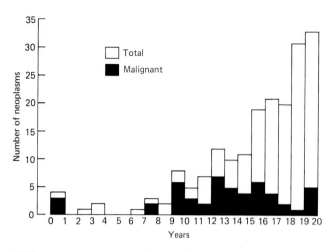

**27.1** Age distribution of ovarian neoplasms in children and adolescents.

symptoms referable to the gastrointestinal or urinary tract. Ascites is occasionally present, both with benign and with malignant tumors. A marked anemia suggests a malignant neoplasm. Leukocytosis may be caused by torsion of the pedicle with infarction or by a malignant neoplasm.

## Paraneoplastic Syndromes

In recent years, considerable attention has been focused on the systemic manifestations of neoplasms, with close to 50 paraneoplastic syndromes having been described.[61,93,137] Expectedly, the great majority of these syndromes occurs in adults and with a variety of histologic types of neoplasms in various primary locations. Many occur with ovarian neoplasms, but extremely few examples have been recognized in children and adolescents. The paraendocrine syndromes are caused by the overproduction of hormones or hormonelike substances by nonendocrine tumors, both benign and malignant. Removal of the neoplasm leads to regression of the syndrome.

Well-recognized paraneoplastic syndromes involving ovarian neoplasms include manifestations of hyperparathyroidism,[51,116] Cushing's syndrome,[93,111] hyperthyroidism,[93] hypoglycemia,[117] Zollinger–Ellison syndrome,[35] aldosteronism,[44] neuropathies and neuromyopathies,[37,42,71] dermatomyositis,[154] migratory thrombophlebitis,[90] erythremia,[61] and hemolytic anemia.[17]

Abnormalities in hormonal blood and urinary levels occur with a number of functioning ovarian neoplasms and with other nonfunctioning tumors, primary and metastatic, because of a functional hyperplasia of the supportive ovarian mesenchyme. Their determinations are of clinical interest and theoretically should be of value in the diagnosis of the different functioning neoplasms, but as yet they are of limited practical value.[159] Roentgenograms are mainly of value in ruling out causes of abdominal enlargement other than ovarian. They may reveal areas of calcification in cystic teratomas or in gonadoblastomas.

## Etiologic Aspects

Very little is known about the etiologic factors in human ovarian neoplasms. It seems obvious, however, that pituitary and/or ovarian hormones play a significant role, particularly in the coelomic epithelial neoplasms and the sex mesenchyme–sex cord tumors. Li et al.,[88] in their assessment of malignant ovarian neoplasms in children and adolescents, found gonadal dysgenesis to be the only congenital defect associated with neoplasia. They found no evidence that prior exposure to ionizing irradiation or chemical agents was of any etiologic significance in the group that they studied.

There are several genetically controlled syndromes, such as the Peutz–Jeghers syndrome[33] and the basal cell nevus syndrome,[16] with which specific types of ovarian neoplasms are associated. A number of examples of familially occurring tumors in the absence of specific genetic syndromes has been reported.[89]

Granulosa–theca cell tumors have been induced in mice subjected to irradiation,[55] in mice by painting the skin with dimethyl benzanthracene,[72] and in hampsters fed methylcholanthrene.[41] Biskind and Biskind[18,19] produced granulosa cell tumors in rats by transplanting ovarian tissue into the spleens of gonadectomized animals. Estrogens produced by the transplants are inactivated by the liver and in response to their absence or low level in the peripheral blood, pituitary gonadotropin output is increased and acts on the transplants, causing hyperplasia and neoplasia. Hormonally dependent papillary neoplasms have been produced in dogs by repeated injections of diethylstilbesterol.[69] Gardner[56] produced ovarian tumors by transplanting ovarian tissue into the testis of mice.

## Classification

The classification of ovarian tumors that best meets the requirements of clinician and pathologist alike is based on our present understanding of the development and normal structure of the ovary.[1,68,135] The primordial germ cells are the direct progeny of the fertilized ovum and can be recognized at about the 12 somite stage in the yolk sac epithelium near its attachment to the hind gut.[48,103,106,126,156] From this location, their migration can be traced to the mesenchymal condensations beneath the posterior coelom, which forms the gonadal folds (ridges). Here they continue to proliferate and acquire a covering of follicular epithelium. By birth, most germ cells have differentiated into oöcytes and primordial follicles, but scattered immature germ cells may be recognized, particularly in premature infants. There is normally no further development of new ova in the postembryonic period.

The coelomic epithelium covering the gonadal primordium thickens at 5 to 6 weeks of fetal life and sends forth cords into the underlying mesenchyme. These persist in the male and form the seminiferous tubules, whereas in the ovary the medullary columns disappear; however, according to Gillman[58] the cortical cords form the follicular epithelium about the germ cells. This concept is in contrast to the theory held by others that the follicular epithelium develops from the ovarian mesenchyme.[126] At birth, the primordial follicles are numerous in the cortex and consist of a central ovum surrounded by flattened epithelial-appearing cells. Later these cells become cuboidal and, still later, stratified. Remnants of the sex cords persist as rete ovarii in the hilum of every ovary and sometimes, particularly in immature infants, remnants can be found in the ovarian cortex.

The sex mesenchyme is relatively inconspicuous in the fetal gonad and is scant at birth and early childhood, increasing progressively in prominence throughout adolescence and the reproductive period. The outer portion assumes a fibrous appearance, the tunica albuginea, and beneath this is the cellular, cytogenic stroma in which the primordial and developing follicles are located. It forms the thecal layers about these structures. Clusters of hilus

**Table 27.1** Relative frequency of ovarian neoplasms in children and adolescents

| Histogenetic category | AFIP series[112] | | Abell–Holtz series[3,4] | |
|---|---|---|---|---|
| | No. | % | No. | % |
| Germ cell | 205 | 58 | 113 | 60 |
| Celomic epithelium | 67 | 19 | 53 | 28 |
| Sex cord–sex mesenchyme | 62 | 18 | 14 | 8 |
| Supportive stroma and miscellaneous | 19 | 5 | 8 | 4 |
| Totals | 353 | 100 | 188 | 100 |

(Leydig) cells are present in the hilum of every ovary. They are inconspicuous in childhood but increase in prominence with age. In addition to the sex mesenchyme, a nonspecific supportive and vascular mesenchyme extends into the primitive gonad from the hilum and forms the mature, supportive, vascular, and neural tissues that the ovary has in common with other glands and organs. Ectopic adrenal cortical tissues, the adrenals of Marchand, are found near the hilum or along the ovarian vessels of 15 to 20% of carefully examined specimens.

# Relative Frequency of Histogenetic Categories

The relative frequency of the four different categories of ovarian tumors in the first two decades of life varies with the type of reporting institution, but in the larger series is fairly similar (Table 27.1). In all such series, the germ cell group of tumors predominates and prior to menarche they comprise the overwhelming majority of tumors.[4] This preponderance in the first and second decades of life is in sharp contrast to an incidence of approximately 15% in adults 20 to 50 years of age. The neoplasms of coelomic epithelium (epithelial–stromal tumors) essentially do not occur prior to menarche but from menarche on they increase progressively in frequency.[1,112] Tumors of sex mesenchyme and sex cord origin are relatively infrequent at all ages but particularly so prior to menarche.

# Germ Cell Neoplasms

The subject of germ cell neoplasms is separately covered in Chapter 26 and in this chapter I endeavor only to describe aspects of germ cell neoplasms as they relate to childhood and adolescence.

Most germ cell tumors of the ovary are benign cystic teratomas, whereas in the testis the vast majority are malignant, particularly after puberty. In our material, 36% of all germ cell tumors of the ovary occurred during the first two decades of life.[1] Approximately one-third of these were malignant or potentially malignant.[4]

## Germinoma (Dysgerminoma, Gonocytoma I, Ovarian Seminoma)

Mueller et al.,[107] in their study of germinoma, found that 45% of the neoplasm occurred in the first two decades of life, 7% in the first, and 38% in the second. Forty-four percent of germinomas in Asadourian and Taylor's series

occurred in patients less than 20 years of age.[9] In our material 6% of all ovarian tumors and 27% of all malignant germ cell neoplasms in children and adolescents were pure germinomas.

### Clinical features

The majority of germinomas occur after menarche; a few appear just before that time. Mueller et al.[107] found only six reported cases 5 years of age or younger. In our material, the age range for children and adolescents was 8 to 19 years.

The presenting symptom is usually abdominal swelling, with some abdominal discomfort or soreness, or a palpable abdominal mass. Menorrhagia is a significant complaint in some of the adolescents. In patients in whom menstrual periods have been established, amenorrhea may occur. This, together with abdominal swelling, often leads to the clinical impression of pregnancy. The presence of ascites does not necessarily indicate peritoneal spread as it may occur with any solid ovarian tumor. If hemorrhagic, however, it must be viewed as suspicious and a search for malignant cells must be made.

In pure germinoma there is usually no evidence of hormonal activity. Virilization or masculinization may accompany amenorrhea and has been attributed to hyperplasia of androgenic Leydig or stromal lutein cells.[63,134,143,149] If increased levels of chorionic gonadotropic hormone (CGH) are found, choriocarcinoma and/or embryonal carcinoma should be sought for in the neoplasm.[91,108]

### Gross features

The majority of germinomas in children and adolescents are confined to one ovary, with no significant adhesions; bilateral lesions are reported in 15% of cases[107] but from our experience this figure is too high. They vary in size from a few centimeters to that of a football, but most lesions are between 8 and 20 cm in greatest diameter when discovered. The capsular surface is generally smooth, opaque, and sometimes bosselated or nodular (Figure 27.2). The cut surface is of lymphoid consistency, soft but rubbery. The color is gray or pinkish gray, often with a slight yellow hue. Focal areas of necrosis and/or hemorrhage may be present in the large tumors. Hemorrhagic infarction from torsion of the pedicle is uncommon.

### Microscopic features

All the tumors are usually histopathologically very similar and are pure germinomas without the suggestion of teratomatous or trophoblastic components. Figure 27.3 shows the characteristic microscopic features. This was

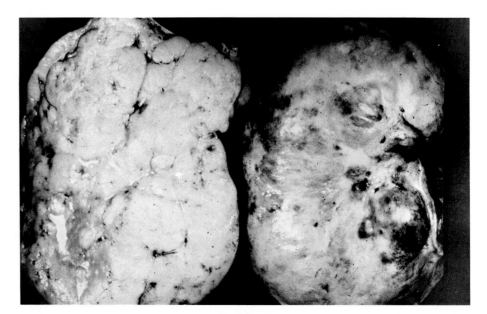

**27.2** Germinoma. A solid lobulated and slightly nodular tumor with subcapsular areas of congestion and hemorrhage.

[Courtesy of Dr. R. D. Hilbert.]

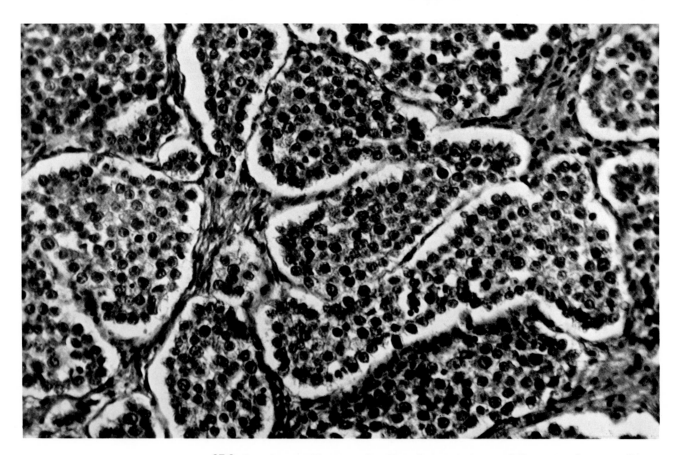

**27.3** Germinoma. Clusters of uniformly appearing, undifferentiated germ cells are separated by thin fibrous septa devoid in this instance of lymphocytes. Hematoxylin–eosin, ×286.

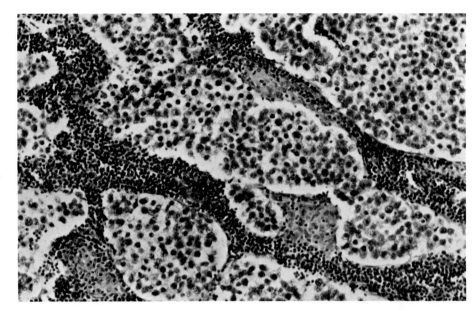

**27.4** Germinoma. Heavy lymphocytic infiltration of septa with several small histiocytic granulomas. Hematoxylin–eosin, ×129.

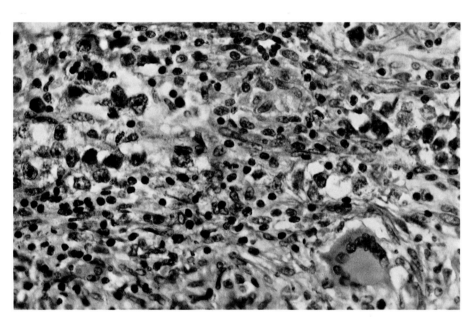

**27.5** Germinoma. Fibrous granulomatous reaction including one Langhan's type of foreign body giant cell. As a result of this reaction it is difficult to recognize the neoplastic cells. Hematoxylin–eosin, ×387.

from a germinoma in a 15-year-old female. Lymphocytes are prominent in most tumors and areas of fibrous and granulomatous reaction are seen frequently. These features are illustrated in Figures 27.4 and 27.5. The latter was a germinoma in a female 14 years of age. Kay *et al.*[80] have found neurosecretory granules in the stromal cells of a dysgerminoma and suggest that they may be the source of hormonal production in the occasional patient who manifests clinical evidence of hormonal activity.

### Treatment and survival information

Careful assessment for any extension of the neoplasm through the capsule into the mesovarium or broad ligament and to lymph nodes, should be made at the time of celiotomy. Fortunately, in children and adolescents most germinomas are confined to one ovary, without any extension beyond it. Hypoplasia of the opposite ovary with focal calcification or a "streak" ovary indicates gonadal dysgenesis. If the neoplasm is confined to one ovary with no penetration of the capsule and the opposite ovary is normal, unilateral salpingo-oophorectomy is adequate and gives a 5-year survival rate of around 90%.[4,9,107] A number of young patients so treated have subsequently had normal pregnancies.[4,9] Evidence of spread beyond the ovary requires postoperative irradiation, which may be curative in that germinomas are very radiosensitive neoplasms. If recurrences appear, they usually do so within 2 years of initial treatment. The prognosis is more favorable if there is a marked lymphocytic and/or granulomatous response in the stroma, whereas a high mitotic count in the tumor cells has an adverse effect on prognosis.

The pathologist has the obligation to examine microscopically all areas of a presumed germinoma that have a different gross appearance. Particular attention should be focused on mucinous microcystic and hemorrhagic areas, to determine whether other germ cell components are present. Impure germinomas with areas of embryonal carcinoma, yolk sac carcinoma, and/or choriocarcinoma have a much poorer prognosis and when found require more aggressive or additive treatment. The occurrence of mature or relatively mature teratomatous areas in an otherwise pure germinoma does not alter the prognosis.

## Embryonal Carcinoma (Teratoblastoma)

Embryonal carcinoma occurs predominately in young women but also appears in infants and young children.[4,110,129] The average age of patients in the series reported by Neubecker and Breen[110] was 20 years. Embryonal carcinoma is more prone to cause local and systemic symptoms than are most germ cell tumors. Abdominal distension, pain, and the finding of an abdominal mass are the initial complaints in most patients. Symptoms are of short duration and when diagnosed the neoplasm has usually spread beyond the confines of the ovary. This is particularly true for infants. Hemorrhagic ascites is frequently present.

Most neoplasms are not associated with any abnormal hormonal manifestations. However, in a few instances, there is the production of chorionic gonadotropins caused in most instances by the presence of foci of trophoblastic tissue, although such are not always found. Luteinization of the supportive ovarian stroma may result in virilization or masculinization.[2] Elevated serum levels of $\alpha$-fetoprotein, a normal globulin of human fetal serum, have been demonstrated in embryonal carcinoma, yolk sac carcinoma, and teratocarcinoma, and in certain non-germ cell tumors and nonneoplastic conditions.[11,47,99,141,153]

Its determination, as with CGH, is of value in monitoring the effect of treatment on metastatic disease.

### Gross features

The majority of neoplasms are unilateral; bilateral primary lesions occur in no more than 5% of cases. The tumors are soft, nodular, and usually range from 5 to 25 cm in diameter (see Figures 26.27 and 26.28). In about one-third of cases, neoplastic nodules involve the external surface, indicating capsular penetration. They tend to fracture readily with handling. The cut surfaces are spongy, wet, gelatinous, microcystic, and variegated in color. Areas of necrosis and hemorrhage are common. They lack the uniform appearance of germinomas and the firmness and variety of tissues of solid teratomas.

### Microscopic appearance

Although these neoplasms show considerable variation in patterns of growth, within individual lesions there is a certain uniformity from tumor to tumor that places them all in the same category. Figure 27.6 shows a section from an embryonal carcinoma from a child 10 years of age. This is a medullary neoplasm that lacks any regularity of arrangement, yet it is characteristic in its appearance. Many of the cells are vacuolated and there are also extracellular vacuoles and globules of homogeneous material. Clumps of more tightly packed and dark-stained cells suggest early attempts at differentiation. Figure 27.7 shows a section from an embryonal carcinoma from a girl 14 years of age. It is a medullary undifferentiated neoplasm consisting of fairly large vacuolated cells with frequent mitotic figures. A clump of darker stained cells suggests an embryoid body (arrow). Hyaline globules are present in the lower central field. An embryonal carcinoma in an infant 11 months of age (Figure 27.8) shows two distinct gland spaces formed by differentiated, columnar epithelium. These are thought to indicate early teratomatous differentiation.

### Survival information

Embryonal carcinomas are exceedingly aggressive, rapidly growing neoplasms and in infant girls are (usually) fatal.[4] The survival figures for adolescents are almost as bad, with most patients dying of metastatic disease within a year. They are not responsive to irradiation therapy. A few neoplasms respond to chemotherapy and the occasional cure is encountered, even when the neoplasm has extended locally beyond the confines of the ovary.

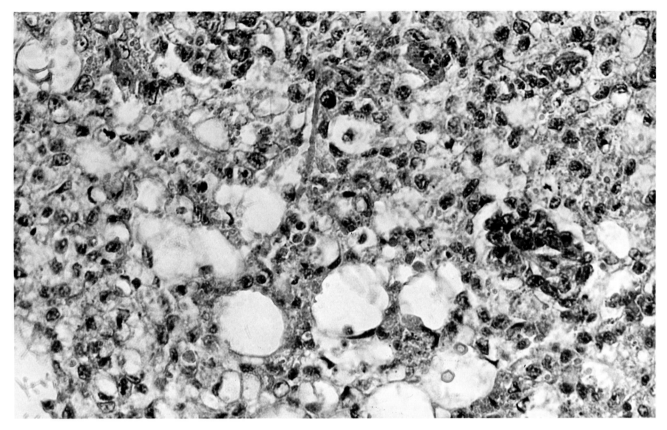

**27.6** Embryonal carcinoma. Sheets of undifferentiated germ cells with scant supportive stroma. Small clusters of darker, more compact cells probably represent attempts at differentiation. Hematoxylin–eosin, ×288.

**27.7** Embryonal carcinoma. Undifferentiated germ cells with scattered hyaline droplets are seen in the upper center field, with one small nest of darker, less undifferentiated neoplastic cells (arrow). Hematoxylin–eosin, ×400.

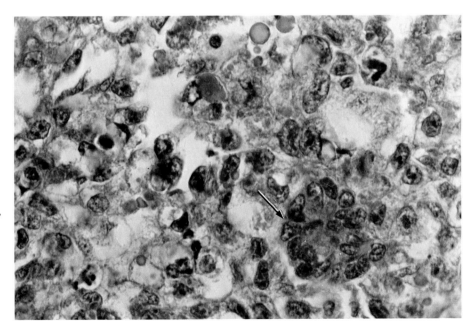

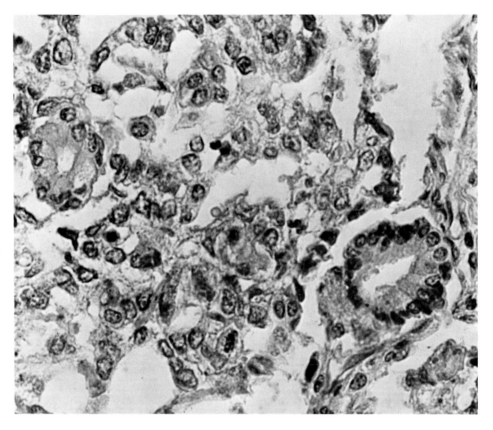

**27.8** Embryonal carcinoma from a 3-month-old infant. Loosely arranged embryonal carcinoma cells are seen with two partially differentiated tubular structures formed by columnar cells. Hematoxylin–eosin, ×480.

## Yolk Sac Carcinoma (Endodermal Sinus Tumor: Vitelline Carcinoma)

This tumor occurs predominantly in infants, children, and adolescents and tends to pursue an aggressive course, much the same as embryonal carcinoma from which it arises.

### Clinical features

Thirteen of the 18 cases of yolk sac carcinoma of the ovary reported by Huntington and Bullock[73] occurred in patients less than 20 years of age, and six patients were under 10 years of age. Two neoplasms occurred in infants. The presenting symptoms and clinical manifestations are essentially the same as for embryonal carcinoma. Some neoplasms give elevated serum levels of α-fetoprotein.[11,141,153] The occasional tumor may develop in a dysgenetic gonad. The gross and microscopic characteristics of the tumor have been described in detail in Chapter 26.

### Treatment and survival information

Yolk sac carcinoma of the ovary pursues essentially the same course as embryonal carcinoma and the survival figures are poor. Only two of the 18 cases reported by Huntington and Bullock[73] survived 5 years. A few neoplasms are responsive to chemotherapy, with sustained remissions and apparent cures.[53] In children and adolescents, conservative instead of radical surgical treatment is generally indicated. Forney et al.[53] reported an example of pure yolk sac carcinoma in a 14-year-old girl with proved peritoneal metastases of a similar nature. A second surgical procedure was done 1 year later after chemotherapy and two excised peritoneal nodules showed only mature squamous epithelium.

## Choriocarcinoma

The majority of teratoid choriocarcinomas occur in children and adolescents. In a review of acceptable cases in the literature and the addition of two personal cases, Marrubini[98] found that 18 of 20 patients were less than 20 years of age. Nine of them were prepubertal. In

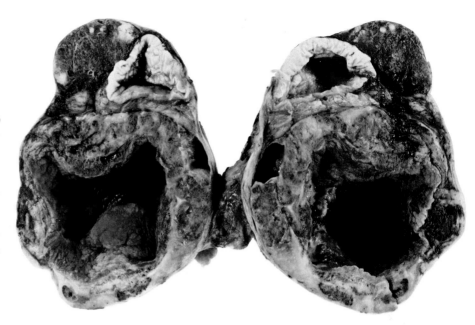

**27.9** Bisected teratocarcinoma of the ovary from a 13-year-old girl. The small, white-appearing cyst at the top is lined by mature skin. The nodule next to it is dysgenetic and gonadoblastomatous tissue. The large, dark, cystic mass is a mixture of embryonal carcinoma and immature somatic tissues. Chromosomal studies after removal of the tumor revealed a Y chromosome, although there was no clinical evidence to suggest dysgenesis.

Sturley's[140] report, 12 of 13 neoplasms occurred in children and adolescents; six patients were less than 10 years of age. Four of eight cases reported by Gerbie *et al.*[57] were adolescents. Schuler and Juhasz[132] reported an example in an infant 7 months of age.

### Survival information

Teratomatous choriocarcinoma is a very aggressive neoplasm, almost inevitably fatal.[98] Metastases occur early and death usually follows in a few months. It does not respond as favorably as gestational choriocarcinoma to chemotherapy.

## Teratocarcinoma (Malignant Teratoma: Malignant Mixed Germ Cell Tumor)

Eight (20%) of 41 malignant germ cell neoplasms in our series in children and adolescents were teratocarcinomas.[4]

### Clinical features

It is estimated that at least 75% of teratocarcinomas occur in children and adolescents, with close to half of these being premenarchal. The presenting symptom is usually abdominal pain and/or a palpable mass. When a neoplasm occurs before puberty, it may cause precocious somatic and sexual development, with enlargement of breasts and spotty vaginal bleeding.[121] There may be increased levels of chorionic gonadotropins in urine and serum. After menarche, clinical manifestations include menstrual irregularities, amenorrhea, and breast enlargement. A few teratocarcinomas have occurred in patients with somatosexual abnormalities, particularly those with a Y chromosome (Figure 27.9).[104,136]

### Pathologic features

Most neoplasms are unilateral and large, varying from 8 to 30 cm in diameter. When diagnosed at celiotomy, approximately 50% of the lesions have penetrated the ovarian capsule and seeded the peritoneum. The gross appearance is dictated by the different germ cell components that the neoplasm contains. Usually there are both cystic and solid areas (Figure 27.10). Soft gray areas suggest germinoma, soft mucoid areas embryonal carcinoma or yolk sac carcinoma, friable hemorrhagic areas choriocarcinoma, and firm solid and cystic areas somatic tissues. Each grossly different area should be carefully sampled; otherwise the true nature of the neoplasm can be missed (Figures 27.11 and 27.12).

### Survival information

Teratocarcinomas of the ovary are very aggressive neoplasms, causing death in a matter of months, irrespective of the type of treatment. Seven of eight children and

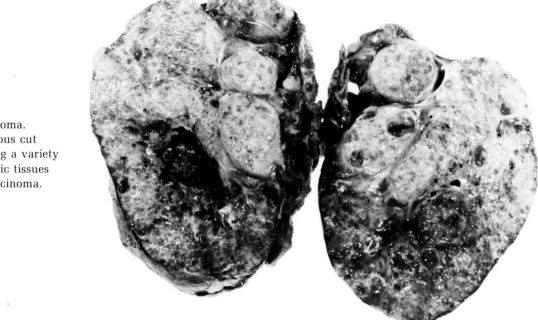

**27.10** Teratocarcinoma. Multicystic gelatinous cut surface representing a variety of immature somatic tissues and embryonal carcinoma.

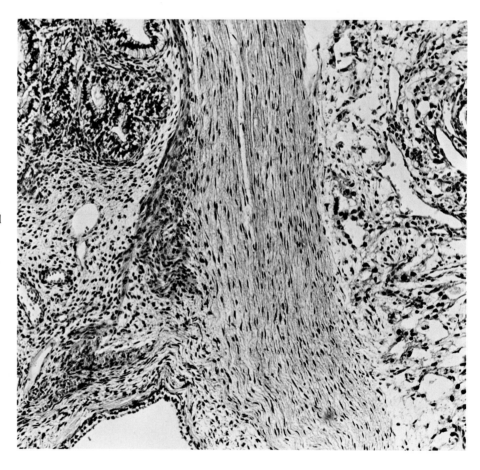

**27.11** Teratocarcinoma. Embryonal carcinoma on the right and partially differentiated teratomatous tissue on the left. Hematoxylin–eosin, ×96.

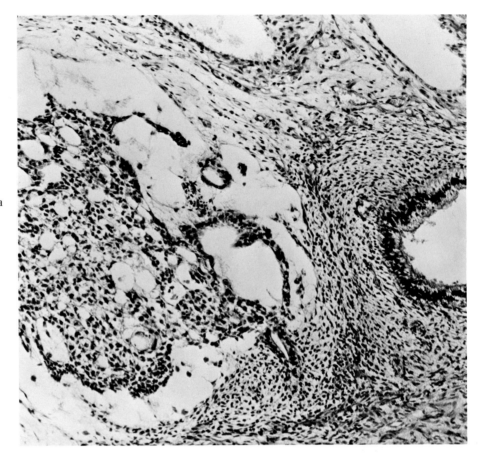

**27.12** Teratocarcinoma. An area of embryonal carcinoma on the left with adjacent teratomatous tissue to the right. Hematoxylin–eosin, ×115.

adolescents with teratocarcinoma that we were able to follow died of disseminated disease within 14 months of diagnosis, with an average survival period of 5.3 months.[4] They resemble embryonal carcinoma in regard to their natural history, which is in sharp contrast to the fairly good prognosis for neoplasms composed solely of immature teratomatous tissues and for germinomas. The neoplasms in reported series of malignant teratomas in which embryonal carcinoma was a significant component pursued the same aggressive course.[21,46,158]

## Immature Teratoma (Complex Teratoma, Solid Teratoma, Fetal Teratoma, Malignant Teratoma, Partially Differentiated Teratoma)

This group of teratomas is characterized by a blend of various immature but readily recognizable tissues, representing the three germ layers. They are devoid of more than a residual trace of embryonal carcinoma and have no extraembryonal carcinoma. They may be viewed as embryonal carcinomas that have matured to various degrees and become less malignant. They are commonly included in reported series of solid teratomas, complex teratomas, and malignant teratomas. Within the category there is considerable variation in the degree of differentiation; some neoplasms are poorly differentiated, whereas others are well differentiated and approach mature teratomas in appearance.

### Clinical features

Immature teratomas occur predominately in children and adolescents. In our series they comprised 12% of all germ cell tumors seen during the first two decades of life. The average age was 14 years, with a range of 10 to 19 years. They occurred slightly later in life on the average than embryonal carcinoma and teratocarcinoma.

The initial symptoms are usually abdominal enlarge-

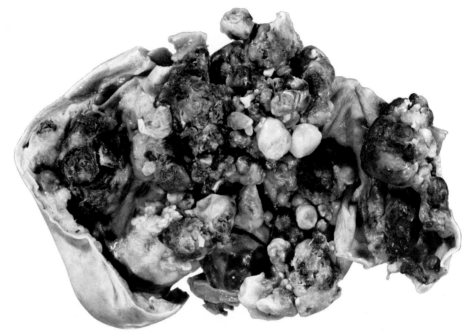

**27.13** Immature teratoma. A solid and cystic neoplasm consisting of a variety of tissues of different color and consistency.

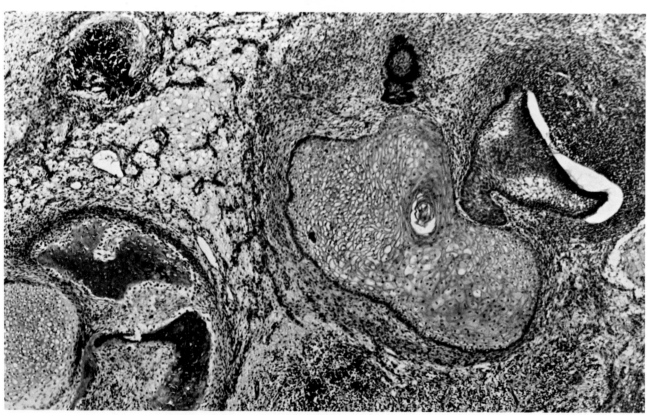

**27.14** Immature teratoma. A variety of nearly mature teratomatous tissues including bone, cartilage, squamous epithelium, tooth bud, and neuroglia. Hematoxylin–eosin, ×65.

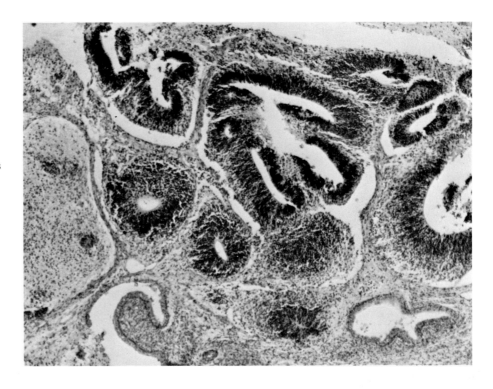

**27.15** Immature teratoma. This field consists predominantly of neuroepithelial structures surrounded by neuroglia. Hematoxylin–eosin, ×85.

ment and a vague, dull abdominal pain. Only occasionally is the pain severe, which suggests torsion or spontaneous rupture. In a few instances, significant symptoms are absent and the tumor is detected by the mother or on routine physical examination.

### Pathologic features

The majority of immature teratomas are unilateral. Occasionally a mature cystic teratoma is present in the opposite ovary.[4,21,155,158] They are frequently lobulated or nodular and generally vary from 10 to 30 cm in diameter. Cystic areas may be seen or felt through the capsule. The cut surfaces display a variety of tissues of differing color and consistency. Although the teratoma is often described as solid, this is only relative, as all have multiple cystic areas of varying size (Figure 27.13). The cysts may contain sebaceous material, hair, or mucin. Cartilage, bone, and neuroectodermal tissues can often be detected. Areas of necrosis and hemorrhage may be present in the softer, less well-differentiated areas, but the possibility that they represent embryonal carcinoma or choriocarcinoma should always be entertained. Between 20 and 30% of patients, when explored surgically, have areas of capsular penetration and/or peritoneal implants, sometimes with a hemorrhagic ascites.

Microscopically there is a plethora of various epithelial and mesenchymal tissues of varying maturity (Figure 27.14). Squamous cell nests and cysts with skin appendages, respiratory and intestinal structures, cartilage, bone, muscle, neuroglia, and neuroepithelium are commonly present (Figures 27.15 and 27.16). Neuroectodermal tissues are frequent and sometimes sufficiently immature that they resemble neuroblastoma or neuroepithelioma. Melanin may be prominent in some of the neuroectodermal structures. The less well-differentiated areas may be recognizable only as epithelium and supportive mesenchyme.

The metastases show the same proclivity for the formation of a variety of tissues. Occasionally one tissue may predominate in the metastases, to the near exclusion of all others. This is often true for the neuroectodermal components which, when they seed the peritoneum, may differentiate to the extent that they form mature glial implants.[155] Other peritoneal implants may consist of mature or nearly mature tissues, such as skin, thyroid, and intestinal epithelium.[14]

### Treatment and survival information

Perusal of the reported cases of malignant teratoma indicate that those neoplasms which are devoid of embryonal carcinoma and choriocarcinoma, i.e., immature

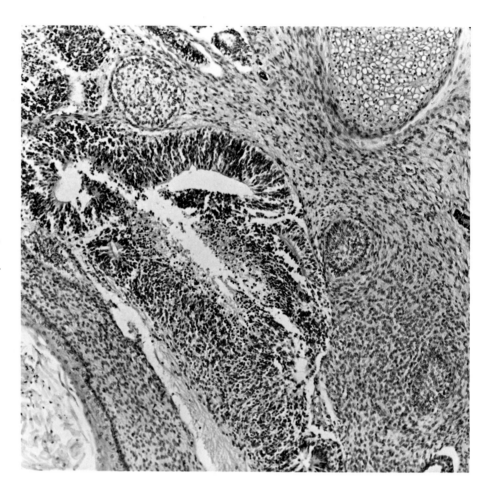

**27.16** Immature teratoma. Neuroepithelium, neuroglia, squamous epithelium, cartilage, small glandular structures and supportive mesenchyme. Hematoxylin–eosin, ×120.

teratomas, are not overly aggressive lesions.[21,146,158] In our material, nine of 12 patients with immature teratomas treated conservatively have now survived more than 5 years without recurrences.[4]

Thurlbeck and Scully[146] offered a system of grading for teratomas on the basis of immaturity of the tissues. This system offers the clinician a guide to treatment and prognosis. It is essential, however, that the pathologist make a very thorough examination of the tumor and sample all of the grossly different areas.

A particularly interesting group of teratomas is that which seeds the peritoneum with neuroglia and neuroepithelium, causing peritoneal gliomatosis. The disease results either from spontaneous rupture of the primary tumor or neoplastic penetration of its capsule. Eleven of 12 patients with peritoneal gliomatoses reported by Robboy and Scully[127] were under 20 years of age, with a range from 16 months to 18 years. The mean age of cases reviewed by Fortt and Mathie[54] was 14.6 years. Although all primary tumors consist of tissues of the three germ layers, neuroepithelium and neuroglia, either mature or immature, commonly predominate. Most of the implants are mature or nearly mature glial tissue but other somatic tissues may be present. In some cases, the evidence suggests that immature neural tissue differentiates once it is implanted on the peritoneum.[49]

The prognosis is good if the glial implants are mature or relatively mature.[54,127] Conservative treatment is indicated unless the implants include primitive neural tissues. The prognosis depends on the maturity of the tissues in the primary tumor and in the peritoneal implants.[54]

## Mature Teratoma (Benign Cystic Teratoma)

Mature teratomas are a compendium of fully differentiated somatic tissues representing the three germ layers. Our present knowledge indicates an origin by neoplastic transformation and differentiation of multipotential germ cells, either directly or by way of embryonal carcinoma.

Pierce *et al.*[125] demonstrated experimentally that embryoid bodies (embryonal carcinoma cells) could differentiate completely, giving rise to benign teratomas. Kleinsmith and Pierce[85] accomplished the same with single embryonal carcinoma cells.

In our material, mature teratomas comprised 38% of all neoplasms in children and adolescents and 64% of the germ cell tumors.[4] Sixteen patients were premenarchial and the youngest was 3 months of age. A familial occurrence is recognized and Feld *et al.*[50] reported bilateral cystic teratomas in all three of a set of probably identical triplets. We have recently seen a benign cystic teratoma in a 12-year-old girl with XY dysgenesis.

## Clinical features

In one-third to one-half of patients, symptoms are insignificant and the neoplasm is found on routine examination or roentgenograms. Some are found in the ovary opposite to a malignant ovarian germ cell tumor. Acute pain generally means torsion of the pedicle. Rupture may cause a fairly severe chemical peritonitis. Rare examples of hemolytic anemia, possibly on an autoimmune basis, have been recorded with relief of the anemia on removal of the tumor.[7,13,101] Extremely rarely masculinization may occur because of stromal luteinization or hyperplasia of hilus (Leydig) cells.[29]

## Gross features

Most mature teratomas are cystic, some are cystic and solid, and a very few are primarily solid (Figure 27.17). Bilateral tumors are present in 10 to 15% of patients. Our cases varied from 1 to 30 cm in diameter, with the majority being between 5 and 10 cm. Occasionally minute teratomas are discovered when grossly normal ovaries are sectioned.[34]

Most teratomas have a heavy feeling and are ovoid or lobulated tumors, encased in an opaque, white capsule in which normal ovarian cortical structures may be recognized. Their cystic nature is evident on palpation and a puttylike or doughy consistency is often appreciated. Firm nodules, representing teeth, cartilage, bone, or other solid structures, may be palpated in the wall of lesions from adolescents but are less common in young children. Adipose tissue and hair may show through a thin capsule.

One large cyst forms the bulk of most cystic teratomas, with smaller cysts often being detected in its thickened wall. In about 12% of lesions, there are two or more cysts roughly equivalent in size and appearance. The contents of

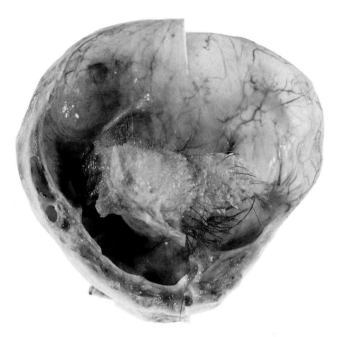

**27.17** Benign cystic teratoma that has been opened and has had the contents removed. The projecting nodule in the center of the cyst is the dermal papilla covered by hair-bearing skin.

most cysts are a rancid mixture of sebaceous material, hair, secretions, and desquamated debris. The lining is skin from which one or more knuckles of solid tissue referred to as dermal or Rokitansky papillae project (Figure 27.18). It is from these structures that most of the hair and the teeth arise and it is in these areas that adipose tissue, skin appendages, thyroid tissue, glia, bone, cartilage, and other formed tissues are found (Figure 27.19). As a result of agitation *in situ,* the hair may form into "hair balls" and the keratin and sebaceous material into "butterballs."

Not all cystic teratomas contain hair and sebaceous material; some cysts are filled with mucin or a clear watery fluid, probably cerebral spinal fluid (Figure 27.20). The latter tumors are usually encountered in young children and may be lined by ependyma. Trites[148] has referred to this type of teratoma as "ovarian hydrocephalus." Large amounts of neural tissue may be present and may be recognized by their brainlike consistency.[4]

Teeth are found in teratomas of adolescents projecting from the dermal papilla or embedded in a bony structure that has been likened by some to a rudimentary mandible or maxilla (Figure 27.21). They are usually incisors or molars; canines are rarely found. Bone formations resembling rudimentary long bones are uncommon.

The term "solid teratoma" is a relative one as many

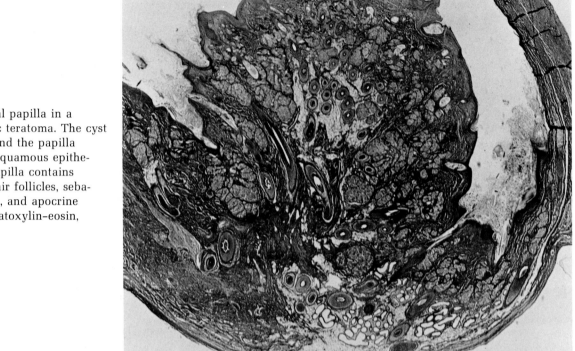

**27.18** Dermal papilla in a benign cystic teratoma. The cyst is lined by and the papilla covered by squamous epithelium. The papilla contains numerous hair follicles, sebaceous glands, and apocrine glands. Hematoxylin–eosin, ×13.

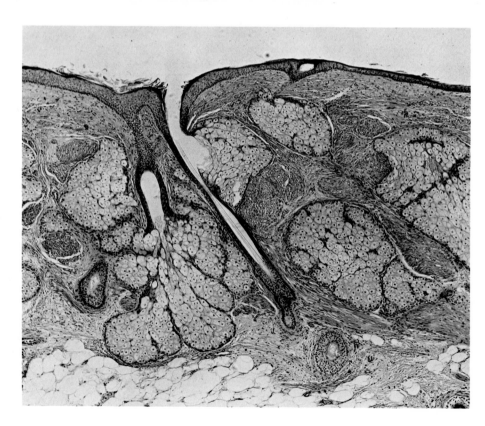

**27.19** Skin of a dermal papilla that includes hair follicles, sebaceous glands, and underlying adipose tissue. Hematoxylin–eosin, ×39.

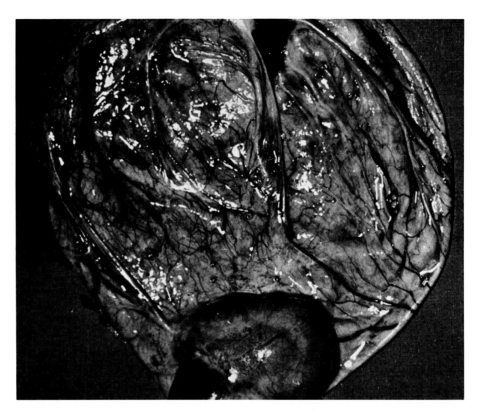

**27.20** Mature teratoma (hydrocephalus ovarii). The cyst contained a clear watery fluid. Its lining was neuroglia and ependyma. The nodule in the lower center field consisted of cerebral tissue.

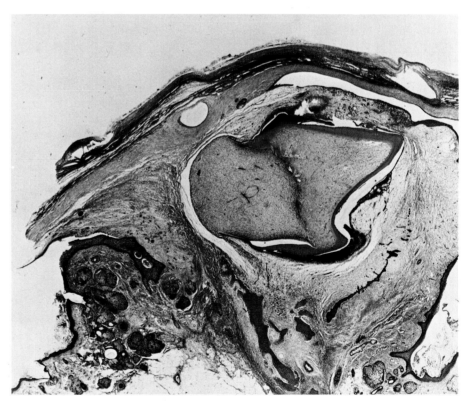

**27.21** Mature teratoma. An unerupted tooth is embedded in the dermal papilla. Hematoxylin–eosin, ×30.

small cysts are usually present; the term "microcystic" may be more appropriate. They show a greater variety of tissue components, with grayish neural tissue being particularly prominent in children.

*Microscopic features*

The histologic sections disclose the expected treasure of tissues (Figures 27.19, 27.21, and 27.22 through 27.24). Proper evaluation demands that multiple blocks of tissue be processed from the dermal knuckle and other thickened areas in the walls, for it is here that the many types of tissues reside. The different tissues encountered in the routine examination of 72 mature cystic teratomas from children and adolescents are given in Table 27.2. This demonstrates the complex nature of these lesions, in contrast to the simple "dermoid" concept.

Ectodermal elements represented by skin and its appendages, hair follicles, sebaceous glands, and sweat glands are present in essentially all lesions (Figures 27.18 and 27.19). The rare exception is the "glioma ovarii," which consists predominantly of neuroglial and neuroepithelial tissues (Figure 27.22). Mesodermal elements represented by smooth muscle, adipose tissue, cartilage, and bone are almost as frequent (Figure 27.23). They tend to be more prevalent in tumors from adults, whereas the neuroglia, ependyma, and nerve cells are more frequent and prominent in the neoplasms from children and adolescents.[4] Occasionally the neurogenous tissue is organized into structures that resemble cerebral and cerebellar convolutions (Figure 27.22). Respiratory and gastrointestinal epithelium are commonly seen and the adjacent mesenchymal tissue may be organized into a recognizable bronchial wall or muscularis propria with a myenteric plexus (Figure 27.24). Salivary gland and thyroid tissue are often closely associated with cartilagenous plates and nodules. Other elements that have been observed infrequently include lung, skeletal muscle, cardiac muscle, pancreas, breast tissue, urinary epithelium, and lymphoid tissue. Kidney, spleen, liver, pituitary, and adrenal and gonadal tissues have rarely been reported.

Teratomas consisting predominantly of thyroid tissue (struma ovarii) rarely occur in children and adolescents, most examples being encountered in adults.[82] Only three of 25 cases of struma ovarii reviewed by Kempers *et al.*[82] occurred in patients less than 20 years of age. The three cases included a 19-year-old girl with hyperthyroidism caused by the struma and two children, ages 7 and 16 years, with follicular adenocarcinoma. The 7-year-old girl died with systemic metastases.

**Table 27.2** Composition of 72 mature cystic teratomas from children and adolescents

| | Number of cases | Percent of total |
|---|---|---|
| Skin and appendages | 70 | 97 |
| Subcutaneous tissue | 65 | 90 |
| Neuroglia | 57 | 80 |
| Nerves and ganglia | 44 | 61 |
| Melanotic pigment | 18 | 25 |
| Respiratory epithelium and glands | 35 | 49 |
| Intestinal epithelium | 11 | 15 |
| Thyroid tissue | 9 | 13 |
| Urinary epithelium | 2 | 3 |
| Smooth muscle | 33 | 46 |
| Bone | 26 | 36 |
| Cartilage | 21 | 29 |
| Skeletal muscle | 2 | 3 |
| Lymphoid follicles | 8 | 11 |
| Teeth | 8 | 11 |
| Foreign body giant cell reaction to hair shafts | 33 | 46 |
| Fat necrosis | 7 | 10 |
| Dystrophic calcific deposits in glial tissue | 8 | 11 |

Several fairly common secondary changes are found in cystic teratomas. The squamous lining of the cysts may become ulcerated and replaced by a granulation tissue containing cholesterol clefts, hemosiderin deposits, and multinucleated foreign body giant cells about dead hair shafts. This reaction occurs to some extent in nearly 50% of teratomas in children and adolescents.[4] Rarely, the entire wall may be replaced by such a granulomatous response and the identification of hair shafts is the only lead to the identity of the lesion. Adipose tissue in cystic teratomas may undergo an aseptic degeneration and necrosis, with the formation of multiple small cystic spaces in and between which there are lipidic foam cells and foreign body giant cells. Neoplasms that have large amounts of neuroglial tissue often show scattered lime salt deposits and in old cystic teratomas that have ceased to grow a sizable proportion of the lesion may have become calcified.

The same tissues described for mature cystic teratomas are found in the more solid microcystic lesions but in greater abundance and more intimately mixed.

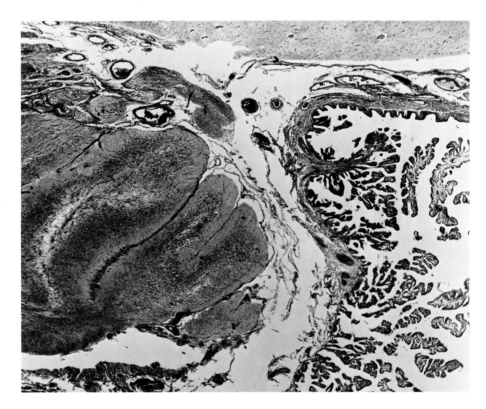

**27.22** Convoluted cerebral cortical tissue, ependyma, and neuroglia in a cystic teratoma of ovary from an infant. Hematoxylin–eosin, ×26.

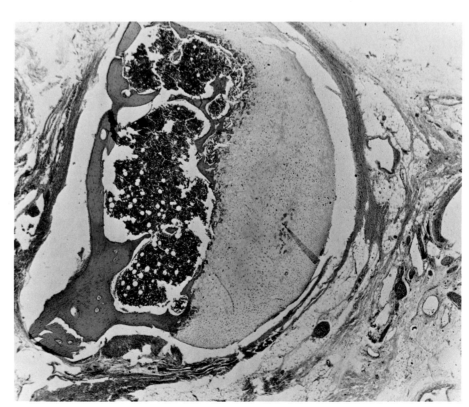

**27.23** Mature teratoma. Cartilage capped bone with joint(?) space. Hematoxylin–eosin, ×26.

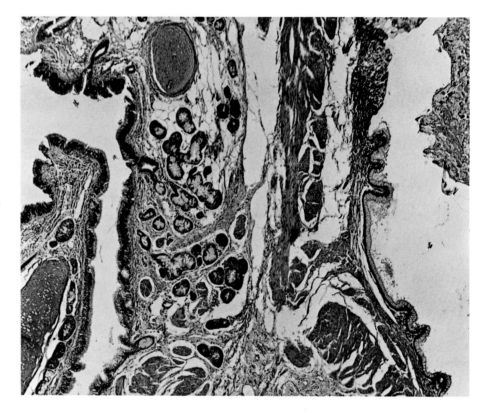

**27.24** This was a bilocular cystic teratoma from a child. One cyst (right) is lined by a mucinous intestinal epithelium; the other on the left is lined by respiratory epithelium and has bronchial glands and cartilage in its wall. Hematoxylin–eosin, ×34.

## Complications

Cystic teratomas may rupture into the peritoneal cavity and on occasion into the intestine, urinary bladder, or vagina, leading to the passage of hair and sebaceous material.[5,84,124,142] The rupture may be explosive, with massive contamination of the peritoneal cavity resulting in a severe chemical peritonitis, or a slow leak may develop, resulting in a localized foreign body reaction, an "oleokeratin," or a "pilar" granuloma.[87,138] With rupture, histologically benign tissues may implant on the peritoneum and grow slowly. Such implants most frequently consist of neural tissues, but we have found skin and intestinal epithelium growing on the pelvic peritoneum.

A variety of second primary neoplasms developing from one of the mature tissues in a teratoma has been recorded, including squamous cell carcinoma, basal cell carcinoma, thyroid carcinoma, leiomyosarcoma, melanoma, and argentaffin carcinoma (carcinoid tumor).[60,81,118,123] Practically all such examples have been in older adults in whom the teratomas have probably been present for many years. The two cases of carcinoma of the thyroid in 7- and 16-year-old girls are exceptions.[82] The only example that we have seen in adolescence was a small carcinoid tumor.

## Mixed Germ Cell Tumors

These are usually seen in children and adolescents. The subject has been thoroughly covered in Chapter 26.

# Coelomic Epithelial Neoplasms (Epithelial–Stromal Neoplasms)

The coelomic epithelial neoplasms arise from the surface epithelium (mesothelium) of the ovary and its inclusions in the cortex. It is also probable that some arise from the rete ovarii, remnants of the primitive sex cords of coelomic epithelial derivation. In their development, this group of tumors expresses the multipotential of the embryonic coelomic epithelium by differentiating into epithelia characteristic of the paramesonephric (Müllerian) system and the mesonephric system. Their epithelial component therefore resembles fallopian tube (serous), endometrium (endometrioid), endocervix (mucinous), and mesonephric tubules (mesonephroid). The epithelium of Brenner tumors represents a neoplastic urothelial differentiation. Two or more types of epithelium may be encountered in some neoplasms, but usually one predominates. In some of the carcinomas the level of differentiation may be such that a more specific diagnosis than undifferentiated or poorly differentiated carcinoma cannot be made. A significant component of ovarian cortical tissue in some tumors results in epithelial–stromal tumors, the cystadenofibromas and adenofibromas. The occasional familial aggregation of epithelial tumors suggests that in some instances there may be transmission as a Mendelian trait.[89]

### Clinical features

In our material, 4% of the coelomic epithelial group of neoplasms occurred in children and adolescents.[1] They comprised 28% of neoplasms in patients under 20 years of age in Jensen's and Norris' series[76] and 19% in ours.[3] In this age group, all of the neoplasms occurred after menarche and consisted of two cell types, serous (tubal) and mucinous (endocervical). The other cell types are rarities in adolescents and the only one that we have encountered has been a Brenner tumor (urothelioma).

The presenting complaint is usually gradual abdominal enlargement, relatively asymptomatic but often with some intermittent discomfort or pain. In adolescents there may be some disturbance in the menstrual cycle, such as oligomenorrhea or hypermenorrhea. Although the stromal component has the potential of increased sex steroid production, it is rarely expressed to the extent that it causes systemic manifestations in children and adolescents.

Most neoplasms in children and adolescents are unilateral and benign. Roughly 10% of patients have simultaneous bilateral primary tumors. Asynchronous bilateral primary tumors are extremely uncommon and none of the patients in our series has so far developed second primary tumors. Of 67 epithelial neoplasms in this age group reported by Jensen and Norris,[76] there were three definite carcinomas and five neoplasms of borderline or low malignant potential (well-differentiated carcinomas). In our series of 54 neoplasms, four were interpreted as carcinomas.[3]

## Serous (Tubal) Cell Neoplasms

The serous cystadenomas are generally not as large as the mucinous tumors; their average diameter is around 10 cm. They have a greater variation in gross appearance than the mucinous tumors, partly because of predominance of a stromal component in some tumors, resulting in cystadenofibromas. The external surface is usually smooth and glistening other than for a few adhesions on the larger tumors. External papillary growths are rare in

children and adolescents. The tumors may be composed of a single cyst but more frequently consist of multiple cysts with nodular fibromatous areas in the cystadenofibromas (Figure 27.25). The contents are watery and clear unless discolored from old or recent hemorrhage. The hallmark grossly is the presence of nodular papillary excrescences scattered over the lining of the cysts (Figure 27.26). These may be few and barely visible or numerous.

Microscopically the cysts are lined by and the papillary processes covered by a single layer of columnar to cuboidal cells (Figures 27.27 and 27.28). Usually a mixture of peg, secretory, and ciliated cells is present. The supportive stroma resembles the collagen-forming fibrous tissue of the tunica albuginea. The stroma of the nodular excrescences is frequently very loose, pale, and edematous. In some neoplasms, there are plump, pale stromal cells that have a distinctly thecal appearance. Electron microscopic studies suggest that these cells are steroid-producing cells.[119]

Neoplasms that have undergone a malignant change show a more extensive and complex papillary pattern with stratification of the epithelial lining (Figures 27.29 and 27.30). The neoplastic cells are less cohesive, with loss of polarity, cellular and nuclear pleomorphism, increased mitotic activity, and stromal invasion. Fingers of neoplastic cells without supportive stroma commonly appear to lie detached adjacent to the lining. The carcinomas in adolescents tend, in general, to be of a lower grade of malignancy than most of those seen in older patients.

There is no evidence to suggest that the serous cell neoplasms in adolescents that rupture and seed the peritoneum or that are carcinomas behave any differently than those in adults of similar type.[3,76]

## Mucinous (Endocervical) Cell Neoplasms

Mucinous cystadenomas are usually unilateral and tend to be larger than the serous cystadenomas. The external surface is smooth, white, or bluish-white, and the tumor is often bosselated or lobulated. They may occasionally be unilocular but the majority are multilocular, with the locules being of varying size (Figure 27.31). The contents are a thick, glary mucin unless discolored by old or recent hemorrhage. The lining of the locules and daughter cysts is smooth and glistening, and intraluminal papillary structures are infrequent: the nodular papillary excrescences characteristic of serous cystadenomas are absent. Cystadenofibromatous tumors of the mucinous type are much less frequent than are those of the serous type.

Microscopically the locules, septa, and budding daughter cysts are lined by tall, columnar, nonciliated cells

**27.25** Multilocular serous cystadenoma from adolescent. Several of the cysts have characteristic nodular papillary excrescences.

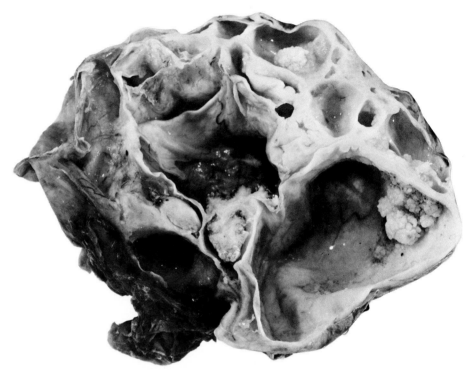

**27.26** Lining of a serous cystadenoma with numerous nodular papillary excrescences. ×3.

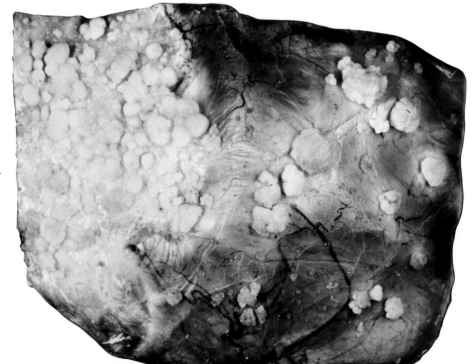

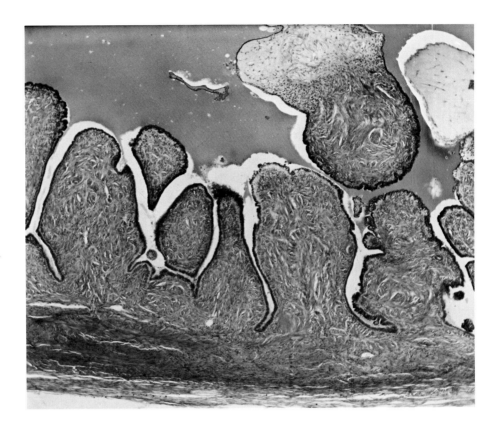

**27.27** Serous cystadenoma. Sessile nodular excrescences consisting largely of a tunica albuginea-like stroma covered by a single layer of epithelial cells. Hematoxylin–eosin, ×49.

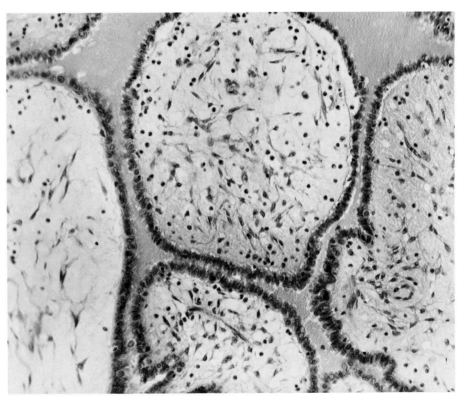

**27.28** Higher magnification of some of the excrescences shown in Figure 27.27. Edematous stroma covered by a single layer of low columnar cells. Hematoxylin–eosin, ×170.

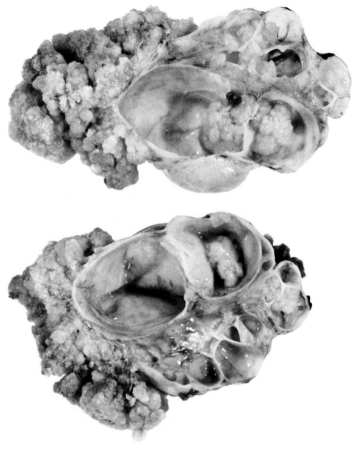

**27.29** Papillary serous cystadenocarcinoma. In addition to extensive intracystic papillary structures, similar formations involve the serosal surfaces.

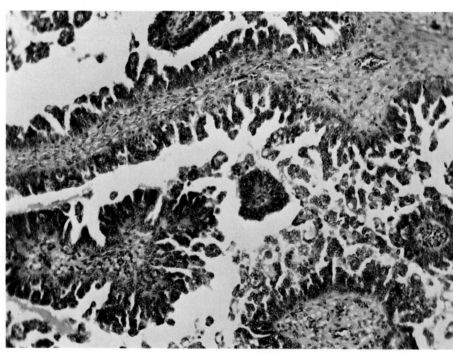

**27.30** Papillary carcinoma. The papillae are covered by several layers of neoplastic cells and loose fingers of similar cells project into the lumen. Hematoxylin–eosin, ×124.

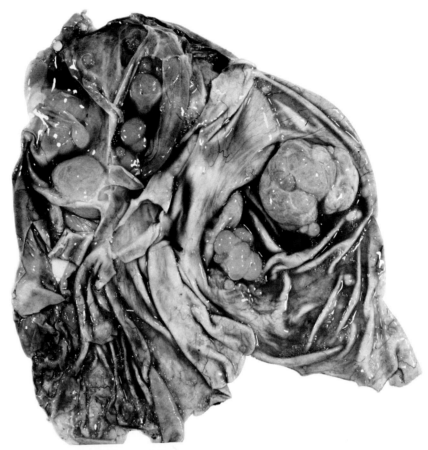

**27.31** Opened mucinous cystadenoma of ovary from a 13-year-old girl. Cut surface shows multiple cysts with smooth linings and multiple small daughter cysts.

**27.32** Mucinous cystadenoma. The folded lining epithelium consists of pale, columnar endocervix-like cells with small, basally placed nuclei. Hematoxylin–eosin, ×234.

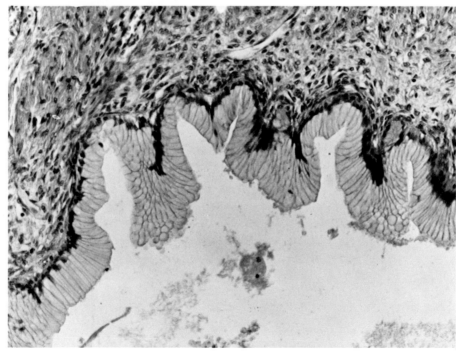

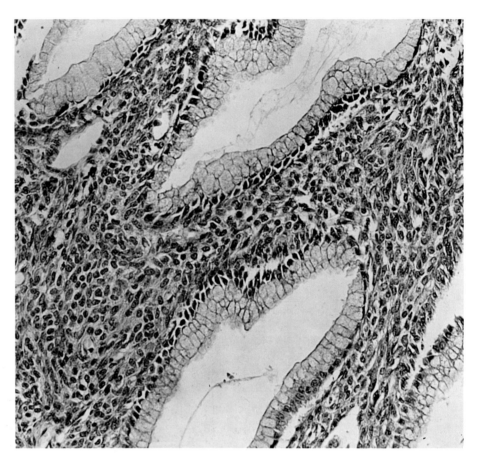

**27.33** Mucinous cystadenoma with plump thecomatous stromal cells which suggest estrogen production. Hematoxylin–eosin, ×144.

(Figure 27.32). The cytoplasm is faintly basophilic and the nuclei are small, dark, and basally placed. In some tumors there are scattered goblet cells that more closely mimic the mucinous cells of the large intestine. Scattered argentaffin cells may be present.[100] The supportive stroma resembles the inner cytogenic cortical stroma and is more cellular than that of the serous tumors, especially adjacent to the epithelium. Commonly, the stromal cells have a thecal and sometimes even a luteal appearance, suggesting steroid production, but in relatively few instances are they functional to a degree that causes systemic manifestations (Figure 27.33).

Malignant neoplasms are characterized by stratification of epithelial cells, loss of nuclear polarity, nuclear pleomorphism, frequent mitotic figures, and stromal invasion. Tumors that grossly have intraluminal papillary or more solid areas must be suspected as being carcinomas.

None of our patients has developed second primary (asynchronous) tumors in the opposite ovaries. Three of 19 mucinous tumors in our series were considered malignant.

# Sex Cord–Sex Mesenchyme Tumors

## Granulosa Cell Tumor

### Clinical features

The ages of patients with granulosa cell tumors range from infancy to the tenth decade. About 5% of tumors are said to occur before puberty,[94] and in one large series only four of 71 granulosa cell tumors occurred prior to 20 years of age.[113] In our material, only three of 188 ovarian tumors in children and adolescents (13, 15, and 19 years of age) were pure granulosa cell tumors[3] (Table 27.3).

Before puberty, granulosa cell tumors may cause a precocious development with maturation of sex characteristics, including increased development of the labia minora, spotty vaginal bleeding, breast enlargement, appearance of pubic and axillary hair, and accelerated growth.[8,145,159] After menarche, the complaints are hyper- and polymenorrhea unless there is the production of androgens, which may cause amenorrhea, hirsutism, and sometimes masculinization.[8] Urinary estrogens may be

**Table 27.3** Sex cord–sex mesenchyme neoplasms in children and adolescents[a]

| | |
|---|---|
| I. Sex cord neoplasms | |
|     Granulosa cell tumor | 3 |
|     Sertoli cell tumor | 3 |
| II. Sex mesenchyme neoplasms | |
|     Thecoma | 3 |
|     Luteoma | 0 |
|     Hilus (Leydig) cell tumor | 0 |
|     Sclerosing stromal tumor | 0 |
| III. Sex cord–sex mesenchyme neoplasms | |
|     Granulosa–theca cell tumor | 2 |
|     Sertoli–Leydig cell tumor | 3 |

[a] Reprinted by permission from M. R. Abell and F. Holtz. Ovarian neoplasms in childhood and adolescence. II. Tumors of non-germ cell origin. *Am. J. Obstet. Gynecol.* 93:850, 1965.

increased and the 17-ketosteroids are usually normal or only slightly elevated.[159]

The manifestations of nonfunctioning granulosa cell neoplasms or tumors that do not function sufficiently to cause an endocrinopathy are those of any slowly growing ovarian neoplasm. Ascites or Demons–Meig's syndrome may be present. The occasional cystic granulosa cell tumor may rupture and result in a massive hematoperitoneum.[59] Associated neoplasms in endometrium and breast encountered in adults do not occur in children and adolescents. In a few instances, granulosa cell tumors may be the cause of virilization or masculinization, presumably because of a luteinized stroma.[8,27,96] We have studied one such tumor in a young girl in which the luteinized lipid-containing stromal cells were probably the source of the androgens.

*Survival information*

It is difficult to say how frequently granulosa cell tumors are malignant in that late recurrences may appear well after 5-year and even at times after 10-year intervals. It is probably around 25% or less. A few lesions are frankly malignant histologically and pursue a more aggressive course.[8] One neoplasm in our series in a 19-year-old patient metastasized throughout the peritoneal cavity and caused death 3 months after diagnosis.[3]

Unilateral salpingo-oophorectomy is adequate treatment, particularly in young patients with encapsulated tumors. More extensive procedures are justified only if there is proved local spread. Pure granulosa cell tumors are moderately radiosensitive.

# Sertoli Cell Tumor (Tubular Androblastoma)

*Clinical features*

Because Sertoli cell tumors have been reported under a variety of names, it is difficult to assess the incidence and age range. It appears that these are similar to granulosa cell tumors. In our series of 188 ovarian neoplasms in patients under 20 years of age, there were three Sertoli cell adenomas.[3]

Prior to puberty, Sertoli cell tumors are prone to cause precocious development of secondary sex characteristics.[3,67,150] After puberty there may be little evidence of endocrine activity other than excessive or irregular uterine bleeding, endometrial hyperplasia, and some enlargement of the breasts.[26] Other symptoms and clinical findings are those common to all neoplasms for the particular age group.

*Survival information*

The majority of cases are perfectly benign histologically and behave so clinically. We have encountered one example in a young child that showed areas of considerable nuclear pleomorphism and mitotic activity and that subsequently metastasized to liver. It may therefore be presumed that malignant variants exist, although they are not as yet defined.

# Thecoma

*Clinical features*

Most thecomas occur during the late reproductive and postmenopausal years and very few occur prior to 20 years of age. Only three of 82 patients with thecomas reported by McGoldrick and Lapp[102] were less than 20 years of age. In our series of 188 ovarian neoplasms in children and adolescents, there were three thecomas, all in adolescents.[3] Their occurrence prior to menarche is extremely unusual, but a few examples causing isosexual precocity have been reported.[4,121] Thecoma may be a cause of Demons–Meig's syndrome.[128]

*Survival information*

The vast majority of thecomas are histologically benign and do not recur or metastasize. Malignant transformation occurs infrequently and nearly always in older patients.[52]

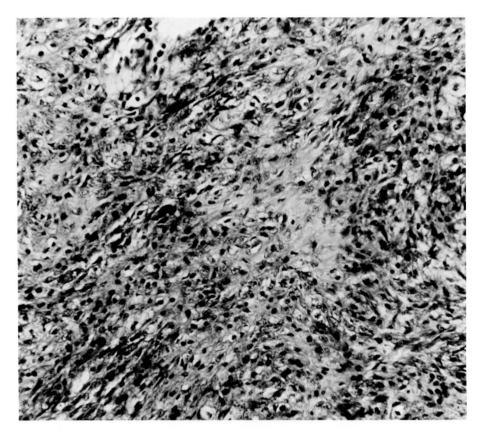

**27.34** Sclerosing stromal tumor. Scattered vacuolated tumor cells in a fibrous hyaline stroma. Hematoxylin–eosin, ×144.

It is characterized by a more crowded nuclear pattern, with large, irregular, hyperchromatic nuclei and frequent mitotic figures.

## Sclerosing Stromal Tumor

Chalvardjian and Scully[31] recently described a characteristic tumor of gonadal stromal origin in which irregular collagen formation was a major component. Four of 10 patients reported by these authors were adolescents 14 to 18 years of age.

### Clinical features

The presenting complaints are menstrual irregularities and in one reported case there was evidence of both estrogen and androgen production.[39]

### Pathologic features

The tumors are unilateral and rubbery firm with smooth, glistening capsular surfaces. The cut surfaces are gray-white with yellow foci and commonly there are areas of cystic degeneration.

Microscopically there are lobular areas of rounded epithelial and spindled cells, separated by irregular areas of dense fibrous and edematous connective tissue (Figures 27.34 and 27.35). The epithelium-appearing stromal cells have clear or finely vacuolated cytoplasm with enlarged nuclei and prominent nucleoli. A few of the cells may have a signet-ring configuration. The cells contain varying amounts of lipid and are PAS negative. Mitotic figures are infrequent. There is abundant reticulin and varying amounts of collagen irregularly interspersed between the neoplastic cells. Areas of edema, necrosis, and cystic degeneration are commonly present. In some neoplasms, small blood vessels are frequent and dilated, almost telangiectatic in nature.

### Survival information

None of the lesions diagnosed as sclerosing stromal tumor has so far proved to be malignant, and no histologically malignant counterpart has, as yet, been recognized.

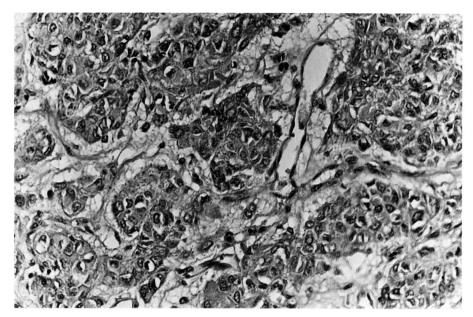

**27.35** Sclerosing stromal tumor. An area in which there are nests of pale, partially vacuolated, epithelium-like cells separated by a pale vascular stroma. Hematoxylin–eosin, ×182.

## Leydig (Hilus) Cell Tumor (Berger's Tumor)

### Clinical features

The clinical manifestations are progressive virilization and masculinization attributed to the excessive production of androgens. The classic end result is marked masculinization of the patient, who has been likened to a chronic alcoholic with gynecomastia by Pedersen and Homburger.[120] Rarely is such a fully expressed syndrome encountered.

Nearly all Leydig cell tumors occur in older adults and in two large series of ovarian tumors in children and adolescents, no Leydig cell tumors were encountered.[3,112] However, in a review of 34 reported examples of Leydig cell tumors by Boivin and Richart,[20] three neoplasms occurred in premenarchial children and one in an older adolescent. Several examples of Leydig cell tumors have been reported to occur in association with gonadal dysgenesis.[151]

In premenarchial children, the tumors usually produce varying degrees of the pure masculinizing syndrome with short stature; growth of pubic, axillary, and facial hair; and hypertrophy of the clitoris. In postmenarchial patients, the initial manifestation is usually oligomenorrhea, followed by amenorrhea, with signs of defeminization and virilization. Most tumors are diagnosed before advanced signs of masculinization are present. Other findings that have been found in some adult patients include polycythemia, hypertension, and impaired glucose tolerance. The urinary 17-ketosteroids are normal or slightly elevated. The serum and urinary testosterone levels may be increased.

### Survival information

Practically all Leydig cell tumors are benign, with no tendency to infiltrate locally or to seed the peritoneum. Following their removal, there is regression of virilized and masculinized signs to varying degrees. This is more complete in children and adolescents than in older adults.

## Sertoli–Leydig Cell Tumor (Arrhenoblastoma, Arrhenoma)

Most Sertoli–Leydig cell tumors occur in young women who have previously had normal menstrual cycles. They rarely occur prior to menarche.[3,15,112] In the O'Hern and Neubecker series[115] six of 31 patients (19%) were less than 20 years of age. The youngest patient was 9 years of age. Eighteen percent of arrhenoblastomas reviewed by Pedowitz and O'Brien[122] were less than 20 years of age.

Classically, the initial complaints are a progressive oligomenorrhea, leading to amenorrhea, followed by loss of feminine body contour, atrophy of breasts, loss of hair, and sterility. Primary amenorrhea is the initial complaint in younger adolescents.[38] Masculinization follows defeminization and includes development of male habitus, deepening and roughening of the voice, prominence of the larynx, facial and body hirsutism, acne, and hypertrophy of the clitoris. These manifestations are attributed to the production of androgens, particularly testosterone.[43] The amount of circulating testosterone need not be great to produce systemic manifestations. In a few patients, there is evidence of estrogen production by the tumor and the patient may present with menorrhagia and endometrial hyperplasia. The clinical findings of Cushing's syndrome occur in a few patients.[28,111] Neoplasms occurring during pregnancy may cause somatosexual abnormalities in the female offspring.[22] Not all patients manifest an endocrinopathy and the presenting complaints in its absence are abdominal enlargement and/or pain. The familial occurrence of arrhenoblastomas, commonly in adolescents with associated thyroid disease, particularly adenomas, has been recorded.[77]

Approximately 25% of Sertoli–Leydig cell tumors are clinically malignant.[75] Most of these belong to the intermediate and, more frequently, the undifferentiated groups. None of the 17 Sertoli–Leydig cell tumors encountered in two large series of ovarian tumors in the first two decades of life were clinically malignant.[3,112] Treatment should be conservative unless there is proved extension beyond the ovary. Regression of the masculinized features may be considerable, particularly in younger patients, but is not always complete. There are a number of examples of patients having normal pregnancies after removal of a Sertoli–Leydig cell tumor.

## Granulosa–Theca Cell Tumor (Thecagranulosa Tumor)

The clinical manifestations do not differ significantly from those caused by granulosa and by Sertoli cell tumors, although there is more likely to be evidence of estrogenic activity. Rare tumors may also cause virilization or masculinization. Most thecagranulosa tumors occur in adults and in our series of 188 ovarian tumors in patients under 20 years of age, only two were thecagranulosa tumors in 13- and 14-year-old girls.[3] There is some evidence to suggest that these neoplasms are less likely to recur or metastasize than the pure granulosa cell tumors.[27]

# Tumors of Nonspecialized Gonadal Mesenchyme

Included in this category is a heterogeneous group of mesenchymal tumors, most of which arise from supportive and vascular tissues that the ovary has in common with other organs. In our series of 188 ovarian neoplasms in children and adolescents, there were eight tumors (4%) in this category.[3] They included three fibromas in patients 15, 18, and 19 years of age; three supportive tissue sarcomas in patients 11, 14, and 17 years of age; and two malignant lymphomas. Other tumors that have been reported in this age group include hemangiomas,[97,130] lymphangioma,[112] a possible ganglioneuroma,[131] fibrosarcomas,[112,145] stromal sarcomas,[10] and teratoid sarcomas.[10]

## Sarcomas

Although supportive tissue sarcomas of the ovary are infrequent neoplasms, a significant proportion occur in older children and adolescents. In our material there were two fibrosarcomas, thought to be of relatively low-grade malignancy microscopically, and a pleomorphic sarcoma that could not be classified. The disease proved aggressive in all three patients and they died of their disease within a year of diagnosis.[3] A similar experience was reported by Thompson et al.[145]; two 14-year-old girls with ovarian fibrosarcomas died within 4 months.

The three sarcomas in our series were large, ill-defined, solid but soft, gray tumor masses that invaded the mesovarium and adjacent adnexal structures. The two fibrosarcomas consisted of small interlacing spindle cells with minimal amounts of fine collagen fibers. The nuclei were hyperchromatic and moderately pleomorphic. Mitotic figures were present but not numerous. The third unclassified sarcoma showed marked cellular and nuclear pleomorphism with numerous mitotic figures.

Azoury and Woodruff[10] reported a series of primary ovarian sarcomas from the Emil Novak Ovarian Tumor Registry. They divided them into three categories; teratoid sarcoma, stromal and mesenchymal sarcomas, and Müllerian sarcomas, including carcinosarcomas. Ten of 47 neoplasms occurred in patients who were less than 20 years of age.

The teratoid sarcomas consisted of an overgrowth of sarcomatous tissue in teratomas and teratocarcinomas. Most of the sarcomatous component was undifferentiated and not classifiable, but in several tumors rhabdomyomatous, leiomyomatous, and chondromatous differentiation was discernible (Figure 27.36). Seven of the 10 patients were 7 to 18 years of age. All patients for whom survival information was available died of their disease within a few months. All apparent sarcomas of the ovary in children and adolescents should be thoroughly examined, both grossly and microscopically to ascertain whether the lesion is a teratoid sarcoma, as the evidence indicates

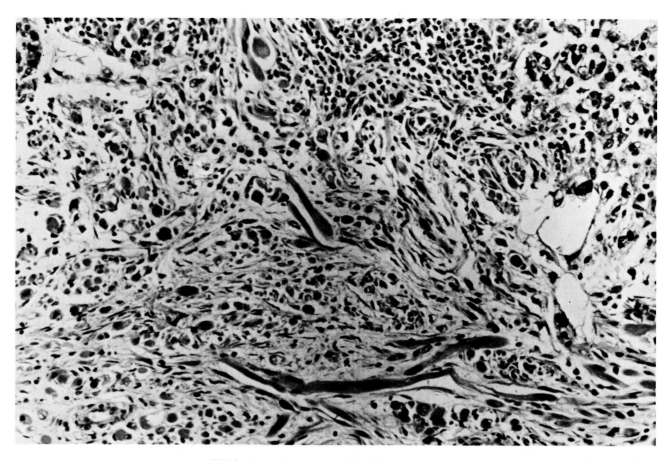

**27.36** Teratoid sarcoma. Rhabdomyosarcoma comprised about two-thirds of this ovarian tumor; the other one-third was teratocarcinoma. Hematoxylin–eosin, ×152.

that they tend to pursue a more aggressive course than certain other types of sarcomas.

Three of seven patients with stromal sarcoma were 11, 13, and 17 years of age.[10] In two of the patients the neoplasms were unilateral and in one they were bilateral. These tumors consisted of spindle and stellate cells with sparse collagen, hyperchromatic nuclei, and frequent mitotic figures. Two patients for whom survival information was available were alive 6 and 14 years later. Their sarcomas were considered to be of low-grade malignancy. There were no children or adolescents in the group of Müllerian sarcomas.

## Malignant Lymphoma

Malignant lymphoma may involve the ovary primarily so that the presenting manifestations are those of a primary ovarian tumor. In nearly every series of ovarian tumors from children and adolescents, there are several examples of malignant lymphoma.[3,112] This is particularly true in certain countries where Burkitt's or African lymphoma is prevalent.[25,40,114] Brew and Jackson[23] stressed the frequency of lymphomatous involvement of the ovaries in young girls; 14 of 16 ovarian tumors excised from young girls were malignant lymphomas. Seven of 35 malignant lymphomas of the ovary reported by Woodruff et al.[157] occurred in patients less than 20 years of age.

In most instances both ovaries were involved, although the disease may predominate in one with little evidence of involvement of the other. The tumors are solid but soft and often somewhat nodular. They are usually gray or pinkish gray in color and sometimes dotted with petechiae (Figure 27.37). Very commonly there is gross extension into the mesovarium and the broad ligament may be infiltrated.

Most ovarian lymphomas in children and adolescents

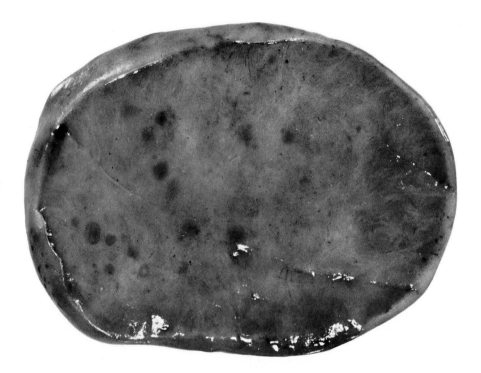

**27.37** Malignant lymphoma of ovary from a 15-year-old girl. Ovarian tissue is replaced by a homogeneous, grayish tumor tissue with dark hemorrhagic foci.

are of the undifferentiated B-lymphocytic type (Burkitt's tumor, African lymphoma) (Figures 27.38 and 27.39). The ovary is replaced by sheets of closely packed primitive lymphocytic cells of fairly uniform size and shape. They have scant rims of amphophilic cytoplasm and relatively large round or oval nuclei with prominent nuclear membranes, coarse chromatin, and commonly one or two small prominent nucleoli. Scattered haphazardly throughout the tumor are large, pale histiocytes with almost clear cytoplasm that give the tissue sections a characteristic starry-sky or water-pot appearance. Ovarian lymphoma is commonly misdiagnosed as granulosa cell tumor, germinoma, or malignant stromal tumor. Initially there is often a favorable response to chemotherapy, but the disease soon recurs, becomes generalized, and results in death.

## Nonneoplastic Tumors of the Ovary

There are several nonneoplastic diseases of the ovary that may result in a sufficiently enlarged mass to be detected clinically. They must be differentiated from true neoplasms and celiotomy may be required to make this differentiation. In many of the reported early series of ovarian tumors in children and adolescents, these lesions, particularly the cysts, comprised a significant percentage.

## Follicle and Luteinized Follicle Cysts in Infants and Children

Cystic follicles are normally present in all ovaries of infants and children. Follicle cysts are infrequent but account for one-third to one-half of clinically significant ovarian enlargements in girls under 15 years of age.[36,144] A common symptom is pain resulting from torsion. There are two peaks in their occurrence, the neonatal and the prepubertal periods. They are all follicle cysts but some show luteinization of granulosa and theca cells and so are referred to as luteinized follicle cysts.

In the newborn infant, follicle cysts may become quite large, 8 to 12 cm in diameter, and rise into the abdominal cavity causing enlargement of the abdomen, sometimes with signs of intestinal obstruction.[24,86,109] The cause is thought to be either an excessive or an altered response to maternal gonadotropins. The cysts have thin translucent walls and usually definite pedicles. The contents are watery and clear or yellow-tinged. The lining is composed of small dark granulosa cells that in some areas may take on a luteinized appearance (Figure 27.40).

In premenarchial children, precocious sexual development may be associated with follicle cysts and is characterized by hypertrophy of the breasts, cyclic vaginal bleeding, enlargement and pigmentation of the labia minora,

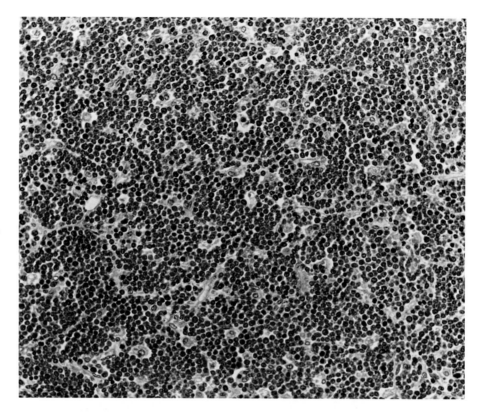

**27.38** Malignant lymphoma of ovary of Burkitt type showing the classic starry-sky appearance. Hematoxylin–eosin, ×162.

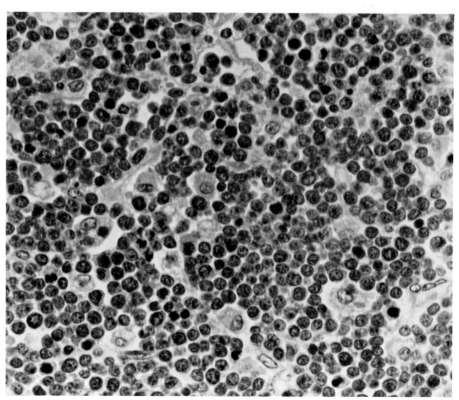

**27.39** Higher magnification of lymphoma illustrated in Figures 27.37 and 27.38. Uniform, enlarged lymphocytes with scant, ill-defined cytoplasm are seen, along with scattered larger pale histiocytic-appearing cells. Hematoxylin–eosin, ×425.

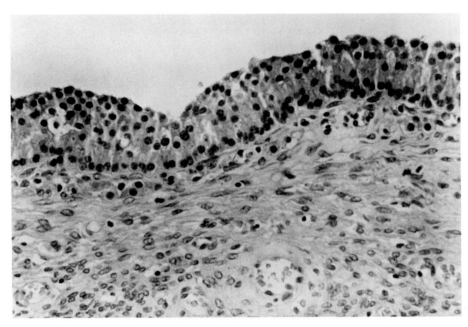

**27.40** Follicle cyst of the ovary of an infant who had clinical signs of estrogen stimulation. The wall is formed by several layers of uniform follicular (granulosa) cells. Hematoxylin–eosin, ×190.

growth of pubic hair, and enlargement of the uterus. In some instances removal of these cysts has resulted in regression of the precocious symptoms,[83,139] whereas in others the precocity has persisted or recurred after a temporary regression.[36,105,144] These observations suggest that there may be two different mechanisms or syndromes involved, one a gonadal precocity and the other a constitutional or pituitary precocity. The follicle cysts of the gonadal form are usually solitary, unilocular, and 4 to 6 cm in diameter, and the opposite ovary is small and has the immature appearance expected for the patient's age. Blood and urine levels of estrogens are elevated but return to normal with removal of the cyst. In the constitutional or pituitary form of the disease the cysts tend to be multiple and both ovaries are enlarged or, when the cysts are limited to one ovary, the other ovary resembles that of a menarchial child. Ovulation may actually occur in this syndrome. Although the cysts are basically follicular, there may be considerable luteinization.

## Follicle and Lutein Cysts in Postmenarchial Children and Adolescents

Follicle and lutein cysts in this age period do not differ from those encountered throughout the reproductive period. They vary from 2.5 to 10 cm in diameter but are not often more than 5 cm. They tend to regress spontaneously and only occasionally is celiotomy indicated for diagnosis. Some are the cause of menstrual irregularities and the large cysts may cause pelvic discomfort or symptoms because of pressure on adjacent organs. Acute pain usually means torsion of the pedicle or rupture.

### Follicle cysts

Follicle cysts are unilocular and spherical, with smooth, glistening linings and thin walls. The contents are watery and clear or yellow and may contain significant levels of estrogen.[6] The lining consists of one to several layers of granulosa (follicular) epithelium supported by a thin fibrous theca.

### Corpus luteum and follicle lutein cysts

Corpus luteum and follicle lutein cysts result from hemorrhage or exudation of serum into the lumen, usually after the rupture of a mature follicle. The cyst is roughly spherical and unilocular, and the contents are water clear, yellow, or blood tinged. The wall consists of a gray, yellow, or orange layer of luteinized cells of varying thickness with an inner thin white coat of young fibrous tissue (Figure 27.41). Microscopically the appearance varies with the age of the lesion. Classically the wall is formed of luteinized granulosa cells with an outer, less well-defined

**27.41** Corpus luteum cyst of the ovary of an adolescent which measured 5 cm in diameter. A layer of gray, luteinized tissue, yellow in the fresh state, is seen within the wall. ×2.4.

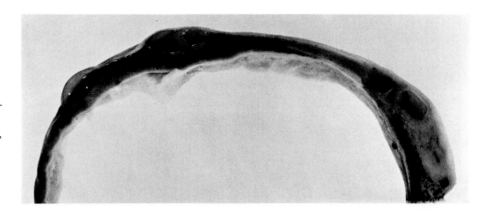

**27.42** Corpus luteum cyst. The inner surface (top) consists of organizing fibrous tissue. Beneath this is a well-defined zone of luteinized granulosa cells. Hematoxylin–eosin, ×113.

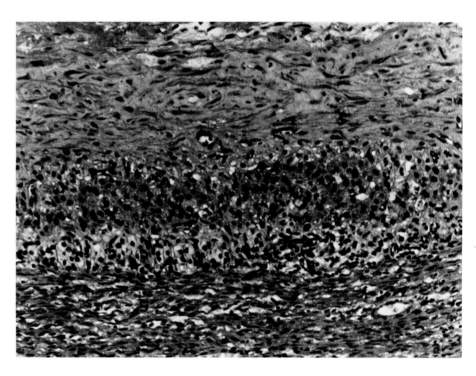

and often patchy zone of theca interna cells luteinized to a lesser degree (Figure 27.42). In the older cysts, the luteinized wall may be thin, irregularly absent, or replaced entirely by a hyaline acellular material. The cyst may then appropriately be termed a corpus albicans cyst, a late variant or a sequel of a corpus luteum cyst.

## Massive Edema of the Ovary

Massive edema caused by partial torsion or kinking of the mesovarium results in a large white, wet ovary, up to 12 cm in diameter (Figure 27.43).[78] Most examples have been encountered in the third decade of life, but examples are seen in children and adolescents. The clinical manifestations are lower abdominal discomfort or pain, sometimes episodic, and the finding of an adnexal pelvic mass. Microscopically, the changes simulate a soft fibroma. There is diffuse edema involving primarily the medulla and the inner cytogenic cortex, with little or no alteration in the tunica albuginea (Figure 27.44). The medullary veins are markedly dilated and there may be a few petechial hemorrhages. Inspection of the mesovarium usually reveals some twisting or kinking. In most instances, there is no evidence of any underlying abnormality in the involved ovary

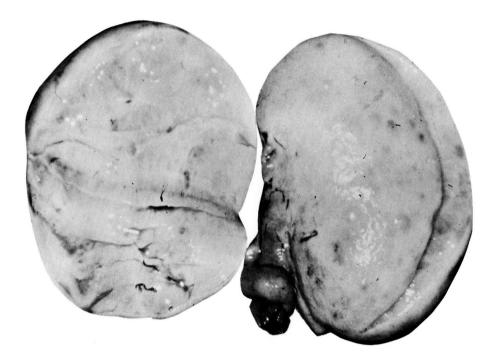

**27.43** Massive edema of the ovary. The large, pale, wet ovary with torsion of the pedicle is visible in the dark area to right of center.

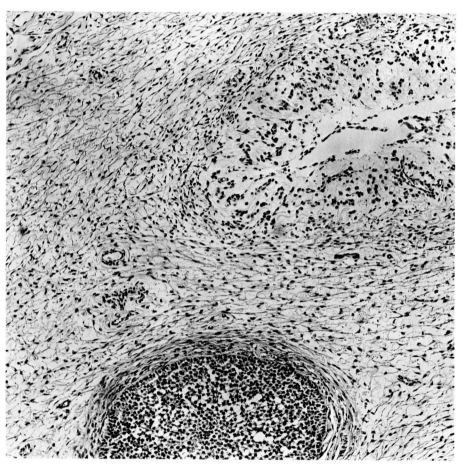

**27.44** Massive edema of the ovary. Stromal cells and cells of follicle are widely separated by edema. Hematoxylin–eosin ×110.

or in the opposite ovary. There is a danger that at celiotomy the solid nature of the ovarian mass may be interpreted as a malignant neoplasm and excessive surgical procedures carried out.

## Massive Hemorrhagic Infarct of the Normal Ovary

In children and adolescents, ovarian cysts and tumors are prone to torsion and hence infarction of the ovary. Massive infarction may also involve a normal ovary or a normal ovary and fallopian tube, particularly in infants and children, in whom these structures are often extremely mobile.[74,133] The classic manifestation is severe acute lower abdominal pain, which may have been preceded by less severe or mild episotic lower abdominal pain or discomfort. Abdominal or rectal examination often discloses either a lower abdominal mass or mass in the pelvis, near or at its brim.

At celiotomy the ovary is enlarged, up to 15 cm, and totally replaced by massive hemorrhage. There may be tears in its capsule, resulting in pelvic hemorrhage. Torsion of the ovarian pedicle is usually clearly visible. The cut surface is a solid mass of blood in which the outlines of scattered cortical structures may be discernible. Microscopically there is massive hemorrhage, with fragmentation of tissues and varying degrees of necrosis and leukocytic infiltration. The hilar vessels may be thrombosed. Careful examination of more solid and viable-appearing areas is essential in order to exclude the possibility of an underlying neoplasm.

Massive edema and massive infarct are variations of the same theme; the differences being dictated by the degree of torsion and the stage at which the disease is diagnosed. One of our patients, a 13-year-old girl, had massive edema of one ovary and massive infarct of the other.[78]

# REFERENCES

1. Abell, M. R. The nature and classification of ovarian neoplasms. *Can. Med. Assoc. J.* 94:1102, 1966.

2. Abell, M. R. Undifferentiated malignant germ cell neoplasm (embryonal carcinoma) of ovary with stromal luteinization and masculinization. *Am. J. Obstet. Gynecol. 101*:570, 1968.

3. Abell, M. R., and Holtz, F. Ovarian neoplasms in childhood and adolescence. II. Tumors of non-germ cell origin. *Am. J. Obstet. Gynecol.* 93:850, 1965.

4. Abell, M. R., Johnson, V. J., and Holtz, F. Ovarian neoplasms in childhood and adolescence. I. Tumors of germ cell origin. *Am. J. Obstet. Gynecol.* 92:1059, 1965.

5. Abitbol, M. M., Pomerance, W., and Mackles, A. Spontaneous intraperitoneal rupture of benign cystic teratomas. Review of literature and report of two cases. *Obstet. Gynecol.* 13:198, 1959.

6. Adair, F. L., and Watts, R. M. A study of the hormonal content of ovarian cyst fluids. *Am. J. Obstet. Gynecol.* 34:799, 1937.

7. Allibone, E. C., and Collins, D. H. Symptomatic haemolytic anaemia associated with ovarian teratoma in a child. *J. Clin. Pathol.* 4:412, 1951.

8. Anderson, W. R., Levine, A. J., and MacMillan, D. Granulosa–theca cell tumors: Clinical and pathologic study. *Am. J. Obstet. Gynecol.* 110:32, 1971.

9. Asadourian, L. A., and Taylor, H. B. Dysgerminoma. An analysis of 105 cases. *Obstet. Gynecol.* 33:370, 1969.

10. Azoury, R. S., and Woodruff, J. D. Primary ovarian sarcomas. Report of 43 cases from the Emil Novak Ovarian Tumor Registry. *Obstet. Gynecol.* 37:920, 1971.

11. Ballas, M. Yolk sac carcinoma of the ovary with alpha fetoprotein in serum and ascitic fluid demonstrated by immunoosmophoresis. *Am. J. Clin. Pathol.* 57:511, 1972.

12. Barber, H. R. K., and Graber, E. A. Gynecological tumors in childhood and adolescence. *Obstet. Gynecol. Surv.* 28(Suppl):357, 1973.

13. Barry, K. G., and Crosby, W. H. Auto-immune hemolytic anemia arrested by removal of an ovarian teratoma: Review of the literature and report of a case. *Ann. Int. Med.* 47:1002, 1957.

14. Benirschke, K., Easterday, C., and Abramson, D. Malignant solid teratoma of the ovary. Report of three cases. *Obstet. Gynecol.* 15:512, 1960.

15. Berendsen, P. B., Smith, E. B., Abell, M. R., and Jaffe, R. B. Fine structure of Leydig cells from an arrhenoblastoma of the ovary. *Am. J. Obstet. Gynecol.* 103:192, 1969.

16. Berlin, N. I., Van Scott, E. J., Clendenning, W. E., et al. Basal cell nevus syndrome. Combined clinical staff conference at the National Institutes of Health. *Ann. Int. Med.* 64:403, 1966.

17. Bernstein, D., Naor, S., Rikover, M., and Menahem, H. Hemolytic anemia related to ovarian tumor. *Obstet. Gynecol.* 43:276, 1974.

18. Biskind, G. R., and Biskind, M. S. Experimental ovarian tumors in rats. *Am. J. Clin. Pathol.* 19:501, 1949.

19. Biskind, M. S., and Biskind, G. R. Development of tumors in the rat ovary after transplantation into the spleen. *Proc. Soc. Exp. Biol. Med.* 55:176, 1944.

20. Boivin, Y., and Richart, R. M. Hilus cell tumors of the ovary. A review with a report of 3 new cases. *Cancer* 18:231, 1965.

21. Breen, J. L., and Neubecker, R. D. Malignant teratoma of the ovary. An analysis of 17 cases. *Obstet. Gynecol.* 21:669, 1963.

22. Brentnall, C. P. A case of arrhenoblastoma complicating pregnancy. *J. Obstet. Gynaecol. Br. Emp.* 52:235, 1945.

23. Brew, D. StJ., and Jackson, J. G. Lymphosarcoma in the ovary in young African girls in Nigeria. *Br. J. Cancer* 14:621, 1960.

24. Brune, W. H., Pulaski, E. J., and Shuey, H. E. Giant ovarian cyst. Report of a case in a premature infant. *N. Engl. J. Med.* 257:876, 1957.

25. Burkitt, D., and O'Conor, G. T. Malignant lymphoma in African children. I. A clinical syndrome. *Cancer* 14:258, 1961.

26. Burslem, R. W., Langley, F. A., and Woodcock, A. S. A clinicopathological study of oestrogenic ovarian tumors. *Cancer* 7:522, 1954.

27. Busby, T., and Anderson, G. W. Feminizing mesenchymomas of the ovary. Includes 107 cases of granulosa–, granu-

losa–theca-cell, and theca-cell tumors. *Am. J. Obstet. Gynecol.* 68:1391, 1954.

28. Canelo, C. K., and Lisser, H. A case of arrhenoblastoma which simulated Cushing's disease. *Endocrinology* 24:838, 1939.

29. Case records of the Massachusetts General Hospital. Case 13-1970. Edited by B. Castleman. *N. Engl. J. Med.* 282:676, 1970.

30. Caspi, E., Schreyer, P., and Bukovsky, J. Ovarian lutein cysts in pregnancy. *Obstet. Gynecol.* 42:388, 1973.

31. Chalvardjian, A., and Scully, R. E. Sclerosing stromal tumors of the ovary. *Cancer* 31:664, 1973.

32. Charache, H. Ovarian tumors in childhood. Report of six new cases and review of the literature. *Arch. Surg.* 79:573, 1959.

33. Christian, C. D. Ovarian tumors: An extension of the Peutz-Jeghers syndrome. *Am. J. Obstet. Gynecol.* 111:529, 1971.

34. Cianfrani, T. Neoplasms in apparently normal ovaries. *Am. J. Obstet. Gynecol.* 51:246, 1946.

35. Cocco, A. E., and Conway, S. J. Zollinger–Ellison Syndrome associated with ovarian mucinous cystadenocarcinoma. *N. Eng. J. Med.* 293:485, 1975.

36. Costin, M. E. Jr., and Kennedy, R. L. J. Ovarian tumors in infants and children. *Am. J. Dis. Child.* 76:127, 1948.

37. Croft, P. B., and Wilkinson, M. The incidence of carcinomatous neuromyopathy in patients with various types of carcinoma. *Brain* 88:427, 1965.

38. Cruikshank, D. P., and Chapler, F. K. Arrhenoblastomas and associated ovarian pathology. *Obstet. Gynecol.* 43:539, 1974.

39. Damjanov, I., Drobnjak, P., Grizelj, V., and Longhino, N. Sclerosing stromal tumor of the ovary. A hormonal and ultrastructural analysis. *Obstet. Gynecol.* 45:675, 1975.

40. Davies, J. N. P. Cancer in Africa. in D. H. Collins, ed., *Modern Trends in Pathology.* Butterworth and Co., London, 1958.

41. Della Porta, G. Induction of intestinal, mammary, and ovarian tumors in hamsters with oral administration of 20-methylcholanthrene. *Cancer Res.* 21:575, 1961.

42. Denny-Brown, D. Primary sensory neuropathy with muscular changes associated with carcinoma. *J. Neurol. Neurosurg. Psychiatry.* 11:73, 1948.

43. Dorfman, R. I. Steroid hormones in gynecology. *Obstet. Gynecol. Surv.* 18:65, 1963.

44. Ehrlich, E. N., Dominguez, O. V., Samuels, L. T., Lynch, D., Oberhelman, H. Jr., and Warner, N. E. Aldosteronism and precocious puberty due to an ovarian androblastoma (Sertoli cell tumor). *J. Clin. Endocrinol.* 23:358, 1963.

45. Ein, S. H. Malignant ovarian tumors in children. *J. Pediatr. Surg.* 8:539, 1973.

46. Ein, S. H., Darte, J. M. M., and Stephens, C. A. Cystic and solid ovarian tumors in children; a 44-year review. *J. Pediatr. Surg.* 5:148, 1970.

47. Esterhay, R. J., Shapiro, H. M., Sutherland, J. C., McIntire, K. R., and Wiernik, P. H. Serum alpha fetoprotein concentration and tumor growth dissociation in a patient with ovarian teratocarcinoma. *Cancer* 31:835, 1973.

48. Falin, L. I. The development of genital glands and the origin of germ cells in human embryogenesis. *Acta Anat.* 72:195, 1969.

49. Favara, B. E., and Franciosi, R. A. Ovarian teratoma and neuroglial implants on the peritoneum. *Cancer* 31:678, 1973.

50. Feld, D., Labes, J., and Nathanson, M. Bilateral ovarian dermoid cysts in triplets. *Obstet. Gynecol.* 27:525, 1966.

51. Ferenczy, A., Okagaki, T., and Richart, R. M. Para-endocrine hypercalcemia in ovarian neoplasms. Report of meso-

nephroma with hypercalcemia and review of literature. *Cancer* 27:427, 1971.

52. Flick, F. H., and Banfield, R. S. Jr. Malignant theca-cell tumors. Two new case reports and review of the eight published cases. *Cancer* 9:731, 1956.

53. Forney, J. P., Di Saia, P. J., and Morrow, C. P. Endodermal sinus tumor. A report of two sustained remissions treated postoperatively with a combination of actinomycin D, 5-fluorouracil, and cyclophosphamide. *Obstet. Gynecol.* 45:186, 1975.

54. Fortt, R. W., and Mathie, I. K. Gliomatosis peritonei caused by ovarian teratoma. *J. Clin. Pathol.* 22:348, 1969.

55. Furth, J., and Butterworth, J. S. Neoplastic diseases occurring among mice subjected to general irradiation with x-rays. II. Ovarian tumors and associated lesions. *Am. J. Cancer* 28:66, 1936.

56. Gardner, W. U. Some studies on ovarian tumorigenesis, in G. E. W. Wolstenholme and M. O'Connor, eds., *CIBA Foundation Colloquia on Endocrinology,* Vol. 12. *Hormone Production in Endocrine Tumours.* Little Brown and Co., Boston, 1958, pp. 153–172.

57. Gerbie, M. V., Brewer, J. I., and Tamimi, H. Primary choriocarcinoma of the ovary. *Obstet. Gynecol.* 46:720, 1975.

58. Gillman, J. The development of the gonads in man, with a consideration of the role of fetal endocrines and the histogenesis of ovarian tumors. *Contrib. Embryol. Carnegie Inst.* 32:81, 1948.

59. Gondos, B., and Monroe, S. A. Cystic granulosa cell tumor with massive hemoperitoneum. Light and electron microscopic study. *Obstet. Gynecol.* 38:683, 1971.

60. Gonzalez-Angulo, A., Kaufman, R. H., Braungardt, C. D., Chapman, F. C., and Hinshaw, A. J. Adenocarcinoma of thyroid arising in struma ovarii (malignant struma ovarii). Report of two cases and review of the literature. *Obstet. Gynecol.* 21:567, 1963.

61. Goodall, C. M. On para-endocrine cancer syndromes: A review. *Int. J. Cancer* 4:1, 1969.

62. Gordon, T., Crittenden, M., and Haenszel, W. Cancer mortality trends in the United States, 1930–1955, in, *United States National Cancer Institute: End Results and Mortality Trends in Cancer,* Monograph No. 6, Washington, D.C., 1961, p. 131.

63. Gough, A. A case of disgerminoma of the ovary associated with masculinity. *J. Obstet. Gynaecol. Br. Emp.* 45:799, 1938.

64. Groeber, W. R. Ovarian tumors during infancy and childhood. *Am. J. Obstet. Gynecol.* 86:1027, 1963.

65. Hain, A. M. An unusual case of precocious puberty associated with ovarian dysgerminoma. *J. Clin. Endocrinol.* 9:1349, 1949.

66. Heald, F. P., Craig, J. M., and Ming, P.-M. L. Ovarian tumors in adolescence: Types and presenting features. *Clin. Pediatr.* 6:401, 1967.

67. Henderson, D. N. Granulosa and theca cell tumors of the ovary: With a report of thirty cases. *Am. J. Obstet. Gynecol.* 43:194, 1942.

68. Hertig, A. T., and Gore, H. Tumors of the ovary and fallopian tube, in *Tumors of the Female Sex Organs, Atlas of Tumor Pathology,* Fasc. 33, Part 3. Washington, D.C., Armed Forces Institute of Pathology, 1961.

69. Hesseltine, H. C., and Smith, R. L. Ovarian malignancy. *Am. J. Obstet. Gynecol.* 72:1326, 1956.

70. Hodgson, J. E., Dockerty, M. B., and Mussey, R. D. Granulosa cell tumor of the ovary. A clinical and pathologic review of sixty-two cases. *Surg. Gynecol. Obstet.* 81:631, 1945.

71. Holt, G. W. Idiopathic neuropathy in cancer. A first sign in multiple system syndromes associated with malignancy. *Am. J. Med. Sci.* 242:93, 1961.

624

72. Howell, J. S., Marchant, J., and Orr, J. W. The induction of ovarian tumours in mice with 9:10-dimethyl-1:2-benzanthracene. *Br. J. Cancer* 8:635, 1954.

73. Huntington, R. W. Jr., and Bullock, W. K. Yolk sac tumors of the ovary. *Cancer* 25:1357, 1970.

74. James, D. F., Barber, H. R. K., and Graber, E. A. Torsion of normal uterine adnexa in children. Report of three cases. *Obstet. Gynecol.* 35:226, 1970.

75. Javert, C. T., and Finn, W. F. Arrhenoblastoma. The incidence of malignancy and the relationship to pregnancy, to sterility, and to treatment. *Cancer* 4:60, 1951.

76. Jensen, R. D., and Norris, H. J. Epithelial tumors of the ovary. Occurrence in children and adolescents less than 20 years of age. *Arch. Pathol.* 94:29, 1972.

77. Jensen, R. D., Norris, H. J., and Fraumeni, J. F. Jr. Familial arrhenoblastoma and thyroid adenoma. *Cancer* 33:218, 1974.

78. Kalstone, C. E., Jaffe, R. B., and Abell, M. R. Massive edema of the ovary simulating fibroma. *Obstet. Gynecol.* 34:564, 1969.

79. Kase, N. Steroid synthesis in abnormal ovaries. II. Granulosa cell tumor. *Am. J. Obstet. Gynecol.* 90:1262, 1964.

80. Kay, S., Silverberg, S. G., and Schatzki, P. F. Ultrastructure of an ovarian dysgerminoma: Report of a case featuring neurosecretory-type granules in stromal cells. *Am. J. Clin. Pathol.* 58:458, 1972.

81. Kelley, R. R., and Scully, R. E. Cancer developing in dermoid cysts of the ovary. A report of 8 cases, including a carcinoid and a leiomyosarcoma. *Cancer* 14:989, 1961.

82. Kempers, R. D., Dockerty, M. B., Hoffman, D. L., and Bartholomew, L. G. Struma ovarii—Ascitic, hyperthyroid, and asymptomatic syndromes. *Ann. Int. Med.* 72:883, 1970.

83. Kimmel, G. C. Sexual precocity and accelerated growth in a child with a follicular cyst of the ovary. *J. Pediatr.* 30:686, 1947.

84. Kistner, R. W. Intraperitoneal rupture of benign cystic teratomas. Review of the literature with a report of two cases. *Obstet. Gynecol. Surv.* 7:603, 1952.

85. Kleinsmith, L. J., and Pierce, G. B. Jr. Multipotentiality of single embryonal carcinoma cells. *Cancer Res.* 24:1554, 1964.

86. Kunstadter, R. H., Schultz, A., and Strauss, A. A. Large ovarian cyst in a newborn infant. *Am. J. Dis. Child.* 80:993, 1950.

87. Kurrein, F., and Fothergill, R. J. Oleo-keratin granuloma in peritoneum: A rare complication of ovarian dermoid. *J. Obstet. Gynaecol. Br. Commonw.* 68:124, 1961.

88. Li, F. P., Fraumeni, J. F. Jr., and Dalager, N. Ovarian cancers in the young. Epidemiologic observations. *Cancer* 32:969, 1973.

89. Li, F. P., Rapoport, A. H., Fraumeni, J. F. Jr., and Jensen, R. D. Familial ovarian carcinoma. *J. Am. Med. Assoc.* 214:1559, 1970.

90. Lieberman, J. S., Borrero, J., Urdaneta, E., and Wright, I. S. Thrombophlebitis and cancer. *J. Am. Med. Assoc.* 177:542, 1961.

91. Liebert, K. I., and Stent, L. Dysgerminoma of the ovary with chorion-epithelioma. *J. Obstet. Gynaecol. Br. Emp.* 67:627, 1960.

92. Lindfors, O. Primary ovarian neoplasms in infants and children. A study of 81 cases diagnosed in Finland and Sweden. *Ann. Chir. Gynaecol. Fenn.* 60:12, 1971, Suppl. 177.

93. Lipsett, M. B., Odell, W. D., Rosenberg, L. E., and Waldmann, T. A. Humoral syndromes associated with nonendocrine tumors. *Ann. Int. Med.* 61:733, 1964.

94. Lyon, F. A., Sinykin, M. B., and McKelvey, J. L. Granulosa-cell tumors of the ovary. Review of 23 cases. *Obstet. Gynecol.* 21:67, 1963.

95. MacAulay, M. A., Weliky, I., and Schulz, R. A. Ultrastructure of a biosynthetically active granulosa cell tumor. *Lab. Invest.* 17:562, 1967.

96. Mackinlay, C. J. Male cells in granulosa cell tumours. *J. Obstet. Gynaecol. Br. Emp.* 64:512, 1957.

97. Mann, L. S., and Metrick, S. Hemangioma of the ovary. Report of a case. *J. Int. Coll. Surg.* 36:500, 1961.

98. Marrubini, G. Primary chorionepithelioma of the ovary. Report of two cases. *Acta Obstet. Gynaecol. Scand.* 28:251, 1949.

99. Masopust, J., Kithier, K., Radl, J., Koutecky, J., and Kotal, L. Occurrence of fetoprotein in patients with neoplasms and non-neoplastic diseases. *Int. J. Cancer* 3:364, 1968.

100. Masson, P. Sur la présence de cellules argentaffines dans les kystes pseudomucineux de l'ovaire. *Union Med Canada* 67:2, 1938.

101. McAndrew, G. M. Haemolytic anaemia associated with ovarian teratoma. *Br. Med. J.* 2:1307, 1964.

102. McGoldrick, J. L., and Lapp, W. A. Theca-cell tumors of the ovary. *Am. J. Obstet. Gynecol.* 48:409, 1944.

103. McKay, D. G., Hertig, A. T., Adams, E. C., and Danziger, S. Histochemical observations on the germ cells of human embryos. *Anat. Rec.* 117:201, 1953.

104. Melicow, M. M., and Uson, A. C. Dysgenetic gonadomas and other gonadal neoplasms in intersexes. Report of 5 cases and review of the literature. *Cancer* 12:552, 1959.

105. Mengert, W. F. Precocious puberty due to an ovarian cyst in a five-year-old girl. *Am. J. Obstet. Gynecol.* 37:485, 1939.

106. Mintz, B. Formation and early development of germ cells. *Symposium on the Germ Cells and Earliest Stages of Development.* Milan, Fondazione A Baselli Instituto Lombardo, 1961.

107. Mueller, C. W., Topkins, P., and Lapp, W. A. Dysgerminoma of the ovary: An analysis of 427 cases. *Am. J. Obstet. Gynecol.* 60:153, 1950.

108. Neigus, I. Ovarian dysgerminoma with chorionepithelioma: Report of a case. *Am. J. Obstet. Gynecol.* 69:838, 1955.

109. Neikirk, W. I., and Hudson, H. W. Jr. Giant ovarian cyst in a newborn infant. *N. Engl. J. Med.* 239:468, 1948.

110. Neubecker, R. D., and Breen, J. L. Embryonal carcinoma of the ovary. *Cancer* 15:546, 1962.

111. Nichols, J., Warren, J. C., and Mantz, F. A. ACTH-like excretion from carcinoma of the ovary. The clinical effect of m, p'-DDD. *J. Am. Med. Assoc.* 182:713, 1962.

112. Norris, H. J., and Jensen, R. D. Relative frequency of ovarian neoplasms in children and adolescents. *Cancer* 30:713, 1972.

113. Novak, E. R., Kutchmeshgi, J., Mupas, R. S., and Woodruff, J. D. Feminizing gonadal stromal tumors. Analysis of the granulosa-theca cell tumors of the ovarian tumor registry. *Obstet. Gynecol.* 38:701, 1971.

114. O'Conor, G. T. Malignant lymphoma in African children. II. A pathological entity. *Cancer* 14:270, 1961.

115. O'Hern, T. M., and Neubecker, R. D. Arrhenoblastoma. *Obstet. Gynecol.* 19:758, 1962.

116. Omenn, G. S., Roth, S. I., and Baker, W. H. Hyperparathyroidism associated with malignant tumors of nonparathyroid origin. *Cancer* 24:1004, 1969.

117. O'Neill, R. T., and Mikuta, J. J. Hypoglycemia associated with serous cystadenocarcinoma of the ovary. *Obstet. Gynecol.* 35:287, 1970.

118. Pantoja, E., Rodriguez-Ibanez, I., Axtmayer, R. W., Noy,

M. A., and Pelegrina, I. Complications of dermoid tumors of the ovary. *Obstet. Gynecol. 45*:89, 1975.

119. Papadaki, L., and Beilby, J. O. W. Ovarian cystadenofibroma: A consideration of the role of estrogen in its pathogenesis. *Am. J. Obstet. Gynecol. 121*:501, 1975.

120. Pedersen, J., and Homburger, C. Virilizing Leydig cell tumour of the ovary. Report of a case with special reference to the hormone excretion. *Acta Endocrinol. 13*:109, 1953.

121. Pedowitz, P., Felmus, L. B., and Mackles, A. Precocious pseudopuberty due to ovarian tumors. *Obstet. Gynecol. Surv. 10*:633, 1955.

122. Pedowitz, P., and O'Brien, F. B. Arrhenoblastoma of the ovary. Review of the literature and report of 2 cases. *Obstet. Gynecol. 16*:62, 1960.

123. Peterson, W. F. Malignant degeneration of benign cystic teratomas of the ovary. A collective review of the literature. *Obstet. Gynecol. Surv. 12*:793, 1957.

124. Peterson, W. F., Prevost, E. C., Edmunds, F. T., Hundley, J. M. Jr., and Morris, F. K. Benign cystic teratomas of the ovary: A clinico-statistical study of 1,007 cases with a review of the literature. *Am. J. Obstet. Gynecol. 70*:368, 1955.

125. Pierce, G. B. Jr., Dixon, F. J. Jr., and Verney, E. L. Teratocarcinogenic and tissue-forming potentials of the cell types comprising neoplastic embryoid bodies. *Lab. Invest. 9*:583, 1960.

126. Pinkerton, J. H. M., McKay, D. G., Adams, E. C., and Hertig, A. T. Development of the human ovary—A study using histochemical technics. *Obstet. Gynecol. 18*:152, 1961.

127. Robboy, S. J., and Scully, R. E. Ovarian teratoma with glial implants on the peritoneum. *Hum. Pathol. 1*:643, 1970.

128. Rubin, I. C., Novak, J., and Squire, J. J. Ovarian fibromas and theca-cell tumors: Report of 78 cases with special reference to production of ascites and hydrothorax (Meigs' syndrome). *Am. J. Obstet. Gynecol. 48*:601, 1944.

129. Santesson, L., and Marrubini, G. Clinical and pathological survey of ovarian embryonal carcinomas, including so-called "mesonephromas" (Schiller), or "mesoblastomas" (Teilum), treated at the radiumhemmet. *Acta Obstet. Gynecol. Scand. 36*:399, 1957.

130. Schaeffer, M. H., and Cancelmo, J. J. Cavernous hemangioma of ovary in a girl twelve years of age. *Am. J. Obstet. Gynecol. 38*:722, 1939.

131. Schmeisser, H. C., and Anderson, W. A. D. Ganglioneuroma of the ovary. *J. Am. Med. Assoc. 111*:2005, 1938.

132. Schuler, D., and Juhasz, J. Choriocarcinoma in a female infant. *Ann. Paediatr.* (Basel) *195*:56, 1960.

133. Schultz, L. R., Newton, W. A. Jr., and Clatworthy, H. W. Jr. Torsion of previously normal tube and ovary in children. *N. Engl. J. Med. 268*:343, 1963.

134. Scully, R. E. Gonadoblastoma. A gonadal tumor related to the dysgerminoma (seminoma) and capable of sex-hormone production. *Cancer 6*:455, 1953.

135. Scully, R. E. Recent progress in ovarian cancer. *Hum. Pathol. 1*:73, 1970.

136. Scully, R. E. Gonadoblastoma. A review of 74 cases. *Cancer 25*:1340, 1970.

137. Shane, J. M., and Naftolin, F. Aberrant hormone activity of tumors of gynecologic importance. *Amer. J. Obstet. Gynecol. 121*:133, 1975.

138. Stein, I. F. Sr., and Kaye, B. M. Granulomatous peritonitis secondary to perforation of dermoid cyst. *Am. J. Obstet. Gynecol. 67*:155, 1954.

139. Steiner, M. M., and Hadawi, S. A. Sexual precocity. Association with follicular cysts of ovary. *Am. J. Dis. Child. 108*:28, 1964.

140. Sturley, R. F. Teratomatous chorionepithelioma of the ovary. Critical review of literature, with report of a new case. *Minn. Med. 25*:629, 1942.

141. Talerman, A., and Haije, W. G. Alpha-fetoprotein and germ cell tumors: A possible role of yolk sac tumor in production of alpha-fetoprotein. *Cancer 34*:1722, 1974.

142. Tancer, M. L., Orron, A., Baker, J. D., and Greenberger, M. E. Spontaneous rupture of ovarian teratoid tumor (dermoid cyst) into the urinary bladder: Review of eleven cases and report of one new case. *Obstet. Gynecol. 6*:668, 1955.

143. Teter, J. A new concept of classification of gonadal tumours arising from germ cell (gonocytoma) and their histogenesis. *Gynaecologia 150*:84, 1960.

144. Thatcher, D. S. Ovarian cysts and tumors in children. *Surg. Gynecol. Obstet. 117*:477, 1963.

145. Thompson, J. P., Dockerty, M. B., Symmonds, R. E., and Hayles, A. B. Ovarian and parovarian tumors in infants and children. *Am. J. Obstet. Gynecol. 97*:1059, 1967.

146. Thurlbeck, W. M., and Scully, R. E. Solid teratoma of the ovary. A clinicopathological analysis of 9 cases. *Cancer 13*:804, 1960.

147. Traut, H. F., and Marchetti, A. A. A consideration of so-called "granulosa" and "theca" cell tumors of the ovary. *Surg. Gynecol. Obstet. 70*:632, 1940.

148. Trites, A. E. W. Benign cystic ovarian teratomas of childhood or "ovarian hydrocephalus". *Canad. Med. Assoc. J. 84*:606, 1961.

149. Usizima, H. Ovarian dysgerminoma associated with masculinization. Report of a case. *Cancer 9*:736, 1956.

150. Waisman, J., Lischke, J. H., Mwasi, L. M., and Dignam, W. J. The ultrastructure of a feminizing granulosa-theca tumor. *Am. J. Obstet. Gynecol. 123*:147, 1975.

151. Warren, J. C., Erkman, B., and Cheatum, S. Hilus-cell adenoma in a dysgenetic gonad with XX/XO mosaicism. *Lancet 1*:141, 1964.

152. White, C. A., and Bradbury, J. T. Ovarian theca lutein cysts. Experimental formation in women prior to repeat cesarean section. *Am. J. Obstet. Gynecol. 92*:973, 1965.

153. Wilkinson, E. J., Friedrich, E. G., and Hosty, T. A. Alpha-fetoprotein and endodermal sinus tumor of the ovary. *Am. J. Obstet. Gynecol. 116*:711, 1973.

154. Williams, R. C. Jr. Dermatomyositis and malignancy: A review of the literature. *Ann. Int. Med. 50*:1174, 1959.

155. Wisniewski, M., and Deppisch, L. M. Solid teratomas of the ovary. *Cancer 32*:440, 1973.

156. Witschi, E. Migration of the germ cells to human embryos from the yolk sac to the primitive gonadal folds. *Contrib. Embryol. Carnegie Inst. 32*:67, 1948.

157. Woodruff, J. D., Noli Castillo, R. D., and Novak, E. R. Lymphoma of the ovary. A study of 35 cases from Ovarian Tumor Registry of the American Gynecological Society. *Am. J. Obstet. Gynecol. 85*:912, 1963.

158. Woodruff, J. D., Protos, P., and Peterson, W. F. Ovarian teratomas. Relationship of histologic and ontogenic factors to prognosis. *Am. J. Obstet. Gynecol. 102*:702, 1968.

159. Zangeneh, F., and Kelley, V. C. Granulosa-theca cell tumor of the ovary in children. *Am. J. Dis. Child. 115*:494, 1968.

Ancel Blaustein, M.D.

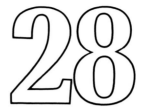

# Metastatic Carcinoma in the Ovary

The ovary is a fairly frequent site of metastasis from certain primary carcinomas; approximately 10% of ovarian tumors are not primary in origin.[5,8,9,18,21] The most common metastasis is from a carcinoma arising in the endometrium. Other primary tumors that have a predilection for metastasis to the ovary are from the gastrointestinal (GI) tract[1] and breast.[4,10] Tumors that metastasize to the ovary much less frequently include those arising in the cervix, fallopian tube, pancreas, gallbladder, lung, and cutaneous melanoma. A study of secondary ovarian carcinoma by Woodruff and Novak[21] demonstrated that at least 50% of the primary tumors giving rise to ovarian metastases were below the diaphragm and 13% above. Metastatic carcinoma to the ovary is bilateral in from 70 to 90% of cases[6,8,21]; unilateral involvement usually is found where metastasis occurs by contiguity. There are, however, instances of unilateral metastases that are difficult to explain, e.g., from the breast or the GI tract.

## Primary Endometrial Carcinoma

There is no doubt that cancer of the endometrium (Figure 28.1) metastasizes to the ovaries, but difficulty may be encountered in distinguishing metastases of an endometrial cancer from a separate primary ovarian tumor. This is particularly true in cases of ovarian endometrioid carcinoma which, according to Scully,[18] is associated with a

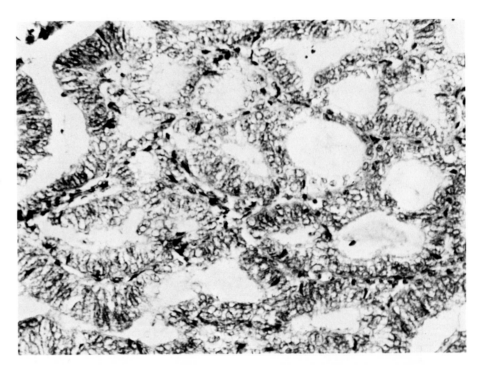

**28.1** Metastasis to the ovary from a well-differentiated carcinoma of the endometrium. Hematoxylin–eosin.

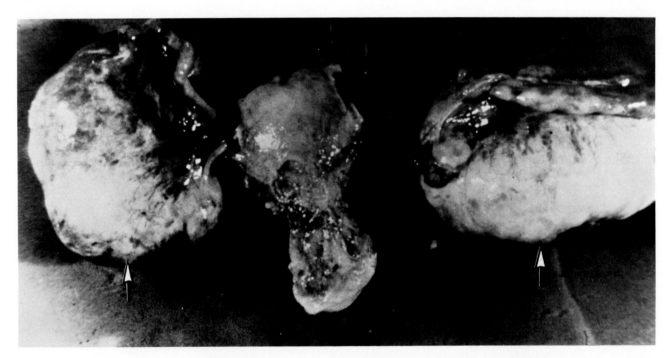

**28.2** Krukenberg tumor. The primary was a superficial spreading carcinoma of the stomach. Note the bilateral, almost uniform enlargement (arrows). The surfaces are smooth and almost spherical.

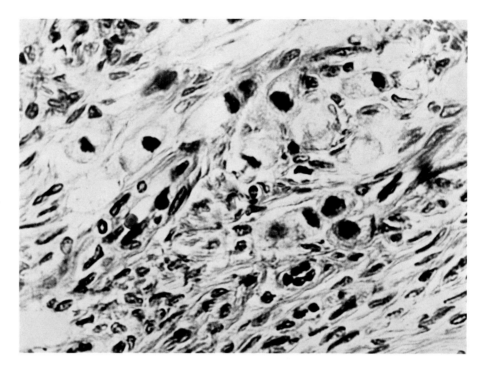

**28.3** Krukenberg tumor (same as in Figure 28.2). The tumor cells have a clear cytoplasm and some have eccentric nuclei. Hematoxylin–eosin.

similar tumor in the endometrium in one-third of cases. The incidence of metastases as reported by Finn[3] is 13%. In the series by Woodruff and Novak,[21] it was 31.5%. Bilateral involvement seems to vary from 29% in Finn's series to 40% in that of Woodruff and Novak.[21] The patients were in the fifth and sixth decades of life.

## Gastrointestinal Tract Primary

Tumors arising in the stomach give rise to bilateral ovarian metastases (Figure 28.2) that are of the signet-ring (mucinous) cell type and are commonly referred to as Krukenberg tumor. Krukenberg[11] described the tumor in 1896. He emphasized the bilateral involvement of the ovaries and the retention of their general shape. The external surface is smooth with a distinct capsule and absence of adhesions. The cut surface is solid and edematous. Occasionally when the tumor is bisected, some mucin may be released and cling to the knife surface. This is a useful clue. The hallmark of the lesion is the presence of signet cells (Figures 28.3 and 28.4). These are epithelial cells that contain mucin in their cytoplasm which tends to compress the nucleus. Mucicarmine stain reveals pink-staining mucin in the cytoplasm. Sometimes well-defined

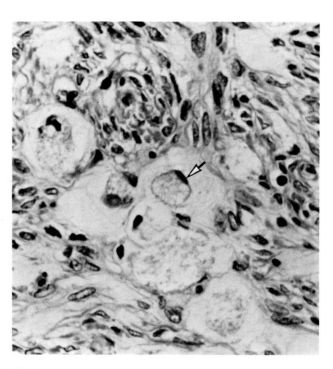

**28.4** Characteristic signet cell (arrow). Above and to the right there is a fibroblastic hyperplasia. Hematoxylin–eosin.

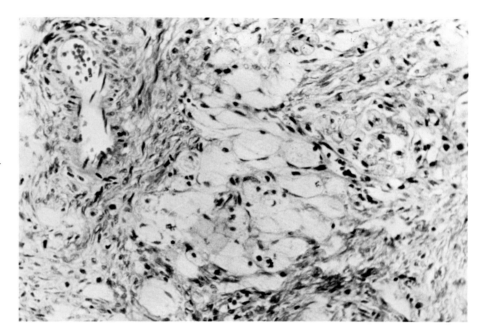

**28.5** Krukenberg tumor. The cells are in clusters and are distended with mucin. Hematoxylin–eosin.

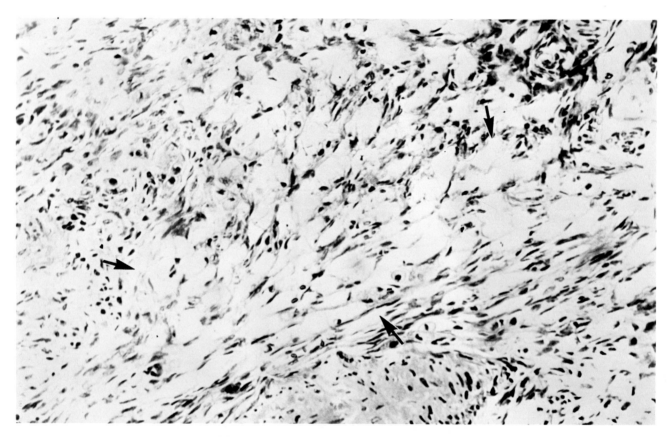

**28.6** Distension of cells by mucin has reached the point where cells rupture (arrows) and release mucin. Hematoxylin–eosin.

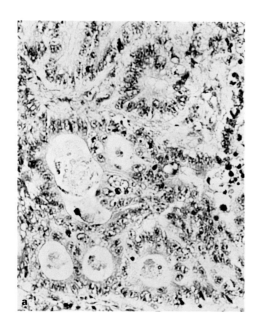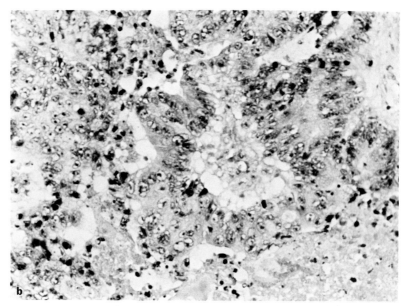

**28.7 a.** Metastasis from an adenocarcinoma of the colon. The tumor retains its glandular structure. Hematoxylin–eosin. **b.** High-power view of glands in the same case. Hematoxylin–eosin.

acini composed of mucin-producing cells (Figures 28.5 and 28.6) are also present. The marked stromal reaction and the scantiness of epithelial elements led Krukenberg[11] erroneously to call the tumor a "sarcoma ovarii mucocellulare." The error was perpetuated for 6 years until Schlagenhaufer,[17] in 1902, recognized the epithelial and metastatic nature of the tumor. The stomach is the primary source in over 90% of cases. Often it may be a superficial or small carcinoma and may elude gross discovery. Less commonly, tumors arising from the colon (Figures 28.7 and 28.8a), gallbladder, or breast produce metastases with similar gross and microscopic changes.[9,14] Woodruff and Novak[21] in their study found ovarian metastases from gastrointestinal tumors in 24 of 120 cases (20%). Burt[1] reported an incidence of 3.5% of ovarian involvement among 493 female patients operated on for carcinoma of the colon. In 13 of his 17 cases with ovarian metastasis, the ovaries were the only grossly visible area of secondary involvement. This would suggest preferential selection of the ovary as a site of spread of colonic cancer. This led Burt[1] to recommend bilateral oophorectomy along with colon resection, in patients over 40, in order to avoid the need for a subsequent laparatomy to remove bulky ovarian metastases. Colon carcinoma, particularly when it involves the ovary by contiguity, results in metastases that closely resemble the primary tumor. Carcinoid

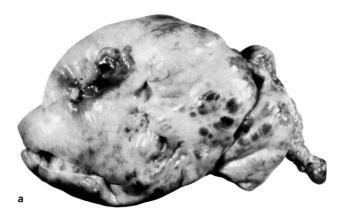

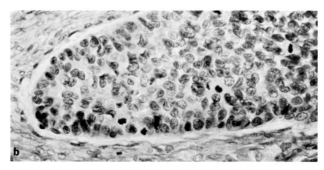

**28.8 a.** Metastasis from carcinoid that originated in the colon. The ovary was large, partly solid, and partly cystic. **b.** Metastasis from carcinoid of colon. Note the uniformity of the cells.

tumors of the gastrointestinal tract can also metastasize to the ovaries.[5,6,7,16,19] Robboy, Scully, and Norris[16] reviewed 35 cases of carcinoid metastatic to the ovary. Twenty-five cases were discovered at laparatomy; the remaining cases were detected only at autopsy as a manifestation of widespread metastasis. Although one ovary was almost always enlarged, the authors emphasized that the opposite ovary was frequently enlarged also. Both ovaries contained tumor with only two exceptions. Abnormal urinary levels of 5-hydroxyindoleacetic acid were often detected within several months after the operation.

The published records of five patients with established intestinal primary tumors described only unilateral ovarian involvement. This apparent discrepancy in four cases was probably a result of inadequate study of the contralateral ovary.[16] In the fifth case the contralateral ovary had been previously resected. This underscores the importance for microscopic examination of both ovaries, even though one appears "normal or is only equivocally enlarged."[16] The prognosis was poor, with one-third of the patients dying within 1 year and two thirds within 4 years after the diagnosis of ovarian involvement. The authors state that metastatic ovarian carcinoid is often misinterpreted as a Brenner tumor or granulosa cell tumor; however, the most difficult diagnosis to exclude is primary carcinoid. They found that primary carcinoid is usually unilateral and associated with the presence of other teratomatous elements within the tumor. An important conclusion drawn by the authors[16] is that, in the absence of a demonstrable intestinal primary tumor, a unilateral ovarian carcinoid is in all probability primary, even though teratomous elements are not demonstrable; however, bilateral carcinoid tumors are metastatic until proved otherwise.

Krukenberg tumors have been found in the ovaries without clinical evidence of a primary site and, in several instances, postmortem examination has not revealed the presence of even a small primary tumor elsewhere. These tumors are then referred to as "primary Krukenberg tumors of the ovary." Confirmation of this diagnosis can only be made by careful postmortem examination. Many are skeptical as to whether this entity exists.

## Primary Breast Carcinoma

The incidence of ovarian involvement by disseminated breast cancer is reported to be about 20% in autopsy series and up to 30% in surgical series. The higher incidence in the surgical series may reflect a more careful microscopic examination of surgically removed ovaries than those examined in a routine autopsy. Alternately, because the surgically castrated patients are premenopausal and are younger than those included in an autopsy study, the higher metastatic incidence in the former group may reflect a greater tendency for breast carcinoma to proliferate successfully in the ovaries of younger women. There is certainly no doubt that ovaries are preferentially selected as a site of growth of disseminated cancer.[12] In the series of Woodruff and Novak[21] 60% of cases showed bilateral involvement. The metastases may be only microscopic but in the majority of cases result in gross enlargement. The microscopic pattern is variable but, in general, tends to retain the appearance of the primary tumor (Figures 28.9 through 28.12).

## Other Primary Sites

In Woodruff and Novak series,[21] metastases were present in the ovary from the following primary sites: lung (Figure 28.15), thyroid, kidney, cervix, fallopian tube (Figures 28.13 and 28.14), Ewing's tumor, choriocarcinoma, melanoma (Figure 28.17), and neural tumors. Martzloff and Manlove[13] reported metastases to the ovary from a hypernephroma of the kidney (Figure 28.16). Bilaterality was much less frequent (35%) than in the major groups.

## Pathways of Spread of the Tumor to the Ovary

There are four possible pathways of spread of tumors to the ovary: (1) direct contiguity—this is readily understood; (2) surface implantation; (3) lymphatic metastasis; and (4) hematogenous spread.

### Surface Implantation

Surface implants are seen with enough frequency to accept transperitoneal spread. The ovaries are a frequent site of metastases where generalized peritoneal carcinomatosis exists. There are instances in which at laparotomy the ovaries appear to be the only organs involved in transperitoneal spread. This is particularly true in some instances of metastasis from breast carcinoma. Willis and other have suggested that perhaps the ovary offers a distinctive milieu in which metastasis can grow.

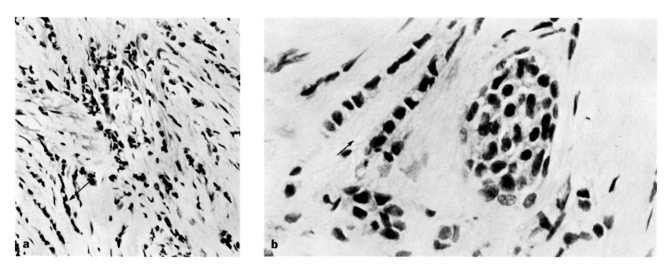

**28.9 a.** Metastasis from scirrhous carcinoma of the breast. Note the Indian-file pattern (arrow) of the tumor cells. Hematoxylin–eosin. **b.** High-power view of cells in the same case. Hematoxylin–eosin.

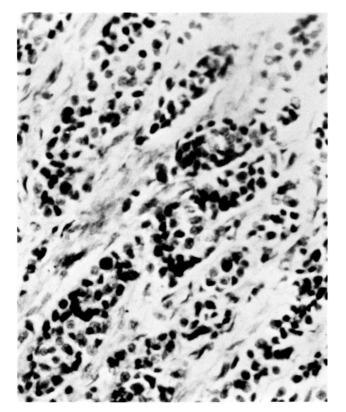

**28.10** Metastasis from breast carcinoma showing a lobular, tubular pattern of spread. Hematoxylin–eosin.

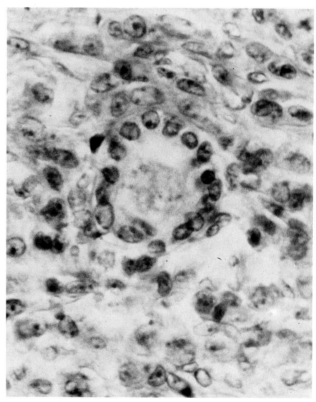

**28.11** Metastasis from breast carcinoma—pseudoglandular or rosette pattern. Hematoxylin–eosin.

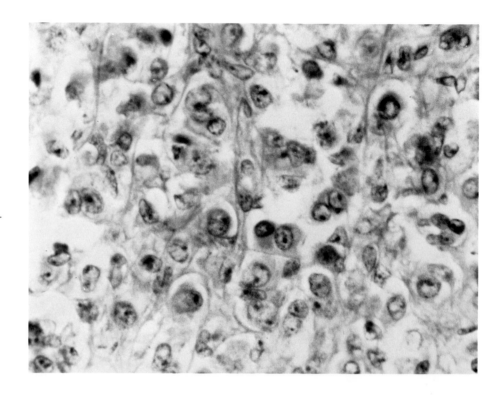

**28.12** Metastasis from breast carcinoma. The primary was poorly differentiated and the metastasis was similar. Hematoxylin–eosin.

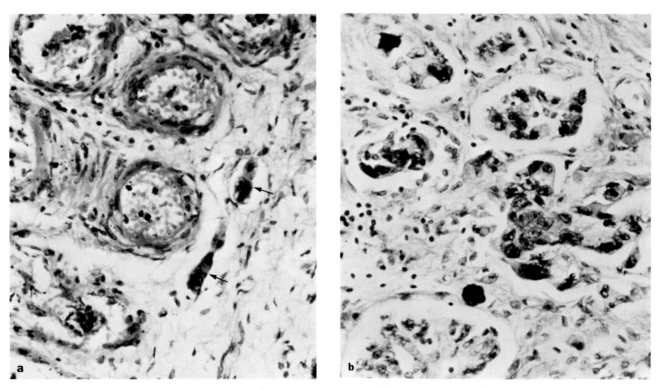

**28.13** Metastasis (arrows) from carcinoma of the fallopian tube found in lymph channels in the hilus of the ovary. Hematoxylin–eosin.

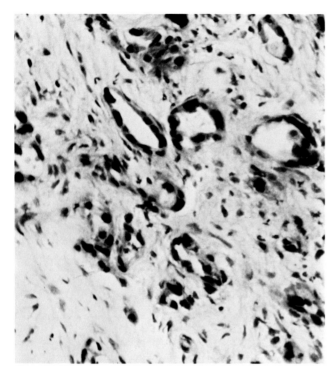

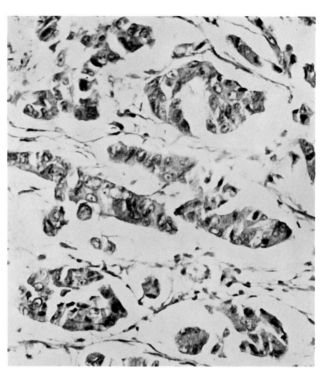

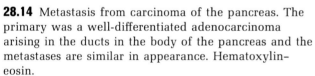

**28.14** Metastasis from carcinoma of the pancreas. The primary was a well-differentiated adenocarcinoma arising in the ducts in the body of the pancreas and the metastases are similar in appearance. Hematoxylin–eosin.

**28.15** Metastases from a peripheral adenocarcinoma of the lung. The glandular structure is maintained in the metastasis. Hematoxylin–eosin.

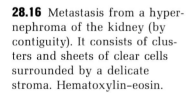

**28.16** Metastasis from a hypernephroma of the kidney (by contiguity). It consists of clusters and sheets of clear cells surrounded by a delicate stroma. Hematoxylin–eosin.

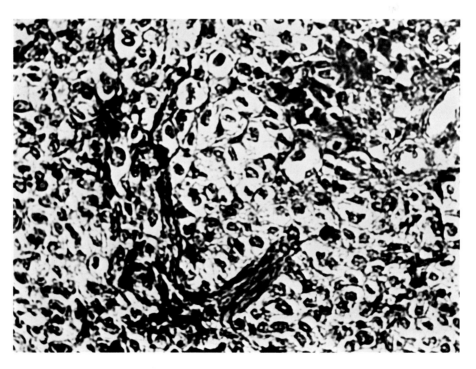

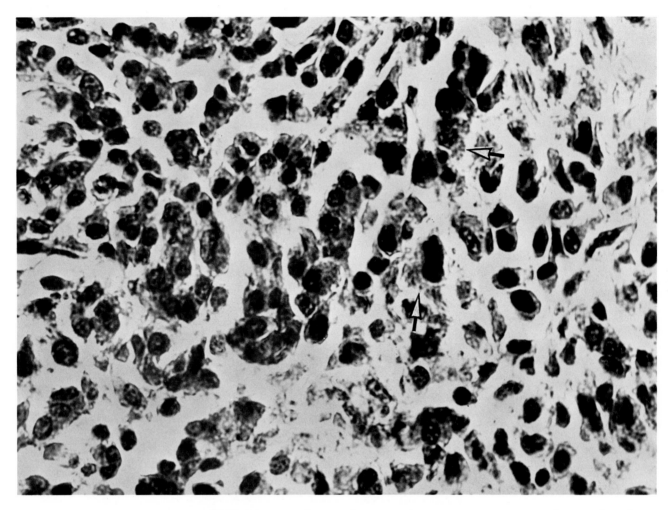

**28.17** Metastasis from malignant melanoma. Arrows point to the granules of melanin pigment in the cell cytoplasm. Hematoxylin–eosin.

## Lymphatic Metastases

This is undoubtedly the commonest pathway for metastases to the ovary. The rich network of lymph nodes and lymphatic channels in the pelvis readily explains the metastatic pathway of tumors to the uterus and contralateral ovary. The rare finding of clusters of tumor cells limited to lymphatics in the medulla of the ovary in cases of breast carcinoma confirm that this is the pathway of spread to the ovary.

As yet, no one has convincingly described the pathway of metastases from a cancer of the stomach to the ovaries, in particular, those arising from superficial spreading carcinoma. It is known that the lymph channels that drain the upper gastrointestinal tract ultimately link up with the lumbar chain of lymph nodes. Ovarian lymphatics drain into the lumbar glands. This could well be the route of spread to the ovaries in these cases. Unfortunately, there are not any good studies available in which exhaustive tissue sectioning of these lymphatics pathways has been made.

## Hemic Metastases

This pathway has been documented in cases of malignant melanoma and choriocarcinoma. Martzloff and Manlove[13] reported venous spread from the renal hypernephroma to the ovary. There are instances, although admittedly not frequent, when a carcinoma of the breast or stomach follows the hemic as well as the lymphatic route.

# Hormonal Activity
# of Metastatic Carcinoma
# to Ovary

Esau,[2] in 1933, described a case of Krukenberg tumor of the ovaries in which there was clinical evidence of virilism. Turenen[20] did urinary estrogen levels both pre- and postoperatively in patients with postmenopausal bleeding in association with Krukenberg tumors. In one patient the estrogen was measured at 400 units per day and this fell to 50 units per day postoperatively. A similar observation was made in a second case. In eight specimens of endometrium (seven patients) which were examined there was cystic hyperplasia. Turenen described large groups of pale cells scattered in the stroma which he felt was thecomatosis. Ober et al.[15] have described virilism in association with Krukenberg tumors and at least nine cases are now documented. In these cases there was also a hyperplasia of thecalike cells. It is conceivable that they produce androgens because they lack the enzymes necessary to proceed to estrogen synthesis. Woodruff et al.[22] have also reported hormonal activity by tumor metastasis in ovaries.

# REFERENCES

1. Burt, C. A. V. Prophylactic oophorectomy with resection of the large bowel for cancer. *Am. J. Surg.* 93:77, 1957.

2. Esau, D. Krukenberg tumoren in der schwangerschaft. Nachtrag zu der arbeit von Dr. Puppel, *Zentvalbl f. Gynak.* 57:1167, May 1933.

3. Finn, W. F. Diagnostic confusion of ovarian metastases from endometrial carcinoma with primary ovarian carcinoma. *Am. J. Obstet. Gynecol.* 62:403, 1951.

4. Haagerson, C. D. *Diseases of the Breast,* 2nd ed. Philadelphia, W. B. Saunders, 1971.

5. Haines, M. Carcinoid tumors of the ovary. *J. Obstet. Gynaecol. Br. Commonw.* 78:1123, 1971.

6. Hall-Allan, R. T. J. Metastatic ovarian carcinoid tumor. *Postgrad. Med. J.* 45:46, 1969.

7. Hopping, R. A., Dockerty, M. B., and Masson, J. C. Carcinoid tumors of the appendix—report of a case in which extensive intraabdominal metastases occurred, including involvement of the right ovary. *Arch. Surg.* 45:613, 1942.

8. Israel, S. S., Helsel, E. V., Jr., and Hausman, D. H. The challenge of metastatic ovarian carcinoma. *Am. J. Obstet. Gynecol.* 93:1094, 1965.

9. Karsh, J. Secondary malignant disease of the ovary. *Am. J. Obstet. Gynecol.* 61:154, 1951.

10. Kasilag, F. B., Jr., and Ruthledge, F. N. Metastatic breast carcinoma of the ovary. *Am. J. Obstet. Gynecol.* 74:989, 1957.

11. Krukenberg, P. Ueben das Fibrosarcoma Ovarii Muco-cellulari (carcinomatoses). *Arch. Gyn. Munch.* 50:287, 1896.

12. Lee, Y. N., and Hori, J. M. Significance of ovarian metastasis in therapeutic oophorectomy for advanced breast cancer. *Cancer* 27:1374, 1971.

13. Martzloff, K. H., and Manlove, C. H. Vaginal and ovarian metastases from hypernephroma: Report of a case and review of literature. *Surg. Gynecol. Obstet.* 88:145, 1949.

14. Munnell, E. W., and Taylor, H. C., Jr. Ovarian carcinoma: Review of 200 primary and 51 secondary cases. *Am. J. Obstet. Gynecol.* 58:943, 1949.

15. Ober, W. B., Pollak, A., Gerstmann, K. E., and Kupperman, H. S. Krukenberg tumor with androgenic and progestational activity. *Am. J. Obstet. Gynecol.* 84:739, 1962.

16. Robboy, S. J., Scully, R. E., and Norris, H. T. Carcinoid—metastatic to the ovary. *Cancer* 33:798, 1974.

17. Schlagenhaufer, F. Uber das Metastatische Ovarialkarzinom Nach Krebs das Magens, Darmes und anderer Bachorgane. *Mschv. Geburtsh Gyak.* 15:485, 1902.

18. Scully, R. E. Recent progress of ovarian cancer. *Hum. Pathol.* 1:73, 1970.

19. Shuster, M., Mendoza-Divino, E., and Joelson, H. Carcinoid tumor metastasizing to the ovaries. *Obstet. Gynecol.* 36:515, 1970.

20. Turenen, K. Hormonal secretion of Krukenberg tumors. *Acta Endocrinol.* 20:50, 1955.

21. Woodruff, J. D., and Novak, E. R. Krukenberg tumors of the ovary. *Obstet. Gynecol.* 15:351, 1960.

22. Woodruff, J. D., Williams, J. J., and Goldberg, B. Hormone activity of the common ovarian neoplasms. *Am. J. Obstet. Gynecol.* 87:679, 1963.

Bradley Bigelow, M.D.

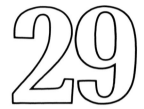

# Fertilization, Implantation, and Placentation

## Site of Fertilization

Fertilization of an ovum by sperm normally occurs in the distal part of the fallopian tube.[14] Cell division and cleavage continue during the transit through the tube. Transit time takes approximately 4 days, a period considered essential in the development of the fertilized ovum in preparation for implantation in the uterus.[14]

## Implantation

Normal implantation in the fundus of the uterus occurs about 7 days after ovulation and fertilization. It corresponds to the twenty-first day in the menstrual cycle, when the endometrium is at the peak of secretory activity. The fertilized ovum, at this time considerably depleted in its nutrition, finds a ready source of glycoproteins and a balanced electrolyte medium.

## Placentation

The early placenta[12] (Figure 29.1) consists of a mass of proliferating trophoblast, which expands rapidly in all directions. Maternal vascular channels are infiltrated by the trophoblast and within hours of implantation, the syncytiotrophoblast is bathed by maternal venous blood.

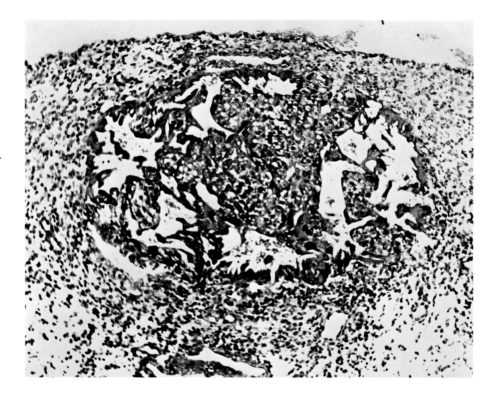

**29.1** An early gestation implanted in the endometrium. It is about 9 days old and has been implanted about 2 days. The level of section does not show the embryonic tissue. Trophoblast is proliferating rapidly in all directions. Villi have not yet appeared.

This supplies the fertilized ovum with nutrition and permits exchange of gases.

At about 12 days gestational age, fetal mesenchyme invaginates the trophoblast with formation of chorionic villi. At this time cells delaminate from the inner surface of the trophoblast to form the amnion.[5,8] Ectoderm continuous with that of the embryonal disc grows out to line the amniotic cavity. The primary yolk sac is formed on this day from endodermal cells of the embryonal disc. Over a period of 5 days (days 13 to 18) mesenchyme condenses and forms the body stalk, which is the precursor of the umbilical cord.

Trophoblastic tissue has differentiated into cytotrophoblast and syncytiotrophoblast cells. Cytotrophoblasts have a single round or oval well-defined nucleus and pale cytoplasm. They are the progenitors of the syncytiotrophoblast, which is a large cell having multiple nuclei and darker staining cytoplasm. These cells produce chorionic gonadotropin,[9,13] chorionic growth hormones, placental lactogen,[7] estrogen,[11,11a] and progesterone, all for the purpose, it is assumed, of developing independence in the production of steroids essential for the maintenance of pregnancy. At 20 days (Figures 29.2, 29.3, and 29.4) chorionic villi are in intimate contact with maternal decidua that is richly supplied with engorged capillaries.

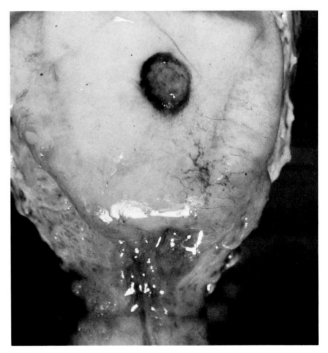

**29.2** Gestation of about 20 days implanted on the mid-posterior surface of the uterus. Note the dark, highly vascular border. The surrounding decidua is thick and velvety.

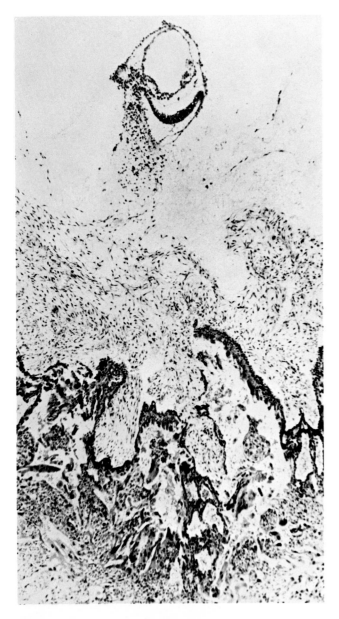

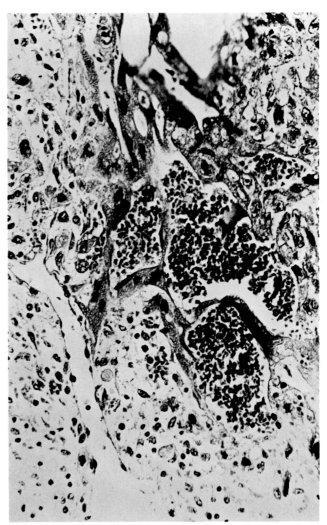

**29.4** High magnification of a deep portion of the 20-day gestation. Multinucleate syncytiotrophoblast invades the decidua at left and bottom. Pools of maternal red blood cells are seen between the syncytiotrophoblast cells near center.

**29.3** Microscopic section of Figure 29.2. The embryonic disc is the dark necklace of cells at top, with primary yolk sac above and amnionic cavity below it. A strand of extraembryonic mesoderm extends downward from it to blend with mesoderm forming the stroma of the early placental villi. Proliferating trophoblast invades maternal decidua at bottom.

Rapid proliferation of the cytotrophoblast serves to anchor the growing placenta to the maternal tissue (Figure 29.5). Trophoblast invades the decidua (Figures 29.6 and 29.7) and uterine veins (Figure 29.8) and can be isolated from the pelvic venous blood.[6] Trophoblasts, as well as villi, have been found as emboli in maternal lungs.[3] This invasive and metastatic character of placental tissue parallels two characteristics of malignant tumor. The factors that control the growth of a normal placenta are the subject of considerable speculation.

At about days 18 to 21, cells delaminate from cytotrophoblast, migrate into the villous stroma, and form capillaries. As the capillaries differentiate they communicate with the umbilical vessels and fetal–placental circulation is

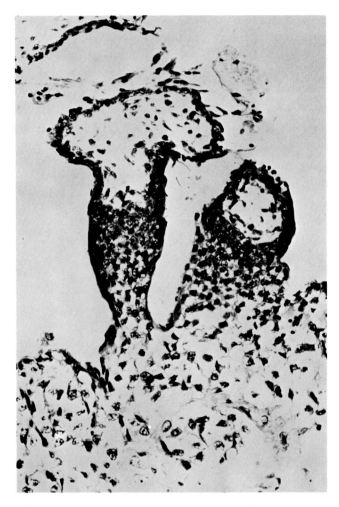

**29.5** Proliferating columns of cytotrophoblast attach early villi to decidua at bottom. These become the so-called anchoring villi.

established. At about 5 weeks, the chorionic villi acquire blood vessels clearly identifiable by light microscopy.

As the fetus grows, the placenta increases in size; villi proliferate and their blood supply proliferates with them. Chorionic villi are anchored to the decidual plate, and from these anchoring villi proliferation of secondary and tertiary villi takes place. Arborescence proceeds in the intervillous space increasing the fetal–maternal interface. Initially the whole chorion is covered with villi but gradually, as the chorion expands, surface pressure and interference with the blood supply result in atrophy of the villi on the chorion leve, the surface lying exposed in the uterine cavity (Figure 29.9). The chorion of the implantation site is called chorion frondosum and here the villi are well preserved.

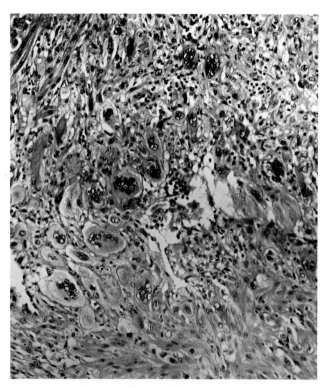

**29.6** Syncytiotrophoblast cells invade the decidua, at top, and extend into the myometrium at bottom.

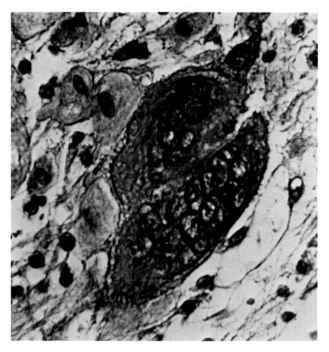

**29.7** Closeup of a multinucleate syncytiotrophoblast surrounded by decidual cells.

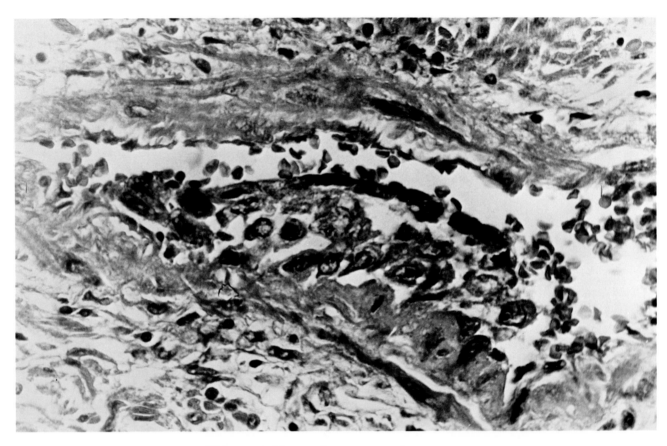

**29.8** Trophoblast within a vein in the myometrium.

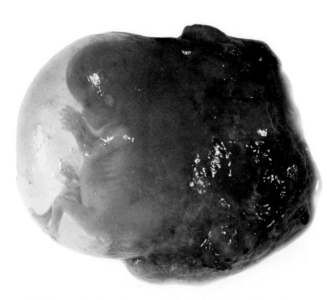

**29.9** Note chorion leve on left and chorion frondosum on the right.

Some time after the fortieth day[4] spiral arterioles penetrate the intervillous space and form arteriovenous shunts that are in contact with the intervillous space (Figure 29.10). Hemodynamic effects exerted on chorionic villi result in the formation of distinct groupings called cotyledons.[10] The mature term placenta consists of 10 to 12 large cotyledons, clearly visible on the maternal surface (see Chapter 37, Figure 37.19). The mature placenta at term is discoid in shape, measures 15 to 20 cm in diameter, and weighs between 400 and 500 g (see Chapter 37, Figure 37.18). The placenta exceeds the fetus in weight up to the fifteenth week or so; the reverse holds true for the rest of the gestation (Figure 29.11). In erythroblastosis and in diabetic patients the placenta may be larger and heavier. The placenta during 9 months of pregnancy undergoes histologic changes. First-trimester villi are relatively large and have a loose stroma and thin-walled vessels (Figure 29.12a). Hofbauer cells[15] (placental macrophages) are

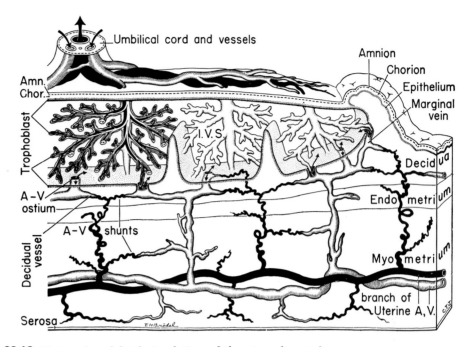

**29.10** Maternal and fetal circulation of the uteroplacental organ.

[Reprinted by permission from C. T. Javert, *Spontaneous and Habitual Abortion*, p. 33. McGraw-Hill, 1957.]

present in the stroma. Villi are covered by an inner layer of cytotrophoblast cells and an outer layer of syncytiotrophoblast cells.[1] The cytotrophoblast is prominent at this stage. In the second trimester, villi are somewhat smaller and increased in number. Stroma is more dense and the fetal vessels are more prominent (Figure 29.12b).

At the commencement of the third trimester cytotrophoblasts are less conspicuous. Syncytial knotting becomes more prominent. The villi decrease in size but the fetal capillaries become more prominent. Hofbauer cells are scant. Syncytiotrophoblast is now a thinned cell mass with prominent nuclear knotting. Fetal capillaries occupy much of the stroma. They are dilated; their walls are thin; and there is now the closest contact with the maternal circulation in the intervillous space (Figure 29.12c). Hofbauer cells are now absent unless infection has occurred. Other changes seen in the placenta relate to its dependence for nutrition on the maternal circulation. Hemorrhage, thrombi, infarction, and fibrin deposition may result from disturbances of the maternal circulation.

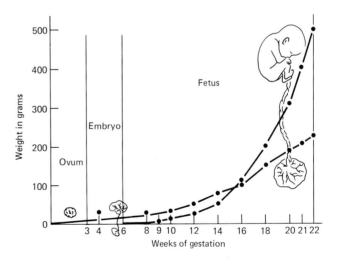

**29.11** Relation of average weights of the ovo–fetus to those of the placenta during 22 weeks of development.

[Reprinted by permission from C. T. Javert, *Spontaneous and Habitual Abortion*, p. 43. McGraw-Hill, 1957.]

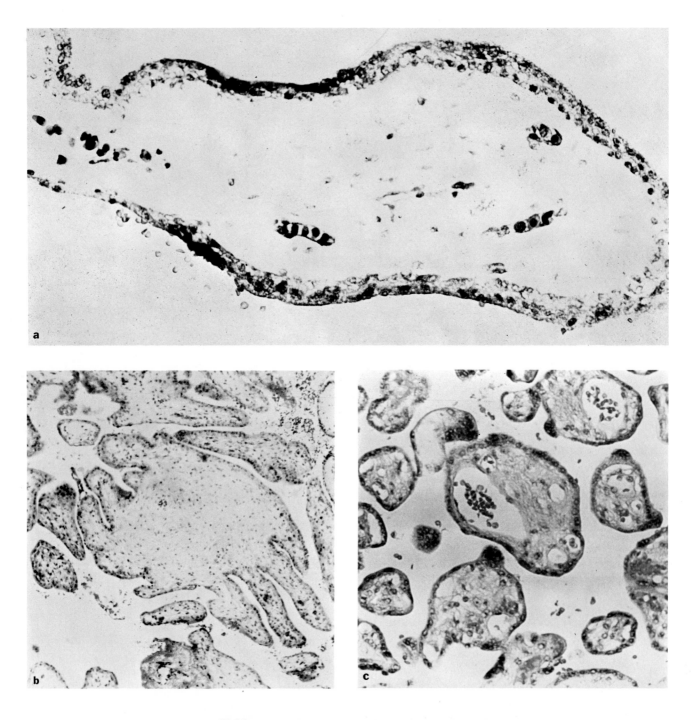

**29.12 a.** A first trimester villus at about 7 weeks gestation. Cytotrophoblast is prominent on the surface. **b.** Second-trimester villi are smaller, stroma is more cellular, and vessels are larger and better developed. **c.** Third-trimester villi, at term, are relatively small with widely dilated vessels. The intervillous, maternal blood is now closely associated with the fetal blood within the villi. The syncytiotrophoblast is prominent, with some "knotting" of the clumped nuclei, and the cytotrophoblast cannot be seen with the light microscope.

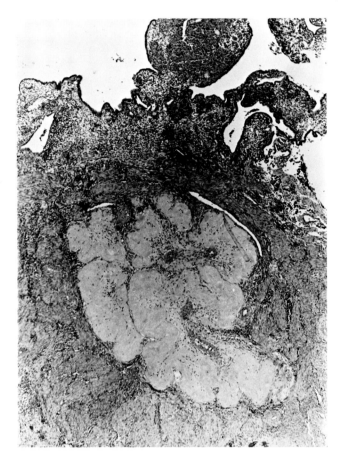

**29.13** Placental site in a uterus removed 13 weeks postpartum. Beneath the somewhat polypoid endometrium (top) is a sharply circumscribed group of blood vessels, with thick and fibrotic walls, which are in the process of involution.

These changes are seen in varying degrees in the normal placenta and to an exaggerated degree in hypertensive disorders of pregnancy.

## Involution of the Placental Site

At delivery, the placenta separates through a plane of cleavage in the maternal decidua lining the fundus of the uterus. Normally the villous tissue is completely delivered with the attached membranes.

The placental site in the uterus undergoes slow involution. Anderson and Davis[2] described the sequence of events in 32 cases. These studies ranged from immediate postpartum to 20 weeks. Hyalinized small arteries (Figure 29.13) are the pathognomonic feature of the organizing placental site. If involution of the vessels fails to occur normally, postpartum hemorrhage may necessitate hysterectomy.

## REFERENCES

1. Adair, F. L., and Thelander, H. A study of the weight and dimensions of the human placenta in its relation to the weight of the newborn infant. *Am. J. Obstet. Gynecol. 10:*172, 1925.

2. Anderson, W. R., and Davis, J. Placental site involution. *Am. J. Obstet. Gynecol. 102:*23, 1968.

3. Attwood, H. D., and Park, W. W. Embolism to the lungs by trophoblast. *J. Obstet. Gynaecol. Br. Commonw. 68:*611, 1961.

4. Boe, F. Studies on the vascularization of the human placenta. *Acta Obstet. Gynecol. Scand. 32*(Suppl.):5, 1953.

5. Bourne, G. L. *The Human Amnion and Chorion.* Chicago, Year Book Medical Publishers, 1962.

6. Douglas, G. W., Thomas, L., Carr, M., Cullen, N. M., and Morris, R. Trophoblast in the circulating blood during pregnancy. *Am. J. Obstet. Gynecol. 78:*960, 1959.

7. Gey, G. O., Segar, G. E., and Hellman, L. M. The production of a gonadotropic substance (prolan) by placental cells in tissue culture. *Science 88:*306, 1938.

8. Mossman, H. W. Comparative morphogenesis of the foetal membranes and accessory uterine structures. *Contrib. Embryol. Carnegie Inst. 26:*129, 1973.

9. Newton, W. N. Hormones and the placenta. *Physiol. Rev. 18:*419, 1938.

10. Reynolds, S. R. M. Formation of fetal cotyledons in the hemochorial placenta. *Am. J. Obstet. Gynecol. 94:*425, 1966.

11. Ryan, K. J. Aromatization of steroids. *J. Biol. Chem. 234:*268, 1959.

11a. Ryan, K. J. Metabolism of C-16-oxygenated steroids by human placenta: The formation of estriol. *J. Biol. Chem. 234:*2006, 1959.

12. Stieve, H. Growth of human placenta. *Anat. Anz. 90:*225, 1940.

13. Thiede, H. A., and Choate, J. W. Chorionic gonadotropin localization in the human placenta by immunofluorescent staining. II. Demonstration of HCG in the trophoblast and amnion epithelium of immature and mature placentas. *Obstet. Gynecol. 22:*433, 1964.

14. Westman, A. Investigations into the transit of ova in man. *J. Obstet. Gynaecol. Br. Emp. 44:*821, 1937.

15. Wynn, R. M. Origin, cytochemistry and ultrastructure of the Hofbauer cells. *Obstet. Gynecol. 25:*425, 1965.

Bradley Bigelow, M.D.

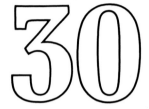

# Abnormalities and Diseases of the Placenta, Membranes, and Umbilical Cord

## Abnormal Sites of Implantation

Implantation normally takes place on the posterior or anterior wall of the uterus. There are, however, instances of implantation in abnormal uterine sites and in extra-uterine locations (Figure 30.1).

### Placenta Previa

Implantation of the placenta across the internal os constitutes a complete placenta previa. Partial and marginal involvement of the os also occurs. The incidence is about 1 in 200 deliveries. Together with placental abruption, previa accounts for most cases of third trimester hemorrhage. Abnormalities of placental architecture, such as placenta membranacea and, probably, succenturiate lobe, are associated with this condition. About 0.2% of cases are reported to have an associated placenta accreta (see next section), according to a review of five series totalling almost 2,000 cases of placenta previa.[26] This figure may be low, however, because the diagnosis of accreta was made only on examination of hysterectomy specimens and did not include cases with placental examination alone.

### Placenta Accreta

A placenta that is attached directly to uterine muscle without intervening decidua is termed accreta or adherent. The condition may be total or partial. Failure of the

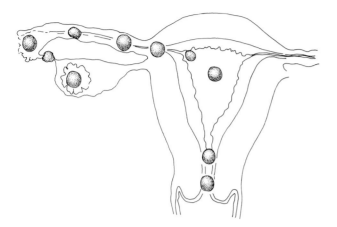

**30.1** Known implantation sites of fertilized ovum.

[Adapted from C. T. Javert, *Spontaneous and Habitual Abortion*, p. 43. McGraw-Hill, 1957.]

placenta to separate through the normal decidual plane can be associated with massive hemorrhage which may necessitate hysterectomy (Figure 30.2). The placenta removed in the face of accreta shows defects on the maternal surface where adherent portions have been retained. The histologic diagnosis requires absence of decidua basalis at the implantation site (Figure 30.3), and is most readily made by examination of the uterus if it is removed. Placental examination alone, however, may show myometrium attached to villi on the material surface, as well as missing areas of retained placenta.

A number of factors have been implicated in the cause of accreta. About 20% are associated with placenta previa,[22] with the failure of decidua formation in the lower uterine segment underlying its development. Other possible causes are primary hypoplasia of decidua, prior endometrial curettage, uterine scars, chronic endometritis, and submucous leiomyomas. Millar[26] has reviewed the subject and concludes that a primary decidual deficiency is the best explanation. Placenta increta and percreta are partial and complete penetration of such a placenta through the uterine wall. They are extremely rare conditions and may be associated with perforation of the uterus, as well as hemorrhage.

## Ectopic Pregnancy

A pregnancy that implants and develops outside of its normal location, on the anterior or posterior surface of the endometrium in the fundus of the uterus, is considered to be an ectopic gestation. The overwhelming majority occur within the fallopian tube. In Breen's review of 654 ectopic

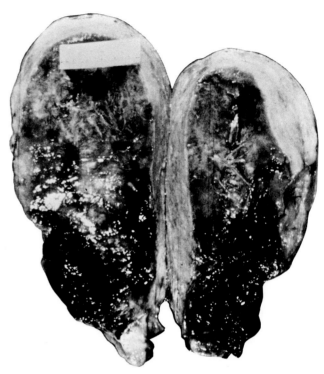

**30.2** Placenta previa and accreta. Vaginal bleeding at term had led to the diagnosis of placenta previa. After caesarean delivery, intractable bleeding was associated with failure of the placenta to separate and necessitated hysterectomy. Most of the placenta has been removed from the bisected uterus shown here. The hemorrhagic area in the lower uterine segment represents adherent placenta that has been implanted across the internal os.

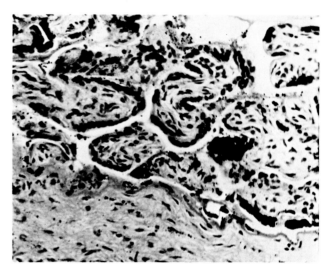

**30.3** Placenta accreta. Chorionic villi at term are attached to the myometrium without intervening decidua.

pregnancies,[12] 96% occurred in the tube, the majority being found in the distal and middle thirds. In the United States the incidence of tubal pregnancy is conservatively estimated to be 1 in 200 live births. While the majority occur in the distal and middle thirds (ampulla) of the fallopian tube, they occur in the following sites in decreasing order of frequency: isthmic, fimbrial, fimbrial-ovarian, abdominal, interstitial, and in the cervix and the ovary.

The commonest symptom of ectopic gestation is pain, occurring in over 90% of cases. Amenorrhea and vaginal bleeding are only slightly less frequent.

### Etiology

The mechanisms responsible for tubal pregnancy are unknown. The human zygote, formed by fertilization of the ovum within the tube, remains there some 4 days before entering the uterine cavity. While delay in entering the uterus is widely believed to predispose to tubal nidation, it is worth considering that zygotes experimentally delayed in the rabbit, guinea pig, and mouse oviducts fail to implant in the tube and, instead, degenerate. Ectopic pregnancy in monkeys is quite uncommon but has been reported in a rhesus colony.[24] The possible mechanisms resulting in tubal pregnancy fall into three broad categories: (1) factors that retard the passage of the conceptus along the tube; (2) factors that increase tubal receptivity; and (3) factors that derive from the conceptus itself.

In the first category, chronic salpingitis is the most frequently incriminated cause. It is usually due to gonococcal or other aerobic or anaerobic infections that may cause interference with a number of normal mechanisms whereby the tube shelters and transports the zygote. Mucosal adhesions and cul de sacs in which nidation may occur are sequelae of infection. Abnormal tubal motility, secondary to pelvic inflammatory disease and tubal adhesions, may cause delayed transportation. It is often extremely difficult for a pathologist to assess the state of a fallopian tube prior to the occurrence of an ectopic pregnancy because the hemorrhage and inflammation, which are secondary to the abortion or tubal rupture, may mask any underlying pathology. It is important, however, to section the tube away from the pregnancy site, in an effort to make such a judgment. A normal section, however, may only mean that the underlying salpingitis was focal and was obscured by the pregnancy itself. While various types of salpingitis have been reported in from 20 to 90% of cases, in nearly 60% of one study no pathologic evidence of prior tubal disease was noted.[28]

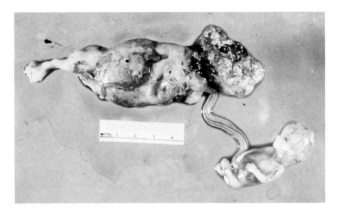

**30.4** Ectopic pregnancy, following tuboplasty. The fetus is attached by the umbilical cord to the placenta, which issues from the distal end of the tube.

Tubal diverticula, possibly of congenital origin, have been suggested as one cause of ectopic pregnancy. Persaud,[30] using a radio-opaque injection technique, found diverticula in 49% of tubes with ectopic nidation and in only 11% of controls. Doubt was cast on their significance, however, because the diverticula appeared to be related to chronic salpingitis and because most were found in the proximal portion of the tube, which is not the commonest site of ectopic pregnancy. In addition, no diverticula were found in the tubes of 50 autopsied stillbirths, infants, and children examined in the same way.

Ectopic pregnancy is of increased incidence following reconstructive procedures on diseased tubes. Such a case is illustrated in Figure 30.4. Space-occupying masses, such as leiomyomas or ovarian or parovarian cysts, may impinge on the tube and arrest the conceptus in some cases.

The second possible underlying factor of increased tubal receptivity refers to the presence of endometriosis or decidual reaction in the tube with the theoretical attraction of the fertilized ovum to this site. Figure 30.5 shows both mucosal adhesions, following salpingitis, and a marked decidual reaction in the proximal portion of the ampulla of a tube harboring a distal ectopic pregnancy. Since decidua in the tube is a frequent accompaniment of intrauterine gestations, and since very little decidua may be found in the vicinity of early tubal pregnancies, as in the case shown in Figures 30.9a,b, this would seem to be an unlikely cause of the condition.

The third major possible cause of ectopic pregnancy relates to the conceptus itself. It has been suggested that the conceptus is either abnormally immature or overly mature at the time of passage down the tube. In the first

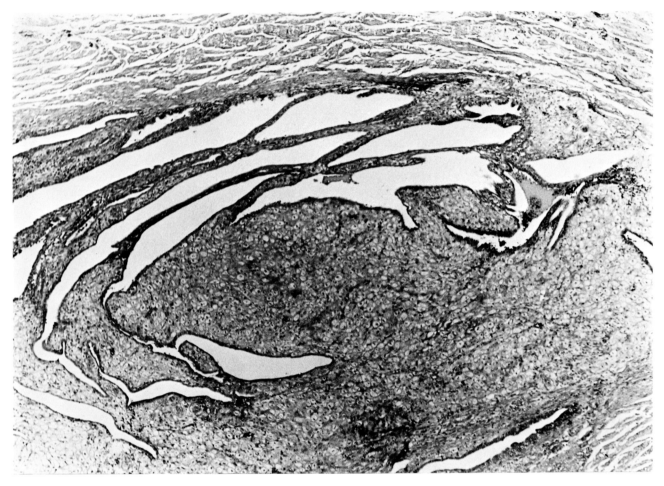

**30.5** Marked decidual reaction in the interadherent mucosa of a fallopian tube. This section was taken proximal to an ectopic pregnancy.

instance, Iffy[21] has suggested that delayed ovulation or delayed fertilization leads to an immature conceptus which, although it reaches the uterine cavity, fails to maintain the corpus luteum, so that menstruation occurs, and regurgitation up the tube is followed by ectopic nidation within it. He derived evidence for this by comparing the size of the fetus recovered from a series of early tubal ectopics with the size expected chronologically, from the date of the last menstrual period. In about 75% of cases, the fetal development was greater than expected and was consistent with fertilization occurring prior to the reported interval since the last period.

An overly mature conceptus, in contrast, might implant in its passage down the tube if it had attained the development reached by a normal intrauterine pregnancy at the time of its implantation. Transmigration of the ovum from the opposite ovary has been suggested as the mechanism for this hypermaturation. Berlind[7] found that the corpus luteum was in the contralateral ovary in 50% of a series of tubal pregnancies. In contrast, in a group of women with intrauterine pregnancies who had only one functional tube, only 8% had the corpus luteum in the ovary opposite the functional tube. In one study of nonmacerated embryos from tubal pregnancies[33] 7 of 40 had a variety of cardiac anomalies. Of 25 successfully karyotyped ectopic pregnancies,[13] one was trisomic and at least 3 were mosaics. Three of the remaining embryos had congenital anomalies but normal karyotypes. No single chromosomal or somatic abnormality predominated.

The highest rate of ectopic pregnancy, from about 8 to 20%,[32] is found in women who have had a previous ectopic. The suggestion that recurrent ectopic pregnancy may be more common after salpingectomy rather than salpingo-oophorectomy remains to be confirmed. It does imply, however, that transmigration with ovum pickup by a contralateral tube may be a factor. Women with intrauterine contraceptive devices who become pregnant are more likely than a control group to have an ectopic pregnancy. If pregnancy does occur, the tube is the implantation site in about 3 to 4%[34] of cases.

The rarely seen intramural pregnancy, within the myometrium, may conceivably occur in an area of adenomyosis or it may also be caused by a prior perforation of the uterus or a prior myomectomy, as suggested by McGowan.[25] The occurrence of a pregnancy after total hysterectomy is extremely rare. In some cases the interval between the hysterectomy and the diagnosis of ectopic pregnancy is so short that it is evident the conception was present in the tube at the time of removal of the uterus. However, in a few cases, including the one reported by Hanes,[17] it is clear that fertilization had followed the operative procedure.

*Pathology*

The fallopian tube, in contrast to the uterus, is ill suited for the development of a pregnancy. It is a thin-walled structure and trophoblast readily penetrates the mucosa and muscle. The tubal mucosa has a very limited ability to undergo decidualization, one of the possible barriers to the penetration of myometrium by villi in normal pregnancy. Ruptured tubal pregnancy is closely analogous to the placenta increta and percreta of an intrauterine pregnancy. Furthermore, the conceptus grows in a lumen which, while distensible, reaches its limit of expansion long before the embryo reaches its full growth. These factors are reflected in the ultimate outcome of most tubal ectopics, namely, abortion (Figure 30.6) or perforation (Figure 30.7). In either event, the blood enters the peritoneal cavity through either the tubal infundibulum or the site of perforation, or both. The surgeon and pathologist should remember that all the gestational tissue may be discharged from the tube, and that the only microscopic proof of pregnancy may be found in a hematoma within the pelvic peritoneal cavity. Any such hematoma should be submitted to the laboratory. Such a situation is illustrated in Figure 30.8.

About 80% of all tubal pregnancies are located in the ampulla, and an additional 5% in the fimbrial end, or infundibulum. Some 13% are in the isthmus and the remainder are interstitial.[12] The clinical importance of the location relates to the early termination, at about 8 weeks,

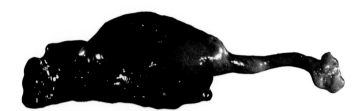

**30.6** Tubal ectopic pregnancy, external view. The fimbriated end is at left. Blood and aborted placenta occupy the distal half of the tube. The wall of the tube is markedly thinned and the blood shows through the serosal surface. Rupture, however, has not occurred.

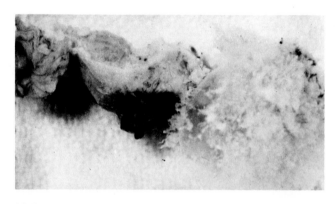

**30.7** Ruptured tubal ectopic pregnancy viewed under water. The fimbriated end is at left; the hemorrhagic site of perforation is at bottom center; and placental tissue, which has ruptured through the wall, is at right.

of ampullary pregnancies, and the late termination, usually by rupture at about 12 or more weeks, of isthmic and interstitial ectopics. An early, asymptomatic tubal pregnancy is shown in Figures 30.9a,b. The chorionic villi and trophoblast are viable, in contrast to the degenerating placental tissue (Figure 30.10) encountered to a variable degree in most aborted ectopics. The associated loss of trophoblast is responsible for the negative pregnancy test in some cases. An unusually advanced ampullary abortion is seen, in Figure 30.11, to contain a fetus whose size indicates at least 14 weeks of age. Although most tubal pregnancies terminate with rapidly developing hemoperitoneum and acute symptomatology, some have a chronic course. Such a case is illustrated in Figure 30.8. Slow leakage of blood, either from the tubal lumen or from a perforation site, accumulates in the cul de sac. The symptomatology may be vague and the differential diagnosis obscure.

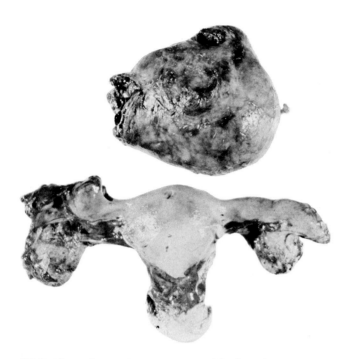

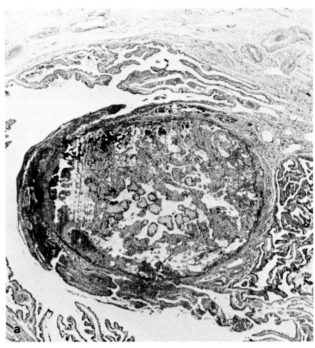

**30.8** Aborted ectopic pregnancy with chronic course. The anterior surface of uterus with attached adnexae is at bottom. There is bilateral chronic salpingitis, with distal occlusion and hydrosalpinx of right tube (on left) and multiple adhesions to right ovary. The left tube (on right) showed mucosal adhesions microscopically, a patent infundibulum, and organizing hemorrhage within its ampullary portion. The mass at top, removed from the pouch of Douglas, was an organizing hematoma in which degenerating placental villi were identified. Although no placental tissue was found in the left tube, one could presume that a pregnancy here had completely aborted into the pelvis. This patient was a diagnostic problem, operated on because of a pelvic mass. The preoperative pregnancy test was negative.

Most ectopic pregnancies terminate by tubal abortion or perforation, and death of the embryo is usual. It seems reasonable, however, that a certain unknown number must degenerate and resorb without detection. Rarely there is progression to fetal viability, probably following the successful transfer of placental growth from a tubal to an extratubal site. A few viable ectopic pregnancies apparently follow primary intraabdominal implantation.[40] Despite the absence of a visible embryo in most tubal pregnancies, microscopic verification of ectopic pregnancy is usually accomplished easily. Chorionic villi may be found penetrating the muscularis (Figure 30.12) and extending close

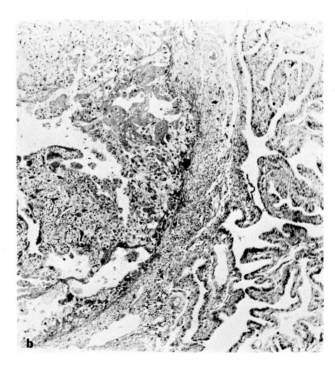

**30.9 a.** Early tubal pregnancy. This was an unsuspected finding in one tube, removed from a 37-year-old patient who underwent bilateral salpingo-oophorectomy for disseminated breast cancer. The pregnancy is intact. **b.** A higher magnification shows early placenta at left and tubal mucosa at right. Very little decidua is present.

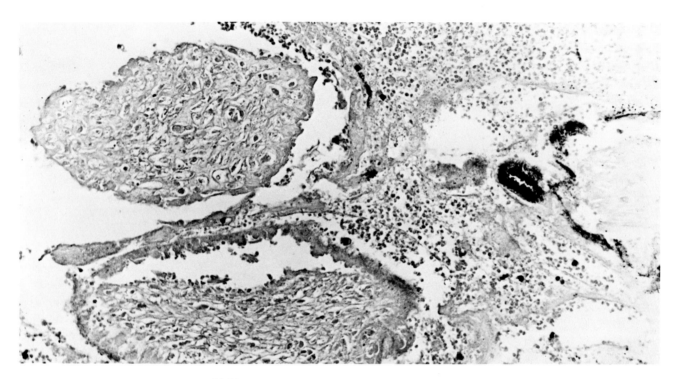

**30.10** Degenerating placental villi in an aborted ectopic pregnancy. No trophoblast can be identified. Fibrin, blood, and leukocytes are seen between the villi. There is calcification at right.

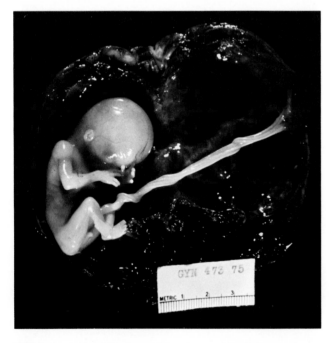

**30.11** An unusually large fetus in a midtubal ectopic pregnancy that aborted at about 14 weeks' gestational age.

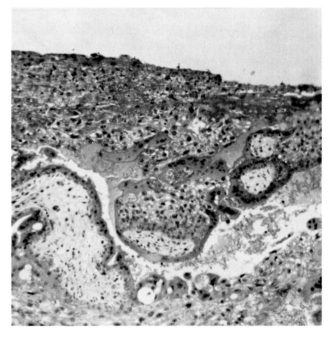

**30.12** Ectopic pregnancy. Chorionic villi of an ectopic pregnancy have all but penetrated to the serosal surface of the tube.

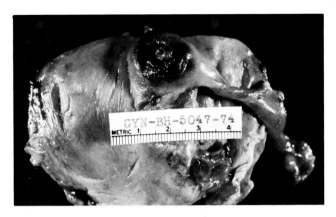

**30.13** A ruptured interstitial ectopic pregnancy. The fetus and some of the placenta had ruptured through the perforation on top of the corpus uteri at center. The associated tube extends to lower right. There was massive hemoperitoneum.

may occur. Rupture or abortion with hemorrhage may be fatal. Repeat ectopics comprises nearly 10% of all ectopic pregnancies.[16] This is presumably due to the frequent bilaterality of predisposing causes. Conservation of the affected tube may be attempted if maximum preservation of tissue is desirable, but the incidence of repeat ectopic pregnancy in the retained tube approaches 15%.[32,39]

### Isthmic and interstitial pregnancies

The less commonly encountered isthmic and interstitial pregnancies are surrounded by a thicker muscular wall and tend to terminate later than the ampullary, usually by rupture at from 10 to 16 weeks (Figures 30.13 and 30.14). In these locations the rupture may occur into the broad ligament rather than into the peritoneal cavity. Interstitial pregnancies may undergo massive hemorrhage and are especially life threatening.

### Ovarian pregnancy

Ovarian pregnancy[11] is extremely rare and must be carefully distinguished from an aborted tubal ectopic. The requirements for an acceptable primary ovarian gestation were originally defined by Spiegelberg[38] in an attempt to exclude a primary tubal site with abortion onto the ovary. A probable ovarian pregnancy is shown in Figure 30.15.

to or through the serosal surface. Decidual reaction at the site of nidation is scanty or absent. Small arteries may show lumenal narrowing by intimal hyperplasia.[10] While the embryo may be well preserved, extensive bleeding at the site of placentation results in fetal death with maceration and consequent difficulty in identifying fetal tissue.

Several important complications of tubal pregnancy

**30.14** A section adjacent to the perforation site in Figure 30.13 shows placenta within the interstitial portion of the fallopian tube.

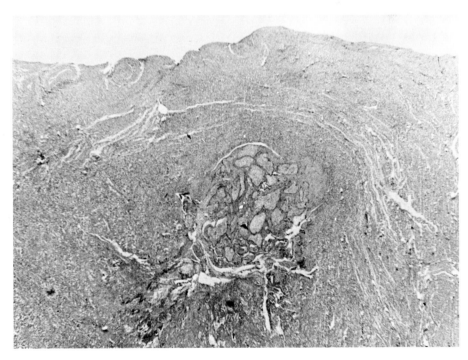

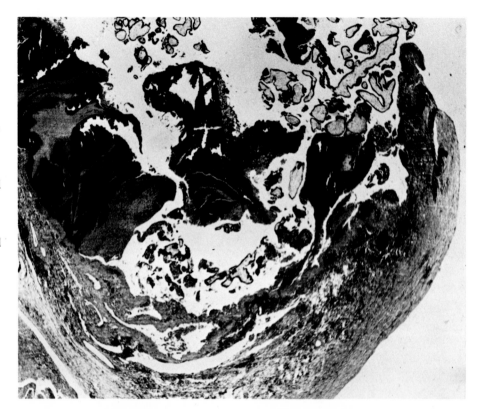

**30.15** Probable primary ovarian pregnancy. Placental tissue and blood occupy a cavity within the ovary. Although the associated tube was not removed, and therefore the possibility of a tubal ectopic aborting onto the ovary could not be eliminated microscopically, the tube looked normal to the surgeon and was described as clearly separate from the ovary.

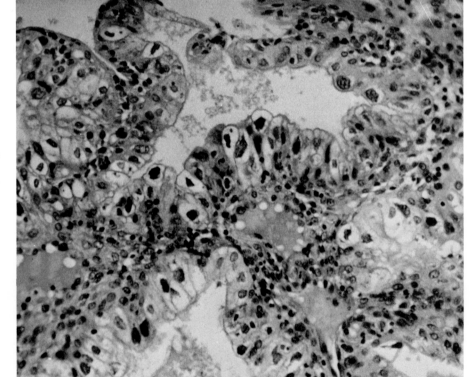

**30.16** Arias–Stella phenomenon. Note the hypersecretory endometrial glands and the pleomorphic nuclei, which are often in an apical location.

*Appearance of endometrium in ectopic pregnancy*

The chorionic gonadotropin levels in ectopic pregnancy are sufficient to give a positive pregnancy test in only about half of those affected. The effect of HCG can result in a piling up of epithelium, loss of polarity, nuclear atypia, and relatively pale cytoplasm (Figure 30.16). This is a hypersecretory response known as the Arias–Stella phenomenon. It is present in nearly 60% of ectopics, and occurs in over 85% where there is good preservation of villi.[8] It should be emphasized, however, that the endometrium may assume any morphology, including all phases of the normal cycle, in the presence of an ectopic pregnancy. Siddall[36] has shown that the frequency of decidual endometrium is inversely related to the duration of the vaginal bleeding. Based on a review totalling 171 cases, a 71% incidence of decidua followed bleeding of less than 1 week duration; whereas only 19% showed decidua after bleeding for more than 4 weeks.

Endometrial curettage can neither establish the diagnosis of ectopic pregnancy nor can it rule it out. If placental tissue is found, it may represent the intrauterine half of a combined, intra- and extrauterine, twin gestation. Although a rare occurrence,[47] this possibility must be kept in mind.

# Umbilical Cord and Major Vessels

The umbilical cord normally contains two arteries and a vein surrounded and protected by a gelatinous substance known as Wharton's jelly. The outer surface of the cord is covered by amnion.

## Length of Cord

The umbilical cord has a mean length in the neighborhood of 60 cm. Long cords are subject to many possible complications. The cord may wrap around the neck or other part of the fetus and result in death or disability. Torsion of the cord may interfere with the fetal blood supply *in utero*. The significance of this is difficult to judge, however, in the absence of thrombosed umbilical vessels. True knots do occur but may be confused with tortuous vessels or varicosities on superficial inspection. Finally, long cords are prone to prolapse at the time of delivery, with a threat to fetal survival.

Short cords may cause traction, leading to premature separation of the placenta (abruption). A further extension of this abnormal traction on the placenta may lead to inversion of the uterus. Disruption of the contained vessels may give rise to cord hemorrhage at the time of delivery. Extremely short cords may be continuous with an umbilical hernia of the fetus, which may contain abdominal viscera.

## Absence of One Umbilical Artery

In about 1% of deliveries, there is only a single umbilical artery. This finding is said to be even more common in spontaneous abortions, twin pregnancies, and especially in acardiac twin pregnancies. The diagnosis can be made grossly by careful examination of the transected cord but should be confirmed microscopically. Some cases show total absence of one artery. In others, muscular or elastic elements suggest the possibility of atrophy of a preexisting artery instead of agenesis. The significance of single umbilical artery lies in the high associated infant mortality and the high incidence of anomalies. A study of Froehlich and Fujikura[15] among approximately 40,000 consecutive single births showed an 0.9% incidence of single artery, an infant mortality of 14%, and malformations in 53% of the dead infants. The anomalies varied widely in the autopsied cases and, in descending frequency, were genitourinary, cardiovascular, cleft palate, musculoskeletal, and omphalocele. Despite the high infant mortality, it is of interest that survivors with a single umbilical artery, who were followed to the age of 4 years, had no clinically detectable anomalies other than inguinal hernia at a higher incidence than a control group of infants.

## Velamentous Insertion of Cord

The cord usually inserts somewhat eccentrically into the surface of the chorion frondosum. Central and marginal insertions are both less common. The rarest position, found in about 1% of placentas, is insertion into the free chorion leve. This is termed velamentous, or membranous, insertion (Figure 30.17). When the exposed cord vessels cross the internal os, in the condition known as vasa previa, rupture and hemorrhage may occur during delivery. Marginal insertion of the cord, so-called battledore placenta, is usually of no clinical significance.

# Placental Membranes

It was mentioned earlier that the amnion develops as early as the twelfth day from cells that originate from the cytotrophoblast. Amniotic fluid accumulates in the cavity and the latter is essentially sealed to the outside until

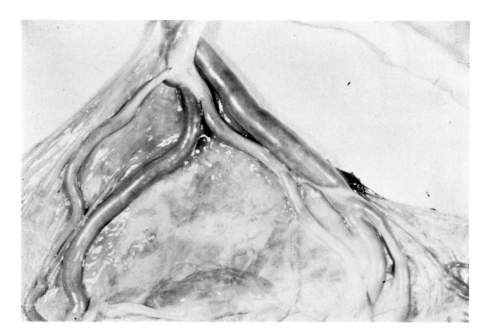

**30.17** Velamentous insertion of the cord. The cord vessels branch within the free membranes, which reflect off the surface of the placenta at the bottom of the photograph.

membranes are ruptured. It is presumed that amniotic fluid is produced by amnion cells either by filtration or by secretion. There is a regular circulation of amniotic fluid. The fetus swallows the fluid, and it is assumed that the water is absorbed through the gut into the bloodstream and some of it then passes into the maternal circulation via the placenta. If esophageal atresia or lack of nervous control of the swallowing reflex, as in anencephaly, is present, the fetus does not swallow amniotic fluid and a condition known as hydramnios, or polyhydramnios, develops, which is an excessive amount of amniotic fluid. When the fetal kidney begins to function, it produces urine that is added to the amniotic fluid. In cases of renal agenesis, too little fluid is present in the cavity and this is oligohydramnios. In summary, amniotic fluid is swallowed by the fetus and excreted in the urine. Chapter 34 discusses in detail the value of studying this fluid by biochemical assay to ascertain fetal maturity and viability. Cytogenetic studies can also be made from amnion cells in order to determine Down's syndrome and other chromosomal abnormalities relatively early in pregnancy. Certain biochemical assays can detect genetic disorders of metabolism.

## Amnionic Bands and Rupture

Amnionic bands may be associated with fetal malformations, usually involving the extremities, such as digital amputations, syndactyly, constriction rings, or clubbed feet (see Figure 37.17a,b). Although often a puzzling phenom-

enon, careful examination of the membranes has shown rupture of the amnion in some cases, with the damage apparently caused by the trauma of constricting strands of membrane.[23] More serious malformations, such as anencephaly and visceral eventration, are also reported in association with rupture of the amnion.[5] Examination of the membranes in suspected cases is, of course, often complicated by trauma to the placenta at delivery. Scrutiny of the amnion under water (see Figure 37.16) may help reveal the rupture site and the bands. Microscopic confirmation should show an area of chorion free from a covering of amnion on the fetal surface. The etiology is unknown, although trauma has been suspected in some cases.

## Meconium

Meconium is excreted from the fetal bowel usually as a result of fetal distress. The surface of the placental membranes shows a green discoloration. Microscopic examination shows pigment-laden macrophages in the subepithelial stroma of the amnion (Figure 30.18). Degeneration of the epithelium itself may follow prolonged contact with meconium.

## Amnion Nodosum

Focal, pale, slightly elevated nodules on the amnionic surface may represent amnion nodosum. Other possibilities are squamous metaplasia (Figure 30.19), or extremely

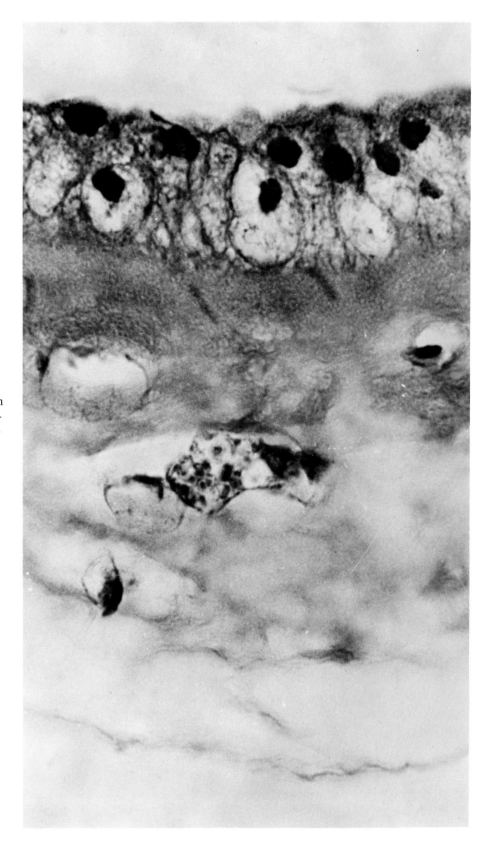

**30.18** Meconium-stained amnion. Pigment granules are seen within the cytoplasm of a macrophage at center. Amnion epithelium is at top.

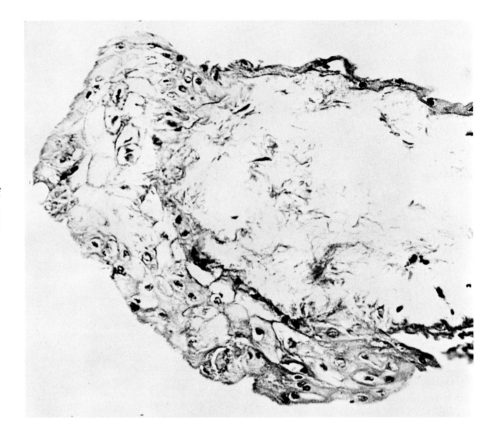

**30.19** Squamous metaplasia of the amnion. The normal single layer of epithelium is replaced by a plaque of squamous epithelium at left.

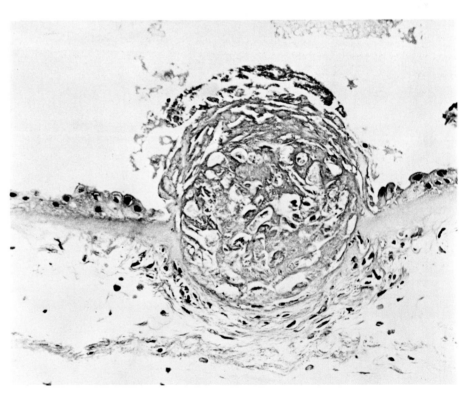

**30.20** Amnion nodosum. This well-circumscribed mixture of amorphous material and poorly defined cells projects above and below the adjacent amnion epithelium.

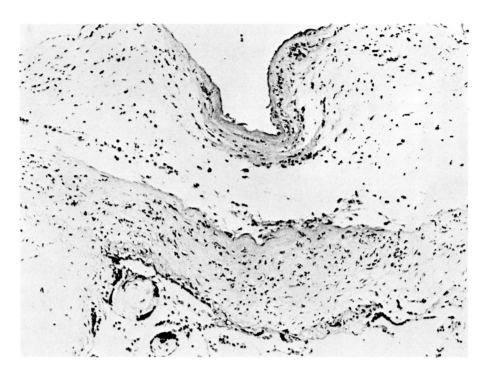

**30.21** Acute chorioamnionitis. Polymorphonuclear leukocytes infiltrate amnion (top) and chorion (bottom).

rarely, tuberculosis. The foci of amnion nodosum are easily detached. Microscopically (Figure 30.20), they are elevated eosinophilic zones composed of a mixture of amorphous material, laminated fibrillary structures, and poorly visualized nuclei. The electron microscope reveals the presence of epithelial cells.[31] This tends to confirm the general belief that they derive from the fetal skin, a theory further buttressed by the finding of lanugo hairs within an occasional nodule. Their presence correlates with oligohydramnios, the close apposition of fetal epidermis to amnion apparently leading to their development. The presence of amnion nodosum can serve to confirm oligohydramnios and should suggest the possibility of a congenital urinary tract abnormality in the fetus.

## Amnionitis and Chorionitis

Bacterial infection of the membranes (Figure 30.21) is a frequent finding, occurring in as many as 10% of all deliveries. It is associated with prematurity of the fetus, respiratory distress and jaundice in the newborn, and increased neonatal mortality. Maternal associations are with premature rupture of the membranes and prolonged labor. Theoretically, infection could reach the membranes directly or could come through the placenta itself via the maternal circulation. The latter route has been implicated in a few cases of maternal septicemia, such as bacterial endocarditis. The usual route, however, is ascent of infection up the birth canal.[4] The most common organisms, *Escherichia coli* and *Staphylococcus,* correspond to the flora usually cultured from the vagina. Inflammation of the cord vessels and of the cord substance itself tends to be less severe and appears to follow the involvement of the membranes (Figure 30.22).

Examination of the membranes and cord has been advocated in order to identify a group of fetuses at risk. Rapid examination of a whole mount of amnion stained with cresyl violet has been suggested[9] as a method for identifying an inflammatory cell infiltrate.

In some instances, microscopically demonstrated chorioamnionitis occurs after otherwise normal pregnancies and deliveries and without morbidity in the newborn infant. Neonatal cultures positive for T-mycoplasma, an organism of low virulence, have been implicated in a sequential group of such cases.[35]

## Twins

Twin placentas are conveniently discussed under the membranes because the number of amnions and chorions surrounding each fetus may establish the zygosity and therefore correlate with some complications of twinning.

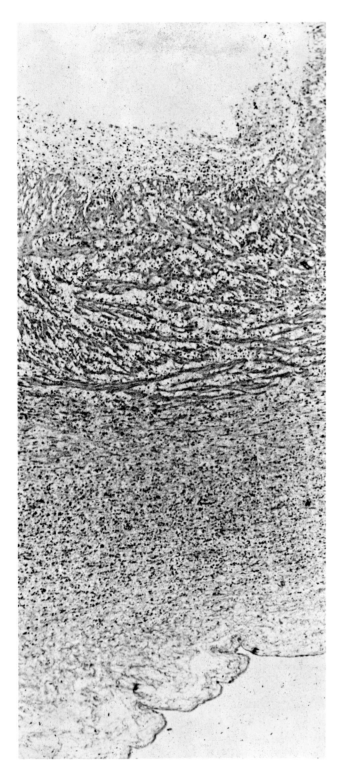

**30.22** Acute funisitis with vasculitis. Neutrophils infiltrate all layers of the vessel as well as the stroma of the umbilical cord.

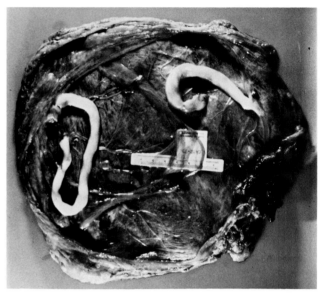

**30.23** Monochorionic, diamnionic twin placenta. The combined membranes are transparent as seen above the ruler.

If a single chorion invests the twins, and no chorion is interspersed between the amnions where the latter are adjacent, the placenta is monochorionic and is always the product of a monozygotic fertilization. Approximately 20% of twin gestations in the United States are monochorionic. The fetuses are of the same sex, are termed identical, and are optimal candidates for organ transplantation in the remote event that it is later indicated. The gross examination of a twin placenta should include careful scrutiny of the combined membranes. In monochorionic twinning, with no chorion between the adjacent amnions, the combined membranes are transparent (Figure 30.23), in contrast to the opaque appearance of the dichorionic variety. Microscopic sections can either be taken of strips of the combined membranes or can assume the shape of an inverted T, in which the crossbar is the fetal surface of the placenta and the vertical bar is represented by the combined membranes inserting into it. In either case, such sections show a monochorionic placenta to have amnion meeting amnion (Figure 30.24).

Vascular anastomoses between the two fetal circulations are present in most monochorionic twin placentas and may be demonstrated by injection studies (Figure 30.25a,b). They are often visible simply on gross examination. They are not present in dichorionic twinning. Such anastomoses form the basis for the transfusion syndrome in which blood is transferred *in utero* from one twin to another.[6]

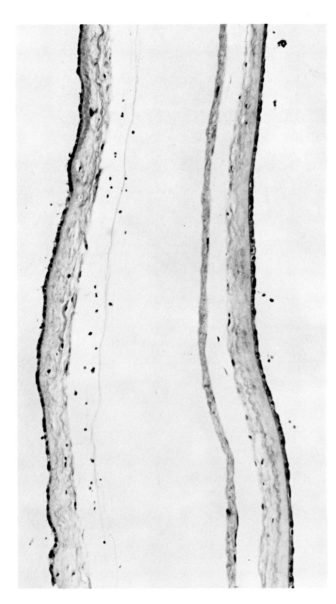

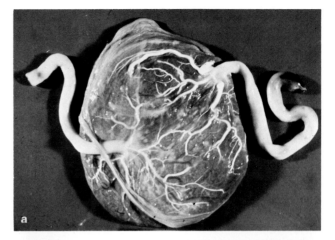

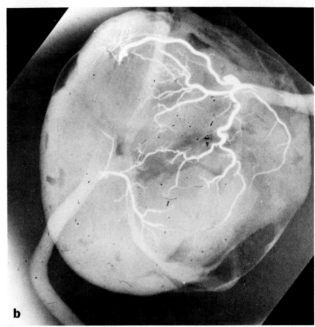

**30.24** Monochorionic, diamnionic twin placenta. This section of the combined membranes shows two amnions without intervening chorions.

Dichorionic placentas, in contrast, occur in about 80% of twin gestations. The fetuses can be either mono- or dizygotic. If the sexes are different, the twins are fraternal. If, however, the sex is the same, the zygosity can only be established by genotypic studies. The combined membranes in dichorionic placentas are opaque and, microscopically, two chorions are interposed between the amnions (Figure 30.26). Vascular anastomoses between the two circulations are absent.

**30.25 a.** This monochorionic twin placenta had radiopaque material injected into the vasculature of the umbilical cord at right. An anastomosis communicating with a vessel of the cord at left is seen directly below center. **b.** X-ray of injected specimen brings out vascular anastomosis.

Monoamnionic twinning is an extremely rare type of monochorionic placentation. An example is shown in Figure 30.27. The fetuses are identical, vascular anastomoses are frequent, and the added hazard of intertwining of the cords leads to the perinatal loss of one or both babies in about 40% of cases.

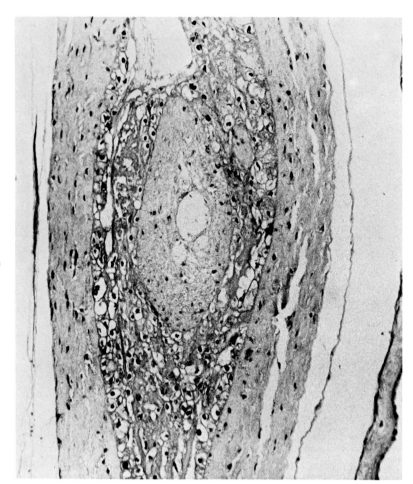

**30.26** Dichorionic, diamnionic twin placenta. Here the combination consist of amnion, chorion, chorion, amnion. Note the degenerate villus in center between the two chorions.

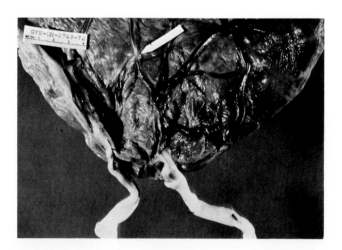

**30.27** Monochorionic, monoamnionic twin placenta. No membrane separates the two umbilical cords, which insert at the placental margin, bottom. An anastomosis between the two circulations is indicated by the pointer. In this case both babies survived.

## Amniotic Fluid Embolism

This condition usually occurs during the first stage of labor, after rupture of the membranes, and is caused by the entrance of amniotic fluid into maternal veins with emboli to the lungs (Figure 30.28). Most common in multiparous patients, it follows rapid labors with strong contractions. Oxytocin stimulation of labor is a frequent precursor. The mother characteristically is dyspneic, goes into shock, and may die within a few minutes. Although considered to be fatal in most cases, it is difficult to document the entity in suspected survivors because the diagnosis depends on the demonstration of amniotic elements within pulmonary vessels.

Postpartum hemorrhage is an important feature of amniotic fluid embolism. It is associated with hypofibrinogenemia and with abnormal blood coagulation that in one well-documented case[3] was primarily characterized by an increase in fibrinolytic activity.

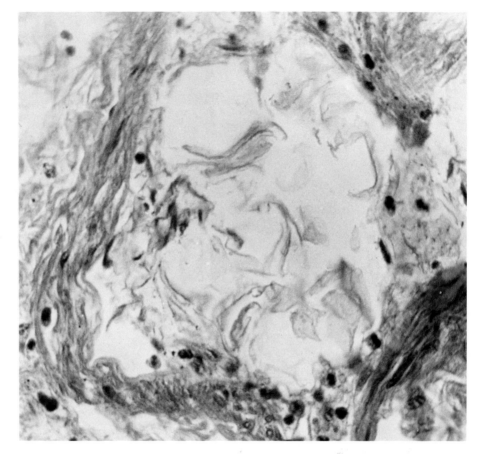

**30.28** Amniotic fluid embolus. Particles of keratin (squames) are within the lumen of a small pulmonary artery.

# Abnormal Placental Architecture

The placenta is subject to innumerable variations in shape and form, many of which are probably of no pathologic significance (bilobed, trilobed, horseshoe-shaped, etc.). A few of the most important are discussed below.

## Succenturiate Lobe

Succenturiate, or accessory, lobes (Figure 30.29) are single or multiple masses of placental tissue, separated from the main part of the placenta and supplied with fetal blood vessels that reach the accessory areas through essentially avillous chorionic tissue. As pointed out by Benirschke and Driscoll,[5] such lobes may be retained in the uterus following the delivery of a placenta that shows no grossly apparent missing portions on the maternal surface. Large fetal vessels, terminating at the edge of a tear in the membranes, suggest this situation. There are only a

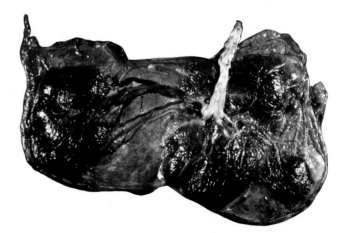

**30.29** Succenturiate lobe. Prominent vessels connect it to the main mass of the placenta at right.

few reports of placenta previa involving a succenturiate lobe; the most recently encountered one[42] includes two cases.

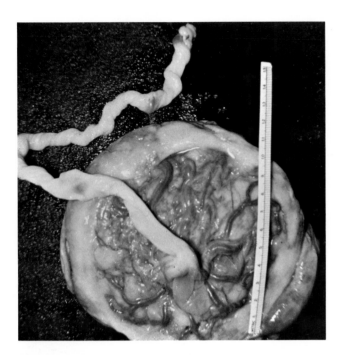

**30.30** Circumvallate placenta. An elevated, pale rim surrounds the fetal surface of the placenta.

## Placenta Membranacea

Placenta membranacea is a rare condition in which most of the fetal membranes are covered by placental tissue. This reduction in the area of free membranes is accompanied by an excessively thin placenta with a large surface area of functional villous tissue. Recognized complications are placenta accreta and placenta previa, with accompanying premature separation. Many theories of origin have been suggested, including abnormally deep implantation and chronic endometritis.[5]

## Circummarginate and Circumvallate Placenta

In these conditions there is a lateral extension of villous tissue beyond the reflection of the chorion leve off the fetal surface of the placenta. In the circummarginate placenta the surface is flat. The circumvallate type is distinguished by an elevated rim at the margin, giving the appearance of a collar button (Figure 30.30).

Both conditions tend to coexist and may be partial or complete. Most observers have associated them with an increased incidence of antepartum hemorrhage. The rim of

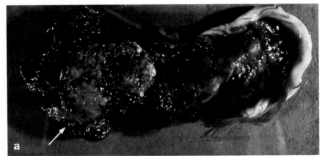

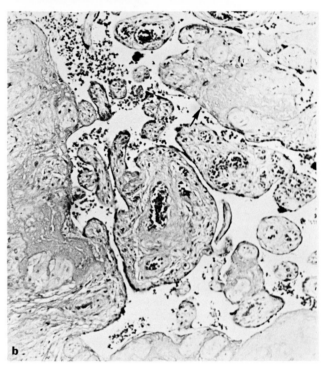

**30.31 a.** Infarct. Seen in cross section, this pale yellow, firm infarct measures about 5 cm in greatest diameter. It occupies almost the entire thickness of the placenta. The umbilical cord inserts into the placenta at top right. **b.** Infarcted villi, at left, are separated by fibrin. The villi at right are viable.

tissue at the margin of the circumvallate placenta contains fibrin and degenerating blood, with or without chorionic villi or decidua. Of the many suggested etiologic factors, the most tenable seems to be that of multiple, small marginal hemorrhages or abruptions.[27]

Leakage of amniotic fluid (hydrorrhea) is also a reported complication.

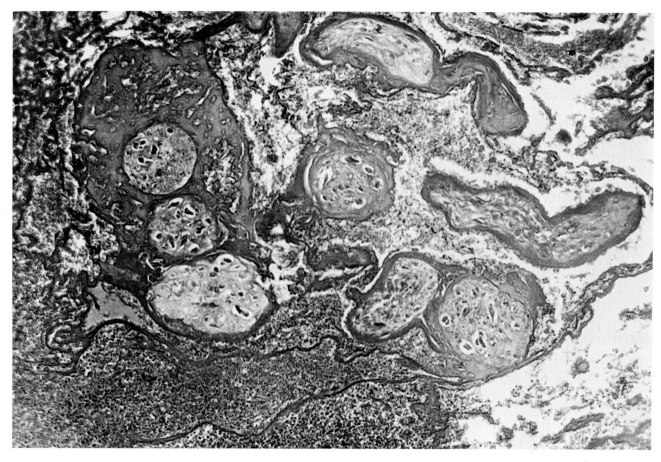

**30.32** Infarcted villi, separated by blood and fibrin, show varying degrees of loss of staining of stromal nuclei. There is no visible trophoblast.

# Disturbances of Circulation

Disturbances in the fetal circulation are associated with effects on the chorionic villi, which are discussed in Chapters 32 and 33 dealing with abortion and gestational trophoblast disease. These effects, however, do not include infarction, which requires interference with the maternal circulation for its occurrence.

## Infarction

Infarcts of the placenta are common and usually occur late in pregnancy. Correlation of their presence with clinical maternal or fetal events is often difficult. They are usually located at the margin of the placenta, vary in size from a few millimeters to several centimeters, and vary in color from deep red, for fresh ones, to yellow-white, for older lesions. They are firm and generally dry when sectioned (Figure 30.31a). Histologically (Figure 30.31b), there is breakdown of the intervillous maternal blood with fibrin deposition. The villi show loss of nuclear staining of all elements, including trophoblast (Figure 30.32) eventuating in the formation of "ghost" villi, totally devoid of viable cells. Although placental infarcts may calcify, organization with the production of granulation tissue and subsequent scarring does not occur and cannot be used to help estimate their age. Zeek and Assali[49] have provided a detailed description of infarcts, with differential features that distinguish them from intervillous fibrin deposits or thrombi and from chorangiomas.

It is now generally agreed that the genesis of infarction of the placenta requires some interference with the mater-

665

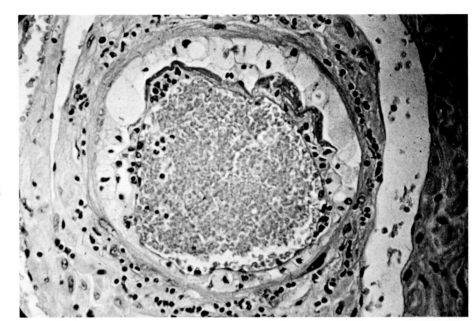

**30.33** Atherosis of a decidual arteriole in toxemia. Large, pale, lipid-filled, subendothelial macrophages surround blood in the center.

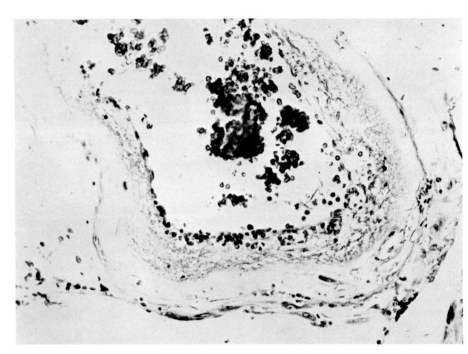

**30.34** Toxemia. Granular deposits of fibrin (fibrinoid) are present beneath the endothelium of this decidual arteriole. Note clumped red blood cells in center.

nal circulation. Placental separation, or abruption, interrupts the normal supply of maternal blood, and infarcts often occur in the vicinity. Infarcts have been produced experimentally by ligation of uteroplacental arteries in pregnant rhesus monkeys.[44] Examination of infarcts in human placentas has implicated thrombosed maternal arteries in their genesis.[43] Frequently, in practice, no maternal vascular lesion can be found, nor can any maternal disease with a vascular component be identified. It is clear, however, that hypertension, toxemia, nephritis, diabetes mellitus, and lupus erythematosus, all with lesions in small maternal arterial branches, are significantly associated with placental infarcts. The examination of the maternal vessels accompanying a specimen of placenta requires a sampling of attached pieces of decidua. This is best done in sections taken at the margin, where a pocket of decidua is often attached in the angle between the reflection of the membranes and the edge of the villous tissue. Additionally, sections of opaque areas on the outside of the chorion leve may show attached decidua vera with contained vessels.

Hertig[19] described lesions of the maternal arterioles in the placental site of toxemics. The lesions included the presence of subendothelial lipid-filled macrophages (Figure 30.33), fibrinoid degeneration (Figure 30.34), and inflammation of arteriolar walls. Dixon and Robertson[14] examined biopsies of the placental bed obtained at caesarean section from 15 normotensive controls and from 18 hypertensive patients, nine of whom were toxemic. They described hyperplasia and hyalinization of arterioles, fibrinoid degeneration, and occasional subendothelial lipophage infiltrates in the hypertensives. They conclude that the lesions are absent from normals, that they are similar in the hypertensives whether or not toxemia is present, and that their extent seems to correlate with the clinical severity of the hypertension.

Predating the descriptions of vascular lesions referred to above was a paper by Tenny and Parker[41] on changes in the syncytiotrophoblast in toxemic placentas. Increased clumping of nuclei, out of proportion to that normally seen in the third trimester placenta approaching term, correlated with the presence of toxemia. They felt that this finding signified premature aging of the placenta. This syncytial "knotting," often referred to as the "Tenny change," is now felt to result from anoxia of the intervillous maternal blood of whatever cause. It is often observed in the chorionic villi adjacent to areas of infarction.

## Abruptio Placentae

Abruptio placentae is defined as premature separation of the normally implanted placenta occurring after 20 weeks' gestation. With placenta previa, it is responsible for most cases of third trimester vaginal bleeding. Abruption can be marginal or central. Marginal abruption (Figure 30.35) is the most common site and is associated with bleeding, which appears vaginally. Central abruption, however, may produce concealed hemorrhage that, if it dissects into the underlying myometrium, leads to the so-called Couvelaire uterus, a large, boggy, deep bluish organ that contracts poorly and then tends to bleed massively postpartum.

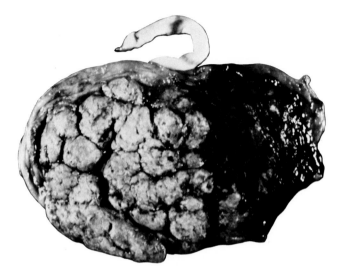

**30.35** Abruptio placentae. The dark area at right, extending to the margin of the maternal surface of the placenta, is the site of premature separation. About one-third of the placenta is involved.

The gross examination of the placenta is of crucial important in the diagnosis of abruption, and it requires great care. Normally the placenta separates by means of a cleavage plane within the maternal decidua, which results in the complete delivery of an intact placenta. A certain amount of blood adheres to the maternal surface of an intact placenta, but it is superficial and does not interrupt the bulging surface of the cotyledons. An area of premature separation, however, occurring before delivery, produces a zone of hemorrhage that extends into the placental tissue and replaces it (Figure 30.36). The microscopic sections add little to the gross examination except, possibly, an assessment of the degree of degeneration of the blood elements in the area of hemorrhage, which may provide an idea of its age. Because placental hemorrhage, like infarction, does not organize in the usual sense, granulation and fibrous tissue do not provide clues to the dating of hemorrhage as they do in other tissues.

There is a significant incidence of toxemia and hypertension in association with abruption. The maternal vascular lesions discussed under infarction, particularly the necrotizing ones, are probably responsible, although it is difficult in practice to relate an area of hemorrhage to disease in an immediately related vessel.

Trauma is responsible for a very small number of cases of premature separation,[20] probably amounting to less than 5%.

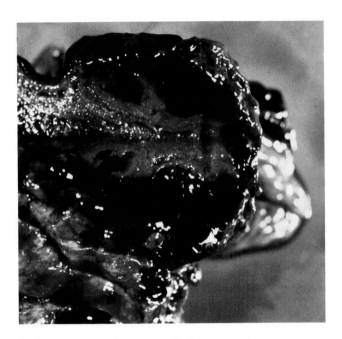

**30.36** Abruptio placentae. The blood has been sectioned through the maternal surface, showing that it extends into, and apparently replaces, placental tissue.

## Toxemia of Pregnancy

Toxemia is also referred to as preeclampsia and hypertensive disorder of pregnancy. In the last trimester of pregnancy, or at the time of delivery, the triad of hypertension, proteinuria, and edema may develop. Some patients have preexisting renal disease and/or hypertension, but in the vast majority of cases there is no underlying disease. The triad described is referred to as preeclampsia, and when convulsive seizures develop it is referred to as eclampsia. The term toxemia of pregnancy is a misnomer that is based on an early postulate that toxins are produced that cause the syndrome. The hallmark of this disorder is hypertension associated with vasospasm. It is a systemic disorder, and small vessels containing fibrin thrombi can be found in the liver, brain, and kidney. The vascular lesions in the maternal decidua, as well as the frequency of placental infarction and abruption, have already been discussed. Although the etiology remains unknown, there is considerable evidence for an initiating factor that originates in the placenta and results from ischemia. Except in those cases where cerebral hemorrhage may occur, the manifestations of this disorder are reversible, and in most cases the blood pressure returns to normotensive levels after evacuation of the placenta.

## Erythroblastosis Fetalis

The fetal morbidity in erythroblastosis results from the hemolysis of fetal red blood cells by maternal antibodies that cross the placenta. Of the three syndromes of kernicterus, anemia, and edema, the most marked placental abnormalities occur in association with fetal edema, or hydrops. As described by Hellman and Hertig,[18] the placenta is a large, heavy, pale organ. Microscopically (Figure 30.37), the villi are large and their stroma is edematous and cellular. Common to all three clinical types of the disease is the finding of dilated fetal capillaries containing many nucleated red blood cells and, on occasion, foci of erythropoiesis. This contrasts with the normal situation in which nucleated red cells are not observed in the villi after midgestation. Finally, in erythroblastosis, the trophoblast is immature relative to the stage of gestation, forming a thick covering of the villi, with the persistence of cytotrophoblast that is visible through the light microscope.

## Chorangioma

Two neoplasms are found in the placenta, choriocarcinoma which is discussed in Chapter 33 and chorangioma which is the subject of this discussion.

Considered by some to be a malformation rather than a true tumor, chorangioma is a focal mixture of blood vessels and fibrous tissue. It varies in color from red toward white, depending on the proportion of these two components (Figures 30.38 and 30.39). Most are located within the placental tissue, although a few have been described attached to the cord or membranes. Although the majority are small, tumors several centimeters in diameter have been reported. Their reported incidence is 1 to 2%, but this figure may be raised by scrupulous gross examination. They are easily mistaken for infarcts or intervillous thrombi.

An association exists between chorangioma, polyhydramnios, and enlargement of the fetal heart. Possibly, the perfusion of the vascular tumor by fetal blood puts a strain on the cardiovascular system analogous to the transfusion syndrome in twins. It is debatable whether fetal circulatory failure precedes and leads to the hydramnios or whether the latter is directly associated with the tumor.

One thorough review of the subject[37] concludes that large tumors tend to be associated with hydramnios and premature births, that toxemia is increased in incidence irrespective of tumor size, and that a possible association of chorangioma with fetal anomalies requires further investigation.

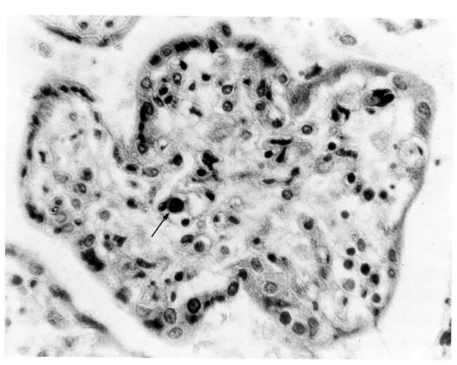

**30.37** Erythroblastosis delivered at 36 weeks. The baby had hydrops fetalis and did not survive. This chorionic villus is immature. The stroma is hypercellular. Nucleated fetal red cells are present in the vessels, with an erythroblast at arrow. There is a prominent surface layer of cytotrophoblast.

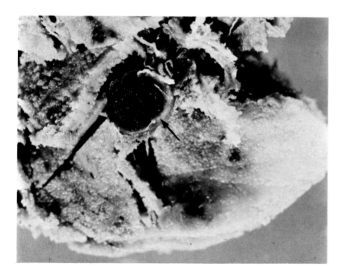

**30.38** Chorangioma. The lesion is dark, sharply circumscribed, and less than 1 cm in diameter.

## Placentitis

The membranes are the part of the placenta most frequently involved by bacterial infection. As already discussed in connection with amnionitis and chorionitis, such infection is usually caused by the ascent of bacteria up the birth canal after premature rupture of the membranes. The villous placental tissue is only secondarily involved, if at all, in this process. *Staphylococcus pyogenes, Escherichia coli,* and other gram-negative organisms are the most common infecting agents.

Three other rare infections of the placenta should be mentioned: tuberculosis, syphilis, and listeriosis. Figure 30.40a,b show the gross and microscopic appearance of tuberculosis. The placenta is involved with extreme rarity, partly because of the infertility of tuberculous patients and partly because miliary spread, apparently a requisite for placental infection in most reported cases, must coincide with gestation. Warthin[45] gives a detailed description of one case, with lesions of the membranes, chorionic blood vessels and villi, and decidua. Granulomata were present except in the decidua, which showed only necrosis and which, the author felt, was incapable of developing a granulomatous response. Lungs and liver are the commonest sites of fetal infection, the former following aspiration of infected amniotic fluid, and the latter resulting from hematogenous spread via chorionic and umbilical vessels.

Syphilitic placentitis has become extremely rare. Classically, the placenta is described as large and pale, with cellular, chronically inflamed villi. Benirschke and Driscoll[5] cast doubt on the specificity of the findings in placental syphilis.

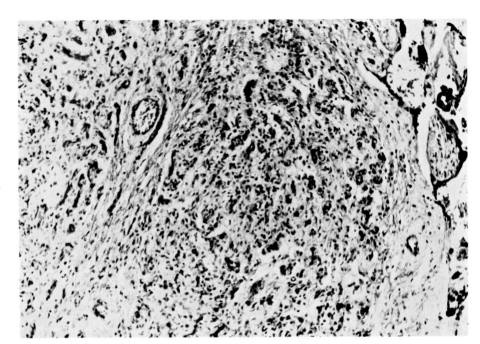

**30.39** Chorangioma. The blood vessels composing it are for the most part extremely small. Normal placenta is at upper right.

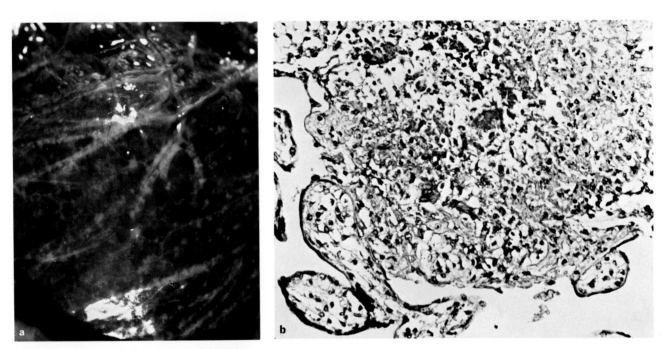

**30.40 a.** Tuberculosis. A 42-year-old black woman, febrile for several weeks, had no prenatal care and came to the hospital in labor. Chest x-ray showed a miliary infiltrate. The fetal surface of the placenta shows miliary white foci. Tubercle bacilli were found on smear and culture of the amniotic fluid. **b.** A moderately well-defined granuloma, with slight central necrosis, apparently involves several chorionic villi. Stainable tubercle bacilli were found in tissue sections. Granulomas were also found in amnion. The infant showed no clinical evidence of tuberculosis and was given prophylactic chemotherapy.

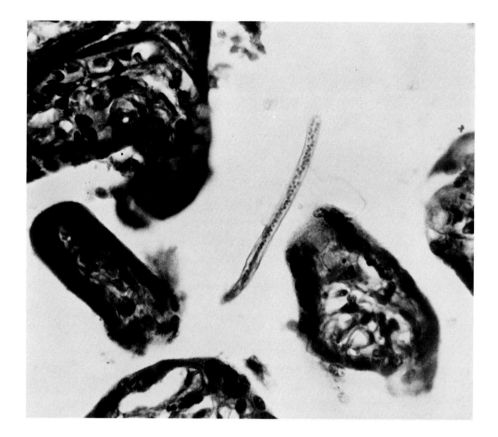

**30.41** Filarial parasite in maternal blood between the chorionic villi of a term placenta.

[Courtesy of Dr. John K. Li.]

Listeriosis[5] is responsible for abortion in cattle, sheep, and goats. Human infection is less common, and reports from Europe exceed those from the United States. Miliary abscesses, containing the *Listeria monocytogenes* bacilli, are found in the membranes, in the placenta proper, and within fetal organs.

The most important parasitic disease of the placenta is toxoplasmosis. Examination of the placenta from cases of congenital toxoplasmosis may reveal focal, chronic inflammatory lesions of the villi, generally nonspecific in nature, with identifiable organisms most often found in sections of the membranes.[46,48]

An incidentally observed filarial parasite in the intervillous blood is seen in Figure 30.41.

A number of maternal virus infections have been shown to involve the placenta and fetus. The best evidence is that the agents pass from the maternal intervillous blood into the villi and thence infect the fetal blood. Rubella, with its documented teratogenic capacity, produces placental lesions in all trimesters of pregnancy, the presence of which tends to correlate with the presence of fetal anomalies. Villous edema, fibrosis, and vasculitis and perivasculitis have been described in a series of induced abortions, as well as areas of villous necrosis, the latter most prominent in the earlier gestations.[29]

Variola, varicella, and vaccinia infections produce necrotizing lesions of placental villi.[5]

Whereas microscopic inflammatory lesions of the villi occur in a variety of known maternal virus infections, such lesions may also be found in placentas from clinically uncomplicated pregnancies. Correlation has been made between the presence of such placental lesions and "dysmature" infants who are small for their gestational age.[2] The suggestion is made that an unrecognized virus infection may be responsible.

# REFERENCES

1. Allen, M. S., and Turner, U. G. Twin birth—identical or fraternal twins? *Obstet. Gynecol.* 37:538, 1971.

2. Altshuler, G., Russell, P., and Ermocilla, R. The placental pathology of small-for-gestational age infants. *Am. J. Obstet. Gynecol.* 121:351, 1975.

3. Beller, F. K., Douglas, G. W., Debrovner, C. H., and

Robinson, R. The fibrinolytic system in amniotic fluid embolism. *Am. J. Obstet. Gynecol.* 87:48, 1963.

4. Benirschke, K. Routes and types of infection in the fetus and the newborn. *Am. J. Dis. Child.* 99:714, 1960.

5. Benirschke, K., and Driscoll, S. G. *The Pathology of the Human Placenta.* New York: Springer-Verlag, 1967.

6. Benirschke, K., and Kim, C. K. Multiple pregnancy. *N. Engl. J. Med.* 288:1276, 1329, 1973.

7. Berlind, M. The contralateral corpus luteum—an important factor in ectopic pregnancies. *Obstet. Gynecol.* 16:51, 1960.

8. Birch, H. W., and Collins, C. G. Atypical changes of genital epithelium associated with ectopic pregnancy. *Am. J. Obstet. Gynecol.* 81:1198, 1961.

9. Blanc, W. A. Pathways of fetal and early neonatal infection. *J. Pediatr.* 59:473, 1961.

10. Blaustein, A., and Shenker, L. Vascular lesions of the uterine tube in ectopic pregnancy. *Obstet. Gynecol.* 30:551, 1967.

11. Boronow, R. C., McElin, T. W., West, R. H., and Buckingham, J. C. Ovarian pregnancy. *Am. J. Obstet. Gynecol.* 91:1095, 1965.

12. Breen, J. L. Ectopic pregnancies: A 21 year survey of 654 ectopic pregnancies. *Am. J. Obstet. Gynecol.* 106:1004, 1970.

13. Busch, D. H., and Benirschke, K. Cytogenetic studies of ectopic pregnancies. *Virchows Arch. B. Coll. Pathol.* 16:319, 1974.

14. Dixon, H. G., and Robertson, W. B. A study of the vessels of the placental bed in normotensive and hypertensive women. *J. Obstet. Gynaecol. Br. Emp.* 65:803, 1958.

15. Froehlich, L. A., and Fujikura, T. Follow-up of infants with single umbilical artery. *Pediatrics* 52:6, 1973.

16. Hallat, J. G. Repeat ectopic pregnancy: A study of 123 consecutive cases. *Am. J. Obstet. Gynecol.* 122:520, 1975.

17. Hanes, M. V. Ectopic pregnancy following total hysterectomy. *Obstet. Gynecol.* 23:882, 1964.

18. Hellman, L. M., and Hertig, A. T. Pathological changes in the placenta associated with erythroblastosis of the fetus. *Am. J. Pathol.* 14:111, 1938.

19. Hertig, A. T. Vascular pathology in the hypertensive albuminuric toxemias of pregnancy. *Clinics* 4:602, 1945.

20. Hertig, A. T., and Sheldon, W. H. Minimal criteria required to prove prima facie case of traumatic abortion or miscarriage. *Ann. Surg.* 117:596, 1943.

21. Iffy, L. Embryologic studies of time of conception in ectopic pregnancy and first-trimester abortion. *Obstet. Gynecol.* 26:490, 1965.

22. Kistner, R. W., Hertig, A. T., and Reid, D. E. Simultaneously occurring placenta previa and placenta accreta. *Surg. Gynecol. Obstet.* 94:141, 1952.

23. Krag, D. Amnionic rupture and birth defects of the extremities. *Hum. Pathol.* 5:69, 1974.

24. Lapin, B. A., and Yakolava, L. A. *Comparative Physiology in Monkeys.* Springfield, Ill., E. E. Thomas, 1963, p. 215.

25. McGowan, L. Intramural pregnancy. *J.A.M.A.* 192:637, 1965.

26. Millar, W. G. A clinical and pathological study of placenta accreta. *J. Obstet. Gynaecol. Br. Emp.* 66:353, 1959.

27. Naftolin, F., Khudr, G., Benirschke, K., and Hutchinson, D. L. The syndrome of chronic abruption placentae, hydrorrhea and circumvallate placenta. *Am. J. Obstet. Gynecol.* 116:347, 1973.

28. Niles, J. H., and Clark, J. F. J. Pathogenesis of tubal pregnancy. *Am. J. Obstet. Gynecol.* 105:1230, 1969.

29. Ornoy, A., Segal, S., Nishmi, M., Simcha, A., and Polishuk, W. Z. Fetal and placental pathology in gestational rubella. *Am. J. Obstet. Gynecol.* 116:949, 1973.

30. Persaud, V. Etiology of tubal ectopic pregnancy. *Obstet. Gynecol.* 36:257, 1970.

31. Salazar, H., and Kanbour, A. I. Amnion nodosum: Ultrastructure and histopathogenesis. *Arch. Pathol.* 98:39, 1974.

32. Schenker, J. G., Eyal, F., and Polishyk, W. Z. Fertility after tubal pregnancy. *Surg. Gynecol. Obstet.* 35:74, 1972.

33. Semba, R., Nakao, Y., Nishiwaki, Y., and Nishimusa, H. High prevalence of cardiac malformation in human embryos arising from tubal pregnancy. *Proc. Congenital Anomalies Research Assoc. Japan* 11:36, 1971.

34. Seward, P. N., Israel, R., and Ballard, C. A. Ectopic pregnancy and intrauterine contraception. *Obstet. Gynecol.* 40:214, 1972.

35. Shurin, P. A., Alpert, S., Rosner, B., Driscoll, S. G., Lee, Y. H., McCormack, W. M., Santamarine, B. A. G., and Kass, E. H. Chorioamnionitis and colonization of the newborn infant with genital mycoplasmas. *New Engl. J. Med.* 293:5, 1975.

36. Siddall, R. S. Occurrence and significance of decidual changes of the endometrium in extrauterine pregnancy. *Am. J. Obstet. Gynecol.* 31:420, 1936.

37. Sieracki, J. C., Panke, T. W., Horvat, B. L., Perrin, E. V., and Nanda, B. Chorangiomas. *Obstet. Gynecol.* 46:155, 1975.

38. Spiegelberg, O. Zur Kasuistik der Ovarialschwangerschaft. *Arch. Gynakol.* 13:73, 1878.

39. Stromme, W. B. Conservative surgery for ectopic pregnancy. *Obstet. Gynecol.* 41:215, 1973.

40. Studdiford, W. E. Primary peritoneal pregnancy. *Am. J. Obstet. Gynecol.* 44:487, 1942.

41. Tenney, B. Jr., and Parker, F. Jr. The placenta in toxemia of pregnancy. *Am. J. Obstet. Gynecol.* 39:1000, 1940.

42. Van Huysen, W. T. Placenta previa of a succenturiate lobe. *N. Engl. J. Med.* 265:284, 1961.

43. Wallenburg, H. C. S., Stolte, L. A. M., and Janssens, J. The pathogenesis of placental infarction. I. A morphologic study in the human placenta. *Am. J. Obstet. Gynecol.* 116:835, 1973.

44. Wallenburg, H. C. S., Hutchinson, D. L., Schuler, H. M., Stolte, L. A. M., and Janssens, J. The pathogenesis of placental infarction. II. An experimental study in the rhesus monkey placenta. *Am. J. Obstet. Gynecol.* 116:841, 1973.

45. Warthin, A. S. Tuberculosis of the placenta. *J. Infect. Dis.* 4:347, 1907.

46. Werner, H., Schmidtke, L., and Thomaschek, G. Toxoplasma-Infektion und Schwangerschaft. Der histologische nachweis intrauterinen infektion sweges. *Klin. Wschr.* 41:91, 1963.

47. Winer, A. E., Bergman, W. D., and Fields, C. Combined intra- and extrauterine pregnancy. *Am. J. Obstet. Gynecol.* 74:170, 1957.

48. Wright, W. H. A summary of the newer knowledge of toxoplasmosis. *Am. J. Clin. Pathol.* 28:1, 1957.

49. Zeek, P. M., and Assali, N. S. The formation, regression, and differential diagnosis of true infarcts of the placenta. *Am. J. Obstet. Gynecol.* 64:1191, 1952.

John Bonnar, M.D., F.R.C.O.G.
and B. L. Sheppard, M.Sc.

31

# The Vascular Supply of the Placenta in Normal and Abnormal Pregnancy

Transmission and scanning electron microscopy have only recently been applied to the study of human pregnancy but the limited work already done has proved of value in elucidating the complex morphologic relationship of the uteroplacental vascular supply. The placenta has also proved to be an ideal organ for electron microscopic studies on cellular function. Most of the early observations involved the fetal part of the placenta. Here, as in other organs and tissues where structure and function are studied together, electron microscopy has increased our understanding of the cellular and syncytial elements of the placenta. New information on the nature of the "placental barrier" was obtained by using electron microscopy for functional studies of placental transport. Earlier work with light microscopy suggested that the syncytium was a simple semipermeable membrane. However, the observations of the first electron microscopists in this field showed that the syncytial trophoblast cytoplasm was too complex to behave as a passive structure for ionic and fluid transport.[4,48] Since this pioneer work extensive studies have been made of the ultrastructure and function of the human trophoblast.[49,50]

The maternal side of the placenta, particularly the ultrastructure of the uteroplacental vasculature, has had relatively little investigation. This vasculature sustains the fetus and placenta throughout pregnancy and study of this area is of importance in understanding the physiologic vascular changes of normal pregnancy and the aberrations that arise when placental function is impaired and fetal health put in jeopardy. Whereas the fetal tissue of the placenta is ideal for most functional morphologic studies, the delivered placenta contains very little maternal component.

In 1958, Dixon and Robertson[13] studied the maternal vasculature by collecting samples of myometrium and decidua at caesarean section by means of punch biopsy forceps. This approach has since been used to study, by light microscopy, the "physiologic" changes in placental bed blood vessels in normal pregnancy[7] and their "pathologic" response to hypertensive pregnancy.[37] This enabled a more detailed histologic picture of the uteroplacental vascular changes than would have been possible from examination of the maternal tissue adherent to the delivered placenta.[34,35,52]

We have used a placental bed biopsy technique that involves the removal of wedge-shaped segments of decidual and myometrial tissue under direct vision at caesarean section. The placental bed biopsies, as well as the delivered placenta, provided the material for an electron microscopic study of the vascular supply of the placenta in normal pregnancy[43,44] and in pregnancies complicated by fetal growth retardation.[2,45]

# Normal Pregnancy

In the uterus during the reproductive years the spiral arteries are the terminal branches of the radial arteries originating just proximal to the junction of the myometrium and endometrium. The radial arteries are branches of the circular arcuate arteries (Figure 31.1). The spiral arteries are tortuous, as their name implies, and this essential feature allows the vessels to adapt to the changes occurring during the menstrual cycle and in pregnancy. They are muscular arteries, 200 to 300 $\mu$ in diameter, with a thin endothelial lining, a well-defined internal elastic lamina that gradually disappears as the spiral artery penetrates the endometrium.[40] The radial arteries also give rise to smaller branches 100 $\mu$ or less in diameter, known as the basal or straight arteries, which supply the inner myometrium and the basal endometrium. The basal arteries appear to be less influenced by the hormonal changes of either the menstrual cycle or pregnancy.

In pregnancy the placenta is supplied by maternal blood via the spiral arteries, which constitute one of the most adaptable vascular systems in the body. There is no analogous physiologic situation in the human vascular tree that necessitates such extensive structural changes as occurs in

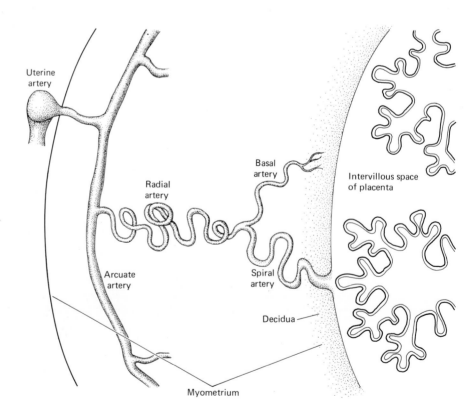

**31.1** Diagram of the arterial supply to the human placenta.

the vascular supply of the placenta. This is required to provide an increase in blood flow from a few milliliters per minute through the spiral arteries to the conceptus at the start of pregnancy to around 600 ml/min to 800 ml/min to the placenta in late pregnancy.[9]

# Early Pregnancy

The pioneer work of Hertig and Rock[25,26] shed much light on early human development following fertilization, but it was not until the work of Hamilton and Boyd[20] that understanding of the uterine vascular changes in early pregnancy emerged. Following implantation of the blastocyst, the maternal vessels in the decidualized endometrium are opened to the lacunae in the trophoblastic shell. The lacunae connect peripherally with maternal capillaries and venules and finally with the decidual terminations of the spiral arteries. Hamilton and Boyd found, as did Harris and Ramsey,[22] that the process of implantation is remarkably orderly with little disturbance of the decidua and a

lack of stromal hemorrhage. The trophoblast at this early stage of placentation appears to replace the endothelium.

About day 15 after implantation the maternal placental circulation fully develops through the intervillous space following invasion of the decidual spiral arteries by the proliferating trophoblast. The endothelium, musculoelastic media, and adventitia of the spiral arteries begin to show structural changes that, as pregnancy progresses, gradually extend from the decidua into the myometrial segments of these placental bed arteries. Simultaneously large mononuclear cells, most numerous at about 12 to 14 weeks of gestation, appear within the lumen of the spiral arteries (Figure 31.2). The cells contain a convoluted nucleus surrounded by a cytoplasm rich in endoplasmic reticulum with attached ribosomes, mitochondria, Golgi complex, and osmiophilic granules. In many of the cells fine fibrils are also evident randomly dispersed within the cytoplasm and the roughened outer cell membrane contains many small microvilli. These cells have been shown to have many of the histologic features of the cytotrophoblast.[3,36,37] Careful consideration of their origin led Ham-

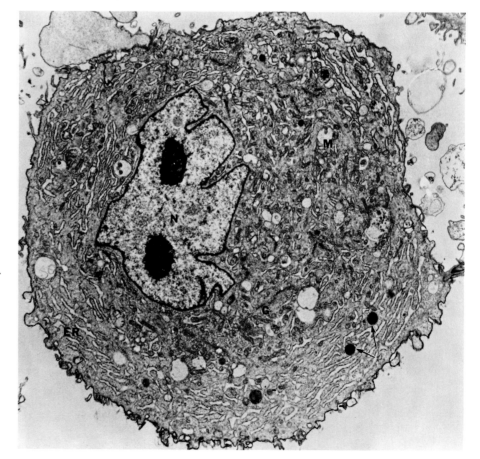

**31.2** An intraluminal cytotrophoblast cell seen at the fourteenth to sixteenth week of pregnancy, containing a convoluted nucleus (N) surrounded by a cytoplasm rich in endoplasmic reticulum (ER), mitochondria (M), Golgi complex (G), and osmiophilic granules (arrows). ×5,810.

[Reprinted by permission from B. L. Sheppard and J. Bonnar, The ultrastructure of the arterial supply of the human placenta in early and late pregnancy, *J. Obstet. Gynaecol. Br. Commonw.* 81:497, 1974.]

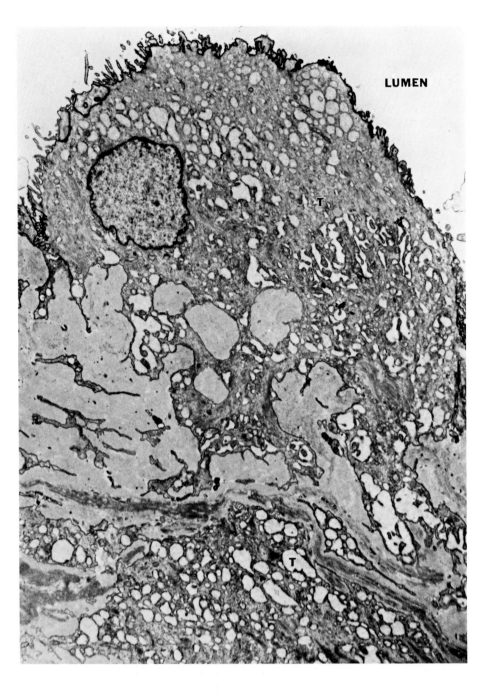

**31.3** Part of the wall of a decidual spiral artery at the fourteenth to sixteenth week of pregnancy. Cytotrophoblast cells (T) are seen both as an intimal lining and within the amorphous material of the media. ×5,395.

[Reprinted by permission from B. L. Sheppard and J. Bonnar, The ultrastructure of the arterial supply of the human placenta in early and late pregnancy, *J. Obstet. Gynaecol. Br. Commonw. 81*:497, 1974.]

ilton and Boyd[20,21] to suggest that these cells were derived from the cytotrophoblastic shell. This suggestion has been accepted by most workers in this field and has been further strengthened on morphologic grounds by electron microscopic studies.[44] The intraluminal cytotrophoblasts can often be so numerous that the lumen may be completely occluded. Hamilton and Boyd[20] considered that reducing the pressure in the vessels was one of the functions of the trophoblast in early pregnancy. Robertson and Dixon[41] suggested that the cells were also responsible for the structural changes that occur in the spiral arteries in early pregnancy and have a continuing function throughout pregnancy.

Trophoblast cells, containing the same cytoplasmic organelles as those seen intraluminally, are also present as an incomplete lining of the decidual spiral arteries (Figure

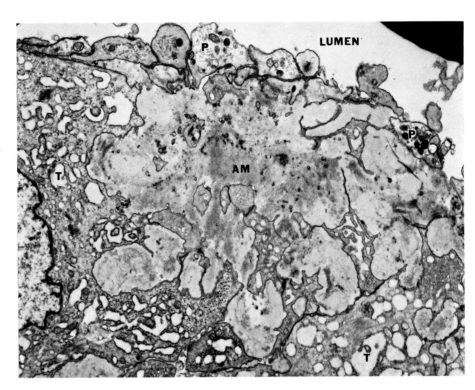

**31.4** Part of the intima of a decidual spiral artery at the fourteenth to sixteenth week of pregnancy. A layer of platelets (P) has formed between two cytotrophoblasts (T) which have formed an incomplete lining in the luminal surface of the vessel. Amorphous material (AM) is visible between the layer of platelets and the cytotrophoblast cells. ×8,000.

[Reprinted by permission from B. L. Sheppard and J. Bonnar, The ultrastructure of the arterial supply of the human placenta in early and late pregnancy, *J. Obstet. Gynaecol. Br. Commonw.* 81:497, 1974.]

31.3). Where gaps occur between these lining trophoblast cells a single layer of platelets or small platelet aggregates complete the lining (Figure 31.4). Small pockets of amorphous material of varying electron density are found within the intima of the vessel wall. In some areas small islands of endothelium remain within the intima but the cells become hypertrophied, often projecting in a striking manner into the vessel lumen.

The tunica media of the decidual spiral arteries shows a dramatic structural change. The normal musculoelastic tissue of the vessel wall is replaced by a matrix containing fibrin and a few trophoblast cells. By electron microscopy it is possible to identify within these cells cytoplasmic organelles similar to those in the intraluminal cells and those forming the intimal lining. These vascular changes not only occur in the decidua but also gradually infiltrate into the myometrial arteries and by the twelfth week are well established in the inner third of the myometrium. By the twenty-eighth week the changes may be found in the distal segments of the radial arteries. In the myometrial arteries proximal to the trophoblast invasion, the spiral arterial wall appears normal except for the absence of a definite internal elastic lamina. Small fragments of elastic tissue are sometimes found but usually only a thin layer of basement membrane is evident between the endothelium and the smooth muscle cells of the media (Figure 31.5). Brosens[5] and Brosens, Robertson, and Dixon[7] have reported in their light microscopic study that this process of cytotrophoblastic cell invasion results in the conversion of the spiral arteries of the placental bed into a series of 100 to 150 distended tortuous funnel-shaped vessels opening into the intervillous space. The loss of the musculoelastic tissue from these vessels undoubtedly reduces the peripheral vascular resistance and lowers the pressure in the blood entering the intervillous space.

## Late Pregnancy

In late pregnancy scanning electron microscopy of the terminal segments of the decidual spiral artery shows that the vessel lumen widens just before opening into the intervillous space of the placenta (Figure 31.6). Blood flowing through the spiral artery meets the large surface area of the placental villi. Several studies have been made, by scanning electron microscopy, of the surface morphology of the syncytiotrophoblast in chorionic villi in both normal and abnormal pregnancy.[14,23,31,32] As yet, these studies have added little to the knowledge that was obtained from light and transmission electron microscopy.

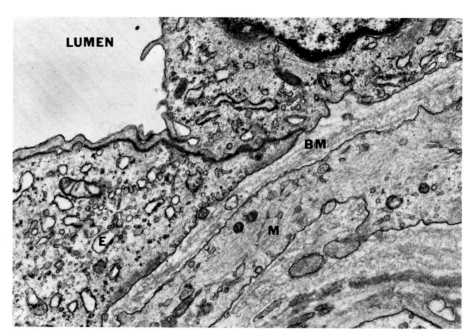

**31.5** Part of a myometrial spiral artery just proximal to the myometrial–decidual junction of the placental bed at the fourteenth to sixteenth week of pregnancy. A thin layer of basement membrane material (BM) is seen between the endothelium (E) and smooth muscle cells (M) of the media. ×20,680.

[Reprinted by permission from B. L. Sheppard and J. Bonnar, The ultrastructure of the arterial supply of the human placenta in early and late pregnancy, *J. Obstet. Gynaecol. Br. Commonw.* 81:497, 1974.]

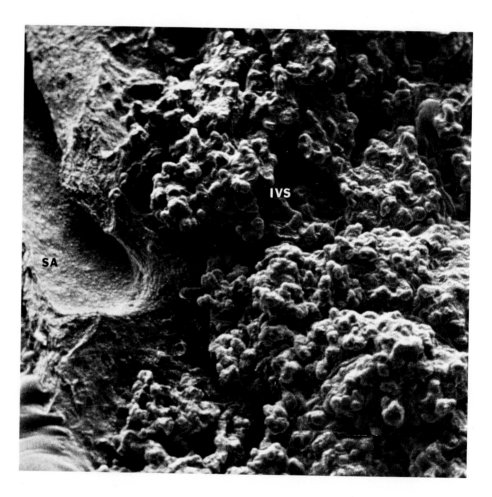

**31.6** A spiral artery (SA), on the maternal surface of a placenta delivered after 38 weeks gestation, bisected longitudinally to show its opening into the intervillous space (IVS). ×62.

[Reprinted by permission from B. L. Sheppard and J. Bonnar, Scanning electron microscopy of the human placenta in early and late pregnancy, *J. Obstet. Gynaecol. Br. Commonw.* 81:20, 1974.]

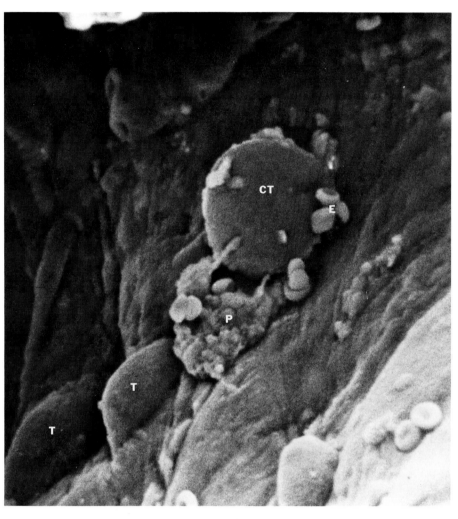

**31.7** Scanning electron microscopy of part of the luminal surface of a spiral artery at 38 weeks gestation shows a lining of cytotrophoblast (T), and an intraluminal cytotrophoblast cell (CT) surrounded by a small platelet thrombus (P) and erythrocytes (E). ×1,500.

[Reprinted by permission from B. L. Sheppard and J. Bonnar, Scanning electron microscopy of the human placenta in early and late pregnancy, *J. Obstet. Gynaecol. Br. Commonw. 81*:20, 1974.]

At term few intraluminal trophoblast cells are visible in the spiral arteries, in contrast to the situation at the 14- to 16-week stage of pregnancy. Occasionally single trophoblast cells are seen within the lumen of the terminal segments of the vessels (Figure 31.7). These cells are usually in association with small platelet thrombi. De Wolf and colleagues[11] have suggested that the vessel intima becomes completely re-endothelialized as pregnancy advances, but our own studies have shown that intimal trophoblast cells as well as endothelial cells are present in the decidual segments of the spiral arteries at term (Figure 31.8a,b).

The trophoblast forming the intimal lining of the decidual spiral arteries flattens considerably as the vessel increases in size. The cells show similar intracellular organelles and an increase in fine fibrils within the cytoplasm, and the luminal surface of the cell still retains many cytoplasmic projections. The structure of the tunica media of these arteries at the thirty-eighth to fortieth week of pregnancy is very similar to that seen at 12 to 16 weeks of pregnancy, but the trophoblasts have taken on the appearance of large fibroblasts with long processes extending from their peripheral hyaloplasm (Figure 31.9). They often contain more than one convoluted nucleus, with uniformly dispersed chromatin. The cytoplasm of the cells is rich in dilated cisternal endoplasmic reticulum. The mitochondria are ovoid with short, blunt cristae. Free ribosomes, glycogen particles, numerous fine filaments, and a very prominent Golgi complex are also evident within the cytoplasm. Desmosomes are often visible between the cell membranes of adjacent trophoblast cytoplasmic processes.

Previously, these trophoblast cells within the vessel wall

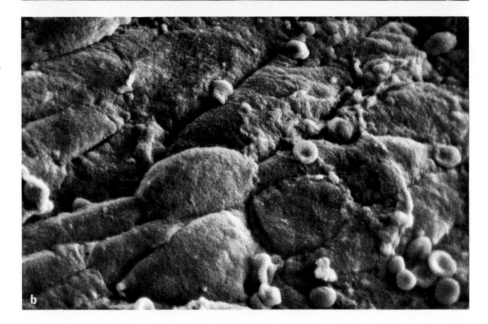

**31.8 a.** An area of the luminal surface of a spiral artery with a lining of normal endothelial cells from a placenta at 38 weeks gestation. ×1,100.
**b.** Another area of the luminal surface of the same spiral artery as shown in (a) where trophoblast cells, much larger in size than endothelium, are seen as an intimal lining. ×1,100.

[Reprinted by permission from B. L. Sheppard and J. Bonnar, Scanning electron microscopy of the human placenta in early and late pregnancy, *J. Obstet. Gynaecol. Br. Commonw.* 81:20, 1974.]

were, by light microscopy, often confused with the decidual cells of maternal origin. Certain ultrastructural features of the decidual cells help to distinguish them from the trophoblast cells (Figure 31.10). The decidual cell contains a single nucleus, with evenly dispersed chromatin, surrounded by cytoplasm with short branches of endoplasmic reticulum and attached ribosomes. The mitochondria are smaller than those in the trophoblast cells but are often elongated or branched with long cristae. Fewer fine fila-

ments are seen in the decidual cell cytoplasm in late pregnancy, whereas the outer cell membrane contains several short projections but never shows any true desmosomal attachments.

The amorphous material surrounding the trophoblasts within the media of the arterial wall contains varying amounts of electron-dense fibers (Figure 31.11a,b). These fibers often exhibit the periodicity of fibrin, 180 to 200 Å (Figure 31.12). The fibrin may be derived from the exuda-

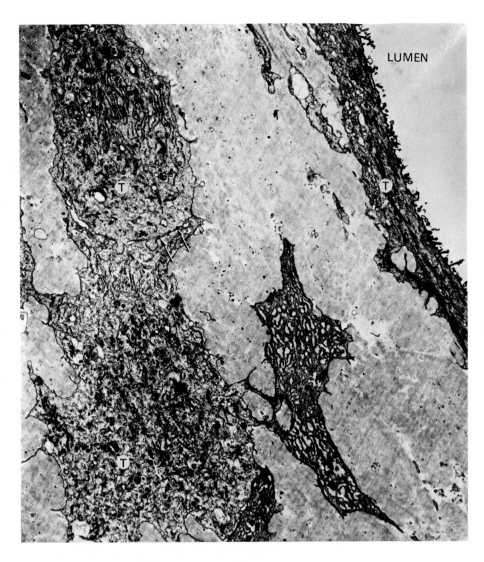

**31.9** Part of the wall of decidual spiral artery at the thirty-eighth to fortieth week of pregnancy. Flattened cytotrophoblast (T) is visible on the intimal surface. Desmosomes (arrows) are evident between the cytotrophoblast within the fibrous matrix of the media. ×1,950.

[Reprinted by permission from B. L. Sheppard and J. Bonnar, The ultrastructure of the arterial supply of the human placenta in early and late pregnancy, *J. Obstet. Gynaecol. Br. Commonw.* 81:497, 1974.]

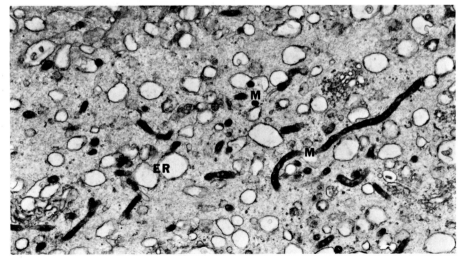

**31.10** In the thirty-eighth to fortieth week of pregnancy the cytoplasm of a decidual cell in the outer wall of a spiral artery contains short branches of dilated endoplasmic reticulum (ER) and narrow, elongated mitochondria (M). ×154,000.

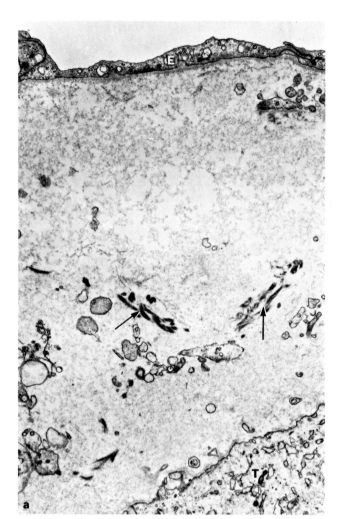
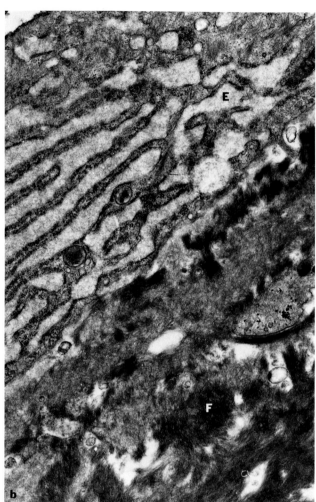

**31.11** Part of a wall of a decidual spiral artery at the thirty-eighth to fortieth week of pregnancy where endothelium (E) is lining the intimal surface.
**a.** Electron-dense fibers (arrows) and cellular debris as well as cytotrophoblast (T) are seen within the amorphous matrix of the media. ×11,340. **b.** Larger amounts of electron dense fibers (F) are sometimes evident below the endothelium. ×23,760.

[Reprinted by permission from B. L. Sheppard and J. Bonnar, The ultrastructure of the arterial supply of the human placenta in early and late pregnancy, *J. Obstet. Gynaecol. Br. Commonw.* 81:497, 1974.]

tion of plasma fibrinogen into the vessel wall. Fibrin does not always exhibit this characteristic periodicity; factors such as degree of polymerization or degradation could influence this banding, and account for the variability in electron density of the amorphous material of the vessel wall. De Wolf *et al.*[11] also suggested that the fibrillar and granular protein of the vessel wall was derived from the filomentous material of degenerating trophoblast.

The presence of fibrin, sometimes large amounts, in the vessel media may be related to the depression of fibrinolytic activity, which is a physiologic feature of pregnancy. The placenta is known to be a potent source of fibrinolytic inhibitor[28] but the source of the inhibitor has not been identified. In the media of the spiral arteries during pregnancy fibrin probably provides the temporary support required in vessels expanding to accommodate an increas-

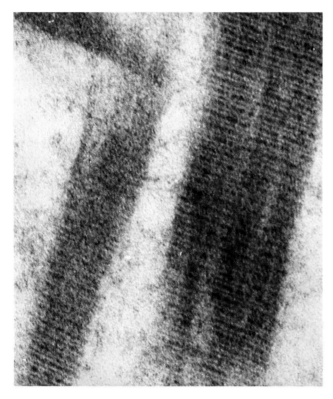

**31.12** Higher magnification of some of the electron-dense fibers within the media of decidual spiral arteries in late pregnancy shows the periodicity of fibrin, 180–200 Å. ×192,000.

ing blood flow. This fibrin support also facilitates the closure of the spiral arteries by the extravascular compression of the myometrium to staunch uteroplacental blood flow following placental separation. The morphologic changes associated with this dilatation of the spiral arteries are evident in the myometrial segments as well as the decidual segments of the vessels. Again, as in the arteries in early pregnancy proximal to trophoblast invasion, the radial and spiral arteries contain no definite internal elastic lamina, only fragments of elastic fibers (Figure 31.13). The internal elastic lamina is a major morphologic characteristic of a distributing artery with pulsatile blood flow and compliance as a major function. The removal of the elastic lamina in the uterine arteries therefore has the effect of reducing vascular resistance to the placental blood flow. In the monkey the persistence of the elastic tissue in spiral arteries, and a lesser degree of trophoblastic activity in the vessel wall, has been shown to be associated with less dilatation of the vessel wall than in the human.[38] The absence of the internal elastic lamina in uteroplacental arteries may be unrelated to trophoblast invasion as it occurs in vessels where the smooth muscle is virtually unchanged and in basal arteries, which are not affected by the trophoblast infiltration in normal pregnancy.[44] However, by light microscopy, an association has been shown between staining properties of a fibrillary element in the amorphous material of the vessel wall surrounding the trophoblast and the fine fibrillary component of the elastic

**31.13** Part of a myometrial spiral artery at the thirty-eighth to fortieth week of pregnancy. The zone between the endothelium (E) and the smooth muscle cells (M) is greater than that seen in early pregnancy. Small elastic fibers (El) and basement membrane material (BM) are seen in this area and between the smooth muscle cells of the media. ×20,900.

[Reprinted by permission from B. L. Sheppard and J. Bonnar, The ultrastructure of the arterial supply of the human placenta in early and late pregnancy, *J. Obstet. Gynaecol. Br. Commonw.* 81:497, 1974.]

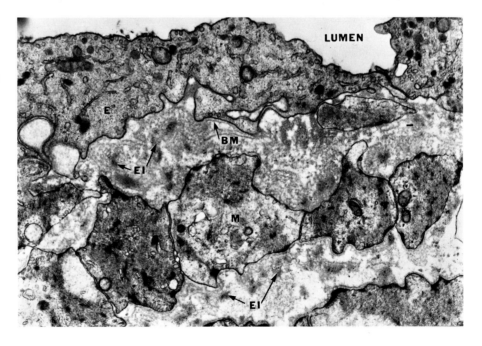

683

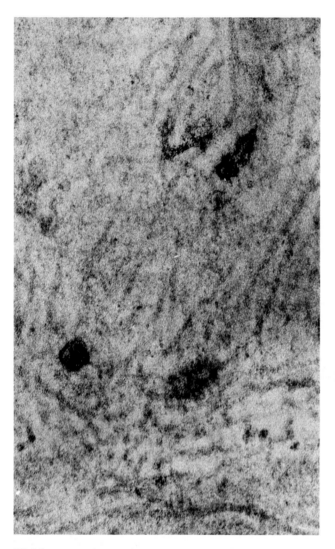

**31.14** In late pregnancy fine fibrils are found within the amorphous material in the media of decidual spiral arteries. ×221,400.

tissue.[33] Indeed, by electron microscopy, fine fibrils of the same dimensions as those usually found surrounding the amorphous, nonelectron-dense, central core of the elastic fibers may be identified around trophoblasts in the media of the decidual spiral arteries (Figure 31.14).

As would be expected from the accumulation of platelets between intimal trophoblasts seen in decidual and myometrial spiral arteries in early pregnancy, numerous mural thrombi are found in varying stages of organization in late pregnancy (Figure 31.15a,b). These thrombi result in an appreciable reduction in the size of the lumen of the vessels, suggesting that the small placental infarcts and areas of ischemia found in association with normal preg-

nancies are most likely the result of thrombotic occlusion of the arterial supply.

In normal pregnancy the *basal arteries* do not exhibit the morphologic changes described in the spiral arteries, with the exception of the loss of an internal elastic lamina. Although trophoblastic cells are evident in the decidua in close proximity to basal arteries, none is visible within the intima or media of the vessel walls. This was one of the factors that led Hamilton and Boyd[21] to conclude that the trophoblast in the spiral arterial walls had migrated from the vessel lumen into the media rather than through the adventitia of the vessels.

Although the modified structure of the uteroplacental arteries as visualized by electron microscopy is in the main uniform, some variation in the response to pregnancy is found. Following their light microscopic studies, Brosens, Robertson, and Dixon[7] introduced the term "physiological" to describe these changes in the morphology of the uteroplacental vasculature in normal pregnancy. This knowledge of the normal appearances of these vessels during pregnancy is essential before any attempt can be made to investigate or understand the pathology of the maternal spiral arteries in such complications as pre-eclampsia and fetal growth retardation.

## Pregnancies Complicated by Fetal Growth Retardation

The severity of fetal growth retardation has been shown to correlate with the degree of placental infarction,[16,30,46,47] and a high incidence of placental infarction has also been reported in pregnancies complicated by essential hypertension, eclampsia, and preeclampsia.[51,52] Greater emphasis is now being placed on the maternal vascular supply as a cause of pathology in the placenta[19] and subsequent fetal growth retardation. Most of the light microscopic studies on the spiral arteries concluded that placental infarction was associated with occlusive vascular lesions as a result of maternal hypertension.[6,8,13,24,27,39,52] Recently, using electron microscopy, we have found similar lesions in placental bed spiral arteries in pregnancies resulting in the birth of severely growth-retarded fetuses where the pregnancy was not complicated by hypertension.[2,45]

Spiral arteries supplying areas of placental infarction show varying degrees of occlusion usually related to the degree of infarction of the placenta. By scanning electron microscopy the occlusive lesions are seen often as plaques on the intimal surface of the spiral artery as they traverse

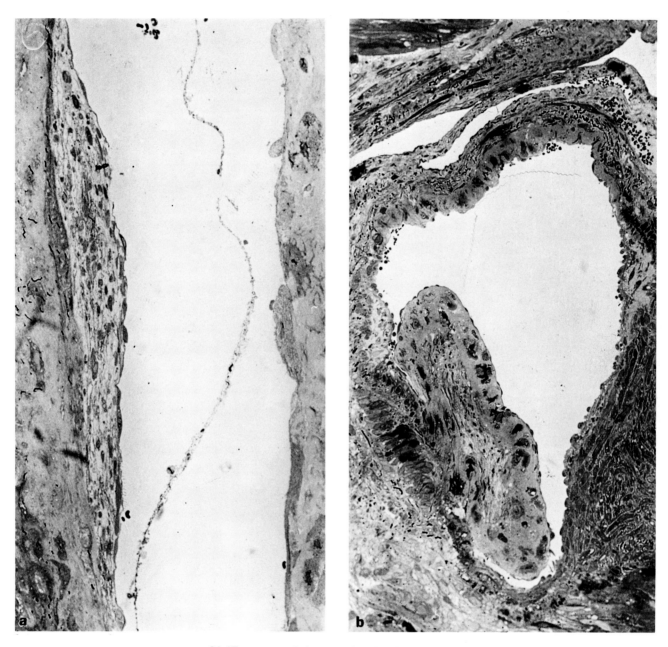

**31.15 a.** Part of the vessel wall of a distal segment of a decidual spiral artery at the thirty-eighth to fortieth week of pregnancy, just before its opening into the intervillous space of the placenta. An organizing thrombus partially occludes the vessel lumen. The thrombus consists mainly of smooth muscle cells covered with endothelium, the remainder of the vessel intima having a lining of trophoblast. ×178. **b.** A spiral artery from the myometrial–decidual junction at the thirty-eighth to fortieth week of pregnancy. A mural thrombus shown in a transverse section through the artery is seen to be lined with endothelium. Both smooth muscle and trophoblastic elements are found within the thrombus and the remainder of the vessel media. ×178.

[Reprinted by permission from B. L. Sheppard and J. Bonnar, The ultrastructure of the arterial supply of the human placenta in early and late pregnancy, *J. Obstet. Gynaecol. Br. Commonw. 81:497, 1974.*]

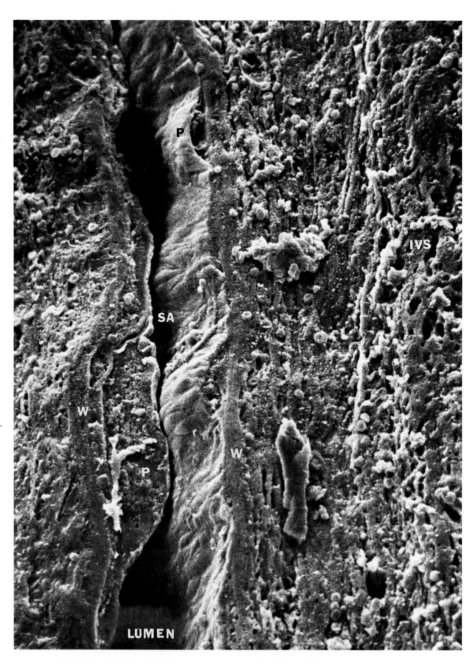

**31.16** Severe hypertension and fetal growth retardation at thirty-sixth week of pregnancy. Scanning electron micrograph of a spiral artery (SA) traversing the decidua just before opening into the intervillous space (IVS) of the placenta. Numerous plaques (P) are visible in the luminal surface of the vessel wall (W) partially occluding the lumen. ×205.

[Reprinted by permission from J. Bonnar, C. W. G. Redman, and B. L. Sheppard, Treatment of fetal growth retardation in utero with heparin and dipyridamole, *Eur. J. Obstet. Gynaecol. Reprod. Biol.* 5:123, 1975.]

the decidua into the intervillous space of the placenta (Figure 31.16). The structures within the plaques consist of mononuclear cells, most of which contain large amounts of lipid, smooth muscle cells, and material of varying electron density, some of which has the periodicity of fibrin (Figure 31.17). The amount of fibrin within the vessel intima and media varies considerably from vessel to vessel and may, in many cases, be the predominant feature of the vessel wall (Figure 31.18). The cells within the wall often contain so much lipid that other organelles are undetectable within their cytoplasm, but small mitochondria, ribosomes, and fragments of endoplasmic reticulum are sometimes visible (Figure 31.19). Trophoblasts, which also may contain lipid droplets, are seen on the intimal surface of these lesions as well as endothelium (Figure 31.20). Pathologic classification of these lesions is compli-

**31.17** Transmission electron micrograph of part of an intimal plaque such as that shown in Figure 31.16. Mononuclear cells (M), some of which contain lipid (L), smooth muscle cells (SM), fibrin (F), and amorphous material (AM) of varying electron density, are seen within the lesion beneath the endothelial lining (E). ×4,350.

[Reprinted by permission from B. L. Sheppard and J. Bonnar, The ultrastructure of the arterial supply of the human placenta in pregnancy complicated by fetal growth retardation, *Br. J. Obstet. Gynaecol.* in press, 1976.]

**31.18** Severe fetal growth retardation in a pregnancy with normal blood pressure delivered at the thirty-fourth week of pregnancy. A longitudinal section has been taken through a decidual spiral artery. Massive fibrin deposition associated with a few lipid-laden cells are visible within the vessel wall. Mononuclear cells are also seen within the surrounding extravascular tissue. ×105.

[Reprinted by permission from J. Bonnar, C. W. G. Redman, and B. L. Sheppard, Treatment of fetal growth retardation in utero with heparin and dipyridamole, *Eur. J. Obstet. Gynaecol. Reprod. Biol.* 5:123, 1975.]

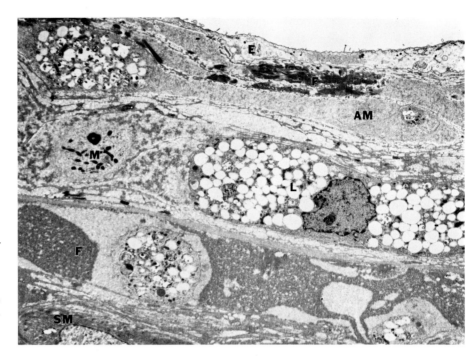

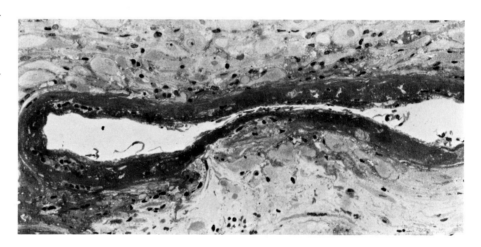

cated by the structural modifications of the vessels which occur in normal pregnancy.

The invasion of the intima and media of the arteries by mononuclear cells containing large amounts of lipid is a predominant feature of the lesion. Mononuclear cells, mostly lymphocytes, and macrophages with the occasional plasma cell are present in the decidua surrounding the vessels; the macrophages may be the origin of the lipid-laden cells seen in the lesions. Some of the cells do exhibit a basement membrane, which is a feature of smooth muscle cells and has been suggested as a feature of trophoblast

cells in spiral arterial walls,[11] but not macrophages. The lesions, in many instances, show similar features to those originally described by Hertig[24] in patients with pre-eclampsia. Zeek and Assali[52] extended these observations by Hertig and introduced the term "acute atherosis," as the lesions resembled atheroma. In their study, Zeek and Assali[52] found that the "atherosis" lesions were localized to certain areas of the uteroplacental vasculature: In 12 out of 13 patients where they were able to study the uterine wall as well as the delivered placenta they found that the atherosis was confined to the decidual portion of the

**31.19** Severe hypertensive pregnancy with proteinuria at 36½ weeks gestation, complicated by fetal growth retardation. Lipid droplets (L) and occasional mitochondria (arrows) are seen surrounding the nucleus (N) within the cytoplasm of the large medial cells of a decidual spiral artery. Fibrin (F) is evident in the inner media and a few smooth muscle cells (M) are in the outer layers of the media. ×3,915.

[Reprinted by permission from B. L. Sheppard and J. Bonnar, The ultrastructure of the arterial supply of the human placenta in pregnancy complicated by fetal growth retardation, *Br. J. Obstet. Gynaecol.* in press, 1976.]

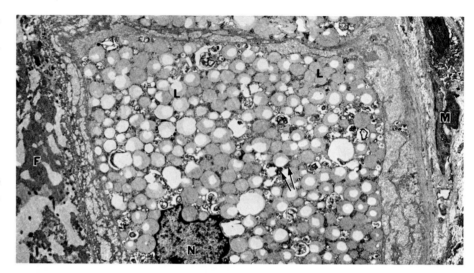

**31.20** Nonhypertensive pregnancy of 33½ weeks gestation resulting in fetal growth retardation. Trophoblast (T) and endothelium (E) are evident lining the intimal surface over the layers of fibrin (F) within the spiral arterial wall. ×8,700.

[Reprinted by permission from B. L. Sheppard and J. Bonnar, The ultrastructure of the arterial supply of the human placenta in pregnancy complicated by fetal growth retardation, *Br. J. Obstet. Gynaecol.* in press, 1976.]

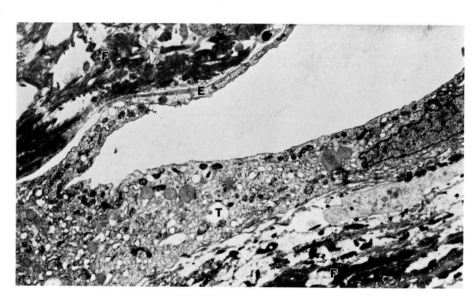

vessels. This also appears to be true of uteroplacental lesions in pregnancies resulting in the delivery of a growth-retarded fetus.[45]

In pregnancies resulting in fetal growth retardation, lesions similar to those seen in spiral arteries are found in the *basal arteries*. This is also the case in hypertensive pregnancies,[39] and the basal artery has been examined in great detail by light microscopy in an effort to explain the pathogenesis of the "acute atherosis" seen in decidual spiral arteries. Morphologic similarities between the basal and spiral arterial lesions do exist, but it is possible that the lesions in the basal arteries are secondary to the placental ischemia and infarction caused by occlusion of the associated spiral artery.

Although in pregnancies resulting in fetal growth retardation the decidual spiral arteries show varying degrees of occlusive lesions, the cell structure of the surrounding decidual tissue appears normal.[45] In contrast, the placental villi supplied by the spiral arteries show ischemia and infarction related to the degree of vascular occlusion. Fox,[15] in a study of placental infarction, has found that if a spiral artery thrombosed as it passes through the basal plate, then the basal plate usually escapes necrosis; if the artery is thrombosed in the decidua some distance from the basal plate, necrosis of this tissue occurs. The damage to the placenta therefore appears to be caused by luminal occlusion of the spiral arteries associated with impaired blood flow to the intervillous space.

The immunologic aspects of trophoblast invasion in the placental bed vasculature are of great interest. In an ultrastructural study of the placental bed in early and late normal pregnancy Robertson and Warner[42] could find no support for the hypothesis that the function of the decidua is to restrict the invasiveness of trophoblast or that placental "fibrinoid" is an effective immunologic barrier. Morphologic evidence suggests that normal pregnancy requires some form of controlled immunologic reaction between maternal and fetal placental tissues, and the lesions found in maternal uteroplacental arteries in pregnancies complicated by preeclampsia could be caused by an "inappropriate immune response."[39] The lesions in the spiral arteries in pregnancies resulting in fetal growth retardation do resemble the vascular changes seen in rejected renal allografts.[10,18] Recently, Kitzmiller and Benirschke[29] have reported some evidence for an immunologic factor in acute atherosis in pregnancies complicated by preeclampsia. They found that antigammaglobulin and anticomplement stains of decidual vessel lesions were positive in women with preeclampsia and negative in decidual vessels from normal pregnancies. This led them to suggest that the lesions may represent an immunopathologic process that could lead to diminished perfusion of the placenta.

Brosens, Robertson, and Dixon[8] have reported that in all the cases of preeclampsia with proteinuria that they have studied the physiologic changes in the placental bed spiral arteries are restricted to the decidua and do not extend into the myometrium despite the presence of trophoblast cells in the latter. They considered that this inadequate response of the vessels to placentation was established in the first half of pregnancy and was likely to be the critical defect in women destined to develop preeclampsia.

Fox[17] explains the basic abnormality in placental insufficiency as an inadequate perfusion of the fetal villi. This was based on a study by light and electron microscopy of the placenta in prolonged pregnancy and similar findings were noted in some cases of fetal growth retardation of unknown etiology. In prolonged pregnancy a decline in placental function occurs coupled with only a minor decrease in maternal blood flow through the placenta.[12] In the histology of these placentas, villous hypovascularity associated with secondary fibrosis and increased syncytial knots were found, but electron microscopy showed no evidence of degeneration of the trophoblast.[17] The lesions in the maternal uterine vasculature undoubtedly explain much of the pathology found in the placenta in pregnancies where the otherwise healthy fetus suffers the spectrum of deprivation, impairment of growth, or death *in utero*. The elucidation of the pathologic changes in the uteroplacental vascular supply are a major research challenge that may hold the key to a therapeutic approach for the improvement of placental blood flow and preservation of fetal wellbeing in pregnancy. Perinatal mortality and morbidity statistics in this area indicate that if we are to reduce the deaths and the incidence of detrimental effects on the surviving infants efforts should be directed at treatment of the problem *in utero*.

## ACKNOWLEDGMENTS

The work reported in this chapter was supported by the Medical Research Council. We also acknowledge the technical assistance of Mrs. Uta Sheppard in the electron microscopic studies.

## REFERENCES

1. Bonnar, J. The blood coagulation and fibrinolytic systems during pregnancy. *Clin. Obstet. Gynaecol.* 2:321, 1975.

2. Bonnar, J., Redman, C. W. G., and Sheppard, B. L. Treatment of fetal growth retardation in utero with heparin and dipyridamole. *Eur. J. Obstet. Gynecol. Reprod. Biol.* 5:123, 1975.

3. Boyd, J. D., and Hamilton, W. J. Cells in the spiral arteries of the human uterus. *J. Anat.* (London). 90:595, 1956.

4. Boyd, J. D., and Hughes, A. F. W. Observations on human chorionic villi using the electron microscope. *J. Anat.* (London) 88:356, 1954.

5. Brosens, I. A study of the spiral arteries of the decidua basalis in normotensive and hypertensive pregnancies. *J. Obstet. Gynaecol. Br. Commonw.* 71:222, 1964.

6. Brosens, I., and Renaer, M. On the pathogenesis of placental infarcts in pre-elampsia. *J. Obstet. Gynaecol. Br. Commonw.* 79:794, 1972.

7. Brosens, I., Robertson, W. B., and Dixon, H. G. The physiological response of the vessels of the placental bed to normotensive pregnancy. *J. Pathol. Bacteriol.* 93:569, 1967.

8. Brosens, I., Robertson, W. B., and Dixon, H. G. The role of the spiral arteries in the pathogenesis of pre-eclampsia, in R. M. Wynn, ed.: *Obstetrics and Gynecology Annual.* New York, Appleton-Century-Crofts, 1972, p. 177.

9. Brown, J. C. M., and Veall, N. The maternal placental blood flow in normotensive and hypertensive women. *J. Obstet. Gynaecol. Br. Emp.* 60:141, 1953.

10. Dempster, W. J., Harrison, C. V., and Shackman, R. Rejection process in human homotransplanted kidneys. *Br. Med. J.* 2:969, 1964.

11. De Wolf, F., de Wolf-Peeters, C., and Brosens, I. Ultrastructure of the spiral arteries in the human placental bed at the end of normal pregnancy. *Am. J. Obstet. Gynecol.* 117:833, 1973.

12. Dixon, H. G., Browne, J. C. Mc., and Davey, D. A. Choriodecidual and myometrial bloodflow. *Lancet* 2:369, 1963.

13. Dixon, H. G., and Robertson, W. B. A study of the vessels of the placental bed in normotensive and hypertensive women. *J. Obstet. Gynaecol. Br. Emp.* 65:803, 1958.

14. Ferenczy, A., and Richart, R. M. Scanning electron microscopic study of normal and molar trophoblast. *Gynecol. Oncol.* 1:95, 1972.

15. Fox, H. White infarcts of the placenta. *J. Obstet. Gynaecol. Br. Commonw.* 70:980, 1963.

16. Fox, H. Pervillous fibrin deposition in the human placenta. *Am. J. Obstet. Gynecol.* 98:245, 1967.

17. Fox, H. The role of the fetal circulation in placental insufficiency, in B. Salvadori, ed.: *Therapy of Feto-Placental Insufficiency.* International Symposium, Parma. Springer-Verlag, Berlin, 1975, p. 109.

18. Goodwin, W. E., Kaufman, J. J., Mims, M. M., Turner, R. D., Glassock, R., Goldman, R., and Maxwell, M. M. Human renal transplantation. I. Clinical experiences with 6 cases of renal homotransplantation. *J. Urol.* 89:13, 1963.

19. Gruenwald, P. Pathology of the deprived fetus and its supply lines, in *Size at Birth.* Symposium 27 (new series), Ciba Foundation. Amsterdam: Associated Scientific Publishers, 1974, p. 3.

20. Hamilton, W. J., and Boyd, J. D. Development of the human placenta in the first three months of gestation. *J. Anat.* (London) 94:297, 1960.

21. Hamilton, W. J., and Boyd, J. D. Trophoblasts in human utero-placental arteries. *Nature* (London) 212:906, 1966.

22. Harris, J. W. S., and Ramsey, E. M. The morphology of the human utero-placental vasculature. *Contrib. Embryol. Carnegie Inst.* 38:43, 1966.

23. Herbst, R., and Multier, A. M. Les microvillosités à la surface des villosités chorioniques du placenta humain. *Gynecol. Obstet.* (Paris) 69(Suppl. 5):609, 1970.

24. Hertig, A. T. Vascular pathology in the hypertensive albuminuric toxemias of pregnancy. *Clinics* 4:602, 1945.

25. Hertig, A. T., and Rock, J. On the development of the early human ovum, with special reference to the trophoblast of the previllous stage. A description of 7 normal and 5 pathologic human ova. *Am. J. Obstet. Gynecol.* 47:149, 1944.

26. Hertig, A. T., Rock, J., and Adams, E. C. A description of 34 human ova within the first 17 days of development. *Am. J. Anat.* 98:435, 1956.

27. Jonas, E. B., and Rewell, R. E. The ethnography of the decidual vasculature in toxaemia of pregnancy. *J. Obstet. Gynaecol. Br. Commonw.* 70:672, 1963.

28. Kawano, T., Morimoto, K., and Uemura, Y. Urokinase inhibitor in human placenta. *Nature* (London) 217:253, 1968.

29. Kitzmiller, J. L., and Benirschke, K. Immunofluorescent study of placental bed vessels in pre-eclampsia of pregnancy. *Am. J. Obstet. Gynecol.* 115:248, 1973.

30. Little, W. A. Placental infarction. *J. Obstet. Gynecol.* 15:109, 1960.

31. Ludwig, H., Junkermann, H., and Klingele, H. Oberflächenstrukturen der menschlichen Placenta im Rasterelektronenmikroskop. *Arch. Gynäkol.* 210:1, 1971.

32. Ludwig, H., and Metzger, H. Das uterine Placentarbett post partum im Rasterelektronenmikroskop, zugleich ein Beitrag zur Frage der extravasalen Fibrinbildung. *Arch. Gynäkol.* 210:251, 1971.

33. Manning, P. J. The staining of elastic tissue and related fibres in uterine blood vessels. *Med. Lab. Technol.* 31:115, 1974.

34. Marais, W. D. Human decidual spiral arterial studies. Part I. Anatomy, circulation and pathology of the placenta. *J. Obstet. Gynaecol. Br. Commonw.* 69:1, 1962.

35. Marais, W. D. Human decidual spiral arteries: ultrastructure of the intima in normal vessels. *J. Obstet. Gynaecol. Br. Commonw.* 75:552, 1968.

36. McKay, D. G., Hertig, A. T., Adams, E. C., and Richardson, M. V. Histochemical observations on the human placenta. *Obstet. Gynecol.* 12:1, 1958.

37. Ortmann, R. Histochemische Untersuchungen an menschlicher Placenta mit besonderer Berucksichtigung der Kernkugeln (Kerneinschlusse) und der Plasmalipoideinschlusse. *Z. Anat. Entwicklungsgesh.* 119:28, 1955.

38. Ramsey, E. M. Vascular anatomy of the uterus, in R. M. Wynn, ed.: *Cellular Biology of the Uterus.* New York, Appleton-Century-Crofts, 1967, p. 33.

39. Robertson, W. B., Brosens, I., and Dixon, H. G. The pathological response of the vessels of the placental bed to hypertensive pregnancy. *J. Pathol. Bacteriol.* 93:581, 1967.

40. Robertson, W. B., Brosens, I., and Dixon, H. G. Utero-placental vascular pathology. *Eur. J. Obstet. Gynecol. Reprod. Biol.* 5:47, 1975.

41. Robertson, W. B., and Dixon, H. G. Utero-placental pathology, in A. Klopper, and E. Diczfalusy, eds.: *Foetus and Placenta.* Oxford, Blackwells, 1969, p. 33.

42. Robertson, W. B., and Warner, B. The ultrastructure of the human placental bed. *J. Pathol.* 112:203, 1974.

43. Sheppard, B. L., and Bonnar, J. Scanning electron microscopy of the human placenta and decidual spiral arteries in normal pregnancy. *J. Obstet. Gynaecol. Br. Commonw.* 81:20, 1974.

44. Sheppard, B. L., and Bonnar, J. The ultrastructure of the arterial supply of the human placenta in early and late pregnancy. *J. Obstet. Gynaecol. Br. Commonw.* 81:497, 1974.

45. Sheppard, B. L., and Bonnar, J. The ultrastructure of the arterial supply of the human placenta in pregnancy complicated by fetal growth retardation. *Br. J. Obstet. Gynaecol.* In press, 1976.

46. Wigglesworth, J. S. Vascular anatomy of the human placenta and its significance for placental pathology. *J. Obstet. Gynaecol. Br. Commonw.* 76:979, 1969.

47. Wilkin, P. *Pathologie du Placenta. Etude Clinique et Anatomo-clinique.* Paris, Masson, 1965, p. 240.

48. Wislock, G. B., and Dempsey, E. W. Electron microscopy of the human placenta. *Anat. Rec.* 123:133, 1955.

49. Wynn, R. M. Cytotrophoblastic specialization. An ultrastructural study of the human placenta. *Am. J. Obstet. Gynecol.* 114:339, 1972.

50. Wynn, R. M. Development and ultrastructural adaptations of the human placenta. *Eur. J. Obstet. Gynecol. Reprod. Biol.* 5:3, 1975.

51. Young, J. The aetiology of eclampsia and albuminuria and their relation to accidental haemorrhage. *J. Obstet. Gynaecol. Br. Emp.* 26:1, 1914.

52. Zeek, P. M., and Assali, N. S. Vascular changes in the decidua associated with eclamptogenic toxemia of pregnancy. *Am. J. Clin. Pathol.* 20:1099, 1950.

Bradley Bigelow, M.D.

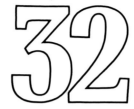

# Abortion

Abortion is defined as the termination of pregnancy before the stage of independent, extrauterine fetal survival. Although there are isolated reports of the survival of extremely immature fetuses, even weighing less than 400 g at a gestational age of about 20 weeks, there is general acceptance of 500 g as the lower limit of survivability.

Abortions may be spontaneous or induced. The latter may be therapeutic, if medically indicated, or may be legal (voluntary) or illegal (criminal) depending on the laws prevailing in the locality. There are other types of abortion, such as threatened abortion, missed abortion, and habitual abortion, and each of these is discussed separately.

## Spontaneous Abortion

Most spontaneous abortions occur in the first trimester of pregnancy. The exact incidence is difficult to judge, especially for very early abortions that may be dismissed by patient and physician as delayed menstruation. A rate of 15 to 20% abortion in the first half of all pregnancies is generally accepted but may be too low.

There is considerable evidence relating the occurence of spontaneous abortion to genetic abnormalities. Warburton and Fraser[16] have described three theoretical genetic bases for abortion: (1) lethal genes, either recessive or mutant dominants in the embryo itself; (2) abortion genes in the gravida herself; and (3) genetically determined antigenic

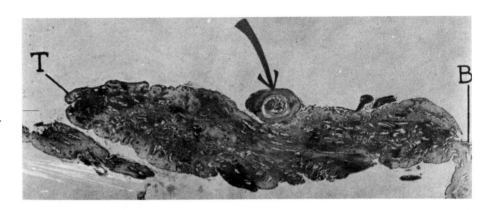

**32.1** Implantation (arrow) on the surface of an endometrial polyp. T, tip of polyp; B, base.

[Reprinted by permission from C. T. Javert, *Spontaneous and Habitual Abortion*, McGraw-Hill, New York, 1957.]

incompatibility of fetus and mother. Hertig and Sheldon[7] examined 1,000 spontaneous abortions and found abnormal or "blighted" ova in 48.9%. The authors described a variety of abnormalities, varying from finding villi only through the additional observation of chorion, amnion, and stunted embryo. Most pathologic ova were one of three types: empty chorionic vesicle (Chapter 37, Figure 37.27); a chorion containing an empty amnion; or a "nodular," disorganized embryo within an amnion and chorion (Chapter 37, Figure 37.28). Cytogenetic studies of spontaneous abortuses have shown a variety of chromosomal abnormalities, supporting the concept of defective germ plasm. These abnormalities include 45XO; triploidy (69 chromosomes) XXY, XXX, XYY; tetraploidy (92 chromosomes) with XXXX, XXYY configurations; and a large variety of single autosomal trisomies (47 chromosomes). Mosaic and translocation patterns have also been reported. The earliest spontaneous abortions demonstrate the most bizarre chromosomal aberrations. Mall and Meyer[11] found fetal malformations to be more common in abortions than in viable births. They classified 396 of 1,000 abortuses as pathologic. These included spina bifida, hydrocephaly, and anencephaly (Chapter 37, Figure 37.30). In recent years there has been a heightened interest in the teratologic effects of drugs, some of which are commonly used by gravid women.

Levine[9] has commented on the relative deficiency of children of blood group A among progeny of group O mothers and group A fathers, suggesting that this may result from a selective diminution of fertility and/or from an increased rate of abortion. He[10] has also reported habitual abortion in women with antibodies to the rare red cell antigen Tj[a].

Maternal infections have been described as possible causes of abortion. *Vibrio fetus,*[15] *Toxoplasma gondii,*[12,17] cytomegalic viral inclusion disease,[5] and rubella[4,14] have all been implicated.

Trauma has been suspected as a rare cause of abortion, but Hertig and Sheldon[7] have felt that it can only rarely be invoked as a cause of abortion, and only if the gestation can be shown to have been anatomically normal prior to trauma and if the events leading to the expulsion of the fetus have begun within minutes to hours after the trauma.

The role of uterine abnormalities has been reviewed by many, particularly the incompetent cervix. Some have described abortions caused by the presence of submucous and/or intramural leiomyomata. Javert[8] reported abortion caused by implantation on an endometrial polyp (Figure 32.1). There is no substantial evidence, however, that uterine factors play a major role in abortion and such factors are usually implicated in abortions occuring after the first trimester of pregnancy or in premature labor.

In most spontaneous abortions the fetus is either grossly abnormal or dies prior to expulsion of the conceptus. The abortion may be complete, but it can be incomplete if some of the products are retained.

Fetal death or fetal circulatory failure produces changes in the placenta unlike those produced by interference with the maternal blood supply. Ischemic necrosis, or infarction, of placental villi is caused by interference with the maternal intervillous blood supply, as is discussed under the subject of infarction (see Chapter 30). Failure of the fetal circulation, however, produces degenerative changes short of infarction. These changes are commonly seen in aborted specimens. One type of alteration, a sclerotic change, is shown in Figure 32.2. The villi are small and their stroma is dense and partially or totally avascular. The covering trophoblast is reduced or absent. A second type of fetal ischemic change is the hydropic swelling, or degeneration, illustrated in Figure 32.3. Here again, the villi show reduced vascularity, but they are swollen and filled with fluid. Trophoblast is reduced or absent. The distinction from hydatidiform mole can be difficult and is essen-

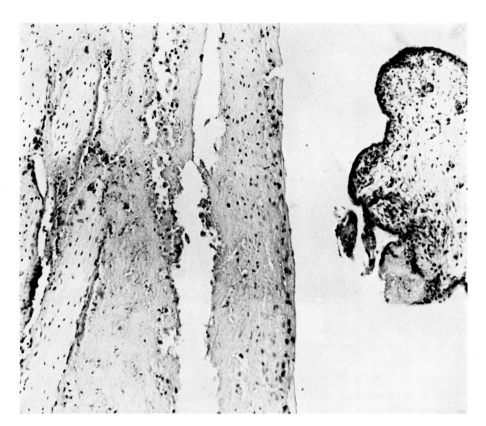

**32.2** Sclerotic villi. The chorionic villi at the extreme left are small and avascular and have dense stroma. Trophoblast is absent. They are separated by fibrin and a strip of chorion from a normal villus at right.

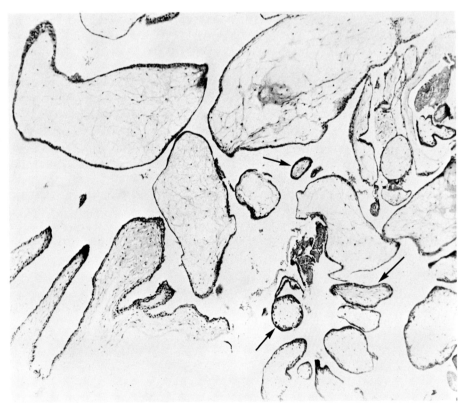

**32.3** Hydropic villi. Several villi are distended with fluid. Blood vessels are present within them, although reduced in number. The covering trophoblast is small in amount. Several small, normal villi are indicated by arrows. This hydropic change can be confused with hydatidiform mole.

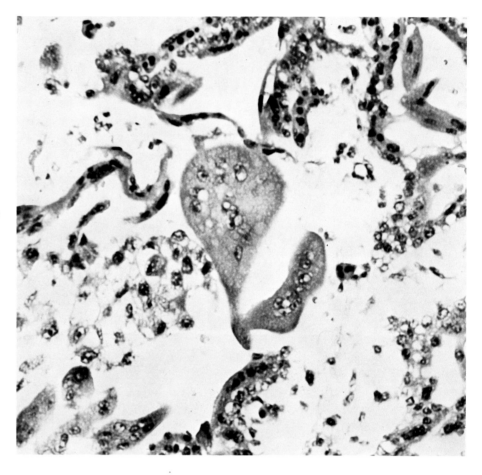

**32.4** Appearance of syncytiotrophoblast in pregnancy. In the center is a multinucleate syncytiotrophoblast with smaller, pale cytotrophoblast cells to its left.

tially based on the requirement for trophoblast proliferation in the case of mole.

Such changes in the placenta are not confined to aborted specimens. They also occur in the villi at the margin of the normal placenta and in those villi attached to the chorion leve, areas poorly perfused with fetal blood.

Degeneration of the placenta occurring *in utero,* especially in the case of missed abortion, may result in hypo- to acellular "ghost" villi recognized by their size, shape, and outline (Chapter 30, Figure 30.32).

In addition to placental tissue, aborted specimens contain considerable blood and inflamed decidua and may contain embryonic tissue that is frequently seen to be abnormal if its degree of maceration does not preclude examination.

The minimum histologic requirement for the diagnosis of pregnancy is the syncytiotrophoblast cell (Figure 32.4). This cell must be carefully distinguished from decidua, as well as from the uterine smooth muscle cells that may appear in curettings and that may be enlarged and pleo

morphic in pregnancy. Cytotrophoblast is difficult to identify with certainty and bears considerable resemblance to decidua.

## Threatened Abortion

Threatened abortion is described as an episode of painless uterine bleeding that may or may not be accompanied by uterine contractions. Hertig and Livingstone[6] found that it affected 16% of recognized pregnancies. In this study 60% of these led to spontaneous abortions.

## Habitual Abortion

Habitual abortion is defined as recurrent pregnancy wastage and is felt to be associated with infection, maternal isoimmunization, chronic maternal vascular diseases, and diabetes mellitus, although it may occur in the ab-

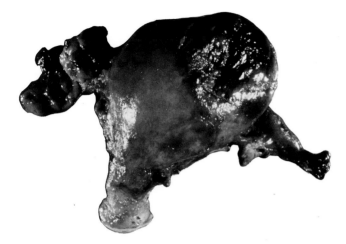

**32.5** Criminal abortion. The perforation seen in this uterus led to generalized peritonitis. The fetus and placenta had been evacuated.

sence of all of these. All previously listed causes of abortion may play a role. Bardewil[1] has studied the role of immune reactions in habitual abortion.

## Missed Abortion

The diagnosis of missed abortion is made when the death of the conceptus antedates its expulsion by at least 8 weeks. Bengtsson[2] states that missed abortion results when there is fetal death with persistence of placental function.

## Induced Abortion

A therapeutic abortion is performed for medical indications that contraindicate continuation of the pregnancy.

Voluntary abortions, performed in response to the mother's desire to terminate the pregnancy, have largely replaced illegal, or criminal, abortions in the United States. The latter, often performed under unsterile conditions and usually following the introduction into the uterus of various instruments or abortifacient substances, resulted in considerable maternal morbidity and mortality. Infection originating in the uterus led to septicemia. Perforation of the uterus, as seen in Figure 32.5, led to peritonitis. In such cases, after hospitalization of the mother, the pathologist was apt to receive curettings that consisted of heavily infected placental or fetal parts or decidua, all showing marked inflammation and necrosis. Gram-negative bacteria

and clostridia were the usual pathogens. If hysterectomy became necessary, the uterus showed infection spreading from the cavity through the myometrium into the parametrium. It might be perforated. If the patient died, the autopsy showed disseminated visceral sepsis, often complicated by endotoxic shock and disseminated intravascular coagulation. This train of events is fortunately becoming a rarity.

The technique of performing therapeutic and voluntary abortions depends on the duration of the pregnancy. Dilatation and curettage, usually with suction technique, are performed prior to the twelfth week. This method is precluded later in pregnancy because of the danger of perforation, hemorrhage, and incomplete removal of the gestation. All the tissue should be submitted to the pathologist, who should verify microscopically that pregnancy products have been removed. Because of the trauma of the suction technique, it is impossible to comment on the completeness of the abortion. The pathologist should keep in mind the possibility of hydatidiform mole, which may be clinically unsuspected but which may be aborted by this technique. The gross diagnosis of mole is rendered difficult because of rupture of the vesicles by the suction. Microscopic examination, however, can confirm the presence of molar villi (Chapter 33, Figure 33.4). It must be recalled that hydropic villi may be attached to the placental margin or the chorion leve in normal gestations. They mimic molar villi and render the diagnosis of mole more difficult. There are two characteristics that aid in the distinction of hydropic and molar change. First, trophoblast proliferation is absent from hydropic villi but present in molar villi. Second, hydropic change tends to involve only a few villi, with the majority normal, whereas molar change tends to be diffuse. The latter distinction is inoperative, however, in a twin gestation in which one twin is molar, where normal and molar villi may be mixed.

On occasion, very little tissue is obtained by the gynecologist attempting an abortion by dilatation and curettage. This may be because there is no intrauterine gestation, or it may be because of incomplete removal of the products of pregnancy. The pathologist should submit all small specimens for microscopic examination. If he finds gestational products, it is probable that the abortion was incomplete. It must be recalled, however, that the rare possibility of a combined intrauterine and extrauterine (ectopic) pregnancy has not been ruled out. If, however, he fails to find products of pregnancy, four possibilities exist. (1) The patient may not be pregnant. (2) The patient may have an intrauterine gestation that the curette has failed to abort. In this case one would expect to see

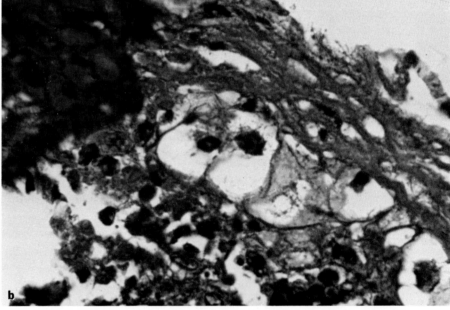

**32.6 a** and **b.** Vacuolar degeneration in cells of the amnion in saline abortion.

[Reprinted by permission from A. Blaustein and L. Shenker, Pathologic findings after hypertonic saline instillation in midtrimester abortion, *Clin. Obstet. Gynecol. 14:*192, 1971.]

decidua with or without the Arias–Stella hypersecretory change. (3) The patient may have an ectopic pregnancy. In a patient who has not had vaginal bleeding, or whose bleeding has been of short duration, one expects to see decidual endometrium in the presence of an ectopic pregnancy. However, endometrium in any phase may coexist with an ectopic pregnancy, and the gynecologist should be promptly informed of the absence of gestational products in order to alert him or her to this possibility. (4) Finally,

a combined intra- and extrauterine twin pregnancy is remotely possible.

After 16 weeks of gestation, when the amniotic sac is accessible, abortion can be performed by the intraamniotic injection of hypertonic solutions. The one most often used is 20% saline. This procedure entails more maternal risk than the curettage abortion technique used earlier in pregnancy. Hypernatremia, consumptive coagulopathy, retained placenta, hemorrhage, and infection are recognized

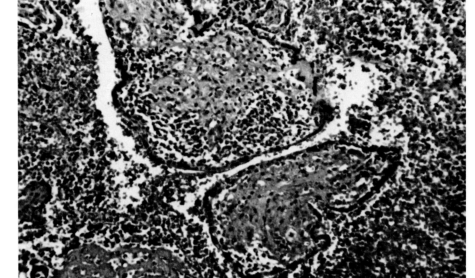

**32.7 a** and **b.** Focal inflammation and necrosis in chorionic villi in saline abortion.

[Reprinted by permission from A. Blaustein and L. Shenker, Pathologic findings after hypertonic saline instillation in midtrimester abortion, *Clin. Obstet. Gynecol. 14*:192, 1971.]

complications of the procedure, albeit rare.[13] The mechanism of saline abortion is not clearly understood. It is probable that fetal death precedes the onset of labor. Because of an interval of hours to days between installation of the saline and delivery, maceration of the fetus is apt to be present. Blaustein and Shenker[3] have described focal and relatively minor changes in the placenta, including vacuolar degeneration (Figure 32.6) of the amnion and chorion and focal inflammation and necrosis of chorionic villi (Figure 32.7).

# REFERENCES

1. Bardewil, W. A., Mitchell, C. W. Jr., McKeough, R. P., and Marchant, D. J. Behaviour of skin homografts in human pregnancy. *Am. J. Obstet. Gynecol. 84*:1284, 1962.

2. Bengtsson, L. P. Missed abortion. The aetiology, endocrinology and treatment. *Lancet 1*:339, 1962.

3. Blaustein, A. and Shenker, L. Pathologic findings after hypertonic saline installation in midtrimester abortion. *Clin. Obstet. Gynecol. 14*:192, 1971.

4. Driscoll, S. G. Histopathologic observations in gestational rubella. *Am. J. Dis. Child. 118*:49, 1969.

5. Goranov, I., and Gaven, S. Fehlgeburt bei Zytomegalie. *Zbl. Gynakol. 85*:1037, 1963.

6. Hertig, A. T., and Livingstone, R. G. Spontaneous, threatened and habitual abortion; their pathogenesis and treatment. *N. Engl. J. Med. 230*:797, 1944.

7. Hertig, A. T., and Sheldon, W. H. Minimal criteria required to prove prima facie case of traumatic abortion or miscarriage. *Ann. Surg. 117*:596, 1943.

8. Javert, C. T. *Spontaneous and Habitual Abortion.* New York, Blakiston, 1957.

9. Levine, P. Serological factors as possible cause of spontaneous abortions. *J. Hered. 34*:71, 1943.

10. Levine, P. The rare human isoagglutinin anti Tj^a and habitual abortion. *Science 120*:239, 1954.

11. Mall, F. P., and Meyer, A. W. Studies on abortions: Survey of pathologic ova in Carnegie Embryological Collection. *Contrib. Embryol. 12*:56, 1921.

12. Remington, J. S. Toxoplasmosis and human abortion. *Prog. Gynecol. 4*:303, 1963.

13. Schiffer, M. A., Pakter, J., and Clahr, J. Mortality associated with hypertonic saline abortion. *Obstet. Gynecol. 42*:759, 1973.

14. Selzen, G. Virus isolation, inclusion bodies, and chromosomes in rubella-infected human embryo. *Lancet ii*:336, 1963.

15. Vinzent, R. An unknown affliction of pregnancy. Placental infection with the vibrio fetus. *Presse Med. 57*:1230, 1949.

16. Warburton, D., and Fraser, F. C. Genetic aspects of abortion. *Clin. Obstet. Gynecol. 2*:22, 1959.

17. Werner, H., Schmidtke, L. and Thomaschek, G. Toxoplasma-Infektion und Schwangerschaft. Der histologische Nachweis intrauterinen infektions weges. *Klin. Wschr. 41*:96, 1963.

Bradley Bigelow, M.D.

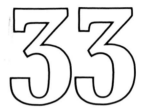

# Gestational Trophoblast Disease

## Introduction

The somewhat awkward title of this final chaper on placental pathology is a reflection of the age-old difficulty in understanding the pathogenesis and predicting the behavior of a very fascinating group of gestational abnormalities. Three conditions are included: hydatidiform mole, invasive mole (chorioadenoma destruens), and choriocarcinoma. They run the gamut from degenerative to neoplastic processes. Although connecting links between them are demonstrable, both in clinical situations and in the laboratory, the unpredictability persists despite years of observation and analysis.

The normal pregnancy has certain very special characteristics that serve to introduce the complexities of this subject. It will be recalled that a gestation is an allograft, with one half of the chromosomes maternal and the other half the foreign contribution of the paternal sperm. Trophoblast normally displays many of the characteristics of malignancy, such as rapid cell division, invasion, and even metastasis. After about 9 months a series of events occur that separates the placental graft from the maternal host. Although the factors that operate to induce normal labor and delivery are not completely understood, the vast majority of pregnancies terminate successfully and the growth of the trophoblast is controlled and stops at term.

Choriocarcinoma represents uncontrolled, truly neoplastic growth of trophoblast. Hydatidiform mole and its

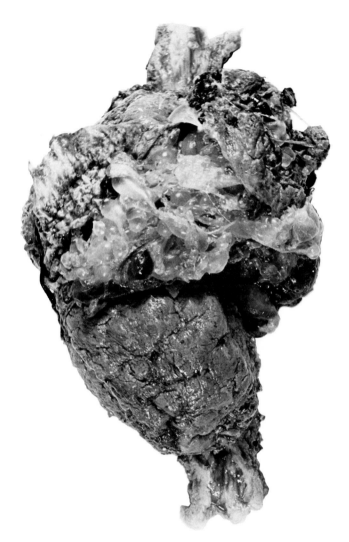

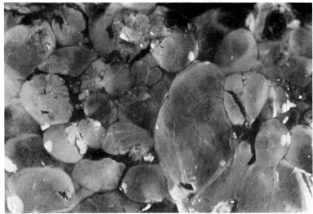

**33.2** Hydatidiform mole. A few vesicles approach 1 cm in diameter. The background is formed by smaller vesicles.

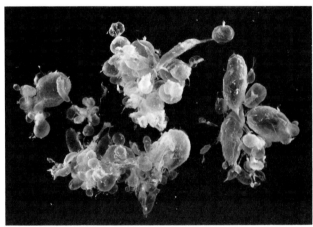

**33.1** Hydatidiform mole within the uterus. Molar tissue is present within this electively removed uterus from a patient in her forties. The uterus has been split laterally, so that the cervix is attached at both top and bottom.

**33.3** Hydatidiform mole photographed under water.

invasive variant, chorioadenoma destruens, fall between degenerative and neoplastic phenomena, and their major importance lies in their relationship to choriocarcinoma.[2,3,8,11,15,16]

## Hydatidiform Mole

We have already referred to the need to distinguish molar change from the hydropic degeneration that can be found both in abortuses and in areas of the normal placenta that are poorly perfused by fetal blood.[27,28] The importance of the recognition of true mole lies in the observation that the most common precursor of choriocarcinoma is the presence of a hydatidiform mole.

Hydatidiform mole, shown in Figures 33.1, 33.2, and 33.3, consists of a mass of vesicles that largely or entirely replace the normal, delicately branching chorionic villi. Each vesicle represents a villus distended with fluid. There may be variation in size, with the larger ones measuring up to an inch in diameter. The diagnosis is obvious grossly if a specimen is delivered largely intact, following either its spontaneous abortion or curettage. However, the diagnosis may be difficult if the amount of tissue is small, if it is mixed with a great deal of blood, or if a suction curette

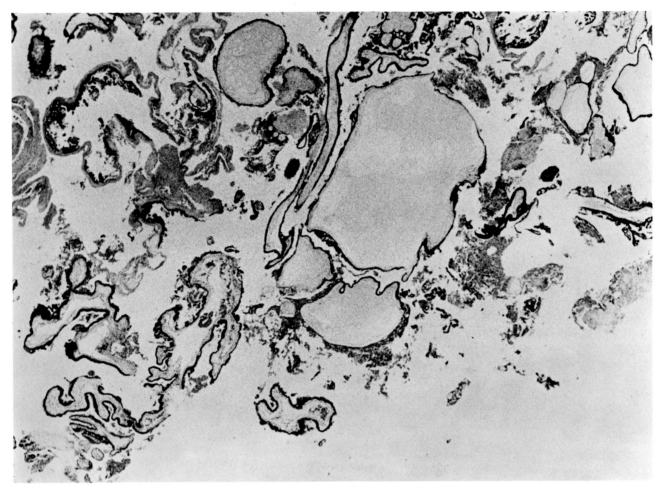

**33.4** Hydatidiform mole aborted by suction curettage. A large, intact vesicle is near the center. Many vesicles, however, have been ruptured and have collapsed.

has caused rupture of many of the vesicles (Figure 33.4). There are three major microscopic criteria for the diagnosis of true mole: first, hydropic swelling of villi; second, complete absence of fetal blood vessels or marked reduction in their number; finally, proliferation of trophoblast (Figure 33.5a,b). The amount of trophoblast may vary considerably in different areas, as it may, incidentally, in sections from voluntarily aborted normal early gestations. Consequently, generous sampling of different areas is indicated.

Hertig and Sheldon[20] reviewed 200 cases of hydatidiform mole. They subdivided them into six groups that varied in stages from benign to malignant, based on the amount and appearance of the trophoblast. In a later publication, Hertig and Mansell[19] reduced the classifica-

tion to three grades, varying from apparently benign to apparently malignant. The authors pointed out the favorable prognosis of most molar pregnancies, with a benign course in 81.5% and with the development of invasive mole in 16.5% and of choriocarcinoma in 2.5%. They concluded that there was a general, although not an absolute, correlation between the morphology of the molar trophoblast and the clinical course. This conclusion, disputed by some, has become less important since the demonstration of the curability of choriocarcinoma by chemotherapy and the extension of the use of chemotherapy, in some quarters, to the prophylactic treatment of moles.

There are two basic theories of pathogenesis of hydatidiform mole. The first, advocated by Hertig, is that molar change results from fetal circulatory inadequacy. Viable

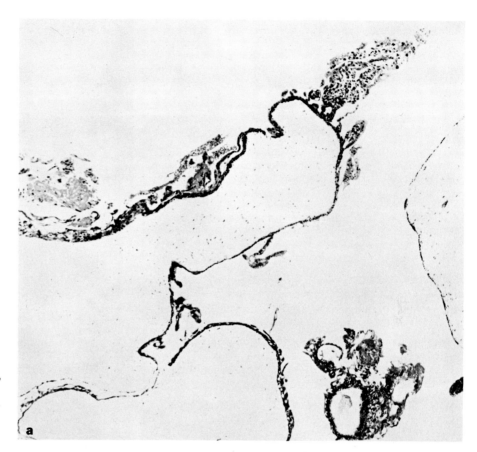

**33.5 a.** Hydatidiform mole. This villus is swollen with fluid, devoid of vessels, and partly covered by proliferating trophoblast. **b.** Closeup of proliferating molar trophoblast. The syncytiotrophoblast has many vacuoles in its cytoplasm.

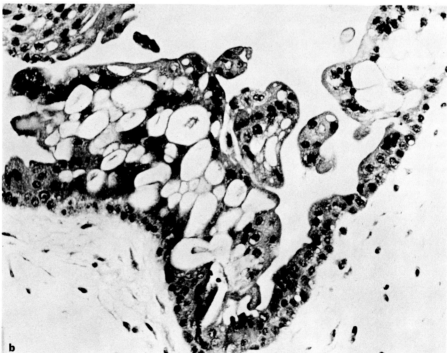

trophoblast transports fluid from the intervillous space into the villous stroma, where it accumulates because of transport failure in the fetal vasculature. Hertig and Edmonds[18] studied a large series of spontaneous abortions and found pathologic ova in 47% at a mean menstrual age of 10.2 weeks. Hydatidiform degeneration, represented by villous swelling of lesser extent and degree than true molar change, was found in 67% of this group. In comparison, the 53% of abortions with nonpathologic ova, at a mean menstrual age of 15.4 weeks, showed hydatidiform degeneration in only 12%. The authors concluded that hydatidiform change resulted from the circulatory inadequacy of a pathologic ovum and that a true mole represented the failure of abortion (missed abortion) of such an ovum, with the hydropic swelling progressing *in utero*. Support for this theory is further derived from Hertig's and Edmonds'[18] additional review of 54 typical moles, in 10 of which either the absence of an embryo was established by finding an empty chorion or, rarely, a markedly abnormal embryo was found. No chorionic cavity was found in the remaining 44 cases. The mean age of abortion of 17.4 weeks for the true moles accords with Hertig's theory of missed abortion of a defective ovum. The defective ovum theory is further substantiated by several chromosomal analyses of moles that have shown a variety of abnormalities.[23,24,31]

The second theory of pathogenesis is a primary abnormality of trophoblast, as advocated by Park.[30] He postulates that the features of mole, blighting or the failure of development of the embryo, hydrops of villi, trophoblast proliferation, and the occasional invasive or autonomous growth, are all secondary to the abnormal trophoblast. Because in the normally developing early gestation the nutrition of the embryo depends on trophoblast and the villous stroma originates from trophoblast, his thesis seems to have great logical merit.

The incidence of hydatidiform mole is approximately one in 2,000 term pregnancies in the United States. It is far commoner in tropical and Asiatic countries. The incidence rises with advancing maternal age and there is a tendency toward repetition of molar gestations, not necessarily consecutively and not necessarily with the same partners.

Most patients present with vaginal bleeding which has started toward the end of the first trimester of pregnancy.[10] The uterus is usually, but not always, larger than expected from the duration of amenorrhea. Molar fragments may be passed in small or massive amount.

The early onset of toxemia should raise the suspicion of a molar pregnancy. As has been discussed in Chapter 30, there is both experimental and other evidence that the

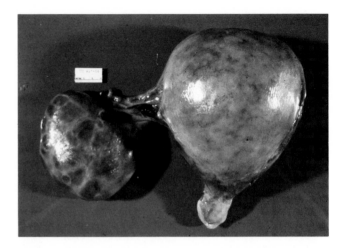

**33.6** Hyperreactio luteinalis. The enlarged ovary, at left, accompanies a hydatidiform mole within the unopened uterus. The other ovary was similarly involved and was left *in situ*.

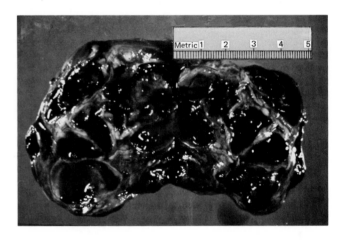

**33.7** Hyperreactio luteinalis. The cut surface of the ovary shows multiple lutein cysts, the walls of which are yellow, and many of which are filled with blood.

development of toxemia is related to ischemia of the placenta. The bulky, irregular mass of intrauterine molar placenta shown in Figure 33.1 assuredly has large areas of reduced exposure to maternal blood in the intervillous space.

Bilateral ovarian enlargement, caused by the presence of multiple lutein cysts, is reported in widely variable incidence (Figures 33.6 and 33.7). Otherwise known as hyperreactio luteinalis, it is most often seen as an accompaniment of molar gestation but it also occurs with invasive mole, choriocarcinoma, multiple normal gestations, single

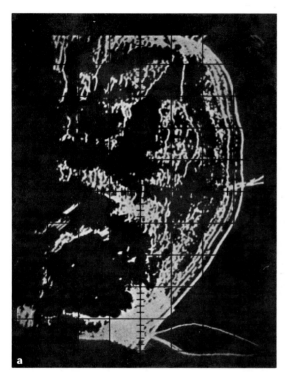

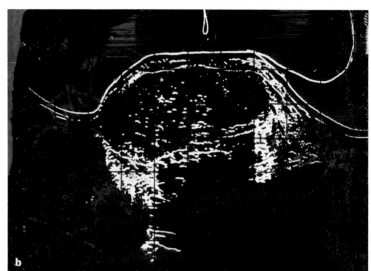

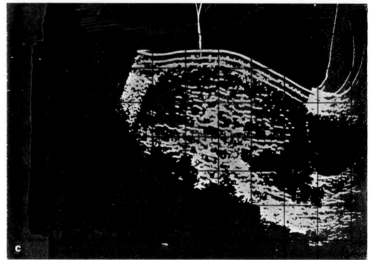

**33.8 a.** Echogram of a normal pregnancy. The chorion is well defined. **b.** Echogram of hydatidiform mole (Figure 33.1). This shows multiple scattered echoes in this enlarged uterus. There are no fetal echoes. This is consistent with a diagnosis of hydatid mole—a diagnosis made preoperatively in a patient who had not yet aborted her mole. **c.** Echogram of hydatidiform mole (Figure 33.1) showing the sunburst pattern.

normal gestations, and erythroblastosis with fetal hydrops.[13] It regresses after elimination of the trophoblast, and the ovaries should not be removed.

Although the diagnosis of mole is obvious with the passage of vesicles, it can be made prior to abortion by special techniques, such as ultrasonography[9,17,26] (Figure 33.8a–c), amniography, or, on occasion, arteriography.[4,15,21] The absence of a fetus, evidenced by failure to detect fetal heart or skeleton, is the general rule. However, in possibly 5% of molar gestations, the presence of a fetus has been reported.[22] In such cases the diagnosis is seldom made prior to abortion or delivery. Most cases probably represent twin pregnancies, one member of which is blighted and accompanies the molar placenta. Usually, in fact, a portion of the molar placenta accompanied by a fetus is free from molar change. A second possibility is

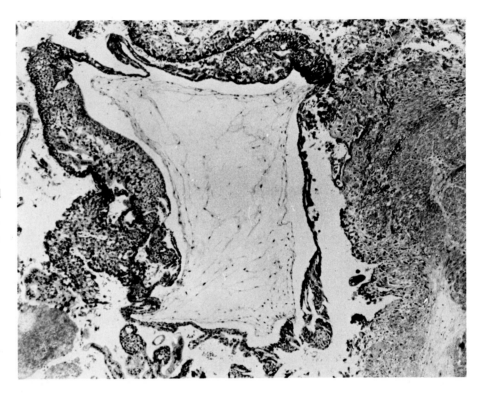

**33.9** Invasive mole (chorioadenoma destruens). An intractable vaginal hemorrhage necessitated hysterectomy. The large molar villus is associated with considerable trophoblast proliferation. It lies within the myometrium, shown at right.

that hydropic degeneration may be misinterpreted as true molar change.

Complications of molar pregnancies[7] include hemorrhage, which may be massive and necessitate hysterectomy. Toxemia of early onset, already mentioned, provides a clue to the diagnosis.

The major concern in this condition is the potential for persistent or progressive trophoblast disease. This occurs in about 20% of cases, most often as invasive mole, rarely as choriocarcinoma. The titer of human chorionic gonadotropin (HCG) provides the best way of monitoring the presence of trophoblast. A valuable refinement has been the development of a radioimmunoassay for the beta subunit of chorion gonadotropin. This permits the distinction of HCG from pituitary luteinizing hormone because there is no cross-reactivity, therefore permitting the detection of smaller levels of HCG than has been possible with the usual pregnancy tests. Assaying the beta subunit[14] is useful in following patients with gestational trophoblast disease when the level of chorionic gonadotropin, as determined by the usual immunologic assay, falls below the level of luteinizing hormone with which the ordinary assay cross-reacts. It is not used as a diagnostic test because the regular immunologic assay serves this purpose.

After the passage of a molar pregnancy the patient must be followed carefully. About 80% of patients have an uncomplicated course. The most reliable indication of persistent trophoblast disease is failure of the level of HCG to drop to normal within 8 weeks of evacuation of the mole. Persistent uterine enlargement or vaginal bleeding represent two other indications.[21]

## Invasive Mole

Originally designated by Ewing as chorioadenoma destruens, this condition is comparable to the increta and percreta extension of a nonmolar placenta. Invasion of the uterine muscle complicates about 16% of molar gestations. Rarely it may result in complete perforation into broad ligament or peritoneum with associated massive hemorrhage. Invasive mole is usually suspected when, after passage of a mole, the chorionic gonadotropin titer fails to drop to normal and vaginal bleeding and uterine enlargement persist. A curettage may or may not produce molar tissue, and it must be emphasized that it is virtually impossible for a pathologist to make the diagnosis of invasive mole from curettings alone. The clearly intramyometrial location of the invasive mole shown in Figure

33.9 can seldom be established in curetted fragments. A biopsy of the corpus uteri obtained at laparotomy may, however, reveal molar vesicles in the myometrium. Park[30] suggests that the invasive portion of a mole shows more proliferation of trophoblast than is seen in noninvasive moles. He also points out that the degree of hydropic swelling of many of the invasive villi may be reduced below that of the classic molar villus. Villi with almost normal stroma may, in fact, be found intramurally. The important point is that the presence of villi removes the lesion from the more ominous category of choriocarcinoma. Rarely, an invasive mole is followed by villous metastases to the vulva, vagina, or lung. The latter may be suggested by pulmonary x-ray findings and a few cases with documentation by lung biopsy have been reported. Here again, the accompaniment of trophoblast by villous stroma distinguishes the lesion from choriocarcinoma.

Although invasive mole is a locally aggressive lesion, the incidence of development of choriocarcinoma is no greater than that following an ordinary mole. Uncontrolled uterine or intraperitoneal hemorrhage may necessitate hysterectomy, however.

## Choriocarcinoma

This rare tumor is usually observed in women of childbearing age as a complication of pregnancy. Accordingly, most choriocarcinomas are of the gestational type. Less often, the tumor appears as a component of a germ cell neoplasm of the gonad in either sex; extremely rarely, such a tumor may be in pure form. This type of choriocarcinoma, the nongestational, markedly worsens the prognosis of the gonadal tumor in which it is found. The response to chemotherapy is less favorable than is that of the gestational type, an unexplained observation of considerable interest.

Choriocarcinoma is a malignant tumor that has been uniformly fatal prior to the advent of chemotherapeutic treatment in 1956.[25] The tumor is an uncontrolled growth of the cyto- and the syncytiotrophoblast. Chorionic villi are absent. The grossly observed tumor tends to be soft, hemorrhagic, and accompanied by necrosis of the tissue surrounding it (Figures 33.10, and 33.11). Microscopically, the diagnosis requires the presence of both types of trophoblast (Figures 33.12–33.15). Cytotrophoblast alone is not diagnostic, mimicking decidua as well as undifferentiated epithelial tumors, and syncytiotrophoblast may be confused with histiocytic giant cells or with tumor giant cells of other derivation. The proportion of cyto- and syncytio-

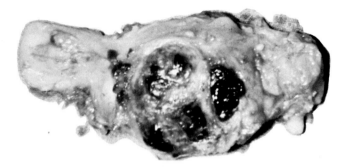

**33.10** Choriocarcinoma. Hemorrhagic masses of tumor stud the inside of this opened uterus. The cervix extends to left and right.

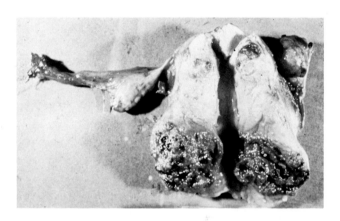

**33.11** Choriocarcinoma. Hemorrhagic tumor occupies the lower uterine segment and cervix. Smaller foci of choriocarcinoma can be seen in left and right fundal walls.

trophoblast may vary in different samples of a given tumor but both must be present to establish the diagnosis. The pleomorphic appearance and the invasive and metastatic capacity of normal trophoblast complicate the pathologist's diagnostic task. As with invasive mole, it is extremely difficult to diagnose choriocarcinoma in uterine curettings. Curetted normal pregnancies and specimens from incomplete abortions may contain microscopic areas of pure trophoblast, without villous stroma, because of random sampling. The ominous presence of trophoblast proliferating in the absence of villi therefore may be erroneously presumed to exist.

Choriocarcinoma is preceded by hydatidiform mole in from one-third to one-half of cases. Those favoring the lower figure suggest that preceding moles may be overdiagnosed. The remaining cases are about equally divided between preceding spontaneous abortions and preceding

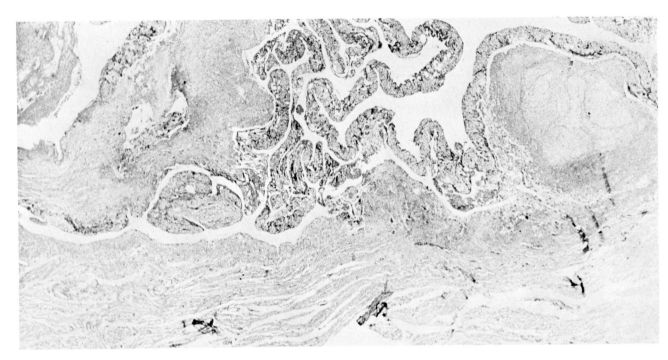

**33.12** Choriocarcinoma. Cords of trophoblast, without associated villous stroma, are mixed with blood. Myometrium is at bottom.

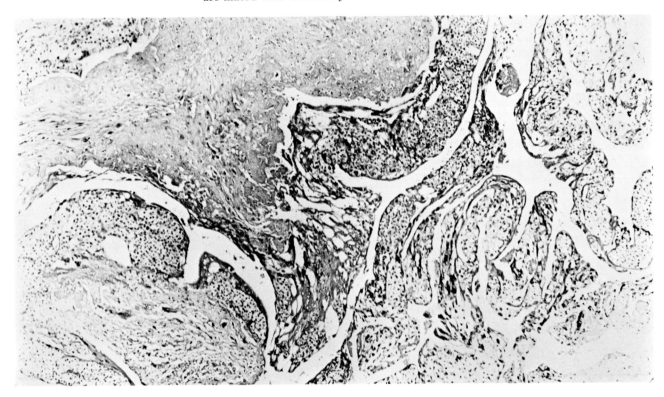

**33.13** Higher magnification of Figure 33.12 shows trophoblast adjacent to partly necrotic muscle at upper left.

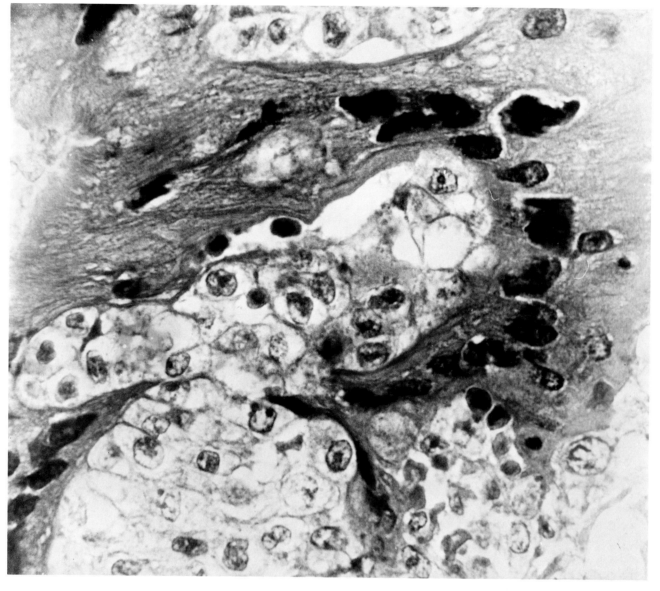

**33.14** High-power view of choriocarcinoma. The central, pale cytotrophoblast is surrounded by syncytiotrophoblast. Nuclei are pleomorphic.

normal pregnancies. A small proportion, in the neighborhood of 2 to 3%, follows ectopic pregnancies.

The behavior of choriocarcinoma is notoriously variable. Usually the disease becomes manifest within 2 years of a preceding molar or nonmolar pregnancy. Extremely long intervals, up to 9 or 10 years, may intervene, however, and there are cases on record of delay in appearance of the tumor until years after hysterectomy or until after the menopause.

Another puzzling feature of the disease is the frequency of extragenital, metastatic choriocarcinoma in the absence of a demonstrable primary lesion in the uterus or in an ectopic site and in the absence of a primary, nongestational choriocarcinoma in the ovary. This situation has been established by careful autopsy examinations, as well as by scrupulous study of excised uteri by surgical pathologists. In several reviews the absence of a primary lesion has been reported in as many as one-third of cases of disseminated

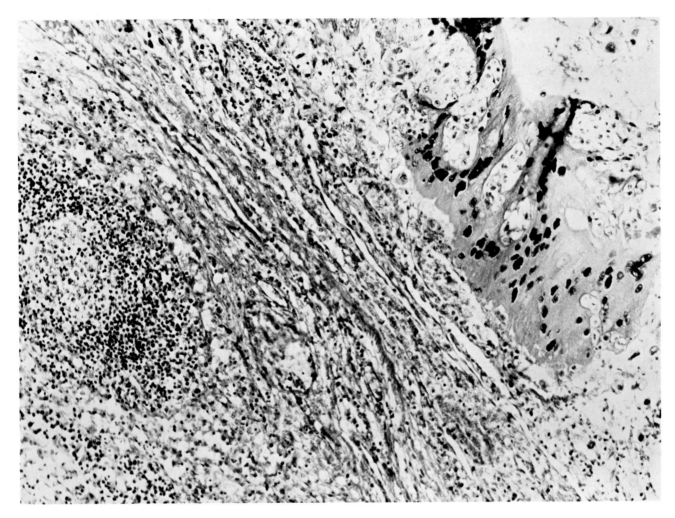

**33.15** Choriocarcinoma metastatic to a lymph node. A germinal center is at left.

choriocarcinoma. The primary lesion may have regressed, as has been suspected to occur, for example, in a significant proportion of disseminated testicular tumors.

Monitoring of the chorionic gonadotropin titer in patients with evacuated hydatidiform moles provides the most reliable method of determining the persistence of proliferating trophoblast, be it caused by residual mole, invasive mole, or choriocarcinoma. Hydatidiform mole provides a warning of the remote possibility of subsequent choriocarcinoma.

In a significant number of cases, however, such warning is not provided, and one may only have a history of normal pregnancy, abortion, or ectopic gestation. The history may be completely negative in the case of a totally unrecognized, very early, spontaneous abortion.

Disseminated choriocarcinoma may involve all parts of the body and may mimic a wide variety of medical and surgical conditions. Lungs are the commonest secondary site, followed by brain and liver. Ober, Edgcomb, and Price,[29] in a detailed review of 44 autopsied cases of gestational choriocarcinoma, reported the lungs to be universally involved, followed in frequency by brain, liver, kidneys, small intestine, spleen, and vagina (see Figure 3.48, Chapter 3). The latter may ulcerate and be a source of severe hemorrhage. As in the primary site, metastatic choriocarcinoma is often extremely hemorrhagic or necrotic, and identifiable tumor may be small in amount and difficult to find microscopically (Figure 33.15).

Further complicating the problem of the genesis of choriocarcinoma is the rare entity of focal choriocarcinoma in an otherwise normal placenta. Brewer and Gerbie[5] described two cases with metastases and fatal outcomes.

They reviewed the two prior reported cases, one of which had metastases and one of which did not. In the few reports, the placenta is described as being nonmolar and normal except for a focal area of marked proliferation of trophoblast. Albeit extremely rare, this apparently represents the very early development of choriocarcinoma. It may explain some cases of metastatic disease following nonmolar pregnancies or abortions. It provides a challenge to pathologists to examine small, focal lesions of the placenta that look like hemorrhage, infarction, or chorangioma.

Since 1956, when Li, Hertz, and Spencer[25] reported response to methotrexate in two cases of metastatic choriocarcinoma, this previously fatal disease has become treatable with chemotherapy. Actinomycin D has also been found effective. The level of the HCG titer is used to monitor response to treatment, reflecting, as it does, the amount of viable trophoblast. Clinical observation has led to the delineation of two classes of patients, the low and the high risk.[21] The high-risk group has one or more of the following: initial HCG titer greater than 100,000 IU per 24 hr; duration of symptoms greater than 4 months before chemotherapeutic treatment; and metastases to brain or liver. Remission rates after chemotherapy are reported to be as high as 100% in the low-risk and 80% in the high-risk group.

Pertinent to a discussion of the uncontrolled growth of trophoblast exhibited by choriocarcinoma is the dilemma of the normal gestation.[12] The half-foreign allograft of normal pregnancy is neither rejected by the mother nor is its invasive and metastasizing potential permitted to proceed unchecked. An understanding of both the toleration and the containment of the normal pregnancy would shed valuable light on the biology of trophoblast disease.

# REFERENCES

1. Bagshawe, K. D. Trophoblastic tumors. Chemotherapy and development. *Br. Med. J.* 2:1303, 1963.
2. Bagshawe, K. D. Hydatidiform mole and choriocarcinoma. *Br. Med. J.* 1:1509, 1966.
3. Barkla, P. C. Hydatidiform mole and chorioepithelioma. *J. Obstet. Gynaecol. Br. Emp.* 62:239, 1955.
4. Borell, U. Hydatidiform mole diagnosed by pelvic angiography. *Acta. Radiol.* 56:113, 1961.
5. Brewer, J. I., and Gerbie, A. B. Early development of choriocarcinoma. *Am. J. Obstet. Gynecol.* 94:692, 1966.
6. Cockshott, W. P., Evans, K. T. E., and De V. Hendrikse, J. P. Arteriography of trophoblastic tumors. *Clin. Radiol.* 15:1, 1964.
7. Coppleson, M. Hydatidiform mole and its complications. *J. Obstet. Gynaecol. Br. Emp.* 65:238, 1958.
8. Corscaden, J. A., and Shettles, L. B. Hydatidiform mole and choriocarcinoma. *Bull. Sloane Hosp. Women* 5:41, 1959.
9. Donald, I., and Brown, T. G. Localization using physical devices, radioisotopes and radiologic methods. I. Demonstration of tissue interfaces within the body by ultrasonic echo sounding. *Br. J. Radiol.* 34:539, 1961.
10. Douglas, G. W. The diagnosis and management of hydatidiform mole. *Surg. Clin. North Am.* 37:379, 1957.
11. Douglas, G. W. Malignant change in trophoblastic tumors. *Am. J. Obstet. Gynecol.* 84:884, 1962.
12. Editorial: The fetus as a homograft. *Lancet II*:535, 1975.
13. Girouard, D. P., Barclay, D. L., and Collins, C. G. Hyperreactio luteinalis. *Obstet. Gynecol.* 23:513, 1964.
14. Goldstein, D. P., and Kosasa, T. S. The subunit radioimmunoassay for HCG—Clinical application, in M. L. Taymor and T. H. Green, Jr., eds.: *Progress in Gynecology.* Grune and Stratton, 1975, Vol. VI, pp. 145–184.
15. Grady, H. G. Hydatidiform mole and choriocarcinoma. *Ann. N.Y. Acad. Sci.* 75:565, 1959.
16. Green, R. R. Chorioadenoma destruens. *Ann. N.Y. Acad. Sci.* 80:143, 1959.
17. Harper, W. F., and McVicar, J. Hydatidiform mole and pregnancy diagnosed by sonar. *Br. Med. J.* 2:1178, 1963.
18. Hertig, A. T., and Edmonds, H. W. Genesis of hydatidiform mole. *Arch. Pathol.* 30:260, 1940.
19. Hertig, A. T., and Mansell, H. *Tumors of the female sex organs.* Part I. Hydatidiform mole and choriocarcinoma. Washington, D.C., Armed Forces Institute of Pathology, 1956.
20. Hertig, A. T., and Sheldon, W. H. Hydatidiform mole—A pathologico-clinical correlation of 200 cases. *Am. J. Obstet. Gynecol.* 53:1, 1947.
21. Hilgers, R. D., and Lewis, J. L. Jr. Gestational trophoblastic neoplasms. *Gynecol. Oncol.* 2:460, 1974.
22. Jones, W. B., and Lauersen, N. H. Hydatidiform mole with coexistent fetus. *Am. J. Obstet. Gynecol.* 122:267, 1975.
23. Klingen, H. P. Points from the discussion in W. M. Davidson and D. R. Smith, eds.: *Human Chromosomal Abnormalities.* Proceedings. London, 1959. London Staples Press, 1961, p. 130.
24. Klingen, H. P., and Atkin, N. B. Sex chromatin studies on hydatidiform moles. *Hum. Chromosome Newsletter* 3:18, 1961.
25. Li, M. C., Hertz, R., and Spencer, D. B. Effect of methotrexate therapy upon choriocarcinoma and chorioadenoma. *Proc. Soc. Exp. Biol. Med.* 93:361, 1956.
26. McVicar, J. Illustrative examples of ultrasonic echograms. *Proc. R. Soc. Med.* 55:638, 1962.
27. Meyer, A. W. Hydatidiform degeneration in tubal pregnancy. *Surg. Gynecol. Obstet.* 28:293, 1919.
28. Nilsson, L. Hydatidiform degeneration in aborted ova. A histopathologic and clinical study. *Acta Obstet. Gynecol. Scand.* 36(Suppl. 7):1, 1957.
29. Ober, W. B., Edgcomb, J. H., and Price, E. B. The pathology of choriocarcinoma. *Ann. N.Y. Acad. Sci.* 172:299, 1971.
30. Park, W. W. *Choriocarcinoma. A Study of Its Pathology.* Philadelphia, F. A. Davis Co., 1971.
31. Szulman, A. E. Chromosomal aberrations in spontaneous human abortions. *N. Engl. J. Med.* 272:811, 1965.

Laszlo Sarkozi, Ph.D.

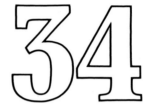

# Amniotic Fluid: Biochemical Assays Relating to Fetal Viability

## Introduction

The selection of this body fluid for inclusion in this book is self-explanatory. This chapter attempts to describe reasons for obtaining the amniotic fluid; its composition, which depends on its origin; and the great wealth of information on the well-being of the fetus obtained by performing biochemical assays of amniotic fluid. References on cytologic, histochemical, and biochemical studies of suspended cells obtained from amniotic fluid are listed and intended as background information in the pursuit of further studies. Most of these studies today are performed only by investigators and some research-oriented laboratories. However, they conduct successful screening programs for the most frequent fetal biochemical disorders and the research tools of yesterday are the routine tests of today. Only 10 years ago, about 20 papers were published annually on amniotic fluid; presently, over 500 publications a year deal with this subject, also several chapters and entire books[39,47,50,88,92,94,186-188,210,213,238,259,282] have been published on amniotic fluid. It was unavoidable that numerous valuable reports concerned with so many separate fields were omitted from this chapter. Detailed discussion of amniotic fluid biochemical assays is restricted to those procedures that are routinely performed by a large number of clinical laboratories, as of 1975.

# Indications for Amniotic Fluid Examination

Examination of amniotic fluid becomes necessary when there is a substantial risk of death or disability for the fetus or newborn. There may be a risk for the mother as well. The list of high-risk factors in pregnancy is expanding rapidly. The Perinatal Section of the Department of Obstetrics and Gynecology of The Mount Sinai Hospital in New York modified the criteria of Reid, Ryan, and Benirschke[281] and Novy[246] as follows:

## High-Risk Identification

I. *Patient characteristics and demographic factors*
   A. Maternal age
      1. Gravida less than 16 years of age
      2. Primigravida 35 years of age or older
      3. Gravida 40 years of age or older
   B. Maternal weight
      1. Underweight, less than 45 kg
      2. Overweight, more than 90 kg
   C. Maternal stature, height less than 1.57 m
   D. Malnutrition
   E. Poor physical fitness
   F. Lower socioeconomic status
   G. Disadvantaged ethnic group

II. *Past pregnancy history*
   A. Reproductive failures: infertility, repetitive abortion, fetal loss, stillbirth, or neonatal death
   B. Antepartum bleeding after 12 weeks' gestation
   C. Premature deliveries or postterm infants
   D. Infants with cerebral palsy, mental retardation, birth trauma, central nervous system disorders, or congenital anomaly
   E. Rh sensitization

III. *Past or present medical history*
   A. Hypertensive disorders
   B. Renal disease
   C. Diabetes mellitus
   D. Cardiovascular disease
   E. Pulmonary disease
   F. Endocrine disorders
   G. Major hemoglobinopathies
   H. Neoplastic disease
   I. Hereditary disorders
   J. Collagen diseases
   K. Epilepsy
   L. Habitual smoking
   M. Alcoholism or addiction
   N. Intercurrent surgery and anesthesia

IV. *Present pregnancy*
   A. Toxemia
   B. Anemia
   C. Placental abnormalities and uterine bleeding
   D. Hydramnios
   E. Multiple pregnancies
   F. Rubella and viral infections
   G. During the first trimester, utilization of unsafe drugs or radiation
   H. Rh sensitization
   I. Abnormalities of fetal or uterine growth
   J. Possible intrauterine death

# Time Dependent Factors

There seems to be an arbitrary but generally accepted division by separate discussion of amniotic fluid obtained in the first and in the second half of the pregnancy. With some overlap, most indications suggest this approach.

The purpose of amniotic fluid examination in early pregnancy is to detect a suspected genetic or metabolic condition of a defective fetus. The birth of affected children, whose prognoses are hopeless today, may be avoided through voluntary therapeutic abortion. Amniocentesis is performed in the second part of the pregnancy to monitor the well-being of the fetus at risk in order to enhance the delivery of a healthy infant.

Origin, circulation, and volume are also time dependent. As late as 25 years ago, amniotic fluid was believed to be a stagnant pool. Experimental evidence indicates that it is in a dynamic equilibrium with the fluids of the fetus and the mother. Figure 34.1 indicates the known and postulated sites of amniotic fluid formation and removal. The exact sites of origin are still controversial.[39,259,272] In early pregnancy the fluid may arise as a transudate of maternal serum across the placenta or fetal membranes, from the umbilical cord, and from fetal urine. The fetal skin and the fetal tracheobronchial tree may contribute to its formation. The concentrations of most biochemical constituents significantly change with advancing gestational age. The two most probable factors responsible for these changes are the keratinization of the fetal skin at about 24 weeks of gestational age[261,314] and the maturation of fetal organs. Amniotic fluid circulates rapidly between the fetal and maternal compartments. It has been

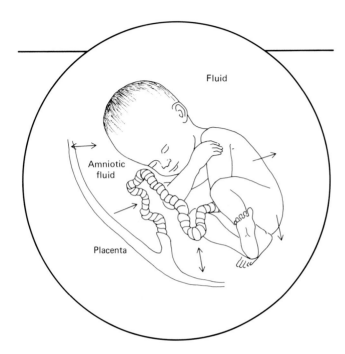

**34.1** Known and postulated sites of amniotic fluid origin and removal near term. Possible pathways for exchange include across the amnion, on the fetal surface, on the placenta, and into fetal vessels between the chorion leve and the amnion.

[After A. E. Seeds, Amniotic fluid and water metabolism, *in* Barnes, A. C., ed.: *Intrauterine Development.* Lea and Febiger, 1968, p. 138.]

reported that the fluid is replaced in about a 3-hr period and the rate of exchange may approach 500 ml/hr at term.[147,271,272] Amniotic fluid may be absorbed through fetal lungs, skin, the cord, and the amnion. Fetal swallowing was also demonstrated.[277] The amniotic volume is estimated at 100 to 300 ml by the end of the first trimester; the range at term may be of the order of 500 to 2,000 ml.[105]

# Obtaining a Specimen for Examination

Amniocentesis is a technique by which amniotic fluid is obtained from the amniotic sac. A needle is inserted into the amniotic cavity, usually through the abdominal wall, and amniotic fluid sample is aspirated. Menees, Miller, and Holly[208] reported the use of amniocentesis in 1930; then Aburel,[2] in 1937, employed the technique for the injection

of hypertonic saline to induce therapeutic abortion. By localizing the placenta and fetus with ultrasonic methods,[29,119] the safety of the procedure has considerably improved. Nadler and Gerbie[235] estimate the risk of maternal and fetal mortality and morbidity well under 1%. In spite of these very favorable developments, it must be emphasized that the obstetrician must weigh the potential value of studying the amniotic fluid to be obtained by amniocentesis against the potential risk of inserting the needle into the amniotic cavity.

# Specimen Handling, Interferences

Prior to performing amniocentesis, it is extremely important that all instructions be available for specimen handling. Because bilirubin is unstable in light, the specimen may have to be protected. Enzymatic decomposition may affect other tests. Therefore, the specimen may have to be refrigerated or frozen if it is not processed immediately. In some instances, centrifugation is recommended. Sterile containers may have to be on hand. The fluid may be contaminated with fetal or maternal blood; it may contain meconium. These contaminations may affect some results or may make analysis completely invalid.

# Fetal Death *in Utero*

Grossly elevated amniotic fluid creatine phosphokinase (CPK) levels were reported by Sarkozi et al.[299] in all tested cases of fetal death *in utero.* The CPK appears to be fetal origin, presumably the result of fetal tissue decomposition.[298] The cessation of fetoplacental circulation precludes subsequent amniotic fluid production. There is apparently no appreciable release through the fetal membranes and this unimpeded accumulation promotes further increase in the concentration of CPK in the amniotic fluid. Serial determinations on an experimental model were performed (Figure 34.2). The time factor was observed by Kerenyi and Sarkozi[155] in confirmed cases of fetal death in utero (Table 34.1).

Although some relevant factors depend on the stage of gestation, e.g., decomposing tissue mass and diluting amniotic fluid volume vary considerably, use of CPK concentration to estimate time elapsed since fetal demise has been promising.

If an amniotic fluid CPK value of 300 to 500 mU/ml is observed, a repeated amniocentesis 3 to 4 days later is recommended and if fetal death has occurred prior to

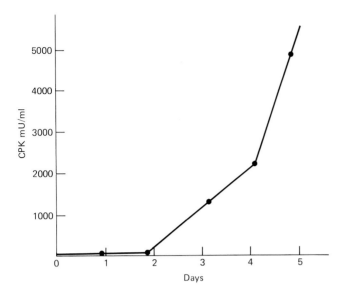

**34.2** Amniotic fluid CPK activities plotted against time elapsed since fetal demise.

[Reprinted by permission from T. Kerenyi and L. Sarkozi, Diagnosis of fetal death in utero by elevated amniotic fluid CPK levels, *Obstet. Gynecol.* 44:215, 1974.]

**Table 34.1** Elevated amniotic fluid CPK levels in confirmed cases of fetal death *in utero*[a]

| Patient | Days after fetal death *in utero* | CPK (mU/ml) |
|---|---|---|
| MF | 1–2 | 10 |
| KB[b] | 1–2 | 35 |
| VJ | 1–2 | 40 |
| WP | 2–3 | 260 |
| KB[b] | 4–5 | 1,000 |
| SA | 4–5 | 1,100 |
| VJ | 4 | 1,700 |
| PE | 4 | 2,000 |
| CF | 4 | 2,500 |
| WA | 5 | 5,200 |
| LE | 5–6 | 5,300 |
| GM | 6 | 6,600 |
| MB | 10 | >8,000 |
| JC | 20–30 | >10,000 |

[a] From T. Kerenyi and L. Sarkozi, *Obstet. Gynecol.* 44:215, 1974.
[b] Same patient.

obtaining the first sample, the CPK activity should be several thousand milliunits per milliliter.

## Early Amniocentesis

Amniotic fluid obtained in the first half of the pregnancy, usually between the twelfth and eighteenth week of gestation, is similar in biochemical composition to the maternal extracellular fluid. However, cells suspended in the amniotic fluid are presumably mostly of fetal origin. Postulated origins of these cells are fetal skin; mouth; upper gastrointestinal, genitourinary, and respiratory tracts; urine; umbilical cord; and amnion.

There are hundreds of reports on predictive diagnoses of affected fetuses. Most of these tests are far from being routine laboratory procedures. In addition, some of the earlier reports are continuously supplemented by additional findings and/or the available information needs further verification. An extensive list of fetal disorders was published by Milunsky and his co-workers.[212,216]

Similar tables compiled by Brock,[47] Dorfman,[88] Nadler and Burton,[232] Seegmiller,[315] and Valenti[357] and the corresponding references demonstrate the complexity of antenatal diagnosis of fetal disorders. These disorders may be classified as:

A. Chromosomal disorders
B. Sex-linked disorders
C. Hereditary biochemical disorders
  1. Lipid metabolism
  2. Mucopolysaccharide metabolism
  3. Amino acid and related disorders
  4. Carbohydrate metabolism
D. Miscellaneous biochemical disorders
E. Congenital malformation

I have compiled and modified the above listed reports on biochemical disorders in Table 34.2.

### Congenital Malformations

The first biochemical test, elevated $\alpha$-fetoprotein levels, for the detection of a central nervous system defect with an open neural tube was reported by Brock and Sutcliffe in 1972.[49] Since then it has been found that these elevated amniotic fluid $\alpha$-fetoprotein levels obtained between the fourteenth and seventeenth weeks of pregnancy reliably predict 85 to 90% of all cases of anencephaly and spina bifida cystica. The undetectable cases have closed or small open lesions.[214,231]

**Table 34.2**  Prenatal diagnosis of fetal biochemical disorders by amniocentesis

| Disorder | Nature[a] | Clinical manifestation | Product (A) in Excess or (B) in Deficiency | Reference |
|---|---|---|---|---|
| Acatalasemia | V | Recurrent and anaerobic infections of gums and oral tissue | (B) Catalase | 169, 336 |
| Adrenogenital syndrome | V | Virilization or pseudohermaphroditism; adrenal insufficiency, with salt loss; hypertensive cardiovascular disease; pregnanetriol and 17-ketosteroids in urine | (B) Failure of C-21, C-11, or steroid hydroxylation | 55, 151, 211, 243, 244, 336 |
| Argininosuccinic acidura | A | Mental retardation; trichorrhexis nodosa; ammonia intoxication | (A) Argininosuccinic acid (B) Argininosuccinase | 5, 149, 181, 320–322 |
| Chediak–Higashi syndrome | V | Photobia; decreased pigmentation of skin, hair, and eyes; increased susceptibility to infections | (A) Cellular inclusions | 36, 76, 367, 368 |
| Citrullinemia | A | Ammonia intoxication; mental retardation | (A) Citrulline (B) Argininosuccinic acid synthetase | 206, 219, 352 |
| Cystathioninuria | A | Normal intellect to mental retardation | (A) Cystathionine (B) Cystathionase | 129, 192, 268, 312, 356 |
| Cystic fibrosis | V | Recurrent pulmonary infection; malabsorption; failure to thrive | (A) Mucopolysaccharide storage or increased production in cultured fibroblasts (B) $\beta$-Glucuronidase deficiency in skin components | 77, 78, 107, 200, 237 |
| Cystinosis | V | Failure to thrive; rickets; glycosuria; aminoaciduria; cystine deposition in tissue | (A) Cystine | 28, 51, 117, 146, 309–311, 316 |
| Erythropoietic porphyria, congenital | V | Photosensitive dermatitis; anemia; splenomegaly; hypertrichosis; and massive porphyrinuria | (A) Uroporphyrin 1 and coproporphyrin 1 in tissues (B) Cosynthetase | 285, 302 |
| Fabry's disease | L | Purple skin papules; renal failure; cardiac and ocular involvement | (A) Ceramidetrihexoside (B) Ceramidetrihexoside galactosidase | 42, 46, 95, 156, 197, 198, 203, 222, 286, 336, 339, 350 |
| Farber's disease | L | Joint swelling; hoarse cry; subcutaneous tissue involvement; progressive neurologic disease | (A) Free ceramide (B) Ceramidase | 95, 222, 339 |
| Fucosidosis | C | Severe progressive cerebral degeneration; intense spasticity; thick skin and excessive sweating; increased salinity of sweat | (A) Fucose containing heteropolysaccharide (B) $\alpha$-Fucosidase | 89, 175, 358, 376 |

**Table 34.2**  Prenatal diagnosis of fetal biochemical disorders by amniocentesis (*cont.*)

| Disorder | Nature[a] | Clinical manifestation | Product (A) in excess or (B) in Deficiency | Reference |
|---|---|---|---|---|
| Galactosemia | C | Cirrhosis, cataracts, mental retardation, and failure to thrive | (A) Galactose<br>(B) Galactose-1-phosphate uridyl transferase | 23, 108, 138, 141, 170, 229, 292 |
| Gaucher's disease | L | Infantile and adult forms; hepatosplenomegaly, erosion of long bones, neurologic involvement, anemia, and thrombocytopenia | (A) Glucocerebroside<br>(B) Glucocerebrosidase | 24, 41, 43–45, 133, 135, 336 |
| $G_{M1}$ gangliosidosis (generalized gangliosidosis, Type I) | L | Mental retardation from birth; unusual facies; hepatosplenomegaly and skeletal changes | (A) $G_{M1}$ ganglioside and ceramide tetrahexoside; visceral mucopolysaccharide of keratin sulfate type and asialomucopolysaccharide<br>(B) $\beta$-Galactosidase B and C | 248, 253, 255, 294, 326–329, 340, 342, 354 |
| $G_{M1}$ gangliosidosis (Juvenile, Type II) | L | Progressive neurologic deterioration after 1 year of age, with decerebrate rigidity seizures and death | (A) $G_{M2}$ ganglioside and its asialo derivative<br>(B) Hexosamidase A | 86, 95, 156, 252, 361, 372 |
| $G_{M2}$ gangliosidosis (Tay–Sachs disease, Type I) | L | Onset at age of 5 to 6 months; degenerative neurologic disorder with cherry-red spot within macula progressing from normal to apathy, hypotonia, profound psychomotor retardation, and death | (A) $G_{M2}$ ganglioside and its asialo derivative<br>(B) Hexosaminidase A | 90, 162, 227, 250–252, 256, 257, 278, 296, 297, 298, 304, 305, 307, 318, 331, 340, 342, 345, 346 |
| $G_{M2}$ gangliosidosis (Sandhoff's disease, Type II) | L | Same as in Tay–Sachs disease | (A) $G_{M2}$ ganglioside and its asialo derivative and visceral globoside<br>(B) Hexosamidase A and B | 283, 297, 347 |
| $G_{M2}$ gangliosidosis (Juvenile, Type III) | L | Progressive neurologic deterioration, with onset 2 to 6 years, ending in decerebrate rigidity, blindness, and death | (A) $G_{M2}$ ganglioside<br>(B) Partial deficiency of hexosaminidase A | 22, 258, 261, 304, 343, 348, 374 |
| Glucose-6-$PO_4$ dehydrogenase deficiency | L | Hemolytic anemia | (B) G-6-$PO_4$ dehydrogenase | 82 |
| Glycogen storage disease (Type II) | C | Failure to thrive; hypotonia; hepatomegaly; cardiomegaly | (A) Glycogen storage<br>(B) $\alpha$-1,4-Glucosidase | 65, 72, 144, 145, 236, 245, 295, 324 |
| Glycogen storage disease (Type III) | C | Hepatomegaly; cardiomegaly; hypoglycemia | (A) Abnormally structured glycogen<br>(B) Amylo-1,6-glucosidase | 52, 56, 96, 99 |
| Glycogen storage disease (Type IV) | C | Familial cirrhosis with splenomegaly | (A) Abnormally structured glycogen<br>(B) Branching enzyme | 7, 140, 148, 325 |

**Table 34.2**  Prenatal diagnosis of fetal biochemical disorders by amniocentesis (*cont.*)

| Disorder | Nature[a] | Clinical manifestation | Product (A) in excess or (B) in Deficiency | Reference |
|---|---|---|---|---|
| Homocystinuria | A | Dislocated lenses; skeletal abnormalities; vascular thrombosis; mental retardation | (A) Methionine and homocystine<br>(B) Cystathionine synthase | 14, 97, 106, 163, 223, 267, 356 |
| Hunter's syndrome | M | Gargoylelike facies less obvious and seen later than in Hurler's syndrome; clear cornea; psychomotor retardation; increased linear growth in first year, will decline later; hepatosplenomegaly; joint stiffness; excessive dermatan sulfate and heparitin sulfate in urine | (A) Dermatan sulfate and heparitin sulfate | 102, 103, 202, 205, 336 |
| Hurler's syndrome | M | Gargoylelike facies; early clouding of cornea; early psychomotor retardation; increased linear growth in first year, then decline to become dwarfed; hepatosplenomegaly; kyphosis; joint stiffness; excessive dermatan sulfate and heparitin sulfate in urine | (A) As in Hunter's syndrome<br>(B) $\alpha$-L-Iduronidase | 18, 20, 48, 53, 75, 79, 80, 87, 98, 103, 134, 193, 199, 202, 204, 205, 215, 241, 262, 336, 359, 360, 370 |
| Hyperammonemia (Type II) | A | Ammonia intoxication; mental retardation | (A) Ammonia, glutamine<br>(B) Ornithine carbamyltransferase | 182, 234, 291 |
| Hyperlysinemia | A | Mental retardation; muscular asthenia (may be normal) | (A) Lysine<br>(B) Lysine–ketoglutarate reductase | 70, 183 |
| Hypervalinemia | A | Mental retardation; failure to thrive | (A) Valine<br>(B) Valine transaminase | 67, 73, 351, 362 |
| Isolencine catabolism disorder | A | Metabolic acidosis with coma precipitated by infection | (B) Defective isolencine oxidation | 81 |
| I cell disease | V | Gargoylelike facies; dwarfism from birth; gingival hyperplasia; psychomotor retardation | (A) Acid mucopolysaccharide and glycolipids<br>(B) Reduced $\beta$-glucuronidase and excessive acid phosphatase | 85, 101, 127, 176, 177, 179, 180, 184, 369 |
| Ketotic hyperglycinemia | A | Ketoacidosis; protein intolerance; developmental retardation | (A) Glycine, proprionic acid<br>(B) Proprionyl CoA carboxylase | 59, 143, 336 |
| Krabbe's disease (globoid cell leukodystrophy) | L | Progressive neurologic deterioration with death before 1 year of age | (A) Ceramide galactoside<br>(B) Galactocerebroside $\beta$-galactosidase | 8, 9, 12, 33, 125, 164, 341, 344, 349 |
| Lactosyl ceramidosis | L | Spasticity, cerebellar ataxia; hepatosplenomegali | (A) Lactosyl ceramide<br>(B) Lactosyl ceramidase | 83, 84, 88 |

**Table 34.2** Prenatal diagnosis of fetal biochemical disorders by amniocentesis (*cont.*)

| Disorder | Nature[a] | Clinical manifestation | Product (A) in excess or (B) in Deficiency | Reference |
|---|---|---|---|---|
| Lesch–Nyhan syndrome | V | Self-mutilation; choreoathetosis; spasticity; mental retardation | (A) Uric acid<br>(B) Hypoxanthine–guanine phosphoribosyltransferase | 21, 68 |
| Lysosomal acid phosphatase deficiency | V | Failure to thrive; progressive neuromuscular involvement; hypoglycemia; seizures and hepatomegaly | (B) Lysosomal acid phosphatase | 228, 230, 233 |
| Mannosidosis | C | Gargoylelike facies; psychomotor retardation; accelerated growth in infancy; hypotonia; mild hepatosplenomegaly | (A) Mannose and glucosamine containing heteropolysaccharide<br>(B) α-Mannosidase | 159, 254 |
| Maple syrup urine disease, severe infantile or intermittent | A | Ketoacidosis; neurologic abnormality; mental retardation; if severe, early death | (A) Valine, leucine, isoleucine, alloisoleucine<br>(B) Branched-chain keto-acid decarboxylase | 69, 71, 74, 115, 116, 118, 174, 209, 218, 313, 317, 333, 365, 366 |
| Marfan's syndrome | L | Connective tissue disorder, with skeletal, cardiovascular, and ocular signs | (A) Hyaluronic acid in cultured fibroblasts | 201 |
| Maroteaux–Lamy syndrome | L | Severe skeletal changes; cloudy corneas; normal intellect; excessive dermatan sulfate in urine | (A) Dermatan sulfate and heparin sulfate | 15, 205 |
| Metachromatic leukodystrophy | L | At least two forms; degenerative neurologic disease progressing from normal to weakness, ataxia, hypotonia, mental retardation, and paralysis; and excessive sulfatide in urine | (A) Sulfatide<br>(B) Arylsulfatase A (sulfatidase) | 10, 11, 17, 40, 120, 124, 132, 150, 152, 178, 207, 225, 226, 265, 266, 273, 274, 275, 276, 303, 338, 371 |
| Methylmalonicaciduria | A | Acidosis; lethargy; failure to thrive; early death | (A) Methylmalonic acid, glycine, homocystine, and cystathionine<br>(B) Methylmalonyl CoA isomerase or vitamin $B_{12}$ coenzyme (decreased carbon dioxide production from propionate) | 142, 189, 194, 195, 220, 221, 223, 247, 289, 290, 334, 337 |
| Morquio's syndrome | M | Severe skeletal changes, with dwarfism; cloudy corneas; aortic regurgitation; intellect usually within normal range; excessive keratan sulfate in urine | (B) Metachromasia | 205, 336 |
| Niemann–Pick disease | L | Four types; hepatosplenomegaly and variable skeletal and neurologic involvement | (A) Sphingomyelin<br>(B) Sphingomyelinase | 41, 43, 66, 93, 137, 306, 330, 355 |

717

**Table 34.2**  Prenatal diagnosis of fetal biochemical disorders by amniocentesis (*cont.*)

| Disorder | Nature[a] | Clinical manifestation | Product (A) in excess or (B) in Deficiency | Reference |
|---|---|---|---|---|
| Ornithine-α-ketoacid transaminase deficiency | A | Liver disease; renal tubular defect; mental retardation | (A) Ornithine<br>(B) Ornithine-α-ketoacid transaminase | 323 |
| Orotic aciduria | V | Infantile megaloblastic anemia; orotic acid in urine | (B) Orotidylic pyrophosphorylase and decarboxylase | 19, 126, 139, 168, 284, 332 |
| Phosphohexose isomerase deficiency | C | Hemolytic anemia | (B) Phosphohexose isomerase | 16, 167, 260, 308 |
| Pyruvate decarboxylase deficiency | C | Intermittent cerebellar ataxia and choreoathetosis, with elevated urinary alanine | (A) Pyruvic acid, alanine and lactate<br>(B) Pyruvate decarboxylase | 34, 35, 191 |
| Refsum's disease | L | Cerebellar ataxia; peripheral polyneuropathy; retinitis pigmentosa; and other cardiac, skin, neurologic, and skeletal changes | (A) Phytanic acid<br>(B) Phytanic acid α-hydroxylase | 130, 131, 153, 287 |
| Sanfilippo syndrome | M | Severe mental retardation; joint stiffness; excessive heparitin sulfate in urine | (A) Dermatan sulfate and heparan sulfate<br>(B) Sanfilippo type A = heparan sulfatase, type B = N-acetyl-α-D-glucosamidase | 102, 165, 202, 205, 242, 249 |
| Scheie's syndrome | M | Coarse facies; stiff joints; usually normal intellect; aortic regurgitation; excessive dermatan sulfate in urine | (A) Dermatan sulfate and heparan sulfate<br>(B) α-L-Iduronidase | 154, 199, 205 |
| Wolman's disease | L | Failure to thrive; steatorrea; hepatosplenomegaly; calcified adrenals; early death | (A) Triglycerides and cholesterol esters<br>(B) Acid lipase | 1, 172, 173, 263, 373, 375 |
| Xeroderma pigmentosum | V | Photosensitive dermatitis and skin cancers | (B) DNA "repair enzyme" | 60, 61, 224, 279, 280 |

[a] Nature of biochemical disorders: A, Amino acid related; C, Carbohydrate metabolism; L, Lipid metabolism; M, Mucopolysaccharide metabolism; V, Various.

# Predelivery Amniocentesis

Amniocentesis performed in the second half of high-risk pregnancies is aimed at obtaining information on the well-being of the fetus in order to determine if the pregnancy should be continued until the proper time arrives for delivery. The composition of the amniotic fluid increasingly reflects the contribution by maturing fetal organs[166] as gestation advances. The presence and concentration of various chemical constituents have been reported extensively.

Most clinical laboratories are able to provide useful information regarding the following questions: (1) the degree of involvement in erythroblastosis fetalis, (2) estimation of fetal maturity, and (3) estimation of fetal lung maturity.

## Erythroblastosis Fetalis

In 1952, Bevis[25] first described the pigmentation of amniotic fluid in isoimmunized pregnancies. This was followed by reports by Walker,[363] Liley,[185] and Freda.[104] Spectrophotometric measurements to assess the degree of disease in the fetuses of sensitized Rh-negative women became routine procedures in most laboratories.

The maternal antibodies return to the fetus through placental transfer and destroy the fetal erythrocytes that contain the antigen. Fetal involvement may range from minimal to very severe, when the infant may die *in utero* suffering from severe anemia resulting in heart failure. Pending on the severity of involvement and on the gestational age, the management ranges from allowing the pregnancy to continue to full-term and spontaneous labor to elective delivery before term or intrauterine transfusion for the replacement of destroyed erythrocytes.

The degree of involvement may be monitored either by chemical determination of the bilirubin concentration or by spectrophotometric analysis. The chemical methods for bilirubin determination are quite specific. Because of the low bilirubin concentration in amniotic fluid, the sensitivity, precision, and accuracy of the selected method is extremely important.[157]

The more commonly used spectrophotometric method is illustrated in Figure 34.3. Other authors also recommend the difference of optical density readings at two wavelengths.[6,38,57,161,217] Bilirubin concentration decreases with advancing gestation. Liley's three-zone chart (Figure 34.4) illustrates those changes.

Deviations in amniotic fluid protein values in erythroblastosis were reported by Cherry and Rosenfield.[58] They attempted to eliminate the effect of amniotic fluid volume changes on the bilirubin content by introducing the ratio of $\Delta$ OD to total protein in grams per deciliter. This ratio is independent of gestational age.

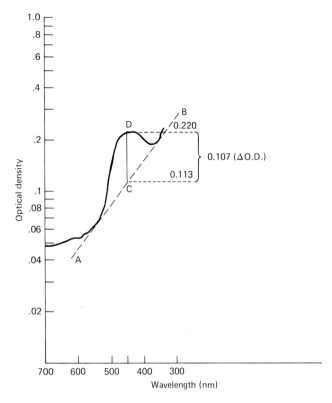

**34.3** $\Delta$O.D. as determined by Liley's method. Note that the ordinate has a logarithmic scale. Tangent (AB) to the spectral absorption curve of the amniotic fluid represents the expected linear curve in the absence of bilirubin pigments. Line DC represents the curve's deviation from linearity at 450 m$\mu$ caused by the bilirubin pigments in the amniotic fluid. Measurement of DC on the ordinate yields the "pigment peak" or $\Delta$O.D.

[Reprinted by permission from F. H. Allen and I. Umansky, Erythroblastosis fetalis, in Reid, D. E., Ryan, K. J., and Benirschke, K., eds.: *Principles and Management of Human Reproduction.* W. B. Saunders, 1972, p. 819.]

## Estimation of Fetal Maturity

There is considerable controversy regarding the value of estimating gestational age (which more or less should correspond with the status of fetal maturity) based on the presence or absence of, or on the concentration of, certain biochemical constituents in amniotic fluid. Sodium, chloride, glucose, urea nitrogen, creatinine, proteins, amino acids, lipids, uric acid, bilirubin, hormones, enzymes, pH and gases, osmolality, and several other features all provide some information about gestational age. However, with the exception of creatinine, in spite of the definite increas-

ing or decreasing trends, no conclusion can be based on a single determination or even on serial determinations. The ranges at any given gestational age are too great and overlapping.

Creatinine excretion by the fetal kidney is a function of glomerular filtration. In normal patients there is a constant rise of amniotic fluid creatinine as pregnancy advances. A concentration greater than 1.8 mg/dl reflects a fetus with the size of 37 weeks or older,[270] as shown in Figure 34.5. The criterion of 1.8 mg/dl creatinine at term or near term is necessary but not sufficient. Premature elevation of amniotic fluid creatinine may be the result of its decreased

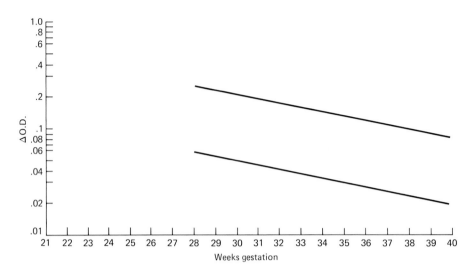

**34.4** Liley's three-zone chart for interpretation of amniotic fluid ΔO.D. A ΔO.D. in the bottom zone is consistent with an unaffected or very mildly affected fetus. A ΔO.D. in the middle zone means the fetus is probably moderately affected; the degree of disease varies with the height of the ΔO.D. in the middle zone. A ΔO.D. in the top zone indicates severe erythroblastosis.

[After F. H. Allen and I. Umansky, Erythroblastosis fetalis, *in* Reid, D. E., Ryan, K. J., and Benirschke, K., eds.: *Principles and Management of Human Reproduction.* W. B. Saunders, 1972, p. 820.]

clearance from the fetal compartment.[288] In diabetes mellitus and in toxemia such possibilities must be considered if amniotic fluid creatinine levels are employed for the estimation of fetal maturity.

## Estimation of Fetal Lung Maturity

When a high-risk pregnancy must be terminated because some complication threatens the life of the fetus or mother, in addition to fetal maturity the pulmonary maturity of the fetus may be questionable. This may occur in pregnancies where mothers have a history of repeated premature births or cervical incompetencies, diabetes, hypertension, familial patterns in the occurrence of hyaline membrane disease, and Rh incompatability.

It has been reported that pulmonary maturity may occur as early as the thirtieth or as late as the thirty-eighth to fortieth week of gestation.

Respiratory distress syndrome (RDS) is caused by a deficiency of some surface tension lowering substances, "surfactants".[13] Phosphatidylcholine (lecithin) has been identified[160] as a major lipid of the "surfactant," a lipoprotein the surface activity of which imparts stability to the normal pulmonary alveolus.

The role, identification, and formation of the surfactants were investigated during a 20-year span.[3,30,111-114,121,122,239,264,301] The first applicable test presented by Gluck and co-workers in 1970[110] became a cornerstone.

### Lecithin: sphingomyelin ratio

It is assumed, with reasonable certainty, that lecithin is the major pulmonary surfactant. Observing that a relatively constant amount of sphingomyelin is present in the amniotic fluid until the last 2 weeks of pregnancy, Gluck quantitated lecithin and sphingomyelin by thin-layer chromatography and expressed the results as lecithin: sphingomyelin (L:S) ratios. If the densitometric ratio is less than 1.5, there is insufficient amount of surfactant present; if the ratio is over 2, the lung is considered matured and ready for extrauterine life. A test for the estimation of pulmonary maturity was long overdue. Thousands of newborns die of RDS every year.

Although it takes many years to collect sufficient patient material to document and verify a test for a rare disease, within 2 years scores of publications have improved, modified, and simplified Gluck's test for L:S

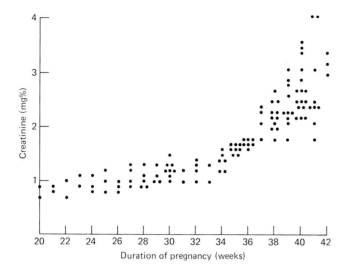

**34.5** Relationship between amniotic fluid creatinine concentration and duration of pregnancy.

[Reprinted by permission from R. M. Pitkin and S. J. Zwirek, Amniotic fluid creatinine, *Am. J. Obstet. Gynecol.* 98:1135, 1967.]

ratio. Moreover, serveral other tests have been published that also indicate the presence and quantity of "surfactants" in amniotic fluid, providing useful prognosis if the fetus needs to be delivered at that time.[32,35,63,64,100,110,128,136,154,171,190,300,319,335]

Blumenfeld[37] reviewed in detail and compared 19 methods or modifications for L:S ratio determinations. His list is only partial and it is continuously expanding. Regardless of the procedures and investigators, there is a general agreement on the usefulness of this procedure as it is shown by Ekelund, Arvidson, and Astedt,[91] who have compiled 975 cases reported from 10 different sources (Table 34.3).

The procedures for L:S ratios are performed by some or all of the following steps.

EXTRACTION OF THE LIPIDS AND CENTRIFUGATION. Most extractions are performed with methanol and chloroform mixtures. Centrifugation time varies from 2 to 10 min and speed from 2,000 to 10,000 rpm (100 to 10,000 $g$).[158,319] Filtering may remove lecithin from the extract.[240] Some methods recommend acetone precipitation of the lecithin before thin-layer chromatography; others omit this step.

THIN-LAYER CHROMATOGRAPHY. Plates employed by the different methods may be homemade or commercial,

**Table 34.3** The validity of L/S ratios[a,b]

| Authors[c] | Number of cases | Lecithin: sphingomyelin | Number of RDS |
|---|---|---|---|
| Whitfield et al. | 10 | Less than 1.5 | 8 |
| (1972) | 16 | 1.5–2 | 4 |
| | 102 | More than 2 | 0 |
| Hobbins et al. | 8 | 1 | 2 |
| (1972) | 41 | More than 1 | 0 |
| Spellacy and Buhl | 18 | Less than 2 | 6 |
| (1972) | 17 | 2.20–4.42 Mean 2.75 | 0 |
| Bryson et al. | 6 | 1.8 or less | 6 |
| (1972) | 161 | 1.66 or more | 0 |
| Sarkozi et al. | 3 | Less than 1.5 | 3 |
| (1972) | 117 | Mean 3.1 Range 1.8–8.6 | 0 |
| Gerbie et al. | 2 | Less than 1.5 | 2 |
| (1972) | 7 | 1.5–1.75 | 0 |
| | 3 | 1.75–2 | 0 |
| | 73 | More than 2 | 0 |
| Lemons and Jaffe | 6 | Less than 2 | 6 |
| (1972) | 87 | More than 2 | 4[d] |
| Harding et al. | 20 | Less than 2 | 6 |
| (1973) | 100 | More than 2 | 0 |
| Nakamura et al. | 47 | Less than 1.5 | 2 |
| (1972) | 43 | More than 1.5 | 0 |
| Schulman et al. | 10 | Less than 1 | 2 |
| (1972) | 5 | More than 1.5 | 0 |
| | 73 | Less than 1.5 | 0 |

[a] From Ekelund, L., Arvidson, G., and Astedt, B., *J. Obstet. Gynaecol. Br. Commonw.* 80:912, 1973.

[b] Reports on the lecithin:sphingomyelin ratio of amniotic fluid as an aid in predicting RDS. The method of Gluck et al.[110] was used by all the authors with the exception of Sarkozi et al.,[300] who omitted acetone precipitation, and Harding et al.,[128] who quantitated the phospholipids by phosphorus determination.

[c] For complete references see article by Ekelund et al. cited in footnote a.

[d] Two mothers had an intrauterine fetal blood transfusion, and two had diabetes mellitus.

silica gel-impregnated glass fiber, glass, plastic, or aluminum-backed silica gel sheets. Developing solvent mixtures may include chloroform:methanol:water, chloroform:methanol:ammonia:water, chloroform:methanol:acetic acid:water, dichloromethane:ethanol:water, and chloroform:ether:water.

DETECTION, VISUALIZATION, AND QUANTITATION. Detection of lipids is possible by ultraviolet light or they may be visualized by heat charring (sulfuric acid, ammonium persulfate) or color reactions (copper acetate, phosphomolybdic acid, bromthymol blue, bismuth nitrate, Rhodamine B dye, ammonium molybdate, molybdenium blue, iodine).

Quantitation of spots may be performed by visual observation, by measuring the surface area of the spots, or by densitometry. Densitometric quantitation appears to be the most reproducible. Chromatograms of two amniotic fluid phospholipids and recordings of their densitometry are shown in Figure 34.6.

One must emphasize that there are two "different" quantitative L:S ratios. Most reports express the L:S as the ratio of the sizes of the spots or as the ratio of the densities (or ratio of integrator trace units). Several reports present weight ratios of lecithin and sphingomyelin. As is shown in Figure 34.7, depending on the method of visualization, in some cases the ratio of the densities of the two spots is less than half the weight ratio. Therefore, some methods may report 4:1 as a ratio, indicating pulmonary maturity of the fetus.

### Other than L:S methods

Before and since the introduction of L:S ratio, several other investigators have suggested tests for the estimation of fetal lung maturity. Biezenski[30] expressed total lecithin as a percentage of the total phospholipids. Nelson[240] observed that if the total phospholipid phosphorus was more than 0.140 mg/dl there was little or no risk of respiratory distress syndrome (RDS). Bhagwanani, Fahmy, and Turnbull[26,27] measured amniotic fluid lecithin as phosphorus, establishing 3.5 mg/dl as an indication of pulmonary maturity. Clements et al.[62] introduced the foam stability or "shake test." Lecithin fatty acids were investigated by Ekelund, Arvidson, and Astedt[91]; lecithin palmitic acid was quantitated by Russell, Miller, and McLain[293]; total palmitic acid was quantitated by Warren, Holton, and Allen[364] and Thom et al.[353]; the palmitic: stearic ratio was determined by Alcindor et al.[4]; and Pfleger and Thomas[269] indicated the role of phosphatidylglycol.

Although the search goes on for more specific tests, one of the least specific but most practical of the above listed tests, the foam stability test, has become widely employed. It is based on the ability of the pulmonary surfactant

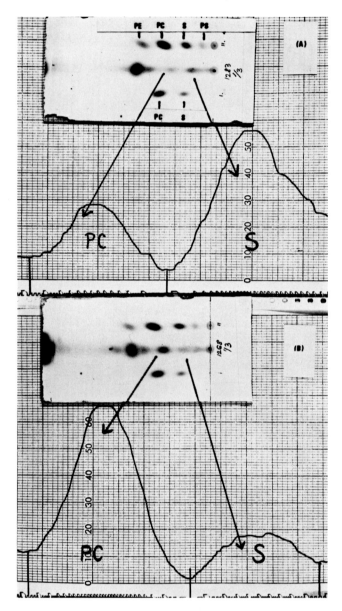

**34.6** Chromatograms of amniotic fluid phospholipids indicating (A) biochemically immature and (B) mature lung. Fluid extracts were applied in the center rows; standard mixtures of phosphatidylserine (PS), sphingomyelin (S), phosphatidylcholine (lecithin) (PC), and phosphatidylethanolamine (PE) on one side; and S and PC on the other side.

[Reprinted by permission from L. Sarkozi, H. N. Kovacs, H. S. Fox, and T. Kerenyi, Modified methods for estimating the phosphatidylcholine:sphingomyelin ratio in amniotic fluid, and its use in the assessment of fetal lung maturity, *Clin. Chem.* 18:956, 1972.]

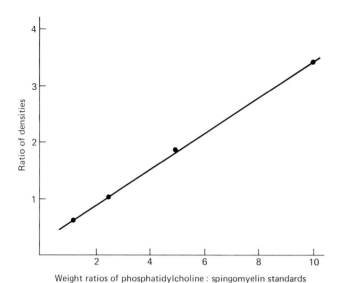

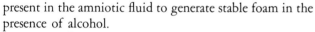

Weight ratios of phosphatidylcholine : spingomyelin standards

**34.7** Weight ratios of lecithin:sphingomyelin versus the ratios of their densities measured as integrator trace units.

[Reprinted by permission from L. Sarkozi, H. N. Kovacs, H. S. Fox, and T. Kerenyi, Modified methods for estimating the phosphatidylcholine:sphingomyelin ratio in amniotic fluid, and its use in the assessment of fetal lung maturity, *Clin. Chem. 18*:956, 1972.]

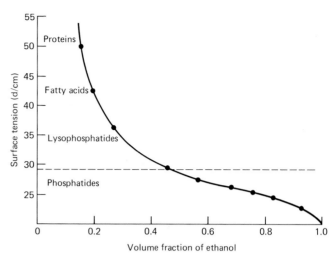

**34.8** Relation of surface tension of ethanol–water mixtures to volume fraction of ethanol at 25°C.

[After Guggenheim[123]. Reprinted by permission from J. A. Clements, A. C. G. Platzker, D. F. Tierney, *et al.*, Assessment of the risk of the respiratory-distress syndrome by a rapid test for surfactant in amniotic fluid, *N. Engl. J. Med. 286*:1077, 1972.]

present in the amniotic fluid to generate stable foam in the presence of alcohol.

Other substances present in amniotic fluid, such as proteins, bile salts, and salts of free fatty acids, can also form a stable foam, but these are eliminated from the surface films by the nonfoaming competitive surfactant ethanol. Guggenheim[123] presented data shown in Figure 34.8 on the relation of surface tension to composition of ethanol–water mixtures. At a surface tension of 29 dyne/cm, which corresponds to a volume fraction of 47.5% ethanol, only double-chain phospholipids compete for the surface film. Clements et al.[62] found that foam formed with unsaturated species breaks down in a few seconds and only foam formed by saturated phosphatidylcholine, the kind that is present in pulmonary surfactant, can be observed for several hours at room temperature.

For a semiquantitative test, 95% ethanol and amniotic fluid diluted with saline at the ratios as 1:1, 1:1.3, 1:2, 1:4, and 1:5 are prepared and shaken for 15 sec; then they

are placed vertically in a rack. After 15 min, the air–fluid interface of each tube is examined. A tube is considered positive if it has a complete ring of bubbles at the meniscus. A clearly negative test—no complete ring of bubbles at the meniscus after 15 minutes at a 1:1 fluid:saline dilution—indicates insufficient surfactant present and is associated with a high risk of RDS. A clearly positive test—complete ring of bubbles at the meniscus after 15 min at 1:2 dilution—was associated with low risk of RDS. Samples negative at 1:1 but positive at 1:1.3 are considered intermediate results and a substantial probability of the infant's experiencing some respiratory difficulty exists.

Although this test is very simple and fast, extreme care with the technique and purity of glassware and reagents are critical. Several investigators compared this test with other tests for the estimation of pulmonary maturity and conducted clinical evaluations. Our experience shows that a positive bubble stability test is a very convincing indication of pulmonary maturity of the fetus, but some intermediate results have appeared to be positive based on L:S ratios.

**Table 34.4**  Selected patients with low and transitional L:S ratios and some other factors possibly affecting the continuation of pulmonary maturation after delivery

| Patient number | Densitometric L:S | 16:0 (rel%) | 18:0 (rel%) | Gestational age (weeks) | Weight (g) | Fetal blood pH | RDS |
|---|---|---|---|---|---|---|---|
| 183 | 1.3 | 38 | 16 | 28 | 980 | 7.33 | No |
| 118 | 1.9 | 62 | 17.6 | 32 | 1,200 | 7.17 | Yes |
| 123 | 0.9 | 58 | 11.5 | 24 | 1,070 | 7.04 | Yes |
| 125 | 1.8 | 53 | 18.2 | 26 | 1,245 | 7.16 | Yes |
| 30 | 2.0 | 68 | 8.7 | 26 | 790 | 7.22 | No |
| 77 | 1.2 | 65 | 7.5 | 25 | 880 | 7.27 | No |

However, intermediate or transitional range of any method may or may not result in respiratory difficulties, depending on other factors affecting the continuing production of pulmonary surfactant, as shown on Table 34.4. Predelivery amniotic fluid samples of these six premature newborns were analyzed. One patient with amniotic fluid L:S ratio of 1.3 but fetal blood pH of 7.33 did not develop RDS, in spite of the estimated gestational age of 28 weeks and a birth weight of 980 g. Fetal blood pH of less than 7.20, combined with low or transitional L:S ratios, resulted in RDS. Two newborns with L:S ratios of 1.2 and 2.0, but fetal pH above 7.20, amniotic fluid lecithin palmitic acid over 64 relative percent, and stearic acid less than 9 relative percent did not develop RDS. The role of acidosis in the development of RDS was confirmed, but the role of most "associated insults" is not known. Considerable overlap of values is possible.

Strict adherence to published and well-documented procedures is imperative. The slightest change in reagents, materials, temperature, and technique requires extensive clinical evaluation.

# REFERENCES

1. Abramov, A., Schore, S., and Wolman, M. Generalized xanthomatosis with calcified adrenals. *Am. J. Dis. Child.* 91:282, 1956.
2. Aburel, M. D. Le declenchement du travail par injections intraamniotique de serum sale hypertonique. *Gynecol. Obstet.* 36:398, 1937.
3. Adams, F. H., Fujiwara, T., Emmanouilides, G. C., and Raiha, N. Lung phospholipids of human fetuses and infants with and without hyaline membrane disease. *J. Pediatr.* 77:833, 1970.
4. Alcindor, L. G., Bereziat, G., Vielh, J. P., and Gautray, J. P. Le rapport de concentration acide palmitique sur acide stearique, indicateur de la maturite pulmonaire foetale. *Clin. Chim. Acta* 50:31, 1974.
5. Allan, J. D., Cusworth, D. C., Dent, C. E., and Wilson, V. K. A disease, probably hereditary, characterized by severe mental deficiency and a constant gross abnormality of amino acid metabolism. *Lancet* i:182, 1958.
6. Alvey, J. P. Obstetrical management of Rh incompatibility based on liquor amnii studies. *Am. J. Obstet. Gynecol.* 90:769, 1964.
7. Andersen, D. H. Studies on glycogen disease with a report of a case in which the glycogen was abnormal, *in* Najjar, V. A., ed.: *Symposium on the Clinical and Biochemical Aspects of Carbohydrate Utilization in Health and Disease.* Baltimore, Johns Hopkins Press, 1952, p. 28.
8. Austin, J. Studies in globoid (Krabbe) leukodystrophy. I. The significance of lipid abnormalities in white matter in 8 globoid and 13 control patients. *Arch. Neurol.* 9:207, 1963.
9. Austin, J. Mental retardation: Globoid (Krabbe) leukodystrophy, *in* Carter, C. H., ed.: *Medical Aspects of Mental Retardation.* Springfield, Ill., Charles C Thomas, 1965, p. 813.
10. Austin, J., Armstrong, D., and Shearer, L. Metachromatic form of diffuse cerebral sclerosis. V. The nature and significance of low sulfatase activity: a controlled study of brain, liver and kidney in four patients with metachromatic leukodystrophy (MLD). *Arch. Neurol.* 13:593, 1965.
11. Austin, J., Armstrong, D., Shearer, L., and McAfee, D. Metachromatic form of diffuse cerebral sclerosis. VI. A rapid test for sulfatase A deficiency in metachromatic leukodystrophy urine. *Arch. Neurol.* 14:259, 1966.
12. Austin, J., Suzuki, K., Armstrong, D., Brady, R., Bachhawat, B. K., Schlenker, J., and Stumpf, D. Studies in globoid (Krabbe) leukodystrophy (GLD). *Arch. Neurol.* 23:502, 1970.
13. Avery, M. E., and Mead, J. Surface properties in relation to atelectasis and hyaline membrane disease. *Am. J. Dis. Child.* 97:517, 1959.
14. Barber, G. W., and Speath, G. L. Pyridoxine therapy in homocystinuria. *Lancet* i:337, 1967.
15. Barton, R. W., and Neufeld, E. F. A distinct biochemical deficit in the Maroteaux-Lamy syndrome (mucopolysaccharidosis VI). *J. Pediatr.* 80:114, 1972.
16. Baughan, M. A., Valentine, W. N., Paglia, D. E., Ways, P. O.,

Simons, E. R., and DeMarsh, A. B. Hereditary hemolytic anemia associated with glucose-phosphate isomerase (GPI) deficiency—a new enzyme defect of human erythrocytes. *Blood 32*:236, 1968.

17. Baum, H., Dodgson, K. S., and Spencer, B. The assay of arylsulfatases A and B in human urine. *Clin. Chim. Acta 4*:453, 1959.

18. Bearn, A. G., ed. Symposium on the mucopolysaccharidoses. *Am. J. Med. 47*:661, 1969.

19. Becroft, D. M. O., and Phillips, L. I. Hereditary orotic aciduria and megaloblastic anaemia: A second case, with response to uridine. *Br. Med. J. 1*:547, 1965.

20. Benson, P. F., Bowser-Riley, F., and Giannelli, F. β-galactosidases in fibroblasts: Hurler and Sanfilippo syndromes. *N. Engl. J. Med. 283*:999, 1970.

21. Berman, P. H. A method for the prenatal diagnosis of congenital hyperuricemia. *J. Pediatr. 75*:488, 1969.

22. Bernheimer, H., and Scitelberger, F. Uber das verhalten der ganglioside im gehirn bei 2 Fallern von spatinfantiler amaurotischer idiotie. *Wien. Klin. Wochenschr. 80*:163, 1968.

23. Beutler, E., Baluda, M. C., Sturgeon, P., and Day, R. A new genetic abnormality resulting in galactose-1-phosphate uridyltransferase deficiency. *Lancet i*:353, 1965.

24. Beutler, E., Kuhl, W., Trinidad, R., Teplitz, R., and Nadler, H. β-Glucosidase activity in fibroblasts from homozygotes and heterozygotes for Gaucher's disease. *Am. J. Hum. Genet. 23*:62, 1971.

25. Bevis, D. C. A. The antenatal prediction of haemolytic disease of the newborn. *Lancet i*:395, 1952.

26. Bhagwanani, S. G., Fahmy, D., and Turnbull, A. C. Prediction of neonatal respiratory distress by estimation of amniotic fluid lecithin. *Lancet i*:159, 1972.

27. Bhagwanani, S. G., Fahmy, D., and Turnbull, A. C. Quick determination of amniotic fluid lecithin concentration for prediction of neonatal respiratory distress. *Lancet ii*:66, 1972.

28. Bickel, H., Baur, H. S., Astley, R., Douglas, A. A., Finch, E., Harris, H., Harvey, C. C., Hickmans, E. M., Philpott, M. G., Smallwood, W. C., Smellie, J. M., and Teall, C. G. Cystine storage disease with amino aciduria and dwarfism (Lignac-Fanconi disease). *Acta Paediatr. (Suppl. 90) 42*:7, 1952.

29. Bieniarz, J. Diagnostic value of ultrasonography in obstetrics and amniotic fluid sampling, *in* Natelson, S., Scommegna, A., and Epstein, M. B., eds.: *Amniotic Fluid*. New York, John Wiley and Sons, 1974, pp. 205–212.

30. Biezenski, J. J. Origin of amniotic fluid lipids. III. Fatty acids. *Proc. Soc. Exper. Biol. Med. 142*:1326, 1973.

31. Biezenski, J. J., Pomerance, W., and Goodman, J. Studies on the origin of amniotic fluid lipids. I. Normal composition. *Am. J. Obstet. Gynecol. 102*:853, 1968.

32. Biggs, J. S. G., Gaffney, T. J., and McGeary, H. M. Evidence that fetal lung fluid and phospholipids pass into amniotic fluid in late human pregnancy. *J. Obstet. Gynecol. 80*:125, 1973.

33. Bischoff, A., and Ulrich, J. Peripheral neuropathy in globoid cell leukodystrophy (Krabbe's disease): Ultrastructural and histochemical findings. *Brain 92*:861, 1969.

34. Blass, J. P., Avigan, J., and Uhlendorf, B. W. A defect in pyruvate decarboxylase in a child with an intermittent movement disorder. *J. Clin. Invest. 49*:423, 1970.

35. Blass, J. P., Thibert, R. J., and Fraisey, T. F. Simple, rapid determination of lecithin and sphingomyelin in amniotic fluid. *Clin. Chem. 19*:1394, 1973.

36. Blume, R. S., Glade, P. R., Gralnick, H. R., Chessin, L. N., Haase, A. T., and Wolff, S. M. The Chediak-Higashi syndrome: Continuous suspension cultures derived from peripheral blood. *Blood 33*:821, 1969.

37. Blumenfeld, T. A. Clinical laboratory tests for fetal lung maturity, *in* Sommers, S. C., ed.: *Pathology Annual*. New York, Appleton-Century-Crofts, 1975, pp. 21–36.

38. Bonsnes, R. W. Model 202. Analysis of bilirubin content of amniotic fluid. *Instrum. News—The Perkin Elmer Corp. 16*:14, 1965.

39. Bonsnes, R. W. The chemistry and physiology of amniotic fluid, *in* Dorfman, A., ed.: *Antenatal Diagnosis*. Chicago, The University of Chicago Press, 1972, pp. 3–16.

40. Brady, R. O. Enzymatic defects in the sphingolipidoses. *Adv. Clin. Chem. 11*:1, 1968.

41. Brady, R. O. Genetics and the sphingolipidoses. *Med. Clin. North Am. 53*:827, 1969.

42. Brady, R. O., Gal, A. I., Bradley, R. M., Martensson, E., Warshaw, A. L., and Laster, L. Enzymatic defect in Fabry's disease: Ceramidetrihexosidase deficiency. *N. Engl. J. Med. 276*:1163, 1967.

43. Brady, R. O., Johnson, W. G., and Uhlendorf, B. W. Identification of heterozygous carriers by lipid storage diseases. *Am. J. Med. 51*:423, 1971.

44. Brady, R. O., Kanfer, J. N., Bradley, R. M., and Shapiro, D. Demonstration of a deficiency of glucocerebroside-cleaving enzyme in Gaucher's disease. *J. Clin. Invest. 45*:1112, 1966.

45. Brady, R. O., Kanfer, J. N., and Shapiro, D. Metabolism of glucocerebrosides. II. Evidence of an enzymatic deficiency in Gaucher's disease. *Biochem. Biophys. Res. Commun. 18*:221, 1965.

46. Brady, R. O., Uhlendorf, B. W., and Jacobson, C. B. Fabry's disease: Antenatal detection. *Science 172*:174, 1971.

47. Brock, D. J. H. Inborn errors of metabolism, *in* Brock, D. J. H., and Mayo, O., eds.: *The Biochemical Genetics of Man*. London, Academic Press, 1972, pp. 385–476.

48. Brock, D. J. H., Gordon, H., Seligman, S., and De H. Lobo, E. Antenatal detection of Hurler's syndrome. *Lancet ii*:1324, 1971.

49. Brock, D. J. H., and Sutcliffe, R. D. α-Fetoprotein in the antenatal diagnosis of anencephaly and spina bifida. *Lancet ii*:197, 1972.

50. Brown, A. K. Constituents of amniotic fluid: Reflections of normal and abnormal fetal maturation, *in* Adamson, K., ed.: *Diagnosis and Treatment of Fetal Disorders*. New York, Springer-Verlag, 1968, pp. 121–140.

51. Brubaker, R. F., Wong, V. G., Schulman, J. D., Seegmiller, J. E., and Kuwabara, T. Benign cystinosis. *Am. J. Med. 49*:546, 1970.

52. Brunberg, J. A., McCormick, W. F., and Schochet, S. S. Type III glycogenosis. *Arch. Neurol. 25*:171, 1971.

53. Cantz, M., Chambach, A., and Neufeld, E. F. Characterization of the factor deficient in the Hunter syndrome by polyacrylamide gel electrophoresis. *Biochem. Biophys. Res. Commun. 39*:936, 1970.

54. Cassidy, G. Amniocentesis, *in* Nesbitt, R. E. L., ed.: *Clinics in Perinatology*. Philadelphia, W. B. Saunders Co., 1974, Vol. 1:1, pp. 87–123.

55. Cathro, D. M., Bertrand, J., and Coyle, M. G. Antenatal diagnosis of adrenocortical hyperplasia. *Lancet i*:732, 1969.

56. Chayoth, R., Moses, S. W., and Steinitz, K. Debrancher enzyme activity in blood cells of families with type III glycogen

storage disease: A method for diagnosis of heterozygotes. *Isr. J. Med. Sci. 3*:433, 1967.

57. Cherry, S. H., Kochwa, S., and Rosenfield, R. E. Bilirubin–protein ratio in amniotic fluid as an index of the severity of erythroblastosis fetalis. *Obstet. Gynecol. 26*:826, 1965.

58. Cherry, S. H., and Rosenfield, R. E. Intrauterine fetal transfusions for the management of erythroblastosis. *Am. J. Obstet. Gynecol. 98*:275, 1967.

59. Childs, B., Nyhan, W. L., Borden, M., Bard, L., and Cooke, R. E. Idiopathic hyperglycinemia and hyperglycinuria: A new disorder of amino acid metabolism. *J. Pediatr. 27*:522, 1961.

60. Cleaver, J. E. Defective repair application of DNA in xeroderma pigmentosum. *Nature (London) 218*:652, 1968.

61. Cleaver, J. E. Xeroderma pigmentosum: A human disease in which an initial stage of DNA repair is defective. *Proc. Natl. Acad. Sci. USA 63*:428, 1969.

62. Clements, J. A., Platzker, A. C. G., Tierney, D. F., Hobel, C. T., Creasy, R. K., Margolis, A. J., Thibeault, D. W., Tooley, W. H., and Oh, W. Assessment of the risk of the respiratory-distress syndrome by a rapid test for surfactant in amniotic fluid. *N. Engl. J. Med. 286*:1077, 1972.

63. Coch, E., and Kessler, G. Rapid TLC separation and detection of lecithin and sphingomyelin in amniotic fluid. *Clin. Chem. 18*:490, 1972.

64. Coch, E., Kessler, G., and Meyer, J. S. Rapid thin-layer chromatographic method for assessing the lecithin/sphingomyelin ratio in amniotic fluid. *Clin. Chem. 20*:1368, 1974.

65. Cox, R. P., Douglas, G., Hutzler, J., Lynfield, J., and Dancis, J. In-utero detection of Pompe's disease. *Lancet i*:893, 1970.

66. Crocker, A. C. The cerebral defect in Tay-Sachs disease and Niemann-Pick disease. *J. Neurochem. 7*:69, 1961.

67. Dancis, J. The antepartum diagnosis of genetic diseases. *J. Pediatr. 72*:301, 1968.

68. Dancis, J., Cox, R. P., Berman, P. H., Jansen, V., and Balis, M. W. Cell population density and phenotypic expression of tissue culture fibroblasts from heterozygotes of Lesch-Nyhan's disease (inosinate pyrophosphorylase deficiency). *Biochem. Genet. 3*:609, 1969.

69. Dancis, J., Hutzler, J., and Cox, R. P. Enzyme defect in skin fibroblasts in intermittent branched-chain ketonuria and in maple syrup urine disease. *Biochem. Med. 2*:407, 1969.

70. Dancis, J., Hutzler, J., Cox, R. P., and Woody, N. C. Familial hyperlysinemia with lysine-ketoglutarate reductase deficiency. *J. Clin. Invest. 48*:1447, 1969.

71. Dancis, J., Hutzler, J., and Levitz, M. Detection of the heterozygote in maple sugar urine disease. *J. Pediatr. 66*:595, 1965.

72. Dancis, J., Hutzler, J., Lynfield, J., and Cox, R. P. Absence of acid maltase in glycogenosis type 2 (Pompe's disease) in tissue culture. *Am. J. Dis. Child. 117*:108, 1969.

73. Dancis, J., Hutzler, J., Tada, K., Wada, Y., Morikawa, T., and Arakawa, T. Hypervalinemia: A defect in valine transamination. *Pediatrics 39*:813, 1967.

74. Dancis, J., Jansen, V., Hutzler, J., and Levitz, M. The metabolism of leucine in tissue culture of skin fibroblasts of maple syrup urine disease. *Biochem. Biophys. Acta 77*:523, 1963.

75. Danes, B. S., and Bearn, A. G. Hurler's syndrome: A genetic study in cell culture. *J. Exp. Med. 123*:1, 1966.

76. Danes, B. S., and Bearn, A. G. Cell culture and the Chediak-Higashi syndrome. *Lancet ii*:65, 1967.

77. Danes, B. S., and Bearn, A. G. A genetic cell marker in cystic fibrosis of the pancreas. *Lancet i*:1061, 1968.

78. Danes, B. S., and Bearn, A. G. Cystic fibrosis of the pancreas: A study in cell culture. *J. Exp. Med. 129*:775, 1969.

79. Danes, B. S., and Bearn, A. G. Correction of cellular metachromasia in cultured fibroblasts in several inherited mucopolysaccharidoses. *Proc. Natl. Acad. Sci. USA 67*:357, 1970.

80. Danes, B. S., Queenan, J. T., Gadow, E. C., and Cederqvist, L. L. Antenatal diagnosis of mucopolysaccharidoses. *Lancet i*:946, 1970.

81. Daum, R. S., Mamer, O. A., Lamm, P. H., and Scriver, C. R. A "new" disorder of isoleucine catabolism. *Lancet ii*:1289, 1971.

82. Davidson, R. G., Nitowsky, H. M., and Childs, B. Demonstration of two populations of cells in the human female heterozygous for glucose-6-phosphate dehydrogenase variants. *Proc. Natl. Acad. Sci. USA 50*:481, 1963.

83. Dawson, G., and Stein, A. O. Lactosyl ceramidosis: Catabolic enzyme defect of glycosphingolipid metabolism. *Science 170*:556, 1970.

84. Dawson, G., and Stein, A. O. Lactosyl ceramidosis: Characterization of a new glycosphingolipidosis, *in* Bernsohn, J., ed.: *Lipid Storage Diseases: Enzymatic Defects and Clinical Implications.* New York, Academic Press, 1971, pp. 183–201.

85. DeMars, R., and Leroy, J. G. The remarkable cells cultured from a human with Hurler's syndrome, *in* Dawe, C. J., ed., *In Vitro, Phenotypic Expression.* Baltimore, Williams and Wilkins, 1966, Vol. 2, pp. 107–118.

86. Derry, D. M., Fawcett, J. S., Andermann, F., and Wolfe, L. S. Late infantile systemic lipidosis. Major monosialogangliosidosis. Delineation of two types. *Neurology 18*:340, 1968.

87. Di Ferrante, N., Donnelly, P. V., and Neri, G. Metabolism of glycosaminoglycans in cultured normal and abnormal human fibroblasts. *Biochem. Med. 5*:269, 1971.

88. Dorfman, A., ed. *Antenatal Diagnosis.* Chicago, University of Chicago Press, 1972.

89. Durand, P., Borrone, C., and Della Cella, G. Fucosidosis. *J. Pediatr. 75*:665, 1969.

90. Eeg-Olofsson, O., Kristensson, K., Sourander, P., and Svennerholm, L. Tay-Sachs disease: A generalized metabolic disorder. *Acta Paediatr. Scand. 55*:546, 1966.

91. Ekelund, L., Arvidson, G., and Astedt, B. Amniotic fluid lecithin and its fatty acid composition in respiratory distress syndrome. *J. Obstet. Gynaecol. Br. Commonw. 80*:912, 1973.

92. Emery, A. E. H. Biochemical analysis of amniotic fluid, *in* Emery, A. E. H., ed.: *Antenatal Diagnosis of Genetic Disease.* Baltimore, Williams and Wilkins Company, 1973, pp. 113–136.

93. Epstein, C. J., Brady, R. O., Schneider, R. M., Bradley, D., and Shapiro, D. In utero diagnosis of Niemann-Pick disease. *Am. J. Hum. Genet. 23*:533, 1971.

94. Fairweather, D. V. I. and Eskes, T. K. A. B., eds. *Amniotic Fluid, Research and Clinical Application.* Amsterdam, Excerpta Medica, 1973.

95. Farber, S., Cohen, J., and Uzman, L. L. Lipogranulomatosis: A new lipoglycoprotein "storage" disease. *J. Mt. Sinai Hosp. 24*:816, 1957.

96. Field, R. A. Glycogen deposition diseases, *in* Stanbury, J. B., Wyngaarden, J. B., and Fredrickson, D. S., eds.: *Metabolic Basis of Inherited Disease,* 2nd ed. New York, McGraw-Hill, 1970, pp. 141–177.

97. Finkelstein, J. D., Mudd, S. H., Irreverre, F., and Laster, L. Homocystinuria due to cystathionine synthetase deficiency: Mode of inheritance. *Science 146*:785, 1964.

98. Fluharty, A. L., Porter, M. T., Lassila, E. L., Trammell, J.,

Carrel, R. E., and Kihara, H. Acid glycosidases in mucopolysaccharidoses' fibroblasts. *Biochem. Med.* 4:110, 1970.

99. Forbes, G. B. Glycogen storage disease. *J. Pediatr.* 42:645, 1953.

100. Foreman, D. T., and Grayson, B. A. Lecithin-sphingomyelin ratio in amniotic fluid. Am. Assoc. Clin. Chem. Symp. Amniotic Fluid, Chicago, May 1973.

101. Forrester, J. S., and Swan, H. J. C. "I-Cell" disease: Leakage of lysosomal enzymes into extracellular fluids. *N. Engl. J. Med.* 285:1090, 1971.

102. Fratantoni, J. C., Hall, C. W., and Neufeld, E. F. The defect in Hurler and Hunter syndromes. II. Deficiency of specific factors involved in mucopolysaccharide degradation. *Proc. Natl. Acad. Sci. USA* 64:360, 1966.

103. Fratantoni, J. C., Neufeld, E. F., Uhlendorf, B. W., and Jacobson, C. B. Intrauterine diagnosis of the Hurler and Hunter syndromes. *N. Engl. J. Med.* 280:686, 1969.

104. Freda, V. The Rh problem in obstetrics and a new concept of its management using amniocentesis and spectrophotometric scanning of amniotic fluid. *Am. J. Obstet. Gynecol.* 92:3, 1965.

105. Fuchs, F. Volume of amniotic fluid at various stages of pregnancy. *Clin. Obstet. Gynecol.* 9:449, 1966.

106. Gerritsen, T., Vaughn, J. G., and Waisman, H. A. The identification of homocystine in the urine. *Biochem. Biophys. Res. Commun.* 9:493, 1962.

107. Gibbs, G. E., and Griffin, G. D. $\beta$-Glucuronidase activity in skin components of children with cystic fibrosis. *Science* 167:983, 1970.

108. Gitzelmann, R. Hereditary galactokinase deficiency, a newly recognized cause of juvenile cataracts. *Pediatr. Res.* 1:14, 1967.

109. Gluck, L., and Kulovich, M. V. Lecithin/sphingomyelin ratios in amniotic fluid in normal and abnormal pregnancy. *Am. J. Obstet. Gynecol.* 115:539, 1973.

110. Gluck, L., Kulovich, M. V., Borer, R. C., Brenner, P. H., Anderson, G. G., and Spellacy, W. N. Diagnosis of respiratory distress syndrome by amniocentesis. *Am. J. Obstet. Gynecol.* 109:440, 1971.

111. Gluck, L., Kulovich, M. V., Eidelman, A. I., Cordero, L., and Khazin, A. Biochemical development of surface activity in mammalian lung. IV. Pulmonary lecithin synthesis in the human fetus and newborn and the etiology of the respiratory distress syndrome. *Pediatr. Res.* 6:81, 1972.

112. Gluck, L., Landowne, R. A., and Kulovich, M. V. Biochemical development of surface activity in mammalian lung. III. Structural changes in lung lecithin during development of the rabbit fetus and newborn. *Pediatr. Res.* 4:352, 1970.

113. Gluck, L., Motoyama, E. K., Smits, H. L., and Kulovich, M. V. The biochemical development of surface activity in mammalian lung. *Pediatr. Res.* 1:237, 1967.

114. Gluck, L., Scibney, M., and Kulovich, M. V. The biochemical development of surface activity in mammalian lung. II. The biosynthesis of phospholipids in the lung of the developing rabbit fetus and newborn. *Pediatr. Res.* 1:247, 1967.

115. Goedde, H. W., and Keller, W. Metabolic pathways in maple syrup urine disease, in Nyhan, W. L., ed.: *Amino Acid Metabolism and Genetic Variation*. New York, McGraw-Hill Book Co., 1967, p. 191.

116. Goedde, H. W., Langebeck, U., and Brackertz, D. Detection of heterozygotes in maple syrup urine disease: role of lymphocyte count. *Humangenetik* 6:189, 1968.

117. Goldman, H., Scriver, C. R., Aaron, K., Delvin, E., and Canlas, Z. Adolescent cystinosis: Comparisons with infantile and adult forms. *Pediatrics* 47:979, 1971.

118. Goodman, S. I., Pollak, S., Miles, B., and O'Brien, D. The treatment of maple syrup urine disease. *Pediatrics* 75:485, 1969.

119. Gottesfeld, K. R., Thompson, H. E., Holmes, J. H., and Taylor, E. S. Ultrasonic placentography: A new method for placental localization. *Am. J. Obstet. Gynecol.* 96:538, 1970.

120. Greene, H. L., Hug, G., and Schubert, W. K. Metachromatic leukodystrophy. Treatment with arylsulfatase-A. *Arch. Neurol.* 20:147, 1969.

121. Gribetz, I., Frank, N. R., and Avery, M. E. Static volume-pressure relations of excised lungs of infants with hyaline membrane disease, newborn and stillborn infants. *J. Clin. Invest.* 38:2168, 1959.

122. Gruenwald, P., Johnson, R. P., Hustead, R. F., and Clements, J. A. Correlation of mechanical properties of infant lungs with surface activity of extracts. *Proc. Soc. Exp. Biol. Med.* 109:369, 1962.

123. Guggenheim, E. A. *Thermodynamics*. Amsterdam, North-Holland Publishing, 1959, p. 267.

124. Hackett, T. N. Jr., Hackett, R. J., Bray, P. F., and Madsen, J. A. Chemical detection of metachromatic leukodystrophy in disease and carrier states. *Am. J. Dis. Child.* 122:223, 1971.

125. Hagberg, B., Kollberg, H., Sourander, P., and Akesson, H. O. Infantile globoid cell leukodystrophy (Krabbe's disease): A clinical and genetic study of 32 Swedish cases, 1953–1967. *Neuropediatrie* 1:75, 1969.

126. Haggard, M. E., and Lockhart, L. H. Megaloblastic anemia and orotic aciduria. A hereditary disorder of pyrimidine metabolism responsive to uridine. *Am. J. Dis. Child.* 113:733, 1967.

127. Hanai, J., Leroy, J. G., and O'Brien, J. S. Ultrastructure of cultured fibroblasts in I-cell disease. *Am. J. Dis. Child.* 122:34, 1971.

128. Harding, P., Possmayer, F., Milne, K., Jaco, N. T., and Walters, J. H. Amniotic fluid phospholipids and fetal maturity. *Am. J. Obstet. Gynecol.* 115:298, 1973.

129. Harris, H., Penrose, L. S., and Thomas, D. H. H. Cystathioninuria. *Ann. Hum. Genet.* 23:442, 1959.

130. Herndon, J. H. Jr., Steinberg, D., and Uhlendorf, B. W. Refsum's disease: Defective oxidation of phytanic acid in tissue cultures derived from homozygotes and heterozygotes. *N. Engl. J. Med.* 281:1034, 1969.

131. Herndon, J. H. Jr., Steinberg, D., Uhlendorf, B. W., and Fales, H. M. Refsum's disease: Characterization of the enzyme defect in cell culture. *J. Clin. Invest.* 48:1017, 1969.

132. Hirose, G., and Bass, N. H. Metachromatic leukodystrophy in the adult. *Neurology* 22:313, 1972.

133. Ho, M. W., and O'Brien, J. S. Gaucher's disease: Deficiency of 'acid' $\beta$-glucosidase and reconstitution of enzyme activity in vitro. *Proc. Natl. Acad. Sci. USA* 68:2810, 1971.

134. Ho, M. W., and O'Brien, J. S. Hurler's syndrome: Deficiency of a specific $\beta$-galactosidase isoenzyme. *Science* 165:611, 1969.

135. Ho, M. W., Seck, J., Schmidt, D., Veath, M. L., Johnson, W., Brady, R. O., and O'Brien, J. S. Adult Gaucher's disease: Kindred studies and demonstration of a deficiency of acid $\beta$-glucosidase in cultured fibroblasts. *Am. J. Hum. Genet.* 24:37, 1972.

136. Hobbins, J. C., Brock, W., Speroff, L., Anderson, G. G., and Caldwell, B. L/S ratio in predicting pulmonary maturity in utero. *Obstet. Gynecol.* 39:660, 1972.

137. Holtz, A. I., Uhlendorf, B. W., and Fredrickson, D. S. Persistence of a lipid defect in tissue cultures derived from patients with Niemann–Pick disease. *Fed. Proc.* 23:129, 1964.

138. Holzel, A. Galactosemia, *in* Gardner, L. I., ed.: *Endocrine and Genetic Diseases of Childhood.* Philadelphia, W. B. Saunders, 1969, p. 823.

139. Howell, R. R. Acatalasia and orotic aciduria, *in* Dorfman, A., ed., *Antenatal Diagnosis.* Chicago, University of Chicago Press, 1972, pp. 145–149.

140. Howell, R. R., Kaback, M. M., and Brown, B. I. Type IV glycogen storage disease: Branching enzyme deficiency in skin fibroblasts and possible heterozygote detection. Presented at the annual meeting of the American Pediatric Society and the Society for Pediatric Research, Atlantic City, N.J., April 29–May 2, 1970.

141. Hsia, D. Y-Y., and Walker, F. A. Variability in the clinical manifestations of galactosemia. *J. Pediatr.* 59:872, 1961.

142. Hsia, Y. E., Lilljeqvist, A. C., and Rosenberg, L. E. Vitamin $B_{12}$ dependent methylmalonicaciduria: Amino acid toxicity, long chain ketonuria, and protective effect of vitamin $B_{12}$. *Pediatrics* 46:497, 1970.

143. Hsia, Y. E., Scully, K. J., and Rosenberg, L. E. Inherited proprionyl-CoA carboxylase deficiency in "ketotic hyperglycinemia." Presented at the annual meeting of the American Pediatric Society and the Society for Pediatric Research, Atlantic City, N.J., April 29–May 2, 1970.

144. Hug, G., Schubert, W. K., and Soukup, S. Electron microscopy of uncultured amniotic fluid cells: In utero diagnosis of Type II glycogenosis. *Abstracts Am. Pediatr. Soc., Soc. Pediatr. Res.,* Atlantic City, April 1971, p. 118.

145. Huijing, F., Van Creveld, S., and Losekoot, G. Diagnosis of generalized glycogen storage disease (Pompe's disease). *J. Pediatr.* 63:984, 1963.

146. Hummler, K., Zajac, B. A., Genel, M., Holtzapple, P. G., and Segal, S. Human cystinosis: Intracellular deposition of cystine. *Science* 168:859, 1970.

147. Hutchinson, D. L., Hunter, C. B., Nelsen, E. D., and Plentl, A. A. The exchange of water and electrolytes in the mechanism of amniotic fluid formation and the relationship to hydramnios. *Surg. Gynecol. Obstet.* 100:391, 1955.

148. Illingworth, B., and Cori, G. T. Structures of glycogens and amylopectins. III. Normal and abnormal human glycogen. *J. Biochem.* 199:653, 1952.

149. Jacoby, L. B., Littlefield, J. W., Milunsky, A., Shih, V. E., and Wilroy, R. S. Argininosuccinase deficiency in cultured human cells. *Am. J. Hum. Genet.* 24:321, 1972.

150. Jatzkewitz, H., and Mehl, E. Cerebroside-sulphatase and arylsulphatase A deficiency in metachromatic leukodystrophy (ML). *J. Neurochem.* 16:19, 1969.

151. Jeffcoate, T. N. A., Fliegner, J. R. H., Russell, S. H., Davis, J. C., and Wade, A. P. Diagnosis of the adrenogenital syndrome before birth. *Lancet* ii:553, 1965.

152. Kaback, M. M. and Howell, R. R. Infantile metachromatic leukodystrophy: Heterozygote detection in skin fibroblasts and possible applications to intrauterine diagnosis. *N. Engl. J. Med.* 282:1336, 1970.

153. Kahlke, W. Heredopathia atactica polyneuritiformis (Refsum's disease), *in* Shettler, G., ed.: *Lipids and Lipidoses.* New York, Springer-Verlag, 1967, pp. 352–381.

154. Kaplan, D. Classification of the mucopolysaccharidoses based on the pattern of mucopolysacchariduria. *Am. J. Med.* 47:721, 1969.

155. Kerenyi, T., and Sarkozi, L. Diagnosis of fetal death in utero by elevated amniotic fluid CPK levels. *Obstet. Gynecol.* 44:215, 1974.

156. Kint, J. A., Dacremont, G., and Vlietinck, R. Type II $G_{M1}$ gangliosidosis? *Lancet* ii:108, 1969.

157. Kish, M. Y., Marko, J., and Letts, H. Bilirubin estimation in amniotic fluid. A comparative study of 60 cases. *Am. J. Obstet. Gynecol.* 106:592, 1970.

158. Kiyasu, J. and Mathur, R. Considerations in determining lecithin/sphingomyelin ratio in amniotic fluid. *Clin. Chem.* 19:1224, 1973.

159. Kjellman, B., Gamstorp, I., Brun, A., Ockerman, P. A., and Palmgren, B. Mannosidosis: A clinical and histopathologic study. *J. Pediatr.* 75:366, 1969.

160. Klaus, M. H., Clements, J. A., and Havel, R. J. Composition of surface-active material isolated from beef lung. *Proc. Natl. Acad. Sci. USA* 47:1858, 1961.

161. Knox, E. G., Fairweather, D. V. I., and Walker, W. Spectrophotometric measurements on liquor amnii in relation to the severity of haemolytic disease of the newborn. *Clin. Sci.* 28:147, 1965.

162. Kolodny, E. G., Uhlendorf, B. W., Quirk, J. M., Jacobson, C. B., and Brady, R. O. Gangliosides in cultured skin fibroblasts: Accumulation in Tay–Sachs disease. Presented at the Twelfth International Congress on Biochemistry of Lipids, Athens, Greece, September 7–11, 1969.

163. Komrower, G. J., Lambert, A. M., Cusworth, D. C., and Westall, R. G. Dietary treatment of homocystinuria. *Arch. Dis. Child.* 41:66, 1966.

164. Krabbe, K. A new familial infantile form of diffuse brain-sclerosis. *Brain* 39:74, 1916.

165. Kresse, H., Wiesmann, U., Cantz, M., Hall, C. W., and Neufeld, E. F. Biochemical heterogeneity of the Sanfilippo syndrome: Preliminary characterization of two deficient factors. *Biochem. Biophys. Res. Commun.* 42:892, 1971.

166. Kretchmer, N., Greenberg, R. E., and Sereni, F. Biochemical basis of immaturity, *in* Degraff, A. C., ed.: *Annual Review of Medicine.* Palo Alto, Calif., Annual Reviews, Inc., 1963, Vol. 14, pp. 407–426.

167. Krone, W., Schneider, G., and Schulz, D. Detection of phosphohexose isomerase deficiency in human fibroblast cultures. *Humangenetik* 10:224, 1970.

168. Krooth, R. S. Properties of diploid cell strains developed from patients with an inherited abnormality of uridine biosynthesis. *Symp. Quant. Biol.* 29:189, 1964.

169. Krooth, R. S., Howell, R. R., and Hamilton, H. B. Properties of acatalasic cells growing in vitro. *J. Exp. Med.* 115:313, 1962.

170. Krooth, R. S., and Weinberg, A. N. Studies on cell lines developed from the tissues of patients with galactosemia. *J. Exp. Med.* 113:1155, 1961.

171. Kulkarni, B. D., Bieniarz, J., Burd, L., and Scommegna, A. Determination of lecithin sphingomyelin ratios in amniotic fluid. *Obstet. Gynecol.* 40:173, 1972.

172. Kyriakides, E. C., Filippone, N., Paul, B., Grattan, W., and Balint, J. A. Lipid studies in Wolman's disease. *Pediatrics* 46:431, 1970.

173. Lake, B. D., and Patrick, A. D. Wolman's disease: deficiency of E600-resistant acid esterase activity with storage of lipids in lysosomes. *J. Pediatr.* 76:262, 1970.

174. Langenbeck, U., Rudiger, H. W., Schulze-Schencking, M., Keller, W., Brackertz, D., and Goedde, H. W. Evaluation of a

heterozygote test for maple syrup urine disease in leucocytes and cultured fibroblasts. *Humangenetik* 11:304, 1971.

175. Leob, H., Tondeur, M., Jonniaux, G., Mockel-Pohl, S., and Vamos-Hurwitz, E. Biochemical and ultrastructural studies in a case of mucopolysaccharidosis "F" (fucosidosis). *Helv. Paediatr. Acta* 36:519, 1969.

176. Leroy, J. G., and DeMars, R. I. Mutant enzymatic and cytological phenotypes in cultured human fibroblasts. *Science* 157:804, 1967.

177. Leroy, J. G., DeMars, R. I., and Optiz, J. M. I-cell disease. The first conference on the clinical delineation of birth defects. Part 4. Skeletal dysplasias. *Birth Defects* (original article series No. 4) 5:174, 1969.

178. Leroy, J. G., Dumon, J., and Radermecker, J. Deficiency of arylsulphatase A in leucocytes and skin fibroblasts in juvenile metachromatic leucodystrophy. *Nature (London)* 226:553, 1970.

179. Leroy, J. G., and Spranger, J. W. I-cell disease. *N. Engl. J. Med.* 283:598, 1970.

180. Leroy, J. G., Spranger, J. W., Feingold, M., Optiz, J. M., and Crocker, A. C. I-cell disease: A clinical picture. *J. Pediatr.* 79:360, 1971.

181. Levin, B. Argininosuccinic aciduria. *Am. J. Dis. Child.* 113:162, 1967.

182. Levin, B., and Russell, A. Treatment of hyperammonemia. *Am. J. Dis. Child.* 113:142, 1967.

183. Levy, H. L., Shih, V. E., and MacCready, R. A. Inborn errors of metabolism and transport: Prenatal and neonatal diagnosis. Proceedings of the 13th International Congress of Pediatrics. *Genetics*, Vol. 1, Vienna, August 29, 1971.

184. Lightbody, J., Wiesmann, U., Hadorn, B., and Herschkowitz, N. N. I-cell disease: Multiple lysosomal-enzyme defect. *Lancet* i:451, 1971.

185. Liley, A. W. Liquor amnii analysis in the management of the pregnancy complicated by rhesus sensitization. *Am. J. Obstet. Gynecol.* 82:1359, 1961.

186. Liley, A. W. Disorders of amniotic fluid, in Assali, N. S., ed.: *Pathophysiology of Gestation*. New York, Academic Press, 1972, Vol. 11, pp. 154–206.

187. Lind, T. Fetal control of fetal fluids, in Hodari, A. A., and Mariona, F., eds.: *Physiological Biochemistry of the Fetus*. Springfield, Ill., Charles C Thomas, 1972, pp. 54–65.

188. Lind, T. The biochemistry of amniotic fluid, in Fairweather, D. V. I., and Eskes, T. K. E., eds.: *Amniotic Fluid, Research and Clinical Application*. Amsterdam, Excerpta Medica, 1973, pp. 60–81.

189. Lindblad, B., Lindblad, B. S., Olin, P., Svanberg, B., and Zetterstrom, R. Methylmalonic acidemia: A disorder associated with acidosis, hyperglycinemia, and hyperlactatemia. *Acta Paediatr. Scand.* 57:417, 1968.

190. Lipshaw, L. A., Weinberg, J. H., Sherman, A. I., and Foa, P. P. A rapid method for measuring the lecithin–sphingomyelin ratio in amniotic fluid. *Obstet. Gynecol.* 42:93, 1973.

191. Lonsdale, E., Faulkner, W. R., Price, J. W., and Smeby, R. R. Intermittent cerebellar ataxia associated with hyperpyruvicemic acidemia, hyperalanemia and hyperalanuria. *Pediatrics* 43:1025, 1969.

192. Lyon, I. C. T., Procopis, P. G., and Turner, B. Cystathioninuria in a well baby population. *Acta Paediatr. Scand.* 60:324, 1971.

193. MacBrinn, M., Okada, S., Woollacott, M., Patel, B., Ho, M. W., Tappel, A. L., and O'Brien, J. S. β-Galactosidase deficiency in the Hurler syndrome. *N. Engl. J. Med.* 281:338, 1969.

194. Mahoney, M. J., Hsia, Y. E., and Rosenberg, L. Abnormalities of vitamin $B_{12}$ metabolism, in Dorfman, A., ed.: *Antenatal Diagnosis*. Chicago, University of Chicago Press, 1972, pp. 95–100.

195. Mahoney, M. J., and Rosenberg, J. E. Defective metabolism of vitamin $B_{12}$ in fibroblasts from children with methylmalonicaciduria. *Biochem. Biophys. Res. Commun.* 44:375, 1971.

196. Mallikarjuneswara, V. R. Lecithin–sphingomyelin ratio in amniotic fluid, as assessed by a modified thin-layer chromatographic method in which a commercial pre-coated plate is used. *Clin. Chem.* 21:260, 1975.

197. Malmqvist, E., Ivemark, B. I., Lindsten, J., Maunsbach, A. B., and Martensson, E. Pathologic lysosomes and increased urinary glycosylceramide excretion in Fabry's disease. *Lab. Invest.* 25:1, 1971.

198. Mapes, C. A., Anderson, R. L., Sweeley, C. C., Desnick, R. J., and Krivit, W. Enzyme replacement in Fabry's disease, an inborn error of metabolism. *Science* 169:987, 1970.

199. Matalon, R., Cifonelli, J. A., and Dorfman, A. L-Iuronidase in cultured human fibroblasts and liver. *Biochem. Biophys. Res. Commun.* 42:340, 1971.

200. Matalon, R., and Dorfman, A. Acid mucopolysaccharides in cultured fibroblasts of cystic fibrosis of the pancreas. *Biochem. Biophys. Res. Commun.* 33:954, 1968.

201. Matalon, R., and Dorfman, A. The accumulation of hyaluronic acid in cultured fibroblasts of the Marfan syndrome. *Biochem. Biophys. Res. Commun.* 32:150, 1968.

202. Matalon, R., and Dorfman, A. Acid mucopolysaccharides in cultured human fibroblasts. *Lancet* ii:838, 1969.

203. Matalon, R., Dorfman, A., Dawson, G., and Sweeley, C. C. Glycolipid and mucopolysaccharide abnormality in fibroblasts of Fabry's disease. *Science* 164:1522, 1969.

204. Matalon, R., Dorfman, A., Nadler, H. L., and Jacobson, C. B. A chemical method for the antenatal diagnosis of mucopolysaccharidoses. *Lancet* i:83, 1970.

205. McKusick, V. A. *Heritable Disorders of Connective Tissue*, 3rd ed. St. Louis, C. V. Mosby, 1966.

206. McMurray, W. C., Mohyuddin, F., Rossiter, R. J., Rathbun, J. C., Valentine, G. H., Koegler, S. J., and Zarfas, D. E. Citrullinuria: A new aminoaciduria associated with mental retardation. *Lancet* i:138, 1962.

207. Mehl, E., and Jatzkewitz, H. Cerebroside 3-sulfate as a physiological substrate of arylsulfatase A. *Biochim. Biophys. Acta* 151:619, 1968.

208. Menees, T. O., Miller, J. D., and Holly, L. E. Amniography. Preliminary report. *Am. J. Roentgenol.* 24:363, 1930.

209. Menkes, J. H., Hurst, P. L., and Craig, J. M. A new syndrome: Progressive familial cerebral dysfunction with an unusual urinary substance. *Pediatrics* 14:462, 1954.

210. Merkatz, I. R., Aladjem, S., and Little, B. The value of biochemical estimations on amniotic fluid in management of the high-risk pregnancy, in Milunsky, A., ed., *Clinics in Perinatology*. Philadelphia, W. B. Saunders Co., 1974, Vol. 1:2, pp. 301–319.

211. Merkatz, I. R., New, M. I., Peterson, R. E., and Seamon, M. P. Prenatal diagnosis of adrenogenital syndrome by amniocentesis. *J. Pediatr.* 75:977, 1969.

212. Milunsky, A. Prenatal genetic diagnosis II. *N. Engl. J. Med.* 283:1441, 1970.

213. Milunsky, A. *The Prenatal Diagnosis of Hereditary Disorders*. Springfield, Ill., Charles C Thomas, 1973, pp. 62–135.

214. Milunsky, A., and Alpert, E. The value of α-fetoprotein in

prenatal diagnosis of neural tube defects. *J. Pediatr.* 84:889, 1974.

215. Milunsky, A., and Littlefield, J. W. Diagnostic limitations of metachromasia. *N. Engl. J. Med.* 281:1128, 1969.

216. Milunsky, A., Littlefield, J. W., Kanfer, J. N., Kolodny, E. H., Shih, V. E., and Atkins, L. Prenatal genetic diagnosis I. *N. Engl. J. Med.* 283:1370, 1970.

217. Misenheimer, H. R. Amniotic fluid analysis in the prenatal diagnosis of erythroblastosis fetalis. *Obstet. Gynecol.* 23:485, 1964.

218. Morris, M. D., Fisher, D. A., and Fiser, R. Late-onset branched-chain ketoaciduria (maple syrup urine disease). *Lancet* 86:149, 1966.

219. Morrow, G. Citrullinemia. *Am. J. Dis. Child.* 113:157, 1967.

220. Morrow, G. III, Mellman, W. J., Barness, L. A., and Dimitrov, N. V. Propionate metabolism in cells cultured from a patient with methylmalonic acidemia. *Pediatr. Res.* 3:217, 1969.

221. Morrow, G. III, Schwarz, R. H., and Hallock, J. A. Prenatal detection of methylmalonic acidemia. *J. Pediatr.* 77:120, 1970.

222. Moser, H. W., Prensky, A. L., Wolfe, H. J., and Rosman, N. P. Farber's lipogranulomatosis—Report of a case and demonstration of an excess of free ceramide and ganglioside. *Am. J. Med.* 47:869, 1969.

223. Mudd, H. S., Uhlendorf, B. W., Hinds, K. R., and Levy, H. L. Deranged $B_{12}$ metabolism: Studies of fibroblasts grown in tissue culture. *Biochem. Med.* 4:215, 1970.

224. Muller, W. E., Jamazaki, Z., Zahn, R. K., Brehm, G., and Korting, G. RNA dependent DNA polymerase in cells of xeroderma pigmentosum. *Biochem. Biophys. Res. Commun.* 44:433, 1971.

225. Murphy, J. V., Wolfe, H. J., Balazs, E. A., and Moser, H. W. A patient with deficiency of arylsulfatases A, B, C and steroid sulfatase, associated with storage of sulfatide, cholesterol sulfate and glycosaminoglycans, in Bernsohn, J., ed.: *Lipid Storage Diseases: Enzymatic Defects and Clinical Implications.* New York, Academic Press, 1971.

226. Murphy, J. V., Wolfe, H. L., and Moser, H. W. Multiple sulfatase deficiencies in a variant form of metachromatic leukodystrophy, in Bernsohn, J., ed.: *Lipid Storage Disease: Enzymatic Defects and Clinical Implications.* New York, Academic Press (in press), 1971.

227. Myrianthopoulos, N. C., and Aronson, S. M. Population dynamics of Tay–Sachs disease. I. Reproductive fitness and selection. *Am. J. Hum. Genet.* 18:313, 1966.

228. Nadler, H. L. Patterns of enzyme development utilizing cultivated human fetal cells derived from amniotic fluid. *Biochem. Genet.* 2:119, 1968.

229. Nadler, H. L. Antenatal detection of hereditary disorders. *Pediatrics* 42:912, 1968.

230. Nadler, H. L. Genetic heterogeneity in acid phosphatase deficiency. *Abstracts Am. Pediat. Soc., Soc. Pediat. Res.*, Atlantic City, April 1971, p. 117.

231. Nadler, H. L. Prenatal Diagnosis of Inborn Defects: A Status Report. *Hosp. Pract.* Vol. 10, 6:41, 1975.

232. Nadler, H. L., and Burton, B. K. Enzymes in the amniotic fluid and the prenatal diagnosis of inborn errors of metabolism, in Fairweather, D. V. I., and Eskes, T. K. A., eds.: *Amniotic Fluid.* Amsterdam, Excerpta Medica, 1973, pp. 223–261.

233. Nadler, H. L., and Egan, T. J. Deficiency of lysosomal acid phosphatase: A new familial metabolic disorder. *N. Engl. J. Med.* 282:302, 1970.

234. Nadler, H. L., and Gerbie, A. B. Enzymes in noncultured amniotic fluid cells. *Am. J. Obstet. Gynecol.* 103:710, 1969.

235. Nadler, H. L., and Gerbie, A. B. Present status of amniocentesis in intrauterine diagnosis of genetic defects. *Obstet. Gynecol.* 38:389, 1971.

236. Nadler, H. L., and Messina, A. M. In-utero detection of type-II glycogenosis (Pompe's disease). *Lancet* ii:1277, 1969.

237. Nadler, H. L., Wodnicki, J. M., Swae, M. A., and O'Flynn, M. E. Cultivated amniotic fluid cells and fibroblasts derived from families with cystic fibrosis. *Lancet* ii:84, 1969.

238. Natelson, S., Scommegna, A., and Epstein, M. B., eds. *Amniotic Fluid.* New York, John Wiley and Sons, 1974.

239. Nelson, G. H. Amniotic fluid phospholipid patterns in normal and abnormal pregnancies. *Am. J. Obstet. Gynecol.* 105:1072, 1969.

240. Nelson, G. H., and Lawson, S. W. Determination of amniotic fluid total phospholipid phosphorus as a test for fetal lung maturity. *Am. J. Obstet. Gynecol.* 115:933, 1973.

241. Neufeld, E. F., and Cantz, M. J. Corrective factors for inborn errors of mucopolysaccharide metabolism. *Ann. N.Y. Acad. Sci.* 179:580, 1971.

242. Neufeld, E. F., and Fratantoni, J. C. Inborn errors of mucopolysaccharide metabolism. *Science* 169:141, 1970.

243. Nichols, J. Antenatal diagnosis of adrenocortical hyperplasia. *Lancet* i:1151, 1969.

244. Nichols, J., and Gibson, G. G. Antenatal diagnosis of the adrenogenital syndrome. *Lancet* ii:1068, 1969.

245. Nitowsky, H. M., and Grunefeld, A. Lysomal, $\alpha$-glucosidase in type-II glycogenosis: Activity in leukocytes and cell cultures in relation to genotype. *J. Lab. Clin. Med.* 69:472, 1967.

246. Novy, M. J. Evaluation and treatment of the fetus at risk, in Behrman, R. E., ed.: *Neonatology. Diseases of the Fetus and Infant.* Saint Louis, The C. V. Mosby Company, 1973, pp. 2–4.

247. Oberholzer, V. G., Levin, B., Burgess, A., and Young, W. F. Methylmalonic aciduria: an inborn error of metabolism leading to chronic metabolic acidosis. *Arch. Dis. Child.* 42:492, 1967.

248. O'Brien, J. Generalized gangliosidosis. *J. Pediatr.* 75:167, 1969.

249. O'Brien, J. S. Sanfilippo syndrome: Profound deficiency of $\alpha$-acetylglucosaminidase activity in organs and skin fibroblasts from type-B patients. *Proc. Natl. Acad. Sci. USA* 69:1720, 1972.

250. O'Brien, J. S., Okada, S., Chen, A., and Fillerup, D. L. Tay–Sachs disease: Detection of heterozygotes and homozygotes by serum hexosaminidase assay. *N. Engl. J. Med.* 283:15, 1970.

251. O'Brien, J. S., Okada, S., Fillerup, D. L., Veath, M. L., Adornato, B., Brenner, P. H., and Leroy, J. G. Tay–Sachs disease: prenatal diagnosis. *Science* 172:61, 1971.

252. O'Brien, J. S., Okada, S., Ho, M. W., Fillerup, D. L., Veath, M. L., and Adams, K. Ganglioside-storage diseases. *Fed. Proc.* 30:956, 1971.

253. O'Brien, J. S., Stern, M. D., Landing, B. H., O'Brien, J. K., and Donnell, G. N. Generalized gangliosidosis: Another inborn error of ganglioside metabolism? *Am. J. Dis. Child.* 109:338, 1965.

254. Ockerman, P. A. Mannosidosis: Isolation of oligosaccharide storage material from brain. *J. Pediatr.* 75:360, 1969.

255. Okada, S., and O'Brien, J. S. Generalized gangliosidosis: $\beta$-Galactosidase deficiency. *Science* 160:1002, 1968.

256. Okada, S., and O'Brien, J. S. Tay-Sachs disease: Generalized absence of a $\beta$-D-N-acetylhexosaminidase component. *Science* 165:698, 1969.

257. Okada, S., Veath, M. L., Leroy, J., and O'Brien, J. S. Ganglioside $G_{M2}$ storage diseases: Hexosaminidase deficiencies in cultured fibroblasts. *Am. J. Hum. Genet.* 23:55, 1971.

258. Okada, S., Veath, M. L., and O'Brien, J. S. Juvenile $G_{M2}$ gangliosidosis: Partial deficiency of hexosaminidase A. *J. Pediatr.* 77:1063, 1970.

259. Ostergard, D. R. The physiology and clinical importance of amniotic fluid: A review. *Obstet. Gynecol. Surv.* 25:297, 1970.

260. Paglia, D. E., Holland, P., Baughan, M. A., and Valentine, W. N. Occurrence of defective hexosephosphate isomerization in human erythrocytes and leukocytes. *N. Engl. J. Med.* 280:66, 1969.

261. Parmley, T., and Seeds, A. E. Permeability of fetal skin to tritated water. *Am. J. Obstet. Gynecol.* 108:128, 1970.

262. Patel, V., Tappel, A. L., and O'Brien, J. S. Hyaluronidase and sulfatase deficiency in Hurler's syndrome. *Biochem. Med.* 3:447, 1970.

263. Patrick, A. D., and Lake, B. D. Deficiency of an acid lipase in Wolman's disease. *Nature* (London) 222:1067, 1969.

264. Pattle, R. E., Claireaux, A. E., Davies, P. A., and Cameron, A. H. Inability to form a lung lining film as a cause of respiratory distress syndrome in the newborn. *Lancet* ii:469, 1962.

265. Percy, A. K., and Brady, R. O. Metachromatic leukodystrophy: Diagnosis with samples of venous blood. *Science* 161:594, 1968.

266. Percy, A. K., and Kaback, M. M. Infantile and adult-onset metachromatic leukodystrophy—Biochemical comparisons and predictive diagnosis. *N. Engl. J. Med.* 285:785, 1971.

267. Perry, T. L., Dunn, H. G., Hansen, S., MacDougall, L., and Warrington, P. D. Early diagnosis and treatment of homocystinuria. *Pediatrics* 37:501, 1966.

268. Perry, T. L., Hardwick, D. F., Hansen, S., Love, D. L., and Israels, S. Cystathioninuria in two healthy siblings. *N. Engl. J. Med.* 278:590, 1968.

269. Pfleger, R. C., and Thomas, H. G. Beagle dog pulmonary surfactant lipids. *Arch. Intern. Med.* 127:863, 1971.

270. Pitkin, R. M., and Zwirek, S. J. Amniotic fluid creatinine. *Am. J. Obstet. Gynecol.* 98:1135, 1967.

271. Plentl, A. A. The dynamics of the amniotic fluid. *Ann. N.Y. Acad. Med.* 75:746, 1959.

272. Plentl, A. A. Formation and circulation of the amniotic fluid. *Clin. Obstet. Gynecol.* 9:427, 1966.

273. Porter, M. T., Fluharty, A. L., Harris, S. E., and Kihara, H. The accumulation of cerebroside sulfates by fibroblasts in culture from patients with late infantile metachromatic leukodystrophy. *Arch. Biochem. Biophys.* 138:646, 1970.

274. Porter, M. T., Fluharty, A. L., and Kihara, H. Metachromatic leukodystrophy: Arylsulfatase-A deficiency in skin fibroblast cultures. *Proc. Natl. Acad. Sci. USA* 62:887, 1969.

275. Porter, M. T., Fluharty, A. L., and Kihara, H. Correction of abnormal cerebroside sulfate metabolism in cultured metachromatic leukodystrophy fibroblasts. *Science* 172:1263, 1971.

276. Porter, M. T., Fluharty, A. L., Trammell, J., and Kihara, H. A correlation of intracellular cerebroside sulfatase activity in fibroblasts with latency in metachromatic leukodystrophy. *Biochem. Biophys. Res. Commun.* 44:660, 1971.

277. Pritchard, J. Deglutition by normal and anancephalic infants. *Obstet. Gynecol.* 25:289, 1965.

278. Rattazzi, M. C., and Davidson, R. G. Limitations of amniocentesis for the antenatal diagnosis of Tay–Sachs disease. *Abstracts Am. Soc. Hum. Genet.* Meeting, Indianapolis, October 11, 1970.

279. Reed, W. B., Landing, B., Sugarman, G., Cleaver, J. E., and McInyk, J. Xeroderma pigmentosum. *JAMA* 207:2073, 1969.

280. Regan, J. D., Setlow, R. B., Kaback, M. M., Howell, R. R., Klein, E., and Burgess, G. Xeroderma pigmentosum: A rapid sensitive method for prenatal diagnosis. *Science* 174:147, 1971.

281. Reid, D. E., Ryan, K. J., and Benirschke, K. *Principles and Management of Human Reproduction.* Philadelphia, W. B. Saunders Company, 1972, p. 410.

282. Reynolds, A. Fetal sources of amniotic fluid: An enigma, in Hodari, A. A., and Mariona, F., eds.: *Physiological Biochemistry of the Fetus.* Springfield, Ill., Charles C Thomas, 1972, pp. 3–31.

283. Robinson, D., and Stirling, J. L. N-Acetyl-$\beta$-glucosaminidases in human spleen. *Biochem. J.* 107:321, 1968.

284. Rogers, L. E., Warford, L. R., Patterson, R. B., and Porter, F. S. Hereditary orotic aciduria I. A new case with family studies. *Pediatrics* 42:415, 1968.

285. Romeo, G., Kaback, M. M., Glenn, B. L., and Levin, E. Y. The enzymatic defect in congenital erythropoietic porphyria: Demonstration in heterozygotes and in nonerythropoietic tissue of homozygotes. Presented at the annual meeting of the American Pediatric Society and the Society for Pediatric Research, Atlantic City, April 29–May 2, 1970.

286. Romeo, G., and Migeon, B. R. Genetic inactivation of the $\alpha$-galactosidase locus in carriers of Fabry's disease. *Science* 170:180, 1970.

287. Ron, M. and Pearce, J. Refsum's syndrome with normal phytate metabolism. *Acta Neurol. Scand.* 47:646, 1971.

288. Roopnarinesingh, S. Amniotic fluid creatinine in normal and abnormal pregnancies. *J. Obstet. Gynaecol. Br. Commonw.* 77:785, 1970.

289. Rosenberg, L. E., Lilljeqvist, A. C., and Hsia, Y. E. Methylmalonic aciduria: an inborn error leading to metabolic acidosis, long-chain ketonuria and intermittent hyperglycinemia. *N. Engl. J. Med.* 278:1319, 1968.

290. Rosenberg, L. E., Lilljeqvist, A. C., Hsia, Y. E., and Rosenbloom, F. E. Vitamin $B_{12}$ dependent methylmalonicaciduria: defective $B_{12}$ metabolism in cultured fibroblasts. *Biochem. Biophys. Res. Commun.* 37:607, 1969.

291. Russel, A., Levin, B., Oberholzer, V. G., and Sinclair, L. Hyperammonaemia: A new instance of an inborn enzymatic defect of the biosynthesis of urea. *Lancet* ii:699, 1962.

292. Russell, J. D. Variation of UDP Glu:$\alpha$-DGal-1-P-uridyl transferase activity during growth of cultured fibroblasts, in Hsia, D. Y.-Y., ed.: *Galactosemia.* Springfield, Ill., Charles C Thomas, 1969, pp. 204–212.

293. Russell, P. T., Miller, W. J., and McLain, C. R. Palmitic acid content of amniotic fluid lecithin as an index to fetal lung maturity. *Clin. Chem.* 20:1431, 1974.

294. Sacrez, R., Juif, J. G., Gigonnet, J. M., and Gruner, J. E. La maladie de Landing: Ou idiotie amaurotique infantile precoce avec gangliosidose generalise de type $G_{M1}$. *Pediatrie* 22:143, 1967.

295. Salafsky, I. S., and Nadler, H. L. $\alpha$-1,4-Glucosidase activity in Pompe's disease. *J. Pediatr.* 79:794, 1971.

296. Sandhoff, K. Variation of $\beta$-N-acetylhexosaminidase-pattern in Tay–Sachs disease. *FEBS Lett.* 4:351, 1969.

297. Sandhoff, K., Andreae, U., and Jatzkewitz, H. Deficient hexosaminidase activity in an exceptional case of Tay–Sachs disease with additional storage of kidney globoside in visceral organs. *Life Sci.* 7:283, 1968.

298. Sarkozi, L., Kerenyi, T., and Jeuell, C. The origin of elevated amniotic fluid CPK levels and experimental verification of the time factor in DIU (Abstr. 101). Presented at the Twenty-fifth National Meeting of the American Association of Clinical Chemists, New York, July 15–20, 1973.

299. Sarkozi, L., Kerenyi, T., Saary, Z., and Hutterer, F. Amniotic fluid CPK and LDH in feto-placental damage and intrauterine death. *Res. Commun. Chem. Pathol. Pharmacol.* 3:189, 1972.

300. Sarkozi, L., Kovacs, H. N., Fox, H. S., and Kerenyi, T. Modified methods for estimating the phosphatidylcholine: sphingomyelin ratio in amniotic fluid, and its use in the assessment of fetal lung maturity. *Clin. Chem.* 18:956, 1972.

301. Scarpelli, E. M. Pulmonary surfactants and their role in lung diseases. *Adv. Pediatr.* 16:177, 1969.

302. Schmid, R. Congenital erythropoietic porphyria, *in* Stanbury, J. B., Wyngaarden, J. B., and Fredrickson, D. S., eds.: *The Metabolic Basis of Inherited Disease*, 2nd ed. New York, McGraw-Hill, 1966, pp. 831–844.

303. Schneck, L., Adachi, M., and Volk, B. W. The fetal aspects of Tay–Sachs disease. *Pediatrics* 49:342, 1972.

304. Schneck, L., Friedland, J., Pourfar, M., Saifer, A., and Volk, B. Hexosaminidase activities in a case of systemic $G_{M2}$ gangliosidosis of late infantile type. *Proc. Soc. Exp. Biol. Med.* 133:997, 1970.

305. Schneck, L., Friedland, J., Valenti, C., Adachi, M., Amsterdam, D., and Volk, B. W. Prenatal diagnosis of Tay–Sachs disease. *Lancet i*:582, 1970.

306. Schenck, L., and Volk, B. W. Clinical manifestations of Tay–Sachs disease and Niemann–Pick disease, *in* Aronson, S. M. and Volk, B. W., eds.: *Inborn Disorders of Sphingolipid Metabolism. Proceedings of the Third International Symposium on the Cerebral Sphingolipidoses*. Oxford, Pergamon Press, 1967, pp. 403–411.

307. Schenck, L., Volk, B. W., and Saifer, A. The gangliosidoses. *Am. J. Med.* 46:245, 1969.

308. Schneider, A. S., Valentine, W. N., Hattori, M., and Heins, H. L. Hereditary hemolytic anemia with triosephosphate isomerase deficiency. *N. Engl. J. Med.* 272:229, 1965.

309. Schneider, J. A., Rosenbloom, F. M., Bradley, K. H., and Seegmiller, J. E. Increased free-cystine content of fibroblasts cultured from patients with cystinosis. *Biochem. Biophys. Res. Commun.* 29:527, 1967.

310. Schneider, J. A., Wong, V. G., Bradley, K., and Seegmiller, J. E. Biochemical comparisons of the adult and childhood forms of cystinosis. *N. Engl. J. Med.* 279:1253, 1968.

311. Schulman, J. D., Wong, V. G., Bradley, K. H., Olson, W. H., and Seegmiller, J. E. Cystinosis: Biochemical, morphological, and clinical studies. *Pediatr. Res.* 4:379, 1970.

312. Scott, C. R., Dassell, S. W., Clark, S. H., Chiang-Teng, C., and Swedberg, K. R. Cystathioninemia: A benign genetic condition. *J. Pediatr.* 76:571, 1970.

313. Scriver, C. R., Mackenzie, S., Clow, C. L., and Devlin, E. Thiamine-responsive maple syrup urine disease. *Lancet i*:310, 1971.

314. Seeds, A. E. Water metabolism of the fetus. *Am. J. Obstet. Gynecol.* 92:727, 1965.

315. Seegmiller, J. E. Amniotic fluid and cells in the diagnosis of genetic disorders, *in* Natelson, S., Scommegna, A., and Epstein, M. B., eds.: *Amniotic Fluid.* New York, John Wiley and Sons, 1974, pp. 291–316.

316. Seegmiller, J. E., Friedmann, T., Harrison, H. E., Wong, V., and Schneider, J. A. Cystinosis. *Ann. Intern. Med.* 68:883, 1968.

317. Seegmiller, J. E., and Westall, R. G. The enzyme defect in maple syrup urine disease (branched chain ketoaciduria). *J. Ment. Defic. Res.* 11:288, 1967.

318. Shaw, R. F., and Smith, A. P. Is Tay–Sachs disease increasing? *Nature* (London) 224:1213, 1969.

319. Shelley, S. A., Takagi, L. R., and Balis, J. U. Assessment of surfactant activity in amniotic fluid in evaluation of fetal lung maturity. *Am. J. Obstet. Gynecol.* 116:369, 1973.

320. Shih, V. E. Early dietary management of an infant with argininosuccinase deficiency. *J. Pediatr.* 80:645, 1972.

321. Shih, V. E., and Littlefield, J. W. Argininosuccinase activity in amniotic fluid cells. *Lancet ii*:45, 1970.

322. Shih, V. E., Littlefield, J. W., and Moser, H. W. Argininosuccinase deficiency in fibroblasts cultured from patients with argininosuccinic aciduria. *Biochem. Genet.* 3:81, 1969.

323. Shih, V. E., and Schulman, J. D. Ornithine-ketoacid transaminase activity in human skin and amniotic fluid cell culture. *Clin. Chim. Acta* 27:73, 1970.

324. Sidbury, J. B. Jr. The glycogenoses, *in* Gardner, L. I., ed.: *Endocrine and Genetic Diseases of Childhood.* Philadelphia, W. B. Saunders, Co., 1969, p. 853.

325. Sidbury, J. B. Jr., Mason, J., Burner, W. B. Jr., and Ruebner, B. H. Type IV glycogenosis: report of a case proven by characterization of glycogen and studied at necropsy. *Bull. Johns Hopkins Hosp.* 111:157, 1962.

326. Singer, H. S., Nankervis, G. A., and Schafer, I. A. Leukocyte $\beta$-galactosidase activity in the diagnosis of generalized $G_{M1}$ gangliosidosis. *Pediatrics* 49:352, 1972.

327. Singer, H. S., and Schafer, I. A. White cell $\beta$-galactosidase activity. *N. Engl. Med.* 282:571, 1970.

328. Sloan, H. R. $\beta$-Galactosidase deficiency in $G_{M1}$ gangliosidosis: Enzymatic and histochemical studies in tissue culture. *Pediatr. Res.* 3:368, 1969.

329. Sloan, H. R., Uhlendorf, B. W., Jacobson, C. B., and Fredrickson, D. S. $\beta$-Galactosidase in tissue culture derived from human skin and bone marrow: Enzyme defect in $G_{M1}$ gangliosidosis. *Pediatr. Res.* 3:532, 1969.

330. Sloan, H. R., Uhlendorf, B. W., Kanfer, J. N., Brady, R. O., and Fredrickson, D. S. Deficiency of sphingomyelin-cleaving enzyme activity in tissue cultures derived from patients with Niemann-Pick disease. *Biochem. Biophys. Res. Commun.* 34:582, 1969.

331. Slome, D. J. Genetic basis of amaurotic family idiocy. *Genetics* 27:363, 1933.

332. Smith, L. H. Jr., Sullivan, M., and Huguley, C. M. Pyrimidine metabolism in man IV. The enzymatic defect of orotic aciduria. *J. Clin. Invest.* 40:656, 1961.

333. Snyderman, S. E. Maple syrup urine disease, *in* Nyhan, W. L., ed.: *Amino Acid Metabolism and Genetic Variation.* New York, McGraw-Hill, 1967, pp. 171–183.

334. Sotos, J. F., Romshe, C. A., Boggs, D. E., and Menking, M. F. Methylmalonic aciduria—Vitamin $B_{12}$ dependent. *Abst. Soc. Ped. Res.*, 39th Annual Meeting, Atlantic City, May, 1969, p.13.

335. Spellacy, W. N., and Buhl, W. C. Amniotic fluid lecithin/sphingomyelin ratio as an index of fetal maturity. *Obstet. Gynecol.* 39:852, 1972.

336. Stanbury, J. B., Wyngaarden, J. B., and Fredrickson, D. S., eds. *The Metabolic Basis of Inherited Disease*, 3rd ed. New York, McGraw-Hill Book Co., 1972.

337. Stokke, O., Eldjarn, L., Norum, K. R., Steen-Johnsen, J., and Halvorsen, S. Methylmalonic acidemia: A new inborn error of metabolism which may cause fatal acidosis in the neonatal period. *Scand. J. Clin. Lab. Invest.* 20:313, 1967.

338. Stumpf, D., and Austin, J. Metachromatic leukodystrophy

(MLD). *Arch. Neurol.* 24:117, 1971.

339. Sugita, M., Dulaney, J., and Moser, H. W. Ceramidase deficiency in Farber's disease (Lipogranulomatosis). *Science* 178:1100, 1972.

340. Suzuki, K., and Chen, G. C. Brain ceramide hexosides in Tay–Sachs disease and generalized gangliosidosis ($G_{M1}$ gangliosidosis). *J. Lipid Res.* 8:105, 1967.

341. Suzuki, K., Schneider, E. L., and Epstein, C. J. In utero diagnosis of globoid cell leukodystrophy (Krabbe's disease). *Biochem. Biophys. Res. Commun.* 45:1363, 1971.

342. Suzuki, K., and Kamoshita, S. Chemical pathology of $G_{M1}$ gangliosidosis (generalized gangliosidosis). *J. Neuropathol. Exp. Neurol.* 28:25, 1969.

343. Suzuki, K., Rapin, I., Suzuki, Y., and Ishii, N. Juvenile $G_{M2}$ gangliosidosis. Clinical variant of Tay–Sachs disease or a new disease. *Neurology* 20:190, 1970.

344. Suzuki, K., and Suzuki, Y. Globoid cell leukodystrophy (Krabbe's disease): deficiency of galactocerebroside $\beta$-galactosidase. *Proc. Natl. Acad. Sci. USA* 66:302, 1970.

345. Suzuki, Y., Berman, P. H., and Suzuki, K. Detection of Tay–Sachs disease heterozygotes by assay of hexosaminidase A in serum and leukocytes. *J. Pediatr.* 78:643, 1971.

346. Suzuki, Y., Jacob, J. C., and Suzuki, K. A case of $G_{M2}$ gangliosidosis with total hexosaminidase deficiency. *Neurology* 20:388, 1970.

347. Suzuki, Y., Jacob, J. C., Suzuki, K., Kutty, K. M., and Suzuki, K. $G_{M2}$ gangliosidosis with total hexosaminidase deficiency. *Neurology* 21:313, 1971.

348. Suzuki, Y., and Suzuki, K. Partial deficiency of hexosaminidase component A in juvenile $G_{M2}$ gangliosidosis. *Neurology* 20:848, 1970.

349. Suzuki, Y., and Suzuki, K. Krabbe's globoid cell leukodystrophy: Deficiency of galactocerebrosidase in serum, leukocytes and fibroblasts. *Science* 171:73, 1971.

350. Sweeley, C. C., and Klionsky, B. Glycolipid lipidosis: Fabry's disease, *in* Stanbury, J. B., Wyngaarden, J. B., and Fredrickson, D. S., eds.: *The Metabolic Basis of Inherited Disease,* 2nd ed. New York, McGraw-Hill, 1966, pp. 618–632.

351. Tada, K., Wada, Y., and Arakawa, T. Hypervalinemia: Its metabolic lesion and therapeutic approach. *Am. J. Dis. Child* 113:64, 1967.

352. Tedesco, T. A., and Mellman, W. J. Argininosuccinate synthetase activity and citrulline metabolism in cells cultured from a citrullinemic subject. *Proc. Natl. Acad. Sci. USA* 57:829, 1967.

353. Thom, H., Dinwiddie, R., Fisher, P. M., Russell, G., and Sutherland, H. W. Palmitic acid concentrations and lecithin/sphingomyelin ratios in amniotic fluid. *Clin. Chim. Acta* 62:143, 1975.

354. Thomas, G. H. $\beta$-D-Galactosidase in human urine: Deficiency in generalized gangliosidosis. *J. Lab. Clin. Med.* 74:725, 1969.

355. Uhlendorf, B. W., Holtz, A. L., Mock, M. B., and Fredrickson, D. S. Persistence of a metabolic defect in tissue culture derived from patients with Niemann–Pick disease. *In* Aronson, S. M. and Volk, B. W., eds. *Inborn Disorders of Sphingolipid Metabolism.* Proceedings of the Third International Symposium on the Cerebral Sphingolipidoses. Oxford, Pergamon Press, 1967, pp. 403–411.

356. Uhlendorf, B. W., and Mudd, S. H. Cystathionine synthase in tissue culture derived from human skin: Enzyme defect in

homocystinuria. *Science* 160:1007, 1968.

357. Valenti, C. Perinatal genetic studies and counseling, *in* Aladjem, S., and Brown, A. K., eds.: *Clinical Perinatology.* Saint Louis, The C. V. Mosby Company, 1974, pp. 87–139.

358. Van Hoof, F., and Hers, H. G. Mucopolysaccharidosis by absence of $\alpha$-fucosidase. *Lancet* i:1198, 1968.

359. Van Hoof, F., and Hers, H. G. The abnormalities of lysosomal enzymes in mucopolysaccharidoses. *Eur. J. Biochem.* 7:34, 1968.

360. Vella, E. E. A chemical method for the antenatal diagnosis of mucopolysaccharidoses. *Lancet* i:798, 1972.

361. Volk, B. W., Adachi, M., Schneck, L., Saifer, A., and Kleinberg, W. $G_5$-ganglioside variant of systemic late infantile lipidosis. Generalized gangliosidosis. *Arch. Pathol.* 87:393, 1969.

362. Wada, Y., Tada, K., Minagawa, A., Yoshida, T., Morikawa, T., and Okamura, T. Idiopathic hypervalinemia. Probably a new entity of inborn error of valine metabolism. *Tohoku J. Exp. Med.* 81:46, 1963.

363. Walker, A. H. C. Liquor amnii studies in the prediction of hemolitic disease of the newborn. *Br. Med. J.* 2:375, 1957.

364. Warren, C., Holton, J. B., and Allen, J. T. A method of assessing amniotic fluid lecithin concentrations and predicting foetal lung maturity, by estimating total palmitic acid concentration using G.L.C. *Ann. Clin. Biochem.* 11:31, 1974.

365. Westall, R. G. Dietary treatment of maple syrup urine disease. *Am. J. Dis. Child.* 113:58, 1967.

366. Westall, R. G., Dancis, J., and Miller, S. Maple sugar urine disease. *Am. J. Dis. Child.* 94:571, 1957.

367. White, J. C. Viruslike particles in the peripheral blood cells of two patients with Chediak–Higashi syndrome. *Cancer* 19:877, 1966.

368. White, J. C. The Chediak–Higashi syndrome: Cytoplasmic sequestration in circulating leukocytes. *Blood* 29:435, 1967.

369. Wiesmann, U. N., Lightbody, J., Vasella, F., and Herschkowitz, N. N. Multiple lysosomal enzyme deficiency due to enzyme leakage? *N. Engl. J. Med.* 284:109, 1971.

370. Wiesmann, U. N., and Neufeld, E. F. Scheie and Hurler syndromes: Apparent identity of the biochemical defect. *Science* 169:72, 1970.

371. Wiesmann, U. N., Rossi, E. E., and Herschkowitz, N. N. Correction of the defective sulfatide degradation in cultured fibroblasts from patients with metachromatic leukodystrophy. *Acta Paediatr. Scand.* 61:296, 1972.

372. Wolfe, L. S., Callahan, J. W., Fawcett, J. S., Andermann, F., and Scriver, C. R. $G_{M1}$ gangliosidosis without chondrodystrophy or visceromegaly. $\beta$-Galactosidase deficiency with gangliosidosis and the excessive excretion of a keratan sulfate. *Neurology* 20:23, 1970.

373. Wolman, M., Sterk, W. V., Gatt, S., and Frenkel, M. Primary familial xanthomatosis with involvement and calcification of the adrenals. *Pediatrics* 28:742, 1961.

374. Young, E. P., Ellis, R. B., Lake, B. D., and Patrick, A. D. Tay–Sachs disease and related disorders: Fractionation of brain N-acetyl-$\beta$-hexosaminidase on DEAE cellulose. *FEBS Lett.* 9:1, 1970.

375. Young, E. P., and Patrick, A. D. Deficiency of acid esterase activity in Wolman's disease. *Arch. Dis. Child.* 45:664, 1970.

376. Zielke, K., Okada, S., and O'Brien, J. S. Fucosidosis: Diagnosis by serum assay of $\alpha$-L-fucosidase. *J. Lab. Clin. Med.* 79:164, 1972.

Charles Debrovner, M.D.

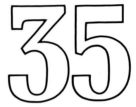

# Pathologic Factors Involved in Infertility

A survey of pathologic factors involved in infertility reveals that in roughly one-quarter of this population the cause is exclusively male and in one-quarter the problem is exclusively female. In a third quarter, there is a dual problem. In some of these cases it is additive and in other cases it is not. An example may be a man who is azospermic and married to a woman with tubal occlusion. In this case they each have a problem, but the problem is not additive. In contrast, a man with a borderline semen may be married to a woman with relatively hostile cervical mucus. In this case, the two problems potentiate each other. If the same man were married to a woman with a very healthy hospitable cervical mucus, pregnancy would probably occur. If the woman were married to a man with a more vigorous sperm population, again, pregnancy would likely occur.

## Physiologic Factors

The last quarter of the infertility population includes couples that are simply impatient but may also include some in which the following factors may be impaired:

1. Sperm capacitation
2. Sperm transport
3. Capacity of the fallopian tube to supply nutrition to the fertilized ovum during the transit period

4. Timing of tubal transport
5. Immunologic capacity to destroy sperm and prevent antisperm antibodies from forming

## Sperm Capacitation

Sperm at the time they are ejaculated are incapable of fertilizing the ovum and must undergo a maturation process referred to as capacitation.[4] This process normally occurs within the lumen of the fallopian tube,[1] although it can also occur in other locations. More is known about this function in animal species. The time required for capacitation is not known in humans; in rabbits it is 8 hr,[1,5] but this sheds no light on the human requirement. The process probably involves either the removal of a coating from the head of the sperm or the activation of an enzymatic site that is necessary for ovum penetration.[43] It has been suggested that there is an enzyme in sperm, called neuroaminidase, that is necessary to dissolve neuroaminic acid in the zona pellucida of the ovum and that it is this enzyme that is either activated or uncovered in capacitation.[14,49]

## Sperm Transport

Sperm transport requires a complex interaction of contractions, fluid currents, ciliary action, and perhaps elimination of anatomic barriers in order to reach the surface of the egg.[12,18,24,25,39,44]

## Capacity of the Fallopian Tube to Supply Nutrition to the Fertilized Ovum during the Transit Period

Once an ovum has been fertilized it is incapable of independent existence[15] and quickly uses up all sources of nutrition that it has carried into the tube with it. In the fallopian tube substances that supply nutrition are secreted by the tubal mucosa.[10,55]

## Timing of Tubal Transport

The fertilized egg must remain in the fallopian tube for 3 days following fertilization.[15] Cell division and cleavage occur until the blastocyst stage is reached. If it remains for less than 3 days, the egg enters the uterine cavity at a time when it is unprepared to survive in the uterus. Implantation occurs on day 21 in the endometrial cycle, when the glands are filled with secretions that are a ready source of nutrition and there is a stroma in which the electrolytes are ideally suited for the blastocyst. Before this day conditions are less than optimal. Delay in transit carries the risk that trophoblast development can lead to embedding of the egg in the fallopian tube. The timing of tubal transit is a complex mixture of both anatomic and physiologic factors that are controlled by both the endocrine and the autonomic nervous systems.[11]

## Immunologic Capacity to Destroy Sperm Antibodies and Prevent Antisperm Antibodies from Forming

The female genital tract is exposed to vast numbers of sperm over a period of many years. Following coitus, sperm that are retained are phagocytized by tissue-fixed macrophages and are apparently in some way rendered immunologically incompetent and destroyed.[7-9]

In some women, apparently, this mechanism for rendering sperm immunologically incompetent is in some way defective and the sperm are carried into the reticulo-endothelial system in an immunologically active form; antibodies can then be produced against the sperm. Because sperm are complex structures, antibodies can be produced against different portions of the sperm and not to the whole system. In rare cases, a woman makes antibodies against her husband's sperm and can theoretically become pregnant by donor sperm. The site of action of these antibodies is not clearly known. Franklin and Dukes[22] demonstrated sperm agglutinating antibodies in the serum of otherwise normal women. Tissue-fixed antibodies have been demonstrated within the tissues lining the genital tract by fluorescent antibody methods. Recently, antibodies that fix and immobilize sperm have been found in cervical mucus. However, not all who have antisperm antibodies secrete them in the cervical mucus. The discovery of antisperm antibodies has elicited a great deal of interest, but it is not yet definitely known whether they interfere with sperm transport, with fertilization, or with implantation.

## Disease Processes

The first four physiologic factors touched on above are not amenable to clinical investigation and they are the subject of continued study. There are, however, a number of disease processes involving the reproductive organs that have infertility as one of their consequences. Many of these disorders are covered in greater detail in other chapters in this text. In the male there may be problems related to semen and these can be studied in clinical laboratories.

## The Semen

Semen analysis is best done on a freshly acquired specimen. If it has to be transported, it should be kept in a scrupulously clean container and kept in a pocket close to the thigh to keep it warm. The volume is measured and the viscosity of the specimen recorded; sperm counts, morphologic examination, and motility studies are then done.[23,34,35] The normal volume of semen measures between 2 and 5 ml. Volumes of less than 1 to 2 ml provide inadequate contact with cervical mucous. Volumes of greater than 5 to 6 ml generally are accompanied by significant dilution of the available sperm by large amounts of seminal plasma and, because sperm swim from semen into cervical mucus across an interface, the greater the density of sperm at that interface, the greater the number of sperm that can enter the cervical mucus. Excessively high volumes of semen diminish this by dilution.[17] MacLeod[34,35] has established criteria in evaluating semen and these appear to be valid and unchallenged.

1. *Good semen* has a volume between 2 and 5 ml and contains 60 million or more sperm per milliliter. Sixty percent of cells should show good motility, graded by some as 3 to 4+. At least 80% of the cells should have normal morphology.
2. *Passable semen.* The volume should be between 2 and 5 ml. It should contain 20 to 60 million sperm per milliliter. Forty to 60% of cells should show good motility, graded at 2 to 3+. Sixty to 80% of cells should be of normal morphology.
3. *Subnormal semen.* This is less than 2 ml in volume and contains fewer than 20 million sperm per milliliter. Motility is present in less than 40% of cells with the grading at less than 2+. Fewer than 50% of cells show normal morphology.

## The Vagina

One problem encountered in the vagina is the occasional finding of a rigid hymen that interferes with penetration. This is amenable to surgical correction. Masters and Johnson[38] have reported a vaginal lethal factor that destroys sperm, but this requires further substantiation.

## The Cervix

The cervix and the mucus it produces play an important role in fertility, and abnormalities of the cervix, both anatomic and physiologic,[36,37,40] play an important role in infertility. It is only at the time of ovulation, under the influence of high doses of estrogen, that the cervical mucus becomes what we consider to be healthy, ovulatory mucus. It is clear, copious, watery, acellular, alkaline, and low in antibody content. This cervical mucus demonstrates a high *spinnbarkeit* when stretched and, when allowed to dry, crystallizes in a fern pattern (see Figure 4.4). It is this mucus that provides an excellent medium for sperm viability and, whereas sperm can live for only 4 to 6 hours in the vaginal environment, they have been demonstrated to be alive in cervical mucus for as long as 6 days.[48]

Chronic cervicitis[52] can result in the production of mucus by the endocervical glands that is thick and tenacious and contains inflammatory cells and products of cell degeneration. The pH may be less alkaline and less conducive to sperm survival and motility.[16] Ectropion may be associated with normal mucus production, but there are cases in which the exposed epithelium is traumatized by exposure to vaginal acidity, becomes inflamed, and produces abnormal secretions despite the absence of infection.

Cervical stenosis has too often been given as a cause of infertility. If hematometria is present, it can certainly be regarded as an index of extreme stenosis that conceivably can be a barrier to impregnation. If, in contrast, menstrual blood can flow freely through the cervix, it must be assumed that sperm can readily be transported in the reverse direction. In many cases, examination of an intrauterine postcoital specimen is desirable. If sperm are abundant in the cervical mucus and yet scant or absent in the intrauterine specimen, it can be postulated that an area of scarring or excessive narrowing may be interfering with the quality or production of cervical mucus at that point. Dilatation should be attempted or the area bypassed by homologous insemination techniques. The collection of an intrauterine specimen, when combined with the modification of the traditional Huhner test as proposed by Davagan,[33] provides an excellent means of evaluating the ability of the cervical mucus to facilitate sperm transport. The technique involves aspiration of a column of cervical mucus in a plastic catheter and selective sectioning of the catheter to evaluate the number of sperm at each level.

Because adequate cervical mucus production requires adequate estrogen levels, it may well be that either total estrogen production is too low or, if the patient is taking drugs that exert an antiestrogenic effect, e.g., Clomiphene citrate, the drug may be effective at the level of the cervix as well as other sites, resulting in the production of inadequate mucus. Other factors that may contribute to infertility include cervical polyps, cervical leiomyomata, and synechiae, all of which may interfere with production of adequate mucus.

Retroversion, with the resultant anteriorly pointing cervix, has been regarded in the past as contributing to infertility. Postcoital examinations of intrauterine secretions are usually found to be normal and, therefore, retroversion without fixation is not a factor in infertility.

## Endometrium

It is, of course, imperative to know whether a woman is having normal menstrual cycles.[21] There are some indirect indices, but an endometrial biopsy performed on day 21 in her given cycle should demonstrate glands filled with secretions and an edematous stroma. Some advocate biopsy on day 1 of the menstrual flow, in order to be sure that a pregnancy has not been interrupted. If on the above days proliferative glands and stroma are found, then it can be considered that the patient has not ovulated. This should be rechecked and confirmed because isolated anovulatory cycles can occur. A number of causes for anovulation may reside in the hypothalamus, the anterior lobe of the pituitary gland, or the ovary itself. Curettage may reveal tuberculous endometritis and this is often associated with similar involvement of the fallopian tubes.

There is a condition referred to as Ascherman's syndrome[2,3,53] in which endometrium may be totally denuded and agglutinative synechiae may virtually obliterate the uterine cavity (Figure 35.1). In its most extreme form, patients are amenorrheic and at best hypomenorrheic. Asherman's syndrome may result in infertility. The diagnosis is often made by hysterogram, which demonstrates adhesive bands. A more recent method is called hysteroscopy and involves direct visualization of the uterine cavity by a lens and light system. The uterine cavity is first filled with either a viscous fluid, such as dextran, or a gas, such as carbon dioxide, in order to distend the cavity and allow visualization.

Endometrial polyps rarely interfere with implantation, but there are instances where a large polyp distorts the uterine cavity and interferes with implantation.

Severe endometritis that may be postabortal, postpartum, or associated with an intrauterine device may occlude the cornual end of the fallopian tube because of granula-

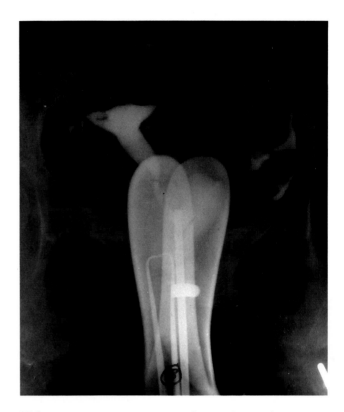

**35.1** Adhesions are present in the uterine cavity.

tion tissue or scar tissue. Occlusion may be total or a flap scar, which acts as a valve over the opening of the tube and which functionally closes an otherwise normal fallopian tube, may be produced.

Leiomyomata can at times result in abortion if they are large and submucus, but rarely do they play a role in inability to conceive.[26,51] Infrequently a large intramural leiomyoma located near the cornu can by compression cause occlusion of this end of the fallopian tube.

Congenital abnormalities, such as uterus didelphys, bicornate uterus, and rudimentary horn, may result in abortion but do not interfere with conception.

## Fallopian Tube

Congenital hypoplasia and atresia are obvious causes of infertility. Extrinsic adhesions caused by manipulative pelvic surgery (Figure 35.2) or following inflammatory reactions in adjacent organs, such as the appendix, may occur. Fimbrial agglutination (Figures 35.3 and 35.4) can result and interfere with ovum pickup and tubal transport. Endosalpingitis (see Chapter 18) can destroy the mucosa

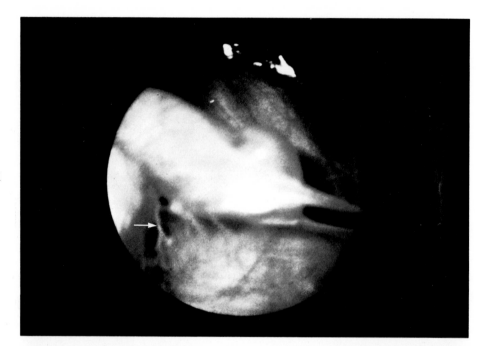

**35.2** Fallopian tube. Laparoscopic view showing adhesions between fimbria and the lateral wall of pelvis (arrow).

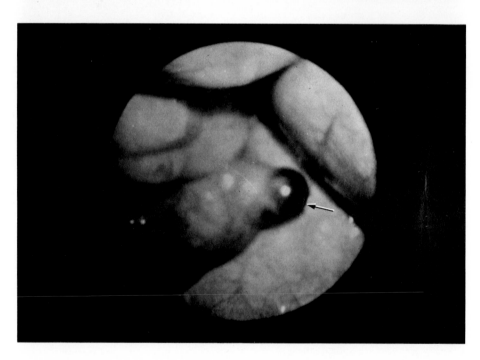

**35.3** Fallopian tube. Laparoscopic view showing retention of dye at site of fimbrial agglutination (arrow).

of the fallopian tube. Infertility or ectopic pregnancy can be the result.

Salpingitis isthmica nodosa (see Chapter 18) may be associated with infertility or, at times, with ectopic pregnancy.

Endometriosis has as its hallmark the production of adhesions, and these may bind tube to ovary and interfere with ovulation and ovum transport.[54]

Diagnostic methods used to study the fallopian tube include tubal insufflation, hysterosalpinography, and endoscopy (culdoscopy or laparoscopy). The finding of both proximal and distal tubal disease rules out the possibility

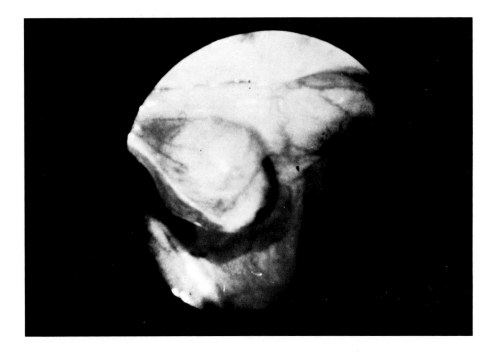

**35.4** Fallopian tube. Laparoscopic view showing hydrosalpinx.

of corrective surgery. Corrective surgery may open the lumen of the fallopian tube but the increased incidence of ectopic pregnancy must be considered in those so treated.

## The Ovary

Pregnancy or the recovery of an ovum from tubal washings are the two absolute indices of ovulation. In clinical practice there is a variety of modalities available to determine whether ovulation has occurred. Regular menstrual cycles, especially if accompanied by breast tenderness and fluid retention, are often an indication that ovulation is preceding monthly bleeding episodes. Physical examination that reveals normally developed secondary sex characteristics at least suggests that estrogen production is present. Basal body temperature studies revealing a biphasic graph, a thermal shift of 0.5°F, and maintenance of temperature elevation for 14 days prior to menstrual flow are an excellent index of ovulation. Temperature graphs that show a luteal phase characterized by a diminished rise, a very slow rise, or one lasting less than 14 days suggest inability of the corpus luteum to adequately produce progesterone and perhaps estrogen.[28,29,47] Endometrial biopsy performed at day 21 or day 1 of menstruation can indicate whether ovulation has occurred. Another observation that is made at times is one in which the glands show

the expected secretory change but the stroma does not. The glands on day 21 or day 1 of menstruation may show uniform subnuclear vacuolation, indicating ovulation but being the endometrium of day 17 in the cycle. These changes are asynchronous, and the fault usually lies in the corpus luteum (Figures 35.5 and 35.6).

Hormone assays for serum estrogen, progesterone, luteinizing hormone (LH), and follicle-stimulating hormone (FSH) can now be accurately and readily assayed by radioimmunoassay. Coupled with urinary pregnendiol levels, these assays can give an accurate view of the endocrine events preceding and after ovulation.

Hypothalamic FSH and LH releasing factors have now been isolated. Their role in the hypothalamic–pituitary–ovary axis is discussed in Chapter 9.

Peri ovarian adhesions may interfere with the ability of the fallopian tube to pick up the ovum following ovulation.[15] At times, surgical removal of the adhesions overcomes this problem.

### Polycystic ovaries

Infertility is one of the complaints associated with the entity known as the Stein–Leventhal syndrome (see Chapter 21). The etiology of this disease is not clearly understood, but at least a contributing factor lies within the ovary because surgical manipulation or wedge resection often results in ovulation and subsequent pregnancy. Med-

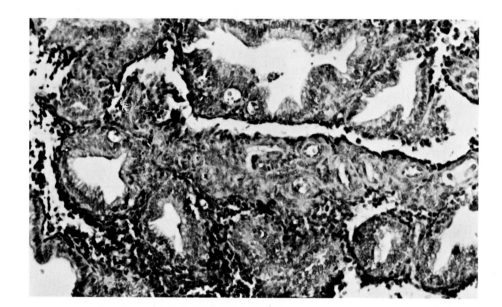

**35.5** Inadequate luteal phase. Glands are day 19 in type. Stroma is compact, now deciduoid.

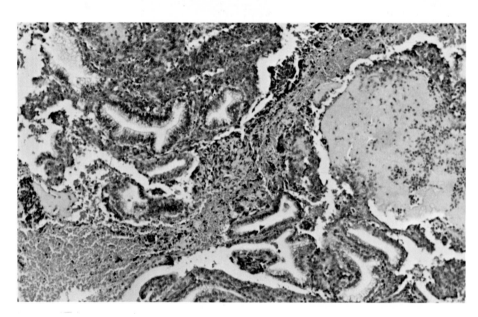

**35.6** Inadequate luteal phase. Sloughing of endometrium at day 19, caused by inadequate corpus luteum that involutes prematurely.

ical management, using injections of an antiestrogen, Clomiphene, may also trigger ovulation that may be followed by successful pregnancy.

The mechanism whereby Clomiphene works is by binding of this substance in the nuclei of cells in the hypothalamus and anterior lobe of the pituitary. Clomiphene occupies estrogen-binding sites and presumably increases FSH releasing factor in the hypothalamus and FSH production in the anterior lobe of the pituitary gland. LH activity rises and ovulation occurs. In some patients, in whom wedge resection does not result in ovulation, the addition of Clomiphene may in combination result in ovulation. Similarly, if medical management with Clomiphene does not suffice, the addition of wedge resection may do so.

## Endometriosis of the Ovary

Endometriosis can interfere with ovarian function in two ways: by producing periovarian adhesions and interfering with ovum pickup and by expansion of an endometrioma interfering with corpus luteum function, result-

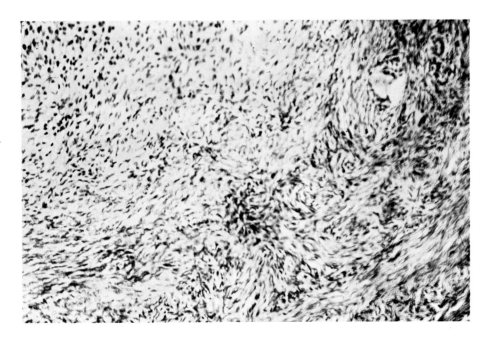

**35.7** Premature ovarian failure. The cortex of the ovary is devoid of follicles or corpora lutea. In the upper right hand corner there is one atretic follicle.

ing in an inadequate luteal phase.[31] The extent of the disease (see Chapter 22) and the degree of adhesions determine what can be done in any given case. There is a new experimental drug, Danazol,[20] that is an inhibitor of gonadotropin activity, peripherally producing a marked, if not total, decrease in ovarian estrogen and progesterone production. Involution of endometrial implants occurs. If the disease is not extensive and is treated early in its development, this drug may be useful. Progestins[32] and methyl testosterone[19] have also been used.

## Gonadal Dysgenesis

Turner's syndrome and testicular feminization are associated with infertility. They are discussed in Chapter 23 in greater detail.

## Premature Ovarian Failure

Ovarian function normally terminates between the ages of 40 and 55 years, with recent data by Blaustein and Shenker[13] suggesting that there is an increase in the number of females that are ovulating longer. In rare instances ovarian function ceases unusually early and is referred to as premature ovarian failure.[6,46] There is no uniform agreement concerning the age at onset other than under the age of 40 years. Some gynecologists accept 30 to 35 years of age as the upper age limit. The clinical history is usually one in which menarche has been normal and the patient exhibits normal secondary sexual characteristics; some patients have had a number of children prior to onset. At some early age amenorrhea may develop or follow oligomenorrhea. The amenorrhea then persists. Serum gonadotropin levels are elevated and remain so. Ovarian biopsy shows normal stroma with few primordial follicles and atretic follicles (Figure 35.7). There have been some cases reported that fit all criteria of premature ovarian failure, in which ovarian biopsy reveals follicles in varying stages of maturation. This is similar to that seen in hypogonadotropic amenorrhea; however, in these cases there is no response to high doses of gonadotropins. Starup and Sele[50] suggest the possibility of an autoimmune reaction in these patients with production of antigonadotropins. Conclusive proof of this phenomenon remains to be demonstrated. There is no single etiologic agent associated with premature ovarian failure. Some cases of Turner's syndrome showing mosaicism have some germ cells in the gonads, and they may ovulate and mestruate but may develop premature ovarian failure, usually during adolescence. The use of irradiation[42] and chemotherapeutic agents in the treatment of lymphomata and neoplasms can result in accelerated follicular atresia and destruction of germ cells. Another possible mechanism involves autoimmunity.[27,30,41,45] Irvine, Chan, and Scarth[27] have demonstrated four clearly distinct immunofluorescent patterns in the corpus luteum of human ovaries when sections of these ovaries are incubated with sera from patients with Addison's disease who have developed premature menopause. The varying staining patterns suggested that there were a multiplicity of antibodies reacting with different antigens in the ovary. The antibodies appeared to be directed against steroid-producing cells. Antibodies were also demonstrated in the adrenal cortex, and they cross-reacted with human corpus luteum. Some cases were found in which there were antibodies to theca interna cells. Recently, Ruehson et al.[45] reported cytoplasmic antibodies in theca and lutein cells in eight patients in a group of 16 cases of premature ovarian failure. They demonstrated ovarian antinuclear antibodies in a ninth patient and in one case of luteal defect. A high incidence of autoantibodies to other tissue antigens was found in a patient with complete ovarian failure, even in the absence of overt immune disorders. These authors postulated an as yet undefined, generalized autoimmune diathesis as one factor in the development of some cases of premature menopause.

The diagnosis of premature ovarian failure may be extremely difficult to establish. The symptomatology, with the exception of the occurrences of hot flushes, is similar to that in secondary hypogonadism caused by pituitary failure. Hot flushes were present in 90% in the series of Ruehson and Jones.[46] However, these authors caution that the flushes are not pathognomic of ovarian failure. Elevated urinary gonadotropins is the most helpful test in the differential diagnosis, but it can, on occasion, give misleading information. Patients may have oscillating levels, and some who have had high levels have proved not to have ovarian failure.

Laparotomy and ovarian biopsy for histopathologic study are indicated if the clinical investigation fails to classify the etiology of amenorrhea. Endoscopic visualization alone cannot differentiate between primary and secondary ovarian failure.

# REFERENCES

1. Addams, C. E., and Chang, M. D. Capacitation of rabbit spermatozoa in the fallopian tube and in the uterus. *J. Exp. Zool.* 151:159, 1962.

2. Asherman, J. G. Amenorrhea traumatica. *J. Obstet. Gynaecol. Br. Emp.* 55:23, 1948.

3. Asherman, J. G. Uterine synechiae. *Bull. Fed. Gynaecol. Obstet. Fran.* 9:490, 1957.

4. Austin, C. R. Observations on the penetration of the sperm into the mammalian egg. *Aust. J. Sci. Res.* 4:581, 1951.

5. Austin, C. R. The capacitation of mammalian sperm. *Nature* (London) 170:326, 1952.

6. Baramki, T. A., and Jones, H. W. Jr. Early premature menopause. *Am. J. Obstet. Gynecol.* 96:990, 1966.

7. Behrman, S. J. Agglutinins, antibodies, and immune reactions. *Clin. Obstet. Gynecol.* 8:91, 1965.

8. Behrman, S. J. *Immunologic Aspects of Fertility and Infertility in Agents Affecting Fertility.* (Biological Council Symposium) London, Churchill, 1965, p. 47.

9. Behrman, S. J. Immunologic phenomenon in infertility: Some clinical applications. *Harper Hosp. Bull.* 24:147, 1966.

10. Bishop, D. W. Metabolic conditions within the oviduct of the rabbit. *Int. J. Fertil.* 2:11, 1957.

11. Black, D. L., and Asdell, S. A. Transport to the rabbit oviduct. *Am. J. Physiol.* 192:63, 1958.

12. Black, D. L., and Asdell, S. A. Mechanism controlling the entry of ova into the rabbit uterus. *Am. J. Physiol.* 197:1275, 1959.

13. Blaustein, A., and Shenker, L. Data to be published, 1975.

14. Brackett, B. G., and Williams, W. L. *In vitro* fertilization of rabbit ova. *J. Exp. Zool.* 160:277, 1965.

15. Burdick, H. O., Whitney, R., and Emerson, B. Observations on the transport of tubal ova. *Endocrinology* 31:100, 1942.

16. Buxton, C. L., and Wong, A. S. H. Spermicidal bacteria in the cervix as a cause of sterility. *Am. J. Obstet. Gynecol.* 64:628, 1952.

17. Chang, M. C. A detrimental effect of seminal plasma of the fertilizing capacity of sperm. *Nature* (London) 285:258, 1957.

18. Clewe, T. H., and Mastroianni, L. Jr. Mechanisms of ovum pick up: One functional capacity of rabbit oviducts ligated near the fimbria. *Fertil. Steril.* 9:13, 1958.

19. Creadick, R. N. Non-surgical treatment of endometriosis—A preliminary report on the use of methyl testosterone. *N.C. Med. J.* 11:576, 1950.

20. Dmowski, W. P., and Cohen, M. R. Treatment of endometriosis with an antigonadotrophin, Danazol. *Obstet. Gynecol.* 46:147, 1975.

21. Foss, B. A., Horne, H. W. Jr., and Hertig, A. T. The endometrium and sterility. *Fertil. Steril.* 9:193, 1958.

22. Franklin, R., and Dukes, C. D. Anti spermatozoa antibody and unexplained infertility. *Am. J. Obstet. Gynecol.* 89:6, 1964.

23. Freund, M. Standards for the rating of human sperm morphology—A cooperative study. *Int. J. Fertil.* (Suppl.) 11:97, 1966.

24. Greenwald, G. S. A study of the transport of ova through the rabbit oviduct. *Fertil. Steril.* 12:80, 1961.

25. Gregoire, A. T., Gongsaldi, D., and Rakoff, A. E. The amino acid content of female rabbit genital tract. *Fertil. Steril.* 12:322, 1961.

26. Ingersall, F. M. Fertility following myomectomy. *Fertil. Steril.* 14:596, 1963.

27. Irvine, W. J., Chan, M. W., and Scarth, L. The further characterization of auto-antibodies reactive with extra-adrenal steroid-producing cells in patients with adrenal disorders. *Clin. Exp. Immunol.* 4:489, 1969.

28. Jones, G. E. S. Luteal phase defects. In Behrman, S. J. and Kistner, R. W., eds. *Progress in Infertility.* Boston, Little Brown, 1968, p. 299.

29. Jones, G. E. S., Woodruff, D. J., and Moszkowskie. The inadequate luteal phase. *Am. J. Obstet. Gynecol.* 83:363, 1962.

30. Jones, H. W. Jr., Ferguson-Smith, M. A., and Heller, R. H. The pathology and cytogenetics of gonadal agenesis. *Am. J. Obstet. Gynecol.* 87:578, 1963.

31. Karnaky, J. K. Endometriosis. *In* Conn, H. T., ed. *Current Therapy.* Philadelphia, W. B. Saunders, 1957, p. 676.

32. Kistner, R. W. New progestins in the treatment of endometriosis. *Am. J. Obstet. Gynecol. 75:*264, 1958.

33. Kunitake, G., and Davagan, V. A new method of evaluating infertility due to cervical mucous spermatazoa incompatibility. *Fertil. Steril. 21:*706, 1970.

34. MacLeod, J. Semen quality in 1,000 men of known fertility and in 800 cases of infertile marriage. *Fertil. Steril. 2:*115, 1951.

35. MacLeod, J. The semen examination. *Clin. Obstet. Gynecol. 8:*115, 1965.

36. Marcus, C. C., and Marcus, S. L. The cervical factor in infertility. *Clin. Obstet. Gynecol. 8:*15, 1965.

37. Marcus, S. L., and Marcus, C. C. Cervical mucous and its relation to infertility. *Obstet. Gynecol. Surv. 18:*749, 1963.

38. Masters, W. H., and Johnson, V. E. *Human Sexual Response.* Boston, Little, Brown, 1966, p. 97.

39. Moghiissi, K. S., Dabich, D., Levine, J., and Neuhaus, O. W. Mechanism of sperm migration. *Fertil. Steril. 15:*15, 1964.

40. Moghissi, K. S., and Neuhaus, O. W. Composition and properties of human cervical mucous. *Am. J. Obstet. Gynecol. 83:*149, 1962.

41. Moraes-Ruehsen, M., and Jones, G. S. Premature ovarian failure. *Acta Obstet. Gynecol. Scand. 52:*259, 1973.

42. Nathanson, I. T., Rice, C., and Meigs, J. V. Hormone studies in artificial menopause produced by roentgen rays. *Am. J. Obstet. Gynecol. 40:*935, 1940.

43. Noyes, R. W. The capacitation of rabbit spermatozoa. *J. Endocrinol. 17:*374, 1958.

44. Noyes, R. W., and Addams, C. E. The transport of spermatozoa into the uterus of the rabbit. *Fertil. Steril. 9:*288, 1958.

45. Ruehson, M. de M., Blizzard, R. M., Garcia-Bunuel, R., and Jones, G. E. S. Auto-immunity and ovarian failure. *Am. J. Obstet. Gynecol. 112:*693, 1972.

46. Ruehson, M. de M., and Jones, G. E. S. Premature ovarian failure. *Fertil. Steril. 18:*440, 1967.

47. Ruehson, M. de M., Jones, G. E. S., Burnett, L. S., and Baramki, T. S. The Aluteal Cycle: A severe form of the luteal phase deficit. *Am. J. Obstet. Gynecol. 103:*1059, 1969.

48. Sobrero, A. J., and MacLeod, J. The immediate post coital test. *Fertil. Steril. 13:*184, 1962.

49. Soupart, P., and Clewe, T. H. Sperm penetration of rabbit zona pellucida inhibited by treatment of ova with neuraminidase. *Fertil. Steril. 16:*677, 1965.

50. Starup, J., and Sele, V. Premature ovarian failure. *Acta Obstet. Gynecol. 52:*259, 1973.

51. Stevenson, C. S. Myomectomy for improvement of fertility. *Fertil. Steril. 15:*367, 1964.

52. Sweeney, W. J. Inflammations in infertility, *in Progress in Infertility.* Boston, Little Brown, 1968, p. 239.

53. Sweeney, W. J. Intrauterine synnechiae. *Obstet. Gynecol. 27:*284, 1966.

54. Westmon, A. Studies of the function of the fallopian tube. *Int J. Fertil. 4:*201, 1949.

55. Zamboni, L, Hongsanand, C. H., and Mastroianni, L. Jr. Influence of tubal secretions on rabbit tubal ova. *Fertil. Steril. 16:*177, 1965.

Felix de Narvaez, M.D.,
and Rita Blaustein, M.D.

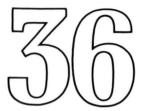

# Cytology of the Female Genital Tract

## General Discussion

Diagnostic cytology is based on the fact that cells exfoliated or collected from the cervix and the vagina reflect features of the tissue from which they arise. The main application of cytology to the female genital tract is in the early diagnosis of precancerous and cancerous lesions. Patients who have been treated for cervical cancer can be followed cytologically for response to radiation and recurrence of the disease.

Assessment of hormonal function is possible if the specimen is obtained properly and if the limitations of cytology are understood by the cytologist and the clinician.

## Normal Components of the Routine Gynecologic Smear

### Epithelial Cells

The components of a smear are related to age, phase of the menstrual cycle, such exogenous influences as inflammation or therapy, and the site from which the material is obtained.[15] The term "normal," therefore, carries the connotation of "compatible with the clinical data." An atrophic smear in a 70-year-old female is compatible with her age. An atrophic smear in a 20-year-old is not compat-

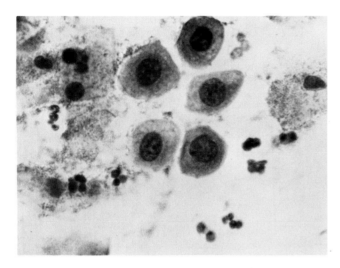

**36.1** Parabasal cells. These small, round, or oval squamous cells have opaque cytoplasm and vesicular nuclei. The nucleocytoplasmic ratio is high. Occasionally they may show cytoplasmic tails. In children and some postmenopausal women, they may constitute the predominant or sole epithelial cell.

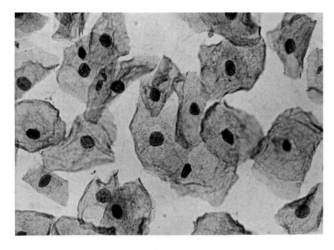

**36.2** Intermediate cells. This group of intermediate cells shows the vesicular nuclei and transparent, abundant cytoplasm that characterize them. Many of the cells show folding of the cytoplasm.

ible with her age. Yet both smears contain "normal" parabasal cells.

The most prominent epithelial cells of the routine cervical–vaginal smear are squamous cells originating from the pars vaginalis of the cervix and from the vagina. Essentially there are three types of cells to be identified.

The parabasal cells (Figure 36.1), as their name implies, originate from the zone immediately above the basal layer of the stratum germinativum. They are round or oval and small, ranging in size from 12 to 30 $\mu$. Their cytoplasm is opaque and usually basophilic and may show vacuolization. Occasionally, when they present in a group, tails of cytoplasm may be seen. The nucleus is round and vesicular; the nucleocytoplasmic ratio is high.

The intermediate cells (Figure 36.2) are polygonal and their cytoplasm is transparent and usually basophilic, but it can be eosinophilic. They are large, measuring up to 50 $\mu$. The nucleus is centrally located and the chromatin is finely distributed, producing a vesicular pattern. Navicular cells are glycogen-containing intermediate cells that characteristically show folding and rolling of their cytoplasmic borders and areas of yellow-orange staining (Papanicolaou stain technique).

The superficial cells (Figure 36.3) originate from the outermost layers of the epithelium. They are large, polyhedral, flat, and waferlike but occasionally may be rolled and appear thin and elongated. The cytoplasm is usually eosinophilic but can be basophilic; it may contain very small, dark granules, so-called keratohyaline granules. The nucleus is small, measuring less than 6 $\mu$ in diameter, with no discernible nuclear structure. This is the "ink dot," karyopyknotic nucleus characteristic of the superficial cell. It is this pyknosis of the nucleus that distinguishes the superficial cell from the large intermediate cell.

In addition to the three types of cells described above, two other types of squamous cells may be noted. If procidentia is present, anucleated and keratinized cells may appear in the smear as flat, orange-staining squamous cells. They may contain a pyknotic nucleus or the nucleus may be absent.[17]

Basal cells may sometimes be seen in a smear, as the result of inflammation or trauma. They are uniform in size, are rounded, and show densely basophilic, opaque cytoplasm. The nuclei appear hyperchromatic and the nucleocytoplasmic ratio is high. It is important to recognize the benign nature of these cells and not confuse them with malignant cervical cells, which may also exhibit nuclear hyperchromatism and a high nucleocytoplasmic ratio. The basal cells display a uniformity of appearance that the malignant cells lack.

The endocervical cells (Figures 36.4 and 36.5) appear as tall columnar cells arranged usually in characteristic groupings, either in parallel rows or, in cross section, forming a honeycomb pattern with clearly defined cell borders. Individual columnar cells are basophilic and their nuclei are basal in position. At the free or luminal edge of

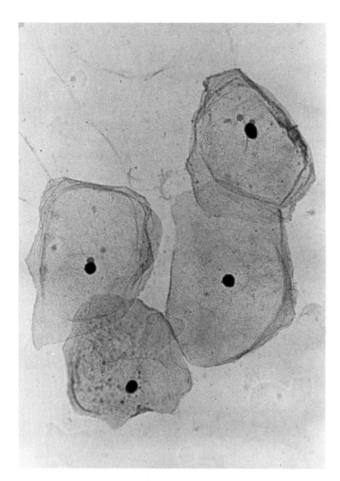

**36.3** Superficial cells. A pyknotic nucleus and abundant, transparent cytoplasm are the characteristics of these large, polyhedral cells. Keratohyalin granules are prominent in the cell at the lower right corner.

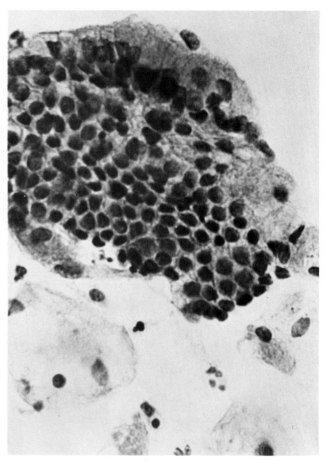

**36.4** Endocervical cells. This sheet of endocervical cells shows both the characteristic "picket fence" arrangement of columnar cells (left border of group) and the "honeycomb" arrangement, wherein the cell borders can be discerned and adequate cytoplasm surrounds each nucleus.

the cell, pink-staining cilia and a terminal bar can occasionally be identified (Papanicolaou stain). The nuclei of these cells are vesicular, round or oval in shape, and they can show considerable variation in size. Small nucleoli may be present. Evidence of secretory activity, in the form of cytoplasmic vacuoles and flattening of a nuclear border, is common. During the height of estrogenic stimulation, a nipplelike nuclear protrusion may be seen.

The endometrial cells are smaller than endocervical cells and when single are difficult to detect in the cervical-vaginal smear. Endometrial cells, occurring as cell balls or clusters (Figure 36.6), can be seen from day 1 to days 10 to 12. These cells usually exhibit a marked degree of degeneration and necrosis. The appearance of endometrial cells in

the cervical–vaginal smear at times other than the first half of the menstrual cycle is abnormal and requires further evaluation, whether the cells show atypia or not.[18]

## Nonepithelial Components of the Smear

Histiocytes are often found in the normal smear.[18] Small histiocytes (Figure 36.7), singly or in clusters, are normally seen during the "exodus" phase, occurring during the first 10 days after menstruation. Their cytoplasm is finely vacuolated or foamy and may contain phagocytosed particulate matter, cellular debris, and blood cells. Larger histiocytes and multinucleated giant cells can measure in excess of $100\,\mu$. Histiocytes frequently exhibit kidney-

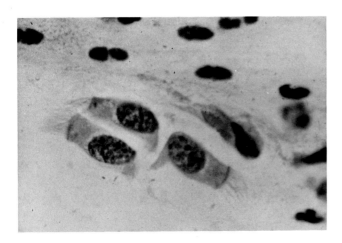

**36.5** Endocervical cells. Cilia and terminal plates are clearly seen. The chromatin is somewhat coarse but it is distributed uniformly in all of the endocervical cells present.

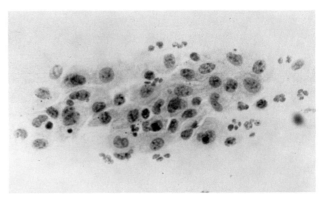

**36.7** Histiocytes. A loosely arranged group of small histiocytes with foamy cytoplasm and poorly delineated cell borders is seen. There is nuclear pleomorphism but the chromatin pattern is quite uniform from cell to cell. Several of the histiocytes exhibit reniform nuclei.

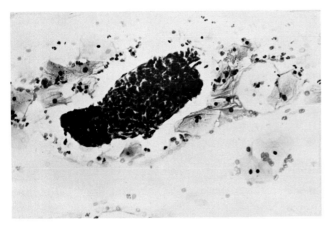

**36.6** Endometrial cells, day 8 of the menstrual cycle. Against a background of superficial and intermediate cells and polymorphonuclear leukocytes, a cluster of overlapping and partly degenerated endometrial cells is seen. The presence of clusters of endometrial cells up to the tenth to twelfth day of the cycle is a normal finding.

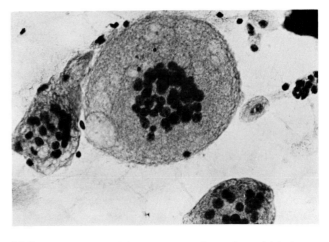

**36.8** Multinucleated histiocyte. Multinucleated histiocytes must be distinguished from multinucleated malignant cells. Typically, the multiple nuclei of histiocytes resemble each other, whereas in the malignant cell, there is marked variation from nucleus to nucleus, in chromatin distribution, hyperchromasia, size, and shape.

shaped nuclei with fine or coarse well-distributed chromatin and occasionally karyosomes. Multinucleated histiocytes (Figure 36.8) must be distinguished from multinucleated malignant cells. Characteristically the multiple nuclei of histiocytes resemble each other, whereas in multinucleated malignant cells there is marked variation from nucleus to nucleus.

Erythrocytes are often seen in the cervical–vaginal smear

at times other than menstrual. Frequently their presence results from slight trauma during gynecologic exploration or from energetic cervical scraping. When bleeding is profuse or the blood is lyzed, the possibility of a pathologic process should be kept in mind.

The presence of a somewhat increased number of leukocytes just prior to or after menstruation is physiologic. With the Papanicolaou stain, it is not possible to distin-

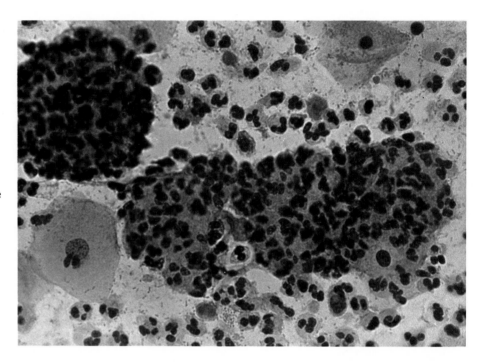

**36.9** Inflammatory exudate. Large numbers of polymorpho-nuclear leukocytes are present, as well as bacteria and cellular debris. When the exudate is so dense as to obscure the epithelial elements, the smear must be considered unsatisfactory and a repeat smear, after the inflammation has cleared, should be requested.

guish the several types of leukocytes because cytoplasmic granules do not stain.

Spermatozoa can be seen in the smear after coitus, often permitting a good evaluation of their morphology.

Powder from surgical gloves, a variety of crystals from unfiltered stains and fixatives, cotton fibers, and pollen granules are frequent contaminants of the smear. Lubricant and anticonceptual jellies produce a deep blue haze so dense at times that they may obscure the cellular components of the smear, thus rendering the material unsatisfactory for evaluation.

## Nonmalignant Disorders

Cytologic atypias are alterations of the normal structure of the squamous and columnar epithelia, resulting in slight departure of the component cells from their normal prototypes. Infection, trauma, and chemical and physical stimuli may produce defensive, destructive, and reparative reactions[18] in the epithelium of the vagina and cervix. The intensity and specificity of this reaction may vary in relation to the agent and the intensity and duration of the stimulus. Most of these benign cellular atypias are nonspecific. However, at times, the alterations may be specific enough to permit a presumptive cytologic diagnosis.

The presence of a few inflammatory cells in the smear does not necessarily reflect a pathologic condition, particularly when the inflammatory cells are seen immediately preceding, during, or immediately following menstruation. During acute or chronic inflammation, there is usually an increased desquamation of epithelial cells, abundant production of mucus, and varying numbers of leukocytes and histiocytes. The inflammatory exudate (Figure 36.9) may be so dense as to obscure the presence of the epithelial elements. When this occurs, the smear may be considered unsatisfactory for reliable evaluation and a repeat smear, after the inflammation has cleared, should be requested.

In response to inflammation, the epithelial elements may exhibit changes in the overall cellular pattern and also in alterations within the individual cells.[27]

### Changes in Cellular Pattern

The proportions of parabasal, intermediate, and superficial cells can be altered by inflammation. The general effect is a wider distribution of the three cell types. In a postmenopausal patient whose smear prior to the occurrence of the inflammation has revealed parabasal cells exclusively, parabasal, intermediate, and superficial cells may all be present simultaneously in varying proportions. Similarly, parabasal cells may appear in the smear of a woman in the childbearing age where previously only superficial and intermediate cells have been expected.

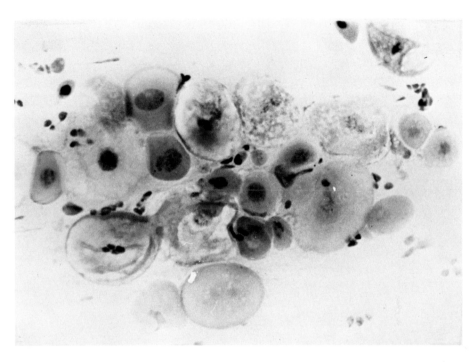

**36.10** Benign atypia. This group of epithelial cells shows cytoplasmic preservation and considerable variation in size and shape. Several nuclei are moderately hyperchromatic, whereas others have undergone karyolysis. Some nuclei show karyorrhexis. The benign nature of these cells is apparent, however, if the even distribution of chromatin within any given intact nucleus and the maintenance of the nucleocytoplasm ratio is noted.

Because inflammation can alter the characteristic cytologic patterns that are associated with normal physiologic changes from birth to the postmenopausal phase, hormonal assessment should not be undertaken on a smear in which an inflammatory process is noted.

## Changes within Epithelial Cells

The epithelial cells may exhibit changes in both nucleus and cytoplasm. The importance of recognizing inflammation-associated changes is twofold: It enables the cytologist to report to the physician the presence of inflammation, often identifying the offending agent, and it enables the cytologist to differentiate between benign abnormalities and malignant changes.

Nucleopyknosis, which is normal in superficial cells, may occur in intermediate and parabasal cells in the presence of inflammation. Some nuclei may exhibit karyorrhexis, (Figure 36.10), the condensation of chromatin into coarse, rounded, darkly staining masses around the periphery of the nucleus. This change must be distinguished from the irregular, coarse, often angular clumping of chromatin that is the most reliable evidence of malignancy. Some nuclei may undergo karyolysis. Nuclear enlargement, binucleation, some coarsening of the chromatin, and hyperchromatism can also be seen with

inflammation. Occasionally a small nucleolus may appear in the nucleus of squamous cells.

Degenerative changes within the cytoplasm may include a poorly defined cell border that is ragged, changes in the staining reaction to an eosinophilic or polychromatia, and the appearance of coarse vacuoles.

In columnar cells of the endocervix, nuclei can show considerable variation in size but usually exhibit a uniformity from nucleus to nucleus in chromatin pattern and in shape. The nucleolus may be more prominent. Multinucleation may be seen; perinuclear vacuolation may also occur. Denuded nuclei are common, and although these nuclei may vary considerably in size, they are usually uniform in shape and chromatin distribution (Figure 36.11).

Cytolysis (Figure 36.12) of intermediate cells by the enzymes of the Döderlein bacilli—a heterogeneous group of lactobacilli—is seen in those situations where intermediate cells predominate, such as pregnancy, the premenarche, or the second half of the menstrual cycle.

## Squamous Metaplasia

Squamous metaplasia (Figures 36.13 and 36.14), another nonmalignant change often encountered in smears from the cervix, may accompany inflammation. It can also be found in cervices where no evidence of inflammation is

**36.11** Acute cervicitis. A group of endocervical cells shows changes caused by inflammation. There are large intracytoplasmic vacuoles, which have pushed the nucleus toward the periphery in some of the cells. Perinuclear halos are visible. The individual cells retain abundant cytoplasm. Polymorphonuclear leukocytes are present. These cellular changes should not be confused with endocervical malignancy. The nuclear chromatin pattern remains uniform and no prominent nucleoli are present.

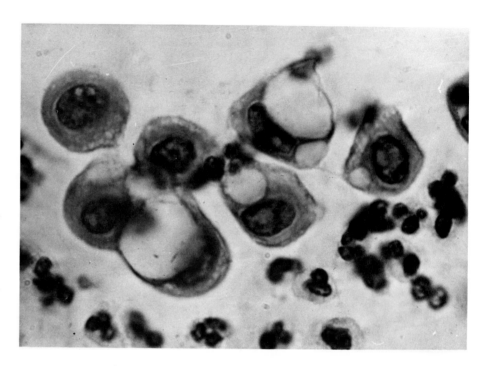

**36.12** Cytolysis. Denuded nuclei, fragments of cytoplasm, and large numbers of Döderlein bacilli are present. In the smear from a pregnant woman, cytolysis of intermediate cells can be marked. In an atrophic smear, the parabasal cells may also exhibit cytolysis and numerous denuded nuclei are present.

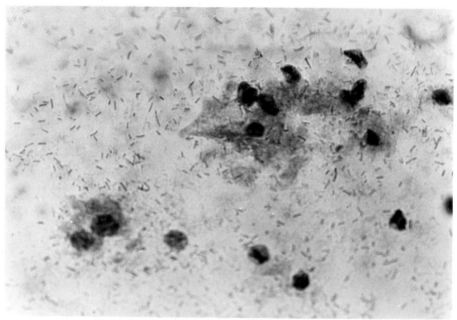

discernible. Koss[15] has defined metaplasia as "the replacement of one type of epithelium by another that is not normally present in a given location." He goes on to explain that "the basis of the process is the ability of the germinative or reserve cells of the endocervix to produce either the typical columnar glandular epithelium or, under abnormal circumstances, squamous epithelium."[15] The metaplastic cells may appear in cervical smears as sheets of elongated and angular cells, often with finely vacuolated cytoplasm. The nuclei are uniformly ovoid, with a delicate

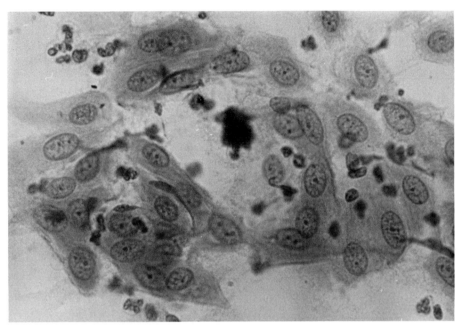

**36.13** Squamous metaplasia. This sheet of elongated cells with vacuolated cytoplasm and large vesicular nuclei represents squamous metaplasia of the reserve cells in the endocervical epithelium. Note the prominent nucleoli. Some inflammatory cells are also present.

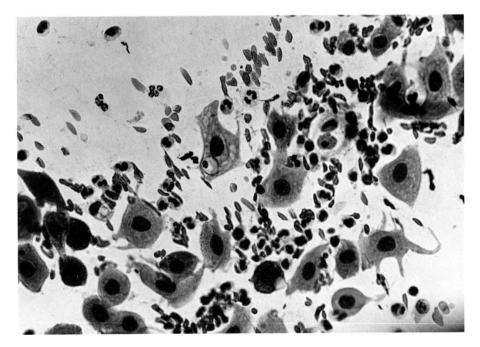

**36.14** Squamous metaplasia. This is a group of metaplastic cells, comparable in size to parabasal cells, with cytoplasm showing some vacuolation. Attenuated tabs of cytoplasm are prominent.

chromatin network and often prominent nucleoli. At times, metaplastic cells (Figure 36.14) may present as a group, comparable in size to parabasal cells, with opaque cytoplasm that shows some vacuolation and occasional infiltration by polymorphonuclear leukocytes. Attenuated tails of cytoplasm are common.

## Specific Inflammations

Bacteria are common components of smears from the cervix and vagina; their presence does not necessarily signify the presence of infection. Coccoid bacteria may be present in large numbers but specific identification can

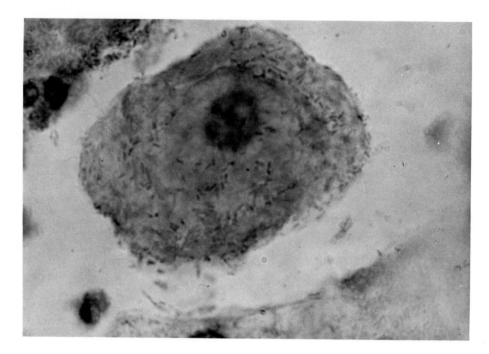

**36.15** "Clue" cell. This large squamous cell is covered with numerous small rods of *Hemophilus vaginalis,* an organism that is responsible for some instances of vaginitis.

only be made by culture. Among the rod forms, *Escherichia coli* is often implicated in the vaginitis of girls and postmenopausal women. *Hemophilus vaginalis (Corynebacterium vaginale),* as the causative agent in some cases of vaginitis, may be suspected when epithelial cells covered by numerous rods are observed. These cells have been tagged "clue" cells (Figure 36.15).

Three specific etiologic agents that are important clinically and that allow for cytologic diagnosis merit special consideration are:

1. *Trichomonas vaginalis,* a parasite
2. *Monilia (Candida albicans),* a fungus
3. *Herpes simplex,* a viral infection

### Trichomonas vaginalis

Cervicitis and vaginitis caused by *Trichomonas vaginalis* is a common clinical occurrence. In the Papanicolaou-stained smear, the protozoa appear as nonmotile, oval, or pear-shaped structures and range in size from a small histiocyte to that of a parabasal cell. The flagella are rarely discernible; therefore, the proper identification of the organism is accomplished by the identification of the small eccentric pale-staining nucleus. Tiny eosinophilic granules are often discernible in the cytoplasm.

In some cases, numerous well-preserved trichomonads (Figure 36.16a) can be seen in the smear, with no discernible inflammatory reaction or cellular atypia. Usually, however, in cases of trichomonal cervicovaginitis the presence of the organism is accompanied by abundant epithelial desquamation, inflammatory exudate, and epithelial atypia. The atypia may be seen in both the squamous and the columnar cells, which show cytolysis, nuclear enlargement, perinuclear "halos," and eosinophilia of the cytoplasm. At times trichomonads are seen parasitizing superficial squamous cells. Vacuolated parabasal cells, either from areas of ulceration or from metaplasia, may be numerous (Figure 36.16b).

### Monilia

The fungus *Candida albicans* appears in smears as long eosinophilic filaments or hyphae and small conidia or yeast bodies (Figure 36.17). Degeneration of polymorphonuclear leukocytes is often striking.

### Herpes simplex

The cytologic findings in *Herpes simplex*[12] are very characteristic. In the early phase of the infection, there is a striking enlargement of the nucleus of the squamous cells, with a "ground-glass" appearance. Multinucleation occurs with a molding of adjacent nuclei (Figure 36.18). The cytoplasm also enlarges, producing very large cells. In

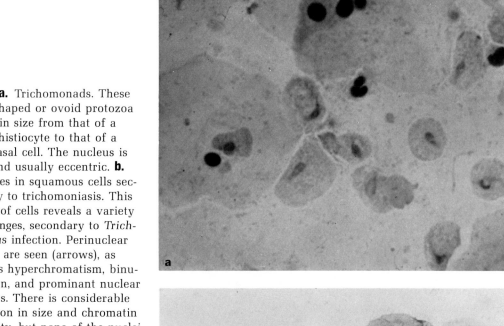

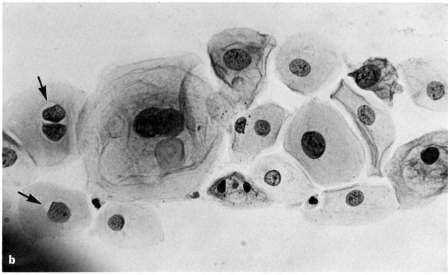

**36.16 a.** Trichomonads. These pear-shaped or ovoid protozoa range in size from that of a small histiocyte to that of a parabasal cell. The nucleus is tiny and usually eccentric. **b.** Changes in squamous cells secondary to trichomoniasis. This group of cells reveals a variety of changes, secondary to *Trichomonas* infection. Perinuclear haloes are seen (arrows), as well as hyperchromatism, binucleation, and prominent nuclear borders. There is considerable variation in size and chromatin intensity, but none of the nuclei exhibits the strikingly abnormal distribution of chromatin seen in malignant cells. The changes seen in this slide are compatible with the diagnosis of "benign atypia."

recurrent herpes, large inclusions (Figure 36.19) may be seen within the nucleus. They are larger than nucleoli and lack the smooth, rounded outline of a nucleolus. A clear "halo" around the inclusion is usually evident.

Genital herpes inflammations[12] are self-limited. Their importance, from a clinical standpoint, is that the virus may be transmitted to the newborn during delivery if the mother has contracted a herpetic infection near term. The infant may develop fatal encephalitis and meningitis. De-

livery by cesarean section provides a viable alternative and a viable infant.

### Other agents

Aberrant genital vaccinia has been described following vaccination or by contact contamination. Cytologic diagnosis depends on the finding of large, eosinophilic, intracytoplasmic inclusions.[12]

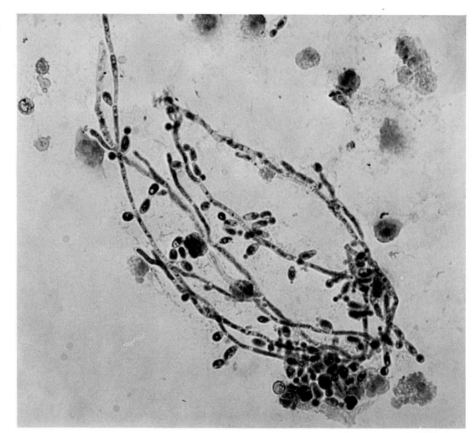

**36.17** *Candida albicans* and trichomonads. Both hyphae and conidia are present in this slide. The hyphae are eosinophilic filaments; the conidia appear as small ovoid structures. Trichomonads are also present, a not uncommon combination of pathogens in the lower genital tract.

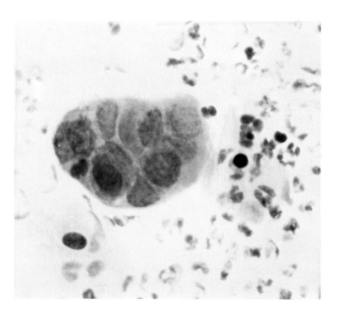

**36.18** *Herpes vaginitis.* A large, multinucleated epithelial cell showing characteristic molding of adjacent nuclei is seen.

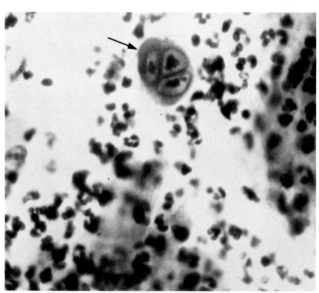

**36.19** *Herpes vaginitis.* Against a background of inflammatory cells, an epithelial cell with several nuclei is visible. There are intranuclear inclusions (arrow), each of which is surrounded by a "halo."

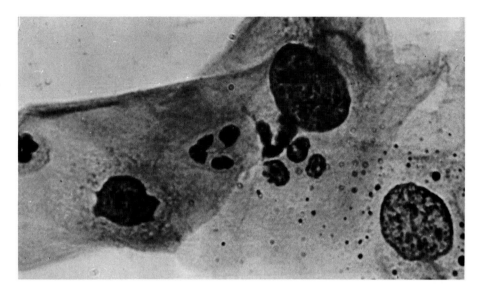

**36.20** Mild dysplasia, dyskaryosis. These squamous cells exhibit abnormal morphology within the nucleus, including chromatin clumping, irregular thickening of the nuclear membrane, and hyperchromatism. The cytoplasm, however, is abundant; the nucleocytoplasmic ratio is low.

In the detection of cytomegalovirus infection,[12] a prominent, single, basophilic intranuclear inclusion surrounded by a clear halo is sought. The term "owl eye" has been given to this finding.

With adenovirus infection,[12] multiple intranuclear inclusions suggest the diagnosis.

Trachoma inclusion conjunctivitis (TRIC), in the female, is believed to be confined to the cervix.[12] The diagnosis is based on the finding of basophilic, intracytoplasmic inclusions in cervical cells.

The diagnosis of condyloma acuminata is one which can usually be made on the basis of the gross findings. The cytologic findings have been described; they include anucleate squames, parakeratosis, enlargement of all the squamous components, molding of nuclei, cytoplasmic vacuolation, and basophilic inclusions in the nuclei.

Other organisms, including *Entamoeba histolytica, Enterobius vermicularis, Ascaris, lumbricoides* and vinegar eels, have been observed occasionally in smears from the female genital tract.[5]

## Intraepithelial Neoplasia of the Cervix[10, 15, 17, 19, 25]

The main objective in cytologic diagnosis is to detect those cellular abnormalities that are the precursors of cancer. A number of terms have been employed to designate those intraepithelial changes that have been considered precancerous. One may subscribe to the International Agreement of 1962,[11] which, following its definitions of

invasive carcinoma and carcinoma in situ, defines dysplasia as "all other disturbances of differentiation of the squamous epithelial lining of surface and glands". Koss[15] has proposed that intraepithelial precancerous changes form a progressive spectrum of abnormalities ranging from slight changes (early borderline lesions or mild dysplasia) to severe changes (carcinoma in situ). Richart[21] has employed the term cervical intraepithelial neoplasia (CIN) to designate all precursors to invasive cervical cancer. For a thorough review of the nature and natural history of cervical intraepithelial lesions, the reader is referred to Chapter 7.

The cytologist can make a major contribution toward eradicating cervical cancer by directing his or her efforts to the detection of abnormalities in the cervical epithelium as they manifest themselves in the cervical smear. Whether the cells under scrutiny are labeled dysplastic, borderline lesions, or intraepithelial neoplasm, the crucial point is that they be recognized and appropriate followup measures be instituted.

## Mild Dysplasia and Dyskaryosis

The smear shows predominantly polygonal superficial and intermediate cells with abundant eosinophilic or basophilic transparent cytoplasm. The cells lie singly or in clusters. There is nuclear enlargement, occasional multinucleation, and slight hyperchromasia (Figure 36.20). The term dyskaryosis has been applied to those cells in which the nucleus exhibits abnormal morphology but in which the cytoplasm is abundant and the nucleocytoplasmic ratio

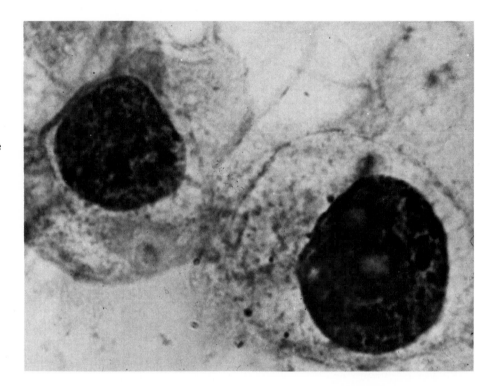

**36.21** Moderate dysplasia. The two cells present in this field both show hyperchromatism, clumping of chromatin, and a high nucleocytoplasmic ratio. Histologic sections revealed moderate intraepithelial neoplasm.

is low. Nucleoli are rarely seen. The background of the smear is usually clean.

Although the cytologic findings show minimal departures from the norm, a followup smear is mandatory because sufficient evidence has been accumulated that a proportion of such lesions progresses to more severe forms of intraepithelial neoplasm.

## Moderate Dysplasia

The smear in moderate dysplasia shows predominantly round or oval cells with basophilic cytoplasm. The nuclei are moderately hyperchromatic. The nucleocytoplasmic ratios may be more strikingly altered but the cytoplasmic width exceeds the diameter of the nucleus (Figure 36.21). A greater number of abnormal cells than in a mild dysplasia is observed. Characteristically, the cells are arranged singly, although loosely arranged groups may be present.

## Severe Dysplasia/Carcinoma in Situ

Histologic differentiation between severe dysplasia and carcinoma in situ has been based on the finding of a layer of flattened cells on the surface of the epithelium in the former, whereas in the latter no differentiation takes place

throughout the entire thickness of the epithelium. In the light of recent exhaustive studies by Richart[21,22] and others, this appears to be an arbitrary distinction. The cytologic findings in severe dysplasia are indistinguishable from the cytologic findings in carcinoma in situ.

The distribution and basic morphology of the cellular content of smears from carcinoma in situ may vary with the method of collection and the anatomic location of the tumor, as well as with the presence of cells from coexistent areas of metaplasia. In general, three smear patterns can be recognized. One pattern is composed mainly of differentiated malignant cells, suggesting origin from squamous epithelium, and the other pattern consists mainly of smaller malignant cells the origin of which is primarily from areas of endocervical metaplasia. Occasionally, it is possible to recognize the highly differentiated keratinizing carcinoma in situ.

A smear from the differentiated squamous type of carcinoma in situ (Figure 36.22a,b) shows a predominance of round cells with a large nucleus and a narrow rim of cytoplasm. The nuclei reveal those characteristics that are the hallmarks of malignancy: the abnormal distribution of chromatin; irregular, often angular outline; variation in size and configuration; and often hyperchromatism. These malignant cells are usually termed "third-type" malignant

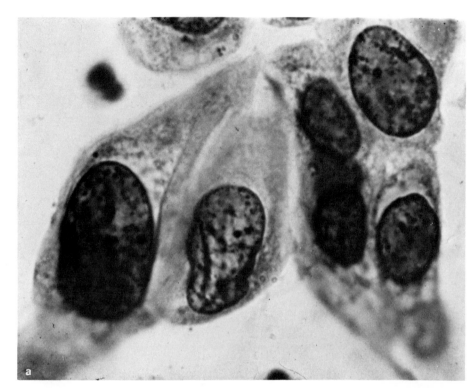

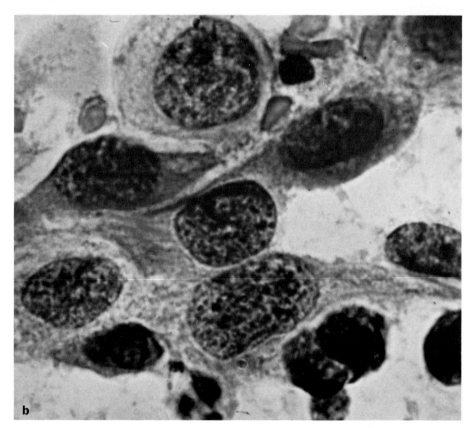

**36.22 a.** Several dysplasia/carcinoma in situ. The coarse clumping of chromatin and the irregular thickening of the nuclear membranes is evident. The nuclei vary in size, shape, and chromatin pattern. The nuclei are surrounded by varying amounts of cytoplasm. **b.** Severe dysplasia/carcinoma in situ. A group of cells in which the chromatin distribution is strikingly abnormal, with coarse clumping and angular masses. In some of the nuclei, a "clearing" in the karyolymph is discernible.

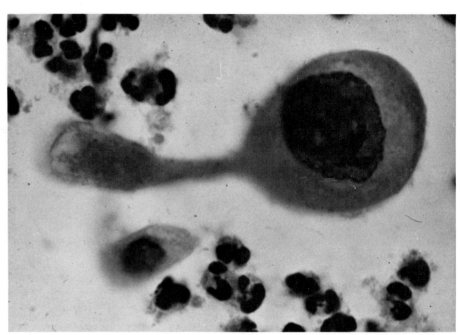

**36.23** Tadpole cell from carcinoma in situ. The head portion of the cell is occupied by a large hyperchromatic nucleus in which coarse chromatin clumping is seen. The tail of cytoplasm shows some vacuolation. Inflammatory cells are evident.

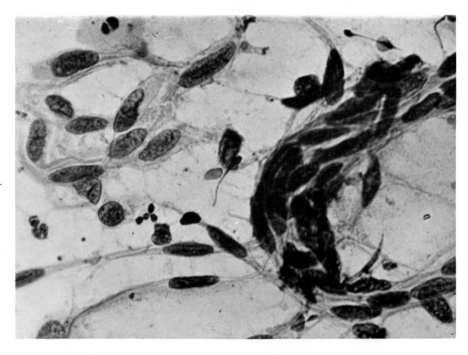

**36.24** Fiber cells from carcinoma in situ. This smear reveals a group of elongated fiber cells the nuclei of which show varying degrees of hyperchromatism and variation in size, as well as irregular chromatin clumping.

cells, distinguishing them from the other two types, which are more bizarre morphologically but are seen less often. The tadpole cell is one in which the "head" contains an enlarged malignant nucleus and the remainder of the cytoplasm appears as an attenuated tail. A fiber cell is an elongated cell in which a malignant nucleus is present (Figures 36.23 and 36.24).

The cytologic findings in the small-cell, anaplastic carcinoma in situ (Figure 36.25) consist of small, poorly differentiated cells, present singly or in loosely arranged

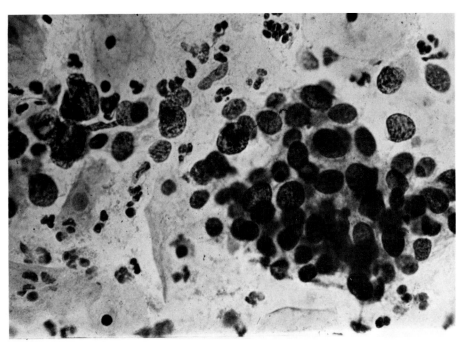

**36.25** Carcinoma in situ. This smear reveals a group of relatively small anaplastic cells with hyperchromatic nuclei that vary somewhat in size and shape but are mainly round or oval. Many of these cells have scant cytoplasm, which presents as a partial rim or fragment. Most of the nuclei are denuded.

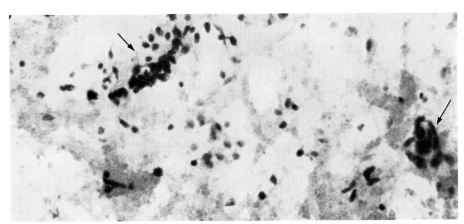

**36.26** Invasive squamous carcinoma of the cervix. Against a background of blood and cellular debris, several groups of small, poorly differentiated, malignant cells can be seen (arrows). The majority of cells have scanty cytoplasm or are totally denuded of cytoplasm.

linear groups. The nuclei occupy most of the cell. Often the cytoplasm may appear as merely an incomplete rim. Nucleoli may be present.

# Invasive Neoplasms of Cervix

## Invasive Squamous Carcinoma of the Cervix

Paradoxically, the cytologic diagnosis of invasive epidermoid carcinoma of the cervix may often prove more difficult than that of the *in situ* lesions (Figure 36.26).

Blood, necrotic material, and leukocytes may obscure the malignant cells, which are frequently poorly preserved. The malignant cells are of a heterogenous mixture, with many extreme abnormalities in both nucleus and cytoplasm. Differentiated malignant squamous cells and undifferentiated malignant cells may coexist throughout the smear. Mutinucleated malignant cells exhibit variation in size and shape and abnormal chromatin patterns from nucleus to nucleus. Fiber cells, with elongated irregular hyperchromatic nuclei, may be found, as well as large, bizarre cells similar to tadpole cells but often exhibiting more extreme nuclear and cytoplasmic aberrations (Figure 36.28). When undifferentiated cells predominate, the

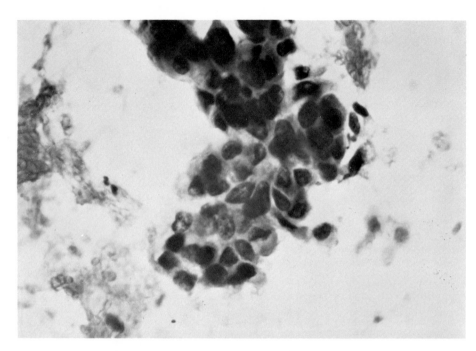

**36.27** Invasive squamous carcinoma of the cervix. The field reveals a loosely arranged group of malignant cells, both differentiated and undifferentiated. Many of the nuclei are markedly hyperchromatic; nuclear detail is difficult to evaluate. However, in a few of the nuclei, the abnormal chromatin is discernible.

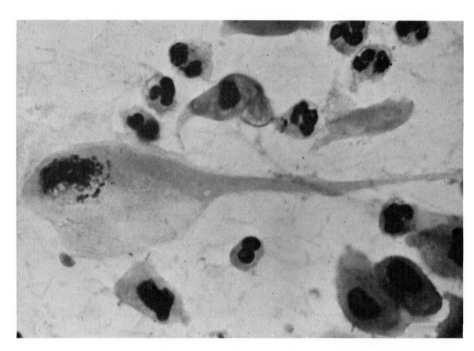

**36.28** Tadpole cell from an invasive squamous carcinoma of the cervix. The nucleus has undergone karyorrhexis. The nuclear membrane is no longer discernible. Several smaller malignant cells and polymorphonuclear leukocytes are present.

smear may be composed mainly of small cells with little cytoplasm (Figure 36.27).

Dysplastic and dyskaryotic cells may be present in the smears of invasive epidermoid carcinoma, a not surprising finding because areas of dyplasia and areas of carcinoma in situ may lie adjacent to the frankly invasive lesion.

## Adenocarcinoma

Adenocarcinoma is a relatively uncommon malignancy of the cervix as compared to the incidence of intraepithelial neoplasms of the squamous epithelium.[24] Abnormal distribution of chromatin is the most significant

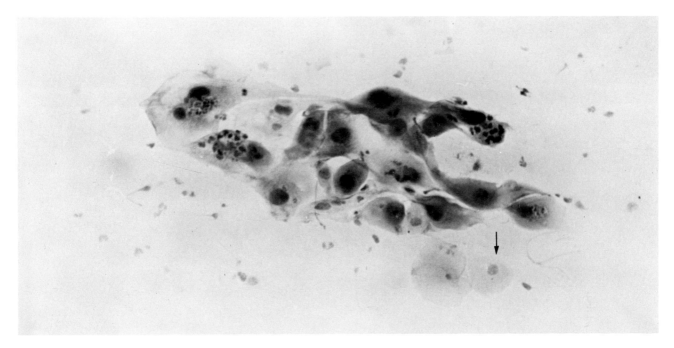

**36.29** Radiation response. There is enlargement of nucleus and cytoplasm. For comparison, observe the normal intermediate cell (arrow). Cytoplasmic vacuolation is present in some of the cells.

feature. The chromatin shows clumping, often with irregular and angular masses. Condensation at the nuclear margins may produce an irregularly thickened nuclear border. Prominent large, pink-staining nucleoli may be present. An eccentric peripheral malignant nucleus within a cytoplasm displaying coarse vacuolation or an elongated columnar form suggests the adenocarcinomatous nature of the lesion. When a group of malignant cells is observed, the nuclei are frequently located peripherally, producing a pseudoacinar appearance. The malignant cells may be undifferentiated, with almost total loss of cytoplasm.

Differentiation of endocervical adenocarcinoma from endometrial adenocarcinoma may not always be possible on a cytologic specimen.

## Changes in Epithelia Secondary to Therapy

### Effects of Radiation

A thorough familiarity with the marked cellular changes that radiation produces in both benign and malignant cells is vital.[7] In the followup smears of patients who have been treated by radiotherapy for cervical cancer, the cytologist must be able to distinguish among benign cells showing radiation effect, malignant cells altered by radiation, and malignant cells unaffected by radiation.

The nonspecific degenerative changes of pyknosis, karyorrhexis, and karyolysis are seen initially, in both benign and malignant cells, and signify cell destruction. In many of the benign cells that retain their structure, that is, cells that have not degenerated, there may be a striking enlargement of both nucleus and cytoplasm (Figure 36.29) with maintenance of the nucleocytoplasmic ratio. At times, cytoplasmic enlargement occurs but the nucleus does not enlarge; consequently the nucleus appears smaller than normal. Within the enlarged nuclei structure remains normal but, as a consequence of the enlargement, the nuclear membrane may appear wrinkled. This wrinkling and folding must be distinguished from malignant intranuclear changes. Multinucleation is also seen.

Vacuolation, both coarse and fine, is seen in the cytoplasm of the benign cells that have responded to radiation (Figure 36.30). Bizarrely shaped benign cells are occasionally seen but the normal structure of their nuclei makes it possible to distinguish them from the bizarrely shaped malignant cells.

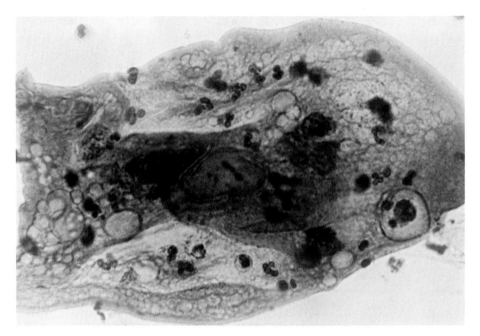

**36.30** Radiation response. The striking cytoplasmic vacuolation that occurs following radiation can produce bizarre morphology.

Malignant cells can also respond to radiation with nuclear and cytoplasmic enlargement but, in these cells, the features that are diagnostic of malignancy are usually still recognizable.

After radiation therapy has been completed, ongoing cytologic studies are essential in detecting residual and recurrent malignancy. The "negative" smear, by which is meant the smear that ultimately proves to be negative for malignancy, may appear abnormal at first glance. Degenerative changes, cytoplasmic vacuolation, multinucleation, cytoplasmic and nuclear enlargement, and the rare bizarre shape may be present in the epithelial cells. However, nuclear chromatin distribution is normal. Commonly the cellular pattern may be atrophic or consist of parabasal and intermediate cells. Large numbers of histiocytes, often multinucleated, are seen and frequently show considerable nuclear activity. Polymorphonuclear leukocytes are also present.

The positive postradiation smears, that is, those containing malignant cells, are seen in patients with persistent disease or in patients in whom the disease has recurred after variable lengths of time.

Ruth Graham[7] has pointed out that the patient with persistent disease is difficult from a cytologic standpoint. If the smear exhibits a predominance of intermediate and superficial cells showing no radiation effect, if histiocytes are absent or few in number, if the background is clean, a very careful search must be made for small, undif-

ferentiated malignant cells. The abnormal chromatin pattern of their nuclei makes it possible to identify them. The smear from a patient with recurrent malignancy usually contains differentiated and undifferentiated malignant cells, often in large numbers.

## Cryosurgery

In recent years, cryosurgery has been used in the treatment of cervicitis. It is incumbent on the cytologist to be familiar with the changes produced by this modality and incumbent on the clinician to inform the cytologist that cryosurgery has been used. Two weeks after treatment, the cervical smear contains cells showing enlargement of nuclei, multinucleation, and karyorhexis. Micro- and macrovacuoles are present in the cytoplasm. If a smear is taken about 3 months after treatment, dysplasia-like changes may be present, particularly parakeratotic changes. Cytoplasmic vacuolation may persist for up to 6 months.

## Folic Acid and/or Vitamin $B_{12}$ Deficiency

Patients with megaloblastic anemia caused by folic acid and/or vitamin $B_{12}$ deficiency may exhibit both nuclear and cellular enlargement of epithelial cells (Figure 36.31). Occasionally, abnormalities in chromatin pattern and the presence of nucleoli may be seen in these enlarged cells, giving rise to diagnostic difficulty. Women who develop

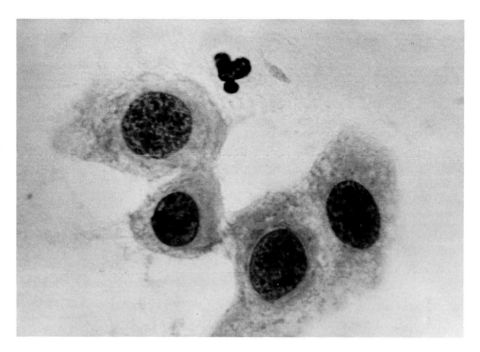

**36.31** Folic acid and/or vitamin $B_{12}$ deficiency. Both cellular and nuclear enlargement may be seen in the squamous cells of patients with megaloblastic anemia caused by folic acid/vitamin $B_{12}$ deficiency. The nuclear chromatin is coarse.

megaloblastic anemia during the course of their pregnancy may display these alterations.

## Alkylating Agents

Koss, Melamed, and Mayer[16] have described the alterations in cervical squamous epithelium that may develop in the course of long-term administration of busulfan (Myleran),[16] an alkylating agent used in the treatment of chronic myelogenous leukemia. These changes closely resemble spontaneously occurring precancerous conditions of the cervix (Figure 36.32). The question has been raised of whether these are cancer-mimetic cellular abnormalities or whether they may represent the early stages of drug-induced human cancer.

# Neoplasms of the Female Genital Tract Other than Cervical

The cytologic detection of endometrial carcinoma in the asymptomatic female does not approach the accuracy or dependability with which cervical neoplasms are diagnosed.[4] When aspiration of the vaginal pool is performed, the yield of diagnostically significant material is greater than that obtained from cervical smears, which are a rather poor source of endometrial cells. Hofmeister[9] has emphasized the important point that in investigating lesions of the endometrium any technique is of value only when positive or atypical and if it alerts the clinician that adequate additional procedures should be carried out. If the technique, be it endometrial biopsy, jet wash, or endomet-

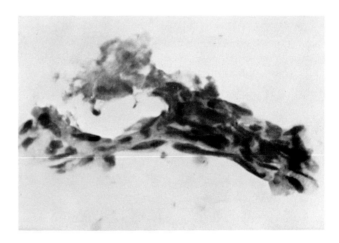

**36.32** Busulfan (Myleran) induced changes in cervical squamous cells. In this sheet of cells enlargement of nuclei can be seen, as well as elongation. The morphology of some of these cells mimics intraepithelial neoplasia.

763

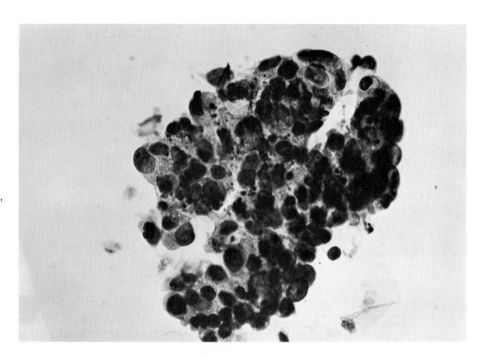

**36.33** Endometrial adenocarcinoma. A cluster of small, overlapping cells is seen. Many show degenerative changes; however, there is sufficient preservation of some of the nuclei so that chromatin clumping, prominent nucleoli, nuclear enlargement, and pleomorphism raise the suspicion of malignancy.

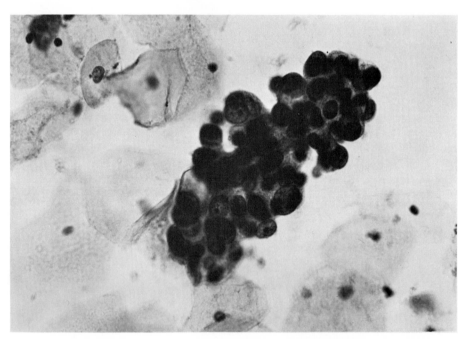

**36.34** Endometrial adenocarcinoma. Cluster of cells from same smear as Figure 36.33. The preservation is better in this group so that abnormal nuclear detail is more obvious. Superficial and intermediate cells are visible in the background.

rial aspiration,[8,9,14,26] is negative and symptoms persist, dilatation and curettage is mandatory.

In premenopausal women, a vaginal smear that contains endometrial cells, singly or more commonly in clusters or balls, after the tenth to twelfth day of the cycle is usually interpreted as an abnormal finding, although not necessar-

ily one suggesting the presence in the endometrium of a malignant lesion. In the smear of an asymptomatic post-menopausal woman, endometrial cells, normal or abnormal, are to be considered an abnormal finding and further investigation is warranted. The finding of marked histiocytic activity or striking maturation of squamous cells

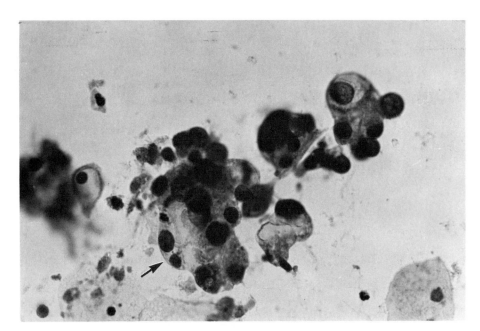

**36.35** Endometrial adenocarcinoma. This grouping of malignant cells suggests an attempt to form an acinar structure (arrow). Prominent nucleoli are visible in some of the cells.

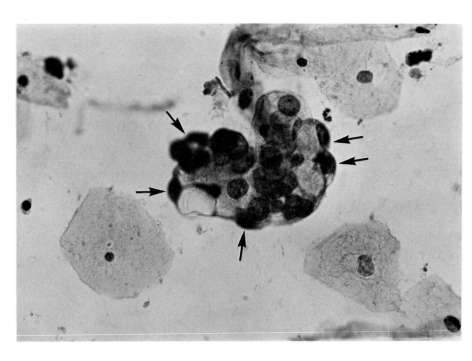

**36.36** Endometrial adenocarcinoma. This aggregate of malignant cells illustrates the peripheral position of many of the nuclei (arrows), a characteristic finding in adenocarcinoma.

similarly signals the necessity for further investigation. In the postmenopausal woman with a history of spotting or bleeding, a careful scrutiny of the smear for abnormal endometrial cells must be carried out. Small cells (Figures 36.33 and 36.34), lying singly or in small clusters, may be detected. The nuclei are slightly enlarged and show abnormal chromatin clumping and clear areas in the karyo-

lymph. Large, prominent, eosinophilic nucleoli, often angular in shape, are a helpful clue to the malignant nature of the cell. The eccentric position of the nucleus is a characteristic feature of adenocarcinoma. Much of the cytoplasm may be absent in the more undifferentiated tumor cells (Figures 36.35 and 36.36).

Adenocarcinoma of the fallopian tube is a rare tumor of

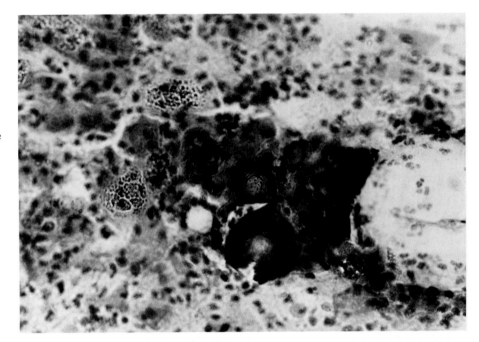

**36.37** Psammoma bodies. These lamellated, calcific granules, so-called psammoma bodies, were found in the vaginal smear of a patient with serous cystadenocarcinoma.

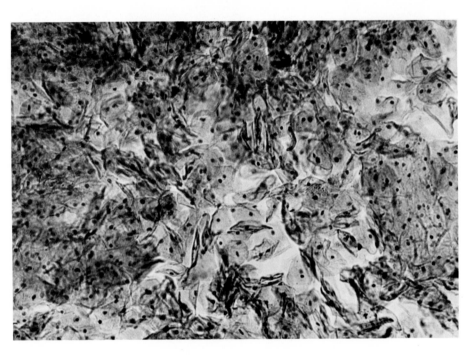

**36.38** Vaginal smear, day 22 of the menstrual cycle. Crowded sheets of overlapping intermediate cells are present. The cytoplasmic borders are folded. Some superficial cells are discernible; they lie flat and show no folding.

the female genital tract. Exfoliated tumor cells may be present in a vaginal smear, where they may be indistinguishable from an endometrial adenocarcinoma.

Rarely, an adenocarcinoma originating in the ovary may shed malignant cells that appear in the vaginal smear.[2,3] If endometrial curettings do not reveal adenocarcinoma, the possibility of an ovarian tumor must be considered (Figure 36.37).

In clear cell adenocarcinoma of the genital tract,[23] a lesion that has been described in young females whose mothers have been administered DES during pregnancy, vaginal smears may reveal tumor cells occurring singly and in clumps. In general, they resemble endocervical cells and nuclear atypia may be seen.

Squamous cell carcinomas of the vagina occurs mainly in elderly women. A smear taken from the vaginal wall, if there is a suspicious area, or from the vaginal pool occasionally yields material that permits a definitive diagnosis to be made. Differentiated and undifferentiated malignant cells may be present; some of the malignant cells may be keratinized.

Occasionally, a cytologic diagnosis of vulvar epidermoid carcinoma may be made. However, the diagnosis is usually made by biopsy of a suspicious site.

# Hormonal Cytology

Cytohormonal evaluation can be useful in investigating disturbances of endocrine function and in assessing the effects of hormone therapy.[29] However, it is essential that the material be suitable and that adequate clinical data be available. The specimen should be taken from the upper third of the vagina or the posterior fornix. The patient's age; menstrual history; and pertinent clinical history, including administration of exogenous hormones and prior surgical or radiation therapy, must be supplied if a valid assessment is to be made.

The vaginal smear reflects the interaction of several hormones, namely, estrogens, progesterones, and androgens. Therefore, at times, it may not be possible to assess whether the changes seen in a smear result from a specific hormonal alteration or from multihormonal factors. Nonhormonal factors, such as inflammation, may also influence the content of the smear. A smear in which there is evidence of inflammation is not suitable for hormonal assessment.

In general, under estrogenic stimulation, the vaginal epithelium undergoes proliferation and maturation. Consequently, the vaginal smear consists of superficial and intermediate cells. When there is unopposed estrogenic stimulation, the smear consists of superficial cells that lie flat and singly on a "clean" background. Because only estrogens can produce this epithelial maturation, such a smear may be taken as evidence of estrogen stimulation, whether endogenous or exogenous.

Progesterone produces proliferation and maturation of the squamous cells but, by itself, it does not produce maturation to superficial cells. The smear, under the influence of progesterone, contains folded intermediate cells, desquamated in large clumps. It is this pattern of exfoliation that is most characteristic of a progesterone effect (Figure 36.38).

Androgens also produce proliferation and maturation of squamous cells to the intermediate cell stage. However, the exfoliated pattern is one of single cells or small groups of folded or flat intermediate cells.

Basically, there are two significant extremes in the main patterns of hormonal cytology. If the smear consists of abundant, single, flat, superficial cells, this can be interpreted as definite estrogenic stimulation. If the smear contains only parabasal cells, it can be interpreted as a lack of estrogenic stimulation. Patterns containing superficial intermediate and parabasal cells may not be used for hormonal assessment because nonhormonal factors may produce this pattern.

## Numerical Indices

Several numerical indices have been proposed to express hormonal cytologic patterns.[15,29] Their major usefulness is in assessing estrogenic activity. The indices are often of questionable value in assessing progesterone effect.

The eosinophilic index measures the relation of mature eosinophilic squamous cells to mature cyanophilic squamous cells, regardless of nuclear appearance.

The karyopyknotic index measures the relation of superficial cells to intermediate cells, regardless of cytoplasmic staining.

The folded index measures the percentage of folded mature squamous cells to flat mature squamous cells, regardless of cytoplasmic staining or of nuclear appearance.

The crowded cell index measures the relation of mature squamous cells in groups or clusters of four or more cells to mature squamous cells lying singly or in clusters of fewer than four cells, regardless of staining reaction or nuclear appearance.

The maturation index[6] measures the relation of superficial, intermediate, and parabasal cells (S/I/P).

Meisels has recommended the use of an assigned numerical value to the different cell types[29] to facilitate communication between cytologists and to make easier the use of digital computers for statistical evaluation in large series. The assigned values are:

| | |
|---|---|
| Superficial eosinophil cell | 1.0 |
| Superficial cyanophilic cell | 0.8 |
| Large intermediate cell | 0.6 |
| Small intermediate cell | 0.5 |
| Parabasal cell | 0.0 |

When the percentage of each of these cells is multiplied by the corresponding numerical factor and the results are added up, a number between 0 and 100 is obtained. This is designated the "maturation value." To compare maturation indices, for example, the newborn is 60 to 70; the menstrual cycle from 60 to 90; pregnancy is from 60 to 69; and menopause is from 0 to 40.

The interpretation of a vaginal smear, regardless of which index is used, ultimately depends on the correlation by the cytologist of the clinical data provided by the clinician and the data obtained from the smear, the proportions of cells present, and their appearance in the smear. The final cytologic report should be in the form of a statement. For example: "The cytohormonal pattern is consistent with . . ." or "The cytohormonal pattern is not compatible with . . ." or "The cytohormonal pattern suggests the possibility of . . . ." It should not be in the form of an isolated numerical index.

## The Vaginal Smear

### At birth and in childhood

At birth, the vaginal smears of mother and child are quite similar, because both are under similar hormonal stimulation. Intermediate cells, usually in groups, predominate, with some admixture of superficial cells. During the next few weeks, these cells disappear gradually from the smear. Parabasal cells become the predominant cell type. Leukocytes and some erythrocytes may be present.

This smear pattern in childhood is stable and alters only in response to infection, to which the thin epithelium is vulnerable, or to endogenous production of estrogens, as from an estrogen-producing ovarian tumor.

### Premenarchial

The early premenarchial period is quite variable. There is a gradually increased steroid stimulation reflected in the vaginal smear by a reduction in the proportion of parabasal cells and an increased intermediate cells. During this transitional period, considerable variation may exist until the normal cycle patterns are established.

### The menstrual cycle

The follicular or proliferative phase extends from the fourth or fifth day to the fourteenth day of a 28-day cycle (in prolonged cycles, the extended phase is the preovulatory one). During the first few days, the smear is composed chiefly of intermediate cells, histiocytes, and clumps or balls of endometrial cells. Gradually, the smear shows an increasing number of single, flat, eosinophilic, karyopyknotic, superficial cells, reflecting the increased growth and maturation of the vaginal epithelium. Histiocytes and polymorphonuclear leukocytes gradually disappear from the smear.

The so-called ovulatory smear pattern consists almost exclusively of flat superficial cells. The background is clean. It should be emphasized that this type of smear, screened as an isolated specimen, cannot be used as definitive evidence that ovulation has occurred. Unopposed estrogen stimulation also produces this type of smear.

During the ensuing secretory phase, there is a gradual decrease in the number of superficial cells and a progressive increase in the number of intermediate cells, which are arranged in clumps and show a fraying or wrinkling of their cytoplasm.

In the premenstrual phase, the number of polymorphonuclear leukocytes increases. Prior to overt menstruation, clumps of endometrial cells may be identified. The vaginal smear in the menstrual phase consists of compact clumps or balls of endometrial cells in a background of blood, leukocytes, and histiocytes.

If vaginal smears are to be utilized to investigate disturbances in the menstrual cycle, serial specimens must be studied, preferably for two or more cycles. Evidence of cycling is sought and this can only be determined by looking for the changing patterns that are associated with the menstrual cycle.

### The menopause and postmenopausal period

Marked individual variations, both clinical and cytologic, are found in the menopause and postmenopausal period. In some women, cessation of menstruation may have occurred, yet some cyclic changes persist in the smears. Anovulation marked by periods of unopposed estrogen production may often occur. Serial smears may reveal a pattern of flat superficial cells. Evidence of cycling is absent.

The general cytologic progression of events is toward a decrease and then disappearance of superficial cells in the vaginal smear. The patterns that emerge eventually are of two types. Intermediate cell predominance consists of intermediate cells showing clumping and cytoplasmic folding, a pattern that may be indistinguishable from the one seen in pregnancy. The administration of small doses of estrogen can resolve this diagnostic problem. In pregnancy, the intermediate cell pattern persists. In the menopausal or postmenopausal woman, a maturation to superficial cells ensues.[13]

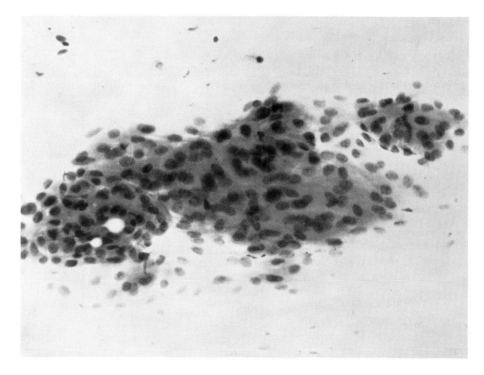

**36.39** "Crowding" in an atrophic smear. Sheets of parabasal cells are seen. The nuclei are regular; no chromatin abnormalities are seen. The denuded nuclei around these sheets are readily identified as parabasal in origin.

The atrophic or parabasal predominant smear reveals sheets of parabasal cells (Figure 36.39) in which some eosinophilic staining of cytoplasm and crowding of nuclei are evident. Parabasal cells may show cytolysis and, occasionally, denuded nuclei appear hyperchromatic and may raise the suspicion of malignancy. However, the uniformity of the nuclear chromatin should dispel this impression. Numerous histiocytes are often present in these smears and giant multinucleated histiocytes are not uncommon. The latter must not be confused with multinucleated malignant cells.

### In pregnancy

In pregnancy, the cyclic changes are absent and the smear consists almost wholly of clumps of intermediate cells that characteristically show folding and thickening of their cytoplasmic borders.[28] The term "navicular" has been used to describe these intermediate cells. Their cytoplasm is rich in glycogen and, with the Papanicolaou stain, shows areas of yellow-orange staining. The nuclei are frequently elongated.

Superficial cells may be present in small numbers. Parabasal cells are rare. A smear in which superficial cells predominate may indicate placental insufficiency.

It must be emphasized that the pattern described is compatible with pregnancy, not diagnostic of pregnancy. Other conditions, such as menopause, can produce a similar pattern.

## Effects of Progestogens on the Vaginal Smear

The overall effect of progestogens on the vaginal smear is the absence of the orderly cyclic changes that accompany a normal menstrual cycle.[20] A predominance of intermediate cells early in the cycle is seen. Folded intermediate cells persist throughout the cycle. Often cytolysis is prominent and Döderlein's bacilli are present. Inflammatory changes are common.

## Hormonal Cytology in the Endocrinopathies

### Primary amenorrheas

In gonadal dysgenesis (Turner's syndrome), the smear is atrophic. Examination of well-preserved nuclei in intermediate cells fails to reveal sex chromatin bodies unless mosaicism is present, in which case sex chromatin bodies may be seen.

In testicular feminization, a disorder in which the patients are genetic males (XY), epithelial maturation is present because female hormones are produced by the undescended testes. Sex chromatin bodies are absent.

In congenital absence of the uterus, ovarian function is present and epithelial maturation occurs.

### Secondary amenorrhea

Aside from the physiologic amenorrhea of pregnancy, secondary amenorrhea is indicative of impairment of ovarian function. The Stein–Leventhal syndrome (polycystic ovarian disease) includes a group of disorders in which follicles persist and become enlarged and cystic. The vaginal smears are generally composed of folded and clustered intermediate cells and superficial cells. Navicular cells with glycogen deposits within the cytoplasm are often seen.[1]

Occasionally, in young girls, periodic vaginal bleeding may occur. Serial vaginal smears in the precocius puberty syndrome often reveal evidence of cycling.

In a child or in a postmenopausal woman whose vaginal smear reveals a high degree of maturation, the possibility of a granulosa cell tumor must be considered. These tumors may produce estrogen-like substances, which act on the vaginal epithelium.

In the Chiari–Frommel syndrome, a condition in which normal lactation continues over a prolonged period, amenorrhea is accompanied by atrophy of the vaginal epithelium. The smear mirrors this atrophy; it is composed of parabasal cells.

# Methods of Obtaining Material from the Female Genital Tract[10,15]

## Cervical Smear

The cervical smear is the method of choice for diagnosis of intraepithelial neoplasms of the cervix:

1. Do not lubricate the speculum. The lubricant can contaminate the smear, producing a basophilic background that can obscure cellular detail.
2. A cotton swab or wooden scraper is applied to the entire portio of the cervix and into the external os so that material is collected from the squamocolumnar junction.
3. The material is immediately and quickly spread onto clean glass slides.
4. The smear must be fixed immediately in order to prevent cellular distortion. Immersion in 95% alcohol

or the use of a coating fixative, either dropped on or sprayed on, are acceptable procedures.
5. Proceed to Papanicolaou staining method.

## Vaginal Smear

The vaginal smear is useful for assessment of hormonal status if the guidelines described in the text are followed:

1. Material is obtained from lateral wall of the upper third of the vagina.
2. Subsequent handling of the material is as in cervical smear.

## Posterior Fornix Aspiration

The posterior fornix aspiration may be useful in the detection of endometrial cancer. It is a poor method for the detection of cervical lesions. A pipette with a suction bulb is employed.

## Endometrial Aspiration

Endometrial aspiration permits a sampling of material from the endometrium directly. Neither the cervical nor the vaginal smear is sufficient in the detection of endometrial cancer. Endometrial aspiration, jet wash, vabra suction, or variants of these techniques are directed to obtaining material directly from the endometrium.

# REFERENCES

1. Bamford, S. B., Mitchell, G. W. Jr., Bardawil, W. A., and Casin, C. M. Vaginal cytology in polycystic ovarian disease. *Acta Cytol.* 9:332, 1965.
2. Benson, P. A. Psammoma bodies found in cervical-vaginal smears. *Acta Cytol.* 17:64, 1973.
3. Beyer-Boon, M. E. Psammoma bodies in cervico-vaginal smears: An indicator of the presence of ovarian carcinoma. *Acta Cytol.* 18:41, 1974.
4. Burk, J. R., Lehman, H. F., and Wolf, F. S. Inadequacy of Papanicolaou smears in the detection of endometrial cancer. *N. Engl. J. Med.* 291:191, 1974.
5. Fentanes de Torres, E., and Benitez-Bribiesca, L. Cytologic detection of vaginal parasitosis. *Acta Cytol.* 17:252, 1973.
6. Frost, J. K. Exfoliative Cytology. In Novak, E. R., and Woodruff, J. D., eds., *Gynecologic and Obstetric Pathology*, 6th ed. Philadelphia, W. B. Saunders Co., 1967.
7. Graham, R. M. *The Cytologic Diagnosis of Cancer*, 2nd ed. Philadelphia, W. B. Saunders Co., 1963.
8. Gravlee, L. C. Jr. Jet irrigation method for the diagnosis of endometrial adenocarcinoma. Its principle and accuracy. *Obstet. Gynecol.* 34:168, 1969.
9. Hofmeister, F. J. Endometrial Biopsy: Another look. *Am. J. Obstet. Gynecol.* 118:773, 1974.

10. Hughes, R. R. Errors in the use of the Pap smear. Southern M. J. *65*:575, 1972.

11. International agreement on histological terminology for the lesions of the uterine cervix. *Acta Cytol. 6*:255, 1962.

12. Josey, Y. W., Nahmias, A., and Naib, Z. M. Viral and virus-like infections of the female genital tract. *Clin. Obstet. Gynecol. 12*:161, 1969.

13. Keebler, C. M., and Wied, G. L. The estrogen test: An aid in differential cyto-diagnosis. *Acta Cytol. 18*:483, 1974.

14. Kohl, G. C., and Larson, C. P. Office endometrial biopsies. *Am. J. Obstet. Gynecol. 118*:406, 1974.

15. Koss, L. G. *Diagnostic Cytology and Its Histopathologic Bases,* 2nd ed. Philadelphia, J. B. Lippincott, 1968.

16. Koss, G. L., Melamed, M. R., and Mayer, K. The effect of busulfan on human epithelia. *Am. J. Clin. Pathol. 44*:385, 1965.

17. Lui, W. *An Introduction to Gynecological Exfoliative Cytology.* Springfield, Ill., Charles C Thomas, 1959.

18. Patten, S. F. Jr. *Diagnostic Cytology of the Uterine Cervix.* Baltimore, Williams and Wilkins, 1969.

19. Reagan, J. W., and Patten, S. F. Jr., eds. The female reproductive tract, in *The Manual for the Atlas of Cytology.* Chicago, Am. Soc. Clin. Pathol., 1967.

20. Reyniak, J. V., Sedlis, A., Stone, D., and Connell, E. Cytohormonal findings in patients using various forms of contraception. *Acta Cytol. 13*:315, 1969.

21. Richart, R. M. Natural history of cervical intraepithelial neoplasia. *Clin. Obstet. Gynecol. 10*:748, 1967.

22. Richart, R. M., and Vaillant, H. W. The irrigation smear: False negative rates in a population with cervical neoplasia. *JAMA 192*:199, 1965.

23. Taft, P. D., Robboy, S., Herbst, A. L., and Scully, R. E. Cytology of clear cell adenocarcinoma of genital tract in young females: Review of 95 cases from the registry. *Acta Cytol. 18*:279, 1974.

24. Tasker, J. T., and Collins, J. A. Adenocarcinoma of the uterine cervix. *Am. J. Obstet. Gynecol. 118*:344, 1974.

25. Te Linde, R. W. Demonstration of the relationship of carcinoma-in-situ to invasive carcinoma of the cervix. *Am. J. Obstet. Gynecol. 115*:1022, 1973.

26. Torres, J. E., Holmquist, N. D., and Danos, M. L. The endometrial irrigation smear in the detection of adenocarcinoma of the endometrium. *Acta Cytol. 13*:163, 1969.

27. Wied, G. L. Interpretation of inflammatory reactions in vagina, cervix and endocervix by means of cytologic smears. *Am. J. Clin. Pathol. 28*:233, 1957.

28. Wied, G. L. Cytology during pregnancy. *in* Greenhill, J. P., ed., *Yearbook of Obstetrics and Gynecology,* Chicago, Year Book Medical Publishers, 1966, pp. 15–33.

29. Wied, G. L., ed. Symposium: Hormonal cytology. *Acta Cytol. 12*:87, 1968.

Ancel Blaustein, M.D.

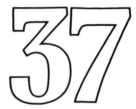

# Gross Description and Processing of Obstetric and Gynecologic Tissue

## General

This chapter offers some guidelines for the study of gross specimens and the processing of these specimens for appropriate microscopic study. All surgical pathology is more meaningfully studied when accurate, pertinent information is submitted with the specimen. With obstetric and gynecologic pathology, receipt of this data is essential. A simple data sheet (Figure 37.1) can be easily filled in by the attending physician or a resident. The information should not be filled out by operating room personnel; this results in too many errors. It should not be filled out prior to surgery, because the procedure may differ from the one originally contemplated.

## Equipment

The grossing room requires certain instruments and supplies (see Appendix I, p. 795). It should be adequate in size, well lit, and well ventilated in order to remove formaldehyde fumes and odors that may emanate from specimens.

Photography, of course, is not essential but can provide a useful visual adjunct to the description of complex radical surgery specimens. A simple rough sketch can, through alphabetical or numerical designation, show precisely from where the sections have come. When the slides are being read, reference to these sketches can, at times, be helpful in interpreting the slide.

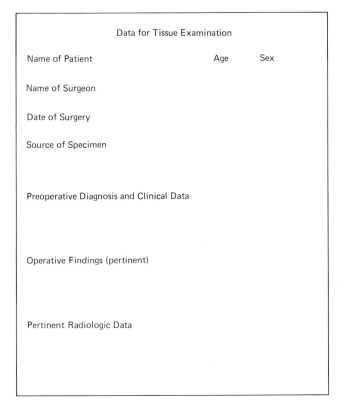

Data for Tissue Examination

Name of Patient                    Age      Sex

Name of Surgeon

Date of Surgery

Source of Specimen

Preoperative Diagnosis and Clinical Data

Operative Findings (pertinent)

Pertinent Radiologic Data

**37.1** Data sheet submitted with surgical specimen.

## Processing of Tissue for Transmission Electron Microscopy

If tissue is to be processed for transmission electron microscopy, it is best that it be fixed in cold buffered glutaraldehyde soon after it has been surgically removed. Several drops of fixative should be placed on a strip of dental wax and small segments of the tissue placed in the glutaraldehyde and cut into 1-mm segments. These should then be placed in a vial containing cold glutaraldehyde and the specimen transported on ice to the electron microscope laboratory. A slip containing information about the case should accompany the specimen.

## Endometrial Curettings

These are often received in gauze and this practice should be discouraged. Some curettings fall into the interstices of the gauze and it is a nuisance to attempt removing them. They are best received in formalin in a container. If scant, they should be placed on filter paper and placed in fixative. Specimens left without fixation, partic-

ularly in a warm room, will undergo some degree of autolysis in a very short period of time. Endometrium should not be sampled; all fragments must be blocked. The only exception to this would be massive amounts of placental tissue from a routine termination of pregnancy. A single block of the spongy villous tissue is sufficient. If large amounts of endometrium are received, they should be poured into a tea strainer and divided into several tea bags for processing. Color, texture, and the presence of polyps should be noted. Polyps should be blocked separately. The volume of curettings is best described as a spherical aggregate with a measured diameter or as normal, scant, or voluminous.

Frozen section examination of endometrial curettings has become common practice in many institutions. The specimen should be described and all the tissue blocked. Sampling is discouraged because normal, hyperplastic, and malignant tissue may at times coexist and sampling has been the main cause for missing tumor at frozen section and finding it later when permanent sections are studied. It is helpful to mount every fifth section until five slides are obtained. Taking sections at different levels minimizes the possibility of missing a tumor. There is a certain amount of contraction and distortion caused by freezing, but cyclic patterns and abnormal changes can still be readily observed. The procedure takes from 10 to 15 min. After the slides are read, the report should be communicated to the surgeon by the pathologist. Communication by a third party is fraught with the possibility of inaccurate reporting. Residual tissue should be defrosted and routinely processed.

## Tissue from Evacuation of a Hydatid Mole

Specimens received following the emptying of the uterus of a hydatidiform mole are usually received in two parts. Part A represents the mass of tissue evacuated, and part B the material from postevacuation curettage. The first part should be examined in a black pan that offers contrast. All tissue should be examined and a rough estimate made of how much vesicular tissue and how much solid tissue is present. Representative sections of vesicles should be taken but the solid material should be thoroughly sampled. Freshly coagulated blood usually can be separated from more firm tissue and discarded.

Part B, the postevacuation curettage specimen, is most important. It is the tissue that has been closest to the myometrium. An energetic curettage usually produces some firm fragments of endomyometrium and these, if present, should be teased from the specimen with a dissecting needle and blocked. Five blocks represent adequate sampling.

## Endocervical Curettings

These should be received on paper towelling or filter paper but never on gauze. They seem to consist solely of mucus. The use of a magnifying glass may enable identification of small flecks of tissue in the mucus, which may be removed with a disecting needle and placed on lens paper. A small drop of 1% eosin on the tissue will help the technician locate it for blocking.

## Cervix

Biopsies may be single or multiple and of varying sizes. Colposcopically directed biopsies tend to be small. Notation should be made of the number of pieces and their size. The magnifying glass is useful in noting granularity, ulceration, and hemorrhage. A dab of eosin on the mucosal surface will help the technician correctly orient the block.

## Cone of the Cervix

A coned cervix is often received with a suture at 12 o'clock. Some pathologists prefer to section the specimen on a clockwise orientation, in order to map the location and extent of the lesion. Information sought is whether there is intraepithelial neoplasia or invasive carcinoma and whether the upper margins and lateral margins are free of tumor. Description of the specimen should include size, the circumference of the mucosal surface, and its appearance. The resected border should be stained with India ink in order to identify its upper limit on the slides. The specimen should be incised at the suture mark, the endocervix described, and the specimen then pinned flat to a cork board (Figure 37.2). The board should be immersed in formalin and left there for several hours before sectioning. The specimen will harden and, with sharp blades, many sections (depending on the size of the cone) 2 to 3 mm in thickness can be cut. They should be serially numbered, blocked, and oriented, so that full thickness of the mucosa is obtained. Some laboratories do frozen section examination of cervical cones.[28] If invasive carcinoma can be ruled out, simple hysterectomy can be performed immediately if desired. Approximately 30 min is required to do the procedure. Two technicians are required, one to section and another to stain, mount, and label the slides. Description of the gross specimen should be followed by placing the opened cervix, pinned to a cork board, in the freezer for 3 to 4 min. This gives the tissue a firmer consistency and renders cutting easier. The resected margins should be stained with India ink. Specimens should be oriented to obtain full thickness sections. Three or four levels should be cut for each block and as many as 30 slides can be prepared and read in 30 min. Specimens should be of good technical quality and overlapping of mucosa avoided. The technique is satisfactory. Following completion of the procedure, the residual tissue should be removed from the cryostat blocks and placed in formalin-filled containers, labeled to correspond with the cryostat sections. They are then routinely processed by the standard paraffin technique with three to four levels for each block.

## Gross Examination of the Uterus

It is important to list the specimens received at the commencement of dictation. Separate resection of the cervix or adnexae should be noted. If the hysterectomy has been total the round ligaments can be used as a point of reference to orient the anterior and posterior surfaces, because they insert on the anterior superior surface of the uterus, just anterior to the fallopian tubes. Left and right adnexae can be clearly designated. The uterus should be weighed and the following measurements taken:

1. Top of the fundus to exocervix
2. Cornu to cornu
3. Thickness of uterus
4. Length of the cervix and its diameter

The adult nonparous uterus measures 7 to 8 cm from top of the fundus to the exocervix, 5 cm from cornu to cornu and 2 to 3 cm in thickness. It varies from 30 to 40 g in weight. Following one or more pregnancies, despite involution, the uterus may become heavier and weigh from 75 to 100 g. The postmenopausal uterus has a diminished amount of muscle and may weigh 20 to 30 g. The shape of the uterus is that of an inverted pear. It may become globular because of adenomyosis or be distorted in shape by subserosal, intramural, and submucous leiomyomata. Both of these disorders can considerably increase the weight of the uterus, particularly leiomyomata. The exocervix should be described for color, erosion, ulceration, or

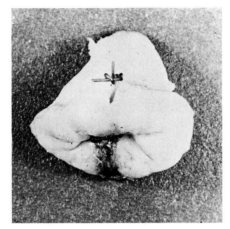

Cone of cervix

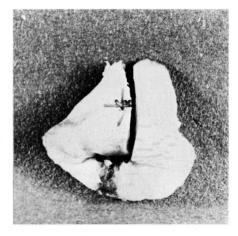

Incised at 12 o'clock

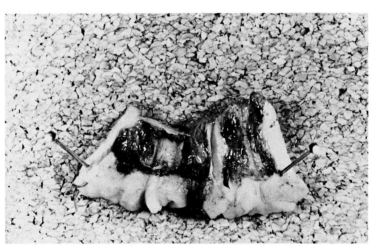

Opened cervix

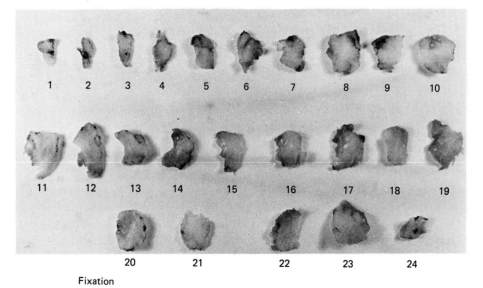

Fixation

**37.2** Method of sectioning a cone of the cervix.

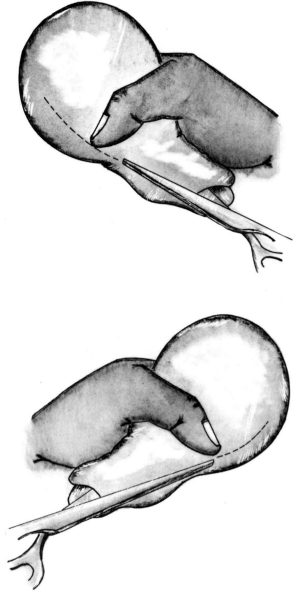

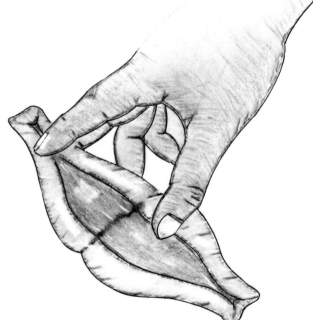

**37.3** Bivalve opening of the uterus.

lacerations and the shape of the external os should be noted. The uterus should then be opened laterally with care to expose the cornua and in order to expose the whole anterior and posterior surface of the endometrium and endocervix (Figure 37.3). The endocervix usually shows a rugal pattern. The presence of Nabothian cysts and polyps should be noted and any tumor, exophytic or endophytic, should be described in detail. The thickness of the endometrium should be measured and its texture and color

noted. Similar observations and measurements should be taken of the myometrium. If myomas are present, their number and location, submucous, intramural, and subserous, should be described and if they are subserous, it should be stated whether they are pedunculated. They should be measured and the appearance of the cut surface described. Myomas usually have a whorled pattern (Figure 37.4) and any deviation from this should be carefully observed. Sarcoma may have a fish-flesh color and be somewhat softer then a myoma. Pushing forms of the tumor show border between tumor and compressed myometrium, whereas infiltrating leiomyosarcoma (Figure 37.5) has no definable border. Hemangiopericytoma[13] may have a fish-flesh appearance too, but there are discrete borders seen between tumor and myometrium (Figure 37.6). Specimens should be examined shortly after removal; delay results in autolysis and color changes that may not arouse the same suspicion as when fresh tissue is seen. When there are multiple tumor masses, each should be transected and the surface pattern observed. Ideally one section should be taken from each tumor but at least those showing hemorrhage or necrosis should be sectioned. It is well to use a rough sketch of the opened uterus (Figure 37.7) to locate the site of the tumors and to designate by

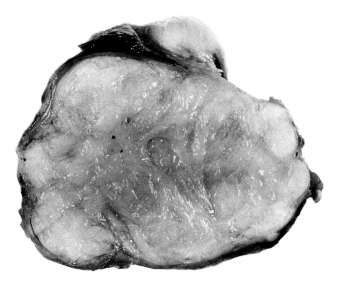

**37.4** Myoma of uterus: whorled pattern.

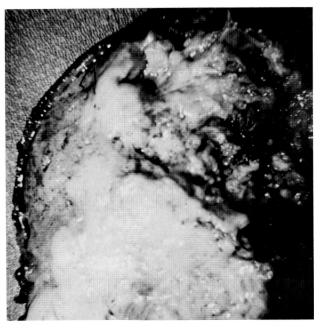

**37.5** Leiomyosarcoma: note the irregular ragged edge of the tumor (arrow).

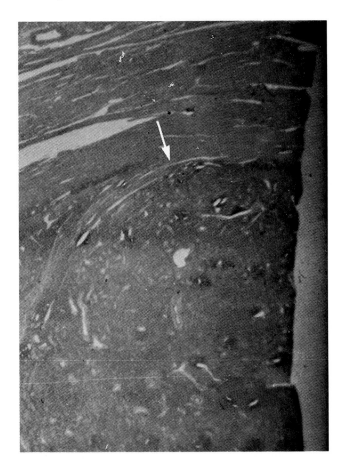

**37.6** Hemangiopericytoma: well-defined border (arrow) separating the tumor from myometrium.

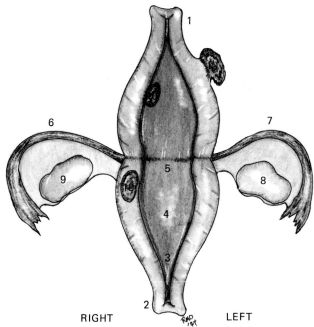

**37.7** Total hysterectomy: routine sites for sectioning. 1, Anterior lip of cervix; 2, posterior lip of cervix; 3, lower uterine segment; 4, upper uterine segment; 5, fundus; 6, right fallopian tube; 7, left fallopian tube; 8, left ovary; 9, right ovary; 10, lymph node.

number from where each section comes. Routine sections of the uterus should include:

1. Anterior lip of the cervix that includes exo- and endo-cervix and vaginal margin
2. Posterior lip of the cervix similarly
3. Lower uterine segment incorporating the internal os
4. Upper uterine segment

Additional sections are dependent on the presence of adnexae and/or specific lesions. At times, one or more submucous and/or intramural leiomyomata can so distort the uterine cavity that it is not possible to open the uterus laterally. The cavity should be probed and incised along the probe in order to visualize the endometrium.

## Tumors of the Cervix

If the tumor is visible, its location and whether it is exophytic or endophytic should be stated. Ulceration, hemorrhage, and/or necrosis should be described. The extent of involvement and the degree of penetration should be gauged; these observations are to be reinforced by microscopic studies. Extension into the body of the uterus and/or vaginal cuff should be noted. Multiple sections should be taken from the junction of the vaginal cuff and cervix. The resected margin of the vaginal mucosa should be painted with india ink for identification on microscopic sections and judgment of whether it is free of tumor. If a radical hysterectomy has been done, the surgeon should make certain that aortic, hypogastric, external iliac, and obturator nodes all are separated and properly labeled, including site of origin. Parametrial lymphatics should be examined by blocking whole segments of parametrium.

## Tumors of the Endometrium

The appearance of the tumor should be described, e.g., whether it is sessile, polypoid, focal, or diffuse. Its dimensions and its location should be noted. The appearance of the uninvolved endometrium should be described. Any gross evidence of myometrial invasion should be described and the depth measured. These observations should be augmented by microscopic study. Spread to the cervix should be noted and sections should be taken from suspected areas. Involvement of the serosa of the uterus or adnexa should be described and adequately sampled. Resected lymph nodes should be labeled as to location.

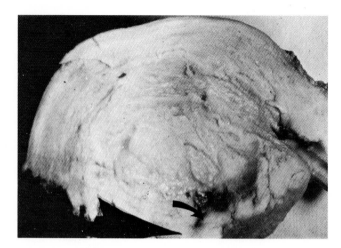

**37.8** Mixed mesenchymal tumor of the uterus: cartilagenous tissue (arrow) is useful in making a gross diagnosis.

## Sarcoma of the Uterus and/or Cervix

They may or may not be grossly distinguished from carcinoma, but with mixed mesodermal tumors there are sometimes clues. At times there may be small cartilagenous deposits (Figure 37.8). If sarcoma is suspected, sections should be fixed in Bouin's solution, for if striated muscle fibers are present, they are best demonstrated with this fixative and may not be visible in formalin-fixed tissue.

# Gross Examination of the Fallopian Tube

Description should include a statement as to whether the whole or only part of the tube is received. Occasionally only small segments are removed at laparoscopy and may only show serosa and muscularis on section. They should be described as "segment of tissue said to be from fallopian tube." The fallopian tube measures about 10-cm in length. The serosa is normally glistening and smooth. Fimbria should be free and nonadherent. The lumen should be probed for patency. The distal portion of the tube can be probed with ease; however, the intramural portion may be curved and may be difficult to probe. The mucosal folds form a stellate pattern, normally wide enough to admit a probe. If the fallopian tube is simply a part of a total hysterectomy, one or two representative sections should be taken. If it is the seat of disease, sections should be taken from the cornual end, isthmus, ampulla, and infundibulum. In an ectopic pregnancy, multisectioning may reveal a preexisting lesion that accounts for the abnormal location of the pregnancy. It is always useful to make a sketch indicating the site of the lesion and where sections have been taken. The site of the ectopic pregnancy should be determined. In chronic salpingitis, where the architecture may be distorted by adhesions and the tube folded on itself or adherent to the ovary, a sketch is often essential in order to relate a slide to the site from which it has been taken.

# Gross Examination of the Ovary

The ovary is an oval, somewhat flattened body that measures 3 to 4 cm in length, 2 to 2.5 cm in breadth, and 1 to 1.5 cm in thickness. The weight varies from 2 to 8 g. Weight and size vary with cyclic activity and pregnancy. At the time of puberty the ovary is large and its surface is smooth. The postmenopausal ovary is a small, coarsely grooved, solid structure the external surface of which resembles brain (Figure 37.9). The color is white-pink, pale blue at the site of surface follicles, reddish-purple where there is a corpus hemorrhagicum, or golden yellow with a corpus luteum. The ovary should be measured and its surface described as to color and presence of adhesions, nodulations, or excrescences. It should be bisected, the cut surface should be described, and sections should be taken that encompass the cortex, medulla, and hilus.

Surface cysts are sometimes confused with large parovarian cysts. There should be no difficulty, if it is recognized that parovarian cysts lie in the mesosalpinx between the fallopian tube and the hilus of the ovary. Serous and follicle cysts are an integral part of the ovary. This seemingly should not require emphasis, but often the surgical slip accompanying the specimen refers to the cyst as an "ovarian" cyst and the novice in pathology proceeds to regard it as such. Some cystic masses are unilocular or multilocular, whereas others may be solid tumors with a cystic component. The outer surface of the cyst should be described for color and vascularity and surface excrescences. The character of the fluid content should be noted, i.e., amber, pale, serous, or mucinous, and the volume measured. The inner surface should be examined for any areas of granularity or excrescence formation. The texture of the latter should be noted; those composed largely of stroma tend to be firmer and are usually benign. Those associated with carcinoma are soft because they are epithe-

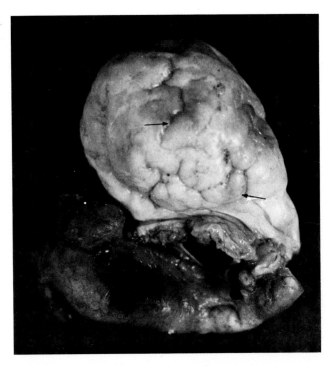

**37.9** Postmenopausal ovary: coarsely grooved surface (arrows).

lial rather than stromal. Mucinous tumors often have a knobby zone that is firm on cut section. This may be the site of malignant alteration, and several sections should be taken. Malignant serous or mucinous tumors, if partly cystic, are usually multiloculated. Both mucinous and serous cystadenocarcinoma frequently coexist with their benign counterparts and, therefore, solid areas and excrescences should be adequately sectioned.

At times, omentum may be received in association with a mucinous or serous tumor and may contain tumor implant (Figure 37.10).

Thin fibrous adhesions on the surface of the ovary are quite common and often relate to previous surgery or infection. Extensive adhesions in association with a cystic mass usually suggest endometriosis. If there are old blood deposits on the surface, this reinforces this diagnosis. Malignant tumors of the ovary may also have surface adhesions that may bind the tumor to adjacent organs.

Other tissues submitted with an ovarian tumor should be listed at the commencement of the description. The size and shape of each mass, as well as its color, should be noted. Special mention should be made as to whether a tumor mass is intact, torn, or received in one or several pieces.

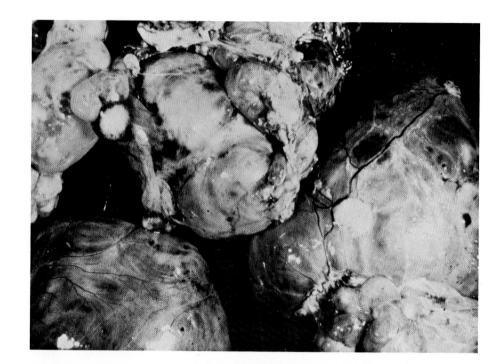

**37.10** Omental implants in myxoma peritonei.

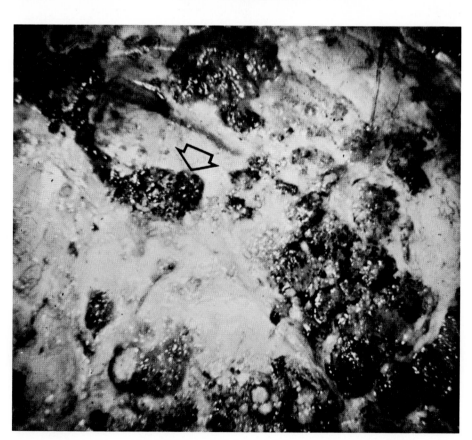

**37.11** Transcapsular spread (arrow) of serous cystadenocarcinoma of ovary.

Adherence or nonadherence to adjacent structures as well as transcapsular spread should be noted (Figure 37.11). Description of the cut surface should include whether the tumor is solid, cystic, or both. The degree of hemorrhage and/or necrosis should be stated. Other tissues removed, if not attached to the tumor mass, should be received in separate containers, each properly labeled, i.e., omentum, peritoneum, lymph nodes.

## Gross Examination of the Vagina

Radical vaginectomy usually results in the removal of the uterus, cervix, fallopian tubes, ovaries, vagina, and frequently the rectum. A rough diagram of the total specimen should be drawn and used to outline the location of the tumor. Its dimensions should be listed. The uterus and cervix should be described and appropriate sections taken. An incision should be made in the vagina (longitudinally) opposite the tumor site and the mass visualized. Its appearance should be described, i.e., whether it is exophytic, endophytic, or ulcerating. The mass should be cut through to determine the depth of infiltration. The total length of the vagina should be measured and the length proximal to and distal from the tumor as well as the distance from the cervix. If the tumor is on the posterior wall, the rectovaginal septum at the tumor site

should be cut through to determine whether infiltration to or through the septum has occurred. The rectum should be opened and the mucosa examined, particularly adjacent to the tumor site. A drop of India ink should be placed on this segment of mucosa and it should be blocked. India ink should be used to mark the resected margins and these should be blocked. Appropriate sections should be taken and their site indicated by number on a rough sketch. All lymph nodes found in the dissection should be blocked and their location similarly indicated in the sketch.

## Gross Examination of the Vulva

The nature of a radical vulvectomy specimen similarly requires the use of a rough sketch (Figure 37.12) to orient the blocks and relate the slides to the total specimen. The lesion should be described, including areas of involvement, e.g., labia majora and minora, clitoris, periurethral tissue, giving dimensions and depth of penetration of tumor. Extratumoral sites should be examined for white keratotic plaques and these should be sectioned separately after their location in the sketch is noted. The margins of the tumor should be marked by India ink and blocks should include tumoral and tumor-free tissue. Where each block comes from should be noted in the sketch. Milbrath and Wilkinson[19a] have found that xerography outlines the borders of

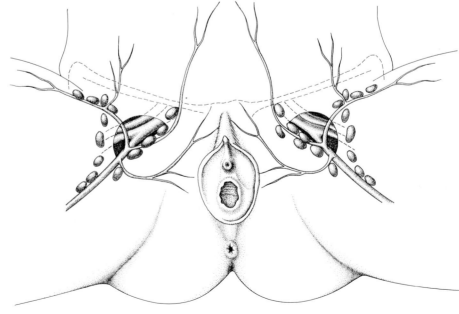

**37.12** Useful diagram for describing vulvectomy specimens.

[Courtesy of Edward J. Wilkinson, M.D., Medical College of Wisconsin.]

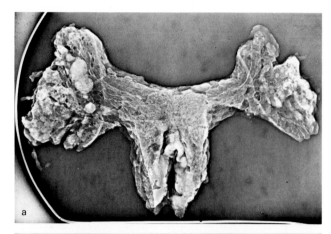

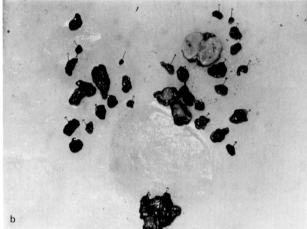

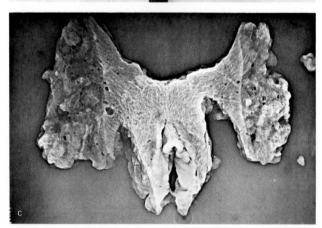

**37.13 a.** Xerogram of radical vulvectomy specimen before dissection. Nodes can be clearly seen. **b.** Lymph nodes dissected from above specimen. **c.** Xerogram of post dissection specimen.

[Figure 37.13a courtesy of J. Milbrath and E. Wilkinson, M.D., Medical College of Wisconsin.]

lymph nodes. They have used this modality to assist the pathologist in locating lymph nodes in the surgical specimen. Xerograms are taken of the fresh tissue (Figure 37.13a). The radiologist notes the sites of lymph nodes and marks them on the xerogram for the pathologist. Orienting the specimens exactly as in the xerogram, the pathologist dissects the lymph nodes (Figure 37.13b). Xerograms are again taken to be sure that all nodes have been removed (Figure 37.13c). Formalin-fixed tissue provides xerograms that are as satisfactory as fresh tissue. Zenker-fixed tissue is unsuitable because small metal densities caused by mercurial deposition register on the xerogram. Very small nodes and those superimposed on others are difficult to identify with xerography. Occasionally hematomas, blood vessels, and adipose tissue may be falsely interpreted as lymph nodes, particularly when they are at the edge of the specimen. As a whole the technique is very useful.

# Examination of the Placenta

## Indications for Examination

There is general agreement that it is not practical to study all placentas. It is good practice to encourage the obstetrical staff to examine the placenta and cord because they are in the best position to select those that should be studied.

These observations should be recorded on an information sheet that is sent with the specimen to the laboratory (Figure 37.14). This information is helpful to the pathologist in determining the extent of his other studies and in issuing a meaningful report (Figure 37.15).

The following list of criteria is widely accepted by obstetricians and pathologists as indications for placental examination:

1. All "high-risk" cases
2. Prematurity (baby weight below 2,500 g)
3. Baby small for the date
4. Postmature cases
5. All babies doing poorly
6. All possible intrauterine infections (viral or parasitic diseases during pregnancy)
7. All instances of premature rupture of membranes
8. Twins
9. Isoimmunization
10. Severe maternal anemia
11. Suspicion of neonatal anemia
12. Preeclampsia, toxemia

**PLACENTA INFORMATION SHEET**

Name: _____ Dr. _____

Age: _____ EDC: By date _____ By examination _____

Prenatal disease:



Labor and delivery:

Birth weight _____

Fetal hypoxia_____ Abnormal fetal hear_____

Rate_____

Meconium_____ Ruptured membranes_____ Duration_____

Amniotic fluid
    Normal            Excessive            Oligohydramnios

Intrapartum bleeding         Intrapartum infection

Infant at birth:

    Good condition                 Apgar
Death intrapartum                   Stillborn

Twins           Mark cord of twin A by tie or suture
                 — preferably before delivery of twin B.

Cord:
    Normal            Prolapse
    True knot         Entanglement

Examination of baby:

Normal
Respiratory disease
Infection
Hyperbilirubinemia
Malformation
Any amputation of fingers, toes, or evidence of abnormal
  rubbing or pressure from amnio-chorionic adhesions.
Other disease

**37.14** Placenta information sheet.

[Modified after P. Gruenwald, M.D.]

13. Maternal diabetes
14. Suspected single umbilical artery
15. Any malformation of baby
16. Stillbirth
17. Bleeding (placenta previa, premature separation, and vas previa)
18. Tumors of the placenta
19. Following uterine procedures during gestation, excluding uncomplicated amniocentesis

Using these criteria,[4,9] between 10 and 15% of placentas will usually be examined. If multiple births were excluded, it would be closer to 10%.

## Procedure

The placenta should be placed in a container in the refrigerator soon after delivery. It is preferable to examine it the same day; the sooner sections are taken and fixed, the better the preservation.[14] However, night deliveries

**37.15** Placenta report form.

```
                          BOOTH MEMORIAL MEDICAL CENTER
                                 Flushing, New York
PLACENTOGRAM                                          DATE _____

_____
       Family name          First name      Middle initial   Room No.   Hosp. No.

_____
          Surgeon                            Age      Date         Lab No.

_____

GROSS EXAMINATION                            Performed by_____

Weight_____ Largest dimension_____ Smallest dimension _____ Thickness_____

Shortest distance from cord insertion to placental margin _____

Cord insertion:     Normal_____ Membranous _____

Number of fetal vessels in cord _____ 2 _____ 3  True knot _____

Insertion of membranes:     Marginal _____ Circumvallate _____ Opaque _____

Thrombosed fetal vessels _____ Describe _____

Maternal surface:    Intact _____ Lacerated _____ Complete _____ Incomplete _____

Depressed area present _____ Size _____
                          Apparently caused by:   Hemorrhage_____ Infarct _____ Other _____

Hemorrhage:  Recent_____ Old _____ Size _____

Cut surface:   Describe _____

Tumor present _____ Describe _____

Hydatid change present _____ Describe _____

Monochorionic _____ Dichorionic _____ Fused _____ Separate _____

Monosmnionic _____ Diamnionic _____ Blood vessel anastomoses _____




PATHOLOGIC DIAGNOSIS:
Lab No.
                                          _____
                                          M.D., Pathologist
```

mitigate against this and refrigeration at least keeps the degree of autolysis to a minimum. Freezing placentas results in artifactual changes and obscures detail. It should be avoided.

If a baby has been born with amputated finger or toes, club feet, clefts, or ulcerations on limbs, the amniotic sac should be distended with water in order to look for amniochorionic adhesions[27] (Figure 37.16). If present they will be seen floating in the water. These are at times seen in monochorial monoamniotic twins. Adhesions can result in damage or loss of a limb (Figure 37.17a,b). If cord insertion is not membranous, membranes should be cut away from the placenta close to its margin.[2] They are laid aside for observation and preparation for sectioning. The location of the cord insertion is then noted and the length of the cord is measured. If membranes have ruptured and

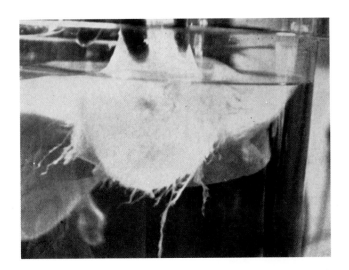

**37.16** Amniotic sac distended by water showing the fibrous strings arising from its outer surface denuded from the chorionic sac.

[Reprinted by permission from R. Torpin, Amniochorionic mesoblastic fibrous strings and amniotic bands. Associated constricting fetal malformations or fetal death, *Am. J. Obstet. Gynecol. 91*:65, 1965.]

**37.17 a.** Damage (arrows) to limb and loss of a finger due to amniochorionic adhesions.
**b.** Monozygotic twins: amniotic adhesions destroying hands (arrows).

[Figure 37.17a reprinted by permission from R. Torpin, Amniochorionic mesoblastic fibrous strings and amnionic bands. Associated constricting fetal malformations or fetal death, *Am. J. Obstet. Gynecol. 91*:65, 1965.]

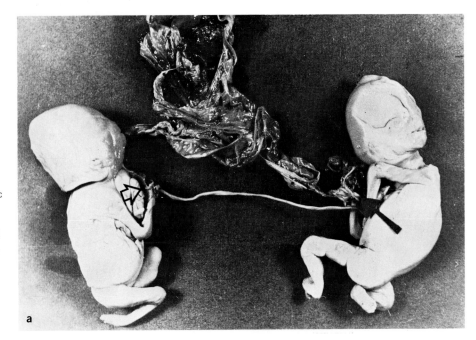

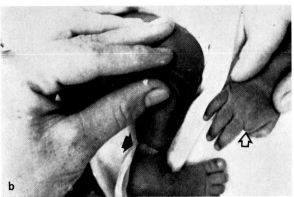

chorioamnionitis may be suspected,[18] frozen section examination of the umbilical cord is useful in detecting leukocytic infiltration.[8,15] The weight of the placenta is important in evaluating fetal development. The normal full-term placenta will weigh approximately 450 to 500 g. With prematurity or an infant small for date, the placenta will weigh less than 450 g. In diabetes mellitus, syphilis, or erythroblastosis, it may weigh considerably more than 500 g and may reach 2,000 g. The normal placenta is discoid in shape (Figure 37.18), measures 15 to 20 cm in diameter, and consists of 15 to 20 large segments (cotyledons) (Figure 37.19). It has two surfaces, one in contact with the uterus (maternal surface) and one in contact with the fetus (fetal surface). Variations of the shape should be recorded.[3] They are, in most instances, of academic interest except for a succenturiate lobe, which may implant on the lower uterine segment or cervix or the opposite wall of the uterus. The maternal surface should be examined to be sure all cotyledons are present. If any are missing and have not been removed separately, the obstetrician should be warned that there is retained placenta. Retroplacental hemorrhage may be diagnosed clinically, but extensive bleeding and hematoma can result in depressions in the maternal surface and be recognized pathologically.

The distribution of vessels on the fetal surface should be studied. Thrombi appear as yellow streaks. The placenta can now be sliced using a large stainless steel knife with a sharp edge (Figure 37.20). Infarcts and intervillous thrombi may be seen. These can be found normally in the placenta but may be present in increased numbers in toxemia. It is time consuming to study each infarct and, in general, it is unrewarding. Driscoll,[10] however, has reported a small choriocarcinoma in a term placenta that resembled an infarct, and occasionally a benign vascular tumor of the placenta can resemble infarctions. There is no simple way to identify a meaningful lesion, but a magnifying glass can be of help in identifying form and structure in a mass that otherwise appears to be a thrombus.

The cut surface of the placenta may be uniformly pale or have zones of pallor. This is exaggerated in erythroblastosis or in the placenta of the affected twin in the transfusion syndrome (see Chapter 30). The amnion should now be examined. If may be stained with meconium if there has been fetal distress. Occasionally yellow nodules may be seen and this is referred to as amnion nodosum. It is usually associated with oligohydramnios. The membranes can now be folded into a sausage-shaped roll and cut into smaller segments that are held together by pins (Figure 37.21). The smaller segments are then placed in fixative

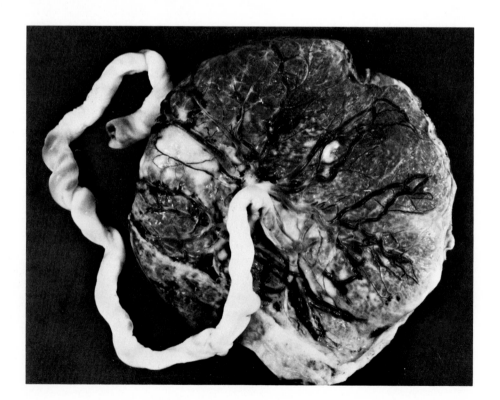

**37.18** Normal placenta, fetal surface.

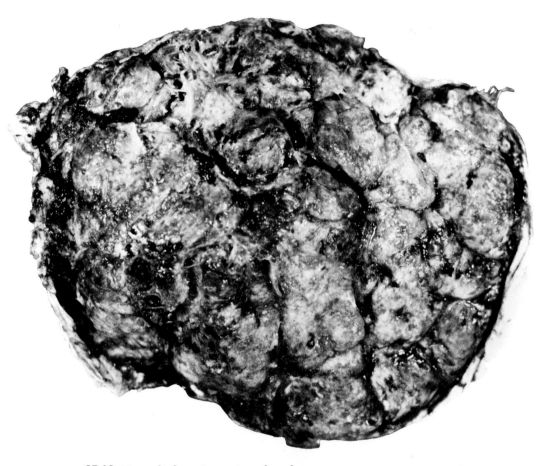

**37.19** Normal placenta, maternal surface.

**37.20** Method of sectioning placenta.

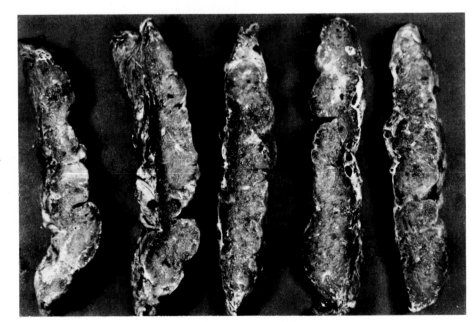

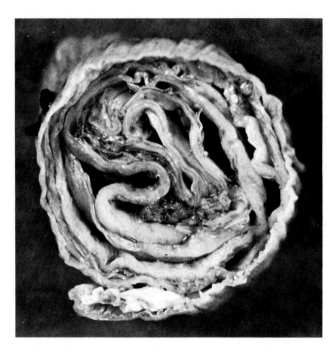

**37.21** Amniochorionic roll.

in preparation for blocking. At the time of embedding in wax, the pin is removed and the roll maintains its shape. This method allows for studying greater amnion–chorion surface and in twinning may be helpful in determining monozygous or dizygous twins.[1,6]

## Umbilical Cord

The normal length of the umbilical cord varies from 30 to 70 cm, with the average at 55 cm. Very long cords are sometimes entangled with parts of the fetus, which may result in death (Figure 37.22) or in cutting off the blood supply to a limb. Javert[17a] states that cords three times the standing length of the fetus are considered long. Conversely they are considered short when they measure less than one-third of fetal standing length. True knots, bleeding, torsion, and cord hemorrhage should be described and sectioned. The cut surface of a normal cord will reveal two arteries and one vein. Occasionally there may be a single artery and this may be associated with congenital anomalies. The umbilical vein should be checked for thrombi.

## Gross Description of the Placenta in Twinning

The gross and histologic examination of the placenta and fetal membranes is directed to determining whether twins are identical (monozygotic) or fraternal (dizygotic).[1,6] If a single chorion is present, the twins are identical. If two chorions are found, the twins may be either identical or fraternal, and further examination of the placenta and membranes is not helpful in differentiating these two. There are gross and microscopic observations that are useful in determining the number of chorions. The gross observations include identifying vascular anas-

**37.22** A long cord is arbitrarily three times the standing height of the fetus.

[Reprinted by permission from C. Javert, *Spontaneous and Habitual Abortion.* New York, McGraw-Hill, 1957, p. 137.]

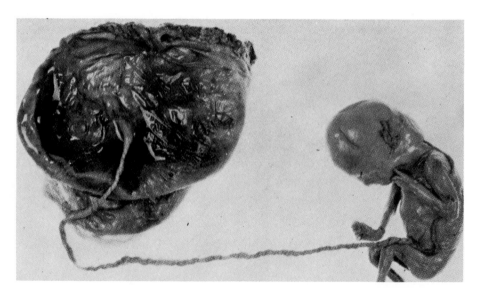

tomoses between the fetal placental circulations (Figure 37.23),[29] examining the placenta or placental masses, and inspecting the septum that separates the fetal cavities. Vascular anastomoses are best studied by injection methods that clearly identify the type of anastomosis, i.e., artery to artery or artery to vein (see Appendix II). A simple method is to see whether air bubbles can be moved from the vessels of one fetal placental circulation into the other. Examination of the placental tissue may reveal separate placentas in which case they are dichorionic. The placental tissue may be a single mass (monochorionic) or represent the fusion of two placentas (dichorionic). Close inspection of the septum between the two fetal cavities is best made by histologic observation of a roll of septum and/or T-zone sections.

In a monochorionic diamnionic twin pregnancy no chorionic tissue extends into the dividing septum between the two fetal cavities (Figure 37.24a). In a dichorionic diamnionic twin pregnancy, chorionic tissue extends between amnions that form the septum between the two fetal cavities (Figure 37.24b). In such instances the twins may be fraternal or identical. If a single placental mass is found which is monoamnionic (Figure 37.24c), the twins are identical.

These gross observations are subject to verification or rejection by histologic sectioning of the rolled segment of septum or the T section of the placenta.[2] If the gross identification of an achorionic septum has been correct, the septum will be seen to consist of two amnions with no chorion between them (Figure 37.25a,c,e). The placenta is monochorionic–diamnionic and the twins are identical. If the septum contains chorionic tissue between the two amnions, the septum will be seen to consist of amnion-chorion–chorion–amnion (Figure 37.25b,d,f). The placenta is diamnionic–dichorionic and the twins may be fraternal or identical.

Gross observations alone should never be relied on but should be combined with histologic study or rolled septal and T-zone sections.

In studying triplet and other multiple pregnancies, the single and fused placentas should be weighed. No attempt to separate fused placentas and to weigh them separately should be made. It is better to take the total weight and compare that figure to the total weight of the babies.

## Examination of Tissue from Spontaneous and Missed Abortion

If bacterial, viral, or cytogenetic studies are to be performed,[16,17,22,23,25,26] the specimen should be handled in a sterile manner in the operating room and placed in a sterile container with no fixative added. If viral studies are

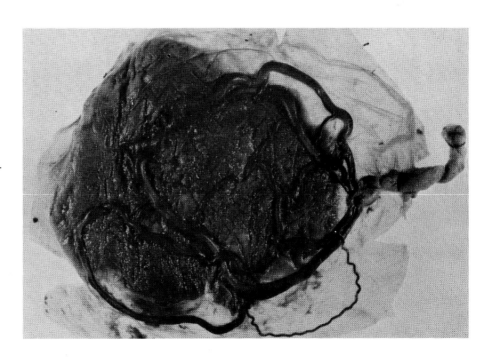

**37.23** Artery to vein anastomosis in monozygotic twins.

[Courtesy of P. Wentworth, M.D.]

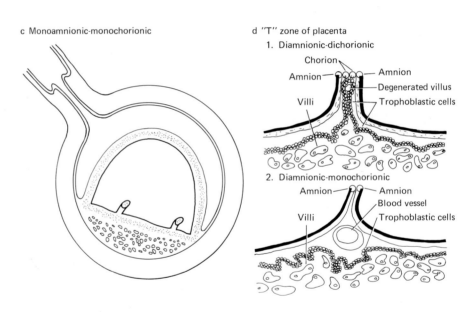

a Diamnionic-Monochorionic

b Diamnionic-dichorionic

"T" zone D2

"T" zone D1

c Monoamnionic-monochorionic

d "T" zone of placenta

1. Diamnionic-dichorionic

Chorion
Amnion — Amnion
Degenerated villus
Trophoblastic cells
Villi

2. Diamnionic-monochorionic

Amnion — Amnion
Blood vessel
Trophoblastic cells
Villi

**37.24 a.** Monochorionic twin pregnancy. No chorionic tissue extends into dividing septum between the two fetal cavities. **b.** Dichorionic twin pregnancy. Chorionic tissue extends between amnions that form the septum between the two fetal cavities. **c.** Rare monoamnionic–monochorionic twin pregnancy. No septum. **d.** Anatomic arrangement of the T zone of a dichorionic placenta (top) as contrasted to a monochorionic placenta (bottom).

[Reprinted by permission from M. Allen and U. C. Turner, Twin births—identical or fraternal twins? *Obstet. Gynecol. 37*(9):4, 1971.]

to be performed,[12,20,21] that portion of the specimen should be stored in −70°C until homogenized and processed in the viral laboratory.

If bacterial cultures are requested,[5,7,11,24] fragments of tissue should be planted in aerobic and anaerobic media and on specific media for TBC or fungae, if these are suspected. Small fragments of tissue, preferably no larger than 5 mm, should be placed in media. Minced fragments are more suitable. Cultures should be taken from both placenta and membranes. Certain types of bacteria grow best in specific media; e.g., TBC grows best in Loeffler's media and fungi on Saboraud's media. Culture media for a wide range of organisms should be kept in the delivery room area and should, of course, be replaced from time to time if not used.

If cytogenetic studies are contemplated, care should be taken to prevent contamination beyond that which occurs from passage per vaginum. This is important if chromosomal studies are to be done; it is not essential for sex chromatin analysis. Sex chromatin studies can be done on

**37.25 a.** Cross section of a rolled segment of the septum (dividing membrane) of a monochorionic twin placenta. No chorion between the two amnions. **b.** Cross section of a rolled segment of the septum (dividing membrane) of a dichorionic twin placenta. Septum is thick chorion between the two amnions. **c.** High magnification of the dividing septum of a monochorionic twin placenta. Septum consists of two amnions (A). **d.** High magnification of the dividing septum of a dichorionic twin placenta. Septum consists of amnion (A) chorion (C) chorion (C) amnion (A). Degenerated villi are seen. **e.** Sections of the T zone of a monochorionic twin placenta. No chorionic tissue extends from the placenta into the dividing septum. **f.** Section of the T zone of a dichorionic twin placenta. Chorionic tissue extends from the placenta into the dividing septum.

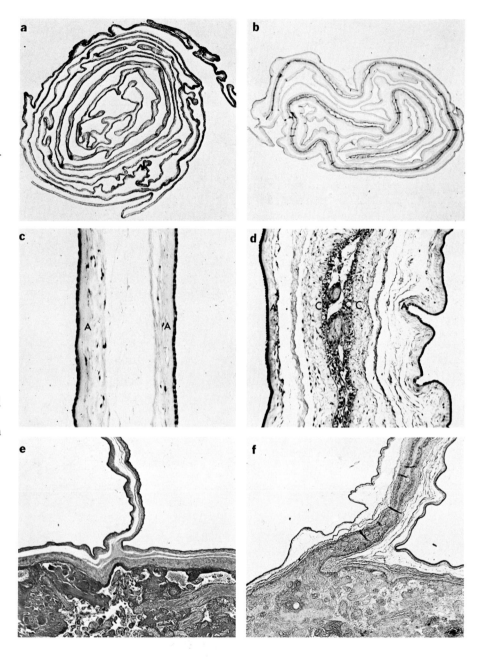

cells from the amnion, peritoneum, or epidermis of the fetus. It is preferable to examine cells from two tissue sites and a record should be kept of the sites studied.

If the fetal tissue is not macerated and is available soon after delivery, liver, kidney, and bone marrow are a good source of mitotic activity. Minced tissue should be added to 10 ml of Hank's balanced salt solution containing 1 mg Colcemid, incubated for 6 hr, and sent for processing to the cytogenetic laboratory. If the tissues are in a good state of preservation this method is simple and useful. It is recommended that more than one tissue site be studied at the same time, because where one preparation may fail, another may be successful.

Short-term cultures (72-hr preparations) from hematopoietic tissue can be useful. Depending on the age of the conceptus, kidney, liver, spleen, lymph node, thymus, and

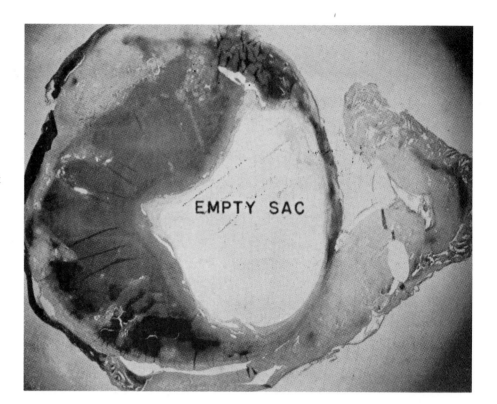

**37.26** Spontaneous abortion: empty sac, absent fetus, absent cord. Pathologic ovum.

[Reprinted by permission from C. Javert, *Spontaneous and Habitual Abortion.* New York, McGraw-Hill, 1957, p. 127.]

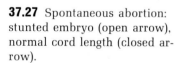

**37.27** Spontaneous abortion: stunted embryo (open arrow), normal cord length (closed arrow).

[Reprinted by permission from C. Javert, *Spontaneous and Habitual Abortion.* New York, McGraw-Hill, 1957, p. 106.]

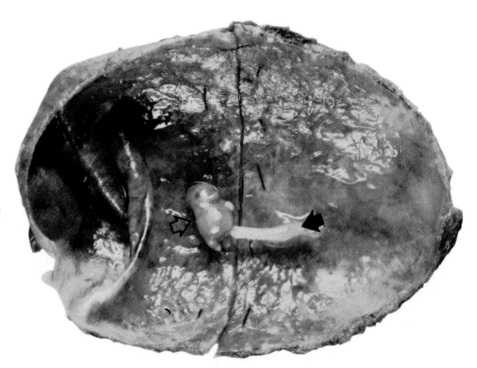

bone marrow yield excellent results when minced in TC-199 media and the cell suspension is incubated with phytohemagglutinin.[16]

Cytogenetic studies are valuable in studying abortion. It appears that 25% of first-trimester abortions show chromosomal abnormalities.

After any of the above have been completed, the material should be examined under saline, using a dissecting microscope,[19] if the specimen is small. A decidual cast should be carefully opened in order to study the enclosed sac, if present. At times it may be empty and devoid of fetus or umbilical cord (Figure 37.26). On occasion, a stump of umbilical cord may be present and it should be sectioned to determine whether all vessels are present. What may appear to the naked eye as a minute yellow fleck may on high magnification with the dissecting microscope have the outlines of an embryo (Figure 37.27).

The fetus may be received separately and have easily recognizable features. It may show varying degrees of maceration but this should not deter further examination. A host of congenital anomalies can be detected in fetuses of varying size. These include meningocoele, spina bifida anencephaly (Figure 37.28), cleft palate (Figure 37.29), absent limb, persistent gill clefts, and deformed ears. If the fetus is small, a magnifying lens should be used to make these observations. The chest, abdomen, and head should be opened and internal anomalies looked for. Javert[17a] noted that there was a far higher incidence of external abnormalities than internal anomalies, a ratio of 20:1. Blanc[5] has emphasized that maceration should not deter examination because one can, at times, assure parents that the cause of abortion was not related to their chromosome makeup.

Some of the fetuses may have umbilical cord looping that may have produced strangulation (Figure 37.30). Loops may wrap around limbs.

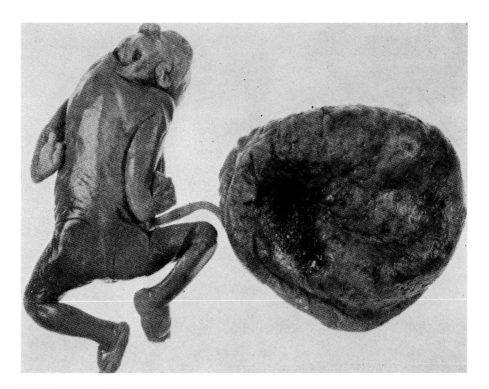

**37.28** Anencephaly.

[Reprinted by permission from C. Javert, *Spontaneous and Habitual Abortion*. New York, McGraw-Hill, 1957, p. 119.]

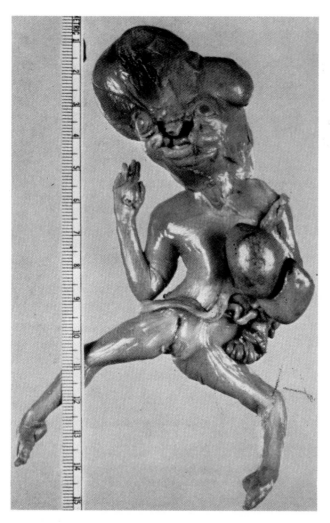

**37.29** Harelip and cleft palate.

[Reprinted by permission from C. Javert, *Spontaneous and Habitual Abortion.* New York, McGraw-Hill, 1957, p. 116.]

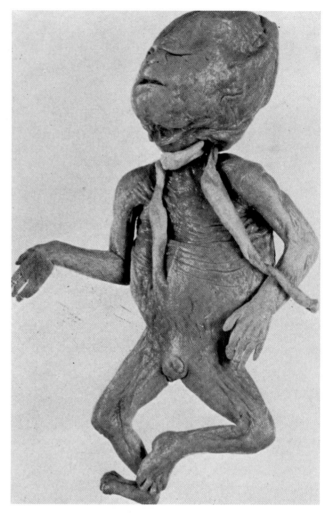

**37.30** Cord strangulation.

[Reprinted by permission from C. Javert, *Spontaneous and Habitual Abortion.* New York, McGraw-Hill, 1957, p. 138.]

**37.31** Injection apparatus used to study fetal vessels.

[Courtesy of P. Wentworth, M.D.]

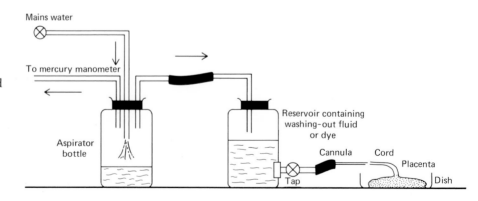

# APPENDIX I: Basic Instruments and Supplies

1. A balance that weighs specimens up to 1 kg and access, when necessary, to a larger one
2. A large, high-quality magnifying glass, preferably mounted on a gooseneck base
3. Aprons
4. Rubber gloves
5. A centimeter ruler
6. Scissors; eye type, medium, and large
7. Toothed forceps, small, medium, and large
8. Probes, of a diameter to enter the lumen of the fallopian tube
9. Surgical blade holders and a supply of disposable blades
10. Large stainless steel knives
11. Tea bags used to hold endometrial curettings
12. Dissecting needles
13. Cork boards and standard pins
14. Dental wax
15. India ink
16. One percent eosin solution
17. Neutral formalin (10%), with a stock of it kept at 4°C
18. Bouin's solution
19. Buffered glutareldehyde (2.5%), kept in a refrigerator at 4°C and replenished each month

# APPENDIX II: Injection Technique for Staining the Fetal Vessel Walls

After blood is washed from the blood vessels, a red dye is injected through a cannula into the umbilical arteries and a blue dye, aniline blue (alcoholic), is injected into the umbilical vein. Both these dyes are insoluable in water but are soluble in ethylene glycol monoethyl ether (Cellosolve). The basis of the technique is to inject the dye, dissolved in Cellosolve, into the vessels and to stain the vessel walls. The dyes do not escape through the vessel walls. The only mixture of dyes occurs in the capillary bed, the main chorionic vessels remaining clearly defined by one dye or the other.

The placenta is placed maternal surface downward in a dish. One of the umbilical arteries is defined by dissection 6 to 10 cm from the placenta and a annula (intravenous drip-set needle) inserted into it and clamped with an artery forceps. A slack ligature is put around the cord and can-

**Table 37.1** Solutions

| | | |
|---|---|---|
| A. Washing solution | | |
| Sodium acetate | | 49 g |
| Water | | 1000 ml |
| B. Red dye | | |
| Stock solution of 2% Fett Rot in Cellosolve | | 20 ml |
| Cellosolve | | 200 ml |
| Liquid formaldehyde | | 10 ml |
| C. Blue dye | | |
| Stock solution of 2% aniline blue (alcoholic) in Cellosolve | | 20 ml |
| Cellosolve | | 200 ml |
| Liquid formaldehyde | | 10 ml |
| D. Fixative | | |
| Liquid formaldehyde | | 500 ml |
| Sodium acetate | | 200 g |
| Water | | 5000 ml |

nula. An incision is made into the umbilical veins just distal to the ligature. The cannula is connected to a reservoir of solution A jointed to an aspirator bottle connected to the main water supply and a mercury manometer (Figure 37.31).

By turning on the water, solution A is fed into the fetal vessels and the blood is washed out from them. The washing is continued until the fluid emerging from the incision in the umbilical veins is almost free of blood. Up to 2 liters of fluid may be used and 15 to 30 min of time to wash out the fetal vessels. The pressure is varied from 100 to 200 mm Hg, the usual figure being 180 mm Hg. The fluid is allowed to remain in the dish throughout the whole process, including the injection with dye, so that as washing proceeds the placenta becomes immersed and pressure on the undersurface is relieved. After washing, the reservoir of solution A is disconnected and replaced by solution B, which is run into the artery at a pressure of 60 mm Hg for 5 min, at the end of which the cannula is removed and the slack ligature tightened to prevent leakage. As a rule it is necessary to connulate only one umbilical artery in order to fill the whole arterial system.

The cannula is now inserted into the incision in the umbilical vein, clamped, and loosely ligated as before and connected to a reservoir of solution C. This solution is also run in for 5 min at 60 mm Hg, at the end of which time the cannula is removed and the slack ligature tightened. The placenta is fixed by immersion in solution D for at least 24 hr. To examine the placenta, the membranes are gently stripped off and the cord and chorionic vessels are inspected either with the naked eye or by the aid of a hand lens. The method is simple and clearly defines the cord and chorion vasculature.

# REFERENCES

1. Allen, M. Shannon, Jr., and Turner, U. C. III. Twin birth—identical or fraternal twins? *Obstet. Gynecol. 37:4*, April 1971.

2. Benirschke, K. Examination of the placenta. *Obstet. Gynecol. 18:*309, 1961.

3. Bergman, P. Accidental discovery of uterus bicornis on examination of placenta. *Obstet. Gynecol. 17:*649, 1961.

4. Blanc, W. A., M.D. Personal communication, 1975.

5. Blanc, W. A. Pathways of Fetal and Early Neonatal Infection. *J. Pediatr. 59:*473, 1961.

6. Bleisch, V. R. Diagnosis of monochorial twin placentation. *Am. J. Clin. Pathol. 42:*277, 1964.

7. Braun, P., Lee, Y. H., Klein, J. O., Marcy, S. M., Klein, J. A., Charles, D., and Kass, H. E. Birthweight and genital mycoplasma in pregnancy. *N. Engl. J. Med. 284:*167, 1971.

8. Dominguez, R., Segal, A. J., and O'Sullivan, J. A. Leukocytic infiltration of the umbilical cord. *J.A.M.A. 173:*346, 1960.

9. Driscoll, S. G., M.D. Personal communication, 1975.

10. Driscoll, S. G. Choriocarcinoma: An "incidental finding" within a term placenta. *Obstet. Gynecol. 21:*96, 1962.

11. Eden, A. Perinatal Mortality Caused by Vibrio Fetus.

12. Garcia, A. G. P. Fetal infection in chicken pox and alastrium with histologic study of the placenta. *Pediatrics 32:*895, 1963.

13. Greene, R. R., Gerbie, A. B., Melorin, V., and Eckman, T. R. Hemangiopericytomas of the uterus. *Am. J. Obstet. Gynecol. 106(7):*1020, 1970.

14. Gruenwald, P. Examination of the placenta by the pathologist. *Arch. Pathol. 77(1):*41, 1964.

15. Hosmer, M. E., and Sprunt, K. Screening for infection after early rupture of membranes. *Pediatrics 49:*283, 1972.

16. Jacobson, C. B. *Reproductive Cytogenetics.* New York, Hoeber, 1967.

17. Jacobson, C. B., and Barter, R. H. Some cytogenetic aspects of habitual abortion. *Am. J. Obstet. Gynecol. 97(5):*666, 1967.

17a. Javert, C. T. *Spontaneous and Habitual Abortion.* New York, McGraw-Hill, 1957.

18. MacVicar, J. Chorioamnionitis. *Clin. Obstet. Gynecol. 13:*272, 1970.

19. Mall, F. P., and Meyers, A. W. Studies on abortions: Survey of pathologic ova in Carnegie embryological collection. *Contrib. Embryol. 12:*56, 1921.

19a. Milbrath, J. R., and Wilkinson, E. Personal communication, 1975.

20. Monif, G. R. G. *Viral Infection of the Human Fetus.* New York, Macmillan, 1969, p. 2.

21. Monif, G. R. G., Sever, J. L., Schiff, G. M., and Traub, R. C. The recovery of rubella virus from productions of conception. *Am. J. Obstet. Gynecol. 91:*1143, 1965.

22. Naujoks, H. Culture of tissue from spontaneous human abortions. *Acta Cytol. 7:*300, 1963.

23. Overbach, A. M., Daniel, S. J., and Cassidy, G. Umbilical cord histology in the management of potential perinatal infection. *J. Pediatr. 76:*22, 1974.

24. Romano, N., Romano, F., and Carollo, F. T strains of *Mycoplasma* in bronchopneumonic lungs of an aborted fetus. *N. Engl. J. Med. 285:*950, 1971.

25. Rosenstein, D. L., and Navorati-Reyner, A. Cytomegalic inclusion disease: Observations of the characteristic inclusion bodies in the placenta. *Am. J. Obstet. Gynecol. 89:*220, 1964.

26. Sever, J. L., Huebner, R. J., Costellano, C. A., and Bell, J. A. *Am. Rev. Respir. Dis. 88*(Suppl):342, 1963.

27. Torpin, R. M. D. Amniochorionic mesoblastic fibrous strings and amniotic bands. *Am. J. Obstet. Gynecol. 91(1):*65, 1965.

28. Wash, T. A., and Davis, F. C. Cryostat examination of the cervical cone. *Am. J. Obstet. Gynecol. 105:*105, 1969.

29. Wentworth, P. Some anomalies of the faetal vessels of the human placenta. *J. Anat. 99(2):*273, 1965.

June Marchant, Ph.D.

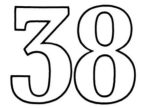

# Animal Models for Tumors of the Ovary and Uterus

## GENERAL INTRODUCTION

The ultimate objective of animal studies of cancer is to achieve a better understanding of factors responsible for human disease in the hope that this may be ultimately eliminated or controlled. In order to establish the basic biologic mechanisms governing the development of human cancer, systematic controlled experiments are required. For practical and ethical reasons, these are impossible to carry out with humans so animal models have to be sought.

Counterparts of many human diseases, including cancer, have been discovered occurring spontaneously in animals. Chapter 39 by E. Cotchin describes naturally occurring tumors of the ovary and uterus in many species. However, these examples are almost always sporadic and usually infrequent in their occurrence, and the most important requirements for cancer models in animals are that they be reproducible and predictable. They should also resemble the human counterpart.

## ANIMAL MODELS FOR TUMORS OF THE OVARY

The first two requirements are best met by disease models that employ highly inbred strains of animals, such as the genetically pure lines of mice established many years ago by

C. C. Little and L. C. Strong by 20 consecutive brother–sister matings. Each pure strain has a different spectrum of spontaneous cancer incidence and different susceptibilities to cancer-inducing agents, as well as to other diseases. Since their pioneering work during the earlier part of this century, pure lines of other species of laboratory animals have been established and proved to be valuable tools in many studies, but the mouse and rat have been the most fully explored species with respect to tumorigenesis.

The third condition, that animal tumor models should resemble the human counterpart, is more difficult to achieve, partly because of the tremendous variation in the gross anatomy of the mammalian female genital tract. Some of these features are illustrated by Figure 38.1.

Comparing the human tract with that of common laboratory animals, one notices that human ovaries lie freely exposed to the general peritoneal cavity; in laboratory mammals, however, the ovaries lie in membranous pouches that partly (rabbit and guinea pig) or completely (rat and mouse) isolate them from the general peritoneal cavity. If the pouch (or bursa) is complete, the internal opening of the oviduct lies within it.[130]

Again, when we look at the uterus, the human species and higher primates have a "simplex" uterus with a single cervix. In the rabbit, however, the uterus is "duplex," having two long separate uterine horns with independent cervical openings into the vagina. Such a condition can occur as a structural anomaly in women on occasion.[63]

The cervix is defined[129] as the "caudal, nongestational portion of the mammalian uterus . . ." whose "epithelial lining is continuous with that of the vagina." The extent of this squamous epithelium into the uterine horns varies considerably in different species.

Another species variation is seen in the relative proportions, one to another, of the different parts of the female genital tract. These variations are matched by complementary variations in the anatomy of the penile structure of the male.[63] This lock and key principle is probably one of nature's ways of keeping different but closely related species distinct from one another.

This chapter considers first ovarian tumor models in laboratory animals. This is followed by animal tumor models of other parts of the female genital tract.

## The Ovary as a Tumor Model

The ovary has many advantages as a model for disease. It is a well-defined entity that can be completely removed without the problem of residual rests. In the mouse, it is often small enough to be transplanted *in toto* back into the ovarian capsules from which it originated (orthotopic transplantation), or it can be exchanged for the ovary of another animal of the same genotype, or of another histocompatible genotype, with a high degree of functional success. With larger ovaries, vascularization of the complete organ is not achieved by this means; however, in such cases the organ can be cut into several fragments, and each fragment contains a full representation of all the different cell types present in the normal organ. Such fragments may be transplanted to a variety of different sites, including the anterior chamber of the eye, where they may become vascularized and remain under constant observation. Function of the transplant can be monitored by taking vaginal smears.

Of the thousands of oocytes present in the normal mouse ovary at birth, only a few are destined to be released during reproductive life. However, reduction in their number occurs by degeneration and this atresia continues throughout life. Its rate varies in different mouse strains and is particularly rapid in CBA mice, which develop a high incidence of spontaneous granulosa cell ovarian tumors in old age.[181] The rate of atresia is retarded when the pituitary is removed[82] and recent results have shown that it is speeded up by neonatal thymectomy, suggesting that a dual control mechanism may be controlling growth and maturation of follicles in postnatal ovarian development.[145] Atretic follicles in the stroma probably come to comprise the interstitial cells in the aging ovary, which are capable of responding to stimulation by pituitary hormones.

The number of oocytes present at birth in the ovaries of mice of different pure strains varies considerably.[83] Oocyte deficiency, which is the prime effect of aging, can lead to tumor development without further intervention, as will be seen later.

In the following pages, we shall examine the evidence in detail and see just how far the present tumor models of the mouse ovary, or the ovaries of other species of laboratory animals, can be made to satisfy the criteria of predictability, reproducibility, and resemblance to the human counterpart as an animal model of human ovarian cancer.

Because the literature is now very cumbersome, only key references are given. The reader desiring a more comprehensive reference list is referred to the excellent reviews by Jull[86] and Murphy.[137]

## Spontaneous Ovarian Tumors in Laboratory Animals

The early report of Slye[174] on autopsies carried out on 22,000 mice suggested that tumors of the mouse ovary are quite uncommon. Only 46 solid ovarian tumors were

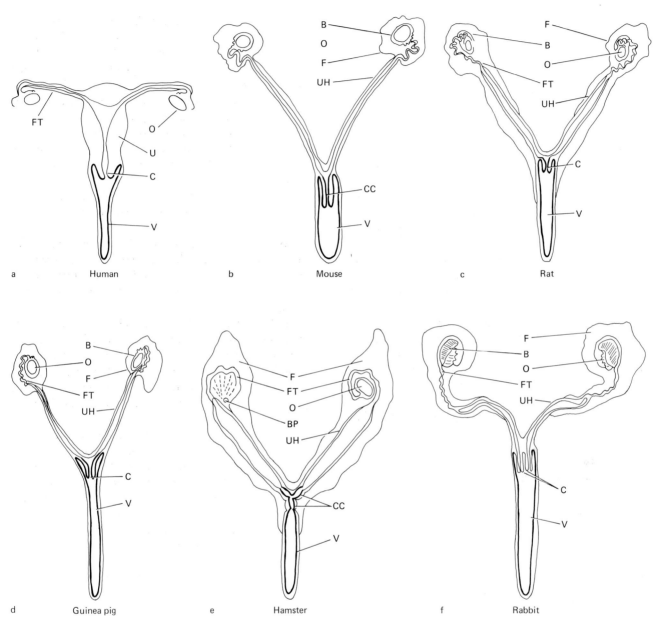

**38.1** Comparative aspects of the female reproductive tract of the human and laboratory animal species. Redrawn and adapted from Hafez[64] and Mossman[130]. B, ovarian bursa; BP, blind pore; C, cervix; CC, cervical canal; F, fat; FT, fallopian tube; O, ovary; U, uterus; UH, uterine horn; and V, vagina. Note the complete (mouse and hamster), almost complete (rat, guinea pig), or partial (rabbit) enclosure of the ovary in a bursa, or pouch, whereas the human ovary remains free in the peritoneum. Also note the different proportions of the various anatomic sites, and the different extents of the vaginal squamous epithelium (heavy line) in the cervical region.

found, together with a small number of simple cysts. A recent report by Carter[19] on the autopsy records of approximately 3,000 female mice, mostly of random-bred Chester Beatty stock with a smaller number of Swiss albino mice and three inbred strains (BALB/c, CBA, and 101), revealed 18 ovarian tumors, only three of which were in untreated animals. He found only three ovarian tumors in 300 autopsies of female rats of the Chester Beatty stock (originally derived from Wistar animals). Reports of spontaneous ovarian tumors in guinea pigs and hamsters are rare and I have not found any report of them in rabbits. They have been reported in cats and monkeys and appear to be quite common in dogs and in fowl (see Chapter 39 by E. Cotchin).

Although it would seem from this that ovarian tumors are uncommon in rats and mice, they are seen much more frequently in research institutes holding certain inbred strains of mice if the animals are allowed to live out their normal life spans. They are not seen in some of the commonly kept strains, possibly because of the competing risks of other diseases; for example, in strains harboring the mammary tumor-inducing or leukemia-inducing viruses, death occurs from these causes at a much earlier age than is usually required for development of ovarian tumors in this species.

Many methods of inducing ovarian tumors in strains of mice in which they are not normally seen have been devised. They are of two types. There are those known as "direct" methods, which have an immediate deleterious effect on the ovary and can bring about tumorigenesis without further intervention. There are also "indirect" methods that do not have such a marked initial effect on the ovary but that bring about a chronic modification of its internal environment. I shall consider the different methods of tumor induction in mouse ovaries in turn and indicate which are applicable to other laboratory species.

## Methods of Inducing Ovarian Tumors in Mice

### Direct methods

X-IRRADIATION. This was the earliest discovered method of inducing ovarian tumors. It was first reported by Furth and Furth[42] that whole-body irradiation of mice with x rays could lead to ovarian tumorigenesis. It has since been confirmed by many investigators and is also an effective method in the rat.

The minimum dose required is around 25 R and the incidence rises with the dose received.[41] Administration of a single dose or chronic exposure to low dose levels, can be effective. By operating and drawing the ovaries out through a lead shield, it was shown that irradiation of the ovaries themselves was all that was required to induce tumors.[104] Conversely, irradiation of the whole body with the ovaries shielded induced no tumors.[28]

Work during the last decade has applied quantitative methods to show that irradiation has an acute effect on the mouse ovary, killing many oocytes within hours. After a dose of 25 R x rays given to 10-day-old mice, the residual oocytes were reduced to zero by the time the animals were 200 to 300 days old, whereas nonirradiated control animals still had several hundred remaining at 600 days.[149] At birth, mouse oocytes are very resistant to irradiation damage, but by 21 days their sensitivity is maximal. Thereafter they become more resistant.[154] At all ages, the smaller oocytes are more vulnerable.

The tumors induced by irradiation of the ovary of rats and mice are predominantly tubular adenomas.

CHEMICAL CARCINOGENS. To avoid confusing the reader with the former names of chemical carcinogens occurring in the older literature and their revised nomenclature, the key in Table 38.1 is appended for those most commonly used in this chapter.

7,12-Dimethylbenz[a]anthracene (DMBA) was the first chemical inducer of mouse ovarian tumors to be recognized. During investigations of mammary tumor induction in mice and rats with various polycyclic hydrocarbon carcinogens, a number of ovarian tumors were also noted in mice that had received DMBA in oily solutions painted on the skin.[73,120]

Since that time there have been many reports of ovarian tumor induction in mice by DMBA administered by a number of different routes: intragastric,[8] intraperitoneal,[96] intravenous,[101] subcutaneous,[172] direct application to the ovary,[97] neonatal injection,[172] as well as after brief *in vitro* exposure of the ovaries to DMBA, followed by reimplantation in the animals from which they had been removed.[87] There is evidence of a dose–response effect of DMBA *in vitro* as well as *in vivo*.[89]

Tumor induction time and incidence rates are influenced by age and strain of the treated mice.[115] Administration of DMBA to immature mice of two strains, induced tumors in all mice by 6 months.[96] Treatment of adult females gives a high incidence in mice of the C3H strain but not in the C57B1 strain.[101]

The experiments in which tumors have developed in reimplanted ovaries after exposure to DMBA *in vitro* suggest that DMBA itself is the effective carcinogen, rather than some metabolite formed by the liver,[89] and recent studies with tritiated DMBA also suggest this.[98] Nevertheless, when three of the metabolites of DMBA were tested, one of them was found to be effective *in vitro*; this was 12-hydroxymethyl-7-methylbenz[a]anthracene.[89]

It has also been shown that the related chemical, TMBA

**Table 38.1**   Chemical carcinogens

| Symbol | Formerly called: | Now called: |
|--------|------------------|-------------|
| BP | 3,4-Benzpyrene | Benzo[a]pyrene |
| DBA | 1,2,5,6-Dibenzanthracene | Dibenz[a,h]anthracene |
| DEN | Diethylnitrosamine | N-Nitrosodiethylamine |
| DMBA | 9,10-Dimethyl-1,2-benzanthracene | 7,12-Dimethylbenz[a]anthracene |
| FAA | 2-Acetylaminofluorene | 2-Fluorenylacetamide |
| MC | 20-Methylcholanthrene | 3-Methylcholanthrene |

(7,8,12-trimethylbenz[a]anthracene) has ovarian tumor-inducing potential comparable with DMBA.[192]

Other polycyclic hydrocarbon carcinogens are relatively poor in inducing ovarian tumors in mice. 3-Methylcholanthrene (MC) is much less effective than DMBA[8] and I have seen very few ovarian tumors in many hundreds of mice treated with this carcinogen. Benzo[a]pyrene (BP) has only weakly carcinogenic action on the mouse ovary.[127]

In many experiments with these chemical carcinogens, particularly DMBA, there are competing risks of development of mammary tumors or leukemia, but if ovaries from a mouse treated with DMBA are grafted orthotopically to a new host of compatible genotype, or if ovaries are treated with DMBA in vitro and then reimplanted, only ovarian tumors are seen and the incidence may be virtually 100%.

Another chemical that can induce ovarian tumors in adult mice is the chemotherapeutic agent triethylene melamine, when injected intraperitoneally.[119]

A chemical method of inducing ovarian tumors that may prove to be very useful in future investigations is the intrauterine exposure of mice to urethane injected into the mother on days 11 and 13 of gestation.[147,197] Tumors induced by this treatment of ICR/J mice were cystadenomas. Ovarian teratomas have also been seen, whereas the vast majority of ovarian tumors induced in adult mice by chemicals are of the granulosa–theca cell series.

Rats respond to DMBA treatment in a different manner from mice. Although development of mammary tumors is frequently seen in both species, development of ovarian tumors does not occur in the rat. Instead, DMBA leads to severe adrenal necrosis in this species.[74] It has been shown that $^{14}$C-DMBA is taken up in similar fashion by the adrenals and ovaries of both rats and mice,[88] so that different susceptibilities of the organs of the two species are not because of a particularly high ability to concentrate the carcinogen. It has, however, recently been shown that DMBA

does have some tumorigenic potential for the rat ovary. Benign tumors arising in intrasplenic ovarian grafts in this species (see p. 802) become malignant and metastasize in many cases if DMBA treatment is also given. Treatment with a different potent carcinogen DEN (diethylnitrosamine, N-nitrosodiethylamine) had no such enhancing effect.[69]

Another chemical having some tumorigenic potential for the rat ovary is 2-acetylaminofluorene (2-fluorenylacetamide, FAA). In combination with the method of parabiosis (see p. 803), granulosa cell tumors were induced in 50% of the intact partners parabiosed to castrates and treated with FAA, whereas no tumors were found in untreated parabionts or in single females given FAA.[9]

An ovarian tumor has been reported arising in the offspring of a mother rat treated during pregnancy with FAA and progesterone. This tumor was classified as a "mucinous ovarian papillary adenocarcinoma." It was transplantable, had a short latent period of 14 days, caused ascites in 40 days, and killed in 60 days with metastases in lymph nodes, lung, and liver.[184] Benign mesovarial leiomyomas have been induced in Charles River CD rats by high and middle doses of mesuprine hydrochloride and soteronol hydrochloride, which are chemically similar and are long-acting, potent, β-adrenergic receptor stimulants.[142]

In guinea pigs and rabbits, DMBA does not give rise to ovarian tumors.[97] In Syrian hamsters, ovarian tumors have been seen after treatment with DMBA or MC, but the incidence is rather low.[70] Occasional tumors have also been seen in hamsters that have received BP or o-aminoazotoluene.

TRANSPLANTATION. Transplantation methods have been exploited in determining the function of different cell types of the ovary, and the relationships of the ovary with other organs have been explored by their use. Transplantation has also been much utilized in studying ovarian tumorigenesis in mice. Once a tumor-inducing method has been discovered, ovarian transplantation (for instance, from a treated animal to an untreated one and vice versa) makes it possible to separate the effects of the inducing agent into direct effects on the ovary itself and indirect effects mediated systemically through the host environment. Also, with the use of $F_1$ hybrids between two strains of differing susceptibilities to an inducing agent, transplantation methods facilitate studies of the factors determining the susceptibility of each of the genotypes.

Despite the advantages of transplantation in the above type of investigation, however, it cannot be regarded as an entirely innocuous procedure. When a mouse ovary is transplanted, even back into its own ovarian capsules, a large part of the tissue breaks down. If vascularization occurs, the grafted organ becomes reconstituted but never fully. There is an early decrease in the number of oocytes and ripening follicles that is associated with a shortening of reproductive life. The diminished amount of functional ovarian tissue may also lead to an imbalance of ovarian and pituitary hormones. Transplantation can, then, be regarded as a method of bringing about premature aging of the ovaries, resulting eventually in ovarian tumorigenesis.

It was observed that ovaries of DBA mice transplanted orthotopically into normal $F_1$ (DBA × C3H) mice became tumorous in five out of nine cases killed 12 to 24 months later.[75] Tumors have also developed in normal ovaries transplanted subcutaneously into castrated hosts of the same genotype.[86] Few tumors were seen if the hosts were ovariectomized females, but up to 80% were seen in some genotypes when the hosts were castrated males. These tumors were almost all tubular adenomas. If grafts came from DMBA-treated donors, however, tumors occurred in many of the castrated hosts of either sex, and they were predominantly of the granulosa–theca cell type.

In experiments with rats, ovarian fragments grafted into the anterior chamber of the eye of gonadectomized hosts all became vascularized after 1 year and many developed into granulosa cell tumors.[99]

OVARIAN VASOLIGATION. In the rat, abnormal ovarian activity can be brought about by ligating ovarian blood vessels temporarily. A continuous estrus is established, but it fails to control the hypophysis and the cytology becomes similar to that of a castrated animal.[35] A ligature of only 30 min was required to produce lasting changes, and ovarian tumors followed 20 months or more afterward.[36] This method of ovarian tumor induction does not seem to have been explored further.

THYMECTOMY. It has been shown, for three different mouse strains and four hybrid genotypes, that thymectomy before 4 days of age (but not at 7 days or later) leads to arrest in ovarian growth in approximately half of the females.[144] It was later observed that in two of the hybrid genotypes, thymectomized at 3 days and allowed to live their normal life spans, unilateral ovarian tumors of the granulosa or tubular adenomatous types developed in about half of them.[146]

There is also a mutant gene "nude" (nu) in mice, among the pleiotrophic effects of which are the absence of a thymus and infertility of both sexes.[151] These observations indicate a relationship between thymus and gonad during differentiation of the latter, which can be manipulated to give rise to ovarian tumors.

GENETIC DELETION. Among the mouse strains particularly susceptible to spontaneous ovarian tumor development are the CBA strain,[181] the CE strain,[29] C3H strain freed from mammary tumor-inducing virus,[27] RIII,[177] and various strains of New Zealand mice.[10] The incidence of ovarian tumors in females of these strains reaching an age of 18 months or more may be very high.

Mutant genes of the W series can lead to a high incidence of spontaneous ovarian tumors in mice carrying them.[139,165] The gonads of $W^vW^v$ mice are deficient in oocytes at birth, because of a failure of the primordial germ cells to multiply between the eighth and twelfth days of fetal life. The animals are sterile and the females develop a 95% incidence of bilateral tubular adenomata of the ovary at about 7 months of age. $F_1$ hybrid (C57B1 × C3H) mice with $W^xW^v$ genes develop tumors by 5 months and they have been shown to have significantly elevated levels (fourfold) of gonadotropins (both luteinizing and follicle stimulating hormones) during the pretumorous period.[140]

Genes of the steel (Sl) series have similar effects.[137] Some of the homozygotes are not viable, because of severe macrocytic anemia, but a high proportion of the less severely affected genotypes, such as $Sl^d/Sl^d$ and $Sl/Sl^d$, survive to adulthood and develop ovarian tumors in old age.

These ovarian tumors of mice represent a constitutional disease dependent to a significant extent on genetic factors of two classes; there are those that result from the action of a single mutant gene, and those with polygenic inheritances that appear spontaneously with characteristic frequencies in different strains of mice.

The disadvantage of using as a model mice whose ovarian tumors arise from a single gene mutation is that these genes have pleiotropic effects. Animals carrying them also have defective hematopoiesis giving rise to macrocytic anemia, and they may not survive to the age when ovarian tumors may develop. Also, as a result of the ovarian dysgenesis, many of the genotypes carrying the mutant genes are sterile, so maintenance of the gene in the population requires complicated breeding programs.

Advantages of using a strain of animals in which the ovarian tumor susceptibility is determined by polygenic inheritance are that many of these strains are quite longlived and there are few problems about breeding them.

### Indirect methods

INTRASPLENIC OVARY GRAFTING TO A CASTRATE. Ovaries transplanted to the spleens of castrated rats by Biskind and Biskind[12] were found to develop into tumors with great regularity. A similar operation in mice was soon shown to have the same effect.[43]

It had already been shown that subcutaneous implants of estrogen pellets in ovariectomized rats induced constant estrus, whereas intrasplenic pellets did not. It was postulated that tumors developing from the intrasplenic ovarian grafts resulted from hormonal imbalance; steroid hormones secreted from the grafts would be destroyed in the liver, just as the estrogen from the intrasplenic pellets, and thus rendered unable to exert their normal feedback inhibition of pituitary gonadotropins. These would be secreted chronically instead of cyclically, at an elevated level that would heighten the stimulation of the ovarian graft in the spleen, giving rise to hyperplasia and eventually neoplasia.

Support for this concept came when it was found that if one ovary remained *in situ* no ovarian tumors developed in the intrasplenic ovary[13] and, further, when it was shown that tumorigenesis could be inhibited by high systemic levels of estrogens or androgens, even when their administration was delayed for 3 or 4 months after transplantation.[103] Ovaries grafted into the pancreas were also found to become tumorous, demonstrating the significance of transplanting into the hepatic portal drainage system. Furthermore, repeated injections of luteotropin (LH) or of pregnant mare's serum were found to increase tumor incidence.[11]

In a recent experiment with rats, levels of both progestins and LH were measured and found to be high, and ovarian tumors developed in all animals bearing intrasplenic ovarian grafts without vascular adhesions. Hormone levels were much lower and no ovarian tumors appeared in such grafts if the animals were given an Eck fistula, which would produce hepatic bypass of the hormones from the intrasplenic ovaries by a portacaval shunt.[102]

Intrasplenic grafting of an ovary to a castrated rat or mouse leads to the appearance of benign "luteomas" after about 6 months, but granulosa cell tumors may appear in them later.[12] Early benign tumors may also be made to become malignant and to metastasize to the liver if DMBA treatment is also given.[68]

In rabbits with intrasplenic ovarian grafts, granulosa cell tumors have been seen after about 18 months.[152] In guinea pigs, large "luteomas" appeared in a similar length of time, but granulosa cell tumors were not seen before 5 years in this species.[121] In Golden hamsters, tumors do not develop in intrasplenic ovarian grafts.[93]

PARABIOSIS WITH A CASTRATE. From what we have seen in the preceding section, one might expect that any way of achieving a persistently high level of gonadotropic hormones might act on residual ovarian tissue to give rise to hyperplasia and subsequent neoplasia in rats and mice and some other species. One method of achieving this is by parabiosis (suturing together side by side) of an intact fe-male with a castrated partner. In this situation, excess gonadotropic hormones circulating in the castrate readily pass over into the circulation of the normal parabiont and stimulate its ovaries to produce larger amounts of estrogens, which are detectable by vaginal smears. However, when an attempt was made to induce ovarian tumors by this method in mice, the high estrogen levels reached, led to hydronephrosis and early death. In one pair that survived 9 months, an ovarian tumor was observed.[132]

Better survival occurs in parabiotic triplets with one intact partner joined to two castrated ones on the same side. In this situation the estrogens passing from the normal partner are metabolized before they can reach the furthest castrate, whose pituitary remains stimulated. Excess gonadotropins produced by this partner are less readily metabolized than the estrogens, and they do reach the normal triplet in elevated amounts.

Parabiosis of an intact female mouse to one or two castrates has been shown to speed up the appearance of ovarian tumors induced by other methods. Induction time for ovarian tumors in irradiated mice has been reduced from around 24 months to 15 by parabiosis to a single castrated partner. It only slightly reduced the 10 months required for tumor induction by intrasplenic ovary grafting, but with two castrate partners, this was reduced to 5 to 6 months.[133]

I have already mentioned the synergistic effect of parabiosis to a castrate combined with administration of FAA in tumor induction in rat ovaries where neither agent alone was effective[9]. Parabiosis of a castrated male or female rat with a hypophysectomized female, a constant estrous female, or an intact male with a grafted ovary will also lead to ovarian tumors in this species.[81]

TRANSPLANTATION OF A GONADOTROPIC PITUITARY TUMOR. It has been reported that transplants of a pituitary tumor secreting FSH and LH produced granulosa cell tumors of the ovary in eight of 146 female A × C rats at a much earlier age than have been the seven spontaneous tumors found in 1,812 old females of this same strain.

Two ovarian tumors so induced were transplanted and showed some degree of dependence on gonadotropins. These ovarian tumors in turn produced estrogenic effects (large uterus, pituitary, and mammary glands) as well as androgenic effects (enlarged clitoris and paraurethral glands). Pituitary hyperplasia led to excessive amounts of prolactin being produced which, together with estrogen from the ovarian tumors, stimulated the mammary glands to become neoplastic.[76] Mammary gland tumors were fast growing compared with ovarian and pituitary ones that preceded them, thus permitting the full chain reaction to occur in a single individual.

NONCYCLIC EXPOSURE TO BRIGHT ILLUMINATION. The incidence of tumors arising in rats with ovarian ligatures was enhanced in animals exposed continually to electric light[36] and 56 out of 60 rats exposed to continuous light from fluorescent lamps for 6 weeks showed persistent vaginal estrus.[173] There was progressive atrophy of the ovaries, which were full of cysts from tertiary follicles. These conditions were reversible and I am not aware of any experiments in which constant bright lighting alone has any tumorigenic effect on mammalian species. It has been observed that Brown Leghorn hens kept in a constant climatic chamber at a temperature of 65°F, relative humidity 60%, with 12 hr of fluorescent lighting but no natural daylight, had no annual cycle of egg laying. Egg production was continuous and gradually fell off over several years and hatchability declined. After 3.5 to 6.8 years, 19 out of 19 died and adenocarcinoma that involved the ovary, oviduct, mesentery, and intestine was seen. A control group in an intensive house, with 12-hr light in winter provided by a 100 W electric bulb, had the usual cyclic phase of molting and decline of egg laying in the winter months and only three developed adenocarcinoma and one a sarcoma in up to $12\frac{1}{2}$ yr.[61] This suggests that under the conditions of bright lighting, without seasonal variation during the year, sustained gonadotropins are produced in these birds leading to the continuous egg-laying and subsequent sterility and neoplasia.

It would appear that in all the four methods of ovarian tumor induction outlined above, a constant elevated level of stimulation of the ovarian tissue by pituitary gonadotropins is being achieved and we must assume that this is the fundamental mechanism of tumorigenesis.

CHRONIC EXPOSURE TO OTHER HORMONES. Chronic exposure to a variety of hormones, both male and female, can lead to tumor induction in laboratory animals.

*Progestational agents.* During chronic treatment of mice with synthetic progestins used as contraceptive agents in women, it was noted that subcutaneous pellets of 19-norprogesterone led to ovarian tumors in four out of 18 BALB/C mice after 13 months or more.[109] A small incidence was seen after implantation of progesterone itself and in two of 24 mice that received norethynodrel (17-ethinyl-5,10-19-nortestosterone); but ovarian tumors occurred in 13 out of 45 mice receiving implants of norethinodrone (17-ethinyl-19-nortestosterone).[106,108]

*Estrogens.* Chronic administration of estrogens to mice leads to hydronephrosis. Stilbestrol administered daily to rats leads to the development of huge cysts in the ovaries, filled with yellow caseous material, and to pyoovarium,

pyometra, and uterine metaplasia.[64] In hamsters, chronic administration of estrogen leads to kidney tumors,[93] but in dogs, stilbestrol administration induces tumors of the ovary;[79] see Chapter 39 by E. Cotchin.

*Androgens.* Normal ovaries grafted subcutaneously or intratesticularly into male mice of the same genotype frequently develop into tumors, whereas subcutaneous grafts into intact females do not.[48] However, the rate of ovarian tumor induction is also high when ovaries are grafted to castrated males. When castrated animals of both sexes are compared, tumor induction occurs more frequently in castrated males than in castrated females.[85] These differences may be caused by sexual differentiation of the hypothalamus that occurs during the neonatal period in rats and mice, giving rise to a tonic (continuous) pattern of gonadotropin secretion in males and cyclic release in females.[57,155]

Administration of testosterone propionate daily to female rats from the age of 3 days to 21 months led to hypertrophy of the clitoris and development of three theca cell ovarian tumors in 10 animals surviving 16 months or more.[72]

*Thyroid hormone.* Thyroid function affects the incidence of tumors developing in ovarian intrasplenic grafts.[126] Addition of thyroid powder to the diet resulted in fewer tumors. Thyroid inhibition with thiouracil or limitation of food intake had no effect.

Recently, proliferative and neoplastic changes have been reported to occur in ovaries of hamsters treated with iodine-131 and methylthiouracil.[21]

INFLUENCE OF HORMONES ON OVARIAN TUMOR INDUCTION BY OTHER AGENTS. Not only does the administration of hormones lead to ovarian tumor induction in some circumstances, but changes in balance of ovarian hormones can also markedly affect ovarian tumor induction by other agents.

Ovaries from DMBA-treated mice will not grow into tumors in the absence of a pituitary in the host, although ovaries of hypophysectomized animals treated with DMBA will do so if transplanted orthotopically.[118] Development of tumors from DMBA-treated ovaries is therefore shown to be dependent on stimulation by pituitary secretions.

DMBA-treated ovaries grafted unilaterally to normal hosts will not develop into tumor,[117] nor will they if grafted subcutaneously to normal females. In the latter situation, removal of the host's own ovaries up to 6 months later will give rise to tumors in the DMBA-treated ovarian graft.[85]

Presence of a normal ovary also prevents tumor development from an irradiated ovary, as in the cases where only one

**Table 38.2** Classification of spontaneous primary tumors reported in the human and other mammalian species[a]

| Species | Total ovarian tumors classified | Cystadenoma | Carcinoma | Granulosa series | Dysgerminoma | Teratoma | Other | No. reports |
|---|---|---|---|---|---|---|---|---|
| Rodents (five species) | 82 | 4 | 2 | 65 | 1 | 4 | 6 | 4 |
| Guinea pig | 3 | 0 | 0 | 1 | 0 | 2 | 0 | 2 |
| Hamster | 5 | 0 | 0 | 5 | 0 | 0 | 0 | 1 |
| Equine | 55 | 11 | 3 | 26 | 0 | 5 | 10 | 4 |
| Sheep | 1 | 0 | 0 | 0 | 0 | 1 | 0 | 1 |
| Swine | 31 | 11 | 3 | 4 | 2 | 2 | 9 | 4 |
| Bovine | 227 | 9 | 46 | 146 | 4 | 7 | 15 | 18 |
| Feline | 14 | 1 | 1 | 6 | 2 | 3 | 1 | 3 |
| Canine | 194 | 61 | 16 | 73 | 33 | 4 | 7 | 12 |
| Monkey | 13 | 4 | 1 | 3 | 0 | 2 | 3 | 2 |
| All mammalian[b] | 624 | 101 (16) | 72 (12) | 329 (52) | 42 (7) | 29 (5) | 51 (8) | 51 |
| Human (two series)[b] | 482 | 252 (52) | 88 (18) | 13 (3) | 4 (1) | 67 (14) | 58 (12) | 1 |

[a] Data condensed from Bonser and Jull.[14]

[b] Numbers in parentheses are percentages.

ovary has been irradiated,[104] and tumors do not appear in intrasplenic ovary grafts if one ovary is left *in situ*.[103]

The ability of ovarian hormones secreted from a normal ovary to prevent the emergence of ovarian tumors in situations where they would otherwise have arisen probably results from their control of pituitary gonadotropin secretion. However, it was not found possible to prevent development of granulosa cell tumors, in mice treated with DMBA, by periodic grafting of a normal ovary.[85] This may be explained by the fact that normal ovarian tissue grafted into intact female mice remains dormant and atrophic unless the host's own ovaries are removed. Normal ovarian grafts require deficiency of ovarian hormones in order to function, and DMBA-treated ovaries similarly require the same in order to develop into tumors. Some ovarian tumors themselves also have the same requirement and can grow only in ovariectomized hosts.

Exogenous administration of estrogens can inhibit tumorigenesis in mouse ovaries. No tumors developed in intrasplenic ovary grafts in castrated mice given regular injections of estradiol benzoate.[103] Injections of progesterone, in contrast, did not have any preventive effect at all.

The male environment has interesting effects on ovarian tumor development. Early observations of transplantable ovarian tumors in mice showed that these frequently grew better in intact males than in intact females. Tumor growth was also promoted by administration of testosterone to castrates.[134] Tumorigenesis was found to occur in subcuta-

neous grafts of normal ovaries to male mice of the same genotype and grafting to the intratesticular site was even more favorable.[46] Subcutaneous ovarian grafts in intact females, however, remain atrophic. When castrated hosts of both sexes were used, the castrated male environment was shown to be far more tumorigenic than the castrated female.[86] Despite the apparent tumor-favoring environment of the male animal, whether intact or castrated, administration of testosterone to mice bearing intrasplenic ovarian grafts inhibits tumorigenesis.[103] If delayed until 10 months after implantation, testosterone did not accelerate the growth of tumor nodules, which were already palpable. It was considered that any accelerating effect of testosterone on tumor growth was counteracted by its inhibiting effect on the pituitary gonadotropins required by the incipient tumors.[103]

# Pathology and Histogenesis of Ovarian Tumors

The most common types of spontaneous ovarian tumors seen in rats and mice are tumors of the granulosa–theca cell series and tubular adenomas. Luteomas, teratomas, and papillary cystadenomas have also been reported but much more rarely.

In other nonhuman mammalian species, the commonest type of ovarian tumor seen is, again, the granulosa cell tumor. Table 38.2 summarizes the distribution of histologic types occurring spontaneously in the various species.

There appears to be no single mammalian species which resembles the human in its distribution of histologic types of ovarian tumor. In the human female, just over half of the ovarian tumors seen are primary epithelial tumors, whereas granulosa cell tumors comprise less than 10%. When all the other mammalian species are taken together, the proportions of these two tumor types are reversed.

Tumors induced in rats and mice by almost all the methods described are classifiable into tumors of the granulosa–theca cell series, luteomas, and tubular adenomas, with the first and last types predominating. Both the induction method and the genotype of the animal have some influence on which of the histologic types predominates.

TUBULAR ADENOMA. This is the most frequent type of tumor seen in mice after irradiation and in mice that have undergone genic deletion of oocytes. It is also the commonest type developing from normal ovaries transplanted into castrated male mice but is much less common in similar subcutaneous grafts in castrated females.[86]

Tubular adenomas are seldom seen after DMBA treatment and seldom arise in subcutaneous implants of ovaries from DMBA-treated donors in castrated hosts of either sex.[86]

Irradiated mice of the C57B1 strain develop tubular adenomas, whereas DBA mice give rise to granulosa cell tumors. "This indicates the importance of the genotype in determining the histology of the tumor."[131]

Tubular adenomas are usually bilateral and do not give evidence of hormonal activity. Transplants sometimes grow, although slowly, but they do so better in gonadectomized hosts.[6]

Tubular adenomas appear to arise from tubular downgrowths of the germinal epithelium that surrounds the ovary. The tubules gradually come to fill the ovary and there may be proliferation of interstitial cells among them that can become luteinized. This probably is the origin of some of the "luteomas" in the literature. Cells budding off from the linings of the tubules may assume the appearance of granulosa cells. Indeed, granulosa cell tumors and luteomas are sometimes a later development from tubular adenomas.

GRANULOSA–THECA CELL TUMORS. These tumors are the predominant type seen after DMBA treatment,[116] even when treated ovaries are residing in castrated male hosts, in which grafts of normal ovaries give rise to tubular adenomas.[86] They are also the commonest type seen in ovaries grafted to the spleen of castrated animals.

Again, certain genotypes are more susceptible than others to their induction, with IF, C3H, and DBA being particularly susceptible and C57B1 and BALB/c resistant. Grafts of ovaries from DMBA-treated females of the resistant strains will develop into granulosa cell tumors if implanted orthotopically in ovariectomized hybrid females[117] or subcutaneously in castrated males.[86] Resistance appears to be caused by a deficiency of pituitary stimulation that exists in the females of resistant strains, but not in the resistant males nor in females of $F_1$ hybrids between resistant and nonresistant strains.

Granulosa cell tumors are usually unilateral, with the ovary on the other side being atrophied. Evidence of secretion of ovarian hormones, such as enlargement of the uterus and constant estrus vaginal smears, is frequently present.

In the histogenesis of granulosa cell tumors after DMBA treatment, the initial event is one of oocyte destruction, with the oocytes of the smaller follicles being most susceptible.[97,116] This is followed by degeneration of granulosa cells and atresia of the follicles. When viable oocytes have gone, theca cells proliferate and undergo luteinization, becoming merged with remnants of old corpora lutea. This luteinized tissue may account for some of the "luteomas" described in the literature. Histogenesis of tumors in intrasplenic ovarian grafts is similar.[62]

Granulosa cell tumors are first recognized microscopically about 5 months after DMBA treatment, appearing as small nodules of basophilic-staining cells with densely stippled nuclei intermingled with acidophil luteinized cells. Tumor nodules are rarely seen in ovaries containing any viable follicles. It is considered that here "granulosa" cell tumor is a misnomer, because these tumors arise not from granulosa cells but probably from theca cells or other stromal elements.

Macroscopically, the early granulosa cell tumors present a pale pink appearance, but as they grow larger they may undergo considerable hemorrhage which gives them a dark purple cystic look. They may also show bright yellow areas of luteinization or be almost an entirely pale yellow.

If vaginal smears are followed during development of granulosa cell tumors following DMBA treatment, it is frequently found that estrous cycles gradually die out during the first months, giving a constant diestrous type of smear for a while. Later, animals usually go into a more or less constant estrus at the time when granulosa cell tumor nodules are first appearing.

Granulosa cell tumors are transplantable, but transplants grow slowly compared with most other types of mouse tumors and often show a preference for male hosts.

LUTEOMAS. Tumors composed of cells resembling those of corpora lutea are much less common in mice than the two previous histologic types mentioned, but they are seen in BALB/c × A F$_1$ mice after reimplantation of ovaries exposed to DMBA in vitro[87] and have also been seen after genic deletion of ovaries, x-irradiation, or intrasplenic grafting.

Transplantability is rare but it has been described.[44] The rareness may be because many of the "luteomas" described in the literature seem to represent a premalignant benign condition that precedes development of granulosa cell tumors, whereas "transplantable luteoma" may be a subsequent development of some granulosa cell tumors as they grow and mature.

Tumorigenesis appears to be much slowed down in castrated guinea pigs with intrasplenic ovarian grafts. These give rise to "luteomas" that may reach a size 50 to 100 times bigger than the normal ovary after about 2 years,[105] but they are not transplantable.[77] Only two granulosa cell tumors were seen in this species. These developed after nearly 5 years, and one metastasized to the liver.[121]

CYSTADENOMAS. Cystadenomas, one of the commonest primary epithelial types of ovarian tumor in the human species, have rarely been seen in animals, so the recent report of their induction in ovaries of ICR/Jcl mice is of great interest. Cystadenomas were seen in ovaries of mice whose mothers were injected with urethane on days 11 and 13 of gestation.[147]

TERATOMAS. Spontaneous ovarian teratomas in animals are extremely rare but they have been seen several times in C3H mice[189] and one of these was transplantable.[34] A case of bilateral teratomas was also seen in a Swiss albino mouse[33] and they have also been reported in CBA and DBA mouse strains.[123] These tumors also occur in guinea pigs[198,200] and have been reported in six ovaries from 1,176 female hares shot in New Zealand, where it is considered that DDT spraying may have been involved in their genesis.[38]

Recently a teratoma has been reported in a mouse exposed to urethane in utero.[148] Ovarian teratoma may also be induced to develop by parthenogenetically activating mouse eggs.[180] It is also of interest that testicular teratoma can be induced in mice of strain 129 by transplantation of 12½-day-old fetal gonadal ridges into adult testes,[179] from mouse egg cylinders,[24] or from displaced visceral yolk sac.[175]

METASTATIC TUMORS TO THE OVARY. The mouse ovary is a very frequent site for metastases from lymphomas. Tissue of the ovary may be almost completely replaced by lymphoma cells without apparent increase in size of the organ, which becomes smooth in outline.[119]

# Assessment of the Present Animal Tumor Models of Ovarian Cancer

We are now in a position to assess whether the present animal tumor models of ovarian cancer make good models for the study of the human disease. The criteria we demanded of a good model were reproducibility, predictability, and resemblance to the human counterpart. How far do animal models of ovarian tumors satisfy these requirements?

There is no doubt at all that highly reproducible and predictable results can be achieved by many of the induction methods described. Some give tumors in virtually all of the animals that survive long enough to develop them, but it is important to avoid competing mortality risks associated with the inducing agent.

It is unfortunate that the most widely explored tumor-inducing agents have given rise to a distribution of histologic type of tumor quite different from the tumors appearing in the human species, although all the tumor types occurring in the human female have been seen developing spontaneously in animals. We have seen that tumors of different histologic types can be induced with a single technique by using mice of different genotypes or sexes. The development of these tumors is therefore probably a reflection of the differing hormonal environments acting on ovarian tissue at the time of action of the inducing agent. (I have personally seen a sequence of quite different histologic types of mammary tumors developing in C57B1 mice exposed to repeated DMBA treatment during the period when their immature ductlike "tree in winter" mammary tissue was being stimulated toward acinar differentiation by the progesterone of pseudopregnancy.) It is possible that deliberate focusing of direct tumor-inducing agents onto the ovary at different stages during its differentiation can yield a much greater variety of tumor types. Induction of cystadenomas and teratomas in recent experiments involving fetal or neonatal exposure to noxious agents or other manipulation seem to indicate that this may be so.

These considerations bring us to ask why the human species is apparently unique in its distribution of spontaneous ovarian tumor types.

The ovary is a highly specialized organ, an intricate complex of different cell types that has evolved from embryologic precursors. Possibly some of the precursors in the human ovary differ from those of other animals. It is of interest in this respect that a recent investigation using immunofluorescent techniques has shown specific intestinal antigenicity in the epithelium and mucin of human ovarian mucinous cystadenomas,[141] suggesting their frequent occurrence might be related to some occasional anomaly of ovarian development in the human fetus that leads to em-

807

bryonic gut cells becoming incorporated in the developing organ. There they may lie undetected until influenced to undergo tumorigenesis, possibly by factors quite different from those giving rise to granulosa cell tumors of other mammalian species.

In contrast, recent induction of cystadenomas in mice by exposure of their mothers to urethane at a certain stage in their fetal development suggests that cystadenomas in human species result from exposure of the human fetus to some unrecognized environmental factor at a certain stage of gestation. Such a factor may be unrecognized because it may have no effect on tissues in later stages of differentiation.

We may also ask what the widely used animal models of ovarian tumors have taught us so far. They have emphasized the dominant role played by oocyte depletion (either induced or under genetic control) and the loss of follicles in the genesis of tumors of the granulosa–theca cell type. All the direct methods of ovarian tumor induction in mice (x-irradiation, chemical, transplantation, neonatal thymectomy, and genic deletion) bring about a premature loss of oocytes and follicles from the ovary. Tumors rarely appear before all viable follicles have gone. In the normal mouse (unlike the human female) oocyte depletion is not usually complete even at the end of the life span, which may be as much as $2\frac{1}{2}$ years. This may explain why spontaneous tumors are rarely seen except in mice of certain genotypes that lose their oocytes more rapidly than is usual.

Follicular disappearance would inevitably lead to changes in the normal cyclic levels of the pituitary gonadotropins, which would feed back in constant elevated amounts on the residual ovarian tissue deprived of its normal target tissue (normal ovarian follicle), stimulating it to hypertrophy and eventually to undergo neoplastic changes, as in the indirect methods of tumor induction (intrasplenic ovary grafting to a castrate, parabiosis to a castrate, transplantation of a gonadotropic pituitary tumor, noncyclic exposure to bright illumination, chronic exposure to steroid hormones).

Although it can be argued that such agents as irradiation and chemical carcinogens may cause mutations in certain ovarian cells that may later go on to form tumors, the apparent indefinite delay of their appearance by the presence of ovarian hormones in the host suggests that development of incipient tumors is completely dependent on continuing gonadotropic stimulation.

It can equally well be argued that continual hormonal stimulation of the ovary, such as is achieved by indirect methods of tumor induction, is the only essential factor in ovarian tumorigenesis in mice. The rodent ovary is, as Jull[86] said, "perhaps the best example of an organ in which hyperstimulation alone can cause tumorigenesis."

# ANIMAL MODELS FOR TUMORS OF THE UTERINE FUNDUS AND PLACENTA

## The Uterus as a Tumor Model

Cancer of the body of the uterus is one of the leading causes of female cancer mortality in developed countries and is geographically associated with various indicators of affluence. Cancer of the uterine cervix, which occurs in the region of the junction of the columnar epithelium of the uterine corpus with the squamous epithelium of the vagina, shows a quite different geographic distribution and is generally associated with low socioeconomic status.

It would seem, then, that cancer of the human uterine cervix and uterine corpus must be regarded as two quite distinct diseases with differing causative factors, and it is unfortunate that cancer mortality rates for some countries do not distinguish between them. In discussing tumor models, I shall endeavor to make the distinction but I shall include the vagina, which is lined by similar squamous epithelium, along with the cervix.

As explained in the introduction, the female genital tract of laboratory (and other) mammals is immensely variable in its gross anatomy and it must be borne in mind that the position of the squamocolumnar epithelial junction is also quite diverse. These factors, together with its much larger size, make the uterus a less convenient organ as a tumor model from the experimenter's point of view.

During the prenatal period, the human uterus undergoes a rapid spurt of growth during the last trimester, under the influence of maternal (possibly placental) hormones. Sudden removal of these hormones at birth causes very rapid involution of the organ during the first two postnatal weeks. These perinatal changes in growth rate occur mainly in the cervix, but the vagina shows similar changes.[25] At this early stage of life, therefore, the sensitivity of the cervix and vagina to female sex hormones is much greater than that of the uterine fundus.

Little attention has been paid to uterine growth in other fetal mammals, but it is known that in adult life there are definite cyclic changes in the histology of the cervix of the mouse,[58] rat,[65] and guinea pig.[90] In the absence of estrogen the transitional zone of the mouse resembles human metaplasia of columnar to stratified epithelium, but estrogen stimulation causes the transitional epithelium to disappear and an abrupt junction results. It seems that stratified epithelial cells of the transitional zone are very malleable and may differentiate to produce either keratinized cells or cells of a uterine type at the surface.[58] An early investigation in seven mouse strains also showed that, with advancing age, the processes sent down by the surface epithelium of vagina and cervix into the underlying connective tissue increased in depth, and this invagination was speeded up by estrogen injection.[182]

Similar changes also occur in rats. However, the vagina and cervix of the rabbit are lined at all stages with columnar epithelium that responds to estrogen by mucification, never by cornification.[25]

It appears, then, that the normal cervix is greatly influenced in its growth and differentiation by female sex hormones—much more so than the body of the uterus—and so it seems likely to respond in a more dramatic fashion to long-term imbalance of sex hormones.

## Spontaneous Uterine Tumors in Laboratory Animals

As Cotchin has shown,[23] no animal species has yet been discovered with a significant incidence of spontaneous cancer of the cervix, suggesting that its common occurrence in women is caused by some specifically human factor.

Human endometrial cancer is less frequent than cancer of the cervix, the proportion being about 1:3 or 1:4 and the majority of patients being postmenopausal. Spontaneous endometrial cancer is uncommon in most animal species except monkeys, cows, and rabbits. These species are discussed in Chapter 39 by E. Cotchin.

In other laboratory species, spontaneous uterine tumors seem to be not infrequent in the rat, where 48 of 489 tumors were reported to be uterine,[18] and in the Golden hamster, where cervical carcinoma and adenocarcinoma, as well as uterine horn adenocarcinoma and leiomyosarcoma, have been seen.[162]

In the mouse, spontaneous tumors of the uterus and vagina are infrequent, except in certain strains and their hybrids. They were found in 13 of 56 exbreeding females of the Pybus Miller (PM) strain. Unfortunately this stock showed high sterility and was later lost. None were seen in six other stocks. Females of the PM strain often had imperforate vaginas and males had few mammary rudiments, suggesting a hormonal imbalance probably existed during fetal life.[51] Some uterine adenocarcinomas have also been seen in mice of the BALB/c strain, as well as in C3H females free from mammary tumor-inducing virus, and their first-generation hybrids. These tumors were transplantable.[30] Spontaneous papillomas and squamous carcinomata of the vulva have also been seen in mice of strain 129.[137] We see again

the importance of genetic and hormonal factors in the etiology of these spontaneous female tumors of laboratory animals.

## Methods of Inducing Tumors of the Uterine Fundus in Laboratory Animals

### Hormone imbalance

ESTROGENS. In an early report, mice of the "Old Buffalo" strain given daily injections of estrogenic hormones (theelol and theelin) for 24 months developed proliferations in the uterus, cervix, and vagina that "in humans would have been considered malignant."[111] In most mice, however, the uterus responds to estrogen administration with hypertrophy leading to septic pyometra. Columnar epithelium of the uterine horns often undergoes squamous metaplasia or is replaced by extension of the squamous cervical epithelium. Carcinoma occurs only occasionally. However, tumors have occurred in high incidence in hybrid (PM × C3H) mice back crossed to PM, and in CBA mice and its hybrids treated with various estrogens.[50] Lesions were adenomas or adenocarcinomas, as well as infiltrative uterocervical epidermoid lesions, some of which were considered to be carcinomas. Hybrid (BALB/c × C3H) mice have given a similar range of tumors after injection of estradiol benzoate.[7]

Rat uteri respond to estrogens in a similar manner to most strains of mice, showing cystic hyperplasia, squamous metaplasia, and sometimes pyometra. Occasional tumors occur but spontaneous ones are not infrequent in this species.[3]

In guinea pigs, prolonged treatment with estrogen injections beginning early in life caused cystic glandular hyperplasia of uterine endometrium in every animal receiving more than 35 days of treatment. At first it was confined to the uterine horns; then it spread to the upper part of the fundus, the cells of which were swollen with glycogen instead of flat as in the cornua. Fibromyomas were seen after 200 days of treatment.[143]

Fibromyomatas were also induced at various other abdominal sites, such as pancreas, kidney, and spleen, by administration of all natural estrogens and by artificial ones. They occurred in castrated females and in intact or castrated males given larger doses. Some of the abdominal tumors invaded liver, pancreas, and muscle but not kidney and spleen. When the estrogen stimulus was withdrawn, they began to regress, undergoing hyalinization and ossification.[110] Spontaneous fibromyomas of women have a much more ordered arrangement of fibrous tissue than does myomata of the guinea pig.

In rabbits, some malignant growths have been described after administration of estrogens.[158] The high incidence of cystic endometrial hyperplasia and uterine tumors seen in old breeding females of some colonies after toxemia of pregnancy is believed to be caused by an excessive concentration of estrogen, resulting from impairment of liver function.[60]

When stilbestrol was given to rabbits with alloxan-induced diabetes, there was no enhancement of the stilbestrol-induced effect, although alloxan on its own produced endometrial hyperplasia and adenomyosis.[125] Examination of the endocrine organs led to the conclusions that estrogen had both direct uterine effects and indirect effects mediated through stimulation of the pituitary basophils and consequent ovarian stimulation. Cancerous animals showed hypertrophy of pituitary, adrenals, and ovaries, with indications of adrenocortical hyperactivity.[176]

Prolonged treatment of 10 squirrel monkeys with diethylstilbestrol led to malignant uterine mesotheliomas, originating from the serosa and presenting sometimes as solid sheets and sometimes in glandular or papillary form, in seven of the treated animals; the other three showed early lesions of the serosa.[122] This would seem to be a species with uteri particularly sensitive to tumor induction by estrogen.

ESTROGENS PLUS ANDROGENS. In all female Syrian hamsters given pellets containing both diethylstilbestrol and testosterone propionate, cystic glandular hyperplasia of the uteri occurred and there were multiple foci of nodular hyperplasia in the muscle of both horns. In addition, six out of 10 had multiple leiomyomas in one or both uterine horns that were indistinguishable histologically from the leiomyomas of the epididymes seen in five out of 11 males similarly treated.[5] Hormone dependency and progress toward autonomy following serial transplantation of similarly induced tumors has been demonstrated.[94]

PROGESTERONES. In an investigation of progesterone and 19-nor-contraceptives in mice, tumors of the endometrial stroma, varying between fibrosarcoma and sarcoma, were produced by progesterone and norethindrone. Another 19-nor-contraceptive, norethynodrel, produced metaplasia of the endometrium and glandular epithelium.[107]

TESTICULAR GRAFTS. Leiomyomas arose in female rats that had received testicular grafts (usually two) from littermates when newborn. By sexual maturity, most animals had constant estrus, and pyometra began after 6 months. The uterus usually ulcerated into the body cavity through the digestive tract, or through the body wall to the exterior, and the animals died. Only 16 of 185 survived more than 3 years and four of these had uterine leiomyomas similar to fibromyomas that frequently occur in women.[156] One rat showing continuous estrus died at $2\frac{1}{4}$ years with a huge typical adenocarcinoma in the left uterine horn and numerous metastases. The pituitary of this animal was enlarged and hemorrhagic.[157]

OVARIAN FRAGMENTATION. About 40 years ago, Lipschutz[105] and his colleagues showed that uterine tumors could be induced in guinea pigs by long-term results of subtotal castration, or "ovarian fragmentation" as he called it. One ovary was completely removed and only a fragment of the other left behind. An irregular sexual cycle reestablished itself with prolonged estrous and diestrous phases. The uterus, sometimes increased up to 10- or even 20-fold its normal weight, showed cystic glandular hyperplasia and metaplasia of the endometrium, as well as polyps filling the uterine cavity. Uterine glands were frequently seen in the myometrium, where some animals showed subserous adenofibromyomas. After 3 years or so, multifocal adenocarcinomas were seen in the small number of survivors.[105] As with prolonged estrogen treatment, other abdominal fibroids were seen. There was also nodular hyperplasia of the adrenal cortex, and a Brenner-type ovarian tumor occurred in one instance. The ovarian fragment contained lutein cysts, sometimes blood filled, and hemorrhagic follicles.[17] These observations and other experimental evidence led to the assumption that the ovarian remnant lost the faculty to control the gonadotropic function of the hypophysis.

PITUITARY GROWTH HORMONE. Daily intraperitoneal injections of pituitary growth hormone in gradually increasing doses gave hypertrophy of the myometrium in all 15 Long Evans rats and glandular cystic hyperplasia in two (one with a polyp). In one animal the entire right horn of the uterus was replaced by a tumor that adhered to the bowel and infiltrated the myometrium extensively.[128]

### Carcinogens

CHEMICALS. *3-Methylcholanthrene (MC)*. Large tumors of the mouse uterus have been induced by implantation of MC crystals, 1% MC in lard, or 1% MC plus 1% estradiol propionate. The mice used were CBA strain or outbred white animals. The implant was secured in place by ligatures above and below. In all, 14 out of 109 developed fibromyosarcomas, which were mostly locally invasive and tended to appear earliest. Twenty out of 109 developed endometrial carcinomas, which were more prevalent in the CBA strain. Immature CBA mice were particularly susceptible to uterine tumor development (12 out of 15).[15]

Another method that has been used to follow early stages in development of adenocarcinoma in the mouse uterus involves using cotton thread, part of which is impregnated with a 1:3 mixture of MC with beeswax. At laparotomy, the thread was inserted with a needle through the lateral wall of one uterine horn and pulled through the tip until the impregnated part lay in contact with the endometrium. Endometrial hyperplasia appeared after 7 weeks and there was fibrous proliferation of stromal tissue. A total of 32 out of 110 mice of the na 2 strain developed adenocarcinoma of the endometrium, three adenoacanthoma, two sarcoma, and two squamous cell carcinoma.[187] This method has been used to study enzyme histochemistry of the lesions.[188]

Tampons of cotton tape or silk strings impregnated with MC in polyvinylchloride and melted paraffin wax induced adenocarcinomas in rabbit uteri and squamous cell carcinoma in mice and rats.[3]

Homburger,[70] reviewing chemical carcinogenesis in Syrian hamsters, reported that in 161 female survivors (of seven different strains) given MC by stomach tube, there were 55 uterine tumors and 82 ovarian and 123 mammary tumors.

*7,12-Dimethylbenz[a]anthracene (DMBA).* In mice, as we have shown earlier in this chapter, DMBA leads to ovarian and breast tumors. In rats, administration of DMBA during early life (fetal, newborn, or 10 days old) to females of a Sprague–Dawley strain resulted in uterine tumors developing over 12 months in 13 out of 31 animals; six were adenocarcinoma, two squamous cell carcinoma, two myosarcoma, one anaplastic, and two mixed. Two metastasized to the lungs and abdominal viscera.[167] One uterine adenocarcinoma that was transplanted had metastases to the lungs when the hosts were injected with medroxyprogesterone acetate.[168]

*2-Fluorenylacetamide (FAA).* Rats of the Buffalo strain given FAA mixed in powdered food for a year, on the average, developed uterine fibrosarcomas in three instances.[183]

*N,N-Fluorenyldiacetamide.* In 10 spayed female A × C rats, this chemical induced cystic hyperplasia of the uterus and three sarcomas. Norethandrolone (17-ethyl-19-nortestosterone) caused endometrial cystic hyperplasia when administered alone, but when administered together with N,N-fluorenyldiacetamide it led to endometrial sarcomas

(possible leiomyosarcomas). They did not appear in intact females so treated. Carcinosarcomas of the salivary glands also developed and had the same induction requirements.[161]

*Vinyl copolymer.* Cotton tampons coated with vinyl copolymer and paraffin wax melted together in a dish and inserted in one uterine horn of MIH Black rats induced marked inflammation of the endometrium and moderate enlargement with pyometra after 4 to 10 months and marked epithelial dysplasia at 10 to 12 months; at 10 to 18 months five out of 12 had squamous cell carcinoma. Controls with strings coated only with paraffin had similar changes, resulting in epithelial dysplasia at 18 months. One leiomyosarcoma was found but no carcinoma.

Tumors seen with the polymer strings were identical in ultrastructure to those seen with strings coated with MC, but the latent period of tumor induction was much longer with the polymer.[4]

INTRAUTERINE DEVICES. In experiments with virgin female Wistar rats, stainless steel or polyethylene loops or springs were sterilized and inserted in both horns of the uterus through a small incision and anchored with silk. After 14 months a sarcoma with widespread metastases throughout the abdomen appeared and after 19 months, when 19 were still alive, six epidermoid cancers appeared in the animals with the stainless steel devices.

With polyethylene devices, the first epidermoid carcinoma appeared at 20 months and a sarcoma occurred at 23 months. Epidermoid carcinomas were considered to be a rare feature in this rat strain.[22]

X-IRRADIATION. In rabbits, where uterine tumors are common in old animals, chronic exposure to low doses (8.8 R) of γ rays induced them in a much shorter period of time.[113]

Implantation of $^{60}$Co wires in the pelvis of female rats for periods from 10 to 200 days induced adenocarcinoma of the uterus in 14 out of 32 females. The tumors were composed of dilated glands with scanty stroma, usually, and the longer exposures gave increased numbers of tumors. It was calculated that the uterus received approximately 16,000 to 961,000 rads, most of these doses being much too high to induce tumors in the ovary, which was often reduced to scar tissue.[71]

VIRUSES. Eight endometrial sarcomas and one leiomyosarcoma were seen to develop in 37% of $F_1$ (C57B1 × DBA) female mice reaching 18 months old or more. They were readily transplantable but did not respond to endogenous or exogenous progesterone; seven of these eight mice had been inoculated with either Friend or Rauscher leukemia virus.[26]

## Methods of Inducing Placental Tumors in Laboratory Animals

### Chemical carcinogens after fetectomy

Malignant tumors of placental origin have been induced in rats, guinea pigs, and rabbits during the past decade. Long Evans rats were mated and the females were fetectomized at 10 to 12 days. Beeswax pellets containing DMBA were placed in the gestation sacs of 144 animals (1,042 sacs). Most of them were also injected with Depo-Provera (medroxyprogesterone acetate) and they were killed at intervals from 7 to 40 weeks later. Sixty-five developed malignant tumors after 12 to 13 weeks, seven of which were choriocarcinomas. Three had pulmonary metastases. Many of the remaining tumors were adenocarcinomas of the endometrium and malignant mesotheliomas.[171]

Tumors histologically resembling human chorioadenoma destruens have been induced in Japanese Hartley guinea pigs following fetectomy at 4 to 5 weeks gestation. The placental mass was left *in situ* and a suspension of *N*-butyl-*N*-nitrosurea in carboxymethyl cellulose instilled into the uterus. Some of the animals received intramuscular injections of human chorionic gonadotropin as well. The tumors were quite proliferative, were composed of bizarre tumor cells that invaded the myometrium, and were seen also as perivascular infiltrates. Pleiomorphic cells resembled malignant cytotrophoblasts. The changes were much more striking in animals not treated with HCG.[170] However, the series is small and the effects of HCG are not certain. The small number was related to the fact that the guinea pig is prone to postoperative infection and only five of the 20 animals survived the procedure.

### Virus after fetectomy

Choriocarcinomas have been induced in Wistar rats after fetectomy at 12 days of gestation and injection of Moloney's mouse sarcoma virus (MSV) followed by Depo-Provera on days 14 and 28. In most animals the injections were made into the placenta, but others were injected intravenously (i.v.) or intraperitoneally (i.p.). Control animals were nonpregnant, with MSV in one horn and control fluid in the other, both ligatured at the bottom to retain the fluid. No tumors were found in controls, but they were seen in 10 out of 29 rats injected with virus *in utero* and in two out of 10 injected i.v. or i.p.[193] Infectious virus could not be isolated from tumor cells, but the presence of the MSV genome could be demonstrated by a direct rescue test. Cytologic appearance supported the yolk sac origin of the tumors.

### Destruction of the hypothalamic nucleus

Tumors resembling human choriocarcinoma were induced in two out of 15 pregnant rabbits after destruction of the hypothalamic nucleus by means of electrocoagulation. Coagulation was carried out at 8 to 14 days postcopulation. Fifty-five animals were treated; 10 died rapidly and 30 failed to show pregnancy. The two successful cases of induction had been treated on the ninth day (just prior to completion of the placenta). No macroscopic metastases were seen, but vascular tumor emboli were seen in the lungs of one of the two animals. No such tumors had been seen in 1,000 pregnant rabbits used for experiments during the previous 10 years.[100]

# ANIMAL MODELS FOR TUMORS OF THE UTERINE CERVIX, VAGINA, AND VULVA

## Methods of Inducing Tumors in Laboratory Animals

### Hormones

ESTROGENS. In a series of publications dating from 1936 to 1959, Gardner and co-workers showed that mouse uterine reactions to high doses of injected estrogens varied markedly according to age. After weaning, estrogen results in hypertrophy of the uterus and pyometria. After birth, the entire uterine epithelium becomes stratified (but not cornified), with metaplasia extending into the uterine ends of the fallopian tubes. The vagina becomes greatly enlarged with increased thickness of the stroma caused by mucoid change.[49] Weekly injections of estrogens, continued for over a year, led to carcinoma of the cervix in 50 to 60%.[1] Mice of all strains responded in this way if they survived long enough, the highest tumor incidence occurring at 450 to 600 days. After cornification, the epithelium might atrophy before the earliest invasive lesions were seen. Grossly the cervices were firm and white with deficient blood supply.[45]

Cervical and vaginal tumors could also be induced in adult mice by pellets of stilbestrol–cholesterol attached to nylon threads, dipped in collodion, and placed in the vagina. They were also seen in some mice after intravaginal instillation of stilbestrol, three times weekly. Several mouse strains were used. Some did not tolerate the treatment well, but epidermoid carcinomas appeared in eight out of 40 BC mice with stilbestrol pellets and another 12 had smaller lesions after 260 days. Estradiol benzoate administered weekly was also effective, and addition of testosterone to estrogen–cholesterol pellets did not diminish the incidence. Other substances under consideration for use in intravaginal contraceptives (urea, adipic acid, and carboxymethyl cellulose) also induced invasive lesions of the vagina after 500 days or more.[47]

Experiments by Dunn confirmed the effectiveness of estrogens administered on the day of birth. Injections of diethylstilbestrol in three mouse strains led to the formation of astonishing concretions in the vagina in 12 out of 30 after 13 months, as well as carcinoma of the cervix and vagina.[32] The antifertility drug Enovid, administered in liquid diet to newborn BALB/c mice, produced similar endometrial changes to estrogens, and some animals continued on Enovid for around 2 years, had lesions of the cervix diagnosed as early cancer.[31] These findings preceded the report that large doses of stilbestrol, given to pregnant women with threatened abortion, could lead to adenocarcinoma of the vagina developing in their daughters 14 to 22 years later.[66]

The early changes seen after treatment of newborn mice with estrogens have been studied and found to be greater with diethylstilbestrol than with the same dose of estradiol.[39] They are not abolished by ovariectomy with or without adrenalectomy or hypophysectomy. Vaginal epithelium continued to proliferate and cornify after transplantation into ovariectomized hosts and frequently showed hyperplastic lesions of the epithelium that occasionally transformed into carcinoma-like tumors after 6 months. Serial transplantation of such vaginas under the abdominal skin of ovariectomized females may result in malignancy, and metastatic cancer has been seen in two instances after the fourth transplant.[186]

TESTOSTERONE. Subcutaneous implants of testosterone pellets twice a week in female (C57Bl × DBA) mice starting at 6 to 13 weeks old induced uterine tumors in 26 out of 42 in 15 to 18 months, mostly in the cervix or unpaired uterine part. Histologically there were large trabeculae of cells next to solid nests; they formed locally branched papillae inside large sinuses, and most infiltrated the uterine wall.

Mice without gross tumors had pink nodules of similar tissue in the stroma of the endometrium. These growths resembled the histologic changes seen in the endometrial stroma during early pregnancy and the hypothesis was advanced that the tumors were related to decidua cells.[194] Many extended into muscle of the uterine wall and some also had lung metastases. Transplants of two tumors grew in androgen castrates, but not in untreated castrates, showing that they were androgen dependent. One of these became autonomous and caused marked atrophy of the ovaries when grafted to intact females.[195]

In another investigation, female BALB/c mice treated neonatally with estrogen or testosterone propionate (at dose levels associated with the induction of persistent vaginal cornification) showed hyperplastic lesions of the vagina resembling epidermoid carcinoma (15 to 17 months later after either hormone). These lesions were reduced in incidence in animals that were ovariectomized around 4 months of age, and there were dose-dependent effects on the epidermization of the middle region of the uterine horns.[92]

### Chemical carcinogens

DIBENZ[a·h]ANTHRACENE (DBA) AND THEELIN. One of the earliest studies in the induction of cancer of the cervix used unpedigreed adolescent female mice, half of which were spayed. Their skin was painted twice a week with DBA solution in benzene and half of each group were also later treated with theelin. Among the great variety of tumors arising was epidermoid cancer of the cervix in three animals that had received treatment with both agents and carcinoma of the uterus and vagina in two that had received similar treatment.[153] These early experiments were soon followed by others using different polycyclic hydrocarbon carcinogens.

BENZO[a]PYRENE (BP). When BP in cholesterol was broken into fragments of about 5 mg and placed into the vagina of 10 mice two or three times a week, tumors appeared in all after 10 to 14 months. They were first seen on the vaginal wall and all were infiltrating squamous cell carcinoma.[37] Similar applications of human smegma from elderly institutionalized men was quite ineffective.

Other methods of applying carcinogens were devised, such as painting acetone solutions on the cervix with cotton-tipped wire loops,[199] later aided by the use of an infant-sized otic speculum,[95] or by impregnating strings that were then threaded into place and secured with knots or stitches at laparotomy.[78] Most experiments with BP, however, have used the direct painting method, and this model has been used to study enzyme histochemistry of changes in the upper vagina,[191] for studies of histogenesis of cervical carcinoma,[163] and for autoradiographic studies of early atypic changes.[164]

All mice treated with BP directly in the vagina develop atypical changes that lead to cancer developing in those surviving long enough. The incidence of cancer induced by this method is high.

Rats appear to be less susceptible than mice to cervical tumor induction by BP painting of the cervix.[178]

3-METHYLCHOLANTHRENE (MC). This carcinogen was shown to induce cervical carcinoma when uteri of young female mice were removed, MC crystals were inserted, and the uterus transplanted subcutaneously on the upper abdomen of hosts (usually brothers or sisters) of the same strain. Of 104 mice of various genetic types, 55 developed 61 tumors (32 carcinomas and 29 sarcomas), the majority appearing by the eighth week. The A strain gave the highest incidence (21 tumors in 16 of 20 mice treated). More tumors occurred in the cervix than in the uterine horns and the tumors included epidermoid carcinoma, adenocarcinoma, adenoacanthoma, and sarcoma.[150]

An investigation using threads with three knots impregnated with MC in beeswax 1:3 and suspended in the vagina of C3H mice led to malignant neoplasms of the cervix developing from 7 weeks onward in the majority of animals. In all the animals with carcinoma, the cervix was involved and there were extensions of tumor into the uterus and upper vagina. A few showed metastases to paraaortic lymph nodes, and adrenal and lung were involved in one case each.[159]

In a review of the subject in 1957, a comparison was made of the string and painting methods with MC and BP in C3H female mice. The highest incidence of cervical tumors was obtained at 11 to 33 weeks by MC and the string method (85%). Then, in order, came BP string, MC painting, and BP painting (50%).[166] With the string method, most tumors were induced in the cervix, but painting gave many vaginal lesions. Many tumors were invasive and extended to pelvic nodes, with metastases seen in lung and liver. It was considered that the mouse anatomy was such that neither method would reach the high site of transition from squamous to columnar epithelium; nevertheless the lesions showed a striking resemblance to human cervical cancer.

MC painting of the cervix of mice has been used to show the evolution of dysplasia of the cervix and vagina.[201] An increased effect of MC on the uterus of spayed females was seen when estrogens were present, and lesser

penetration of the stroma was seen if progesterone was injected in addition to estrogen.[91] More recent experiments showed that when progesterone was given in addition to MC treatment of the cervix, the tumors were significantly increased in number, giving a mucoepidermoid type of invasive carcinoma in the endocervix but having no maturational effect on tumors of the exocervix or vagina.[160]

Limited exposure to MC-impregnated threads gave increasing numbers of tumors as exposure increased from 2 to 4 weeks, and the addition of a diethylstilbestrol (DES) pellet increased the incidence. There were strain variations in susceptibility to both MC and DES effects.[136] Castration after-exposure to MC threads (knotted or unknotted to give high or low doses) markedly decreased the incidence of invasive cervical carcinoma (from 100 to 62% in A strain mice after a high dose of MC), thus showing the promoting effect of estrogen on cervical cancer.[138] This model has also been used to show the relationship of carcinogenesis with epidermization (spread of benign stratified squamous epithelium within the uterus),[59] as well as the histochemistry of the cervical epithelium during carcinogenesis,[114] the effect of anticancer drugs,[185] and the effect of neonatal treatment with estradiol on cervical carcinoma induction.[40]

The MC string method has also been used to induce carcinoma of the cervix in rabbits and here it seems to be uninfluenced by the addition of estradiol or progesterone.[2]

DIMETHYLBENZ[a]ANTHRACENE (DMBA). DMBA was first used by the knotted string method to induce carcinoma of the cervix in rats.[196] Eleven of 39 female Wistar rats surviving the operation developed gross tumors and two more had microtumors. Sometimes invasion into parametrial and endocervical tissue was detected, but no metastases were seen. The endocervix of 12 out of 13 rats with neoplasia was dilated and filled with keratin. In the walls, papillomas formed that ultimately transformed to epidermoid carcinoma.

This observation was followed by a long series of papers by Cherry and Glucksman in which female hooded Lister rats painted intravaginally with 1% DMBA in acetone were used as the model to study the role of the ovary, the effect of endocrine changes, the effect of castration with additional steroid or other hormones, and the effect of irradiation.[53] Their general conclusions were that the effect of these agents on cervical carcinogenesis by DMBA differed from their effects on normal target tissue of the cervicovaginal tract. For example, estrogens (which stimulated the growth of the cervicovaginal stroma, induced the multiplication of epithelial cells, and promoted keratinization) inhibited the development of sarcomas in a dose-dependent way in both intact and spayed females. Similarly, testosterone, cortisone, methylthiouracil, L-thyroxine, or repeated whole-body x rays (which do not stimulate stromal growth or epithelial keratinization) increased the rate of growth of tumors induced by DMBA. These apparently anomalous results may be complicated by the fact that DMBA itself has progesterone-mimetic effects.[84] They also noted that the histologic type of tumor that was induced was influenced to some extent by the various hormonal treatments.

These authors have shown similar results in mice treated with DMBA by the cervical painting method. Ovariectomy significantly increased the incidence of mucoepidermoid carcinoma of the cervix. Spayed females treated with progesterone had an increased adenocarcinomatous component, whereas stilbestrol gave only squamous cell carcinoma.[55]

Carcinogen paintings of the cervix and vagina often result in contamination of the vulva and this leads to marked hyperplasia, papillomas, and finally squamous carcinoma, all changes similar to those induced in normal skin with carcinogen painting. In mice it was shown that ovariectomy, which had little effect on cervical tumors induced by DMBA, increased the incidence of vulval tumors significantly.[56]

Induction of vulval tumors in rats painted with DMBA was not influenced by estrogen administration, ovariectomy,[54] or irradiation, but the incidence did increase with the dose of DMBA used.[20] In another experiment, castration promoted progression of vulval papillomas to carcinoma.[56]

Experiments have also been performed in mice with DMBA-impregnated knotted silk, with and without estrogen or androgen. Testosterone accelerated tumor appearance; ovariectomy lowered the incidence, as did estrogen treatment of intact females. The majority of tumors seen were squamous cell carcinoma; there were also a few cases of adenocarcinoma and myosarcoma, but no particular group had a preponderance of one kind of tumor.[124] Cytogenetic analysis of these tumors has been made.[80] It was found to vary considerably, in contrast with that of thymic lymphomas induced by DMBA.

CARBOWAX 1000 (POLYETHYLENE GLYCOL). In testing spermicidal contraceptives for possible carcinogenesis in mice, test substances were dissolved in Carbowax 1000 and introduced into the vagina twice a week using a syringe with a blunt needle. Eighteen months later, tumors of the cervix and vagina were seen in five out of 11 control animals, which received only the carbowax. All the tumors were carcinoma. DMBA added to the Carbowax resulted in nine tumors in 10 animals in a period of 12 months.[16]

N, N[1]-DIMETHYL-N-NITROSOUREA. Administration of this chemical by subcutaneous injection once a week to young adult Syrian hamsters, after 18 injections, resulted in adenoacanthomas of the uterus in 86% of test animals.[69]

### Virus

Viruslike particles have been seen in examination of the ultrastructure of cervical carcinomas induced in (C3H X A) mice by treatment with BP. These particles were indistinguishable from those described in mammary tumors of these strains. They were not seen in any of the normal tissues of the mice that were examined and it was speculated that the virus particles seen in the tumors might be a result, rather than a cause, of the carcinomatous process.[190]

HERPESVIRUS TYPE 2 (HSV-2). Experiments have been done in order to attempt to induce cervical cancers in animals with this virus. The animals were infected by applying the virus on cotton wool swabs to the cervix. It is reported that rabbits treated in this way die with paralysis and encephalitis.[169] BALB/c mice treated with hormones (estrogen, progesterone, or Enovid) and with HSV-2 intravaginally (twice at the beginning and again after 10 months) show characteristic cytologic changes of herpes infection in 40%. No significant difference was seen in the frequency of cancerous or precancerous lesions of the cervix or vagina between those receiving HSV-2 with hormone and those receiving hormone alone. However, in 19 animals on HSV-2 alone, two cancers and one precancerous lesion were seen. One of these cancers was transplanted with success.[135]

Treatment of various nonhuman primates has also been tried. Rhesus and squirrel monkeys could not be infected. Baboons could be infected but did not show lesions. Marmosets could be infected but soon died. However, *Cebus* monkeys (*albifrons* or *apella*) were susceptible to genital infection and survived. Twelve strains of HSV-2 were used, each on at least two monkeys, and 11 of the strains caused genital infection. Five strains produced tumor. In a total of 89 female *Cebus* monkeys exposed to HSV-2 infection, 50% developed lesions on the vulva, the cervix, and occasionally on the mouth. Nineteen males were exposed to the infected females and cross-infection by venereal infection was noted in two. One had penile lesions similar to those in humans.[112]

## Assessment of the Animal Tumor Models for Cancer of the Uterus

On the whole, the administration of steroid hormones to adult female animals is not a very effective way of obtaining a specific type of uterine tumor. These hormones have a multitude of target organs and tissues, leading to many unwanted side effects that may kill the animal before tumors have had time to develop at the desired uterine site. As with ovarian tumors, species and genotypes are important factors in determining the outcome. The age at which experimental treatment begins is also of importance and greater specificity of action can sometimes be obtained by treatment at very early ages, even *in utero*.

Induction methods using carcinogens are generally to be preferred. Chemical carcinogens can be made to deliver a much more localized and continuous action on the target tissue when knotted threads impregnated with them are sewn into a particular part of the reproductive tract. When they (or oncogenic viruses) are injected directly into exposed fetectomy sites, their action is also localized and effective in inducing only the desired tumor type.

Although spontaneous tumors of the female genital tract (particularly of the cervix) are uncommon in most animal species, they can be induced with varying degrees of reliability in laboratory animals and virtually all types of tumors seen in the human female have been encountered in one species or another. In describing their induction methods I have tried to show that chemical factors (chemical carcinogens); physical factors (irridiation, intrauterine devices); and biologic factors, both intrinsic (genetic factors, age, hormones) and extrinsic (viruses), may all play their part in causing cancer of the female reproductive tract. None of them can be neglected in the search for etiologic factors in the human species.

## LABORATORY ANIMALS AS HOSTS FOR HUMAN TUMORS

The experimentally minded gynecologic oncologist may be interested in the utilization of laboratory animals as hosts for human tumor transplants. This enables study of the hormone dependence of a tumor to be made or the tumor's susceptibility to inhibition by drugs to be examined.

One system that allows such transplants to be maintained is the hamster cheek pouch. Transplantation of human trophoblastic tumors to this immunologically privileged site has shown profound inhibition of tumor growth by methotrexate.[67]

Another system is the immune-suppressed mouse, either genetically determined as in the "nude" athymic mice or induced as a result of neonatal thymectomy. In a recent investigation of 19 human malignant tumors inoculated into male and female "nude" hosts, nine showed exclusive or preferential growth in one sex only, suggesting a hormonal influence on a wide variety of human tumors.[52]

It is hoped that further study along these lines can lead to more effective treatment of human malignant disease.

## REFERENCES

1. Allen, E., and Gardner, W. U. Cancer of the cervix of the uterus in hybrid mice following long-continued administration of estrogen. *Cancer Res.* 1:359, 1941.

2. Alvizouri, M., and de Pita, V. R. Experimental carcinoma of the cervix. Hormonal influences. *Am. J. Obstet. Gynecol.* 89:940, 1964.

3. Baba, N., and von Haam, E. Experimental carcinoma of the endometrium. Adenocarcinoma in rabbits and squamous cell carcinoma in rats and mice. *Prog. Exp. Tumor Res.* 9:192, 1967.

4. Baba, N., and von Haam, E. Squamous cell carcinoma of the rat endometrium produced by insertion of strings coated with paraffin and polymer. *J. Natl. Cancer Inst.* 47:675, 1971.

5. Bacon, R. R. Tumors of the epididymis and of the uterus in hamsters treated with diethylstilbestrol and testosterone propionate. *Cancer Res.* 12:246, 1952.

6. Bali, T., and Furth, J. Morphological and biological characteristics of X-ray induced transplantable ovarian tumors. *Cancer Res.* 9:449, 1949.

7. Barbieri, G., Olivi, M., and Sacco, O. Lesioni microscopiche nel' uteri di topi (BALB/C$_f$, C3H/CB/Se substrain) trattati con benzoato di estradiolo. *Lav. Ist. Anat. Istol. Patol. Perugia* 18:165, 1958.

8. Biancifiori, C., Bonser, G. M., and Caschera, F. Ovarian and mammary tumours in intact C3Hb virgin mice following a limited dose of four carcinogenic chemicals. *Br. J. Cancer* 15:270, 1961.

9. Bielschowsky, F., and Hall, W. H. Carcinogenesis in parabiotic rats. Tumours of the ovary induced by acetylaminofluorene in intact females joined to gonadectomised littermates and the reaction of their pituitaries to endogenous oestrogens. *Br. J. Cancer* 5:331, 1951.

10. Bielschowsy, M., and D'Ath, E. F. Spontaneous granulosa cell tumours of mice of strain NZC-Bi, NZO-Bi, NZY-Bi and NZB-Bi. *Pathology* 5:303, 1973.

11. Biskind, G. R., Bernstein, D. E., and Gospe, S. M. The effect of

exogenous gonadotrophins on the development of experimental ovarian tumors in rats. *Cancer Res.* 13:216, 1953.

12. Biskind, G. R., and Biskind, M. S. Experimental ovarian tumors in rats. *Am. J. Clin. Pathol.* 19:501, 1949.

13. Biskind, G. R., Kordan, B., and Biskind, M. S. Ovary transplanted to spleen in rats: The effect of unilateral castration, pregnancy and subsequent castration. *Cancer Res.* 10:309, 1950.

14. Bonser, G. M., and Jull, J. W. Tumours of the Ovary. Personal communication, 1974.

15. Bonser, G. M., and Robson, J. M. The induction of tumours following the direct implantation of 20-methylcholanthrene in the uterus of mice. *Br. J. Cancer* 4:196, 1950.

16. Boyland, E., Charles, R. T., and Gowing, N. F. C. The induction of tumours in mice by intravaginal application of chemical compounds. *Br. J. Cancer* 15:252, 1961.

17. Bruzzone, S., and Lipschutz, A. Endometrial adenocarcinoma and extragenital tumours in guinea-pigs with 'ovarian fragmentation'. *Br. J. Cancer* 8:613, 1954.

18. Bullock, F. D., and Curtis, M. R. Spontaneous tumors of the rat. *J. Cancer Res.* 14:1, 1930.

19. Carter, R. L. Pathology of ovarian neoplasms in rats and mice. *Eur. J. Cancer* 3:537, 1968.

20. Cherry, C. P., and Glucksman, A. The effect of endocrine changes, of irradiation and of additional treatment of the skin on the induction of tumours in the female genital tract of rats by chemical carcinogens. *Br. J. Cancer* 14:489, 1960.

21. Christov, K., and Raichev, R. Proliferative and neoplastic changes in the ovaries of hamsters treated with 131-iodine and methylthiouracil. *Neoplasma* 20:511, 1973.

22. Corfman, P. A., and Richart, R. M. Induction in rats of uterine epidermoid carcinomas by plastic and stainless steel intrauterine devices. *Am. J. Obstet. Gynecol.* 98:987, 1967.

23. Cotchin, E. Spontaneous uterine cancer in animals. *Br. J. Cancer* 18:209, 1964.

24. Damjanov, I., and Solter, D. Host related factors determine outgrowth of terato-carcinomas from mouse egg-cylinders. *Z. Krebsforsch.* 81:63, 1974.

25. Davies, J., and Kusama, H. Developmental aspects of the human cervix. *Ann. N.Y. Acad. Sci.* 97:534, 1962.

26. Dawson, P. J., Brooks, R. E., and Fieldsteel, A. H. Unusual occurrence of endometrial sarcomas in hybrid mice. *J. Natl. Cancer Inst.* 52:207, 1974.

27. Deringer, M. K. Occurrence of tumors, particularly mammary tumors, in agent-free strain C3HeB mice. *J. Natl. Cancer Inst.* 22:995, 1959.

28. Deringer, M. K., Lorenz, E., and Uphoff, D. E. Fertility and tumor development in (C57L × A)F$_1$ hybrid mice receiving X radiation to ovaries only, to whole body, and to whole body with ovaries shielded. *J. Natl. Cancer Inst.* 15:931, 1954.

29. Dickie, M. M. The use of F$_1$ hybrid and backcross generations to reveal new and/or uncommon tumour types. *J. Natl. Cancer Inst.* 15:791, 1954.

30. Dunn, T. B. The importance of differences in morphology in inbred strains. *J. Natl. Cancer. Inst.* 15:573, 1954.

31. Dunn, T. B. Cancer of the uterine cervix in mice fed a liquid diet containing anti-fertility drug. *J. Natl. Cancer Inst.* 43:671, 1969.

32. Dunn, T. B., and Green, A. W. Cysts of the epididymis, cancer of the cervix, granular cell myoblastoma, and other lesions after estrogen injection in newborn mice. *J. Natl. Cancer Inst.* 31:425, 1963.

33. Fawcett, D. W. Bilateral ovarian teratomas in a mouse. *Cancer Res.* 10:705, 1950.

34. Fekete, E., and Ferrigno, M. A. Studies on a transplantable teratoma of the mouse. *Cancer Res.* 12:438, 1952.

35. Fels, E. Effet de la ligature tubaire sur la fonction ovarienne chez le rat. *C. R. Soc. Biol.* 148:1666, 1954.

36. Fels, E. Aspectos morfológicos y funcionales de los tumores experimentales del ovario. *Rev. Arg. Endocrinol. Metab.* 2:1, 1956.

37. Fishman, M., Shear, M. J., Friedman, H. F., and Stewart, H. L. Studies in carcinogenesis. XVII. Local effect of repeated application of 3,4-Benzpyrene and of human smegma to the vagina and cervix of mice. *J. Natl. Cancer Inst.* 2:361, 1941–2.

38. Flux, J. E. C. Incidence of ovarian tumors in hares in New Zealand. *J. Wildlife Mgmnt.* 29:622, 1965.

39. Forsber, J. G. Estrogen, vaginal cancer and vaginal development. *Am. J. Obstet. Gynecol.* 113:83, 1972.

40. Forsberg, J. C., and Breitstein, L. S. Carcinogenesis with 3-methylcholanthrene in uterine cervix of mice treated neonatally with estrogen. *J. Natl. Cancer Inst.* 49:155, 1972.

41. Furth, J., and Boon, M. C. Induction of ovarian tumors in mice by X-rays. *Cancer Res.* 7:241, 1947.

42. Furth, J., and Furth, O. B. Neoplastic diseases produced in mice by general irradiation with X-rays. *Am. J. Cancer* 28:54, 1936.

43. Furth, J., and Sobel, H. Neoplastic transformations of granulosa cells in grafts of normal ovaries into spleens of gonadectomised mice. *J. Natl. Cancer Inst.* 8:7, 1947.

44. Furth, J., and Sobel, H. Transplantable luteoma in mice and associated secondary changes. *Cancer Res.* 7:246, 1947.

45. Gardner, W. U. Studies on steroid hormones in experimental carcinogenesis. *Rec. Prog. Horm. Res.* 1:217, 1947.

46. Gardner, W. U. Further studies on experimental ovarian tumorigenesis. *Proc. Am. Assoc. Cancer Res.* 2:300, 1958.

47. Gardner, W. U. Carcinoma of the uterine cervix and upper vagina: Induction under experimental conditions in mice. *Ann. N.Y. Acad. Sci.* 75:543, 1959.

48. Gardner, W. U. Tumorigenesis in transplanted irradiated and nonirradiated ovaries. *J. Natl. Cancer Inst.* 26:829, 1961.

49. Gardner, W. U., Allan, E., and Strong, L. C. Atypical uterine and vaginal changes in mice receiving large doses of estrogenic hormone. *Anat. Rec.* 64:17, Suppl. 3 (Abstract), 1936.

50. Gardner, W. U., and Ferrigno, M. Unusual neoplastic lesions of the uterine horns of estrogen-treated mice. *J. Natl. Cancer Inst.* 17:601, 1956.

51. Gardner, W. U., and Pan, S. C. Malignant tumors of the uterus and vagina in untreated mice of the PM stock. *Cancer Res.* 8:241, 1948.

52. Giovanella, B. C., and Stehlin, J. S. Influence of the host's sex on the growth of human tumors heterotransplanted in "nude" thymusless mice. *Am. Assoc. Cancer Res.,* 15, Abstract 92, 1974.

53. Glucksman, A. Some effects of steroid hormones on carcinogenesis in rats: Effects of oestrogens on the induction of tumours in the cervico-vaginal tract and in the salivary glands, in Williams, D. C., and Briggs, M. C., eds.: *Some Implications of Steroid Hormones in Cancer.* London, Heinemann Medical Books, 1971, pp. 70–78.

54. Glucksman, A., and Cherry, C. P. The role of the ovary in the induction of tumours by the local application of 9,10-dimethyl-1,2-benzanthracene to the genital tract of rats. *Br. J. Cancer* 12:32, 1958.

55. Glucksman, A., and Cherry, C. P. The effect of castration and of additional hormonal treatments on the induction of cervical and vulval tumours in mice. *Br. J. Cancer* 16:634, 1962.

56. Glucksman, A., and Cherry, C. P. The effect of increased numbers of carcinogenic treatments on the induction of cervico-vaginal and vulval tumours in intact and castrate rats. Br. J. Cancer 24:333, 1970.

57. Gorski, R. A., and Wagner, J. W. Gonadal activity and sexual differentiation of the hypothalamus. Endocrinology 76:226, 1965.

58. Graham, C. E. Cyclic changes in the squamo-columnar junction of the mouse cervix uteri. Anat. Rec. 155:251, 1966.

59. Graham, C. E. Relationship of carcinogenesis and epidermization during 20-methylcholanthrene treatment of the mouse uterine cervix. Am. J. Obstet. Gynecol. 103:1084, 1969.

60. Greene, H. S. N. Adenocarcinoma of the uterine fundus in the rabbit. Ann. N.Y. Acad. Sci. 75:535, 1959.

61. Greenwood, A. W. Controlled environments and cancer incidence in the domestic fowl, in Shives, A. A., ed.: Racial and Geographical Factors in Tumour Incidence. Medical Monograph 2. Edinburgh, University Press, 1967, pp. 241–249.

62. Guthrie, M. J. Tumorigenesis in intrasplenic ovaries in mice. Cancer, N.Y. 10:190, 1957.

63. Hafez, E. S. E. The comparative anatomy of the mammalian cervix in Blandau, R. J., and Moghissi, K., eds.: The Biology of the Cervix. Chicago, Chicago University Press, 1973, Ch. 3.

64. Hale, H. B., and Weichert, C. K. Ovarian tumors in adult rats following prepuberal administration of estrogens. Proc. Soc. Exp. Biol. Med. 55:201, 1944.

65. Hamilton, C. E. The cervix uteri of the rat. Anat. Rec. 97:47, 1947.

66. Herbst, A. L., Ulfelder, H., and Poskanzer, D. C. Adenocarcinoma of the vagina—association of maternal stilboestrol therapy with the tumor appearance in young women. N. Engl. J. Med. 284:878, 1971.

67. Hertz, R. Biological aspects of gestational neoplasms derived from trophoblast. Ann. N.Y. Acad. Sci. 172:279, 1971.

68. Hilfrich, J. A new model for inducing malignant ovarian tumours in rats. Br. J. Cancer 28:46, 1973.

69. Hiraki, S. Carcinogenic effect of N,N'-dimethylnitrosourea on Syrian hamsters. Gann 62:321, 1971.

70. Homburger, F. Chemical carcinogenesis in Syrian hamsters. Prog. Exp. Tumor Res. 16:152, 1972.

71. Hori, C. G., Warren, S., Patterson, W. B., and Chute, R. N. Gamma ray induction of malignant tumors in rats. Am. J. Pathol. 65:279, 1971.

72. Horning, E. S. Carcinogenic action of androgens. Br. J. Cancer 64:414, 1958.

73. Howell, J. S., Marchant, J., and Orr, J. W. The induction of ovarian tumors in mice with 9:10-dimethyl-1;2-benzanthracene. Br. J. Cancer 8:635, 1954.

74. Huggins, C. B., and Sugiyama, T. Production and prevention of two distinctive kinds of destruction of the adrenal cortex. Nature (London) 206:1310, 1965.

75. Hummel, K. P. Induced ovarian tumors. J. Natl. Cancer Inst. 15:711, 1954.

76. Iglesias, R. Newer concepts in pathogenesis. Secondary endocrine and mammary malignancies as main signs of hormonal syndromes produced by endocrine tumors. Ann. N.Y. Acad. Sci. 230:500, 1974.

77. Iglesias, R., Mardones, E., and Lipschutz, A. Evolution of luteoma in intrasplenic ovarian grafts in the guinea-pig. Br. J. Cancer 7:214, 1953.

78. Iijima, H., Nasu, K., and Taki, I. Comparative study of carcinogenesis in squamous columnar epithelium of mouse uterus by string method of producing cervical carcinoma. Am. J. Obstet. Gynecol. 89:946, 1964.

79. Jabara, A. G. Induction of canine ovarian tumours by diethylstilboestrol and progesterone. Aust. J. Exp. Biol. Med. Sci. 40:139, 1962.

80. Joneja, M. J., and Coulson, D. B. Histopathology and cytogenetics of tumors induced by the application of 7,12-dimethylbenz[a]anthracene (DMBA) in mouse cervix. Eur. J. Cancer 9:367, 1973.

81. Jones, D. C., and Witschi, E. Endocrinology of ovarian tumor formation in parabiotic rats. Cancer Res. 21:783, 1961.

82. Jones, E. C., and Krohn, P. L. Influence of the anterior pituitary on the ageing process in the ovary. Nature (London) 183:1155, 1959.

83. Jones, E. C., and Krohn, P. L. The relationships between age, numbers of oocytes and fertility in virgin and multiparous mice. J. Endocrinol. 21:469, 1961.

84. Jull, J. W. Hormones as promoting agents in mammary carcinogenesis. Acta Un. Int. Cancer (Louvain) 12:653, 1956.

85. Jull, J. W. Mechanism of induction of ovarian tumors in the mouse by 7,12-dimethylbenz[a]anthracene. VI Effect of normal ovarian tissue on tumor development. J. Natl. Cancer Inst. 42:967, 1969.

86. Jull, J. W. Ovarian tumorigenesis. Methods Cancer Res. 7:131, 1973.

87. Jull, J. W., Hawryluk, A., and Russell, A. Mechanism of induction of ovarian tumors in the mouse by 7,12-dimethylbenz[a]anthracene. III Tumor induction in organ culture. J. Natl. Cancer Inst. 40:687, 1968.

88. Jull, J. W., and Jellink, P. H. Mechanism of induction of ovarian tumors in the mouse by 7,12-dimethylbenz[a]anthracene. IV Uptake and retention of $C^{14}$—DMBA by mouse and rat tissues. J. Natl. Cancer Inst. 40:707, 1968.

89. Jull, J. W., and Russell, A. Mechanism of induction of ovarian tumors in the mouse by 7,12-dimethylbenz[a]anthracene. VII Relative activities of parent hydrocarbon and some of its metabolites. J. Natl. Cancer Inst. 44:841, 1970.

90. Jurow, H. N. Cyclic variations in the cervix of the guinea-pig. Am. J. Obstet. Gynecol. 45:762, 1943.

91. Kaminetzky, H. A. Methylcholanthrene-induced cervical dysplasia and the sex steroids. Obstet. Gynecol. 27:489, 1966.

92. Kimura, T., and Nandi, S. Nature of induced persistent vaginal cornification in mice. IV Changes in the vaginal epithelium of old mice treated neonatally with estradiol or testosterone. J. Natl. Cancer Inst. 39:75, 1967.

93. Kirkman, H. Hormone-related tumors in Syrian hamsters. Prog. Exp. Tumor Res. 16:201, 1972.

94. Kirkman, H., and Algard, F. T. Characteristics of an androgen/estrogen induced uterine smooth muscle tumor of the Syrian hamster. Cancer Res. 30:794, 1970.

95. Koprowska, I., Bogacz, J., Pentikas, C., and Stypulkowski, W. Induced cervical carcinoma of the mouse. A quantitative cytological method for evaluation of the neoplastic process. Cancer Res. 18:1186, 1958.

96. Krarup, T. 9:10-dimethyl-1:2-benzanthracene induced ovarian tumours in mice. Acta Pathol. Microbiol. Scand. 70:241, 1967.

97. Krarup, T. Oocyte destruction and ovarian tumorigenesis

after direct application of a chemical carcinogen (9:10-dimethyl-1:2-benzanthracene) to the mouse ovary. *Intl. J. Cancer* 4:61, 1969.

98. Krarup, T., and Loft, H. Presence of DMBA-³H in the mouse ovary and its relation to ovarian tumour induction. *Acta Pathol. Microbiol. Scand. A* 79:139, 1971.

99. Kullander, S. On tumor formation in gonadal and hypophyseal transplants into the anterior eye chambers of gonadectomised rats. *Cancer Res.* 20:1079, 1960.

100. Kushima, K., Noda, K., and Makita, M. Experimental production of chorionic tumor in rabbits. *Tohuko J. Med.* 91:209, 1967.

101. Kuwahara, I. Experimental induction of ovarian tumors in mice treated with single administration of 7,12-dimethylbenz[a]anthracene, and its pathological observation. *Gann* 58:253, 1967.

102. Lee, S., Condon, J. K., Chandler, J. G., Koopmans, H., Ehara, Y., Yen, S. S., and Orloff, M. J. The effect of Eck fistula upon intrasplenic ovarian neoplasm formation. *Surg. Forum* 23:110, 1972.

103. Li, M. H., and Gardner, W. U. Further studies on the pathogenesis of ovarian tumors in mice. *Cancer Res.* 9:35, 1949.

104. Lick, L., Kirschbaum, A., and Mixer, H. Mechanism of induction of ovarian tumors by X-rays. *Cancer Res.* 9:532, 1949.

105. Lipschutz, A. *Steroid Homeostasis. Hypophysis and Tumorigenesis.* Cambridge, Heffer and Sons, 1957.

106. Lipschutz, A., Iglesias, R., Panasevich, V. I., and Salinas, S. Granulosa-cell tumours induced in mice by progesterone. *Br. J. Cancer* 21:144, 1967.

107. Lipschutz, A., Iglesias, R., Panasevich, V. I., and Salinas, S. Pathological changes induced in the uterus of mice with the prolonged administration of progesterone and 19-nor-contraceptives. *Br. J. Cancer* 21:160, 1967.

108. Lipschutz, A., Iglesias, R., Panasevich, V. I., and Socorro, S. Ovarian tumours and other ovarian changes induced in mice by two 19-nor-contraceptives. *Br. J. Cancer* 21:153, 1967.

109. Lipschutz, A., Iglesias, R., Salinas, S., and Panasevich, V. I. Experimental conditions under which contraceptive steroids may become toxic. *Nature (London)* 212:686, 1966.

110. Lipschutz, A., and Vargas, L. Structure and origin of uterine and extragenital fibroids induced experimentally in the guinea-pig by prolonged administration of estrogens. *Cancer Res.* 1:236, 1941.

111. Loeb, L., Burns, E. L., Suntzeff, V., and Moskop, M. Carcinoma-like proliferations in vagina, cervix and uterus of mouse treated with estrogens. *Proc. Soc. Exp. Biol. Med.* 35:320, 1936.

112. London, W. T., Nahmias, A. J., Naib, Z. M., Fucillo, D. A., Ellenberg, J. H., and Sever, J. L. A nonhuman primate model for the study of the cervical oncogenic potential of *Herpes simplex* virus type 2. *Cancer Res.* 34:1118, 1974.

113. Lorenz, E. Some biologic effects of long continued radiation. *Am. J. Roentgenol Radium Ther. Nucl. Med.* 63:176, 1950.

114. Manocha, S. L., and Graham, C. E. Histochemistry of mouse cervical epithelium during chemical carcinogenesis. *Histochem. J.* 2:357, 1970.

115. Marchant, J. Influence of the strain of ovarian grafts on the induction of breast and ovarian tumours in F₁ (C57B1 × IF) hybrid mice by 9:10-dimethyl-1:2-benzanthracene. *Br. J. Cancer* 13:306, 1959.

116. Marchant, J. Changes in the ovaries of mice treated with dimethylbenzanthracene and observations on the subsequent development of tumours in ovaries and breasts. *Br. J. Cancer* 13:652, 1959.

117. Marchant, J. The development of ovarian tumours in ova-

ries grafted from mice pretreated with dimethylbenzanthracene. Inhibition by the presence of normal ovarian tissue. *Br. J. Cancer* 14:514, 1960.

118. Marchant, J. The effect of hypophysectomy on the development of ovarian tumours in mice treated with dimethylbenzanthracene. *Br. J. Cancer* 15:821, 1961.

119. Marchant, J. Personal observation, 1960.

120. Marchant, J., Orr, J. W., and Woodhouse, D. L. Induction of ovarian tumors with 9:10-dimethyl-1:2-benzanthracene. *Nature (London)* 173:307, 1954.

121. Mardones, E., Iglesias, R., and Lipschutz, A. Granulosa cell tumours in intrasplenic ovarian grafts, with intrahepatic metastases, in guinea-pigs at five years after grafting. *Br. J. Cancer* 9:409, 1955.

122. McClure, H. M., and Graham, C. E. Malignant uterine mesotheliomas in squirrel monkeys following diethylstilboestrol administration. *Lab. Anim. Sci.* 23:493, 1973.

123. Meier, H., Myers, D. D., Fox, R. R., and Laird, C. W. Occurrence, pathological features, and propagation of gonadal teratomas in inbred mice and rabbits. *Cancer Res.* 30:30, 1970.

124. Meisels, A. Effect of sex hormones on the carcinogenic action of dimethylbenzanthracene on the uterus of intact and castrated mice. *Cancer Res.* 26:757, 1966.

125. Meissner, W. A., Sommers, S. C., and Sherman, G. Endometrial hyperplasia, endometrial carcinoma, and endometriosis produced experimentally by estrogen. *Cancer, N.Y.* 10:500, 1957.

126. Miller, O. J., and Gardner, W. U. The role of thyroid function and food intake in experimental ovarian tumorigenesis in mice. *Cancer Res.* 14:220, 1954.

127. Mody, J. K. The action of four carcinogenic hydrocarbons on the ovaries of IF mice and the histogenesis of induced tumours. *Br. J. Cancer* 14:256, 1960.

128. Moon, H. D., Simpson, M. E., Li, C. H., and Evans, H. M. Neoplasms in rats and mice treated with pituitary growth hormone. III Reproductive organs. *Cancer Res.* 10:549, 1950.

129. Mossman, H. W. The embryology of the cervix. In Blandau, R. J., and Moghissi, K. eds.: *The Biology of the Cervix.* Chicago, Chicago University Press, 1973, Ch. 2.

130. Mossman, H. W., and Duke, K. L. *Comparative Morphology of the Mammalian Ovary.* Madison University of Wisconsin Press, 1973.

131. Mühlbock, O. Hormonale ovariumtumoren na Röntgenbestraling. *Ned. Tijdsch. v. Geneesk.,* 95:915, 1951.

132. Mühlbock, O. Ovarian tumours in mice in parabiotic union. *Acta Endocrinol.* Copenhagen. 12:105, 1953.

133. Mühlbock, O. On the genesis of ovarian tumours. Experiments with mice in parabiotic union. *Acta Un. Int. Cancr (Louvain)* 10:141, 1954.

134. Mühlbock, O., van Nie, R., and Bosch, L. The production of oestrogenic hormones by granulosa cell tumours in mice, in *Hormone Production in Endocrine Tumours,* Ciba Found. Colloq. Endocrinol., 1958, Vol. 12, p. 78.

135. Muñoz, N. Effect of Herpesvirus Type 2 and hormonal imbalance on the uterine cervix of the mouse. *Cancer Res.* 33:1504, 1973.

136. Murphy, E. D. Carcinogenesis of the uterine cervix in mice: Effect of diethylstilbestrol after limited application of 3-methylcholanthrene. *J. Natl. Cancer Inst.* 27:611, 1961.

137. Murphy, E. D. Characteristic tumors, in Green, E. L., ed:

Jackson Laboratory. *Biology of the Laboratory Mouse,* 2nd ed. New York, McGraw Hill, 1966, Ch. 27.

138. Murphy, E. D. Carcinogenesis of the uterine cervix in mice: Effect of castration after limited application of 3-methylcholanthrene. *J. Natl. Cancer Inst.* 41:1111, 1968.

139. Murphy, E. D. Hyperplastic and early neoplastic changes in the ovaries of mice after genic deletion of germ cells. *J. Natl. Cancer Inst.* 48:1283, 1972.

140. Murphy, E. D., and Beamer, W. G. Plasma gonadotropin levels during early stages of ovarian tumorigenesis in mice of the W$^x$/W$^v$ genotype. *Cancer Res.* 33:721, 1973.

141. Nairn, R. C., Wallace, A. C., and Guli, E. P. Intestinal antigenicity of ovarian mucinous cystadenomas. *Br. J. Cancer* 25:276, 1971.

142. Nelson, L. W., Kelly, W. A., and Weikel, J. H. Mesovarial leiomyomas in rats in a chronic toxicity study of mesuprine hydrochloride. *Toxicol. Appl. Pharmacol.* 23:731, 1972.

143. Nelson, W. O. Atypical uterine growths produced by prolonged administration of estrogenic hormones. *Endocrinology* 24:50, 1939.

144. Nishizuka, Y., and Sakakura, T. Ovarian dysgenesis induced by neonatal thymectomy in the mouse. *Endocrinology* 89:886, 1971.

145. Nishizuka, Y., and Sakakura, T. Effect of combined removal of thymus and pituitary on post-natal ovarian follicular development in the mouse. *Endocrinology* 89:902, 1971.

146. Nishizuka, Y., Tanaka, Y., Sakakura, T., and Kojma, A. Frequent development of ovarian tumors from dysgenetic ovaries of neonatally thymectomised mice. *Gann* 63:139, 1972.

147. Nomura, T. Carcinogenesis by urethane via mother's milk and its enhancement of transplacental carcinogenesis in mice. *Cancer Res.* 33:1677, 1973.

148. Nomura, T., Okamoto, E., and Manabe, H. Ovarian teratoma found in an offspring of mothers (ICR-JCL mice) treated with urethane. *Med. J. Osaka Univ.* 23:121, 1972.

149. Oakberg, E. F. Effect of 25R of X-rays at 10 days of age on oocyte numbers and fertility of female mice, in Lindop, D. J., and Sacher, G. A., eds.: *Radiation and Ageing.* London, Taylor and Francis, 1966, pp. 293–306.

150. Pan, S. C., and Gardner, W. U. Induction of malignant tumors by methylcholanthrene in transplanted uterine cornua and cervixes of mice. *Cancer Res.* 8:613, 1948.

151. Pantelouris, E. M. Athymic development in the mouse. *Differentiation* 1:437, 1973.

152. Peckham, B. M., and Greene, R. R. Experimentally produced granulosa-cell tumors in rabbits. *Cancer Res.* 12:654, 1952.

153. Perry, I. H., and Ginzton, L. L. The development of tumors in female mice treated with 1;2;5;6-dibenzanthracene and theelin. *Am. J. Cancer* 29:680, 1937.

154. Peters, H. Effects of radiation in early life on the morphology and reproductive function of the mouse ovary. *Adv. Reprod. Physiol.* 4:149, 1969.

155. Pfeiffer, C. A. Sexual differences of the hypophysis and their determination by the gonads. *Am. J. Anat.* 58:195, 1936.

156. Pfeiffer, C. A. Development of leiomyomas in female rats with an endocrine imbalance. *Cancer Res.* 9:277, 1949.

157. Pfeiffer, C. A. Adenocarcinoma in the uterus of an endocrine imbalance female rat. *Cancer Res.* 9:347, 1949.

158. Pierson, H. Experimental production of uterine enlargement with cancer through ovarian hormone. *Ztschr. Krebsforsch.* 41:103, 1934.

159. Reagen, J. W., Wentz, B. W., and Hachico, N. Induced cancer of the mouse. *Arch. Pathol.* 6:451, 1955.

160. Reboud, S., and Pageant, G. Co-carcinogenic effect of progesterone on 20-methylcholanthrene-induced cervical carcinoma in mice. *Nature (London)* 241:398, 1973.

161. Reuber, M. D. Endometrial sarcomas of the uterus and carcinosarcoma of the submaxillary salivary gland in castrated A × C strain female rats receiving N,N′-fluorenyldiacetamide and norethandrolone. *J. Natl. Cancer Inst.* 25:1141, 1960.

162. Roberts, D. C. Transplanted tumours of the Golden hamster (*Mesocricetus auratus*) used in research 1964–1970. *Prog. Exp. Tumor. Res.* 16:558, 1972.

163. Rubio, C. A., and Lagelöf, B. Studies on the histogenesis of experimentally induced cervical carcinoma. *Acta Pathol. Microbiol. Scand. A* 82:153, 1974.

164. Rubio, C. A., and Lagelöf, B. Autoradiographic studies of experimentally induced atypias in the cervical epithelium of mice. *Acta Pathol. Microbiol. Scand. A* 82:475, 1974.

165. Russell, E. S., and Fekete, E. Analysis of W-series pleiotropism in the mouse: Effect of W$^v$W$^v$ substitution on definitive germ cells and on ovarian tumorigenesis. *J. Natl. Cancer Inst.* 21:365, 1958.

166. Scarpelli, D. G., and von Haam, E. Experimental carcinoma of the uterine cervix in the mouse. *Am. J. Pathol.* 33:1059, 1957.

167. Sekiya, S., Takamizawa, H., Wang, F., Takane, T., and Kuwata, T. In vivo and in vitro studies on uterine adenocarcinoma of the rat induced by 7,12-dimethylbenz[a]anthracene. *Am. J. Obstet. Gynecol.* 113:691, 1972.

168. Sekiya, S., Yam, A., and Takamizawa, H. Enhancement of tumor growth and metastases by medroxyprogesterone acetate in transplanted uterine adenocarcinoma cells of the rat. *J. Natl. Cancer Inst.* 52:297, 1974.

169. Sever, J. L. Herpes virus and cervical cancer studies in experimental animals. *Cancer Res.* 33:1509, 1973.

170. Shen, C. N. Experimental induction of placental tumor in the guinea pig. *Nagoya Med. J.* 17:33, 1971.

171. Shintani, S., Glass, L. E., and Page, E. W. Studies of induced malignant tumors of placental and uterine origin in the rat. II Induced tumors and pathogenesis. *Am. J. Obstet. Gynecol.* 95:550, 1966.

172. Shisa, H., and Nishizuka, Y. Unilateral development of ovarian tumour in thymectomized Swiss mice following a single injection of 7,12-dimethylbenz[a]anthracene at neonatal stage. *Br. J. Cancer* 22:70, 1968.

173. Singh, K. B. Induction of polycystic ovarian disease in rats by continuous light. I. The reproductive cycle, organ weights and histology of the ovaries. *Am. J. Obstet. Gynecol.* 103:1078, 1969.

174. Slye, M., Holmes, M. F., and Wells, H. G. Primary spontaneous tumors of the ovary in mice. *J. Cancer Res.* 5:205, 1920.

175. Sobis, H., and Vandeputte, M. Development of teratomas from displaced visceral yolk sac. *Intl. J. Cancer* 13:444, 1974.

176. Sommers, S. C., and Meissner. W. A. Host relationship in experimental endometrial carcinoma. *Cancer, N.Y.* 10:510, 1957.

177. Staats, J. Standardised nomenclature for inbred strains of mice. Third listing. *Cancer Res.* 24:147, 1964.

178. Stein-Werblowsky, R. Induction of cancer of the cervix in relation to the oestrus cycle. *Br. J. Cancer* 14:300, 1960.

179. Stevens, L. C. Experimental production of testicular teratomas in mice. *Proc. Natl. Acad. Sci. USA* 52:654, 1964.

180. Stevens, L. C., and Varnum, D. S. The development of teratomas from parthenogenetically activated ovarian mouse eggs. *Dev. Biol.* 37:369, 1974.

181. Strong, L. C., Gardner, W. U., and Hill, R. T. Production of estrogenic hormone by a transplantable ovarian carcinoma. *Endocrinology* 21:268, 1937.

182. Suntzeff, V., Burns, E. L., Moskop, M., and Loeb, L. On proliferative changes taking place in epithelium of vagina and cervix of mice with advancing age and under influence of experimentally administered estrogenic hormones. *Am. J. Cancer* 32:256, 1938.

183. Symeonides, A. Tumors induced by 2-acetylaminofluorene in virgin and breeding females of five strains of rats and in their offspring. *J. Natl. Cancer Inst.* 15:539, 1954.

184. Symeonides, A., and Mori-Chavez, P. A transplantable ovarian papillary adenocarcinoma of the rat with ascites implants in the ovary. *J. Natl. Cancer Inst.* 13:409, 1952.

185. Takamizawa, H., and Wong, K. Effect of anticancer drugs on uterine carcinogenesis. *Obstet. Gynecol.* 41:701, 1973.

186. Takasugi, N. Carcinogenesis by vaginal transplants from ovariectomized, neonatally-estrogenized mice into ovariectomized normal host. *Gann* 63:73, 1972.

187. Taki, I., and Iijima, H. A new method of producing endometrial cancer in mice. *Am. J. Obstet. Gynecol.* 87:926, 1963.

188. Taki, I., Iijima, H., Doi, T., Uetsuki, Y., and Masahiko, M. Histochemistry of hydrolytic and oxydative enzymes in the human and experimentally induced adenocarcinoma of the endometrium. *Am. J. Obstet. Gynecol.* 94:86, 1966.

189. Thiery, M. Ovarian teratoma in the mouse. *Br. J. Cancer* 17:231, 1936.

190. Thiery, M., De Groodt, M., De Rom, F., Sebryns, M., and Lagasse, A. Viruslike particles in chemically-induced carcinoma of the uterine cervix. *Nature (London)* 183:694, 1959.

191. Thiery, M., and Willighagen, R. G. J. Enzyme histochemistry of induced and transplanted squamous cell carcinoma of the uterine cervix. *Br. J. Cancer* 18:582, 1964.

192. Uematsu, K., and Huggins, C. B. Induction of leukaemia and ovarian tumors in mice by pulse-doses of aromatic hydrocarbons. *Mol. Pharmacol.* 4:427, 1968.

193. Vandeputte, M., Sobis, H., Billiau, A., van de Maele, B., and Leyten R. *In utero* tumor induction by murine sarcoma virus (Maloney) in the rat. I. Biological characteristics. *Intl. J. Cancer* 11:536, 1973.

194. van Nie, R., Benedetti, E. L., and Mühlbock, O. A carcinogenic action of testosterone, provoking uterine tumours in mice. *Nature (London)* 192:1303, 1961.

195. van Nie, R., Smit, G. M. J., and Mühlbock, O. The induction of uterine tumours in mice treated with testosterone. *Acta Un. Int. Cancer* 18:194, 1962.

196. Vellios, F., and Griffin, J. The pathogenesis of dimethyl-benzanthracene-induced carcinoma of the cervix in rats. *Cancer Res.* 17:364, 1955.

197. Vesselinovich, S. D., Mihailovich, N., Rao, K. V., and Itze, L. Perinatal carcinogenesis by urethane. *Cancer Res.* 31:2143, 1971.

198. Vink, H. H. Ovarian teratomas in guinea pigs: A report of ten cases. *J. Pathol.* 102:180, 1970.

199. von Haam, E., and Scarpielli, D. G. Experimental carcinoma of the cervix: A comparative cytologic and histologic study. *Cancer Res.* 15:449, 1955.

200. Willis, R. A. Ovarian teratomas in guinea pigs. *J. Pathol. Bacteriol.* 84:237, 1962.

201. Yong, H. Y., and Campbell, J. S. Evolution of dysplasia of the uterine cervix and vagina induced by low dosages of carcinogen in mice. *Obstet. Gynecol.* 26:91, 1965.

E. Cotchin,
D.Sc., F.R.C.V.S., F.R.C. Path.

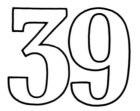

# Spontaneous Tumors of the Uterus and Ovaries in Animals

## General Introduction

In this chapter, a survey is made of the spontaneous tumors of the uterus and ovaries in animals. The bulk of information is about such tumors in domesticated animals, but some reference is also made to tumors in laboratory animals, wild animals, and animals in zoos. This is not a fully comprehensive bibliographic review but highlights the features of these tumors that appear to me, a veterinary pathologist, to be of most interest.

A note of caution may be sounded for those who are approaching the subject of spontaneous tumors in animals for the first time. Information about such tumors is inferior in quantity, and sometimes in quality, to that about tumors in humans.[40] Most of the reported studies of material from domesticated animals have been based on the histopathologic examination of biopsy or autopsy specimens in laboratories servicing the clinics in veterinary schools or examining material submitted by practitioners, although information has also been obtained from studies of abattoir material. As regards material from clinics and private practices, a considerable element of selection bias arises because the affected animal is not even brought in for surgical treatment or autopsy unless the owner, or the referring practitioner, so chooses. Again much information available in veterinary pathologic laboratories is never published and even then may be restricted to rare or unusual cases. However, with the advent of indexing and computerized recording, a start is being made to bring such unpublished material to light, as, for example, in Priester's valuable surveys of material in 12 North American veterinary schools.[165]

Although a number of veterinary school studies of animal tumors have been published, their statistical value has been diminished by the absence of information about the background animal population. This situation is being remedied (cf. the Alameda County surveys in California[52-54]). The common practice of spaying cats and the increasingly common practice of spaying bitches will even here distort the true picture of the incidence of uterine and ovarian tumors.

Abattoir surveys are not easy to organize, but they can provide valuable information, as in the case of the federally inspected abattoirs in the United States,[21] the British survey by Anderson, Sandison, and Jarrett,[7] and a recent survey in Australia.[192] It must be remembered that food animals are slaughtered at an early age, in contrast to domestic pets and horses, which are more often allowed to live out something closer to an expected lifespan.

A considerable advance in the study of animal neoplasms was the establishment of the Registry of Veterinary Pathology at the Armed Forces Institute of Pathology in Washington, D.C. Computerized recording of tumors in animals in zoos is also developing,[10] and neoplasms in lower animals are being studied at the Registry of Tumors in the Lower Animals (RTLA) at the Smithsonian Institution, also in Washington, D.C.

A basic need in studying tumors of animals is for some standardized nomenclature, preferably in harmony with that of human neoplasms. The World Health Organization has interested itself in this problem and has recently published[214] its first set of classifications of tumors in six domesticated mammalian species, horse, ox, pig, sheep, dog, and cat. The classification of tumors of the female genital system should appear shortly.[123,161]

Attention may finally be drawn to what might be termed the "negative" significance of studying *spontaneous* tumors in animals. The "positive" significance is clear: A study of tumors occurring commonly in animals may provide epidemiologic or other clues to their etiology,[42] and the tumors provide opportunities for etiologic, biologic, and therapeutic investigation. For example, there is in some stocks of rabbits a high incidence of endometrial glandular tumors, which allows histogenetic and genetic analyses of considerable comparative oncologic interest. The "negative" significance may arise if careful study indicates that certain tumors of importance in humans are rarely if ever seen in animals.[43] For example, the observation that carcinoma of the uterine cervix is reported only very rarely as a spontaneous tumor in animals and that

choriocarcinoma is reliably reported even more rarely may add weight to the proposition that factors that are more or less specific to the human patient are involved in the etiology of these particular tumors.

# Spontaneous Tumors of the Uterus

In a detailed literature review 10 years ago,[41] I showed that endometrial carcinoma is significant only in cows and rabbits, and that carcinoma of the uterine cervix is rarely encountered in animals. Most examples of bovine uterine carcinoma have been reported in the United States, at least in recent years, and most endometrial tumors of rabbits have been seen in three colonies in that country. In no domesticated species has choriocarcinoma been convincingly diagnosed.

The main part of this section is concerned with endometrial tumors in cows and in rabbits. Before these are dealt with, however, a brief survey is made of uterine tumors in other domesticated animals (horse, sheep, goat, pig, dog, cat, fowl), laboratory animals, and wild and zoo animals and birds.

## Domesticated Animals: General Survey

### Mare (*Equus caballus*)

Carcinoma of the uterine corpus or cervix has been rarely recorded in mares, and detailed pathologic reports are lacking. Myometrial tumors may be more important than endometrial tumors. Malignant as well as benign muscle tumors have been encountered. Jennings[41] found a probable leiomyosarcoma in the uterus of a 12-year-old mare, and Grant[79] reported a curious case of a leiomyoma of the right uterine cornu of a 12-year-old thoroughbred mare: The foal present showed extensive deformities of the extremities of all four limbs.

Records of epidermoid carcinoma of the vagina, vulva,[196] and clitoris of the mare are more common. These tumors resemble, in their papilliform structure and slow metastasizing course, the more common epidermoid carcinoma of the glans penis of the castrated male horse, and it is possible that the carcinomas have a common etiology (smegma ?, virus ?) in the two sexes.

### Ewe (*Ovis aries*)

Practically all reported tumors of the genital tract of the ewe have been leiomyomas of the uterus or fibromas of the vagina.[21] There is one report of a probable endometrial carcinoma in a 5-year-old crossbred ewe by Terlecki and Watson,[195] who have found a poorly differentiated mucus-secreting adenocarcinoma of the uterine wall.

### Goat (Capra hircus)

The total number of tumors of any kind whatever that have been reported in goats is very small. In Kronberger's survey[117] there are listed 24 caprine tumors, which include one fibroma of the uterus, one adenoma of the vagina and vulva, and three fibromas of the vagina and vulva. Riedel[168] reported a sclerosing metastasizing adenocarcinoma in the region of the uterus of a 12-year-old goat that had not been pregnant for some years. Brandly[41] had also seen a caprine uterine adenocarcinoma, and Barboni[41] reported a mucous cystadenocarcinoma of the uterine cervix.

### Sow (Sus scrofa)

No convincing report of uterine or cervical carcinoma in the sow has come to my notice. Most reported tumors are myomas or fibromas, some affecting the uterus and vagina and some the broad ligament. For example, Winterfeldt[213] found a leiomyoma measuring 53 by 38 by 17 cm and weighing 20.62 kg in the broad ligament of the right cornu of an old sow.

### Dog (Canis familiaris)

The number of reported cases of adenocarcinoma of the canine uterus is quite small.[41,75] The unwary pathologist may be deceived by the development of hyperplastic glandular changes, which may be quite localized, in cases of the common condition of "pyometra," or by the apparent myometrial invasion in adenomyosis uteri.[34,181] This may be the true diagnosis of the lesion reported as a uterine adenocarcinoma by Joshi et al.[109]

However, acceptable cases of canine endometrial carcinoma are on record. In one case,[5] the tumor affected the right uterine cornu, with metastases in the lungs, bronchial nodes, liver, spleen, pericardium, gastrointestinal tract, kidneys, and pancreas. It is probable that this was a spontaneous tumor but the host, dying at 10 years of age, was a Beagle bitch that, in an experimental lifespan evaluation of the effects of irradiation, had received whole-body exposures of 75 rads each at 7-day intervals at the age of 11 months. The bitch had produced two litters, at 96 and 130 weeks of age, and had shown false estrus or anestrus for 1,300 days before death.

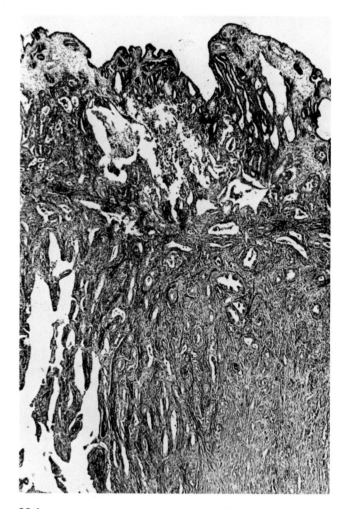

**39.1** Adenocarcinoma of the uterus of a 10-year-old Persian cat, showing endometrial origin and deep invasion of myometrium. $\times 32$.

Carcinoma of the uterine cervix seems to be as great a rarity in the bitch as it is in other domesticated mammals. Dämmrich and Lettow[45] reported an adenocarcinoma, possibly arising from cervical glands, in a 14-year-old Dachshund bitch.

There is no convincing record of a choriocarcinoma in a bitch; the most likely example is that recorded by Christopher[33] in a 2½-year-old Alsatian bitch. Two sorts of cell were described in the lesion—large round cells, and syncytial cells—which probably occupied a placental site.

The common tumor of the canine female genital tract is a leiomyoma or other mesodermal tumor of the vagina.[11,127]

In a series of 3,073 tumor-bearing dogs, Brodey and Roszel[22] found 96 tumors of the uterus, vagina, and vulva

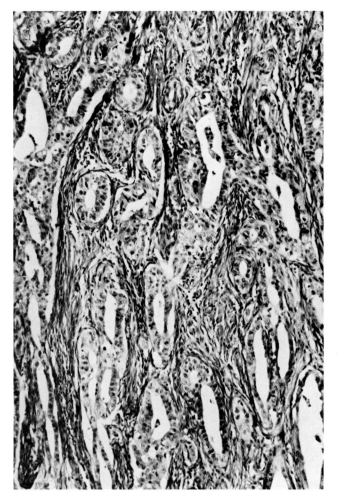

**39.2** Same tumor as in Figure 39.1, showing well-differentiated glandular pattern. ×127.

in 90 bitches. The commonest tumor was a leiomyoma, 76 such tumors being found in 70 dogs (66 affecting the vagina and vulva and only 10 the uterus). Affected bitches averaged 10.8 years of age. Most of the myomas affected the vestibule of the vulva, growth being extraluminal or intraluminal. In this series, there were also three leiomyosarcomas.

## Cat (*Felis catus*)

Female cats are frequently subjected to ovariohysterectomy. Since my 1964 review, Preiser[164] and Belter, Crawford, and Bates[18] have described endometrial adenocarcinomas in cats, both aged 11 years. I have seen one case of endometrial adenocarcinoma (Figures 39.1 and

39.2), as well as a possible carcinoleiomyosarcoma. O'Rourke and Geib,[157] who state that only eight uterine carcinomas have been recorded in cats, described a case in a 12-year-old domestic short-haired cat. Dystocia was noted 2 months previously. One month later a blackish green vaginal discharge developed. The cat showed incoordination, and there was bilateral retinal hemorrhage and detachment. Metastases from the endometrial carcinoma were found in the ovaries, adrenal, lung, brain, and eyes.

Squamous cell carcinoma of the uterine cervix seems to be as rare in cats as in other domesticated animals, but squamous metaplasia may be found in some endometrial carcinomas.[139]

## Fowl (*Gallus domesticus*)

Although the fowl oviduct differs structurally and functionally from the mammalian uterus, it is worth drawing attention to the remarkable incidence of carcinoma of the oviduct that has recently been encountered in the United Kingdom. Goodchild and Cooper,[77] for example, in a flock of Light Sussex hens 66 to 68 weeks old, found that 84 (37.7%) of 223 birds examined had macroscopic tumors in the magnum of the single (left) oviduct. Metastases were noted macroscopically in three hens.

The tumor is diffuse or nodular and is generally multifocal in origin, being more pronounced toward the cranial end of the oviduct.[76] It affects active and regressed oviducts and it can affect the normally nonpersistent right oviduct.

# Laboratory Animals: General Survey

## Primates

In their survey of tumors in nonhuman primates, O'Gara and Adamson[156] stated that 41 tumors of female sex organs have been reported in 39 primates.

In a survey of neoplasms and proliferative lesions in 1,065 nonhuman primate necropsies, Seibold and Wolf[182] recorded leiomyoma of the uterus in three *Pan troglodytes* (aged 23, 44, and over 44 years, respectively) and in two *Macaca mulatta* (both adult, one multiparous). An old multiparous *M. mulatta* showed adenomatous hyperplasia of the endocervical glands, developing in the everted mucosa of the posterior lip of the cervix and the posterior fornix. Seibold and Wolf also refer to six cases (in 317 female *M. mulatta*) of endometriosis, or extrauterine occurrence of tissue resembling the uterine mucous membrane. One monkey, killed after signs of abdominal distress, showed intestinal adhesions from endometrial proliferations in the peritoneal cavity.

An account of endometriosis in rhesus monkeys is given by McCann and Myers.[138] Twenty-one of 69 mature females examined had such lesions, which increased in incidence with parity, age, increasing number of hysterotomies, and increased time since last pregnancy. The lesions are described and their incidence analyzed in detail, and it is concluded that "there exist basic differences in the pathogenesis and the pattern of pathology of this disease in the monkey as compared to that in man. It would thus appear that theories of pathogenesis of this disease valid for monkey may not necessarily be valid for man" (p. 583).

Recently, Strozier et al.[190] have described lesions in a female *M. mulatta,* approximately 15 years old, that died after an extended period of diarrhea and weight loss. At autopsy, there were found cystic endometrial hyperplasia and foci of endometrial tissue in the uterine wall, colon, and a regional lymph node. A focus of adenocarcinoma was found in the proliferated endometrium. The endometrial cavity contained purulent fluid from which a pure culture of *Escherichia coli* was isolated.

Special mention may be made of the metastasizing cervical carcinoma that Hisaw and Hisaw[96] found in an old female *M. mulatta,* and the cervical carcinoma *in situ* that Sternberg[185] found in a young adult of the same species.

Digiacomo and McCann[51] also found a case of carcinoma *in situ* of the cervix in one of 63 female *M. mulatta.* Hertig and MacKey[94] examined the complete genital tracts of 11 adult female crab-eating monkeys, *M. fascicularis,* and the same number of adult chimpanzees, *Pan troglodytes.* In one of the monkeys, a mature individual whose endometrium was in the preovulatory phase, the cervix showed an extensive squamous cell carcinoma *in situ,* involving the ventral portion of the glandular mucosa of the inner endocervix and the outer endocervix, the area most exposed to the vaginal environment in this species. There was no histologic contiguity with the normal squamous epithelium of the exocervix (the endocervix and the exocervix in this species are separated by an encircling fornix). Eight of the other 10 monkeys showed squamous metaplasia of the endocervix or of the exocervix or (in two animals) of both. One of the chimpanzees, 22 to 23 years old, showed three leiomyomas of the uterine fundus and corpus. In sections of endomyometrium of the corpus there were changes classified as proliferative endometrium, a focus of adenomatous hyperplasia, and a focus of adenocarcinoma *in situ.*

Moreland and Woodard[144] described a possible uterine

hamartoma in an adult cottontop marmoset [*Saguinus (Oepomidas) oedipus*]. Of particular interest is the report by Lindsey et al.[121] of what they considered to be the only reported case of choriocarcinoma in a nonhuman primate. A rhesus monkey became pregnant in the laboratory. It was subsequently given norethindrone enanthate daily except at weekends for 1 month, but it is not thought that this was involved in the occurrence of the tumor. The monkey died, but no fetus was found in the uterus, which contained a thick yellow material with ragged brown fragments. A large uterine mass was diagnosed as a choriocarcinoma, with extensive metastases in the lungs. In the trophoblastic tumor, cells of cytotrophoblast predominated. Granulomatous lesions, possibly tuberculous, were superimposed on the lung lesions.

In passing, mention may be made of the choriocarcinoma found in a pregnant nine-banded armadillo,[133] which had been given 100 mg thalidomide per kilogram of body weight per day for 10 days and was killed 17 days after the first dose. This mammal possesses a hemochorial placenta which resembles that of man in its maternal–fetal border.

## Mouse

Spontaneous carcinomas and sarcomas of the mouse uterus[175] have been reported by a few authors.[41] Age-related uterine leiomyomas or leiomyosarcomas were studied by Malinin and Malinin[132] and Chouroulinkov, Guillon, and Guérin[31] surveyed 130 cases of endometrial sarcomas. Gardner and Pan[72] found 13 of 56 female mice of Pybus Miller stock, 200 days old or older, had cervical or vaginal tumors at the time of death (five carcinomas of the vagina or uterine cervix, seven probably of epithelial origin, and one spindle cell sarcoma).

## Rat

A variety of uterine tumors[41,175] has been reported in rats, including adenocarcinomas and sarcomas (some of which were leiomyosarcomas). The tumors are not very frequently encountered but sometimes they achieve a moderate importance. For example, Schulze[180] found 23 uterine carcinomas among 34 spontaneous tumors of the uterus and ovaries in 66 tumors in 1,373 autopsied Sprague–Dawley and Bethesda Black rats.

Recent reports include those by Snell,[184] Jacobs and Huseby,[106] and Schardein et al.[177] In rats examined in the Laboratory of Pathology of the National Cancer Institute Snell[184] recorded that nearly two-thirds of the animals of F344 strain and one-third of those of the M520 strain over

20 months of age had endometrial tumors. Only a few OM, ACI, and BUF rats had similar tumors, and none were found in WN rats. In the strains with high incidence, but not in others, the tumors were more often found in virgins than in breeders. Most of the tumors were adenomatous polyps, a few were angiosarcomas. One BUF and two ACI rats showed endometrial adenocarcinomas, and one BUF rat had a uterine horn, lined with squamous cells, and showing two foci of squamous cell carcinoma. One 24-month-old F344 rat had a uterine myoma. The only cervical tumor noted was a polyp in a 27-month-old OM breeder. Yang[218] recorded a remarkable keratinizing metaplasia in a virgin 22-month-old Sprague–Dawley rat—one cornu (right) was completely affected, whereas the other showed only two microscopic foci.

Jacobs and Huseby[106] found macroscopic tumors of the uterine horns in 21 of 95 autopsied female Fischer rats. They occurred at an average age of 669 days, including some rats less than 1 year old. The tumors, often multiple, were polypoid glandular structures, mostly covered by endometrial epithelium. One consisted of very cellular sarcomatous tissue and three others showed sarcomatous change. All four sarcomas were transplanted, as were five benign polyps. It was concluded that the sarcomas were not of smooth muscle origin but arose from the lamina propria of the endometrial polyps. Schardein, Fitzgerald, and Kaump[177] found four Holtzman-source rats with well-differentiated adenomatous endometrial polyps with an average latent period of 467 days. Thompson et al.[199] have described similar tumors in a 2-year-old Sprague–Dawley rat, as well as cases of leiomyosarcoma of the uterus and fibrovascular polyp of the cervix.

Gellatly[74] has drawn attention to the need for histologic study in the diagnosis of uterine tumors in rats—a misdiagnosis of pyometra can occur. In a series of some 50 25-month-old virgin Wistar rats, the uterus was the organ most often affected by tumors; half the tumors were fibroadenomas, the next most common being a highly malignant adenocarcinoma. Some tumors were squamous cell carcinomas, which could sometimes be traced to originate from preexisting areas of squamous metaplasia of the endometrium (present in 28% of this series of rats), and in a few animals such metaplasia, with squamous cell carcinoma formation, was found on the surface of a fibroadenoma.

### Guinea pig

Lipschutz et al.[124] found two leiomyomas of the uterus in animals over 5 years of age, and two (histologic) adenocarcinomas in animals 3½ and 5 years old. Rogers and

Blumenthal[172] listed the following uterine tumors: four fibro- and leiomyomas, one adenomyoma, three fibro- and leiomyosarcomas, and one mesenchymal mixed tumor.

### Hamster

In a colony of Chinese hamsters (*Cricetulus griseus*) Ward and Moore[204] found uterine tumors in 30 of 120 females. These were adenocarcinomas, firm whitish nodular growths that always appeared to have included the cervical area, although they did not necessarily originate in the cervix. Implantations were not infrequent on visceral and parietal peritoneum, and three animals showed lung secondaries when examined histologically. The lesions showed extensive stromal fibrosis. The tumors usually occurred in the second year of life. The authors refer to a personal communication from Yerganian who stated that the incidence of such lesions could be enhanced by radiation.

### Gerbil

Rowe et al.[173] found 44 neoplasms at necropsy in 37 of 115 gerbils from a colony which contained wild-caught and first or second generation laboratory-raised gerbils (mostly *Meriones* species). The tumors included a moderately differentiated adenocarcinoma of the oviduct in *M. lybicus,* and endometrial adenocarcinoma in *M. tristrami* and the *M. shawi* × *M. lybicus* hybrid. (Both these latter animals also had granulosa cell tumors of the ovary.) Two other gerbils (*M. shawi* and *Pachyuromys duprisi*) had uterine leiomyosarcomas.

## Wild Animals, Animals in Zoos, and Birds: General Survey

In her impressive bibliographic survey of references to diseases in wild and zoo mammals and birds, Halloran[90] includes references to the following tumors of the uterus:

Fibroma: armadillo, agouti, axis deer, yak, nylghaie, blesbok, antelope
Fibroid: agouti, black leopard, lion, elephant
Fibromyoma: squirrel, lion
Myoma: lion, elephant
Carcinoma: coypu, mink, lion, wild swine, bontebok, gemsbok, sable antelope

Other tumors of the uterus referred to include: chorionic epithelioma and chorioma in porcupines; uterine tumor in an aardwolf; adenoma of cervix in the lion; cystic tumor in the jaguar; fibroadenoma in a jaguar. A tumor of the oviduct in Psittaciformes is listed. "A tumor was reported in the vagina of a hyena" (p. 200).

A female gray seal, shot at an estimated age of 44 years, had uterine squamous cell carcinomas and leiomyomas.[137]

Rewell and Willis[167] examined a uterine fibromyoma, 4 cm across, from a whale.

## Domesticated Animals: Detailed Account

Attention may now be concentrated on the two species in which uterine endometrial adenocarcinoma has been encountered in significant numbers—the cow and the rabbit.

### Cow (Bos taurus)

Although carcinoma of the bovine uterus has been recorded in a number of countries,[41,111,142,201] it is noteworthy that in recent years the majority of such tumors have been encountered in cows in federally inspected abattoirs in the United States. There is a strong possibility that such tumors are overlooked in many abattoirs elsewhere, since butchers commonly discard the uterus after only the most casual inspection. However, even in the careful abattoir survey by Anderson and Sandison[6] of tumors encountered in 1.3 million cattle at abattoirs in Great Britain, no tumors of the uterine corpus or cornu were found (there were three squamous cell carcinomas of the cervix in cows 6 to 8 years old). A search is still worth making—I have recently examined a metastasizing bovine uterine adenocarcinoma from a London abattoir.

The key papers on bovine uterine adenocarcinoma are those based on findings in American abattoirs.[21,141,143] In fact, these tumors are almost always abattoir findings. A clinical case was described by Lingard and Dickinson:[122] A 4-year-old Hereford cow with metastases in the lungs, liver, and bronchial, mediastinal, and internal iliac nodes was pregnant with a 100-day fetus in the right cornu, which showed, on its lesser curvature, a firm discoid carcinoma, 8 by 3 cm. That uterine carcinoma is not incompatible with pregnancy in cows has long been known. Wyssmann[216] found an affected cow with twin calves, and three of the 79 cases of Migaki et al.[141] were pregnant. This is consistent with the observation that the ovaries and the nonneoplastic endometrium showed no significant deviation from normal cyclic changes in the cows examined by Monlux et al.[143]

The relative incidence of bovine uterine carcinoma in American abattoirs is indicated by Brandly and Migaki.[21]

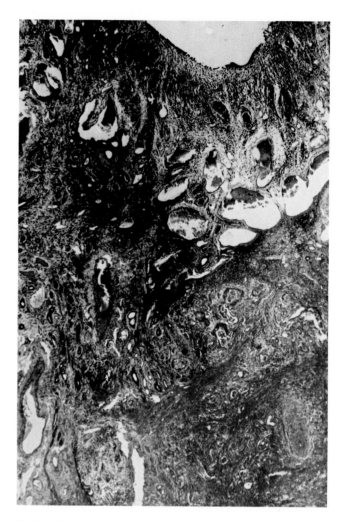

**39.3** Adenocarcinoma of the uterus of an 11-year-old cow, showing deep origin in endometrium. Metastases were present in regional nodes, lungs, kidney, heart, bronchial, and mediastinal nodes. ×32.

[From a section kindly provided by Dr. George Migaki (4004-AFIP 1448288).]

In a total of 737 tumors of all kinds (484 malignant, 253 benign) examined in less than 10 years, this was the second most common tumor submitted for histologic examination—lymphosarcoma 177, uterine carcinoma 166.

Affected cows[141] range from 2 to 12 years of age, most being over 6 years. There is no indication of breed susceptibility. The carcinoma is usually a single lesion, although occasionally two or three separate primary tumors may be present. The lesion is generally located in the free rather than the common part (body) of the uterine horns. It is generally firm and fibrous; white, whitish-yellow, or yel-

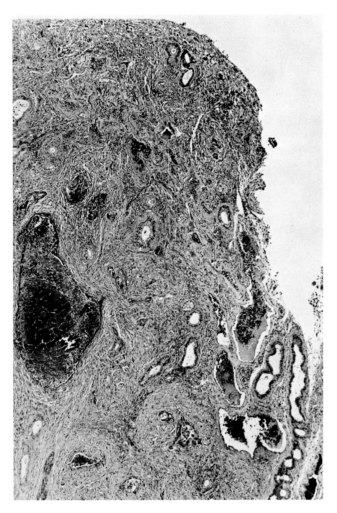

**39.4** Adenocarcinoma of the uterus of a cow from London abattoir, showing endometrial tumor. ×32.

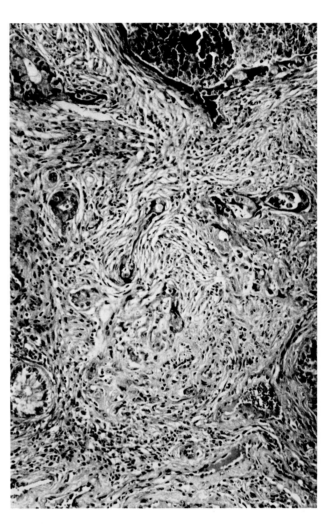

**39.5** Same tumor as Figure 39.4, showing sclerosing primary endometrial carcinoma. ×127.

low; and sometimes calcified. Small tumors can easily be overlooked. The thickening of the wall is rather diffuse and may be outwardly umbilicated. The tumor appears to develop deep in the endometrium (Figures 39.3 and 39.4) and the endometrial and serosal surfaces may appear grossly uninvolved. The tumor is typically accompanied by the abundant formation of dense fibrous tissue (Figure 39.5), which may lead to the incorrect diagnosis of sarcoma or even of mixed tumor. The tendency to marked sclerosis is also a feature of metastases, but in them the glandular conformation is usually retained (Figure 39.6).

The endometrial tumor extends locally to the serosa and the ovaries, this being accompanied by the local formation of a dense mat of fibrous tissue, the presence of

which, as Trotter[200] recognized, as an abattoir finding, points strongly to the presence of a uterine carcinoma. The visceral and parietal peritoneum may show neoplastic spread, especially near the uterus, and metastases may be found in the nodes and viscera. In one series of 26 cases, Monlux et al.[143] found metastases in lung (22), bronchial node (12), mediastinal node (14), sublumbar node (15), internal iliac node (17), and ovary (5), as well as on peritoneal surfaces. The metastatic growths, in lymph nodes particularly, are firm, white, or yellow and may be calcified; they therefore resemble granulomas, such as tuberculosis. Once pulmonary deposits have formed, they may increase in number by local "closed-circuit" lymphatic–vascular spread.

829

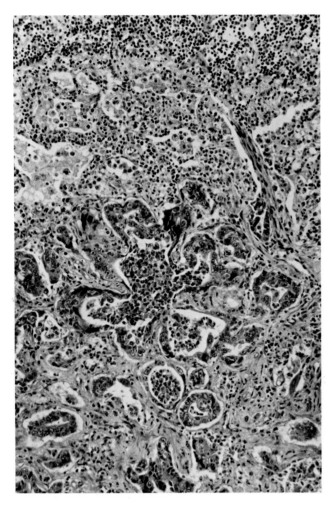

**39.6** Same tumor as Figure 39.4, showing retention of glandular conformation in a pulmonary metastasis. ×127.

Since Ottosen[160] suggested that the uterus might be an important site of origin for deposits of adenocarcinoma metastases in the bovine lung, Monlux et al.[143] have carefully described the histology of pulmonary metastases of known primary uterine adenocarcinomas in cows, stressing their retention of differentiated structure and the marked fibrous sclerosis. Hartigan and Flynn[93] in Eire have described pulmonary lesions in a cow that fulfilled these histologic criteria for a carcinoma of uterine origin. (In passing, it is worth noting that the bovine endometrium is sometimes the site of lymphosarcoma.)

Few cases of uterine cervical carcinoma have been described in cows.[6,41]

A variety of other tumors have been reported in the bovine female genital tract, including leiomyomas, fibromas, and fibromyomas. Most of these occur in the vaginal wall. My own series of vaginal tumors[38] included seven fibromas, seven lipomas, three fibromyomas, and two leiomyomas. Some uterine myomas may become fantastically large; Vandeplasche and Thoonen[202] recorded a weight of 200 kg. Some smooth muscle tumors are malignant. Maeda et al.[130] found a leiomyosarcoma of low-grade malignancy. Noordsy et al.[150] reported a leiomyosarcoma of the uterus in an 8-year-old Holstein cow, with secondaries on the omentum, diaphragm, and peritoneum and in the mesenteric lymph nodes, lungs, pleura, and myocardium. The primary tumor measured 75 by 50 by 30 cm and (together with the uterus) weighed 75 kg. The lesion in an extirpated uterine mass (weighing 110 kg) reported by Keindorf[113] was a partially cartilaginous mesenchymal tumor. It is not known whether uterine mixed tumors occur in cows.

Mention should be made of a curious vascular mesenchymal lesion of the bovine fetal placenta, which has been called a "choriohemangioma." Karlson and Kelly[112] found such a lesion in a 2-year-old cow that had given birth to a healthy calf. The lesion, attached to the fetal surface of the allantochorion by a narrow pedicle, measured 6 by 3 by 3 cm. It was the only such lesion found in a study of 550 membranes. Drieux and Le Coustumier[56] found a similar but larger lesion in a 3-year-old Montbéliard cow. A still larger tumor (30 by 20 by 7.5 cm) was examined by Corcoran and Murphy:[35] The fourth calf of a 6-year-old crossbred Hereford cow, a male, was born alive, followed by the tumor, composed of capillaries in a loose embryonal stroma. This lesion was accompanied by a remarkable degree of hydramnios. That such placental tumors are hamartomas rather than true neoplasms is supported by the observation by Kirkbride, Bicknell, and Robl[115] of a lesion of the placenta of a cow, when the calf, aborted at about 8 months gestation, showed angiomatous masses of the skin of the left forelimb and on the ventrolateral surface of the tongue.

## Laboratory Animal: Detailed Account

### Rabbit (Oryctolagus cuniculus)

There are several reports of uterine endometrial epithelial tumors in rabbits.[41] Greene[84] has summarized his outstanding pioneer work on these tumors, and a valuable illustrated summary account is given by Weisbroth.[207] Their value as animal models for the study of human endometrial adenocarcinomas has been discussed by Baba and von Haam.[13] The tumors have been reported in

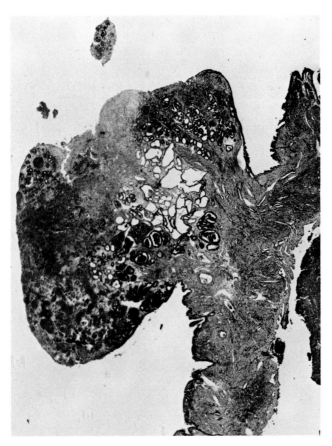

**39.7** Adenocarcinoma of the uterus of a rabbit, showing polypoid endometrial tumor with invasion of myometrium. ×25.

[Photograph kindly provided by the Imperial Cancer Research Fund, Tumor Reference Collection 145, Polson's case.]

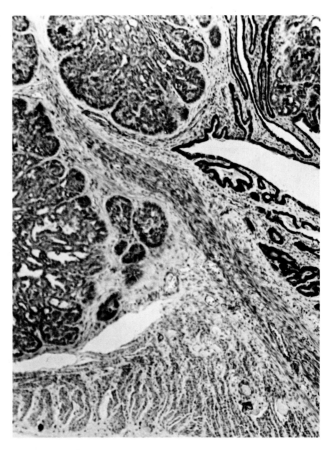

**39.8** Adenocarcinoma of the uterus of a rabbit, showing morphology and myometrial invasion. ×108.

[Photograph kindly provided by the Imperial Cancer Research Fund, Tumor Reference Collection 145, Polson's case.]

Europe (Figures 39.7 and 39.8) as well as America, but most of them have been in three rabbit colonies: those studied by Greene and his colleagues in the Rockefeller Institute rabbitry following a move from New York to Princeton; those in the Henry Phipps Institute colony of the University of Pennsylvania, studied by Ingalls et al.[102]; and those in the Dutch rabbits in the Ohio State University colony, studied by Baba and von Haam themselves. As summarized by Baba and von Haam,[13] Greene and his colleagues found 142 adenomas and adenocarcinomas of the endometrium in a colony of 849 rabbits observed for 9 years. Ingalls et al. found 353 uterine tumors in 1,735 rabbits in a colony observed for 30 years. Baba and von Haam[13] found 16 adenocarcinomas (two *in situ*) in the uteruses of 83 out of 117 Dutch rabbits studied for 30 months.

The salient feature of uterine endometrial tumors in rabbits is that they tend to occur with increasing frequency in older animals.[102] Burrows[25] found that 50% of his noninbred rabbits surviving to the age of 2½ years had endometrial tumors, and such tumors may occur in animals 7 or even 9 years of age.

In the Rockefeller Institute colony, following its move from New York to Princeton,[80] Greene and Saxton[87] found 83 rabbits with uterine endometrial tumors—adenomas and adenocarcinomas were not readily distinguishable—in a colony of about 500 breeding does in a 4-year period. Eight of the rabbits died of metastases. The tumors were discovered, either by palpation or at autopsy, at an average age of 45 months. They were confined to breeding females but disturbances of reproductive function, such as reduction of litter size, fertility, and maternal care, preceded the detection and probably the initiation of the tumors. The early lesions were either single or often multiple and might affect one or both horns. They appeared as pedunculated growths, or small thickenings of the endometrium, usually on the endometrial folds adjacent to the mesometrial insertion. The tumors might remain small or reach the size of a hen's egg in 6 months. Metastases were somewhat delayed, considering the early signs of vascular invasion, but they were found in all cases in which the known duration of the tumor was over 1 year. A possibly significant observation was, that prior to metastasis, the primary tumor might undergo obvious regressive changes.

Greene,[83] noting the similar breed susceptibility to uterine tumors and to what he called "toxaemia of pregnancy,"[80,81] suggested that liver damage associated with this condition (of unknown origin) might lead to failure by that organ to inactivate estrogen, and this could result in tumor formation. Indeed, histologic alterations that Greene noted in the thyroid, adrenal, pituitary, and mammary glands of the affected rabbits were similar to those seen in estrogen-treated mice, and Meissner et al.[140] have indeed described the experimental production of uterine adenocarcinoma in rabbits by the administration of estrogen. Greene[82] and Greene and Saxton[87] were able to transplant the uterine tumors auto-, homo-, and heterologously (guinea pig eye), but such tumors were not accompanied by the pituitary, thyroid, or adrenal changes accompanying the primary tumors, suggesting that these changes were an indication of the cause rather than the result of the tumors. Greene and Newton[85] showed that the morphologic and transplantation characteristics of the tumors progressed from nonmalignant to malignant states.

Ingalls et al.[102] surveyed the incidence of uterine tumors found by autopsy, abdominal palpation, or laparotomy in the Henry Phipps rabbit colony. They concluded that the dominant factor in the development of uterine carcinomas in these rabbits was age: Of animals dead at 2½ to 3 years of age 8.8% had tumors, whereas of those over 4 years old at death about 60% had tumors. Although there was no significant difference in tumor incidence in breeding and nonbreeding females, there was a difference in strains that had been bred for increased susceptibility to tuberculosis. The possibility that a virus might be involved is mentioned.

Further interesting reports on rabbit endometrial adenocarcinoma, this time in the Ohio State University rabbit colony, are given by Baba and von Haam.[13] Here again, the incidence of tumors increased with age. No association was noted with cystic or glandular endometrial hyperplasia and, in fact, administration of estrogen to aged Dutch

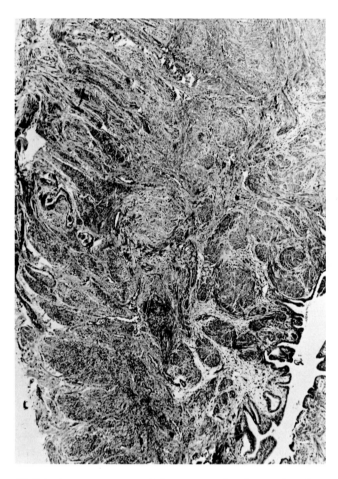

**39.9** Leiomyosarcoma of the uterus of a domestic rabbit. ×32.

rabbits reduced the incidence of endometrial carcinomas from 17 to 3%. The tumors were shown by electron microscopy[12] to contain cells resembling those of the deeper endometrial glands.

In commenting on the value of the rabbit endometrial carcinoma as an animal model for the study of the human tumor, Baba and von Haam[13] mentioned that the three major rabbit colonies concerned were no longer maintained. However, they noted that rabbits of the Dutch breed, which they found to be susceptible to such tumors, are commercially available and that investigators could expect to find a number of uterine tumors developing within 1 to 2 years. It is of interest too that the endometrial carcinoma reported by Flatt[67] occurred in an adult multiparous New Zealand rabbit killed for meat purposes. Lombard's[126] three cases in France were in white Angora rabbits.

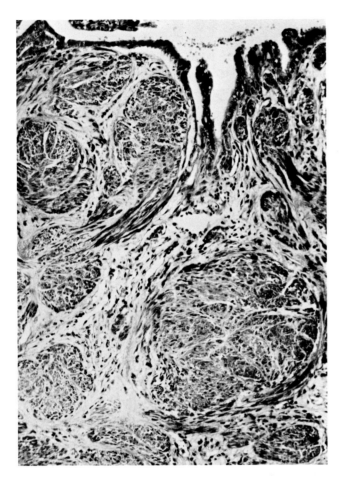

**39.10** Same tumor as Figure 39.9, showing multiple origin of the tumor in the myometrium. ×127.

Not all uterine tumors in rabbits are epithelial in nature. Greene and Strauss[88] showed that their uterine carcinomas might be accompanied by uterine myomas and myosarcomas, and Polson[163] and Baba and von Haam[13] also found myosarcomas. I too have seen a metastasizing uterine myosarcoma (Figures 39.9 and 39.10).

Greene, Newton, and Fisk[86] found three cases of squamous cell carcinomas of the columnar–squamous epithelial junction in the vagina of rabbits (all three animals also had uterine carcinomas).

## Spontaneous Tumors of the Ovary

Neoplasms of the ovary[161] have been mostly encountered in the cow, the bitch, and the domestic fowl and to a lesser extent in the mare and the cat. The few examples of ovarian tumors in species other than these five will be briefly referred to in domesticated animals (ewe, goat, sow, buffalo), laboratory animals (nonhuman primates, mouse, rat, guinea pig, hamster, gerbil, ferret), and wild animals. The abbreviation GCT will be used throughout for granulosa cell tumor(s). For an account of the comparative morphology of the mammalian ovary see Mossman and Duke.[146]

### Domesticated Animals with Infrequently Reported Tumors

#### Ewe

Neoplasms of the ovary of sheep are rarely recorded. Anderson and Sandison,[6] in their abattoir survey of tumors from 4.5 million sheep in Great Britain, found none and Brandly and Migaki,[21] in their United States abattoir material, found only one, a teratoma. The tumor described by Di Domizio[50] as an arrhenoblastoma could well be a Sertoliform GCT.

#### Goat

No reference to ovarian tumors in goats has been noted, apart from the "ovarioblastoma sarcomatodes" reported by Hilsdorf,[95] a tumor of uncertain nature.

#### Sow

According to Nelson et al.,[149] Dobberstein stated that of 188 recorded porcine neoplasms, 18 affected the ovary: 10 cystadenomas, five sarcomas, two teratomas, and one fibroma. They refer to other records of cavernous hemangioma and cystadenocarcinoma and report two hemangiomas (in 52,000 sows), one papillary cystadenoma, and one case of bilateral GCT. The report of hemangioma is interesting, for Maeda et al.[131] found two sows (multiparous Berkshire–Yorkshire cross) with ovarian hemangiomas, and Davis et al.[46] found one. In their abattoir survey in Great Britain, Anderson and Sandison[6] recorded two serous cystadenomas, one GCT, and one leiomyoma. Lombard and Havet[129] saw bilateral metastasizing tumors in a 5-year-old Large White sow. They illustrate the lesion, which they designate "seminoma," but this is in any case a difficult diagnosis to substantiate. The lesion reported as an arrhenoblastoma in a 3-year-old pig by Guarda[89] is more likely to be an abdominal testis in a hermaphrodite. The head-sized "fibromyxosarcoma" of the left ovary of a 9-month-old sow reported by

Schlegel[179] was apparently diagnosed from macroscopic appearance only.

### Buffalo

Polding and Lall[162] found teratomas containing hairs in the ovary of four buffaloes.

## Laboratory Animals

### Primates

A few previously reported ovarian tumors in subhuman primates are tabulated by Martin et al.[134] and by Kraemer and Vera Cruz.[116] Martin et al. themselves report a papillary serous cystadenoma, histologically of low-grade malignancy; a benign cystic teratoma (dermoid cyst); and a cavernous hemangioma. These three cases were found among approximately 75 animals subjected to one or more laparotomies or to autopsy over a 5-year period. The teratoma was in a female that had received 50 rads or less of x irradiation, which was thought to be unlikely to have been of etiologic significance in relation to the dermoid cyst.

The ultrastructural features of a surface papilloma and serous cystadenofibroma, respectively, found incidentally in the ovaries of a 2-year-old rhesus monkey were described by Amin et al.[4] The papilloma contained many ciliated epithelial cells, similar to those of the oviduct epithelium; nonciliated cells resembled the celomic covering of the ovary. In the cystadenoma, there were secretory, ciliated, and "peg" cells, like those of the oviduct epithelium.

Seibold and Wolf,[182] in their series of 1,065 nonhuman primate necropsies, found one case of ovarian adenocarcinoma in an adult *Cebus albifrons;* there was extensive peritoneal implantation. Crews et al.[44] found a mixed lesion, dermoid cyst and papillary cystadenoma, in a young adult rhesus monkey. Weston[209] referred in passing to a thecoma. Rewell[166] found bilateral GCT (and uterine fibromas) in a senile squirrel monkey (*Saimiri sciurea*) that had been in the Lister Institute in London for at least 20 years.

### Mouse

A range of tumor types occurs sporadically in the ovary of the mouse.[98,175] In a period of about 15 years, in the Chester Beatty stock mice, 18 ovarian tumors were found[28] in about 3,000 female mice: 13 GCT, two adenocarcinomas, one cystadenoma, one teratoma, and one

fibrosarcoma. Some have been found to be transplantable, as with the GCT in a CBA mouse demonstrated by Strong, Gardner, and Hill.[189] Whiteley and Horton[210] found a transplantable hormonally inactive GCT in a 2¼-year-old CBA mouse. A spontaneous carcinoma in the ovary of a C3H mouse was transplantable intraperitoneally[63] into C3HeB/FeJ mice and proved useful in demonstrating the role of lymphatic obstruction in the diaphragm in the development of ascites. C3HeB mice have been studied particularly by Deringer,[48] who found mainly GCT and tubular adenomas but also luteomas and a mixed tumor. She quotes Woolley and Little as having seen a 33% incidence of ovarian tumors in strain CE mice, and Dickie as noting a 52% incidence of ovarian tumors in CE backcross mice. Bielschowsky and d'Ath[20] have drawn attention to what may be a suitable animal model of GCT, which occurred with some frequency in three of four inbred strains of mice they studied in New Zealand. In mice surviving the age of the first tumor-bearing animals, routine histologic sectioning of ovaries revealed GCT in NZC (virgins, 15 out of 45; breeders, eight out of 39), NZO (virgins, nine out of 199; breeders, seven out of 45) and NZY (virgins, three out of 82; breeders, four out of 183), but no such tumors were found in NZB mice, whose median age was lower than for the other three strains. The two chief tumor patterns were cylindromatous and follicular. Eight tumors were classified as diffuse (malignant). The tumors in NZO mice appeared to be nonfunctional, and although hyperplasia of the endometrium was present in each NZC tumor-bearing mouse, cystic endometrial hyperplasia was present in practically all animals in the second year of life. Gardner, Strong, and Smith[73] in a 695-day-old Strong E1 mouse, found a chromophobe adenoma of the pituitary, bilateral ovarian GCT, endometrial hyperplasia, and multiple, small mammary adenocarcinomas. Hooker and Strong[97] found a GCT in a hermaphrodite.

Jackson and Brues[105] found an embryoma in a C3H mouse which could be transplanted subcutaneously, intrasplenically, and intrahepatically. Fawcett[58] found bilateral ovarian teratomas in a Swiss mouse, and Fekete and Ferrigno[62] reported a transplantable teratoma in a C3H mouse (see also Thiery[197]). Scheuler and Ediger[178] found a unilateral teratoma of the ovary in a C3H/HeN clinically normal breeder mouse. They illustrate a focus of epithelial cells suggestive of malignant transformation.

Particular interest attaches to the reports[147,148,174] of the development of tubular adenomas of the ovary of mice of the (C57B1/6J × C3H/HeJ) $F_1$ $W^x/W^x$ genotype. Such mice have few oocytes at birth, and their number

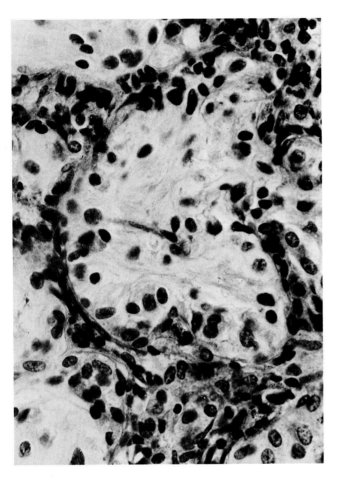

**39.11** Rat ovary, showing Sertoliform tubules. Note "grooved" nuclei. ×813.

[From a section kindly provided by D. S. G. Patton.]

progressively diminishes. The mice develop a 95% incidence of bilateral complex tubular adenomas of the ovary by 5 months of age.

It is of interest that Andervont and Dunn[8] found nine GCT among 98 tumors they saw in 225 wild house mice—seven in 99 autopsied breeding females, and two in 72 autopsied virgin females.

### Rat

Ovarian neoplasms occur with some frequency in certain strains of rat. Katherine Snell[184] reported the incidence of tumors of various kinds in six inbred strains of rat in the laboratory of Pathology of the National Cancer Institute in Bethesda, Maryland (ACI, BUF, F344, OM, M520 and WN). GCT were found in about one-third of

the OM rats over 18 months of age, only a few being found in ACI, M520 and, WN rats and none in BUF and F344. A few OM rats had simple papillary cystadenocarcinoma of the ovary. (Snell[184] refers to other reports of ovarian GCT, fibromas, adenomas, sarcomas, and carcinomas in rats.)

Lingeman[123] stated that the Registry of Experimental Cancers of the National Cancer Institute lists epithelial neoplasms in the ovaries of five untreated rats; of these, four were papillary cystadenocarcinomas, two of which contained foci of chondrosarcoma and had given widespread implantation peritoneal metastases.

In a period of 15 years, three ovarian tumors (excluding lymphomas) were found[28] in about 300 female Chester Beatty stock rats, including one GCT, one cystadenoma, and one anaplastic sarcoma. One of the most interesting recorded ovarian neoplasms in rats[175] is the spontaneous hormone-producing metastasizing GCT discovered by Iglesias et al.[100,101] in a female A × C rat. Symeonidis and Mori-Chavez[193] found a transplantable papillary adenocarcinoma in a 9-month-old OM rat. Other authors have recorded GCT in rats, e.g., Kullander,[118] who saw two GCT, along with one mixed androblastoma and GCT and one androblastoma; Thompson and Hunt[198] (see for review of literature) found one GCT and one papillary adenocarcinoma. In view of the peculiar Sertoliform structure of some bovine and canine GCT, the report by Engle[57] of the occurrence of testislike tubules and tubular adenomas in the ovaries of aged Wistar rats (Figures 39.11, 39.12, and 39.13), shrew,[211] and other mammals[211] (for references see Weir[206]) are relevant, even if they have no human counterpart.[123]

### Guinea pig

Although GCT may occur,[107] the most interesting ovarian tumor of the guinea pig is the teratoma.[92,205] Willis[212] described a teratoma measuring 2 cm in a 9-week-old guinea pig and another 8.5 by 5.5 by 3 cm in a 1-year-old animal. Vink[203] also saw two ovarian teratomas in approximately 13,000 autopsies. Mosinger[145] refers to ovarian embryoma and to chorioepitheliomatous-like nodules described by Loeb;[125] they have limited duration, being destroyed and replaced by fibrous tissue.

### Hamster

Handler[91] referred in his review of spontaneous lesions in Syrian hamsters to reports by Fortner[69] and by Kirkman of thecoma of the ovary.

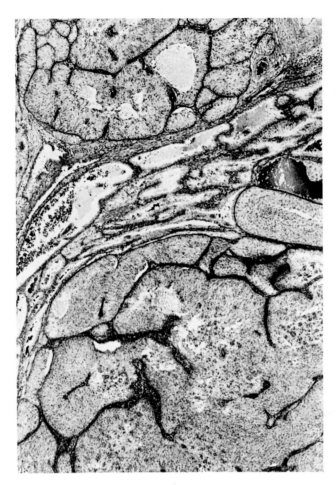

**39.12** Tubular adenoma of the ovary of a rat. ×32. [From a section kindly provided by D. S. G. Patton.]

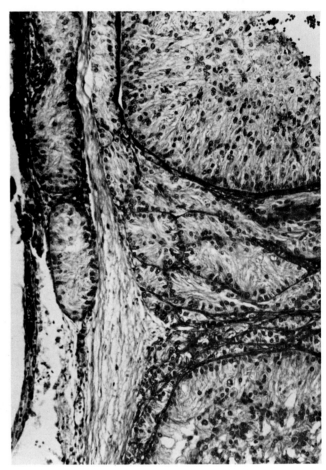

**39.13** Same tumor as Figure 39.12, showing Sertoliform morphology. ×127.

[From a section kindly provided by D. S. G. Patton.]

*Gerbil*

Rowe et al.[173] found GCT in three of their gerbils; one also had a uterine leiomyosarcoma and showed bilateral symmetrical alopecia. The other two also had endometrial adenocarcinoma. One *M. shawi* had a bilateral granulosa-theca cell ovarian tumor as well as a unilateral ovarian papillary cystadenoma. Two gerbils, *M. shawi* and *G. hesperinus,* had leiomyomas of the ovary.

*Ferret*

In a stock of 123 female ferrets over 1 year of age, Chesterman and Pomerance[30] found bilateral ovarian thecomas; the endometrium had marked glandular hyperplasia. They also reported bilateral ovarian fibromyomas in

a ferret, aged 5 years 4 months, which had been on a hepatotoxic diet for a short time about 4 years before its death.

*Mastomys*

Lingeman[123] reported a personal communication from Katherine Snell that malignant granulosa cell tumors are frequent in mastomys [*Praomys (Mastomys) natalensis*].

## Wild Animals, Animals in Zoos, and Birds

Goyon[78] found a metastasizing teratoma in the left ovary of a hare, and Lombard[128] diagnosed a peculiar lesion in the ovary of a young hare as a seminoma. Flux[68] records some interesting findings in the ovaries of female

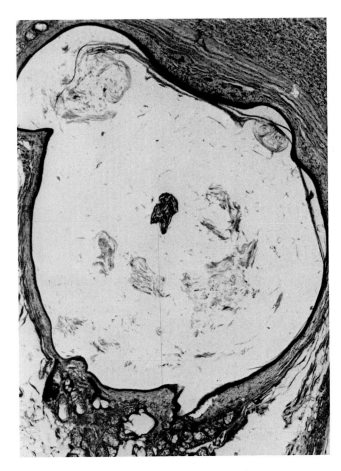

**39.14** Teratoma of the ovary of a hare, showing cyst containing keratin and lined by stratified squamous epithelium, and groups of sebaceous glands (bottom). ×32.

[From material kindly provided by Dr. J. E. Flux.]

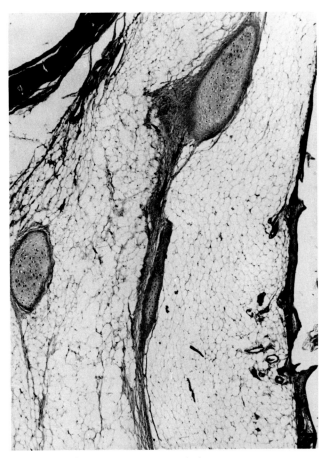

**39.15** Teratoma of the ovary of a hare (same tumor as Figure 39.14), showing the wall of the epidermoid cyst (right), adipose tissue, and cartilage plates. ×32.

[From material kindly provided by Dr. J. E. Flux.]

hares (*Lepus europaeus*) shot in New Zealand. Of 1,176 ovaries from adult hares, 48 contained cysts. Most of these cysts were filled with clear or opaque jelly or white, yellow, or green greasy sebaceous material. Six hares had true teratomas (Figures 39.14 through 39.18), containing teeth or bone (in four ovaries) and hair (in three). All six also had cysts filled with sebaceous material. The original liberation of hares in New Zealand in 1851 numbered only a few animals; the possibility is mentioned that a genetic susceptibility might be involved or an effect resulting from DDT spraying.

Dehner et al.[47] recorded a teratoma and a dysgerminoma in a ground squirrel, and Nowotny[155] a GCT in a squirrel (*Sciuris vulgaris* L.). In a chamois goat showing signs of masculinization, Dewalque[49] found a GCT of the left ovary which was surgically removed. Signs of

masculinization reappeared 7 months later. The endometrium was hyperplastic and a histologic metastasis was found in one uterine cornu. In a koala (*Phascolarctos cinereus*), an Australian marsupial, Finckh and Bolliger[65] found a serous cystadenoma which appeared to arise from ovarian surface epithelium. Weir[206] found bilateral ovarian papillomata in an agouti (a dasyproctid member of the rodent suborder Hystricomorpha). The left ovary of a southern elephant seal (*Mirounga leonina*) contained what was taken to be a malignant GCT.[136] In their small series of tumors from whales, Rewell and Willis[167] reported a mucinous cystadenoma of the ovary, about 12 inches across, in a blue whale (*Balaenoptera musculus*) and presumed GCT in a pregnant blue whale and in two fin whales (*B. physalus*), one of which was pregnant.

Halloran[90] lists references to the following tumors in

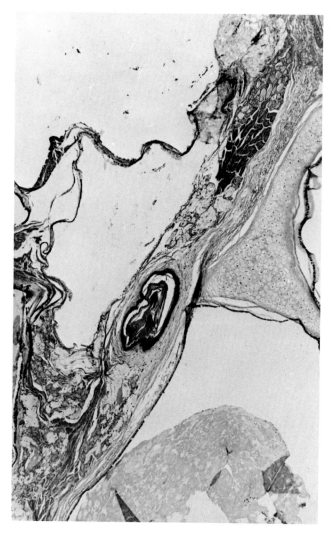

**39.16** Teratoma of the ovary of a hare, showing cysts, salivary gland tissue (lower left), keratin (center), and cartilage (right). ×32.

[From material kindly provided by Dr. J. E. Flux.]

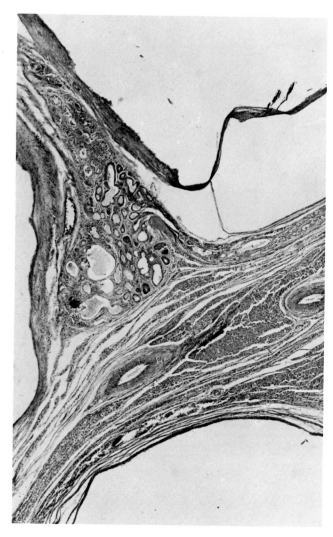

**39.17** Teratoma of the ovary of a hare, showing cysts and glandular tissue. ×32.

[From material kindly provided by Dr. J. E. Flux.]

birds: ovarian tumor in a pelican; fibrosarcoma of ovary in Charadriiformes; sarcoma of ovary in Psittaciformes; and carcinoma and adenoma of ovary in Passeriformes.

Streett,[188] dissecting an adult female *Rana pipiens,* found a teratoma in the posterior pole of the right ovary, measuring 12 by 8 by 8 mm. Representative tissues of all three germ layers were present, including cartilage, bone, bone marrow, gut, and skin. A tumor in a *R. pipiens,* which was illustrated by Abrams,[2] was considered to be an ovarian cystadenocarcinoma (the kidney, the common site of tumors in this species, was free of tumor).

According to Balls and Clothier,[15] Plehn in 1906 reported an ovarian carcinoma in *R. esculenta.*

In a survey of 44 avian and 11 mammalian cases of neoplasia in free-living wild mammals and birds in Britain, Jennings[108] found the following ovarian tumors: dysgerminoma in a mallard (*Anas platyrhynchos*), GCT also in a mallard, cystadenoma in a black-headed gull (*Larus ridibundus*), and arrhenoblastoma in a pheasant (*Phasianus colchicus*).

West[208] found a gonadal tumor, with an epithelial tubular structure, in the position of the ovary in a chukar

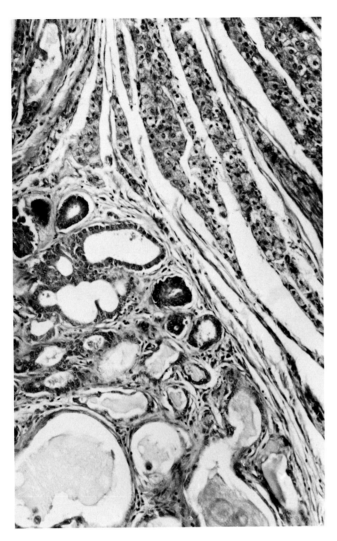

**39.18** Teratoma of the ovary of a hare (same tumor as Figure 39.17), showing glandular tissue. ×127.

[From material kindly provided by Dr. J. E. Flux.]

partridge from a game farm. The bird was typically female in appearance. The oviduct was present but incompletely mature.

## Insect Study

Mention may be made of ovarian lesions in *Drosophila melanogaster*. King[114] states that "Two recessive mutations that render homozygous females sterile, because ovarian tumors are produced, have been extensively studied. The tumorous chambers seen in the ovaries of homozygotes contain cells resembling germarial cystocytes. Such chambers grow slowly by mitosis and some eventually contain as many as 10,000 cells. Cell division continues when tumors are transplanted to new hosts. However, the tumors do not invade nonovarian tissues and apparently have little effect on the viability of the donor or the host" (p. 325).

## Domesticated Animals with Most Frequently Reported Tumors

Most information about ovarian tumors in domesticated animals refers to the mare, cow, cat, fowl, and bitch, and these species are now considered.

### Mare

Ovarian tumors are not very rare in horses. Most of them are GCT (Figures 39.19 through 39.22) and most occur in young adults (see Finocchio and Johnson[66] for colored photographs, Mastronardi and Potena[135] for photomicrographs, and Burghardt[24] for ovarian cysts). It is uncertain what type of tumor affected the ovary of a foal reported by Christl[32] as no histologic support for the macroscopic diagnosis of cystadenoma was given. Among the reports of GCT are those by Howard,[99] Wurster,[215] and Leopold[120] (who also reviewed previous cases of GCT in mares and cows) and by Fessler and Brobst.[64] In the Fessler and Brobst case, the neoplastic left ovary, weighing over 1 kg, was removed from a 9-year-old mare that was infertile, showed anestrus, and developed malelike appearance and behavior. These signs regressed after the operation.

Teratomas appear to affect the ovary less frequently than the testis in the horse. Abraham[1] found the right ovary of a 10-year-old Quarter Horse mare to contain a tumor, approximately 12 by 10 by 10 cm, with cystic spaces lined by stratified squamous epithelium and filled with hair. The mare was multiparous but had failed to breed at three successive cycles. A teratoma in the right ovary of a 6-year-old Percheron mare[70] was located as a projection in a unilocular pseudomucinous cystadenoma.

The key papers on ovarian tumors in mares are those by Norris et al.[153] and by Cordes.[36] It is of interest that in the series of GCT in six horses and one Peruvian wild ass reported by the former, none were known to cause endocrine abnormality. The affected animals ranged from 4 to 31 years of age, and the tumors weighed 1 to 8 kg. They were yellowish, usually multicystic masses, with focal ne-

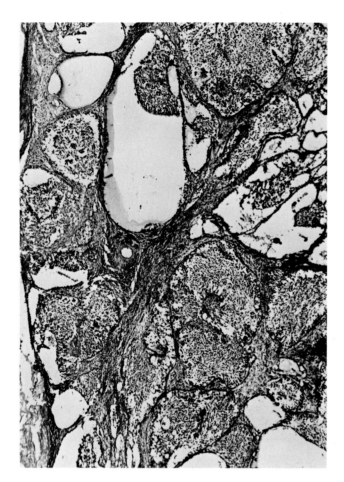

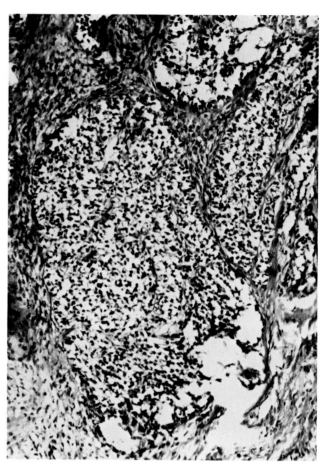

**39.19** GCT of the ovary of a 13-year-old mare, showing tubular pattern. ×32.

**39.20** Same tumor as Figure 39.19. ×127.

crosis and hemorrhage. Histologically, the tumors showed prominent microcysts and tubules, with cells at the periphery of the cysts in double-paired layers, with basally oriented nuclei. These cells resembled the cells at the periphery of developing follicles and the Sertoli cells of the testis. A prominent stroma of spindle cells, possibly representing a thecal component, was present in all the tumors.

Cordes[36] studied nine cases of GCT in mares. All the tumors were removed surgically, eight from racehorse mares and one from a pony mare. The age (known for five mares) ranged from 7 to 16 years. Three tumors affected the right ovary and four the left. They were in mares with prolonged estrus (in one case there were clinical signs of masculinization) and were detected by rectal palpation. One grew from approximately 7 to 23 cm in 10 months. Eight were multicystic, the largest cyst being 3 cm in diameter. The tumor cells were chiefly in a follicular

pattern, and theca cells were prominent. Some of these mares had given birth to foals prior to the neoplasms being detected, and they usually returned to normal after an operation.

### Cow

The incidence of ovarian neoplasms in cows has been variously estimated. Although Davis, Leeper, and Shelton,[46] in their Denver abattoir survey, reported that five of the six ovarian tumors they recorded in cows were carcinomas (the sixth was diagnosed as a hypernephroma), the commonest form seems to be the GCT, of which Lagerlöf and Boyd[119] found 13 examples (including three carcinomas and three GCT) in the examination of 6,286 bovine genital tracts. Brandly and Migaki[21] found 13 GCT in 1,000 chronologically received tumors from veter-

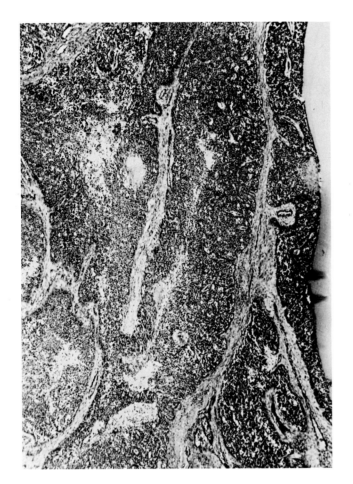

**39.21** GCT of the ovary of a 30-year-old pony mare, showing solid pattern. ×32.

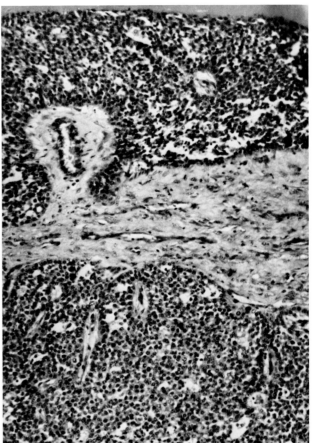

**39.22** Same tumor as Figure 39.21. ×127.

inary meat inspectors. Anderson et al.,[7] in their British abattoir survey, found 302 tumors of all kinds from about 1.3 million cattle. There were 11 ovarian tumors—seven carcinomas (three serous cystadenocarcinomas, three mucinous adenocarcinomas,[191] one adenoacanthoma), two GCT, one combined teratoma–GCT, and one fibroma. In his abattoir survey in Holland, Misdorp[142] found 21 ovarian tumors in cows—10 GCT, seven carcinomas, and four thecomas.

The ages of affected cattle with GCT range from newborn[110] to 21 years[217] but the majority of tumors have been reported in animals of about 2 or 3 years of age. An interesting endocrinologic analysis was made by Short et al.[183] of a case of GCT in a Friesian heifer. At the age of 2 years 2 months, the heifer was noted to be showing enlargement of the udder. She developed certain behavior changes—mounting other animals in the herd but being seldom mounted herself. Her voice became more bull-like, and she pawed and horned the ground as a bull would. The tail head was found to be raised and the neck somewhat thickened, but the sacroiliac ligaments were not relaxed. When the heifer was sexually excited, an erectile structure, a fold of dorsal vaginal mucosa, appeared at the vulva. Lactation was noted. Rectal examination showed an enlarged left ovary and the heifer was destroyed. The ovarian tumor, approximately 15 cm in diameter, contained many cystic spaces and was a typical GCT, without luteinized cells. The endometrium showed signs of excessive progestational stimulation. The fluid in the tumor cysts contained progesterone, 20β-hydroxypregn-4-en-3-one, possibly a trace of 17α-hydroxyprogesterone, and estradiol-17β. It is suggested that the estradiol-17β came from normal theca interna cells, which surrounded some of the cystic follicles, or was being produced by neoplastic granulosa cells. The further comment is made that although the progesterone:estradiol-17β ratio was only 6:1, the tumor appeared to have caused normal mammary development and lactation.

Bovine GCT may be large tumors; the largest of Baumann's[17] five cases was 48 cm long and weighed 17.10 kg.

An important paper on bovine ovarian tumors is that by Norris, Taylor, and Garner,[154] who have studied the cases on file at the AFIP Registry of Veterinary Pathology. They classify the tumors as in the following tabulation.

| Tumor type | No. |
| --- | --- |
| Ovarian stromal tumors | 26 |
|   Granulosa type | 13 |
|   Sertoli type | 13 |
| Teratoma | 3 |
| Carcinoma, primary site uncertain | 3 |
| Sarcoma, unclassified | 2 |
| Mixed mesodermal tumor | 1 |
| Metastatic lymphoma | 1 |
| Unclassified | 3 |
| Total | 39 |

The main contribution these authors have made is to draw attention to the possible clinical significance of distinguishing typical GCT, composed of cells resembling typical granulosa cells, from what they term "Sertoli-type" ovarian stromal tumors; the former are much more prone to produce metastases.

Typical GCT occurred in animals 1.2 to 9 years of age (median 5 years). Two of the cows had nymphomania, and a third would not accept service by the bull. The tumors showed a consistent microfollicular pattern. Nine of the 13 cases of GCT of granulosa type showed metastases. The metastases occurred mainly to the broad ligament, to pelvic and abdominal peritoneal surfaces, and along the lumbar aorta. Two tumors had metastasized to the spleen and one to the lung. It was possible to examine the endometrium histologically in two cows: one showed a metastatic GCT and the other a pyometra.

The Sertoliform GCT arose in cows 4 to 12 years of age (median 8 years). Eleven were incidental findings. One cow had persistent pyometra, and one had shown an abdominal mass and estrus lasting 1 year. Hemorrhage and necrosis occurred in only three tumors, in contrast with the granulosa cell type. The tubular Sertolian arrangement was accompanied, in five tumors, by small areas of typical

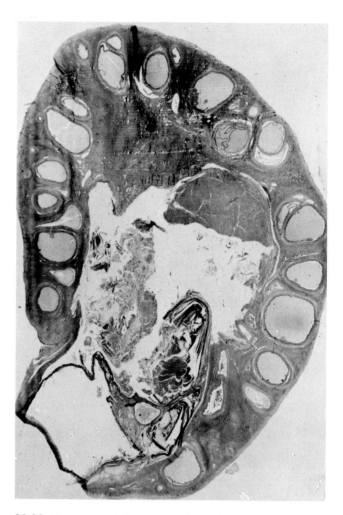

**39.23** Teratoma of the ovary of a Zebu cow, showing keratin-filled cysts in depth of ovary (center lower left), and a superficial zone of Graafian follicles. Entire ovary.

[From material kindly provided by Dr. Silney A. Costa.]

granulosa cell pattern. The authors describe and picture cells resembling Sertoli cells in the peripheral layer of early bovine granulosa follicles, prior to and during antrum formation.

Through the kindness of Dr. S. A. Costa, of Goiania, Brazil, I have been able to examine cases of peculiar cystic ovarian lesions he found in 13 of 4,008 slaughtered Zebu (Brahman) cattle. The lesions take the form of "dermoid cysts" and appear to be truly teratomatous in nature. The cysts, which vary in number from one to five in the sections I have studied, are rarely more than 2 cm across and are usually much smaller. They usually lie deep in the ovary (Figures 39.23 through 39.25) but in one instance

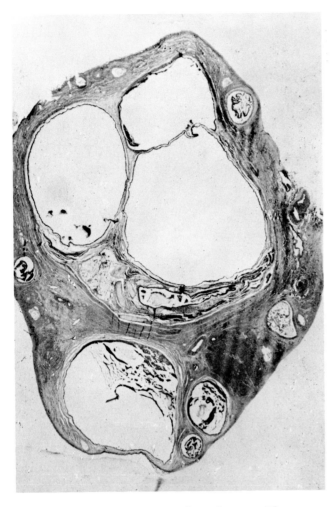

**39.24** Teratoma of the ovary of a Zebu cow. There are four large deep cysts and, in the center, a focus of glands and cartilage. Entire ovary.

[From material kindly provided by Dr. Silney A. Costa.]

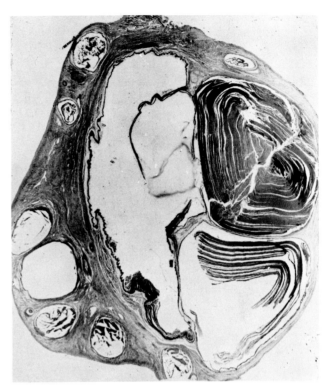

**39.25** Teratoma of the ovary of a Zebu cow. There are four deep cysts, two filled with keratin.

[From material kindly provided by Dr. Silney A. Costa.]

the cyst is located no deeper than the Graafian follicles present. The cysts contain fluid or a colloid material or are more or less filled with keratinized squamous or dense keratin material. The typical cyst lining is stratified epithelium, from two to six or more cells thick, with keratin varying from scanty to massive. In one ovary there are patches of pseudostratified ciliated epithelium intermingled with the stratified epithelium, and in places goblet cells lie superficially on the stratified epithelium (Figure 39.26). In three ovaries the stratified epithelium is pigmented by melanin. In four ovaries from three cows, cartilage plates are present in the cyst walls (Figure 39.27). Three ovaries contain salivary glandlike tissue (Figure

39.27); one shows simple tubular glands; one has hair follicles, sebaceous, and sweat glands; one has sweat glands; and one has hair follicles. In two ovaries one and two neuronlike cells, respectively, are present.

The presence of hair follicles and of pigment allows these cysts to be called "dermoid" instead of "epidermoid." The presence of melanin and of salivary glandlike tissue and of possible neurons supports the diagnosis of teratoma. The histogenesis of the cysts is obscure. There is a hint in the superficial location of the cyst in one tumor, in the presence of keratin, squamous and possible squamous epithelium in the lining of a Graafian follicle in another, and the apparent continuity with structures resembling egg cords (or SES) in two sites in the wall of one cyst in a third (Figure 39.28) that they may originate from the Graafian follicles. Study of further such tumors may help decide the question.

### Cat

Few ovarian tumors have been reported in cats, but in assessing the significance of this, the common practice of

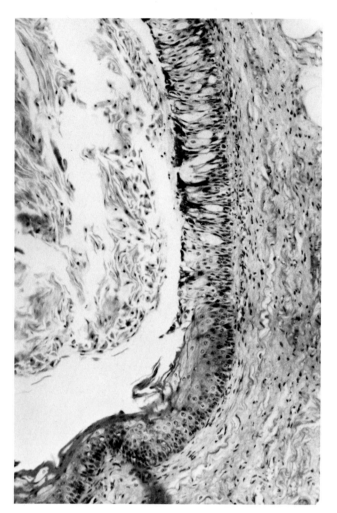

**39.26** Teratoma of the ovary of a Zebu cow. Part of the wall of the cyst, showing stratified squamous and goblet cell epithelium merging. Same tumor as Figure 39.23. ×127.

[From material kindly provided by Dr. Silney A. Costa.]

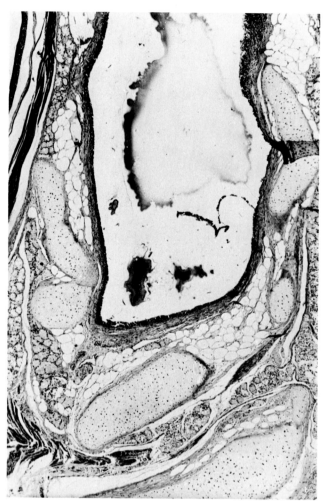

**39.27** Teratoma of the ovary of a Zebu cow, showing cartilage plates in the wall of the cyst and salivary gland tissue. ×32.

[From material kindly provided by Dr. Silney A. Costa.]

spaying female cats must be remembered. The key paper is by Norris, Garner, and Taylor.[151] Other reports include those by Federer[59]; by Di Domizio[50] of GCT with lung and liver metastases; by Fukushima and Konishi[71] of GCT in a 3-year-old cat, with omental and kidney metastases; by Baker[14] of GCT; by Sbernardori and Nava[176] of dysgerminoma of the right ovary of a 7-year-old plurigravid cat; and by Dehner et al.[47] of two dysgerminomas (one metastasizing), one teratoma, and one mixed dysgerminoma and teratoma.

Norris et al.[151] studied 12 ovarian neoplasms from 10 cats and one lion (a leiomyoma). Six GCT were found in

five cats of mixed domestic breed. All five cats showed signs of estrogen stimulation; two had prolonged estrus, thinning of coat, and loss of hair and three had endometrial hyperplasia. One cat also had a mammary carcinoma. Four tumors were unilateral. Three were 6 cm or more across, and three extended beyond the ovary. They were usually yellow cystic tumors with areas of hemorrhage, and were composed of small cells with hyperchromatic nuclei devoid of nuclear grooves; the arrangement was typically microfollicular and Call–Exner bodies were present in two tumors. Four neoplasms showed a minor theca cell component. A virilized 9-year-old cat had a lipid cell tumor;

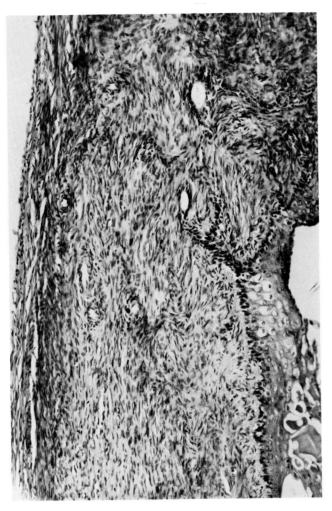

**39.28** Teratoma of a Zebu ovary, showing apparent continuity of the epithelium lining the cyst and a subsurface epithelial structure. Surface of ovary on left. ×127.

[From material kindly provided by Dr. Silney A. Costa.]

the endometrium was cystic. There were two ovarian teratomas: The smaller had well-differentiated tissues, including cartilage, glial tissues, glandular epithelium, hair, keratin, and squamous epithelium, whereas the larger tumor had cells resembling those of human dysgerminoma in some areas. One tumor was a metastasizing adenocarcinoma, and the tenth cat, a 10-year-old Persian, showed metastasis of an endometrial carcinoma to both ovaries and elsewhere.

Norris et al.[151] comment on the absence of a Sertoliform pattern in feline GCT. They also state that ovarian capsular epithelium of the cat, unlike that of dog and man, shows little tendency toward hyperplasia with inclusion cyst formation.

### Fowl

An extensive account of ovarian tumors in domestic fowl is given by Campbell,[26,27] which may be summarized as follows: Although formerly frequent, advanced adenocarcinoma of the hen's ovary is now comparatively rare because of the policy of discarding hens after their first or second year of reproductive life. Ovarian tumors of the granulosa–thecal–luteal type are not uncommon in broiler chickens aged 10 weeks or less. Ovarian adenocarcinomas are common in older hens and may have a high incidence in hens reared in a constant environment. The tumor, which may appear as a serous or mucous-secreting cystadenocarcinoma, may have an extensive plain muscle component and tends to form serosal implantation metastases.

Other tumors described by Campbell[26] include theca cell tumors, Brenner tumor, lipoid cell tumor, and hemangioma. Surgical removal of the left or functional ovary almost invariably leads to the development of an ovotestis in the right rudimentary ovary, from which tumors may later develop, including Sertoli cell adenoma or arrhenoblastoma and dysgerminoma.

Sparse reports of ovarian and oviductal tumors in Anatidae are reviewed by Rigdon,[169] who has observed a teratoma of the ovary region in two of 17 hermaphrodites which resulted from mating male Muscovy and female white Pekin ducks.

### Dog

TYPES OF CANINE OVARIAN TUMORS. The types of canine ovarian tumors encountered in four collections are summarized in Table 39.1.

The source of material in these reports varied. Dow's[55] material was collected at the Glasgow Veterinary School from histologically examined ovaries of 400 unselected autopsied bitches. Of these, 93 had a total of 127 tumors of various types in one or more sites. Twenty-five bitches (18 of which were nulliparous, ranging from 5 to 15 years of age) had primary ovarian tumors. One in 16 of the bitches therefore had an ovarian tumor. From the nature of the survey, no strong correlation with genital system symptoms would be expected. Dow's findings may be compared with those of Zaldivar.[219] In a series of Beagles in the Argonne colonies, he found spontaneous malignant tumors in 540 dogs: of these two were of ovarian origin

**Table 39.1**  Canine ovarian tumors in four collections

| Tumor type | Investigator | | | | |
|---|---|---|---|---|---|
| | Dow[a] | Cotchin[b] | Ishmael[c] | Norris et al.[d] and Dehner et al.[e] | Total |
| Group 1 | 11 | 25 | 14 | 33 | 83 |
| Papilloma and | | | | | |
| Adenoma | 10 | 20 | 8 | 20 | |
| Carcinoma | 1 | 5 | 6 | 3 | |
| Intermediate | | | | 10 | |
| Group 2 | 13 | 30 | 5 | 26 | 74 |
| GCT | 13 | 15 | 5 | 15 | |
| Sertoliform | | 15 | | 6 | |
| Nonspecific | | | | 5 | |
| Group 3 | 0 | 9 | 3 | 13 | 25 |
| Seminoma | | 8 | 1 | 11 | |
| Teratoma | | 1 | 2 | 2 | |
| Group 4 | | | | | 14 |
| Miscellaneous | | | | | |
| and undiagnosed | 1 | 5 | 2 | 6 | |
| Total | 25 | 69 | 24 | 78 | 196 |

[a] Located in Glasgow; see Ref. 55.

[b] Located in London; see Ref. 39.

[c] Located in Liverpool; see Ref. 103.

[d] Located at Armed Forces Institute of Pathology, Washington, D.C.; see Ref. 152.

[e] Located at Armed Forces Institute of Pathology, Washington, D.C.; see Ref. 47.

(in 264 females), adenocarcinoma and granulosa cell carcinoma in 10-year-old animals. My own material[39] was a mixture of specimens obtained during surgery and at autopsy and therefore exaggerates the number of tumors coming from bitches with genital system symptoms. Ishmael's[103] series included material examined in the pathology laboratory of the Liverpool Veterinary School. The material reported by Norris et al.[152] (the dysgerminomas and teratomas being reported in detail by Dehner et al.[47]) was comprised of the 78 primary canine ovarian tumors on file in the Armed Forces Institute of Pathology Registry of Animal Pathology, again a selective collection.

The separation of tumors into different groups in Table 39.1 reflects my concept of their histogenesis. In Group 1 are included tumors of epithelial type, which develop from surface epithelium (papillomas) or from its extensions below the surface (adenomas). Some tumors are predominantly if not entirely papillomatous and there is often some adenomatous component. In Group 2 are included what Norris et al.[152] call gonadal stromal tumors but which are more commonly called by veterinary pathologists, especially in the United Kingdom, granulosa cell tumors. Group 3 includes tumors that morphologically resemble canine testicular seminomas, and teratomas. These are classed by Dehner et al.[47] as germ cell tumors. Group 4 includes miscellaneous tumors and tumors of uncertain type.

The following account of the various types of canine ovarian tumors is mainly based on my own report.[39]

*Group 1: Papilloma and adenoma.* The ages of 19 of my 20 bitches ranged from 4 to 15 years, with an average of 9.4 years (in Dow's series, the 10 animals were 6 to 13 years of age). In six of 13 bitches for which information was available, both ovaries were affected; the other tumors involved the left (five) or right (two) ovary alone. Six of the 20 bitches showed signs of hormonal disturbance ("pyometra" in four; cystic endometrial hyperplasia in two). Six other bitches showed signs of an enlarged abdominal mass.

Not unexpectedly, the tumors in Dow's autopsy series

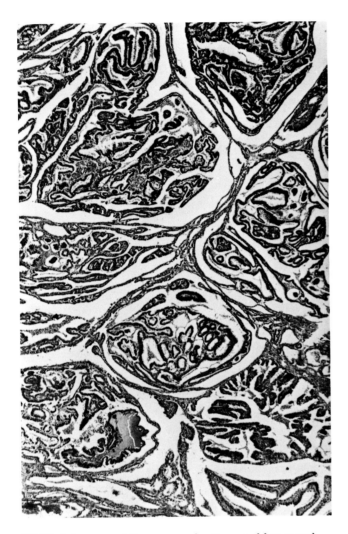

**39.29** Adenoma of the ovary of a 9-year-old mongrel bitch. ×32.

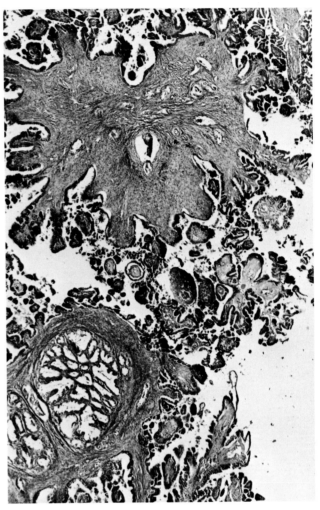

**39.30** Papilloma and adenoma of the ovary of a 14-year-old crossbred bitch. ×32.

were generally small, ranging from 0.8 to 1.5 cm in diameter, although four of them (including two pseudomucinous cystadenomas) were from 6 to 10 cm diameter. In my series, one adenoma was a histologic finding in a bitch with a vaginal fibroma, the other tumors ranging from 1.5 to 17 cm in length (average 7 cm).

The macroscopic appearance of the tumors varied according to whether surface papilloma formation was present (five out of 20 dogs) or not. In at least six dogs, and probably in more, the tumor lay in an intact but distended bursa. The surface (apart from papillomatous tumors, which had a fine coxcomblike surface) was smooth but nodular or bosselated, and variably gray, yellowish, or hemorrhagic. The cut surface was partly solid and partly

cystic. The solid areas were mostly grayish or pinkish white, and usually finely lobulated or papillary. The cysts varied in size and contained clear watery fluid, sometimes brown or bloodstained.

The histologic structure was predominantly that of a papillary cystadenoma (Figure 39.29) (cf. Fedrigo[60]) with a variable superficial papillary component (Figure 39.30). The cyst contents were hyaline. They were lined by one or sometimes more layers of cuboidal or columnar cells with basal or central nuclei; the papillae were supported by a connective tissue stroma, varying from fine to edematous, hyaline (Figure 39.31), and hemorrhagic. In five tumors, the prominent superficial papillomatous growths appeared in places to be continuous with the surface epithelium. In

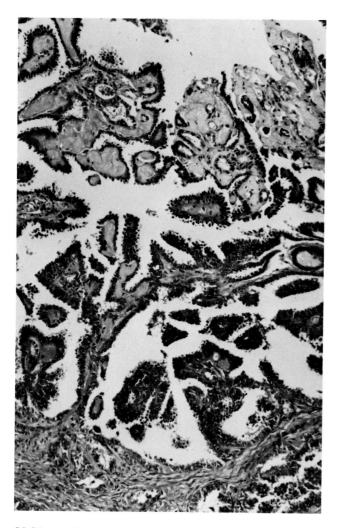

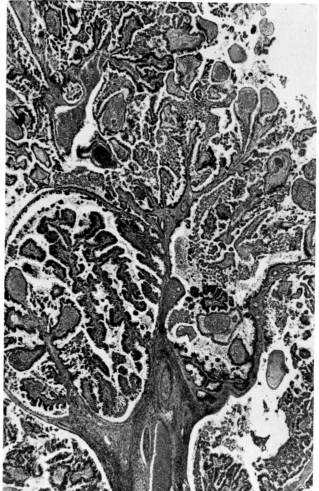

**39.31** Papilloma of the ovary of a 10-year-old Alsatian bitch, showing hyalin cores of papillae. ×32.

**39.32** Papillary carcinoma of the ovary of a 15-year-old bitch. ×32.

six tumors, there were areas resembling GCT. Two of Dow's 10 cases were of the pseudomucinous type.

A sufficiently detailed histochemical analysis has not been made of my series, but the main if not the only type appears to be the serous cystadenoma.

*Carcinoma.* Carcinomas are less common in the bitch ovary than are adenomas. Dow has found one metastasizing carcinoma as against 10 adenomas; in my series, there have been five against 20; in the Norris et al.[152] series, even if the 10 intermediate tumors are classed as carcinomas, they form in total 13 against 20 adenomas. In my series, the average age of the affected dogs (9.5 years) was the same as for the bitches with ovarian adenoma (9.4

years). Four of the five bitches showed signs of hormonal disturbance ("pyometra," two; cystic endometrial hyperplasia, one; vaginal hemorrhage, one).

The tumors, from 3 to 10 cm long, showed a smooth, nodular surface, covering a homogenous or finely cystic whitish or yellowish tissue. They were histologically predominantly intracystic papillary tumors (Figure 39.32) with areas of compressed tubular structures and of anaplasia (Figure 39.33). Mitoses were present and lymphatic permeation was noted. Two of the affected bitches showed metastases; in both, the greater omentum was involved and fluid was present in excess in the abdomen. One of the bitches also showed, in addition to implantation metastases, lymph nodal and pulmonary deposits.

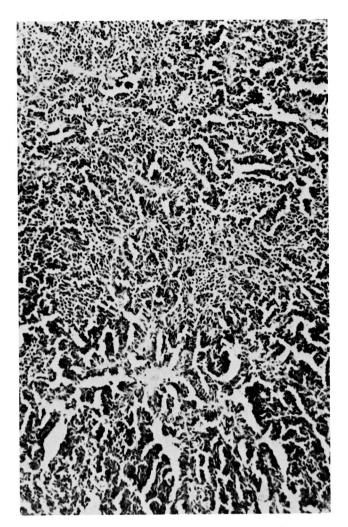

**39.33** Anaplastic adenocarcinoma of the ovary of a 7-year-old hound-type bitch. ×127.

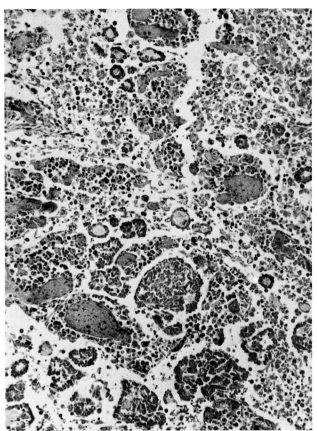

**39.34** Nodal deposit, with globular epithelial formations, from an ovarian adenocarcinoma in a 9-year-old Terrier bitch. ×127.

Fedrigo and Rugiati[61] described the use of Papanicolaou smears to identify tumor cells in the ascitic fluid of a 4-year-old Alsatian bitch with a recurrent papillary adenocarcinoma of the right ovary. Chromosomal abnormalities (number and morphology) were demonstrated in the tumor cells. Addis and Baglioni[3] found apparent neoplastic elements in rosettes in May–Grunwald–Giemsa smears of recurrent ascitic fluid in a 6-year-old Alsatian bitch with an ovarian papillary "cystoadenoma" (sic). I have seen similar globes of tumor cells in a nodal deposit of a bitch with adenocarcinoma (Figure 39.34), and Case and Small[29] also illustrate such structures in the right iliac node of a 1½-year-old English Setter bitch with adenocarcinoma of the right ovary. In view of the presence of

eosinophils in some ovarian tumors, it is of interest that Cork[37] found an elevated blood eosinophilia (up to 4.5%) in an 8-year-old mixed-breed bitch with a cystadenocarcinoma of the right ovary.

*Group 2: Granulosa cell tumor (GCT).* In their account of gonadal stromal tumors, Norris et al.[152] have separated (not solely on morphologic grounds) from the classic GCT a group that they call Sertoli pattern tumors (for which I use the adjective, Sertoliform) and another of nonspecific type. It appears possible that these are in fact all of granulosa cell or related origin. In my own series of 30 tumors classified as GCT, at least 15 had some more or less pronounced histologic resemblance to the canine Sertoli cell tumor (SCT).

The age range in my series of dogs with GCT (including Sertoliform tumors) was 1½ to 12 years, average 8.0. The Norris et al.[152] "granulosa" (non-Sertoliform) tumors

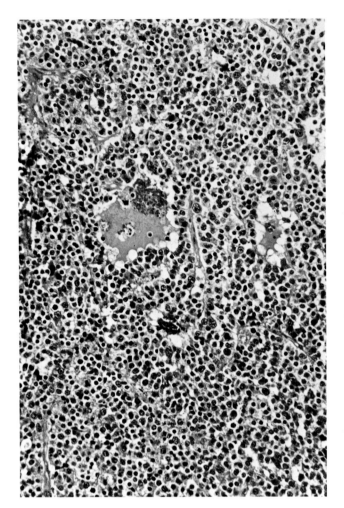

**39.35** GCT of the ovary of an 11-year-old Labrador bitch, showing sheets of cells, follicular fluid pools, and fine connective tissue septa. ×127.

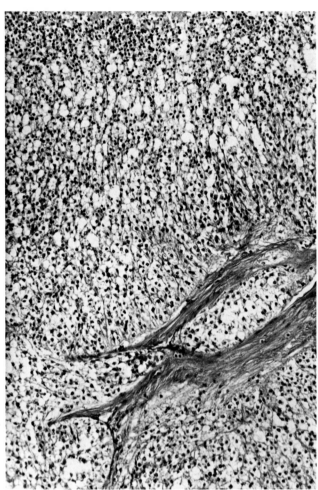

**39.36** GCT of the ovary of a 5-year-old Alsatian bitch, showing coarse and fine stromal septa. ×127.

were found in bitches 4 to 12 years of age (median 7 years) but their six Sertoliform tumors were in dogs from 10 to 15 years of age (median 12 years). In both series, there is an indication of a tendency for Bulldogs and Boxers to be affected more often than other breeds. Twenty-three of my series of 30 bitches showed signs of hormonal disturbance: 19 had "pyometra," three had cystic endometrial hyperplasia, and one, which had shown no true estrus for 2 years, had remained persistently attractive to male dogs.

The tumors were large, varying from 5 to 11 cm in length with an average of 7 cm. They lay wholly or partly in a distended ovarian bursa. The surface was smooth, nodular, or bossellated and the color was gray or blue (from hemorrhage). The cut surface was partly solid and partly cystic, commonly with areas of hemorrhage.

Two of my cases showed metastases, one mainly as retroperitoneal extension and the other to nodes and viscera, including lung. Three of the Norris et al[152] "granulosa" tumors had local extension or metastasis; none of their six Sertoliform tumors had metastasized or extended locally beyond the ovary.

Histologically, the usual pattern was of connective tissue septa of varying thickness, usually broad, dividing the tumor cells into large groups (Figures 39.35 and 39.36) that were in turn divided into smaller groups by finer connective tissue septa. The tumor cells resembled either mature granulosa cells with rounded nuclei and eosinophilic or sometimes foamy, clear, or granular cytoplasm, sometimes arranged in a tubular pattern (Figure 39.37) or were more elongated and arranged in a Sertoli-

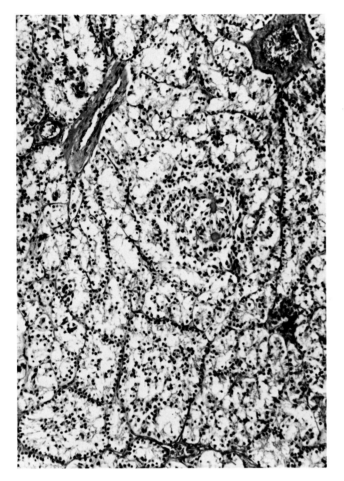

**39.37** GCT of the ovary of a 10-year-old Retriever bitch, showing clear cells in tubular arrangement. ×127.

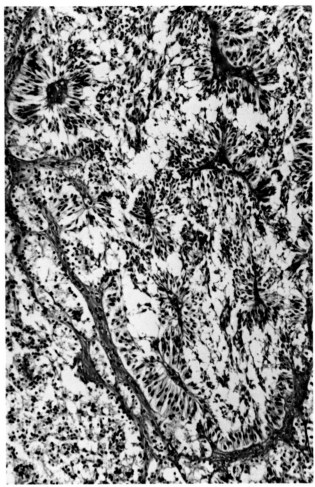

**39.38** Sertoliform GCT of the ovary of a bitch (same tumor as Figure 39.37). ×127.

form fashion (Figures 39.38 and 39.39). Mitoses were sometimes readily found in the typical granulosa cell regions but were not readily found in Sertoliform areas. The presence of Call–Exner-like bodies (Figure 39.40) was not constant, but they were found in three of my cases. In some tumors, a marked perithelial arrangement was seen. Pools or lakes of hyaline material resembling follicular fluid were typically present.

There was a clear suggestion, in a least five tumors, that the granulosa-cell pattern was mixing (Figure 39.41) smoothly with a papillary or tubular adenoma, and a transition between typical granulosa cell and typical Sertoliform areas was also noted in some tumors.

*Group 3: Seminoma (dysgerminoma).* I have reported eight cases of a seminoma-like tumor of the canine ovary, Dehner et al.[47] have found 11, and Andrews et al.[9] have

found two. The tumors bear a close histologic resemblance to canine testicular seminoma (see Buergelt[23]). It would be desirable that electron microscopic examinations be made to see whether this similarity exists at the ultrastructural level.

The bitches in my series ranged from 6 to 16 years of age, with an average of 10.5, which is a little above the average age for other forms of ovarian tumors. In this group, the dogs studied by Dehner et al.[47] were, on the average, considerably older (13 years) than their dogs[152] with GCT (7 years) and a little older than their dogs with Sertoliform tumors. Indeed Taylor and Dorn[194] saw a dysgerminoma in a 20-year-old Alsatian bitch. Signs of hormonal disturbance accompanied at least four of my eight seminomas—"pyometra" in two bitches, cystic en-

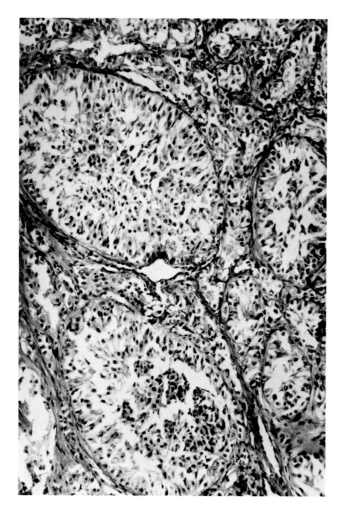

**39.39** Sertoliform GCT of the ovary of an 8-year-old Spaniel bitch. ×127.

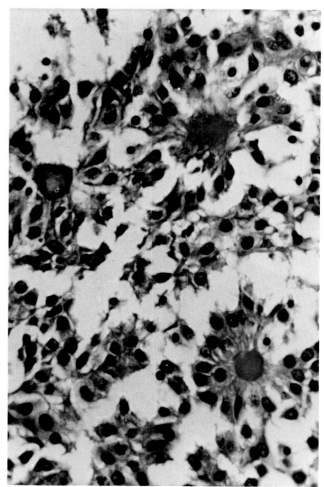

**39.40** Call–Exner-like bodies in GCT of the ovary of a bitch (same tumor as Figure 39.37). ×813.

dometrial hyperplasia in one, and vaginal hemorrhage in one. Four of the Dehner et al.[47] dogs had a sanguinopurulent vaginal discharge.

The tumors had smooth, variably bulging surfaces and were of a gray, reddish, or bluish color with hemorrhagic areas. The typical tumor tissue was grayish white and rather soft, closely resembling the typical canine testicular seminoma.

On histologic examination, the tumors also resembled testicular seminomas. The tumor cells, which were large, rounded, angular, or polygonal, had large central chromatic nuclei, with a prominent nucleolus. The cytoplasm was eosinophilic or amphophilic or sometimes clear. Exceptionally large single nuclei and bi-, tri-, or multinucleated cells, as in canine testicular seminomas, were also

seen. The resemblance was made still closer by the presence of clear spaces, often containing shrunken or ghost cells (Figure 39.42), and of spotty necrosis with karyorrhexis. Mitoses were numerous and sometimes abnormal.

The amount of stroma was usually small, and lymphocytic foci or granulomatous reactions were either not seen or were rare.[47]

*Teratomas.* Typical mature teratomas occur occasionally in dogs. Dehner et al.[47] described two instances, in dogs 2 and 8 years of age: One dog, which was emaciated, had an abdominal mass which on x ray films showed focal calcification; the other, with similar radiologic findings, also showed intermittent episodes of intestinal obstruction.

Storm[186] described a hair-bearing dermoid cyst 15 cm

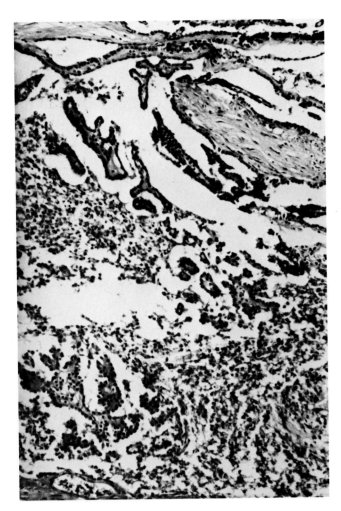

**39.41** GCT of the ovary of an 8-year-old Spaniel bitch, showing diffuse granulosa cell areas and epithelial conformations. ×127.

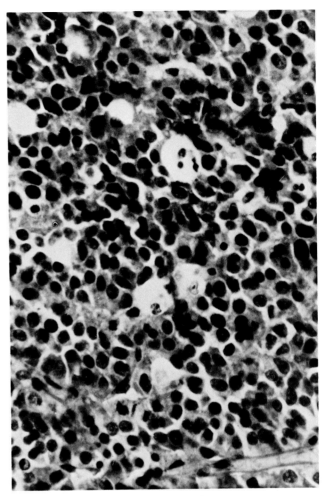

**39.42** Seminoma of the ovary of a 10-year-old Scottish terrier bitch, showing multinucleate cells and clear spaces containing shrunken cells. ×813.

long in the left ovary of an 8-year-old Collie bitch and Riser et al.[170] described an almost equally large hair-bearing teratoma in the left ovary of a 5-year-old Pointer bitch. Benesch[19] found a teratoma filled with hair and weighing 2½ kg in the ovary of an 18-month-old Alsatian bitch. Röcken[171] has published a good account of a teratoma of the ovary in a 6-year-old Boxer bitch.

GENERAL DISCUSSION OF CANINE OVARIAN TUMORS. There are three matters of interest raised by this study of canine ovarian tumors: first, their endocrine activity; second, their histogenesis; and third, their etiology. There is no doubt that some of these ovarian tumors are responsible for the hormonal effects that accompany their presence,

for these signs regress when the tumors are surgically removed. However, a closer analysis of the particular hormones involved would be worthwhile. The indications are that the development of tumors of most kinds may lead to such conditions as pyometra, cystic endometrial hyperplasia, or vaginal hemorrhage. That such signs should accompany GCT is not surprising. Their relation to epithelial tumors and to dysgerminomas, however, is not easily understood, particularly in the latter instance.

As regards the histogenesis of canine ovarian tumors, it is not possible to give a completely satisfactory explanation. As a working hypothesis, however, I suggest the following: Papillomas, adenomas, papillary carcinomas, and adenocarcinomas are derived from the surface epithe-

853

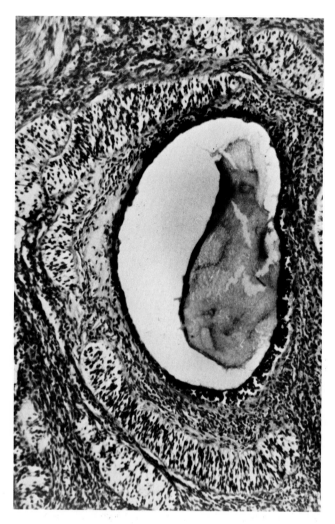

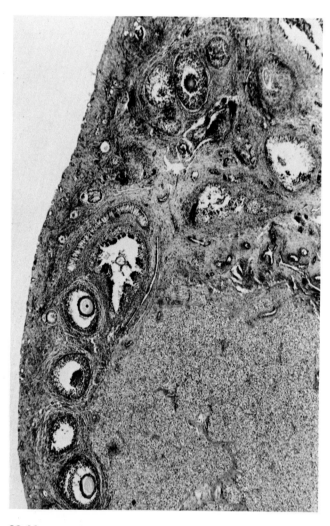

**39.43** Sertoliform tubule around an atretic follicle in the ovary of a 12-year-old Miniature Poodle bitch. ×127.

**39.44** Part of the ovary of a 1-year-old Fox Terrier bitch, showing a Sertoliform tubule (left center) arching over a Graafian follicle, with a folded granulosa layer. ×32.

lium of the ovary, or from the epithelial cords that lie under the surface epithelium, or from both epithelia. In some of my tumors, the papillomatous conformation predominates, and it may be that these tumors are derived mainly if not wholly from the surface epithelium. However, some tumors appear to consist entirely of subsurface epithelial structures, and these may not contain a pure surface epithelial component.

There is some evidence for this view. Hormone-dependent epithelial proliferations were induced in bitches by the administration of diethylstilbestrol[104]; these lesions were reasonably interpretable as metastasizing carcinomas, some at least being hormone dependent. O'Shea and Jabara[158] produced histologic and histochemical evidence

that these proliferative lesions were derived mainly from the surface epithelium but that some came from subsurface epithelial structures (SES), in which O'Shea had demonstrated characteristic sialic acid-containing mucinous secretion and intracytoplasmic droplets. O'Shea and Jabara[159] also found proliferative lesions of the serosa of the uterus in ovariectomized females treated with stilbestrol.

O'Shea and Jabara[158] were of the opinion that SES did not give rise to follicles, including oocytes, in adult dogs, but the coincident occurrence in canine ovarian tumors of tissues of undoubted granulosa cell origin and of epithelial tumor tissue with apparently smooth transitions between

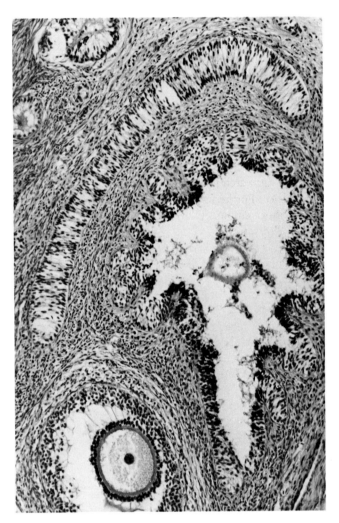

**39.45** High power view of the Sertoliform tubule and follicle shown in Figure 39.44, showing apparent outward budding of granulosa layer. ×127.

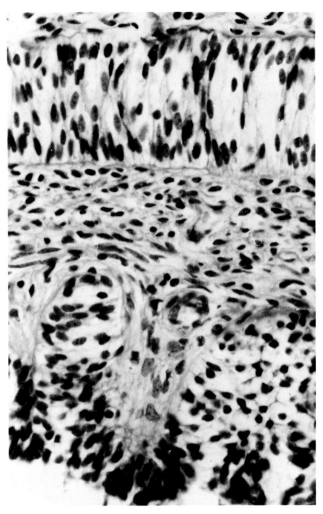

**39.46** Closer view of the granulosa "buddings" and Sertoliform tubule seen in Figures 39.44 and 39.45. ×813.

the two, and also of tubular adenomas resembling the Sertoliform GCT in continuity with papillomas, suggests that the question needs further study.

As regards GCT, there is no difficulty in accepting that typical tumors are derived from the follicular granulosa layer. The problem is to account for the Sertoliform tumors, which are such a feature in the bitch but which are also found in man, cow, rat, and possibly other species. Anyone accustomed to examining the ovaries of the bitch will be struck by the common presence of small tubular structures, closely resembling immature testis tubules, lined by Sertoli-like cells (Figures 39.43 through 39.46). Sometimes these tubules are short and sometimes, in any

one section, they are long. They occur at any level of the ovarian cortex and also in the hilus near the rete ovarii. Some are demonstrably continuous with the granulosa cell layer of follicles in which ova may still be present.

These tubules may partly be explained as being the "granulosa cell islands" described by Stott.[187] He states that germinal epithelial cells in the bitch are known to be mitotically active throughout life. Balls or cords of cells migrate into the cortex of the ovary from the germinal epithelium and, seemingly, invaginating germinal epithelial cells become granulosa cells. In the ovaries of 115 bitches, including 83 Beagles, ranging from 1 day to 19 years of age, he noted that at the appearance of the first signs of estrus (5 to 7 months of age) SES were seen in the outer cortex. Some SES had a lumen. Beneath the tunica albuginea, groups of SES containing primordial follicles were seen, as well as primary and growing follicles. Because many more follicles began to grow than reached maturity, follicular remnants were commonly seen in the ovary at this stage. From the fibroblast invasion of large atretic follicles, isolated granulosa cell islands (GCI) were formed. These GCI were more numerous in older bitches, especially those over 5 years old. It was noted that early or advanced proliferation of granulosa cells in GCI occurred, and this could result in GCT formation. Stott[187] illustrates tubular adenomas, one resembling a Sertoliform tumor, which could have arisen from SES.

Although this study by Stott[187] is very satisfying in providing an explanation of some Sertoliform GCT, the appearance in some canine ovaries of long Sertoli-like tubules is not easily directly attributable to follicular atresia; however, these tubules could of course have developed from GCI by a process of hyperplastic proliferation. Further study may show that at least some of these "testis cords" are, as defined by Mossman and Duke,[146] medullary cords persisting in adult ovaries and have the appearance of an immature seminiferous tubule or of the seminiferous tubule of a cryptorchid testis, but their possible relationship to "epithelial cords" derived from germinal epithelium (see Barton[16]) also needs study.

Dehner et al.[47] classify seminomas and teratomas as germ cell tumors and present a diagrammatic representation of their possible origin and relationship. They figure the dysgerminoma as a derivative of the primordial germ cells, which remains at the primordial level of histogenetic differentiation. A slight degree of differentiation produces an embryonal carcinoma (so far unidentified in dogs). From this stage trophoblastic differentiation would result in choriocarcinoma formation (so far unidentified in dogs), whereas somatic differentiation would result in the formation of a teratocarcinoma (so far unidentified in dogs), which, when completely differentiated, would form a mature teratoma (the typical form in the dog).

## Summary

Inquiring readers will be able to pursue their studies further by reading in detail the various papers referred to in the references, but a few points are worth reemphasis.

In the case of uterine tumors, a striking fact is that carcinoma of the cervix is rarely reported in animals, and this is in accord with the concept that the cause of this cancer in women is likely to be specifically related to the human tumor. Again, if the apparent relative lack of bovine endometrial carcinomas in countries other than the United States can be confirmed, this may lead to a search for possible etiologic factors peculiar to that country. The apparent common occurrence of endometrial adenocarcinoma in some stocks of aged rabbits provides a useful model for study, for example, to search for a possible causal virus, or an unusual hormonal stimulus, or some specific genetic background. Similarly, the high incidence of carcinoma of the oviduct in domestic hens ought to facilitate the search for a possible causal agent or hormonal disturbance. Furthermore, the extreme rarity of endometrial choriocarcinoma in animals may be a significant "negative" observation.

In the case of ovarian tumors, there is an apparent important incidence of GCT in animals, and the not rare occurrence of this type of tumor in the bitch, for example, may permit more detailed hormonal and other functional analyses that may well have human relevance. Again, the occurrence of ovarian teratomas in Zebu cattle and in hares, for example, may facilitate histogenetic and other investigations of comparative medical importance.

If this chapter has alerted the medical oncologist to possible lines of inquiry in animals, it has served its purpose.

# REFERENCES

1. Abraham, R. Equine ovarian teratoma. A case report. *Iowa State Univ. Vet.* 30:42, 1968.

2. Abrams, G. C. Diseases in an amphibian colony, in Mizell, M., ed.: *Biology of Amphibian Tumors.* New York, Springer-Verlag, 1965, p. 419.

3. Addis, M., and Baglioni, T. Sur un cas de cysto-adenoma papillaire de l'ovaire chez la chienne. *Proceedings of the 16th International Veterinary Congress* 11:271, 1959.

4. Amin, H. K., Ferenczy, A., and Richart, R. M. The ultrastructural features of a surface papilloma and serous cystadenofibroma respectively found incidentally in the ovaries of a two-year-old rhesus monkey. *J. Comp. Pathol.* 84:161, 1974.

5. Anderson, A. C. Carcinoma of the uterus in a Beagle. *J. Amer. Vet. Med. Assoc.* 143:500, 1963.

6. Anderson, L. J. and Sandison, A. T. Tumours of the female genitalia in cattle, sheep, and pigs found in a British abattoir survey. *J. Comp. Pathol.* 79:53, 1969.

7. Anderson, L. J., Sandison, A. T., and Jarrett, W. F. H. A British abattoir survey of tumours in cattle, sheep and pigs. *Vet. Rec.* 84:547, 1969.

8. Andervont, H. B., and Dunn, T. B. Occurrence of tumors in wild house mice. *J. Natl. Cancer Inst.* 28:1153, 1962.

9. Andrews, E. J., Stookey, J. L., Holland, D. R., and Slaughter, J. J. A histopathological study of canine and feline ovarian dysgerminomas. *Can. J. Comp. Med.* 38:85, 1974.

10. Appleby, E. C. Proceedings of the "Centennial Symposium on Science and Research" of the Philadelphia Zoological Society, November 1974 (in press).

11. Arbeiter, K. Der Scheidentumor bei der Hündin und seine operative Behandlung. *Wien. Tierärztl. Mschr. 48*:750, 1961.

12. Baba, N., and von Haam, E. Ultramicroscopic changes in the endometrial cells of spontaneous adenocarcinoma of rabbits. *J. Natl. Cancer Inst. 38*:657, 1967.

13. Baba, N., and von Haam, E. Spontaneous carcinoma in aged rabbits. *Am. J. Pathol. 68*:653, 1972.

14. Baker, E. Malignant granulosa cell tumor in a cat. *J. Am. Vet. Med. Assoc. 129*:322, 1956.

15. Balls, M. and Clothier, R. N. Spontaneous tumours in amphibia. *Oncology 29*:501, 1974.

16. Barton, E. P. The cyclic changes of epithelial cords in the dog ovary. *J. Morphol. 77*:317, 1945.

17. Baumann, R. Zur pathologischen Anatomie der Granulosazelltumoren des Eierstockes. *Wien. Tierärztl. Mschr. 22*:193, 1935.

18. Belter, I. F., Crawford, E. M., and Bates, H. R. Endometrial adenocarcinoma in a cat. *Pathol. Vet. 5*:429, 1968.

19. Benesch, F. 2½ Kg. schwere Dermoïdzyste des Ovariums bei einer Schäferhündin. *Wien. Tierärztl. Mschr. 22*:265, 1935.

20. Bielschowsky, M., and D'Ath, E. F. Spontaneous granulosa cell tumours in mice of strains NZC/B1, NZO/B1, NZY/B1 and NZO/B1. *Pathology 5*:303, 1973.

21. Brandly, P. J., and Migaki, G. Types of tumors found by Federal meat inspectors in an eight-year survey. *Ann. N.Y. Acad. Sci. 108*:872, 1963.

22. Brodey, R. S., and Roszel, J. F. Neoplasms of the canine uterus, vagina and vulva: A clinicopathologic survey of 90 cases. *J. Am. Vet. Med. Assoc. 151*:1294, 1967.

23. Buergelt, C. D. Dysgerminomas in two dogs. *J. Am. Vet. Med. Assoc. 153*:553, 1968.

24. Burghardt, R. Zur pathologischen Anatomie des Stuteneierstockes. *Arch. Wiss. Prakt. Tierheilk. 37*:455, 1911.

25. Burrows, H. Spontaneous uterine and mammary tumours in the rabbit. *J. Pathol. Bacteriol. 51*:385, 1940.

26. Campbell, J. G. Some unusual gonadal tumours of the fowl. *Br. J. Cancer 5*:69, 1951.

27. Campbell, J. G. *Tumours of the fowl*. London, Heinemann, 1969.

28. Carter, R. L. Pathology of ovarian neoplasms in rats and mice. *Eur. J. Cancer 3*:537, 1968.

29. Case, M. T., and Small, E. Ovarian carcinoma in a young dog. *Illinois Vet. 10*:6, 1967.

30. Chesterman, F. C., and Pomerance, A. Spontaneous neoplasms in ferrets and polecats. *J. Pathol. Bacteriol. 89*:529, 1965.

31. Chouroulinkov, I., Guillon, J. C., and Guérin, M. Endometrial sarcomas in mice: A survey of 130 cases. *J. Natl. Cancer Inst. 42*:593, 1969.

32. Christl, H. Ein angeborenes Ovarioblastom als Geburtshindernis. *Tierärztl. Umschau. 5*:276, 1950.

33. Christopher, J. Chorio-carcinoma in a bitch: A note. *Indian J. Anim. Sci. 42*:731, 1972.

34. Colombo, G. Neoformazione uterina nell cagna referibile ad adenomiosi. *Zootec. e Vet. 19*:240, 1964.

35. Corcoran, C. J., and Murphy, E. C. Rare bovine placental tumour—a case report. *Vet. Rec. 77*:1234, 1965.

36. Cordes, D. O. Equine granulosa tumours. *Vet. Rec. 85*:186, 1969.

37. Cork, L. Ovarian cystadenocarcinoma in a bitch. *Southwest Vet. 23*:243, 1970.

38. Cotchin, E. Tumours of farm animals: A survey of tumours examined at the Royal Veterinary College during 1950–1960. *Vet. Rec. 72*:816, 1960.

39. Cotchin, E. Canine ovarian neoplasms. *Res. Vet. Sci. 2*:133, 1961.

40. Cotchin, E. Problems of comparative oncology with special reference to the veterinary aspects. *Bull. WHO 26*:633, 1962.

41. Cotchin, E. Spontaneous uterine tumours in animals. *Br. J. Cancer 18*:209, 1964.

42. Cotchin, E. Some aetiological aspects of tumours in domesticated animals. *Ann. R. Coll. Surg. Engl. 38*:92, 1966.

43. Cotchin, E. Comparative oncology. Neoplasms of domesticated animals of interest to medical and veterinary pathologists. *Pesquisa Agropecuaria, Brasileira, Série Veterinaria, 7*(Suppl.):1, 1972.

44. Crews, L. M., Kerber, W. T., and Feinman, H. An ovarian tumor of dual nature in a rhesus monkey. *Pathol. Vet. 4*:157, 1967.

45. Dämmrich, K., and Lettow, E. Adenokarzinom der Cervix uteri bei einer Hündin. *Berl. Münch. tierärztl. Wschr. 61*:51, 1968.

46. Davis, C. L., Leeper, R. S., and Shelton, J. E. Neoplasms encountered in federally inspected establishments in Denver, Colorado. *J. Am. Vet. Med. Assoc. 83*:229, 1933.

47. Dehner, L. P., Norris, H. J., Garner, F. M., and Taylor, H. B. Comparative pathology of ovarian neoplasms. III. Germ cell tumours of canine, bovine, feline, rodent and human species. *J. Comp. Pathol. 80*:299, 1970.

48. Deringer, M. K. Occurrence of tumors, particularly of mammary tumors, in agent-free strain C3HeB mice. *J. Natl. Cancer Inst. 22*:995, 1959.

49. Dewalque, J. Tumeur ovarienne et masculinisation chez une chèvre chamoisée. *Ann. Méd. Vét. 107*:322, 1963.

50. Di Domizio, G. Tumori ormonoattivi degli animali domestici. *Atti Soc. Ital. Sci. Vet. 1*:220, 1947.

51. Digiacomo, R. F., and McCann, T. O. Gynecologic pathology in the *Macaca mulatta*. Part I. *Am. J. Obstet. Gynecol. 108*:538, 1970.

52. Dorn, C. R., Taylor, D. O. N., and Chaulk, L. E. The prevalence of spontaneous neoplasms in a defined canine population. *Am. J. Public Health 56*:254, 1966.

53. Dorn, C. R., Taylor, D. O. N., and Frye, F. L. Survey of animal neoplasms in Alameda and Contra Costa Counties, California. I. Methodology and description of cases. *J. Natl. Cancer Inst. 40*:295, 1968.

54. Dorn, C. R., Taylor, D. O. N., Schneider, R., Hibbard, H. H., and Klauber, M. R. Survey of animal neoplasms in Alameda and Contra Costa Counties. II. Cancer morbidity in dogs and cats from Alameda County. *J. Natl. Cancer Inst. 40*:307, 1968.

55. Dow, C. Ovarian abnormalities in the bitch. *J. Comp. Pathol. 70*:59, 1960.

56. Drieux, H., and Le Coustumier. Hémangiome du chorion foetal chez la vache. *Rec. Méd. Vét. 142*:293, 1966.

57. Engle, E. T. Tubular adenoma and testis-like tubules of the ovaries of aged rats. *Cancer Res. 6*:578, 1946.

58. Fawcett, D. W. Bilateral ovarian teratomas in a mouse. *Cancer Res. 10*:705, 1950.

59. Federer, Otto. Über hormonal wirksame Ovarialblastome bei Hund und Katze. Inaugural-Dissertation, Berne, 1958, p. 24.

60. Fedrigo, M. Cistoadenocarcinoma papillare sieroso un-

differenziato dell'ovaio in una cagna. Aspetto clinico e terapeutico. *Veterinaria, 17:22, 1968.*

61. Fedrigo, M., and Rugiati, S. Alterazioni cromasomiche in une carcinoma ovarico di cagna. *Atti Soc. Ital. Sci. Vet. 21:359, 1967.*

62. Fekete, E., and Ferrigno, M. A. Studies on a transplantable teratoma of the mouse. *Cancer Res. 12:438, 1952.*

63. Feldman, G. B., Knapp, R. C., Order, S. E., and Hellman, S. The role of lymphatic obstruction in the formation of ascites in a murine ovarian carcinoma. *Cancer Res. 32:1663, 1972.*

64. Fessler, J. F., and Brobst, D. F. Granulosa cell tumor. *Cornell Vet. 62:110, 1972.*

65. Finckh, E. S. and Bolliger, A. Serous cystadenomata of the ovary in the koala. *J. Pathol. Bacteriol. 85:526, 1963.*

66. Finocchio, E. J., and Johnson, J. H. Granulosa cell tumor in a mare. *Vet. Med. 64:322, 1969.*

67. Flatt, R. E. Pyometra and uterine adenocarcinoma in a rabbit. *Lab. Anim. Care 19:398, 1969.*

68. Flux, J. E. C. Incidence of ovarian tumors in hares in New Zealand. *J. Wildlife Mgmt. 29:622, 1965.*

69. Fortner, J. G. Spontaneous tumors including gastrointestinal neoplasms and malignant melanomas in the Syrian hamster. *Cancer 10:1153, 1957.*

70. Fujimoto, Y., and Sakai, T. On a case of an ovarian cystadenoma associated with a teratoma(dermoid) in horse. *Jap. J. Vet. Res. 3:8, 1955.*

71. Fukushima, A., and Konishi, Y. A case report of feline ovarian tumor. *J. Jap. Vet. Med. Assoc. 23:481, 1970.*

72. Gardner, W. U., and Pan. S. C. Malignant tumors of the uterus and vagina in untreated mice of the PM stock. *Cancer Res. 8:241, 1948.*

73. Gardner, W. U., Strong, L. C., and Smith, G. M. An observation of primary tumors of the pituitary, ovaries and mammary glands in a mouse. *Am. J. Cancer 26:541, 1936.*

74. Gellatly, J. B. M. Normal and pathological anatomy and histology of the genital tract of rats and mice, in Cotchin, E., and Roe, F. C. J., eds.: *Pathology of Laboratory Rats and Mice.* Oxford and Edinburgh, Blackwell Scientific Publications, 1967, p. 498.

75. Gilmore, C. E. Tumors of the female reproductive tract. *Calif. Vet. 19:12, 1965.*

76. Goodchild, W. M. Personal communication, 1975.

77. Goodchild, W. M., and Cooper, D. M. Oviduct adenocarcinoma in laying hens. *Vet. Rec. 82:389, 1968.*

78. Goyon, M. Tératome ovarien avec métastases pulmonaires chez la hase. *Rec. Méd. Vét. 135:651, 1959.*

79. Grant, D. L. Uterine tumour in a mare—leio-myoma. *Vet. Rec. 76:474, 1964.*

80. Greene, H. S. N. Toxaemia of pregnancy in the rabbit. I. Clinical manifestations and pathology. *J. Exp. Med. 65:809, 1937.*

81. Greene, H. S. N. Toxaemia of pregnancy in the rabbit. II. Etiological considerations with special reference to hereditary factors. *J. Exp. Med. 67:369, 1938.*

82. Greene, H. S. N. Uterine adenomata in the rabbit. II. Homologous transplantation experiments. *J. Exp. Med. 69:447, 1939.*

83. Greene, H. S. N. Uterine adenomata in the rabbit. III. Susceptibility as a function of constitutional factors. *J. Exp. Med. 73:273, 1941.*

84. Greene, H. S. N. Diseases of the rabbit, in Ribelin, W. E. and McCoy, J. R., eds.: *The Pathology of Laboratory Animals.* Springfield, Charles C Thomas, 330, 1965.

85. Greene, H. S. N. and Newton, B. L. Evolution of cancer of the uterine fundus in the rabbit. *Cancer 1:82, 1948.*

86. Greene, H. S. N., Newton, B. L., and Fisk, A. A. Carcinoma of the vaginal wall in the rabbit. *Cancer Res. 7:502, 1947.*

87. Greene, H. S. N., and Saxton, J. A., Jr. Uterine adenomata in the rabbit. I. Clinical history, pathology and preliminary transplantation experiments. *J. Exp. Med. 67:691, 1938.*

88. Greene, H. S. N., and Strauss, J. S. Multiple primary tumors in the rabbit. *Cancer 2:673, 1949.*

89. Guarda, F. Contributo allo studio dei tumori ovarici. L'arrenoblastoma nella varietà di adenoma tubulare nel suino. *Ann. Fac. Med. Vet. Torino 8:9, 1958.*

90. Halloran, P. O'C. A bibliography of references to diseases in wild mammals and birds. *Am. J. Vet. Res. 16(2):1, 1955.*

91. Handler, A. H. Spontaneous lesions of the hamster, in Ribelin, W. E. and McCoy, J. R., eds.: *The Pathology of Laboratory Animals.* Springfield Ill. Charles C Thomas, 1965, p. 210.

92. Haranghy, L., Gyergyay, F., Antalffy, A., and Mérei, Gy. Meerschweinchentumoren. *Acta Morphol. 4:301, 1954.*

93. Hartigan, P. J., and Flynn, J. A. A scirrhous adenocarcinoma in the lungs of a slaughtered cow. *Irish Vet. J. 27:161, 1973.*

94. Hertig, A. T., and MacKey, J. J. Carcinoma *in situ* of the primate uterus: Comparative observations on the cervix of the crab-eating monkey, *Macaca fascicularis,* the endometrium of the chimpanzee, *Pan troglodytes,* and on similar lesions in the human patient. *Gynecol. Oncol. 1:165, 1973.*

95. Hilsdorf, L. Beitrag zur Kenntnis der Ovarialhyperplasien und—Geschwülste bei Rind, Schwein, Ziege und Hündin. *Münch. Tierärztl. Wschr. 77:271, 1926.*

96. Hisaw, F. L., and Hisaw, F. L., Jr. Spontaneous carcinoma of the cervix uteri in a monkey (*Macaca mulatta*). *Cancer 11:810, 1958.*

97. Hooker, C. W., and Strong, L. C. An ovarian tumor in a hermaphrodite mouse. *Cancer Res. 9:550, 1949.*

98. Horn, H. A., and Stewart, H. L. A review of some spontaneous tumors of noninbred mice. *J. Natl. Cancer Inst. 13:591, 1952–1953.*

99. Howard, F. A. Granulosa cell tumor of the equine ovary—a case report. *J. Am. Vet. Med. Assoc. 114:134, 1949.*

100. Iglesias, R., and Mardones, E. The influence of the gonads and of certain steroid hormones on the growth of the spontaneous and transplantable ovarian tumor in A × C rats. *Cancer Res. 16:756, 1956.*

101. Iglesias, R., Sternberg, W. H., and Segaloff, A. A functional ovarian tumor occurring spontaneously in a rat. *Cancer Res. 10:226, 1950.*

102. Ingalls, T. H., Adams, W. M., Lurie, M. B., and Ipsen, J. Natural history of adenocarcinoma of the uterus in the Phipps rabbit colony. *J. Natl. Cancer Inst. 33:799, 1964.*

103. Ishmael, J. Dysgerminoma of the ovary in a bitch. *J. Small Anim. Pract. 11:697, 1970.*

104. Jabara, A. G. Induction of canine ovarian tumours by diethylstilboestrol and progesterone. *Aust. J. Exp. Biol. Med. Sci. 40:139, 1962.*

105. Jackson, E. B., and Brues, A. M. Studies on a transplantable embryoma of the mouse. *Cancer Res. 1:494, 1941.*

106. Jacobs, B. B., and Huseby, R. A. Neoplasms occurring in aged Fischer rats, with special reference to testicular, uterine and thyroid tumors. *J. Natl. Cancer Inst. 39:*303, 1967.

107. Jain, S. K., Singh, D. K., and Rae, U. R. K. Granulosa cell tumour in a guinea pig. *Indian Vet. J. 47:*563, 1970.

108. Jennings, A. R. Tumours of free-living wild mammals and birds in Great Britain. *Symp. Zool. Soc. Lond.* No. 24, 273, 1968.

109. Joshi, K. V., Sardeshpande, P. D., Jalnapurkar, B. V., and Ajinkyo, S. M. A case of uterine adenocarcinoma in a dog. *Indian Vet. J. 44:*114, 1967.

110. Kanagawa, H., Kawata, K., Nakao, N., and Sung, W. K. A case of granulosa cell tumor of the ovary in a newborn calf. *Jap. J. Vet. Res. 12:*7, 1964.

111. Karetta, F. Über ein skirrhöses Karzinom des Uterus beim Rind. *Wien. Tierärztl. Mschr. 15:*625, 1928.

112. Karlson, A. G., and Kelly, M. D. Choriohemangioma of the bovine allantois-chorion. *J. Am. Vet. Med. Assoc. 99:*133, 1941.

113. Keindorf, H. J. Ein Uterusmischgeschwulst beim Rind-Ätiologische und differentialdiagnostische Betrachtungen. *Mh. Vet. Med. 26:*522, 1971.

114. King, R. C. Hereditary ovarian tumors of *Drosophila melanogaster*, in C. J. Dawe and J. C. Harshberger, eds.: *Neoplasms and Related Disorders of Invertebrates and Lower Vertebrate Animals*, Monograph 31. Washington, D.C., Natl. Cancer Inst., 1969, p. 323.

115. Kirkbride, C. A., Bicknell, E. J., and Robl, M. G. Hemangiomas of a bovine fetus with chorioangioma of the placenta. *Vet. Pathol. 10:*238, 1973.

116. Kraemer, D. C., and Vera Cruz, N. C. The female reproductive system, in R. N. T.-W.-Fiennes, ed.: *Pathology of Simian Primates. Part 1: General Pathology.* Karger, Basel, 1972, p. 841.

117. Kronberger, H. Spontane Geschwülste bei Haussäugetieren. *Mh. Vet. Med. 15:*730, 1961.

118. Kullander, S. Studies on spayed rats with ovarian tissue autotransplanted into the spleen. *Acta Endocrinol. 24:*307, 1957.

119. Lagerlöf, N., and Boyd, H. Ovarian hypoplasia and other abnormal conditions in the sexual organs of cattle of the Swedish Highland breed: Results of post-mortem examination of over 6,000 cows. *Cornell Vet. 43:*64, 1953.

120. Leopold, A. Tumore a cellule della granulosa dell'ovaio destro in una cavalla. *Nuova Vet. 43:*168, 1967.

121. Lindsey, J. R., Wharton, L. R., Woodruff, J. D., and Baker, H. J. Intrauterine choriocarcinoma in a rhesus monkey. *Path. Vet. 6:*378, 1969.

122. Lingard, D. R., and Dickinson, E. O. Uterine adenocarcinoma with metastasis in the cow. *J. Am. Vet. Med. Assoc. 148:*913, 1966.

123. Lingeman, C. H. Etiology of cancer of the human ovary: A review. *J. Natl. Cancer Inst. 53:*1603, 1974.

124. Lipschutz, A., Iglesias, R., Rojas, G., and Cerisola, H. Spontaneous tumorigenesis in aged guinea-pigs. *Br. J. Cancer 13:*486, 1959.

125. Loeb, L. Ueber chorionepitheliomartige Gebilde im Ovarium des Meerschweinchens und über ihre wahrscheinliche Entstehung aus parthogenetisch sich entwickelnden Eiern. *Z. Krebsforsch. 11:*259, 1912.

126. Lombard, C. Nouvelle observation de cancer utérin chez la lapine. *Bull. Acad. Vét. Fr. 32:*447, 1959.

127. Lombard, C. Contribution à l'étude des tumeurs de l'appareil génital, chez les mammifères domestiques. *Rev. Méd. Vét. 112:*509 and 598, 1961.

128. Lombard, C. Deux cas de tumeurs de gibier. *Bull. Acad. Vét. Fr. 35:*39, 1962.

129. Lombard, C., and Havet, J. Premier cas de seminoma ovarien chez la truie. *Bull. Acad. Vét. Fr. 35:*135, 1962.

130. Maeda, T., Hayashi, T., Sasaki, H., and Tsumura, I. Tumors of the genital organs in domestic animals. I. Uterine and vaginal tumors in cows and a sow. *J. Jap. Vet. Med. Assoc. 24:*226, 1971.

131. Maeda, T., Tsumura, I., Sasaki, H., Osugi, T., Omura, Y., and Kido, H. Tumors of genital organs in domestic animals. II. Seven cases of ovarian tumors in cows and sows. *J. Jap. Vet. Med. Assoc. 26:*134, 1973.

132. Malinin, G. I., and Malinin, I. M. Age-related spontaneous uterine lesions in mice. *J. Gerontol. 27:*193, 1972.

133. Marin-Padilla, M. and Benirschke, K. Thalidomide induced alterations in the blastocyst and placenta of the armadillo, *Dasypus novemcinctus mexicanus*, including a choriocarcinoma. *Am. J. Pathol. 43:*999, 1963.

134. Martin, C. B. Jr., Misenhimer, H. R., and Ramsey, E. M. Ovarian tumors in rhesus monkeys (*Macaca mulatta*): Report of three cases. *Lab. Anim. Care 20:*686, 1970.

135. Mastronardi, M., and Potena, A. Contributo alla conoscenze dei tumori ovarici nella cavalla. *Acta Med. Vet. 12:*171, 1966.

136. Mawdesley-Thomas, L. E. An ovarian tumour in a southern elephant seal (*Mirounga leonina*). *Vet. Pathol. 8:*9, 1971.

137. Mawdesley-Thomas, L. E., and Bonner, W. N. Uterine tumours in a grey seal (*Halichoerus grypus*). *J. Pathol. 103:*205, 1971.

138. McCann, T. O., and Myers, R. E. Endometriosis in rhesus monkeys. *Am. J. Obstet. Gynecol. 106:*516, 1970.

139. Meier, H. Carcinoma of the uterus in the cat: Two cases. *Cornell Vet. 46:*188, 1956.

140. Meissner, W. A., Sommers, S. C., and Sherman, G. Endometrial hyperplasia, endometrial carcinoma, and endometriosis produced experimentally by estrogen. *Cancer 10:*500, 1957.

141. Migaki, G., Carey, A. M., Turnquest, R. U., and Garner, F. M. Pathology of bovine uterine adenocarcinoma. *J. Am. Vet. Med. Assoc. 157:*1577, 1970.

142. Misdorp, W. Tumours in large domestic animals in the Netherlands. *J. Comp. Pathol. 77:*211, 1967.

143. Monlux, A. W., Anderson, W. A., Davis, C. L., and Monlux, W. S. Adenocarcinoma of the uterus of the cow—differentiation of its pulmonary metastases from primary lung tumors. *Am. J. Vet. Res. 17:*45, 1956.

144. Moreland, A. F., and Woodard, J. C. A spontaneous uterine tumor in a New World primate *Saguinus* (*Oedipomidas*) *oedipus*. *Pathol. Vet. 5:*193, 1968.

145. Mosinger, M. Sur la carcinorésistance du cobaye. Première partie. Les tumeurs spontanées du cobaye. *Bull. Assoc. Franç. Cancer 48:*235, 1961.

146. Mossman, H. W., and Duke, K. L. *Comparative Morphology of the Mammalian Ovary.* Madison, University of Wisconsin Press, 1973.

147. Murphy, E. D. Hyperplastic and early neoplastic changes

in the ovaries of mice after genetic deletion of germ cells. *J. Natl. Cancer Inst.* 48:1283, 1972.

148. Murphy, E. D., and Beamer, W. G. Plasma gonadotropin levels during early stages of ovarian tumorigenesis in mice of the $W^x/W^v$ genotype. *Cancer Res.* 33:721, 1973.

149. Nelson, L. W., Todd, G. G., and Migaki, G. Ovarian neoplasms in swine. *J. Amer. Vet. Med. Assoc.* 151:1331, 1967.

150. Noordsy, J. L., Leipold, H. W., Cook, J. E., and Downing, C. W. Leiomyosarcoma of the uterus in a Holstein cow. *Vet. Med.* 68:176, 1973.

151. Norris, H. J., Garner, F. M., and Taylor, H. B. Pathology of feline ovarian neoplasms. *J. Pathol.* 97:138, 1969.

152. Norris, H. J., Garner, F. M. and Taylor, H. B. Comparative pathology of ovarian neoplasms. IV. Gonadal stromal tumours of canine species. *J. Comp. Pathol.* 80:399, 1970.

153. Norris, H. J., Taylor, H. B., and Garner, F. M. Equine ovarian granulosa tumours. *Vet. Rec.* 82:419, 1968.

154. Norris, H. J., Taylor, H. B., and Garner, F. M. Comparative pathology of ovarian neoplasms. II. Gonadal stromal tumors of bovine species. *Pathol. Vet.* 6:45, 1969.

155. Nowotny, F. Granulosazelltumor bei einem Eichhörnchen (*Sciurus vulgaris* L.) *Wien. Tierärztl. Mschr.* 49:158, 1962.

156. O'Gara, R. W., and Adamson, R. H. Spontaneous and induced neoplasms in nonhuman primates, *in* R. N. T.-W.-Fiennes, ed.: *Pathology of Simian Primates.* Part 1. General Pathology. Basel, Karger, 1972, p. 190.

157. O'Rourke, M. D., and Geib, L. W. Endometrial adenocarcinoma in a cat. *Cornell Vet.* 60:598, 1970.

158. O'Shea, J. D., and Jabara, A. G. The histogenesis of canine ovarian tumours induced by stilboestrol administration. *Pathol. Vet.* 4:137, 1967.

159. O'Shea, J. D., and Jabara, A. G. Proliferative lesions of serous membranes in ovariectomised female and entire male dogs after stilboestrol administration. *Vet. Pathol.* 8:81, 1971.

160. Ottosen, H. E. Scirrhøse adenokarcinomer i Uterus hos Køer. *Skand. Vet. Tidskr.* 33:473, 1943.

161. Parodi, A. L. *Tumeurs spontanées de l'ovaire chez l'animal. Revue Générale.* Extrait des XXVII^es Assises Françaises de Gynécologie sur Les Tumeurs de l'Ovaire. Masson et Cie, Paris, 1975, p. 7.

162. Polding, J. B., and Lall, H. K. Some genital abnormalities of the Indian cow and buffalo with reference to anatomical differences in their genital organs. *Indian J. Vet. Sci.* 15:178, 1945.

163. Polson, C. J. Tumours of the rabbit. *J. Pathol. Bacteriol.* 30:603, 1927.

164. Preiser, H. Endometrial adenocarcinoma in a cat. *Pathol. Vet.* 1:485, 1964.

165. Priester, S. W., and Mantel, N. Occurrence of tumors in domestic animals. Data from 12 United States and Canadian Colleges of Veterinary Medicine. *J. Natl. Cancer Inst.* 47:1333, 1971.

166. Rewell, R. E. Uterine fibromas and bilateral ovarian granulosa-cell tumours in a senile squirrel monkey, *Saimiri sciurea. J. Pathol. Bacteriol.* 68:291, 1954.

167. Rewell, R. E., and Willis, R. A. Some tumours found in whales. *J. Pathol. Bacteriol.* 61:454, 1949.

168. Riedel, W. Ein metastasierendes Uteruskarzinom einer Ziege. *Berl. Münch. Tierärztl. Wschr.* 77:395, 1964.

169. Rigdon, R. H. Tumors in the duck (family Anatidae): A review. *J. Natl. Cancer Inst.* 49:467, 1972.

170. Riser, W. H., Marcus, J. F., Guibor, E. C., and Oldt, C. C. Dermoid cyst of the canine ovary. *J. Am. Vet. Med. Assoc.* 134:27, 1959.

171. Röcken, H. Bildbericht: Teratombildung und gleichzeitige Trächtigkeit beim Hund. *Berl. Münch. Tierärztl. Wschr.* 86:74, 1973.

172. Rogers, J. B., and Blumenthal, H. T. Studies of guinea-pig tumors. I. Report of fourteen spontaneous guinea-pig tumors with a review of the literature. *Cancer Res.* 20:191, 1960.

173. Rowe, S. E., Simmons, J. L., Ringler, D. H., and Lay, D. M. Spontaneous neoplasms in aging Gerbillinae. A summary of forty-four neoplasms. *Vet. Pathol.* 11:38, 1974.

174. Russell, E. S., and Fekete, E. Analysis of W-series pleiotropism in the mouse. Effect of $W^vW^v$ substitution on definitive germ cells and on ovarian tumorigenesis. *J. Natl. Cancer Inst.* 21:365, 1958.

175. Russfield, A. B. Pathology of the endocrine glands, ovary and testis of rats and mice, *in* Cotchin, E. and Roe, F. C. J., eds.: *Pathology of Laboratory Rats and Mice.* Oxford and Edinburgh, Blackwell Scientific Publications, 1967, p. 391.

176. Sbernardori, U., and Nava, A. Disgerminoma dell'ovaio nella gatta. *Clin. Vet. Milano* 91:333, 1968.

177. Schardein, J. L., Fitzgerald, J. E., and Kaump, D. H. Spontaneous tumors in Holtzman-source rats of various ages. *Path. Vet.* 5:238, 1968.

178. Scheuler, R. L., and Ediger, R. Murine ovarian teratoma. *Amer. J. Vet. Res.* 36:341, 1975.

179. Schlegel, M. Bedeutung, Vorkommen, und Charakteristik der Ovarialtumoren bei den Haustieren. *Berl. Tierärztl. Wschr.* 31:589, 1915.

180. Schulze, F. Spontantumoren der Schädelhöhle und Genitalorgane bei Sprague–Dawley und Bethesda-Black Ratten. *Z. Krebsforsch.* 64:78, 1968.

181. Sedlmeier, H. Drei bemerkenswerte Fälle von Uterustumoren. *Münch. Tierärztl. Wschr.* 81:89, 1930.

182. Seibold, H. R., and Wolf, R. H. Neoplasms and proliferative lesions in 1065 nonhuman primate necropsies. *Lab. Anim. Sci.* 23:533, 1973.

183. Short, R. V., Shorter, D. R., and Linzell, J. L. Granulosa cell tumour of the ovary in a virgin heifer. *J. Endocrinol.* 27:327, 1963.

184. Snell, K. Spontaneous lesions of the rat, *in* Ribelin, W. E., and McCoy, J. R., eds.: *The Pathology of Laboratory Animals.* Springfield, Ill., Charles C Thomas, 1965, p. 241–300.

185. Sternberg, S. S. Carcinoma *in situ* of the cervix in a monkey (*Macaca mulatta*). *Amer. J. Obstet. Gynecol.* 82:96, 1961.

186. Storm, R. E. Dermoid cyst of the ovary. *N. Am. Vet.* 28:30, 1947.

187. Stott, G. G. Granulosa-cell islands in the canine ovary: Histogenesis, histopathologic features, and fate. *Am. J. Vet. Res.* 35:1351, 1974.

188. Streett, J. J. A note on a teratoma occurring in the Leopard frog. *Tex. J. Sci.* 16:493, 1964.

189. Strong, L. C., Gardner, W. U., and Hill, R. T. Production of estrogenic hormone by a transplantable ovarian carcinoma. *Endocrinology* 21:269, 1937.

190. Strozier, L. M., McClure, H. M., Keeling, M. E., and

Cummins, L. B. Endometrial adenocarcinoma, endometriosis, and pyometra in a rhesus monkey. *J. Am. Vet. Med. Assoc. 161:*704, 1972.

191. Studer, E. Mucinous adenocarcinoma of the bovine ovary. *J. Am. Vet. Med. Assoc. 151:*438, 1967.

192. Summers, P. M. An abattoir study of the genital pathology of cows in Northern Australia. *Aust. Vet. J. 50:*403, 1974.

193. Symeonidis, A., and Mori-Chavez, P. A. A transplantable ovarian papillary adenocarcinoma of the rat with ascites implants in the ovary. *J. Natl. Cancer Inst. 13:*409, 1952–1953.

194. Taylor, D. O. N., and Dorn, C. R. Dysgerminoma in a 20-year-old female German Shepherd dog. *Am. J. Vet. Res. 28:*587, 1967.

195. Terlecki, A., and Watson, W. A. Adenocarcinoma of the uterus of a ewe. *Vet. Rec. 80:*516, 1967.

196. Teutscher, R. Ein Plattenepithelkrebs der Schamlippe der Stute. *Dtsch. Tierärztl. Wschr. 66:*567, 1959.

197. Thiery, M. Ovarian teratoma in the mouse. *Br. J. Cancer 17:*231, 1963.

198. Thompson, S. W., and Hunt, R. D. Spontaneous tumors in the Sprague-Dawley rat. *Ann. N.Y. Acad. Sci. 108:*832, 1963.

199. Thompson, S. W., Huseby, R. A., Fox, M. A., Davis, C. L., and Hunt, R. D. Spontaneous tumors in the Sprague-Dawley rat. *J. Natl. Cancer Inst. 27:*1037, 1961.

200. Trotter, A. M. Carcinoma of the uterus of a cow. *J. Comp. Pathol. 19:*41, 1906.

201. Trotter, A. M. Malignant diseases in bovines. *J. Comp. Pathol. 24:*1, 1911.

202. Vandeplasche, M. and Thoonen, J. Reuze tumoren in de baarmoeder bij een koe. *Vlaam. Diergeneesk. Tijdschr. 19:*157, 1950.

203. Vink, H. H. Ovarian teratomas in guineapigs. A report of ten cases. *J. Pathol. 102:*180, 1970.

204. Ward, B. C., and Moore, W., Jr. Spontaneous lesions in a colony of Chinese hamsters, *Cricetulus griseus. Lab. Anim. Care 19:*516, 1969.

205. Warren, S., and Gates, O. Spontaneous and induced tumors of the guinea pig. *Cancer Res. 1:*65, 1941.

206. Weir, B. J. Some observations on reproduction in the female agouti. *J. Reprod. Fertil. 24:*203, 1971.

207. Weisbroth, S. H. Neoplastic diseases, in Weisbroth, S. H., Flatt, R. E., and Kraus, A. L. eds.: *The Biology of the Laboratory Rabbit.* New York, Academic Press, 1974, Ch. 14, 331.

208. West, J. L. Arrhenoblastoma in a chukar partridge. *Avian Dis. 18:*258, 1974.

209. Weston, J. K. Spontaneous lesions in monkeys, in Ribelin, W. E., and McCoy, J. B., eds.: *The Pathology of Laboratory Animals.* Springfield, Ill., Charles C Thomas, 1965, p. 351.

210. Whiteley, H. J., and Horton, D. L. A spontaneous transplantable ovarian tumour of the CBA mouse. *Br. J. Cancer 17:*252, 1964.

211. Wilcox, D. E., and Mossman, H. W. The common occurrence of "testis" cords in the ovaries of a shrew (*Sorex vagrans,* Baird). *Anat. Rec. 92:*183, 1945.

212. Willis, R. A. Ovarian teratomas in guineapigs. *J. Pathol. Bacteriol. 84:*237, 1962.

213. Winterfeldt, K. V. Ein Leiomyom des Ligamentum latum uteri eines Schweines. *Dtsch. Tierärztl. Wschr. 71:*70, 1964.

214. World Health Organization. International histological classification of tumours of domestic animals. *Bull. WHO 50:*1, 1974.

215. Wurster, A. C. Granulosa cell tumor in the ovary of a mare. *Southwest Vet. 17:*149, 1964.

216. Wyssmann, E. Uteruskrebs als Ursache der Nichtöffnung des Cervix uteri int. bein einer Kälbin. *Schweiz. Archiv. Tierheilk. 54:*8, 1912.

217. Yamauchi, S. A histological study of ovaries of aged cows. *Jap. J. Vet. Sci. 25:*315, 1963.

218. Yang, Y. H. Endometrial metaplasia in an albino rat. *Pathol. Vet. 1:*491, 1964.

219. Zaldivar, R. Incidence of spontaneous neoplasms in beagles. *J. Am. Vet. Med. Assoc. 151:*1319, 1967.

# Index

# Index

# Index

Index

# Contributors

**Murray R. Abell**, M.D., Ph.D.
Professor of Pathology
University of Michigan - Medical School
Ann Arbor, Michigan 48109

**Bradley Bigelow**, M.D.
Associate Professor of Pathology
New York University Medical Center
School of Medicine
New York, New York 10016

**Ancel Blaustein**, M.D.
Clinical Professor of Pathology
New York University Medical Center
School of Medicine
New York, New York 10016

**Rita Blaustein**, M.D.
Attending Cytopathologist
Department of Pathology
Booth Memorial Medical Center
Flushing, New York 11355

**John Bonnar**, M.A., M.D., F.R.C.O.G.
Professor and Head
Department of Obstetrics and Gynecology
University of Dublin
Trinity College Medical School
Rotunda Hospital
Dublin 1
Ireland

**Herbert J. Buchsbaum**, M.D.
Professor of Obstetrics and Gynecology
Director Gynecologic Oncology Service
University of Iowa Medical Center
Iowa City, Iowa 52242

# Contributors

**E. Cotchin,** D.Sc., F.R.C.V.S., F.R.C. Path.
Department of Pathology
Royal Veterinary College
University of London
Camden Town
London NW1, OTU
England

**Bernard Czernobilsky,** M.D.
Chief, Department of Pathology
Kaplan Hospital
Rehovot
Israel
Associate Professor of Pathology
Medical School of the Hebrew University
Jerusalem
Israel

**Charles H. Debrovner,** M.D.
Clinical Associate Professor of Obstetrics and Gynecology
New York University School of Medicine
New York, New York 10016

**Rita Demopoulos,** M.D.
Assistant Professor of Pathology
Department of Pathology
New York University School of Medicine
New York, New York 10016

**Felix de Narvaez,** M.D.
Adjunct Associate Professor
Department of Pathology
New York University
Director of Central Cytopathology Laboratory
Public Health Department
New York, New York 10016

**Alex Ferenczy,** M.D.
Assistant Professor of Pathology
Department of Pathology
Jewish General Hospital
Montreal H3T 1E2, Quebec
Canada

**Eduard G. Friedrich, Jr.,** M.D.
Associate Professor of Gynecology and Obstetrics
Department of Gynecology and Obstetrics
The Medical College of Wisconsin
Milwaukee, Wisconsin 53226

**Arthur L. Herbst,** M.D.
Professor and Chairman
Department of Obstetrics and Gynecology
University of Chicago
Chicago, Illinois 60637

**Jan Langman,** M.D., Ph.D.
Professor and Chairman
Department of Anatomy
School of Medicine
University of Virginia
Charlottesville, Virginia 22901

**June Marchant,** Ph.D.
Senior Lecturer in the Biology of Cancer
Regional Cancer Registry
Queen Elizabeth Medical Centre
Birmingham B15 2TH
England

**Luigi Mastroianni, Jr.,** M.D.
Professor and Chairman
Department of Obstetrics and Gynecology
Hospital of the University of Pennsylvania
University of Pennsylvania
Philadelphia, Pennsylvania 19104

**Lila E. Nachtigall,** M.D.
Associate Professor of Obstetrics and Gynecology
New York University Medical Center
New York, New York 10016

**Stanley Robboy,** M.D.
Assistant Professor of Pathology
Department of Pathology
Massachusetts General Hospital
Boston, Massachusetts 02114

**Laszlo Sarkozi,** Ph.D.
Director, Henry Dazian Department of Chemistry
The Mount Sinai Hospital
New York, New York
Associate Professor of Clinical Pathology
Mount Sinai School of Medicine of the
    City University of New York
New York, New York

**Robert E. Scully,** M.D.
Professor of Pathology
Department of Pathology
Harvard Medical School
Massachusetts General Hospital
Boston, Massachusetts 02114

**Lawrence R. Shapiro,** M.D.
Director of Cytogenetics
Letchworth Village Developmental Center
Thiells, New York 10984
Clinical Associate Professor of Pediatrics
    and Pathology
New York Medical College
Valhalla, New York 10595
Consultant in Genetics
Westchester County Medical Center
Valhalla, New York 10595

**Lewis Shenker,** M.D.
Professor of Obstetrics and Gynecology
New York University School of Medicine
New York, New York 10016

**B. L. Sheppard,** M.Sc. (Oxon)
Head of Electron Microscopy
Department of Obstetrics and Gynaecology
University of Dublin
Trinity College Medical School
Rotunda Hospital
Dublin 1
Ireland

**A. Talerman,** M.D., M.R.C. Path.
Department of Pathology
Institute of Pathology
Institute of Radiotherapy
Postbox 5201
Rotterdam
The Netherlands

**James E. Wheeler,** M.D.
Assistant Professor of Pathology at the
  University of Pennsylvania School of Medicine
Division of Surgical Pathology
Hospital of the University of Pennsylvania
Philadelphia, Pennsylvania 19104

**A. J. White,** M.D., F.A.C.O.G., F.A.C.S.
Gynecology and Gynecologic Oncology
306 Oak Hills Medical Building
San Antonio, Texas 78229

**Edward J. Wilkinson,** M.D., F.A.C.O.G., F.A.S.C.P.
Assistant Professor of Pathology and Gynecology
Department of Pathology
The Medical College of Wisconsin
Milwaukee, Wisconsin 53226